Pharmacotherapeutics for Advanced Practice

A Practical Approach

THIRD EDITION

Pharmacotherapeutics for Advanced Practice

A Practical Approach

THIRD EDITION

Editors

VIRGINIA POOLE ARCANGELO, PhD, CRNP

Family Nurse Practitioner
Avocare Gigliotti Family Medicine
Berlin, New Jersey

ANDREW M. PETERSON, PharmD, PhD

Dean, Mayes College of Healthcare Business and Policy
Associate Professor of Clinical Pharmacy and Health Policy
University of Sciences in Philadelphia
Philadelphia, Pennsylvania

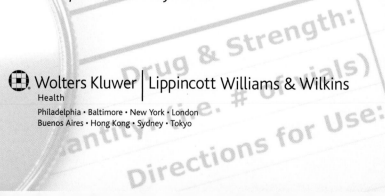

Wolters Kluwer | Lippincott Williams & Wilkins
Health

Philadelphia • Baltimore • New York • London
Buenos Aires • Hong Kong • Sydney • Tokyo

Acquisitions Editor
Bill Lamsback

Product Director
David Moreau

Product Manager
Rosanne Hallowell

Copy Editor
Amy Furman

Proofreader
Christine Dahlin

Editorial Assistants
Karen J. Kirk, Jeri O'Shea, Linda K. Ruhf

Creative Director
Doug Smock

Cover Designer
David Levy

Vendor Managers
Beth Martz and Karyn Crislip

Manufacturing Manager
Beth J. Welsh

Production and Indexing Services
SPi Global

Printed in China

PAP3E010112-040614

Library of Congress Cataloging-in-Publication Data
Pharmacotherapeutics for advanced practice: a practical approach /
[edited by] Andrew M. Peterson, Virginia Poole Arcangelo. — 3rd ed.
    p. ; cm.
  Includes bibliographical references and index.
  ISBN 978-1-4511-1197-2 (pbk.)
  1. Chemotherapy. I. Peterson, Andrew M. II. Arcangelo, Virginia Poole.
  [DNLM: 1. Drug Therapy—methods. 2. Pharmaceutical Preparations—administration & dosage. WB 330]
  RM262.P4685   2011
  615.5'8—dc22

                                        2011012201

This book is in memory of Tony. Without your love and support, this book would never have happened. You will always be remembered and will live in our hearts forever.

*Death leaves a heartache no one can heal,
love leaves a memory no one can steal.*

—From a headstone in Ireland

Pharmacotherapeutics for Advanced Practice originated from our combined experience in teaching nurse practitioners. As a nurse practitioner and educator herself, Virginia saw a need for practical exposure to the general principles of prescribing and monitoring drug therapy, particularly in the Family Practice arena. As a PharmD, Andrew saw a need to be able to teach new prescribers how to think about prescribing systematically, regardless of the disease state. We both found no suitable book that combined the practical with the systematic—most of the textbooks dedicated to this topic provided too much basic pharmacology with too little therapeutics. This book not only gives the basics on the pharmacology of the drugs, it also provides a process through which learners can begin to think pharmacotherapeutically—that is, learners will begin to identify a disease, review the drugs used to treat the disease, select treatment based on goals of therapy and special patient considerations, and learn how to adjust therapy if it fails to meet goals.

This is a book that meets the needs of both students and practitioners in a practical approach that is user friendly. It teaches the practitioner how to prescribe and manage drug therapy in primary care. The design of the book is based on input from both academicians and practitioners. Contributors were selected from academia and practice to provide a combination of evidence-based medicine and practical experience. The text considers disease- and patient-specific information. With each chapter, there are tables and algorithms that are practical and easy to read and that complement the text.

Additionally, the text guides the practitioner to a choice of second- and third-line therapy when the first line of therapy fails. Since new drugs are being marketed at all times, drug categories are discussed and information can be applied to the new drugs. Each chapter ends with a simple case study designed to prompt the learner to think and the teacher to ask critical questions. Also, each case study asks the same questions, reinforcing a clinical decision-making process. There are no answers to the questions since the authors believe the purpose of the case studies is to promote discussion, and that there may be more than one correct answer to each question, especially as new drugs are developed. What's more, the questions appear in the order in which they would be asked by a practitioner as he or she prescribes a medication.

ORGANIZATION OF THE BOOK

Unit 1—Principles of Therapeutics

The first chapter introduces the prescribing process, including how to avoid medication errors. The next chapter provides the traditional, and necessary, information on the pharmacokinetics and pharmacodynamics of drugs. Using this foundation, the subsequent chapters apply this information to drug–drug and drug–food interactions, and discuss the changes in these parameters in pediatric, geriatric, and pregnant patients. The remaining chapters in the Principles unit give overviews of drugs that are used across many disease states: pain medications and antibiotics. These chapters discuss the principles of pain management and infectious disease therapy, so that the reader can learn how these concepts are applied to the disorders discussed in the following units. A full chapter on Complementary and Alternative Medicine (CAM) is included in this unit, recognizing continued use of these modalities and attempting to meet the ever-growing need for information related to this aspect of patient care. New to this unit is a full chapter on Pharmacogenomics—the study of the human genes, effect on drug behavior. The addition of this chapter reflects the rapidly growing need for the clinician to understand how small variations in a person's genetic makeup can greatly affect how that person responds to drug therapy. While this chapter presents a general overview of this area of study, several of the disorders chapters incorporate this information directly into the clinical decision-making process.

Units 2 through 12—Disorders

This section of the book, consisting of 40 chapters, reviews commonly seen disorders in the primary care setting. Although not all-inclusive, the array of disorders allows the reader to gain an understanding of how to approach the pharmacotherapeutic treatment of any disorder. The chapters are designed to give a brief overview of the disease process, including the causes and pathophysiology, with an emphasis placed on how drug therapy can alter the pathologic state. Diagnostic Criteria and Goals of Therapy are discussed and underlie the basic principles of treating patients with drugs.

The drug sections review the agents' uses, mechanism of action, contraindications and drug interactions, adverse effects, and monitoring parameters. This discussion is organized primarily by drug class, with notation to specific drugs within the text and the tables. The tables provide the reader with quick access to generic and trade names and dosages, adverse events, contraindications, and special considerations. Used together, the text and tables provide the reader with sufficient information to begin to choose a drug therapy for a patient.

The section on Selecting the Most Appropriate Agent aids the reader in deciding which agent to choose for a given patient. This section contains information on first-line, second-line, and third-line therapies, with rationales for why agents are classified in these categories. Accompanying this section is an algorithm outlining the thought process by which clinicians select an initial drug therapy. Again, the text organization and the illustrative algorithms provide readers with a means of thinking through the process of selecting drugs for patients. In the third edition, we have kept the Recommended Order of Treatment tables and updated them, along with the algorithms and drug tables, to reflect current knowledge. Each chapter has been updated to reflect the most current guidelines available at the time of writing. However, medicine and pharmacotherapy are constantly changing, and it remains the clinician's responsibility to determine the most current information.

Included in each chapter is a section on monitoring a patient's response. This encompasses clinical and laboratory parameters, times when these items should be monitored, and actions to take in case the parameters do not meet the specified goals of therapy. In addition, special patient populations are discussed when appropriate. These discussions include pediatric and geriatric patients, but may also include ethnic- or sex-related considerations. Last, this section includes a discussion of patient education material relevant to the disease and drugs chosen. In each chapter there is a patient education section that includes information on CAM related to that disorder as well as sections on external information for patients and practitioners.

Each of the case studies has been reviewed and updated as appropriate. However, the pedagogical style of reasoning remains the same. Answers to these case studies are not supplied since the purpose is to promote discussion and evoke a thought process. Also, as time changes, so do therapies. The cases are short, compelling the learner to ask questions about the patient and allowing flexibility for multiple "right" answers to be developed by the instructor as they work through the clinical decision-making process.

Unit 13—Pharmacotherapy in Health Promotion

This unit discusses several areas of interest for promoting health or maintaining a healthy lifestyle using medications, including smoking cessation, immunizations, weight management, and contraception. A new chapter to this section is Travel Medicine. This is a growing area, and we felt readers of this text need to have an understanding of the complexity of world travel and how it affects pharmacotherapy.

Unit 14—Women's Health

This is a new unit in the third edition. We felt that there is a growing emphasis on Women's Health and that compiling the chapters relevant to this area of study would assist the learner in recognizing the special nature of care that this population deserves.

Unit 15—Integrative Approach to Patient Care

While there are only two chapters in this unit, they represent the culmination of the text. Practitioners need to have an understanding of the economics of pharmacotherapeutics in order to effectively prescribe medications and treat patients.

With the ever-increasing costs of pharmaceuticals and the introduction of far-sweeping legislation, such as Medicare Part D, the practitioner needs to be fully aware of the systems in place that facilitate, or hinder, a patient's access to medications. This chapter discusses the economics of therapeutics, including formularies, co-pays, prior authorizations, and Medicare as well as managed care as it applies to prescribing medications.

The last chapter, Integrative Approaches to Pharmacotherapy, is an attempt to examine real-life, complex cases. Each case addresses the nine questions posed in the individual chapter case studies, but now provides the reader with examples of how to approach the case studies and examines issues to consider when presented with more than one diagnosis. These cases are more complex, requiring the reader to think through multiple diseases and therapies instead of a single disorder in isolation. Within this chapter we do offer potential answers to the cases. These may not be the only answers, but indicate some of the thought processes that go into the decision-making process in the pharmacologic management of a problem.

Chapter Organization

The book offers a consistent approach throughout each disorder chapter. The chapter format begins with the background and pathophysiology of the disorder, followed by a discussion of the relevant classes of drugs. These broad categories are then integrated in the section on Selecting the Most Appropriate Agent.

Drug overview tables are also organized consistently, giving the reader much information on each drug, including the usual dose, contraindications and side effects, and any special considerations a prescriber should be aware of during therapy. All of this information is supported by the significant text.

Algorithms provide the reader with a visual cue on how to approach treating a patient.

Recommended order of treatment tables provide the reader with basic drug therapy selection, from first-line to third-line therapies for each disorder. These, coupled with the algorithms and the drug tables, are the core of the text.

A **case study** is provided for each disorder discussed. These short cases are designed to stimulate discussion among students and with instructors. The nine questions at the end of each case are tailored to each disorder, but remain similar across all cases to reinforce the process of thinking pharmacotherapeutically.

Pharmacotherapeutics for Advanced Practice is intended to provide primary care students with a reasoned approach to learning pharmacotherapeutics and to serve as a reference for the seasoned practitioner. As experienced educators and practitioners, we are dedicated to providing you with a textbook that will meet your needs.

Virginia Poole Arcangelo
Andrew M. Peterson

CONTRIBUTORS

Angela A. Allerman, PharmD, BCPS
Clinical Pharmacy Specialist
Department of Defense Pharmacoeconomic Center
Fort Sam Houston, TX
Chapter 49: Anticoagulation Disturbances

Kelly Barranger, MSN, RN, CRNP
Department of Veteran's Affairs
Philadelphia, PA
Chapter 19: Hypertension
Chapter 50: Anemias Anemias

John Barron, BS Pharmacy, PharmD
Executive Director
Health Plan Research
HealthCore, Inc.
Wilmington, DE
Chapter 20: Hyperlipidemia

Laura L. Bio, PharmD, BCPS
Assistant Professor in Clinical Pharmacy, Pediatrics
Department of Pharmacy Practice and Pharmacy
　Administration
University of the Sciences
Philadelphia, PA
Clinical Pediatric Pharmacy Specialist
Department of Pharmacy
Cooper University Hospital
Camden, NJ
Chapter 18: Otitis Media and Otitis Externa

Tim A. Briscoe, PharmD, CDE
Clinical Pharmacist Specialist
Columbus Regional Health System
Columbus, GA
*Chapter 3: Impact of Drug Interactions and Adverse Events
　on Therapeutics*

Debra Carroll, MSN, CRNP
Gerontological Nurse Practitioner
Tri-Valley Primary Care
Telford, PA
*Chapter 6: Principles of Pharmacotherapy in Elderly
　Patients*

Quinn A. Czosnowski, PharmD, BCPS
Assistant Professor of Clinical Pharmacy
Pharmacy Practice and Pharmacy Administration
Philadelphia College of Pharmacy
University of the Sciences
Philadelphia, PA
Clinical Pharmacist, Intensive Care Unit
Cooper University Hospital
Camden, NJ
Chapter 39: Seizure Disorders

Lauren M. Czosnowski, PharmD, BCPS
Assistant Professor of Clinical Pharmacy
Department of Pharmacy Practice/Pharmacy Administration
Philadelphia College of Pharmacy
University of the Sciences
Internal Medicine Clinical Specialist Pharmacy
Hospital of the University of Pennsylvania
Philadelphia, PA
Chapter 47: Allergies and Allergic Reactions

Elyse L. Dishler, MD
Karen S. Harkaway Dermatology
Delran, NJ
Chapter 38: Headaches

Amy M. Egras, PharmD, BCPS
Assistant Professor
Department of Pharmacy Practice
Thomas Jefferson University, Jefferson School of
　Pharmacy
Clinical Pharmacist
Jefferson Family Medicine Associates
Thomas Jefferson University Hospital
Philadelphia, PA
Chapter 54: Weight Loss

Heather E. Fean, MSN, APN-C
Nurse Practitioner
Advocare Gigliotti Family Medicine
Berlin, NJ
Chapter 22: Heart Failure

Kelleen N. Flaherty, MS
Assistant Professor
Biomedical Writing
University of the Sciences in Philadelphia
Philadelphia, PA
Chapter 38: Headaches

Maria Foy, PharmD, CPE
Clinical Coordinator, Pharmacy Department
Abington Memorial Hospital
Abington, PA
  Chapter 7: Principles of Pharmacology in Pain Management
  Chapter 14: Bacterial Infections of the Skin

Stephanie A. Gaber, PharmD, CDE
Clinical Coordinator
Department of Pharmacy
Thomas Jefferson University Hospital—Methodist Division
Philadelphia, PA
  *Chapter 5: Principles of Pharmacotherapy in Pregnancy and
    Lactation*

Jomy M. George, PharmD, BCPS
Assistant Professor in Clinical Pharmacy
Department of Pharmacy Practice and Pharmacy
  Administration
University of the Sciences
Philadelphia, PA
Clinical Pharmacist—Infectious Disease/HIV
Department of Pharmacy
Cooper University Hospital
Camden, NJ
  Chapter 18: Otitis Media and Otitis Externa

Steven P. Gelone, PharmD
Vice President, Clinical Development
ViroPharma Incorporated
Exton, PA
  Chapter 8: Principles of Antimicrobial Therapy

Ellen Boxer Goldfarb, CRNP
Outpatient Coordinator
Jefferson Antithrombic Services
Thomas Jefferson Internal Medicine Associates
Philadelphia, PA
  Chapter 49: Anticoagulation Disturbances

Andrew J. Grimone, PharmD, RPh, BCPS
Assistant Professor
Department of Nursing
Clarion University of Pennsylvania
Oil City, PA
Clinical Pharmacy Manager
Department of Pharmacy
Saint Vincent Health Center
Erie, PA
  Chapter 8: Principles of Antimicrobial Therapy

Emily R. Hajjar, PharmD, BCPS, CGP
Associate Professor
Jefferson School of Pharmacy
Thomas Jefferson University
Philadelphia, PA
  Chapter 44: Alzheimer's Disease

Andrea M. Heise, MSN, APN-C
Nurse Practitioner
Advocare Gigliotti Family Medicine
Berlin, NJ
  Chapter 22: Heart Failure

Lauren K. McCluggage, PharmD, BCPS
Assistant Professor
Department of Pharmacy Practice and Pharmacy
  Administration
Philadelphia College of Pharmacy, University of the Sciences
Clinical Pharmacy Specialist—Internal Medicine
Department of Pharmacy
Hospital of the University of Pennsylvania
Philadelphia, PA
  Chapter 36: Osteoarthritis and Rheumatoid Arthritis

Carol Gullo Mest, PhD, RN, ANP-BC
Associate Professor
Director of Graduate Nursing Programs
DeSales University
Center Valley, PA
  Chapter 36: Osteoarthritis and Rheumatoid Arthritis

Samir K. Mistry, PharmD
Corporate Vice President of Pharmacy
Aveta, Inc.
Fort Lee, NJ
  Chapter 59: The Economics of Pharmacotherapeutics

Angela Cafiero Moroney, PharmD
Senior Clinical Science Manager
Global Pharmaceutical Research and Development
Abbott Laboratories
Abbott Park, IL
  Chapter 44: Alzheimer's Disease

Betty E. Naimoli, MSN, CRNP
Adjunct Professor
Frances M. Maguire School of Nursing
Gwynedd-Mercy College
Gwynedd Valley, PA
Nurse Practitioner
Health Physicians Network
Abington Memorial Hospital
Abington, PA
  Chapter 37: Fibromyalgia

Judith A. O'Donnell, MD, FIDSA
Associate Professor of Clinical Medicine
Division of Infectious Diseases
Perelman School of Medicine at the University of
  Pennsylvania
Chief, Division of Infectious Diseases
Hospital Epidemiologist and Director, Department of
  Infection Prevention & Control
Penn Presbyterian Medical Center
Philadelphia, PA
  Chapter 8: Principles of Antimicrobial Therapy

Jessica O'Hara, PharmD
Medical Writer
Aston, PA
  Chapter 54: Weight Loss

Staci Pacetti, PharmD
Clinical Professor
University of Medicine and Dentistry
Schools of Nursing and Osteopathic Medicine
Stratford, NJ
  Chapter 8: Principles of Antimicrobial Therapy

Dharmi Patel, PharmD
Clinical Pharmacist
Home Solutions
Horsham, PA
  *Chapter 43: Attention-Deficit/Hyperactivity
  Disorder*

Jeegisha R. Patel, PharmD
Assistant Professor of Clinical Pharmacy
Philadelphia College of Pharmacy
University of the Sciences in Philadelphia
  Chapter 52: Smoking Cessation

Louis R. Petrone, MD
Clinical Assistant Professor
Family and Community Medicine
Jefferson Medical College
Attending Physician
Family and Community Medicine
Thomas Jefferson University Hospital
Philadelphia, PA
  Chapter 46: Thyroid Disorders

Jennifer A. Reinhold, BA, PharmD, BCPS
Assistant Professor of Clinical Pharmacy
Department of Pharmacy Practice/Pharmacy
  Administration
Philadelphia College of Pharmacy
University of the Sciences
Philadelphia, PA
Clinical Pharmacist
Quality Family Physicians
Hockessin, DE
  Chapter 34: Overactive Bladder
  Chapter 40: Major Depressive Disorder

Alicia M. Reese, PharmD, MS, BCPS
Assistant Professor of Clinical Pharmacy
Philadelphia College of Pharmacy
University of the Sciences
Philadelphia, PA
  Chapter 21: Chronic Stable Angina

Cynthia A. Sanoski, BS, PharmD, BCPS, FCCP
Chair and Associate Professor
Department of Pharmacy Practice
Jefferson School of Pharmacy
Thomas Jefferson University
Philadelphia, PA
  Chapter 23: Arrhythmias

Matthew Sarnes, PharmD
Vice President
Xcenda
Palm Harbor, FL
  *Chapter 3: Impact of Drug Interactions and Adverse Events
  on Therapeutics*

Jason J. Schafer, PharmD, BCPS, AAHIVE
Assistant Professor
Department of Pharmacy Practice
Jefferson School of Pharmacy
Thomas Jefferson University
Philadelphia, PA
  Chapter 14: Bacterial Infections of the Skin

Susan M. Schrand, MSN, CRNP
Executive Director
Pennsylvania Coalition of Nurse Practitioners
Jenkintown, PA
  Chapter 37: Fibromyalgia

Henry M. Schwartz, BSc Pharm, PharmD, CDE
Assistant Professor of Clinical Pharmacy
Director of Community Pharmacy Experiences
Pharmacy Practice and Pharmacy Administration
Philadelphia College of Pharmacy
University of the Sciences
Philadelphia, PA
  Chapter 53: Travel Medicine

Anita Siu, PharmD
Clinical Associate Professor
Pharmacy Practice and Administration
Ernest Mario School of Pharmacy
Rutgers, The State University of New Jersey
Piscataway, NJ
Neonatal/Pediatric Pharmacotherapy Specialist
Department of Pharmacy
K. Hovnanian Children's Hospital at Jersey Shore University
  Medical Center
Neptune, NJ
  Chapter 4: Principles of Pharmacotherapy in Pediatrics

Joshua J. Spooner, PharmD, MS
Assistant Dean for Student Affairs
College of Pharmacy
Western New England University
Springfield, MA
  Chapter 17: Ophthalmic Disorders
  Chapter 59: The Economics of Pharmacotherapeutics

Linda M. Spooner, PharmD, BCPS
Associate Professor of Pharmacy Practice
Department of Pharmacy Practice
Massachusetts College of Pharmacy and Health Sciences
Boston, MA
Clinical Pharmacy Specialist in infectious Diseases
Department of Pharmacy
Saint Vincent Hospital
Worcester, MA
    Chapter 48: Human Immunodeficiency Virus

Liza Takiya, PharmD, BCPS
Associate Director
U.S. Medical Information
Pfizer, Inc
Collegeville, PA
    Chapter 31: Inflammatory Bowel Disease

Jim Thigpen, PharmD, BCPS
Assistant Professor
Department of Pharmacy Practice
Bill Gatton College of Pharmacy
East Tennessee State University
Clinical Pharmacist
Department of Pharmacy Services
Niswonger Children's Hospital
Johnson City, TN
    Chapter 4: Principles of Pharmacotherapy in Pediatrics

Tyan F. Thomas, PharmD, BCPS
Assistant Professor of Clinical Pharmacy
Pharmacy Practice and Pharmacy Administration
Philadelphia College of Pharmacy
University of the Sciences
Clinical Pharmacist
Philadelphia Veterans' Affairs Medical Center
Philadelphia, PA
    Chapter 52: Smoking Cessation

Craig B. Whitman, PharmD, BCPS
Assistant Professor of Clinical Pharmacy
Pharmacy Practice and Pharmacy Administration
Philadelphia College of Pharmacy
University of the Sciences
Philadelphia, PA
Clinical Pharmacist, Intensive Care Unit
Cooper University Hospital
Camden, NJ
    Chapter 39: Seizure Disorders

Veronica F. Wilbur, PhD, FNP-BC
Chair, Nurse Practitioner Program
College of Health Professions—Graduate Nursing
Wilmington University
New Castle, DE
    Chapter 30: Constipation, Diarrhea, and Irritable Bowel Syndrome
    Chapter 42: Insomnia and Sleep Disorders
    Chapter 45: Diabetes Mellitus

Eric T. Wittbrodt, PharmD
Field Scientific Lead
Scientific Strategies
Takeda Pharmaceuticals America, Inc.
Deerfield, IL
    Chapter 27: Bronchitis and Pneumonia

ACKNOWLEDGMENTS

We would like to thank the following reviewers, who provided valuable feedback on several chapters in the third edition:

Lynda K. Ball, MSN, RN, CNN
Quality Improvement Director
Northwest Renal Network
Seattle, Washington

Barbara A. Broome, PhD, RN, FAAN
Associate Dean College of Nursing and Chair Community/
    Mental Health
University of South Alabama – College of Nursing
Mobile, Alabama

Shelley Yerger Hawkins, DSN, APRN-BC, FNP, GNP, FAANP
Senior Director, Clinical Team
Celgene Corporation
Los Angeles, California

Linda Ludwig, RN, BS, MEd
Clinical Consultant
Kingfisher, Oklahoma

Diane Orlov, CNP, RN, BS, MS
Nurse Practitioner
The Ohio State University Medical Center
Division of Infectious Diseases
Columbus, Ohio

We would also like to thank the people at Lippincott Williams & Wilkins, including Bill Lamsback and Rosanne Hallowell, as well as Amy Furman, Copy Editor. We are also forever indebted to the contributors and reviewers who spent countless hours working on this project. Without them, this would never have become a reality.

In addition, we would like to thank our families who supported us throughout the project and understand of the importance of this book to us.

CONTENTS

UNIT 1

Principles of Therapeutics

Issues for the Practitioner in Drug Therapy

Drug therapy is often the mainstay of treatment of acute and chronic diseases. An important role of health care practitioners is to develop a treatment plan with the patient; an integral part of the treatment plan of disease and health promotion is drug therapy. According to the National Ambulatory Medical Care Survey (Cherry, et al., 2008), in 2006 there were 1.9 billion drugs prescribed during office visits, 247.7 million drugs prescribed during visits to a hospital outpatient department, and 212.1 million drugs prescribed during visits to a hospital emergency department. The percentage of patient visits involving drug therapy was approximately 75% in all three locations.

In developing a treatment plan that includes drug therapy, the prescribing practitioner considers many issues in achieving the goal of safe, appropriate, and effective therapy. Among them are drug safety and product safeguards, the practitioner's role and responsibilities, the step-by-step process of prescribing therapy and writing the prescription, and follow-up measures. Particularly important are promoting adherence to the therapeutic regimen and keeping up-to-date with the latest developments in drug therapy.

DRUG SAFETY AND MARKET SAFEGUARDS

In the United States drug safety is ensured in many ways, but primarily by the U.S. Food and Drug Administration (FDA), which is the federal agency charged with conducting and monitoring clinical trials, approving new drugs for market and manufacture, and ensuring safe drugs for public consumption. Although the federal government provides guidelines for a pure and safe drug product, guidelines for prescribers of drug therapy are dictated both by state and federal governments and licensing bodies in each state.

Clinical Trials

Various legislated mechanisms are in place to ensure pure and safe drug products. One of these mechanisms is the clinical trial process by which new drug development is carefully monitored by the FDA. Every new drug must successfully pass through several stages of development. The first stage is preclinical trials, which involve testing in animals and monitoring efficacy, toxic effects, and untoward reactions. Application to the FDA for investigational use of a drug is made only after this portion of research is completed.

Clinical trials, which begin only after the FDA grants approval for investigation, consist of four phases and may last up to 9 years before a drug is approved for general use. During clinical trials, performed on informed volunteers, data are gathered about the proposed drug's purity, bioavailability, potency, efficacy, safety, and toxicity.

Phase I of clinical trials is the initial evaluation of the drug. It involves supervised studies on 20 to 100 healthy people and focuses on absorption, distribution, metabolism (sometimes interchangeable with biotransformation), and elimination of the drug. In phase I, the most effective administration routes and dosage ranges are determined. During phase II, up to several hundred patients with the disease for which the drug is intended are subjects. The testing focus is the same as in phase I, except that drug effects are monitored on people with disease.

Phase III begins once the FDA determines that the drug causes no apparent serious adverse effects and that the dosage range is appropriate. Double-blind research methods (in which neither the study and control subjects nor the investigators know who is receiving the test drug and who is not) are used for data collection in this phase, and the proposed drug is compared with one already proven to be effective. Usually several thousand subjects are involved in this phase, which lasts several years and during which most risks of the proposed drug are discovered. At the completion of phase III, the FDA evaluates data presented and accepts or rejects the application for the new drug. Approval of the application means that the drug can be marketed—but only by the company seeking the approval.

Once on the market, the drug enters phase IV trials. Initially, the drug is released on a limited basis, then later on a more widespread basis. Everyone who takes the drug is monitored. Adverse drug reactions are reported and investigated. In late phase III and phase IV studies, the pharmaceutical companies have two objectives:

- To compare the drug with other drugs already available
- To monitor long-term effectiveness and impact on quality of life

BOX 1.1

Scheduled Drugs

Schedule 1 drugs have a high potential for abuse. There ...

... These drugs contain a combination of controlled and ...ances. Use of these drugs can ... to low physiologic dependence ...ological dependence. A verbal ... the pharmacy and the prescrip-...up to five times within 6 months. ...ertain narcotics (codeine) and ...tives.

... a low potential for abuse. They ...ogical dependency but limited ...ncy. Examples include nonnar-...d antianxiety agents, such as

... e least potential for abuse. They ...amount of opioids and are used ...es and antidiarrheals. Examples ... and antidiarrheals with small ...s.

...ll health plans and health care clear-...in the administrative and financial ...er HIPAA. The NPI is a 10-posi-...neric identifier (10-digit number). ...other information about the health ...health care provider's specialty or ...s. The NPI must be used in lieu of ...in HIPAA standard transactions. ...so share their NPI with other pro-...nghouses, and any entity that may ....

...IPI is to uniquely identify a health ...transactions such as health care ...sed to identify health care providers ...al files to link proprietary provider ...other information, in coordination ...plans, in patient medical record sys-...files, and in other ways. HIPAA ...ies (i.e., health plans, health care ...health care providers who trans-...electronic form in connection with ...e Secretary of Health and Human ...dard) use NPIs in standard transac-...health care provider identifier that ...nsactions by covered entities.

...may apply for an NPI through a ...ocess at https://nppes.cms.hhs.gov ...ng a paper application to the NPI ...application (CMS-10114), which ...ator's mailing address, is available

---

[Overlaid letter:]

- details the principles of therapeutics for a wide range of disorders
- provides clear, concise guidelines for prescribing and monitoring drug therapy
- includes new chapters and the most current information to keep you up to date
- features algorithms, tables, and charts for at-a-glance guidance

It's really quite simple. Try **Pharmacotherapeutics for Advanced Practice, Third Edition** risk FREE, and see how this standard in therapeutics will help you ...

- make the best drug choices
- avoid medication errors
- provide optimal patient care

I'm sure you'll find this new edition to be a valuable resource in your every day practice.

Sincerely,

Joan M. Robinson

Joan M. Robinson, RN, MSN
Clinical Director

P.S. Please take a moment to review the enclosed flyer for more details on this actionable resource.

Wolters Kluwer Health

Two Commerce Square, 2001 Market Street, Philadelphia, PA 19103

upon request through the NPI Enumerator at 1-800-465-3203, TTY 1-800-692-2326.

When applying for an NPI, providers are asked to include their Medicare identifiers as well as those issued by other health plans. A Medicaid identification number must include the associated state name. The legacy identifier information is critical for health plans to aid in the transition to the NPI. When the NPI application information has been submitted and the NPI assigned, NPPES sends the health care provider a notification that includes their NPI. This notification is proof of NPI enumeration and helps to verify a health care provider's NPI.

Prescription Versus Nonprescription Drugs

Some drugs may be obtained without a prescription. Although they are commonly and legally obtained over the counter (OTC) without a prescription, these drugs also must have approval from the FDA for specific uses in specific doses. At one time, many of these drugs were available only by prescription. Currently, however, they are available in lower doses (i.e., the lowest effective dose) without a prescription.

These drugs carry user warnings on the labels. Many have the potential for interacting adversely with prescribed drugs or complicating existing disease. The self-prescribed use of OTC drugs may delay diagnosis and treatment of potentially serious problems. On the other hand, the use of OTC drugs can be beneficial for treatment of self-limiting disorders that are not serious.

Generic Drugs Versus Brand Name Drugs

Substituting a generic drug for a brand name drug is a common practice. In many states, it is required. When the patent on a brand name drug expires, other drug manufacturers can then produce the same drug formula under its generic name (the generic name and formula of a drug are always the same; only the brand names change). This practice not only benefits the manufacturer but decreases the cost to the consumer.

To ensure safety, the FDA must grant approval for these drugs, and rigorous testing is again required to ensure that all generic drugs meet specifications for quality, purity, strength, and potency. Generic drugs must demonstrate therapeutic equivalence to the brand name equivalent. They must be manufactured under the same strict standards and meet the same batch requirements for identity, strength, purity, and quality as the brand name drug. Bioavailability can only differ from the brand name by less than 4%.

To obtain FDA approval, the generic drug is administered in a single dose to at least 18 healthy human subjects. Next, peak serum concentration and the area under the plasma concentration curve (AUC) are measured. The values obtained for the generic drug must be within 80% to 125% of those obtained for the brand name drug. Most generic drugs have a mean AUC within 3% of the brand name drug. There has been no reported therapeutic difference of a serious nature between brand name products and FDA-approved generic products. For more information, see **Table 1.1**, which presents FDA equivalency ratings for brand name and generic drugs.

TABLE 1.1	**FDA Therapeutic Equivalence Ratings**
Rating Scale	**Definition**
A	Therapeutically Equivalent
AA	Products in conventional dosage forms not presenting bioequivalence problems
AB	Products meeting necessary bioequivalence requirements
AN	Solutions and powders for aerosolization
AO	Injectable oil solutions
AP	Injectable aqueous solutions and, in certain instances, intravenous nonaqueous solutions
AT	Topical products
B	Not Therapeutically Equivalent
BB	Drug products requiring further FDA investigation and review to determine therapeutic equivalence
BC	Extended-release dosage forms (capsules, injectables, and tablets)
BD	Active ingredients and dosage forms with documented bioequivalence problems
BE	Delayed-release oral dosage forms
BN	Products in aerosol–nebulizer drug delivery systems
BP	Active ingredients and dosage forms with potential bioequivalence problems
BR	Suppositories or enemas that deliver drugs for systemic absorption
BS	Products having drug standard deficiencies
BT	Topical products with bioequivalence issues
BX	Drug products for which the data are insufficient to determine therapeutic equivalence
AB	Potential equivalence problems have been resolved with adequate in vivo or in vitro evidence supporting bioequivalence

U.S. Department of Health and Human Services, Food and Drug Administration, Center for Drug Evaluation and Research, Office of Pharmaceutical Science, Office of Generic Drugs. (2010). *Approved drug products with therapeutic equivalence evaluation* (30th ed.).

Complementary and Alternative Medicine

In the United States, the use of herbal preparations as treatments for disease and disease prevention has increased tremendously. Historically, herbs were the first healing system used. Herbal medicines are derived from plants and thought by many to be harmless because they are products of nature. Some prescription drugs in current use, however, such as digitalis, are also "natural," which is not synonymous with "harmless." Before 1962, herbal preparations were considered to be drugs, but now they are sold as foods or supplements and therefore do not require FDA approval as drugs. Hence, there are no legislated standards on purity or quantity of active ingredients in herbal preparations. The value of herbal therapy is usually measured by anecdotal reports and not verified by research. Like synthetic products, herbal preparations may interact with other drugs and may produce undesirable side effects as well.

In the United States, approximately 38% of adults (about 4 in 10) and approximately 12% of children (about 1 in 9) are using some form of complementary and alternative medicine (CAM). In December 2008, the National Center for Complementary and Alternative Medicine and the National Center for Health Statistics (part of the Centers for Disease Control and Prevention) released new findings on Americans' use of CAM. The findings are from the 2007 National Health Interview Survey, an annual in-person survey of Americans (Barnes, Bloom, & Nahin, 2008). A national survey conducted in 2007 found that 17.7% of American adults had used "natural products" (i.e., dietary supplements other than vitamins and minerals) in the past 12 months. The most popular products used by adults for health reasons in the past 30 days were fish oil/omega 3/DHA (37.4%) and glucosamine, a substance found in the fluid around joints and used by the body to make and repair cartilage. Glucosamine in dietary supplements is made in the laboratory or from shrimp, lobster, and crab shells (19.9%), Echinacea (19.8%), flaxseed oil or pills (15.9%), and ginseng (14.1%). In another, earlier national survey covering all types of dietary supplements, approximately 52% of adult respondents said they had used some type of supplement in the last 30 days; the most commonly reported were multivitamins/minerals (35%), vitamins E and C (12% to 13%), calcium (10%), and B-complex vitamins (5%) (http://nccam.nih.gov/health/supplements/wiseuse.htm#use).

The Dietary Supplement Health and Education Act (1994) requires labeling about the effect of herbal products on the body and requires the statement that the herbal product has not been reviewed by the FDA and is not intended to be used as a drug. CAM is discussed in Chapter 9.

Foreign Medications

Today, patients may come from many countries or may get their drugs from other countries because they are less expensive. There may be different active ingredients in the medications, or the names are not recognizable. They present with a medication for a chronic condition that was prescribed in another country and ask for a refill. To learn more about foreign medications, the prescriber can go to www.pharmj.com/noticeboard/info/pip/foreignmedicines.html.

Disposal of Medications

Many medications can be potentially harmful if taken by someone other than the person for whom they are prescribed. Almost all medicines can be safely disposed of if they are mixed with an undesirable substance, such as cat litter or coffee grounds, and placed in a closed container. Any personal information should be removed from the container by using a black marker or duct tape. Many communities have a drug take-back program for disposal, or drugs can be disposed of when the community collects hazardous material. Drugs should not be flushed down the toilet or drain unless the dispensing directions say this is permitted. Drugs permitted to be flushed can be found on the website http://www.fda.gov/Drugs/ResourcesForYou/Consumers/BuyingUsingMedicineSafely/EnsuringSafeUseofMedicine/SafeDisposalofMedicines/ucm186187.htm.

PRACTITIONER'S ROLE AND RESPONSIBILITIES IN PRESCRIBING

Before prescribing therapy, the practitioner has a responsibility to gather data by taking a thorough history and performing a physical examination. Once the data are gathered and evaluated, one or more diagnoses are formulated and a treatment plan established. As noted, the most frequently used treatment modality is drug therapy, usually with a prescription drug.

If a drug is deemed necessary for therapy, it is essential for the practitioner to understand the responsibility involved in prescribing that drug or drugs and to consider seriously which class of medication is most appropriate for the patient. The decision is reached based on a thorough knowledge of diagnosis and treatment.

Drug Selection

To determine which therapy is best for the patient, the practitioner conducts a risk–benefit analysis, evaluating the therapeutic value versus the risk associated with each drug to be prescribed. The practitioner then selects from a vast number of pharmacologic agents used for treating the specific medical problem. Factors to consider when selecting the drug or drugs are the subtle or significant differences in action, side effects, interactions, convenience, storage needs, route of administration, efficacy, and cost. Another factor in the decision may involve the patient pressuring the practitioner to prescribe a medication (because that is the expectation of many patients at the beginning of a health care encounter). Clearly, many responsibilities are inherent in prescribing a medication, and serious consequences may result if these responsibilities are not taken seriously and the prescription is prepared incorrectly.

BOX 1.2

Questions to Address When Prescribing a Medication

- Is there a need for the drug in treating the presenting problem?
- Is this the best drug for the presenting problem?
- Are there no contraindications to this drug with this patient?
- Is the dosage correct? Or is it too high or too low?
- Does the patient have allergies or sensitivities to the drug?
- What drug treatment modalities does the patient currently use, and will the potential new drug interact with the patient's other drugs or treatments?
- Is there a problem with storage of the drug?
- Does the dosage regimen (schedule) interfere with the patient's lifestyle? For example, if a child is in school, a drug with a once- or twice-daily dosing schedule is more realistic than one with a four-times-daily schedule.
- Is the route of administration the most appropriate one?
- Is the proposed duration of treatment too short or too long?
- Can the patient take the prescribed drug?
- Has the patient been informed of possible side effects and what to do if they occur?
- Is there a genetic component to consider?
- What is the cost of the drug?
- What, if any, prescription plan does the patient have?

Initial questions to ask when selecting drug therapy include "Is there a need for this drug in treating the presenting problem or disease?" and "Is this the best drug for the presenting problem or disease?" Additional questions are listed in **Box 1.2.**

Concerns Related to Ethics and Practice

Certain ethical and practical issues must be considered as well. One overriding issue may be the lack of a clinical indication for using a medication. As mentioned, many patients visit a practitioner with the sole purpose of obtaining a prescription. In seeking medical attention, the ill patient expects the health care provider to promote relief from symptoms. In today's world, an abundance of information available in books, magazines, television, Web sites, and other media suggests that the health care provider can do this by prescribing a special medication. This expectation that a magic pill or potion—the

prescription—is the ticket that will relieve reflux, kill germs, end pain, and restore health puts pressure on the practitioner to prescribe for the sake of prescribing. A common example of this involves the patient with a cold who seeks an antibiotic, such as penicillin. In such a situation, the practitioner has a responsibility to prescribe only medications that are necessary for the well-being of the patient and that will be effective in treating the problem. In the example of the patient with an uncomplicated head cold, an antibiotic would not be effective, and the responsible practitioner must be prepared to make an ethical and judicious decision and explain it to the patient.

Patient Education

An integral part of the practitioner's role and responsibility is educating the patient about drug therapy and its intended therapeutic effect, potential side effects, and strategies for dealing with possible adverse drug reactions. This may be explained verbally, with written instructions given, when appropriate. Instructions that are printed and handed to the patient must be readable and in a language that the patient can understand. If side effects are discussed in advance, the patient will know what to expect and will contact the prescriber with symptoms. There may be less likelihood that the patient will discontinue the drug before discussing it with the prescriber.

Medications can also have a placebo effect. Patients must believe that the drug will work for them to be committed to taking it as recommended. If that belief is not instilled in patients, the drug may not be perceived as effective and may not be taken as directed.

The practitioner may want to advise the patient to use only one pharmacy when filling prescriptions. The choice of only one pharmacy has several advantages, which include maintaining a record of all medications that the patient currently receives and serving as a double check for drug–drug interactions.

Prescriptive Authority

Prescribing practices of each practitioner are regulated by the state in which he or she practices. Each state determines practice parameters by statutes (laws enacted by the legislature) and rules and regulations (administrative policies determined by regulatory agencies). Each practitioner is responsible for knowing the laws and regulations in the state of practice. For instance, some states require a physician's signature on all prescriptions; other states require a physician's signature just on prescriptions for controlled substances.

Prescriptive authority is regulated by the State Board of Nursing, Board of Medicine, or Board of Pharmacy, depending on the state. States allow independent practice, collaborative practice, supervised practice, or delegated practice. Independent practice has no requirements for mandatory physician collaboration or supervision. Collaborative practice requires a formal agreement with a collaborating physician, ensuring a referral–consultant relationship. Supervised practice is overseen or directed by a supervisory physician. Delegated practice means that prescription writing is a delegated medical act. Regulations can be gotten from the Board of Nursing in each state.

Related to prescriptive authority issues is the issue of drug samples. Most drug companies engage in the promotional practice of distributing sample drugs to practitioners for use by patients. The Prescription Drug Marketing Act (PDMA), which was enacted in 1988 to protect the American consumer from ineffective drugs, also affects the receipt and dispensing of sample drugs. Prescription drugs can be distributed only to licensed practitioners (one licensed by the state to prescribe drugs) and health care entity pharmacies at the request of a licensed practitioner. PDMA protects the public in several ways. It forbids foreign countries to reimport prescription drugs; bans the sale, trade, and purchase of drug samples; prohibits resale of prescription drugs purchased by hospitals, health care entities, and charitable organizations; requests practitioners to ask for drug samples in writing; and regulates wholesale distributors of prescription drugs by requiring licensing in states where facilities are located. There are penalties for violation of the act. This act affects the distribution and use of pharmaceutical samples.

Because these samples are freely available, it might be assumed that they can be distributed by all practitioners, but this is not the case. The practitioner must be aware of the rules that govern requesting, receiving, and distributing these agents because the rules vary from state to state.

Specific procedures are required with drug samples. The pharmaceutical representative's Sample Request Form must be signed. It includes the name, strength, and quantity of the sample. The sample must be then recorded on the Record of Receipt of Drug Sample sheet. The samples must be stored away from other drug inventory and where unauthorized access is not allowed or in a locked cabinet or closet in a public area. Samples are to be inspected monthly for expiration dates, proper labeling and storage, presence of intact packaging and labeling, and appropriateness for the practice. If a sample has expired, it must be disposed of in a manner that prevents accessibility to the general public. They cannot be disposed into the trash.

When distributing samples, each must be labeled with the patient's name, clear directions for use, and cautions. They are to be dispensed free of charge along with pertinent information. The medication is then documented in the patient's chart with dose, quantity, and directions.

ADVERSE DRUG EVENTS

When prescribing a drug, there is the risk of the patient experiencing an adverse drug event (ADE). Some ADEs can be very harmful. It is estimated that 7.6% of all outpatient prescriptions contain errors, with 3% of them being preventable (Gandhi, et al., 2005). An estimated 2.5% of emergency department visits are due to ADEs (Budnitz, et al., 2005). It is estimated that there are more than 700,000 visits to emergency

departments for ADEs each year in the United States. Nearly 120,000 of these patients need to be hospitalized for further treatment. This is an important patient safety problem, but many of these ADEs are preventable (http://www.cdc.gov/features/medicinesafety/).

Moreover, an estimated 3.1% to 6.2% of all admissions are likely due to ADEs. Deaths from ADEs have been estimated at over 100,000 a year (Moore, Cohen & Furberg, 2007).

Lack of Drug Knowledge

There can be a lack of knowledge about indications and contraindications for drugs. This includes underuse, overuse, and misuse of drugs. An example of underuse is failure to prescribe an inhaled corticosteroid for an asthmatic patient who uses his albuterol daily. An example of overuse is prescribing an antibiotic for a cold or prescribing an antihypertensive drug for someone whose blood pressure is elevated because he is taking Sudafed. An example of misuse is prescribing hydrochlorothiazide to someone who is allergic to sulfa.

Dosing errors occur when a larger dose is prescribed than needed. Starting someone on 30 mg paroxetine instead of 20 mg may increase anxiety.

Lack of knowledge about drug–drug interactions can cause errors. For example, many drugs interfere with warfarin and cause increased bleeding if taken together.

Lack of Patient Information

A common error in prescribing is failure to obtain an adequate history from the patient. Often an adequate drug history is not obtained and the provider does not specifically inquire about OTC medications. Also information on allergies to medications is not always obtained. In addition to allergies, it is imperative to ascertain the reaction to the medication. Nausea is not considered an allergic reaction. An allergy history should be taken and documented at each visit before a new medication is prescribed.

Poor Communication

Poor communication can be a result of poor handwriting, incorrect abbreviations, misplaced decimals, and misunderstanding of verbal prescriptions. Poor communication also results when the prescriber fails to discuss potential side effects or ask about side effects at subsequent visits.

SPECIAL POPULATION CONSIDERATIONS

Doses for children are usually based on weight in kilograms. The prescriber has a responsibility to calculate the dose and write the correct dose, rather than relying on the pharmacist to calculate the dose.

Elderly patients may have some difficulty hearing or reading small print. Additionally, they may be taking multiple prescription medications and OTC medications. The prescriber needs to be specific about when the patient should take each medication and if one drug cannot be taken with others. When the practitioner prescribes for the elderly, he or she must consider renal function because some medications can cause toxicity, even in small doses, with decreased renal function.

PHARMACOGENOMICS

Recently, pharmacogenomics has gained importance in prescribing medication. The way a person responds to a drug is influenced by many different genes. Without knowing all of the genes involved in drug response, it has not been possible to develop genetic tests that could predict a person's response to a particular drug. Knowing that people's genes show small variations in the DNA base makes genetic testing for predicting drug response possible. Genetic factors can account for 20% to 95% variability of the patient's reaction to a drug. Pharmacogenomics examines the inherited variations in genes that dictate drug response and explores the ways these variations can be used to predict the response a patient will have to a drug. Pharmacogenetic testing may enable providers to understand why patients react differently to various drugs and to make better decisions about therapy. This understanding may allow for highly individualized therapeutic regimens. This concept will be discussed in detail in Chapter 10.

STEPS OF THE PRESCRIBING PROCESS

At each visit, a medication history is obtained with the name of the drug, dosage, and frequency of administration. Information on any allergies should also be obtained. It is also helpful if the patient brings his or her actual drugs to the visit.

Multiple steps **(Figure 1-1)** are involved in prescribing drugs and evaluating their effectiveness. Again, the first step is determining an accurate diagnosis based on the patient's history, physical examination, and pertinent test findings.

Next, in selecting the best agent, the practitioner thoroughly evaluates the patient's condition, taking into consideration the effect that various medications may have on the patient and the disorder, the expected outcomes of therapy, and other variables **(Box 1.3).** When prescribing any drug therapy, the practitioner must have a solid knowledge and background in the pathophysiology of disease, pharmacotherapeutics,

FIGURE 1–1 Process for prescribing.

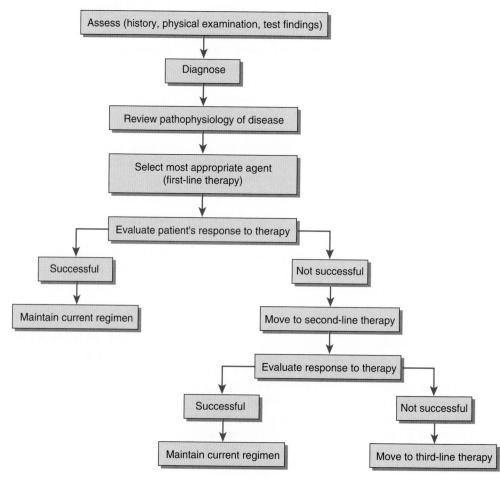

Variables to Consider in Prescribing a Medication

Age
Sex
Race
Weight
Culture
Allergies
Pharmacogenomics
Other diseases or conditions
Other therapies
   Prescription medications
   Over-the-counter medicines
   Alternative therapies
Previous therapies
   Effectiveness
   Adverse effects
   Adherence
Socioeconomic issues
   Insurance status
   Income level
   Daily schedule
   Living environment
   Support systems
Health beliefs

pharmacokinetics, pharmacodynamics, and any interactions (see Chapter 3).

The practitioner needs to be knowledgeable about the best class of drugs for the diagnosed disorder or presenting problem, the recommended dosage, potential side effects, possible interactions with other drugs, and special prescribing considerations, such as required laboratory tests, contraindications, and patient instructions. To select the correct medication, the practitioner must thoroughly understand the pathophysiology of the condition being treated and the natural history of the disease. This information allows the practitioner to decide at which point in the disease process intervention with drug therapy is indicated because in many diseases or disorders, nonpharmacologic therapies are tried before drug therapy is initiated.

Next, the practitioner sets goals for therapy. Goals need to be realistic and outcomes measurable. All interventions, nonpharmacologic and pharmacologic, are initiated to meet these goals, and evaluation of the therapy's efficacy is based on these goals.

Lines of Therapy

For most disease entities, there is a recommended first-line therapy—that is, research shows certain agents to be more effective than others. Once initiated, the first-line therapy is evaluated and either continued or changed. If the desired goals are not achieved, or if an adverse reaction occurs, second-line therapy is initiated. The second-line therapy is then evaluated. If this therapy is not tolerated or efficacious, a third-line therapy is initiated, and so on. The practitioner continually evaluates the patient's response to therapy and maintains current therapy or changes it as indicated by the patient's response. For more information, see the case study outlining the prescribing process in **Box 1.4**. Case studies such as this one are used throughout the text.

Consideration of Special Populations

Another step in prescribing drugs is considering specific concerns related to special populations, such as children, pregnant or breast-feeding women, and the elderly. Cultural beliefs are also considered to ensure that the drug regimen honors individual and family customs and preferences. Pharmacogenomics are gaining in popularity when considering which drug to prescribe.

Identifying Outcomes

Expected outcomes can include improvement in clinical symptoms or pathologic signs or changes in biochemistry as determined by laboratory tests. To assess whether expected outcomes have been achieved, the practitioner reviews data collected on subsequent visits, evaluates the effectiveness of drug therapy, and investigates any adverse reactions.

The frequency of follow-up visits is determined by the disease and the patient's response to treatment. While outcomes are being assessed, the practitioner educates the patient about the outcomes of therapy as well. Topics for discussion include drug benefits, side effects, dosage adjustments, and monitoring parameters.

The patient as well as the practitioner must be informed about any undesirable outcomes of therapy with a prescription drug. Reactions that may be expected and must be discussed include side effects, drug or food interactions, and toxicity. Unexpected reactions include allergic reactions or intolerance to a drug. If a patient experiences a serious adverse drug reaction, the practitioner files a report with the FDA's MedWatch program on a special form obtainable from MedWatch (5600 Fishers Lane, Rockville, MD 20852-9787 or can be reported online at https://www.accessdata.fda.gov/scripts/medwatch/; see Chapter 4 for a sample of the MedWatch form). Similarly, adverse reactions to vaccines are reported through the Vaccine Adverse Event Reporting System (VAERS) online at http://vaers.hhs.gov/esub/index#Online or by mail by completing a VAERS form requested by calling 1-800-822-7967 and mailing it to VAERS, P.O. Box 1100, Rockville, MD 20849-1100. Adverse events are discussed in Chapter 4.

WRITING THE PRESCRIPTION

The prescription is a form of communication between the practitioner and the pharmacist. It is also the basis for written

BOX **1.4**

A.J. is a 16-year-old who has just started soccer practice at school. She complains of increased shortness of breath with exercise, and describes having a hard time catching her breath when she runs, which she does 5 to 6 times a week. She does not wake up at night with a cough or shortness of breath, and has no problems at any other time except in the spring when the trees start to blossom. The soccer coach advised A.J.'s mother to seek health care because A.J. had a very difficult time breathing at practice that afternoon. A.J. also has a history of eczema and seasonal allergies for which she takes an over-the counter antihistamine when symptoms get severe.

Social History: Nonsmoker. Lives in an urban area with mother, father, and brother. Does not use street drugs.

Family History: Father has a history of asthma.

Physical examination:

  Nose: Mucosa pale and boggy bilaterally

  Lungs: Respirations 26 and shallow; diffuse expiratory wheezing; peak flow 340

Diagnosis: Mild persistent asthma

DISCUSSION

1. List specific goals of therapy for A.J.

   • Prevent troublesome symptoms (coughing, breathlessness on exertion)
   • Maintain normal activity levels
   • Prevent exacerbations of asthma

2. What drug therapy would you prescribe and why?
   A low-dose inhaled corticosteroid (ICS) is recommended with a short-acting beta agonist (SABA) as needed. This is the recommendation because there is an inflammation of the airways that is causing the persistent symptoms. The SABA is used for quick relief of symptoms, whereas the ICS provides long-term relief of symptoms.

3. What are the parameters for monitoring success of the therapy?
   Use of the SABA less than 2 times a week would indicate success. A follow-up visit in 1 month is recommended, with the patient bringing a log of times symptoms appeared and peak flow records. After the first visit, if A.J. is stable, visits are recommended every 1 to 6 months to ensure proper control.

4. Discuss specific patient education based on the prescribed therapy.
   A.J. should be encouraged to keep a log. An action plan should be developed by A.J. and the practitioner. A.J. must be taught to use an inhaler and a peak flow meter. A plan should be developed for treatment in school. A.J. should be taught to rinse her mouth after using the ICS.

5. List one or two adverse reactions for the selected agent that would cause you to change therapy.
   There are few adverse reactions associated with either ICS or SABA. A sign that therapy is not successful would be the use of the SABA more than 2 times a week or being awakened at night with symptoms more than 2 times a month.

6. What would be the choice for second-line therapy?
   The second-line therapy would be the use of a medium-dose ICS.

directions to patients, and it is a legal document. Each prescription should be clearly written to avoid errors of misinterpretation in filling the prescription. Although potentially serious errors occur infrequently, they are avoidable and should not occur at all.

An early step in the prescribing process involves ensuring that common but potentially serious errors are not made. The first is failure to identify a patient's allergies, particularly to a medication. In identifying a drug allergy, the practitioner should also investigate the kind of reaction experienced with the medication to differentiate between a true, life-threatening drug allergy and less serious drug sensitivity. Some cross-sensitivities must also be considered. Another error is failure to instruct the patient to stop a previously prescribed medication that treats the same condition. In some instances, an additional medication may be prescribed to increase the effect for the same problem, but the patient must be made aware of this. Otherwise, the original medication must be canceled. Failure to recognize the effect of a prescribed drug on other diseases or drugs can lead to potentially serious effects. There are now programs that can do multiple checks for interactions. One of these is Epocrates for PDAs and desktops.

Date, Name, Address, and Date of Birth

There are standard components of any prescription. One is the date and another is the full name, address, and date of birth of the patient. The name should be the patient's given name (the one on the medical record) and not a nickname. If a different name is used each time, the patient could have multiple records in pharmacy record-keeping systems. The address should be the current home address of the patient and not a work address or a post office box.

Prescriber's Name, Address, and Phone Number

The next components are the name, address, and phone number of the prescriber and the collaborating physician if required by state law or regulations. This enables the pharmacist to contact the prescriber if there is a question about the prescription.

Name of Drug

Of course, the name of the drug is the most essential part of the prescription. Ideally, the generic name (with the trade or brand name in parentheses) is used. The name must be legible to avoid errors in filling the prescription correctly. For instance, some drugs have names that are commonly confused or misread, such as Norvasc and Navane, Prilosec and Prozac, carboplatin and cisplatin, and Levoxine and Lanoxin. Severe problems may result if the wrong drug is supplied erroneously. Adding the diagnosis to the prescription, although optional, can help the pharmacist avoid misinterpreting the prescribed drug.

Dose, Dosage Regimen, and Route of Administration

The drug dose is essential because many drugs are available in various strengths. The dose is written in numerals. If the dose is a fraction of 1, it is written in decimal form with a zero to the left of the decimal point (e.g., 0.75). However, a whole number should not be followed by a decimal point (10.0 could be misinterpreted as 100). The numeric dose is followed by the correct metric specification such as milligram (mg), gram (g), milliliter (mL), or microgram (mcg). Many practitioners spell out *microgram* to avoid confusion with *milligram*. Some drugs are manufactured in units that should be specified, and the term *unit* should be written out (insulin 10 units, not 10 U). Usually, the strength of drugs that are combination products or that are manufactured only in one strength do not need to be included. The route of the drug is specified as well. (Routes of administration are discussed in Chapter 3.)

The prescription also specifies how frequently the drug is to be taken. A drug prescribed to be taken as needed is termed a *prn* drug. For example, dosage frequency can be written as "prn every 4 hours" (or another appropriate interval) for the problem for which the drug is prescribed (e.g., "as needed for nausea"). It is good practice to write out the number (10–ten), especially with controlled substances. Any special instructions, such as "after meals," "at bedtime," or "with food," also should be specified. If the dose is once a day it is safer practice to write out daily than to write OD because this can be confused with every other day.

The prescription also includes the number of pills, vials, suppositories, or containers or amount in milliliters or ounces to be dispensed. Many prescription reimbursement or health care insurance programs allow only a 1-month supply to be dispensed at a time, so it is good practice to be knowledgeable about the rules of various prescription plans. The prescription indicates whether the prescription may be refilled and the number of refills permitted.

When prescribing a new drug for a patient, the practitioner may want to consider prescribing just a few doses or a 7-day supply initially. Alternatively, samples may be provided, if allowed by law or regulations, to determine if the patient can tolerate the drug and if it is effective. When deciding on the number of refills, the practitioner may decide when the patient should return for a follow-up visit and allow just the number of refills that will take the patient until the next visit to ensure that the patient returns. Some drug prescriptions cannot be refilled. For all Schedule 2 drugs, for example, a new prescription must be written each time.

Allowable Substitutions

There are many generic equivalents for brand name drugs. Indication of whether a substitution is allowed is a part of the prescription. A generic drug substitute must have the same chemical composition and dosage as the brand name drug originally prescribed. In many states, a generic drug will automatically be substituted for a brand name drug. If there is a medical reason to require a brand name drug (that has a generic equivalent), "Brand Medically Necessary" must be written on the prescription.

Prescriber's Signature and License Number

The signature of the prescriber is required. It should be legible and should be the person's legal signature. The license number of the prescriber or the collaborating physician is required on the prescription. In some instances, the DEA number of the prescriber is also required, especially when prescribing between states or prescribing a controlled substance. **Figure 1-2** illustrates a blank prescription and a completed prescription. Each state has specific requirements for components on a printed prescription. The practitioner must be in compliance with state regulations and may prescribe only in the state in which he or she holds

Sally Jones, FNP
111 High Street
Hometown, NH 00440
555-432-1111

Serial #00001
NPIH 1234567890

Patient's Name _____ Date _____

Patient's Address _____

_____

Date of Birth _____

Drug _____ Dosage _____

Number _____

Directions _____

Number of refills _____

Generic substitution   yes _____ no _____

Signature _____

License Number _____

DEA Number (if required) _____

Sally Jones, FNP
111 High Street
Hometown, NH 00440
555-432-1111

Serial #00001
NPIH 1234567890

Patient's Name   John Smith   Date 6/29/00

Patient's Address   13 Comstock Street

Newtown, NH 33300

Date of Birth   1/2/33

Enalapril (Vasotec)   5 mg

#30

Take one daily

Number of refills 5

Substitution   yes X   no

Signature *Sally Jones, FNP*

License Number RN0000033

DEA Number (if required)   *012345-E*

FIGURE 1–2   Example of a blank prescription form (*left*) and a completed form (*right*).

a license. Although the prescription may be filled in another state (if allowed by state regulations), a DEA number is usually required. If the practitioner is a federal employee, he or she may prescribe in any federal facility. An NPI number must be on each prescription along with a serial number of the prescription form.

Any drug prescribed should be clearly documented in the medical record with date of order, dosage, amount prescribed, and number of refills. It is helpful to have a specific area in the record to record all drugs taken by the patient—prescription, OTC, and CAM—for ease of audit, reference, and communication among health care professionals.

Electronic Prescriptions

Electronic prescribing has become increasingly popular. Health care technology reduces medication errors with the use of drug-checking software, which checks the medication dose, potential interactions with other medications the patient may be taking, and the patient's known allergies. This drug-checking software may be part of the electronic health record (EHR) or of a freestanding e-prescribing system. Integrated EHRs can calculate dosing based on a patient's weight and carry out other contextual medication checking against a patient's laboratory results, age, and disease states. In addition, computer systems provide pick lists of each clinician's favorite medications with a pre-calculated dose, frequency, and route, reducing the opportunity for clinicians to

order inappropriate amounts of medications with the wrong frequency and route.

E-Prescribing improves the legibility of prescriptions and the rate of completed prescriptions. Patients no longer need to carry paper copies of a prescription to a pharmacy and are more likely to have formulary-compliant medications prescribed for them and to find their prescriptions waiting for them when they arrive at the pharmacy. This leads to greater patient convenience, shorter wait times, and increased compliance with formulary requirements. Electronic prescribing has been said to show a 12% to 20% decrease in ADEs (Figge, 2009).

With electronically generated prescriptions, there are no handwriting misinterpretations and no manual data entry. Correct dosages are built into the software. They assist with formulary requirements based on the patient's insurance and maintain allergy profiles and ADEs. They also serve to decrease drug-drug interactions.

There is an integration among the prescriber, patient, pharmacist, and insurance company. Additionally, medications prescribed by other providers are included in the electronic record.

ADHERENCE ISSUES

A prescribed drug must be used correctly to produce optimal benefits. Patient nonadherence to a prescribed regimen leads to less-than-optimal outcomes, such as progression of the

---

BOX 1.5

Factors Influencing the Patient's Adherence to a Medication Regimen

- Approachability of the health care provider
- Perception of respect with which he or she is treated by the practitioner
- Belief that the therapy is beneficial
- Belief that the benefits of therapy outweigh the risks or side effects
- Degree to which the patient participates in developing the treatment regimen
- Cost of the regimen
- Simplicity of the regimen
- Understanding of the treatment regimen
- Degree to which the patient feels that expectations are being met
- Degree to which the patient perceives his or her concerns are important and being addressed
- Degree to which the practitioner motivates the patient to adhere to the regimen
- Degree to which the regimen is compatible with the patient's lifestyle

---

Of patients with 10 or more prior medications, 20% were adherent.

Karter (2009) studied 27,329 subjects prescribed new medications. Pharmacy utilization data were used. It was found that 22% of patients had the prescription filled zero or one times. The proportion of newly prescribed patients that never became ongoing users was eight times greater than the proportion who maintained ongoing use, but with inadequate adherence. Four percent of those who had the prescription filled at least two times discontinued therapy during the 24-month follow-up. Non-adherence was significantly associated with high out-of-pocket costs and clinical response to therapy.

Several variables are associated with improved adherence to a drug regimen. These include variables associated with the patient's perception of the encounter and of the benefit of the treatment. If a patient is nonadherent to the prescribed regimen, it is important to document that in the chart. The risks of nonadherence are discussed and that discussion is documented. It is essential to ask why the patient is not following the prescribed treatment, and actions to rectify the problem should be taken. All of this is documented. One issue may be that the patient is unable to swallow the pill. The medicine may be available in liquid form or the pill may be split or crushed. The practitioner needs to review and understand the factors that affect adherence to a regimen (**Box 1.5**).

UPDATING DRUG INFORMATION

Many sources of drug information can be accessed by practitioners who must keep current on changes in drug therapy and continually update their fund of knowledge. Resources include reference books, pharmacists (who are expertly informed about drugs, interactions, dosages, etc.), easy-to-carry drug handbooks and pocket guides for quick reference, and on-line databases and programs for PDAs and handheld computers (**Tables 1.2** and **1.3**).

disease state and an increased incidence of hospitalizations. Studies demonstrate that the more complex the treatment regimen, the less likely the patient is to follow it. Benner (2009) studied 5,759 patients taking antihypertensive and lipid-lowering drugs. In patients with 0, 1, and 2 prior medications, 41%, 35%, and 30% of patients were adherent, respectively, to antihypertensive and lipid-lowering therapy.

TABLE 1.2	Common Drug Reference Books
Reference	**Features**
American Hospital Formulary Service. Bethesda, MD: American Society of Health System Pharmacists.	Drug entries are indexed by generic and brand names and organized by pharmacologic–therapeutic class.
Drug Facts and Comparisons Philadelphia: Wolters Kluwer Health.	Drugs are indexed by generic and brand names and organized by major classes of drugs. Updates are issued monthly (in print and CD-ROM).
Physician's Desk Reference (PDR) Montvale, NJ: Medical Economics.	Drugs are indexed by manufacturer, brand name, generic name, and product category. Volume contains product identification section. Information replicates the official package insert from the drug manufacturer.

TABLE 1.3	On-Line Drug Reference Data	
Reference	**Address**	**Features**
AHCPR Guidelines	www.ahrq.gov	Guidelines for clinical practice from the Agency for Health Care Policy and Research
Center Watch Clinical Trials	www.centerwatch.com	Lists clinical research trials and drug therapy newly approved by the U.S. FDA and the FDA New Drug Listing Service
Coreynahman	www.coreynahman.com	Pharmaceutical news and information Gives a choice of many sites for information
Epocrates	www.epocrates.com	Software for PDA with drug information, interactions, etc.
Healthtouch Drug Information	www.healthtouch.com	Information for patient and provider
Mediconsult	www.mediconsult.com	Professional- and consumer-focused Detailed medical and drug information
Medscape	www.medscape.com	Drug search database Links to on-line journals
Pharmaceutical Information Network	www.pharminfo.com	Information about treatment and drug therapy Articles from clinical publications, symposium information, and new drug information
RxList—The Internet Drug Index	www.rxlist.com	Cross-index of U.S. prescription products

BIBLIOGRAPHY

*Starred references are cited in the text.

Adler, K. G. (2009). E-prescribing: Why the fuss. *Family Practice Management, 16*(1), 22–27.

Atwater, A., Bednar, S., Hassman, D., & Khouri, J. (2008). Nurse practitioners and physician assistants in primary care. *Disease-a-Month, 54*(11), 728–744.

*Barnes P. M., Bloom, B., & Nahin R. (2008). CDC National Health Statistics Report #12. Complementary and Alternative Medicine Use Among Adults and Children: United States, 2007.

Belle, D. G., & Singh, H. (2008). Genetic factors in drug metabolism. *American Family Physician, 77*(11), 1553–1168.

*Benner, J. S. (2009). Association between prescription burden and medication adherence in patients initiating antihypertensive and lipid-lowering therapy. *American Journal of Health System Pharmacies, 66*(16), 1471–1477.

*Budnitz, D. S., Pollock, D. A., Weidenbach, K. N., et al. (2005). National surveillance of emergency department visits for outpatient adverse drug events. *JAMA, 296,* 1858–1866.

*Cherry, M. S., Hing, E., Woodwell, D. A., & Rechtsteinen, E. A. (2008). National Ambulatory Medical Care Survey: 2006 summary. National health statistics reports; no 3. Hyattsville, MD: National Center for Health Statistics.

Court, M. H. (2007). A pharmacogenomics primer. *Journal of Clinical Pharmacology, 47*(9), 1087–1103.

Cusack, C. M. (2008). Electronic health records and electronic prescribing: Promise and pitfalls. *Obstetric and Gynecology Clinics of North America, 35*(1), 63–79.

DiPiro, J. T., Talbert, R. L., Hayes, P. E., et al. (Eds.). (2008). *Pharmacotherapy: A pathophysiologic approach* (7th ed.). New York, NY: McGraw-Hill Medical.

Doherty, K., Segal, A., & McKinney, P. (2004). The 10 most common prescribing errors: Tips on avoiding the pitfalls. *Consultant, 44*(2), 173–182.

*Figge, H. (2009). Electronic prescribing in the ambulatory care setting. *American Journal of Health System Pharmacy, 66*(1), 16–18,

*Gandhi T. K., Weingart S. N., Seger A. C., et al. (2005). Outpatient prescribing errors and the impact of computerized prescribing. *Journal of General Internal Medicine, 20,* 837–841.

*Karter, A. J. (2009). New prescription medication gaps: A comprehensive measure of adherence to new prescriptions. *Health Service Research, 44*(5 Pt. 1), 1640–1661.

Keohane, C. A., & Bates, D. W. (2008). Medication safety. *Obstetrics and Gynecology Clinics, 35*(1), 37–52.

Mahoney, D. F. (2010). More than a prescriber: Gerontological nurse practitioners' perspectives on prescribing and pharmaceutical marketing. *Geriatric Nursing, 31*(1), 17–27.

*Moore, T. J., Cohen M. R., & Furberg C. D. (2007). Serious adverse drug events reported to the Food and Drug Administration, 1998–2005. *Archives of Internal Medicine, 167,* 1752–1759.

National Center for Complementary and Alternative Medicine. [on-line: retrieved July 14, 2010]. http://nccam.nih.gov/health/supplements/wiseuse.htm#use.

O'Connor, N. R. (2010). FDA boxed warnings: How to prescribe drugs safely. *American Family Physician, 81*(3), 298–303.

Pollock, M., Bazaldua, O., & Dobbie, A. (2007). Appropriate prescribing of medications: An eight-step approach. *American Family Physician, 75*(2), 231–236.

Sadee, W. (2008). Drug therapy and personalized health care: Pharmacogenomics in perspective. *Pharmacology Research, 25*(12), 2713–2719.

Weber, W. W. (2008). Pharmacogenomics: From description to prediction. *Clinics in Laboratory Medicine, 28*(4), 499–511.

Pharmacokinetic Basis of Therapeutics and Pharmacodynamic Principles

The art and science of clinical practice is based on understanding the relationship between the person and the disease and determining the most appropriate means for alleviating symptoms, curing disease, or preventing severe morbidity or even mortality. Very often, medications are prescribed to accomplish one or more of these goals.

Underpinning this treatment process is the intricate relationship between the body and the medication. Often, practitioners seek to understand the effect a drug has on the body (whether therapeutic or harmful) but neglect to consider the effect that the body has on the drug—even though one cannot be understood without the other. How the body acts on a drug and how the drug acts on the body are the subjects of this chapter.

Pharmacokinetics refers to the movement of the drug through the body—in essence, how the body affects the drug. This involves how the drug is administered, absorbed, distributed, and eventually eliminated from the body. *Pharmacodynamics* refers to how the drug affects the body—that is, how the drug initiates its therapeutic or toxic effect, both at the cellular level and systemically. **Box 2.1** lists terms and definitions used throughout this chapter.

The purpose of pharmacokinetic processes is to get the drug to the site of action where it can produce its pharmacodynamic effect. There is a minimum amount of drug needed at the site of action to produce the desired effect. Although the amount of drug concentrated at the site of action is difficult to measure, the amount of drug in the blood can be measured. The relationship between the concentration of drug in the blood and the concentration at the site of action (i.e., the drug receptor) is different for each drug and each person. Therefore, measuring blood concentrations is only a surrogate marker, an indication of concentration at the receptor (i.e., the site of action). **Figure 2-1** shows the relationship between pharmacokinetics and pharmacodynamics.

PHARMACOKINETICS

Pharmacokinetics relates to how the drug is absorbed, distributed, and eliminated from the body. In reality, it is the study of the fate of medications administered to a person. It is sometimes described as *what the body does to the drug*. In theory, pharmacokinetics not only deals with medications, it deals with the disposition of all substances administered externally to any living organism. Pharmacokinetics can help the clinician determine the onset and duration of a drug's action as well as determine blood levels that would produce therapeutic and toxic effects. As such, one can determine the blood levels necessary to produce a desired effect. This target drug concentration is key to monitoring the effects of many medications. Assuming that the magnitude of the drug concentration at the site of action influences the drug effect, whether desired or undesired, it can be inferred that a range of drug levels produces a range of effects (**Figure 2-2**). Below a specific level, or threshold, the drug exerts little to no therapeutic effect. Above this threshold, the concentration of drug in the blood is sufficient to produce a therapeutic effect at the site of action. However, as the drug concentration increases in the blood, so does the concentration at the site of action. Above a specific level, an increased therapeutic effect may no longer occur. Instead, an unacceptable toxicity may exist because the drug concentration is too high. Between these two levels—the minimally effective level and the toxic level—is the *therapeutic window*. The therapeutic window is the range of blood drug concentration that yields a sufficient therapeutic response without excessively toxic reactions. This range should not be considered absolute because it varies from individual to individual and therefore serves only as a guide to the practitioner.

Absorption

The first aspect of pharmacokinetics to consider is how drugs are administered, how they are absorbed into the body, and how they eventually reach the bloodstream. Merely introducing the drug into the body does not ensure that the compound will reach all tissues uniformly or even that the drug will reach the target site. Commonly recognized methods of absorption include enteral absorption (after the drug is administered by the oral or rectal route) and parenteral absorption (associated with drugs administered intramuscularly [IM], subcutaneously, or topically). The various administration routes and other factors affect a drug's ability to enter the bloodstream.

The extent to which the drug reaches the systemic circulation is referred to as *bioavailability*, or F, which is defined as the fraction or percentage of the drug that reaches the

BOX **2.1**

Definitions of Terms Related to Pharmacokinetics and Pharmacodynamics

Affinity: The attraction between a drug and a receptor.

Allosteric site: A binding site for substrates not active in initiating a response; a substrate that binds to an allosteric site may induce a conformational change in the structure of the active site, rendering it more or less susceptible to response from a substrate.

Bioavailability (F): The fraction or percentage of a drug that reaches the systemic circulation.

Biotransformation: Metabolism or degradation of a drug from an active form to an inactive form.

Chirality: Special configuration or shape of a drug; most drugs exist in two shapes.

Clearance: Removal of a drug from the plasma or organs.

Downregulation: Decreased availability of drug receptors.

Enantiomer (also called isomer): A mirror-image spatial arrangement, or shape, of a drug that suits it for binding with a drug receptor.

Enterohepatic recirculation: The process by which a drug excreted in the bile flows into the gastrointestinal tract, where it is reabsorbed and returned to the general circulation.

First-pass effect: The phenomenon by which a drug first passes through the liver for degradation before distribution to the tissues.

Half-life ($t_{1/2}$): The time required for half of a total drug amount to be eliminated from the body.

Hepatic extraction ratio: A comparison of the percentage of drug extracted and the percentage of drug remaining active after metabolism in the liver.

Pharmacodynamics: Processes through which drugs affect the body.

Pharmacokinetics: Processes through which the body affects drugs.

Prodrug: A drug that is transformed from an inactive parent drug into an active metabolite; in effect, a precursor to the active drug.

Receptor: The site of drug action.

Second messenger: A chemical produced intracellularly in response to a receptor signal; this second messenger initiates a change in the intracellular response.

Therapeutic window: The range of drug concentration in the blood between a minimally effective level and a toxic level.

Threshold: The level below which a drug exerts little to no therapeutic effect and above which a drug produces a therapeutic effect at the site of action.

Upregulation: Increased availability of receptors.

Volume of distribution (V_d): The extent of distribution of a drug in the body.

---

systemic circulation. Drugs administered intravenously are 100% bioavailable. Drugs administered by other routes (e.g., oral, IM) may be 100% bioavailable, but more often they are less than 100% bioavailable. Therefore, bioavailability depends on the route of administration and, equally important, the drug's ability to pass through membranes or barriers in the body. **Box 2.2** discusses the specific case of oral bioavailability.

Factors Affecting Absorption

A variety of factors affect absorption, such as the presence or absence of food in the stomach, blood flow to the area for

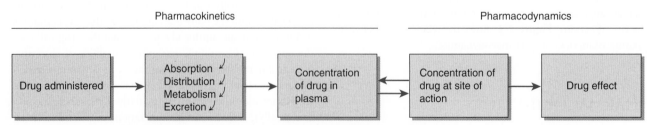

FIGURE 2–1   Relationship between pharmacokinetics and pharmacodynamics. Note the two-way relationship between the concentration of drug in the plasma and the concentration of drug at the site of action, depicting the interrelationship between pharmacokinetics and pharmacodynamics.

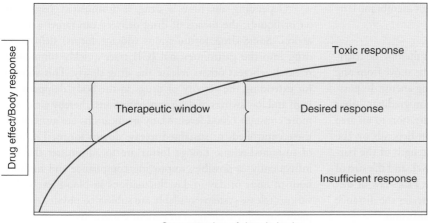

FIGURE 2–2 Therapeutic window: concentration versus response. The concentration of the drug in the body produces specific effects. A low concentration is considered subtherapeutic, producing an insufficient response. As the concentration increases, the desired effect is produced at a given drug level. A drug concentration that exceeds the upper limit of the desired response may produce a toxic reaction. The concentration range within which a desired response occurs is the therapeutic window.

absorption, and the dosage form of the drug. The following sections discuss some of the major factors affecting absorption.

Movement Through Membranes and Drug Solubility

Throughout the body, biologic membranes act as barriers, blocking or permitting the passage of various substances. These membranes protect certain areas of the body from harmful chemicals and allow other areas to be accessed as needed.

Biologic membranes composed of cells serve as barriers primarily because of the structure and function of the cells that make up the membrane. Cell membranes are composed of lipids and proteins, creating a phospholipid bilayer. This bilayer acts as a barrier that is almost impermeable to water, other hydrophilic (water-loving) substances, and ionized substances. However, the bilayer does allow most lipid-soluble (hydrophobic) compounds to pass through readily. Interspersed throughout this bilayer are protein molecules and small openings, or pores. The proteins may act as carrier molecules, bringing molecules through the barrier. The pores allow hydrophilic molecules to pass through if they are small enough. Therefore,

---

BOX 2.2

Oral Bioavailability and the First-Pass Effect

Drugs given by the oral route may be subject to the first-pass effect, by which drugs are metabolized by the liver before passing into circulation. After absorption from the alimentary canal, drugs go directly to the liver through the portal vein. In the liver, hepatic enzymes act on the drug, reducing the amount of active drug reaching the bloodstream and decreasing the amount available to the body. The fraction (or percentage) of medication reaching systemic circulation after the first pass through the liver is referred to as the drug's bioavailability (F).

The first-pass effect is not the only factor contributing to the oral bioavailability of a drug. Poorly soluble drugs and drugs adversely affected by gastric pH or other presystemic factors can also have a low bioavailability.

Drugs not usually subject to the liver's first-pass effect are known as drugs with a low hepatic extraction ratio because the liver does not extract a large percentage of the drug before releasing it into the circulation. Usually, drugs with a low extraction ratio have high oral bioavailability. In contrast, drugs with a high extraction ratio have low oral bioavailability. For example, lidocaine has a hepatic extraction ratio of 0.7; that is, the liver metabolizes 70% of the drug before the drug reaches the circulation and, as such, only 30% remains available systemically. (This is one reason lidocaine is administered parenterally.) In other words, the first-pass effect for lidocaine is of such magnitude that an alternative route of administration is required. Giving large oral doses of a drug to compensate for the high extraction ratio is often an alternative to parenteral administration. For example, because of the high extraction ratio of propranolol, a 1-mg dose administered intravenously is approximately equivalent to a 40-mg dose administered orally.

Examples of drugs with a high hepatic extraction ratio (70% or more) are imipramine (Tofranil), lidocaine (Xylocaine), and meperidine (Demerol); drugs with intermediate rankings are codeine, nortriptyline (Aventyl), and quinidine (Quinaglute); and some drugs with a low extraction ratio (30% or less) are barbiturates, diazepam (Valium), theophylline (Theo-Dur), tolbutamide (Orinase), and warfarin (Coumadin).

drugs and other compounds that pass through membrane barriers can do so by passive and active means.

Passive Diffusion Drugs can pass through membrane barriers by diffusion. In passive diffusion, molecules move from one side of a barrier to another without expending energy. In passing, the molecules move down a concentration gradient—that is, they move from an area of higher concentration to an area of lower concentration. The rate of diffusion depends on the differences in concentrations, the relative strength of the barrier, the distance that the molecules must travel, and the size of the molecules. This relationship is known as Fick's law of diffusion. In essence, Fick's law states that the greater the distance and the larger the molecule, the slower the diffusion.

Another major barrier to the absorption of a drug is its solubility. To facilitate drug absorption, the solubility of the administered drug must match the cellular constituents of the absorption site. Lipid-soluble drugs can penetrate fatty cells; water-soluble drugs cannot. For example, a water-soluble drug such as penicillin cannot easily pass through the barrier between the blood and brain, whereas a highly lipid-soluble drug such as diazepam (Valium) can. The relative strength of the barrier is important because the barrier must be permeable to the diffusing substance. Drugs diffuse more readily through the lipid bilayer if they are in their neutral, non-ionized form. Most drugs are weak acids or weak bases, which have the potential for becoming positively or negatively charged. This potential is created through the pH of certain body fluids. In the plasma and in most other fluids, most drugs remain non-ionized. However, in the gastric acid of the stomach, weak bases become ionized and are more difficult to absorb. As this weak base progresses through the alkaline environment of the small intestines, it becomes non-ionized and therefore more easily absorbed. Similarly, weak acids remain non-ionized in the stomach and become ionized in the small intestines. The result is reduced absorption by the intestines.

Active Transport In active transport, membrane proteins act as carrier molecules to transport substances across cell membranes. The role of active transport in moving drugs across cell membranes is limited. To be carried through by a protein, the drug must share molecular similarities with an endogenous substance the transport system routinely carries. Cells can accomplish this through the process of endocytosis. In this process, the cell forms a vesicle surrounding the molecule, and it is subsequently invaginated in the cell. Once inside the cell, the vesicle releases the molecule into the cytoplasm of the cell.

Pharmaceutical Preparation

Drugs are formulated and administered in such a way as to produce either local or systemic effects. Local effects (e.g., antiseptic, anti-inflammatory, and local anesthetic effects) are confined to one area of the body. Systemic effects occur when the drug is absorbed and delivered to body tissues by way of the circulatory system.

Depending on how a drug is formulated (e.g., tablet or liquid), the means of drug delivery can target a site of action. Some drug formulations (dosage forms) deliver the drug into the gastrointestinal (GI) tract quickly (immediate release), whereas others release the drug slowly. This strategy for extending the activity of drugs in the body dampens the high and low swings of drug concentrations, thereby yielding a more constant blood level. Many medications are available in these controlled- or sustained-release dosage forms. The aims of sustained-release dosage forms are to administer them as infrequently as possible, improving compliance and minimal hour-to-hour or day-to-day fluctuations in blood levels. The various release systems available are subject to physiologic and pathophysiologic changes in patient conditions.

Blood Flow

Blood flow ensures that the concentration across a gradient is continually in favor of passive diffusion—that is, as blood flows through an area, it continually removes the drug from the area, thereby maintaining a positive concentration gradient. Many hydrophobic–lipophilic drugs can readily pass through membranes and be absorbed. However, if the blood flow to that area is limited, the extent of absorption is limited. Because of the minimal vascularization in the subcutaneous layer compared with the greater vascularity of the musculature, drugs injected subcutaneously may undergo limited absorption compared with drugs delivered by IM injection.

Gastrointestinal Motility

High-fat meals and solid foods affect GI transit time by delaying gastric emptying, which in turn delays initial drug delivery to intestinal absorption surfaces. The administration of agents that delay or slow intestinal motility (e.g., anticholinergic agents) prolongs the contact time. This increased contact time secondary to prolonged intestinal transit time may increase total drug absorption. Conversely, laxatives and diarrhea can shorten an agent's contact time with the small intestine, which may decrease drug absorption.

Enteral Absorption

Enteral absorption, with the oral route of administration being the most common and probably the most preferred, occurs anywhere throughout the GI tract by passive or active transport of the drug through the cells of the GI tract.

Following Fick's law, low-molecular-weight, non-ionized drugs diffuse passively down a concentration gradient from the higher concentration (in the GI tract) to the lower concentration (in the blood). Active transport across the GI tract occurs more frequently with larger, usually ionized, molecules. These active mechanisms include binding of the drug to carrier molecules in the cell membrane. The molecules carry the drug across the lipid bilayer of the cells. However, most drugs are absorbed passively.

Oral Administration

The oral route of administration refers to any medication that is taken by mouth (*per os*, or PO). The ability to swallow is implicit in oral administration; however, many practitioners consider local action, in which absorption does not occur, also to be "oral" (e.g., troches for fungal infections of the mouth). Common dosage forms administered by mouth include tablets, capsules, caplets, solutions, suspensions, troches, lozenges, and powders.

Absorption after oral administration usually occurs in the lower GI tract (small or large intestine), is usually slow, and depends on the patient's gastric emptying time, the presence or absence of food, and the gastric or intestinal pH. Variations in one or more of these factors can affect the stability of the drug, the contact time with the walls of the GI tract, or the blood flow to the GI tract and hence the ability of the drug to cross the epithelial lining of the GI tract. Most of the absorption occurs in the small intestine, where the large surface area enhances and controls drug entry into the body.

Drugs administered orally must be relatively lipid soluble to cross the GI mucosa into the bloodstream. The diffusion rate, a function of the lipid solubility of a drug across the GI mucosa, is a major factor in determining the rate of absorption of a drug. The acid pH of the stomach and the nearly neutral pH of the intestines can degrade some medications before they are absorbed. In addition, bacteria in various parts of the intestines secrete enzymes that also can break down drugs before absorption.

Although the GI tract is generally resistant to a variety of noxious agents, considerable irritation and discomfort can arise from certain medications in some people. Nausea, vomiting, diarrhea, and less often mucosal damage are common side effects of medications, and the practitioner should monitor all patients for these effects.

Sublingual Administration

Sublingual (SL, *under the tongue*) drug administration relies on absorption through the oral mucosa into the veins that drain those vascular beds. These veins carry the drug to the superior vena cava and eventually the heart. Drugs administered this way are not subject to the first-pass effect (see **Box 2.2**). This method of administration is limited by the amount of drug that can be placed sublingually and the drug's ability to pass through the oral mucosa into the venous system. Buccal administration, in which the drug is absorbed through the mucous membranes of the mouth, is similar to sublingual administration.

Rectal Administration

Drugs administered rectally (PR, *per rectum*) include suppositories and enemas. Primarily used in the treatment of local conditions (e.g., hemorrhoids) and inflammatory bowel disease, this method is less effective than other enteral routes of administration because of the erratic absorption of most agents. Bowel irritation, early evacuation, and minimal surface area contribute to erratic absorption and poor tolerability of

this route. Advantages, however, include the ability to administer a medication to an unconscious or nauseated patient.

Parenteral Absorption

All routes of administration not involving the GI tract are considered parenteral. Parenteral routes include inhalation, all forms of injection, and topical and transdermal administration.

Inhalation

Drugs that are gaseous or sprayable in small particles may be delivered by inhalation. The lungs provide a large surface area for absorption and quick entry into the bloodstream. Inhaled medications bypass the first-pass effect and therefore may have a high bioavailability. Examples of inhalants are anesthetic gases and beta-adrenergic agonists (e.g., albuterol) used in treating asthma. Conversely, agents such as inhaled corticosteroids are intended for local action in the lung tissue. Regardless of the intent of inhaled medications, the disadvantages include irritation to the alveolar space and the need for good coordination during self-administration, such as with metered-dose inhalers.

Intravenous Administration

The intravenous (IV) route provides rapid access to the circulatory system with a known quantity of drug. Bypassing the first-pass effect and any GI metabolism or degradation, drug absorption by this route is considered the gold standard with regard to bioavailability. IV bolus injections allow for large amounts of medication to be administered quickly for a high peak drug level and a rapid effect. However, adverse effects from these high levels of medications also occur with this form of administration. Repeated bolus doses of medications, at designated intervals, can produce large fluctuations in peak and trough (lowest concentration before next dose) levels. Although over time these peaks and troughs produce average desired concentrations, significant peak and trough fluctuations may not be desirable in some patients. Continuous administration by an infusion can minimize or eliminate these fluctuations and produce a consistent, steady-state concentration.

Like IV administration, intra-arterial administration produces a rapid effect. However, because the drug is directly instilled in an organ, this route is considered more dangerous than the IV route. Therefore, intra-arterial administration is usually reserved for a time when injection into a specific tissue is indicated (e.g., anticancer treatment for a specific tumor).

Subcutaneous Administration

Subcutaneous (SC or SQ) administration produces a slower, more prolonged release of medication into the bloodstream. Injected directly beneath the skin, a drug must diffuse through layers of fat and muscle to encounter sufficient blood vessels for entry into the systemic circulation. This route is limited by the quantity of the liquid suitable for administration (usually 2 to 3 mL). Caution must also be taken because dermal irritation, or even necrosis, may occur. More recent technological advances allow the practitioner to implant drug-releasing mechanisms under the skin, providing a reservoir of drug for long-term absorption. Levonorgestrel (Norplant), a hormonal contraceptive, is administered in this manner.

Intramuscular Administration

Injecting medications into the highly vascularized skeletal muscle is a way of administering drugs quickly and avoiding the relatively large changes in plasma levels seen with IV administration. Local pain and muscle soreness are drawbacks to this method, as is the wide variability in the rate of absorption resulting from injections given in different muscles and in different patients. Blood flow to the area is the major factor in determining the rate of absorption. This is considered a safe way to administer irritating drugs, although not all IM injections are truly IM: in grossly obese patients, presumed IM injections may actually be intralipomatous, which decreases the rate of absorption because of the lower vascularity of fatty tissue.

Topical Administration

Topical drug administration involves applying drugs, in various vehicles (e.g., liquids, powders), to the site of action, primarily the skin. Topical ointments, creams, drops, and gels typically produce a local effect. Ointments are occlusive, preventing water absorption or evaporation, and therefore have a hydrating effect and typically produce greater local effects than their cream counterparts. Creams are water soluble and therefore can be washed from the skin more readily than ointments. In hairy areas, creams are preferred over ointments because creams are hydrophilic and hence easier to apply and wash off. Gels, the most water-soluble topical dosage form, allow medication to be spread more easily over a larger area.

Transdermal Administration

Transdermal (*across the skin*) administration refers to the systemic delivery of medication through the skin. Several transdermal drug delivery systems are available for a wide range of medications, including nitroglycerin (Transderm Nitro®), estrogens (Estraderm®), and fentanyl (Duragesic®). In general, this method continuously delivers medication to achieve a constant blood level. The consistent delivery of drug throughout the dosing interval minimizes the peak-to-trough fluctuations seen with other forms of drug administration, thereby minimizing the toxicity associated with high blood levels while maintaining therapeutic concentrations.

Distribution

A discussion of the routes of administration offers the opportunity to consider the factors affecting drug absorption and bioavailability; once the medication is in the body, however, it must distribute to the site of action to be effective.

Distribution of an absorbed drug in the body depends on several factors: blood flow to an area, lipid or water solubility, and protein binding. For an absorbed drug to distribute from the blood to a specific site of action, there must be adequate blood flow to that area. In patients with compromised blood flow (e.g., from shock), relying on the blood to deliver a drug to a site of action, such as the kidney, may be risky.

In addition, drug distribution may be affected by obesity, both immediately after absorption and after achieving an equilibrium or steady state in the body. Lipid-soluble drugs readily distribute into the fatty tissues, where they may be stored and even concentrated. Water-soluble drugs, however, tend to remain in the highly vascularized spaces of the skeletal muscle. Ideal body weight is usually considered the standard for determining drug dosage, which is often adjusted for obese or cachectic patients.

Protein Binding

After absorption into the blood (and lymph), a drug may circulate throughout the body unbound (*free drug*) or bound to carrier proteins such as albumin. The extent of drug binding to carrier proteins depends on the affinity of the drug for the carrier protein and the concentrations of both the drug and the proteins. Acidic drugs commonly bind to albumin and basic drugs commonly bind to alpha$_1$-acid glycoprotein or lipoproteins.

Plasma protein binding is typically a reversible phenomenon, with binding and unbinding occurring within milliseconds. Therefore, the bound and unbound forms of the drug can be assumed to be at equilibrium at all times. As such, the degree of binding to plasma proteins can be expressed as a percentage of bound drug to total concentration (bound plus unbound). It is only the unbound or free drug that can exert a pharmacologic effect. If the drug becomes bound, it becomes inactive because it cannot leave the bloodstream or bind to an enzyme or receptor and exert its therapeutic action (**Figure 2-3**).

Once the free drug is eliminated from the body through metabolism or excretion, the bound drug can be released from the protein to become active. In essence, the bound drug may serve as a storage site or reservoir of the drug. The percentage of the free drug usually is constant for a single drug and varies among drugs. Patient-specific factors, such as nutritional status, renal function, and levels of circulating protein or albumin, can change the percentage of the free drug.

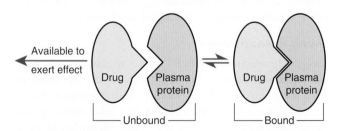

FIGURE 2–3 Relationship between bound and unbound drugs and plasma proteins.

Volume of Distribution

The amount of drug in the human body can never be directly measured. Observations are made of the concentration of drug in plasma or sometimes in blood. Over time, the concentration of drug in the plasma depends on the rate and extent of drug distribution to the tissues and on how rapidly the drug is eliminated. For most drugs, distribution occurs more rapidly than elimination. The resultant plasma concentration after distribution depends on the dose and the extent of distribution into the tissues. This extent of distribution can be determined by relating the concentration obtained with a known amount of administered drug.

For example, if 100 mg of an IV drug is administered to a person and remains only in the blood, and if that person's total blood volume measures 5 L, the resulting measured concentration of drug would be 20 mg/L [concentration = dose/volume: 100 mg/5 L]. However, in reality, few drugs distribute solely in the plasma, and many bind to plasma proteins. Drugs commonly bind not only to plasma proteins but also to tissue-binding sites on fat and muscle. In addition, drugs translocate into other "compartments" or spaces throughout the body. The apparent volume into which a drug distributes in the body at equilibrium is called the (apparent) volume of distribution (V_d). This volume does not refer to a real volume; rather, it is a mathematically calculated volume (**Box 2.3**). The V_d is a direct measure of the extent of distribution of a drug in the body and represents the apparent volume that a drug must distribute to contain the amount of drug homogenously.

Drugs that are highly water soluble or highly bound to plasma proteins remain in the blood compartment and do not distribute or bind to fatty tissue. These drugs have a low V_d, usually less than the volume of total body water (approximately 50 L, or 0.7 L/kg). Drugs with a low V_d usually circulate at high levels in the blood. In contrast, drugs that are not highly protein bound and are highly lipophilic have a high V_d

(150 L, which is greater than the volume of total body water). These drugs distribute widely throughout the body and may even cross the blood–brain barrier.

Elimination

All drugs must eventually be eliminated from the body to terminate their effect. Drugs can be eliminated through metabolism (or biotransformation) of the drug from an active form to an inactive form. Drugs can also be eliminated by excretion from the body. Therefore, elimination is a combination of the metabolism and excretion of drugs from the body. Important concepts in understanding drug elimination are half-life, steady state, and clearance. Knowledge of these phenomena in any given patient helps practitioners understand how long a drug will last in the body and how much should be given to maintain therapeutic levels and therefore helps in determining the appropriate dose and dosing intervals.

Metabolism

Metabolism is a function of the body designed to change substances into water-soluble, more readily excreted forms. The liver primarily performs the body's metabolic functions because of its high concentration of metabolic enzymes. This is why the first-pass effect is significant to the bioavailability of a drug administered orally.

Other organs, such as the kidneys and intestines, as well as circulating enzyme systems, also contribute to the metabolism of drugs. Metabolic processes are used to detoxify drugs and other foreign substances as well as endogenous substances. Drugs may be metabolized from active components into inactive or less active ones. Some drugs, however, may be biologically transformed from an inactive parent drug into an active metabolite. This type of drug is called a prodrug because it is a precursor to the active drug (**Table 2.1**). Not all drugs are metabolized to the same extent or by the same means. In fact, some drugs, such as the aminoglycosides (e.g., gentamicin [Garamycin]), are not metabolized at all.

Enzyme actions are the primary means for metabolizing drugs, and these actions are broadly classified as phase 1 and phase 2 enzymatic processes. Phase 1 enzymatic processes involve oxidation or reduction, by which a drug is changed to form a more polar or water-soluble compound. Phase 2 processes involve adding a conjugate (e.g., a glucuronide) to the parent drug or the phase 1–metabolized drug to further increase water solubility and enhance excretion.

BOX **2.3**

Calculating the Apparent Volume of Distribution (V_d)

$$V_d = \frac{\text{Amount in body}}{\text{Plasma drug concentration}}$$

V_d is usually measured in liters (L); *amount in body* is usually measured in milligrams (mg); and *plasma drug concentration* is usually measured in milligrams per liter (mg/L).

The apparent volume of distribution is a theoretical parameter calculated by determining the amount of drug in the body (usually the dose administered) divided by the concentration of drug in the plasma taken at an appropriate time interval after administration.

TABLE 2.1	Selected Prodrugs and Metabolites
Parent Drug (Prodrug)	**Active Metabolite**
allopurinol	oxypurinol
codeine	morphine
enalapril	enalaprilat
prednisone	prednisolone
sulindac	sulindac sulfide

TABLE 2.2	Key Cytochrome P450 Families and Isoforms in Drug Metabolism	
Family	Isoform	Example of Drugs Metabolized
CYP1	CYP1A2	theophylline
CYP2	CYP2C	omeprazole
	CYP2D6	dextromethorphan
	CYP2E1	acetaminophen
CYP3	CYP3A4	quinidine

The oxidative process of phase 1 metabolism is catalyzed by a superfamily of more than 100 enzymes called the cytochrome P450 system (CYP). Three families and five isoforms of the CYP are important contributors to drug metabolism. The common feature of these enzymes is their lipid solubility. Most lipophilic drugs are substrates for one or more of the CYP enzymes (**Table 2.2**).

Some drugs can induce or stimulate the production of one or more isoforms of the enzymes by a process called enzyme induction, which increases the amount of enzyme available to metabolize drugs. The result of enzyme induction is an increased metabolism of other drugs, thereby decreasing the amount of drug circulating throughout the body.

Conversely, some drugs inhibit the production of CYP enzymes and thereby decrease the metabolism of drugs and increase circulating levels. This is known as enzyme inhibition. Both enzyme induction and inhibition are the basis of metabolically mediated drug–drug interactions. See Chapter 3 for further discussion of induction and inhibition and their role in drug–drug interactions.

Although the liver is regarded as the primary site of drug metabolism, other tissues also possess the enzymes necessary for metabolism. The kidneys, for example, have several enzymes needed for drug metabolism and can serve as the site of drug inactivation. The GI tract is also known to possess several of the CYP isoforms, contributing to the extrahepatic metabolism of drugs.

The nature, function, and amount of any drug-metabolizing enzyme can be different, resulting in differing drug disposition among patients. Disease-induced changes can affect drug metabolism as well. For example, alterations in liver function induced by long-standing cirrhotic changes can reduce the production of necessary enzymes, resulting in increased concentrations of drugs typically metabolized in the liver. Also, decreased blood flow to the liver, as occurring in congestive heart failure, can decrease the delivery of drug to metabolic sites in the liver. Cigarette smoking on the other hand, can increase the levels of enzymes responsible for drug metabolism, resulting in increased metabolic rates and the need for higher doses of drugs (e.g., theophylline) in smokers than in nonsmokers.

Drug Excretion

Metabolism eliminates a drug from the body by changing the drug molecule into something else, but drugs also can be eliminated from the body by excretion. Excretory organs include the kidneys, lower GI tract, lungs, and skin. Other structures, such as the sweat, salivary, and mammary glands, are active in excretion as well. Drugs may also be removed forcibly by dialysis.

The primary route of excretion is the kidney. After the drug is metabolized, the resultant metabolite may be filtered by the glomerulus. As the drug continues through the proximal tubule, loop of Henle, and distal tubule, several things may occur: the drug may exert action (as in the case of diuretics), be reabsorbed into the bloodstream, or remain in the nephron, eventually reaching the collecting ducts, from which it ultimately leaves the body in the patient's urine. This filtration works well for hydrophilic, ionized compounds and is a common route of elimination. Conversely, active secretion of drugs occurs in the proximal tubule. Two different systems exist, one for organic acids (e.g., uric acid) and one for organic bases (e.g., histamine). Once ionized by the acidic pH of the urine, organic bases are not reabsorbed back into the bloodstream. If the pH rises, then more of the organic base becomes non-ionized and becomes more readily reabsorbed. Similarly, changes in urine pH can alter the reabsorption of organic acids, increasing or decreasing the circulating levels as the pH changes. Drugs such as penicillin are excreted by the organic acid system.

Drugs are excreted by the liver into the gallbladder, resulting in biliary elimination. Biliary elimination can sometimes result in drug reabsorption. For example, if a drug is excreted in the bile, it goes into the GI tract, where it may be reabsorbed and returned to the general circulation. This is called *enterohepatic recirculation* (**Figure 2-4**). The result of

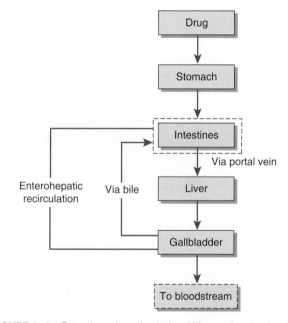

FIGURE 2–4 Enterohepatic recirculation. When a drug is absorbed from the intestine, travels to the liver and gallbladder, and into the bile unchanged, it has the potential for being reintroduced into the intestine and therefore reabsorbed. This is known as enterohepatic recirculation.

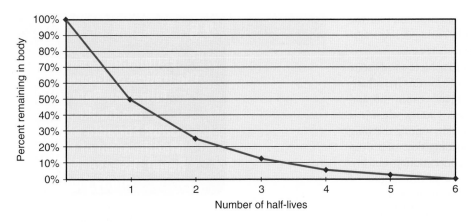

FIGURE 2–5 Drug elimination based on half-life ($t_{1/2}$).

significant enterohepatic recirculation is a measurable increase in the plasma concentration of a drug and a delay in its elimination from the body.

Half-Life

The time required for a drug to be eliminated from the body varies according to the drug and the individual. However, useful generalizations can be made that help practitioners estimate how long a drug will remain in the body. The first generalization has to do with the elimination half-life ($t_{1/2}$), which is the time required for half of the total drug amount to be eliminated from the body. Assuming 100% of a drug exists in the body at time X, then one half-life later, 50% of the original amount would remain in the body. An additional half-life later, 25% would remain. For example, theophylline (Theo-Dur) has a $t_{1/2}$ of approximately 8 hours in nonsmokers. If the theophylline concentration in a patient's body is 15 mg/L, then it would take 8 hours to decline to 7.5 mg/L, another 8 hours (16 hours total) to fall to 3.75 mg/L, and so on. The actual rate of elimination of a drug remains constant, but as can be seen in **Figure 2-5,** the actual amount of drug eliminated is proportional to the concentration of the drug—that is, the more drug there is, the faster it is eliminated. This phenomenon, known as first-order kinetics, applies to most drugs. Rate processes can also be independent of concentration, and fixed amounts of drugs, rather than a fractional proportion, are eliminated at a constant rate. This phenomenon is called zero-order kinetics. Alcohol undergoes zero-order elimination.

After five half-lives, according to first-order kinetics, approximately 97% (96.875%) of the drug is eliminated from the body. Even after three half-lives, nearly 90% (87.5%) of the drug is eliminated. In most cases, after three to five half-lives, the amount of drug remaining is too low to exert any pharmacologic effect, and the drug is considered essentially eliminated. Understanding this concept is useful for practitioners in many situations. For example, if a drug reaches a toxic level, the practitioner knows that it will take three to five half-lives for the drug to be essentially eliminated from the body. The practitioner also can estimate when the drug level will approach a minimally effective concentration and can then calculate when to administer another dose of medication to reach a therapeutic drug level.

Steady State

In reality, patients take medications on a consistent basis usually somewhere between one and four times daily. By doing so, they are absorbing and eliminating the drug throughout the day. Because the rate of elimination is proportional to the concentration, at some point equilibrium is reached. **Figure 2-6** demonstrates how doses of a drug with a half-life of 8 hours produce this equilibrium. Note that after approximately three to five half-lives, the curve levels off. This demonstrates equilibrium between the amount of drug entering the body and the amount leaving the body. This point, which is called *steady state*, reflects a constant mean concentration of drug in the body. At steady state, even though the blood levels of a drug

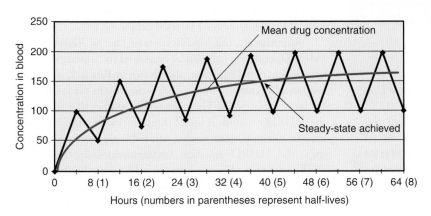

FIGURE 2–6 Steady state achieved with regular dosing (half-life = 8 hours).

fluctuate above and below this mean concentration and the drug level tends to have peaks and troughs during dosing intervals, the fluctuations remain within a constant range.

For some drugs, the time required to achieve steady state may be very long. For example, digoxin (Lanoxin) has a half-life of 39 hours (1.6 days), meaning that between 4.8 and 8 days are needed to achieve steady state. Clearly, when it is imperative to gain a therapeutic level quickly, waiting this long is unacceptable. Therefore, an initial loading dose of a drug is needed to reach the desired blood concentration quickly. The loading dose is based on the volume of distribution of the drug, independent of the half-life. The maintenance dose, however, is based on the half-life of the drug. Maintenance doses of the drug are given at scheduled intervals to replace the amount of drug eliminated.

Clearance

The concept of clearance, which refers to the removal of a drug from the plasma or organ, is the final element in the process of elimination. Drugs with high clearances are removed rapidly; those with low clearances are removed slowly. Drugs can be cleared by biliary, hepatic, and renal means. The following discussion highlights renal clearance.

Clearance is related to the volume of distribution and the half-life (**Box 2.4**). Clearance of a drug from the body depends directly on the apparent volume of distribution and is inversely related to the elimination half-life: the greater the volume of distribution and the shorter the half-life, the faster the clearance.

Because most drugs are "cleared" through the kidney, estimating the renal elimination rate or clearance can help the practitioner to understand how fast a drug is being eliminated in an individual patient. The kidney's ability to clear drugs is estimated through a surrogate substrate: creatinine. Creatinine, which is produced through the continual breakdown of muscle tissue and eliminated largely by glomerular filtration, is not

---

BOX **2.4**

Relationship Between Apparent Volume of Distribution, Clearance, and Half-Life

$$\text{Clearance} = \frac{0.693 \times V_d}{t_{1/2}}$$

Clearance is usually expressed as L/hour; V_d is in L; $t_{1/2}$ is usually in hours.

Clearance of a drug is directly dependent on the apparent volume of distribution and inversely related to the elimination half-life. The larger the V_d, the faster the clearance. Also, the smaller the $t_{1/2}$, the faster the clearance.

BOX **2.5**

Estimating Creatinine Clearance or Glomerular Filtration Rate (GFR) —the Cockroft and Gault Formula and the Modification of Diet in Renal Disease (MDRD) Study Equation

Cockroft and Gault: $CrCl_{est} = \dfrac{[140 - age\ (y)] \times IBW}{Scr \times 72}$

MDRD: $GFR = 175 \times (\text{Standardized } S_{cr})^{-1.154} \times (age)^{-0.203} \times (0.742 \text{ if female}) \times (1.212 \text{ if African American})$

Note: GFR is expressed in mL/min per 1.73 m^2, S_{cr} is serum creatinine expressed in mg/dL, and age is expressed in years.

Multiply $CrCl_{est}$ by 0.85 for women.

$CrCl_{est}$ = estimated creatinine clearance

Scr = serum creatinine (mg/dL)

IBW = ideal body weight in kilograms (kg; 2.2 lb = 1 kg)

---

significantly secreted or reabsorbed. Therefore, in estimating the creatinine clearance, the practitioner can also estimate the glomerular filtration rate (GFR). The level of creatinine is usually measured through a blood test (serum creatinine), with normal values ranging from 0.8 to 1.2 mg/dL. By combining this information with a patient's ideal body weight and age, the practitioner can use the formula of Cockroft and Gault to evaluate creatinine clearance and evaluate the kidney's ability to function and eliminate drugs (**Box 2.5**). For example, for a 40-year-old man of average height weighing 70 kg (154 lb) and having a serum creatinine level of 1 mg/dL, the estimated creatinine clearance is 97 mL/min. (This is only an estimate of this patient's creatinine clearance. The best method of determining the actual value is by a 24-hour urine specimen collection and measurement of excreted creatinine.)

Alternatively, the Modification of Diet in Renal Disease (MDRD) equation can also be employed to estimate the GFR of a patient. This equation, also shown in **Box 2.5,** should be used in adults only. This equation estimates the GFR adjusting for body surface area. There are several studies that show that the MDRD equation is useful in patients with chronic kidney disease, but in patients with a true GFR greater than 90 mL/min, the MDRD equation underestimates the true GFR (National Kidney Disease Education Program, 2010).

In either case, creatinine clearance or GFR values below 50 mL/min suggest significant impairment of renal function and thus possible impairment of renal drug elimination. This may result in administered drugs having longer half-lives and higher steady-state concentrations, which may result in toxicity if the dose is not decreased or the length of time between doses is not increased.

Not every patient needs to have creatinine clearance estimated. Two rules of thumb are useful for the practitioner: patients older than age 65 or those with a serum creatinine value greater than 1.5 mg/dL may be at risk for accumulating drug (and therefore toxicity) because of decreased renal function. In patients with either of these characteristics, a baseline and routine evaluation of renal function (e.g., serum creatinine determination) should be performed.

PHARMACODYNAMICS

Pharmacodynamics refers to the set of processes by which drugs produce specific biochemical or physiologic changes in the body. Most often, pharmacodynamic effects occur because a drug interacts with a receptor. Receptors may be cell membrane proteins, extracellular enzymes, cytoplasmic enzymes, or intracellular proteins. A receptor is the component of the cell (or an enzyme) to which an endogenous substance binds, or attaches, initiating a chain of biochemical events. This chain of

biochemical events culminates in a change in the physiologic function of the cell or activity of the enzyme. Like endogenous substances, drugs can initiate the biochemical chain of events. For example, a drug stimulating a receptor on the surface of an artery may ultimately cause vasoconstriction or vasodilation; or the drug's binding to a receptor may produce a change in cell wall permeability, thus allowing other substances to enter or leave a cell, such as occurs in nerve cells; or the drug attached to a receptor may initiate an increase or decrease in the production of an enzyme, thereby changing the amount of enzymatic activity for a given process.

Any chemical, endogenous or exogenous, that interacts with a receptor is called a *ligand*. Regardless of the ligand, or the actual interaction type, a substance can only alter or modify a cell or process, not impart a new function.

Drug Receptors

The capacity of a drug to bind to a receptor depends on the size and shape of the drug and the receptor. The drug acts as a "key" that fits into only a certain receptor or receptor type (**Figure 2-7**). Once the drug fits into the receptor, it may act to "unlock" the activity of the receptor, thus initiating the biochemical chain of events, much like an ignition key initiates the chain of events that starts a car.

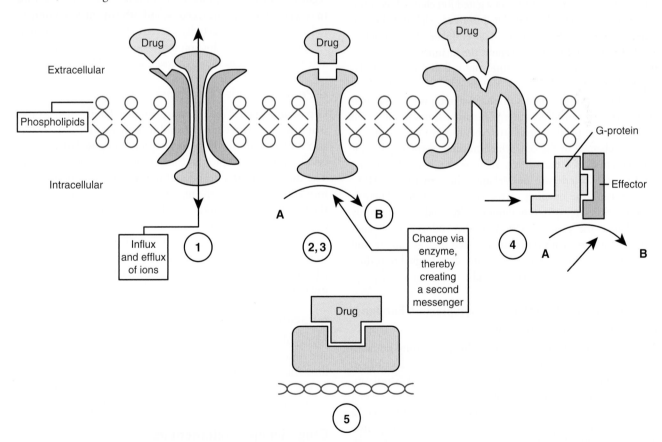

FIGURE 2–7 Drug and drug receptor interaction and signal transduction. The five primary receptors and their mechanisms of signal transduction include (1) gated ion channels; (2,3) transmembranous receptors—cytoplasmic enzyme and tyrosine kinase activated; (4) G-protein—coupled receptors; and (5) intracellular receptors.

Drug receptors are commonly classified by the effect they produce. Some drugs interact with several receptors, causing multiple effects, whereas others interact with only a specific receptor, eliciting a single response. Epinephrine, for example, interacts with the alpha and beta receptors of the sympathetic nervous system. As a result, epinephrine produces vasoconstriction (alpha receptor action) and an increase in heart rate (beta receptor action). Various molecules or enzymes can serve as drug receptors, such as ion channels (calcium channels), enzymes (angiotensin-converting enzyme [ACE]), and even receptors that generate intracellular second messengers (substances that interact with other intracellular components).

There are four known types of receptors: gated ion channels, transmembranous receptors, G-protein–coupled receptors, and intracellular receptors (see **Figure 2-7**). Understanding these receptors and the signals they generate is central to understanding the actions of many drugs.

Gated Ion Channels

The function of gated ion channel receptors is to open or close channels to allow certain ions to pass through the cell membrane. Binding of ligands to these receptors produces a conformational change that widens or narrows the channel, thereby regulating the access of soluble ions. The nicotinic acetylcholine receptor is a good example of a gated ion channel receptor. Its function is to translate the signal from acetylcholine into an electrical signal at the neuromuscular endplate. As such, when acetylcholine binds to this receptor, the channel opens, allowing sodium or potassium to enter the cell and cause cellular depolarization.

Other types of gated ion channel receptors are associated with the neurotransmitters. Gamma-aminobutyric acid (GABA$_A$), the primary inhibitory neurotransmitter, opens a chloride channel in the cell, which minimizes the depolarization potential. Certain drugs, such as the benzodiazepines, bind to an allosteric site and enhance the activity of GABA$_A$ by increasing the opening of the chloride channel. There is no intrinsic activity at the allosteric site, and it serves only to enhance the primary action of the endogenous ligand. Other excitatory neurotransmitters, such as L-glutamate and L-aspartate, operate by this mechanism, called signal transduction, which transfers the signal quickly.

Transmembranous Receptors—Cytoplasmic Enzyme or Tyrosine Kinase Activated

A transmembranous receptor has its ligand-binding domain, the specific region to which ligands bind, on the cell's surface. The enzymatic portion of the receptor is in the cell cytoplasm. When a ligand binds to a transmembranous receptor, several things may occur. The receptor–ligand complex produces a conformational change in the receptor and triggers a response. Alternatively, the ligand–receptor complex can pass through the cell membrane and trigger an intracellular response directly. This intracellular response often is a change in enzymatic activity. A key feature of the transmembranous receptor

response is the downregulation of the receptors or a decrease in the number of receptors available for response. The opposite of this is upregulation, which does not occur as frequently. The nature of the signal depends on the specific ligand–receptor interaction, but it commonly results in the generation of second messengers. A second messenger is an intracellular chemical that interacts with other intracellular components. Ions such as calcium and potassium, along with cyclic adenosine monophosphate, are common second messengers. Hormones and other endogenous substances, such as growth factors and insulin, often operate with this signaling mechanism.

The receptor tyrosine kinase signaling pathway can bind with a polypeptide hormone or growth factor at the receptor's extracellular domain. This results in enzymatically active tyrosine kinase domains that phosphorylate each other, allowing a single receptor to activate multiple biochemical processes. For example, insulin works by stimulating the uptake of glucose as well as amino acids, resulting in changes in glycogen content within the cell. Alternatively, inhibition of tyrosine kinase processes through blockage of the external receptor can result in a decrease in stimulation of growth factors within the cell. This is particularly important in cancer treatments, when inhibiting the growth of the cell is key to treatment success.

A drawback of this system is the potential for downregulation of the receptors. Activation of these receptors leads to an endocytosis of the receptor and subsequent receptor degradation. When this activity exceeds the production of new receptors, there is a reduction in the number of receptors available for stimulation, thus a decrease in the cell's activity.

G-Protein–Coupled Receptors

G-protein–coupled receptors are another family of receptors that generate intracellular second messengers. These receptors also exist as transmembranous receptors composed of an extracellular protein receptor and an intracellular type G protein. The interaction of a ligand and the receptor produces a conformational change in the receptor, bringing it in contact with the G protein. This contact results in activation of an enzyme or opening of an ion channel in the cell and, in turn, increased levels of the second messenger. It is the second messenger that triggers a change in the function of the cell. Alpha- and beta-adrenergic receptors, along with several hormone receptors, use G proteins to affect cell function.

Intracellular Receptors

Lipid-soluble drugs can traverse the lipid bilayer of the cell and enter the cytoplasm. Once inside, these drugs attach to intracellular receptors and initiate direct changes in the cell by affecting DNA transcription. Glucocorticoids and sex hormones are known to act by way of this signaling mechanism.

Drug–Receptor Interactions

The ability of a drug to bind to any receptor is dictated by factors such as the size and shape of the drug relative to the configuration of the binding site on the receptor. The electrostatic attraction between the drug and the receptor may also be important in determining the extent to which the drug binds to the receptor.

Affinity

A drug attracted to a receptor displays an *affinity* for that receptor. This affinity, the degree to which a drug is attracted to a receptor, is related to the concentration of drug required to occupy a receptor site. Drugs displaying a high affinity for a given receptor require only a small concentration in the circulation to elicit a response, whereas those with a low affinity require higher circulating concentrations. There exists equilibrium between the blood concentration of a drug, the concentration of drug at the site of action (i.e., near the receptor), and the amount of drug bound to a receptor. The magnitude of a drug's effect can be explained by the receptor occupancy theory—that is, a response from a cell (or group of cells) depends on the fraction of receptors occupied by a drug or endogenous substance. Therefore, one can infer a relationship between the minimally and maximally effective concentrations needed at the site of action and the minimum and maximum blood concentrations.

Chirality

The shape of a drug can influence its interaction with a receptor. Most drugs display chirality—that is, they exist in two forms with mirror-image spatial arrangements called enantiomers, or isomers. Each enantiomer is distinguished from the other through its ability to rotate polarized light in pure solution to the right or left. This results in a dextrorotary, or *d*-enantiomer, and a levorotary, or *l*-companion.

A pair of enantiomers is like a left and a right hand. As such, enantiomeric pairs may not fit into a receptor equally well, just as a right hand does not fit well into a left-hand glove. This is called stereoselectivity; one enantiomer may fit better into a receptor than the other and, hence, be more active. For example, the drug dextromethorphan (Robitussin DM) is the *d*-isomer of a compound. This *d*-isomer is a common cough suppressant found in most over-the-counter medications. Its *l*-isomer counterpart, levorphanol (Levo-Dromoran), is an extremely potent narcotic analgesic. Although the *l*-isomer also possesses cough suppressant activity, the *d*-isomer is essentially devoid of analgesic activity at commonly used doses. This similarity coincident with dissimilarity illustrates the importance of isomers in pharmacodynamics.

Agonists and Antagonists

Not all drugs with an affinity for a receptor elicit a response. Drugs that display a degree of affinity for a receptor and stimulate a response are considered agonists. Others that display an affinity and do not elicit a response are called antagonists. Antagonists do not have intrinsic activity; they can only block the activity of the endogenous agonist. An antagonist may be viewed as a key that fits into the lock, but because of its different configuration cannot be turned. Because an antagonist can occupy, or fit into, a receptor, it competes with agonists for that receptor, thereby blocking the effect of the agonist. Antagonists with a high

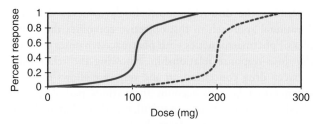

FIGURE 2–8 Two drugs with differing receptor affinities produce similar effects at different dosage ranges. The drug with the greater affinity (*solid line*) requires less drug to produce the same effect as a drug with less affinity (*dotted line*). This demonstrates the relationship between receptor affinity and drug potency.

affinity for a receptor may be able to "bump" an agonist off the receptor and reverse the agonist activity. Antagonists usually are used to block the activity of an endogenous substance, but they also can be used to block the activity of exogenously administered drugs. For example, when naloxone (Narcan) is given to a patient taking opioid drugs, the analgesic (and adverse) effects of the opioid are reversed within 1 to 2 minutes. In most cases, naloxone has a higher affinity for the opioid receptor than the opioid itself. This rough explanation of drug–receptor interactions serves only as a basis for understanding the complexity of this interplay.

Dose–Response Relationships

For many drugs, the relationship between the dose and the response is obvious: lower doses produce smaller responses, whereas higher doses increase the response. This correlation is based on the amount of drug occupying specific receptors. As the amount of drug exceeds the number of available receptors, the response reaches a plateau, so that further increases in dose do not increase response. However, dose–response relationships such as these clearly depend on the affinity of a drug for a receptor: a drug with a high affinity for a receptor needs a significantly lower concentration to achieve the same effect compared with a drug with a lower affinity.

This difference in affinity accounts for the varying "potency" of drugs. For example, drugs such as hydromorphone (Dilaudid) and morphine produce the same effect: analgesia. However, hydromorphone is more potent than morphine and therefore requires a smaller concentration to elicit a similar level of analgesia. **Figure 2-8** demonstrates a typical dose–response relationship.

FACTORS AFFECTING PHARMACOKINETICS AND PHARMACODYNAMICS

The goal of pharmacotherapeutics is to achieve a desired beneficial effect with minimal adverse effects. Once a medication has been selected for a patient, the practitioner must determine the dose that most closely achieves this goal. A rational approach to this objective combines the principles of pharmacokinetics with pharmacodynamics to clarify the dose–response relationship. Knowing the relationship between drug concentration and response allows the practitioner to take into account the various pathologic and physiologic features of a particular patient that make his or her response different from the average person's response to a drug.

Patient Variables

A host of variables affect the disposition of a drug in the body and the reaction the body has to the drug. People vary in their body type, weight, diet, ethnicity, and genetic makeup. These factors, individually and combined, contribute to significant variation in the response to drug therapy. For example, the genetic makeup of the people of Japan is known to affect the expression of certain hepatic enzymes involved in the metabolism of drugs. This suggests that, at least pharmacokinetically, some people of Japanese heritage respond differently to certain drugs. The same logic applies to people who are overweight and underweight, people of varying ages, people with various pathophysiologic problems, and even people with different diets and nutritional habits.

Pathophysiology

Structural or functional damage to an organ or tissue responsible for drug metabolism or excretion presents an obvious problem in pharmacology. Diseases that initiate changes in tissue function or blood flow to specific organs can dramatically affect the elimination of various drugs. Certain diseases may also impair the absorption and distribution of the drug, complicating the problem of individualized response. The role of disease in affecting the patient's response is crucial because the response to the medication may be affected by the same pathologic process that the drug is being used to treat. For instance, renal excretion of antibiotics, such as aminoglycosides, is altered radically in many types of bacterial infection, but these drugs are typically administered to treat the same infections that alter their own excretion. Consequently, great care must be taken to adjust the dosage accordingly when administering medications to patients with conditions in which drug elimination may be altered.

Genetics

Genetic differences are a major factor in determining the way that people metabolize specific compounds. Genetic variations may result in abnormal or absent drug-metabolizing enzymes. The anomaly can be harmful or even fatal if the drug cannot be metabolized and therefore exerts a toxic effect from accumulation or prolonged pharmacologic activity. Some people, for example, lack the enzyme that breaks down acetylcholine. In these people, a drug such as succinylcholine (Anectine, an acetylcholine-like drug) is not degraded and therefore accumulates. The result is respiratory paralysis because the undegraded, accumulated succinylcholine has an increased half-life, causing it to remain active longer.

Age

The influence of age on pharmacokinetics and pharmacodynamics is well known. Developmental differences in the neonate, toddler, and young child, for instance, influence how drugs are handled by the GI tract, liver, and kidneys. Of equal importance is how these children respond to drugs in light of the presence or absence of receptors at different stages of development. For example, drug-metabolizing enzymes are deficient in the fetus and premature infant. The fetus can metabolize drugs early in its development, but its expression of drug-metabolizing enzymes differs from that of the adult and is usually less efficient.

Children can metabolize many drugs more rapidly than adults, and as children approach puberty, the rate of drug metabolism approaches that of adults. Similarly, older adults undergo physiologic changes that affect the absorption, distribution, and elimination of many agents. The pharmacodynamic changes imparted by age as well as accompanying diseases pose a greater challenge for the practitioner in understanding the impact a single agent has on a patient's health and well-being. Chapter 4 discusses pediatric considerations, and Chapter 6 discusses geriatric considerations in more depth.

Sex

The role of sex as a distinct patient variable is recognized by some but poorly understood by most. Most of the published clinical drug studies use male subjects as the primary study population, and clinicians then extrapolate the data to women. However, women in general have a higher percentage of body fat, which could ultimately alter the pharmacokinetic disposition of certain drugs. Similarly, the pharmacodynamic response of women may be different because of the presence or absence of hormones such as estrogen and testosterone.

Ethnicity

Ethnicity is a significant factor in both the pharmacokinetic and pharmacodynamic responses of patients. The genetic makeup of various ethnic populations governs the levels of hepatic enzymes expressed in these groups. Equally important are the habits and traditions of certain groups, such as diet or the use of home remedies.

Pharmacodynamically, ethnically based differences exist in the responses to agents. An example is the minimal response of African-American patients to monotherapy with some drugs, such as ACE inhibitors. African Americans produce a low level of renin, a key component in the renin–angiotensin–aldosterone system by which the ACE inhibitors work. This low level of renin makes this system untouchable by the ACE inhibitor, thereby negating its effect.

Diet and Nutrition

Diet affects the metabolism of and response to many drugs. Animal and human studies indicate that total caloric intake and the percentage of calories obtained from different sources (carbohydrates, proteins, and fats) influence drug pharmacokinetics. Specific dietary constituents, such as cruciferous vegetables and charcoal-broiled beef, can also alter drug metabolism. Fortunately, most food–drug interactions are not serious and do not alter the clinical effects of the drug. However, a few well-known food and drug combinations should be avoided because of their potentially serious interactions. For instance, certain tyramine-containing foods, such as fermented cheese and wine, should not be ingested with drugs that inhibit the monoamine oxidase enzyme (MAO) inhibitors. Tyramine-rich foods stimulate the body to release catecholamines (norepinephrine, epinephrine). MAO-inhibiting drugs work by suppressing the destruction of catecholamines, thereby allowing higher levels of norepinephrine and epinephrine to accumulate. Consequently, when MAO inhibitors are taken with tyramine-containing foods, excessive catecholamine levels may develop and lead to a dangerous increase in blood pressure (hypertensive crisis). Practitioners should be aware of this and should be on the alert for other such interactions as new drugs arrive on the market.

BIBLIOGRAPHY

Starred references are cited in the text.

Goodman, L. S., Gilman, A., Hardman, J. G., Gilman, A.G., & Limbird, L. E. (Eds.). (1996). *Goodman and Gilman's the pharmacological basis of therapeutics* (9th ed.). New York, NY: McGraw-Hill.

Gunaratna, C. (2000). Drug metabolism and pharmacokinetics in drug discovery: A primer for bioanalytical chemists, Part I. *Current Separations, 19*(1), 17–23.

Gunaratna, C. (2001). Drug metabolism and pharmacokinetics in drug discovery: A primer for bioanalytical chemists, Part II. *Current Separations, 19*(2), 87–92.

Katzung, B. G. (Ed.). (2001). *Basic and clinical pharmacology* (8th ed.). New York, NY: McGraw-Hill.

*National Kidney Disease Education Program. (2010). http://www.nkdep.nih.gov/professionals/drug-dosing-information.htm#recommended-approach. Viewed, 7/21/2010.

Rowland, M., & Tozer, T. N. (Eds.). (1995). *Clinical pharmacokinetics: Concepts and applications* (3rd ed.). Philadelphia, PA: J. B. Lippincott.

Smith, C. M., & Reynard, A. M. (Eds.). (1992). *Textbook of pharmacology.* Philadelphia, PA: W. B. Saunders.

Williams, B. R., & Baer, C. L. (Eds.). (1998). *Essentials of clinical pharmacology in nursing* (3rd ed.). Spring House, PA: Springhouse Corp.

CHAPTER 3

Tim A. Briscoe
Matthew Sarnes
Andrew M. Peterson

Impact of Drug Interactions and Adverse Events on Therapeutics

As the quantity and types of pharmacologic agents continue to expand, the likelihood of drug interactions and adverse reactions increases. Currently, more than 8,000 drugs are available to treat various conditions. Each agent is designed to alter the homeostasis of the human body to some degree, and individual responses to these agents can be unpredictable.

In a meta-analysis, Lazarou, Pomeranz, and Corey (1998) found that 6.7% of hospitalizations were due to serious adverse drug reactions (ADRs), of which 0.32% resulted in death. Based on 1996 hospitalization rates, that accounts for approximately 100,000 deaths and more than 2 million serious ADRs (National Center for Health Statistics, 1996). It has been reported that the incidence of hospital admissions secondary to ADRs in the elderly was 8.37 per 100 admissions (Olivier, et al., 2009). In hospitalized children, the overall incidence of ADRs has been reported to be 9.5% with a rate of hospital admissions of 2.09% (Impicciatore, et al., 2001). ADRs present an alarming problem that warrants significant attention from health care practitioners. Not only do ADRs affect morbidity and mortality, they also dramatically increase health care costs. Estimates suggest that an additional $1.56 to $4 billion is spent in direct hospital costs precipitated by ADRs (Bates, et al., 1997; Classen, et al., 1997).

Similarly, drug interactions are potentially preventable ADRs posing a significant problem to the health care community. It has been reported that approximately 10% to 20% of hospital admissions are drug related and about 1% of these are secondary to drug interactions. Others have reported that drug interactions are responsible for up to 3% of hospital admissions (Bjerrum, et al., 2008). In addition, the prevalence of a first dispensing of drug–drug interactions in people older than age 70 has been reported to have increased from 10.5% in 1992 to 19.2% in 2005 (Becker, et al., 2008). Therefore, a thorough understanding of how drug–drug interactions occur and how they relate to ADRs should help decrease the rate of occurrence and the associated morbidity/mortality. This chapter discusses the mechanisms of drug interactions and their potential consequences. For the purpose of this chapter, these interactions are broken down into four major categories: drug–drug interactions, drug–food interactions, drug–herb interactions, and drug–disease interactions. Each of the interaction categories can affect the drug's pharmacokinetic or pharmacodynamic profile. The definition, identification, and management of ADRs are discussed at the end of the chapter.

DRUG–DRUG INTERACTIONS

When a person takes two or more medications concomitantly, the potential exists for one or more drugs to change the effect of other drugs. The drug whose effect is altered by another drug is termed the *object* or *target* drug. Although minor interactions between drugs probably occur frequently, these interactions may not be significant enough to alter the effect of either drug. However, it is important for the practitioner to understand the mechanisms behind these interactions to predict more accurately when clinically significant (and potentially fatal) drug interactions may occur.

Pharmacokinetic Interactions

Absorption

Because most medications in the ambulatory care setting are administered orally, this route is the focus of discussion. For a drug to exert its effect, it must reach its site of action. Normally, this requires access to the bloodstream. As discussed in Chapter 2, drugs administered orally must be absorbed into the portal vein, through the intestinal wall, to reach the systemic circulation. The oral tablet must dissolve in the gastrointestinal (GI) tract before it can penetrate the intestinal wall.

Acidity (pH)

For some drugs, this process depends on the acidity in the GI tract. Therefore, if a drug that alters the gastric pH is administered concomitantly with a drug that depends on a normal gastric pH for dissolution, the absorption of the object drug will be affected. An example of this type of interaction is the concurrent administration of a histamine-2 (H$_2$) receptor antagonist (e.g., ranitidine) and ketoconazole, an imidazole antifungal agent. Ketoconazole is the object drug that requires an acidic pH for absorption. When ranitidine is administered along with ketoconazole, the increase in gastric pH hinders the dissolution of ketoconazole and, therefore, decreases its absorption. Similarly, this change in pH can increase the absorption of other drugs that require a more alkaline environment for absorption.

Adsorption

Another mechanism of absorptive drug–drug interactions is adsorption. Adsorption occurs when one agent binds the other to its surface to form a complex. The most common agents associated with this type of interaction are divalent and trivalent cations (Mg^{2+}, Ca^{2+}, Al^{3+}, found in antacids and some vitamin preparations) and anionic binding resins (colestipol, cholestyramine). This type of interaction occurs when certain medications such as tetracyclines or fluoroquinolones are given with antacids. The metal ions in the antacid chelate (form a complex with) the antibiotic, preventing absorption of both components (ion and antibiotic). Adsorbents can interact with a variety of drugs; therefore, appropriate intervals between doses of the interacting medications are warranted. In general, with agents known to interact in this manner, the object drug should be administered at least 2 hours before or 4 to 6 hours after the interacting agent.

Gastrointestinal Motility and Rate of Absorption

Drugs that affect the motility of the GI tract produce a less common absorption-altering mechanism. These agents tend to affect the rate of absorption and not the amount of drug absorbed. Any agent—for example, metoclopramide—that stimulates peristalsis and increases gastric emptying time can affect the rate of absorption of other medications. In most cases, an increase in the rate of absorption occurs because the target drug reaches the duodenum faster, allowing absorption to occur sooner. However, in some cases such as with metoclopramide and digoxin, a decrease in digoxin concentrations may occur (American Society of Health-System Pharmacists, 2008).

Conversely, anticholinergic agents and opiates decrease gastric motility, thereby decreasing the rate of absorption of object drugs. Because this type of interaction does not usually affect the amount of drug absorbed, it is usually clinically insignificant.

GI Flora and Absorption

The bacteria present in the GI tract are also responsible for a portion of the metabolism of some agents. An example of this is digoxin; concomitant administration with antibiotics (such as erythromycin or tetracycline) may alter the normal bacterial flora and reduce digoxin metabolism, thereby increasing bioavailability and serum concentrations in some patients (Susla, 2005). To the contrary, GI bacteria produce enzymes that deconjugate inactive unabsorbable ethinyl estradiol metabolites of oral contraceptives that have been excreted into the GI tract via the bile. Deconjugation allows reabsorption of active ethinyl estradiol back into the bloodstream. By disrupting the GI flora, anti-infectives may decrease or eliminate reabsorption of active ethinyl estradiol, thereby decreasing plasma concentrations and the effectiveness of oral contraceptives (Weaver & Glasier, 1999).

Table 3.1 summarizes some of the major drug interactions that occur in the absorptive process.

Distribution

After drugs are absorbed into the bloodstream, most of them, to some degree, are bound to plasma protein such as albumin or α_1-acid glycoprotein. As described in Chapter 2, only an unbound drug is free to interact with its target receptor site and is therefore active. The percentage of drug that binds to plasma proteins depends on the affinity of that drug for the protein-binding site. If two drugs with high affinity for circulating proteins are administered together, they may compete for a single binding site on the protein. In fact, one drug may displace the other from the binding site with the result being an increase in the unbound (free) fraction of the displaced drug. This increase in free drug may trigger an exaggerated pharmacodynamic response or toxic reaction. However, because the excess unbound drug is now subject to elimination processes, the increases in both free drug fraction and the effects produced are usually transient.

Clinically significant drug displacement interactions normally occur only when drugs are more than 90% protein bound and have a narrow therapeutic index (Rolan, 1994). For example, warfarin is 99% protein bound, and therefore only 1% of the drug in the bloodstream is free to induce a pharmacodynamic response (inhibition of clotting factors). If a second drug is administered that displaces even 1% of the warfarin bound to albumin, the amount of free warfarin is doubled, to 2% free. This can result in a significant increase in its pharmacodynamic action, leading to excessive bleeding. **Table 3.2** lists examples of several displacement interactions.

Metabolism

Lipophilicity (fat solubility) enables drug molecules to be absorbed and reach their site of action. However, lipophilic drugs are difficult for the body to excrete. Therefore, they must be transformed by the body to more hydrophilic (water-soluble) molecules. This is accomplished primarily through phase I, or oxidation, reactions. The main sites of metabolism in the body are the liver (hepatocytes) and small intestine (enterocytes). Other tissues, such as the kidneys, lungs, and brain, play a minor role in the metabolism of drug molecules (Michalets, 1998). These sites of metabolism contain enzymes called cytochrome P450 isoenzymes. This group of isoenzymes has been identified as the major catalyst of phase I metabolic reactions in humans.

The nomenclature of the cytochrome P450 system classifies the isoenzymes (designated CYP) according to family (>36% homology in amino acid sequence), subfamily (77% homology), and individual gene (Brosen, 1990; Guengerich, 1994; Nebert, et al., 1987). For example, the isoenzyme CYP3A4 belongs to family 3, subfamily A, and gene 4. As one moves down the classification system from family to gene, the structures of the isoenzymes become more similar.

TABLE 3.1   Drugs Affecting Absorption

	Mechanism of Action	Object Drug	Results
Absorption Inhibitors			
activated charcoal	Binding agent	digoxin	Decreased absorption
aluminum hydroxide	Unknown	allopurinol	Decreased absorption
antacids (Mg^{2+}, Ca^{2+}, Al^{3+})	Chelating agent	quinolones, tetracyclines, levodopa, levothyroxine	Decreased absorption
aluminum and Mg hydroxide	Binding agent	digoxin	Decreased absorption
bismuth (Pepto-Bismol)	Binding agent	tetracycline, doxycycline	Decreased absorption
antibiotics (i.e., erythromycin, tetracycline	Altered GI flora	digoxin	Increased absorption
	Altered GI flora	oral contraceptives	Decreased reabsorption, decreased enterhepatic recycling
anticholinergics	Decreases gastric emptying	acetaminophen, atenolol, levodopa	Decreased absorption
cholestyramine	Binding agent	acetaminophen, diclofenac, digoxin, glipizide, furosemide, iron, levothyroxine, lorazepam, methotrexate, metronidazole, piroxicam	Decreased absorption
colestipol	Binding agent	carbamazepine, diclofenac, furosemide, tetracycline, thiazides	Decreased absorption
desipramine	Decreases GI motility	phenylbutazone	Decreased absorption
didanosine	Binding agent	ciprofloxacin	Decreased absorption
	Increases gastric pH	imidazole, antifungals	Decreased absorption
ferrous sulfate	Chelating agent	quinolones, tetracyclines, levodopa, levothyroxine	Decreased absorption
histamine-2 receptor antagonists/ proton pump inhibitors	Increases gastric pH	imidazole, antifungals, enoxacin	Decreased absorption
phenytoin	Unknown	furosemide	Decreased absorption
sucralfate	Binding agent	quinolones, tetracyclines, phenytoin, levothyroxine	Decreased absorption
sulfasalazine	Unknown	digoxin	Decreased absorption
Absorption Enhancers			
cisapride	Increases gastric emptying	disopyramide	Increased absorption
histamine-2 receptor antagonists	Increases gastric pH	pravastatin, glipizide, dihydropyridine, calcium antagonists	Increased absorption
metoclopramide	Increases gastric motility	cyclosporine	Increased absorption
	Increases GI motility	acetaminophen, cefprozil, ethanol	Increased absorption

GI, gastrointestinal.

This enzyme system has evolved to form new isoenzymes that metabolize foreign substrates (i.e., drugs) that are presented to the body. These enzymes are structured to recognize and bind to molecular entities on substrates. Many different substrates may have molecular structures that differ only slightly; therefore, an isoenzyme can bind to any one of these substrates. Although several different substrates may compete for the same enzyme receptor, the substrate with the highest affinity binds most often. The converse of this is also true. Two isoenzymes can bind to the same substrate (**Figure 3-1**), but the substrate binds more often to the isoenzyme to which it has the most affinity. However, not every drug molecule ("substrate") can be metabolized by every enzyme with which it binds; therefore, it

is not a true substrate. These concepts form the backbone for the drug interactions that are expanded on later.

Six isoenzymes have been determined to be responsible for most metabolism-related drug interactions. They are the isoforms CYP1A2, CYP2C9, CYP2C19, CYP2D6, CYP2E1, and CYP3A4. The CYP3A4 isoform is responsible for 40% to 45% of drug metabolism, the CYP2D6 for the next 20% to 30%, CYP2C9 about 10%, and CYP2E1 and CYP1A2 each responsible for about 5% (Ingelman-Sundberg, 2004). The remaining 5% to 20% is accounted for by several lesser important isoforms. Because there are so few enzymes that transform a multitude of substrates, it is easy to see how there would be a great potential for interactions.

TABLE 3.2	Distribution Drug Interactions
Displacing Agent	**Object Drug**
aspirin	meclofenamate tolmetin
salicylates	methotrexate
TMP–SMZ	
sulfaphenazole	phenytoin
tolbutamide	
valproic acid	
halofenate	sulfonylureas
quinidine	digoxin
aspirin	warfarin
chloral hydrate	
diazoxide	
etodolac	
fenoprofen	
lovastatin	
nalidixic acid	
phenylbutazone	
phenytoin	
sulfapyrazone	

TMP-SMZ, Trimethophein–sulfamethoxazole

There are some genetic variations with respect to the distribution of the enzymes. For example, about 10% of Europeans lack the CYP2D6 enzyme and are therefore considered poor metabolizers of drugs using this pathway for biotransformation. These individuals are at greater risk for ADRs related to drugs metabolized by CYP2D6. In addition, prodrugs requiring this enzyme for activation (e.g., codeine, tamoxifen) may be less effective or have no effect. In contrast, about 5% of this population are considered ultra-metabolizers, have too rapid metabolism, and may show little to no response related to drugs metabolized by the CYP2D6 pathway (Ingelman-Sundberg, 2004). Similarly, there is variability within the CYP2C19 isoform, with about 14% of Chinese, 2% of Whites, and 4% of Blacks being poor metabolizers (Xie, et al., 2001). The effectiveness of certain prodrugs (e.g., clopidogrel) that require metabolic activation by this enzyme system may be reduced (Holmes, et al., 2010).

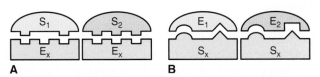

FIGURE 3–1 Substrate binding. **A.** Different substrates: Although Enzyme X (E_x) can bind to both Substrate 1 (S_1) and Substrate 2 (S_2), S_2 has greater affinity for E_x than S_1. Therefore E_x will bind to S_2 most often. **B.** Different enzymes. Although Substrate X (S_x) can bind to both Enzyme 1 (E_1) and Enzyme 2 (E_2), E_1 has a greater affinity for S_x than E_2. Therefore S_x will bind to E_1 most often.

There has been increasing interest in genetic testing to identify strategies to reduce the risk of ADRs and to optimize therapy for individuals. Pharmacogenomic information has been incorporated into about 10% of labels for drugs approved by the U.S. Food and Drug Administration (FDA) in an effort to identify responders and non-responders, avoid toxicity, and adjust doses of medications to optimize efficacy and ensure safety (FDA table of genomic markers accessed July 2010). In addition, regulatory authorities have recently recommended genetic testing to aid the clinician in determining if an agent is safe and effective in certain individuals (e.g., carbamazepine, abacavir, clopidogrel) (Tegretol [carbamazepine] Label accessed July 2010, FDA Drug Safety Communication: Plavix [clopidogrel] accessed July 2010, Highlights of Prescribing Information: Ziagen [abacavir sulfate] accessed July 2010). While commercial assays are available for genetic testing, turn-around time for the results vary, testing can be expensive, data on the validation of techniques used and reliability and reproducibility are limited, and to date there is limited evidence-based data on which to develop specific recommendations on the role of genetic testing in routine care (Holmes, et al., 2010).

There are two types of metabolic drug interactions: drugs that inhibit the action of an enzyme and those that induce the activity of the enzyme.

Inhibition

Inhibition of drug metabolism occurs through competitive and noncompetitive inhibition. When two drugs, administered concurrently, are metabolized by the same isoenzyme, they are defined as competitive inhibitors of each other. In essence, they compete for the same binding site on an enzyme to be metabolized.

Noncompetitive inhibition also occurs when both drugs compete for the same binding site, but one drug is metabolized by that isoenzyme and the other drug is not. The best known example of a noncompetitive inhibitor is quinidine. Quinidine is metabolized by the CYP3A4 isoenzyme but can also bind to the CYP2D6 enzyme. Therefore, although quinidine does not compete for metabolism by the CYP2D6 isoenzyme, it does compete for the CYP2D6 isoenzyme binding site.

In both competitive and noncompetitive inhibition, the drug with the greatest affinity for the isoenzyme receptor is usually the inhibiting drug because it binds in the receptor site, preventing the other drug from being bound and metabolized (**Figure 3-2**). The significance of the drug interaction depends on several characteristics of the inhibiting drug.

Affinity The first characteristic, affinity, has already been mentioned. Many drugs may inhibit the same isoenzyme but not to the same extent. The greater the affinity of an inhibiting drug for an enzyme, the more it blocks binding of other drug molecules.

Half-Life Along with affinity, the half-life (t½) of the inhibiting drug determines the duration of the interaction. The longer the half-life of the inhibiting drug, the longer the

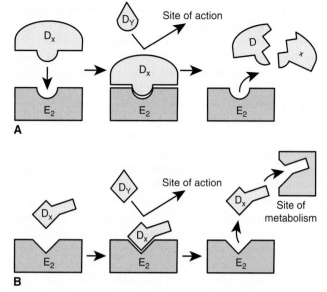

FIGURE 3–2 Inhibition. **A.** Competitive inhibition. Drug X (D_X) and Drug Y (D_Y) are both metabolized by Enzyme 2 (E_2). **B.** Noncompetitive inhibition. Although D_X and D_Y compete for the binding site on E_2, only D_Y is metabolized by E_2. Therefore D_X noncompetitively inhibits D_Y.

drug interaction lasts. For example, after a regimen of keto-conazole ($t\frac{1}{2}$ = 8 hours) is discontinued, its ability to inhibit the CYP3A4 enzyme lasts until it is eliminated, in three to five half-lives or approximately 1 day. However, the inhibiting effect of amiodarone, with a $t\frac{1}{2}$ of approximately 53 days, lasts for weeks to months after its discontinuation.

Concentration The third major factor contributing to a drug's ability to inhibit hepatic enzymes is the concentration of the inhibiting drug. A threshold concentration must be reached or exceeded to inhibit an enzyme. This is similar to the threshold concentration discussed in Chapter 2 regarding minimally effective concentrations and therapeutic responses. This minimally effective threshold concentration, or concentration-dependent inhibition, is exhibited by a variety of drugs. The dose yielding this concentration-dependent inhibition varies based on volume of distribution, drug and receptor affinity, and characteristics of the individual patient. An example of a dose- or concentration-dependent inhibitor is cimetidine. In most patients, a dose of 400 mg/d results in only weak enzyme inhibition. However, at higher doses, it interacts significantly with both the CYP2D6 and CYP1A2 isoenzymes (Shinn, 1992).

Some enzyme inhibitors may affect one enzyme at a smaller concentration and more than one isoenzyme at higher concentrations. These enzyme inhibitors demonstrate that some isoenzymes have differing thresholds. For example, fluconazole at a dose of 200 mg/d significantly inhibits only the 2C9 isoenzyme, but as the dose increases above 400 mg/d, it also inhibits the 3A4 isoenzyme (Hansten, 1998; Kivisto, Neuvonen, & Koltz, 1994).

Toxic Potential Another consideration with regard to inhibition interactions is the toxic potential of the object drug. For example, nonsedating antihistamines (i.e., terfenadine and astemizole) are metabolized by the CYP3A4 isoenzyme to a nontoxic metabolite. The parent compound of both drugs is cardiotoxic. If a potent CYP3A4 inhibitor (e.g., erythromycin) is administered concurrently with these agents, the parent compound accumulates in the body and causes a potentially fatal arrhythmia, such as torsades de pointes (Mathews, et al., 1991; Woosley, 1996). Because of their serious toxic potential, both terfenadine and astemizole have been removed from the market.

Efficacy An additional consideration related to inhibition interactions is the effectiveness of the object drug. This is particularly important for prodrugs that require cytochrome P450 metabolism to the active metabolite in order for the drug to be effective. An example of this is clopidogrel, an antiplatelet agent, which requires CYP2C19 enzymes to be metabolized to the active form. When administered with omeprazole, a CYP2C19 inhibitor, a reduction in plasma concentrations of the active metabolite of clopidogrel as well as reduced platelet function occur (clopidogrel prescribing information). In addition, tamoxifen, an agent used for breast cancer, is converted to its active metabolite by CYP2D6. Women may have a higher risk of breast cancer recurrence if they take tamoxifen in combination with CYP2D6 inhibitors such as the serotonin reuptake inhibitors paroxetine, fluoxetine, or sertraline (The Medical Letter, 2009).

Not all inhibition reactions result in harmful effects, however. Some interactions may be inconsequential or even beneficial. For example, ketoconazole (a potent inhibitor of the CYP3A4 isoenzyme) can be given with cyclosporine. The consequent interaction enables practitioners to give less cyclosporine to achieve the same immunosuppressive response (Hansten & Horn, 1997).

The cytochrome P450 system is complex, but an understanding of the basic concepts of inhibitory interactions leads to the ability to anticipate which agents are likely to interact. The affinity, half-life, and drug concentration determine the potency of the inhibiting drug. A potent enzyme inhibitor inhibits most drugs metabolized by that enzyme. A clinically significant drug interaction also depends on the toxic potential of the drug being inhibited. **Table 3.3** lists several enzyme inhibitors.

Induction

Drug–drug interactions can also result from the action of one drug (inducer) stimulating the metabolism of an object drug (substrate). This enhanced metabolism is thought to be produced by an increase in hepatic blood flow or an increase in the formation of hepatic enzymes. This process, known as *enzyme induction*, increases the amount of enzymes available to metabolize drug molecules, thereby decreasing the concentration and pharmacodynamic effect of the object drug.

| TABLE 3.3 | Drugs Affecting Metabolism Through Cytochrome P450 Isoenzymes | | | | |

Inhibitors	Inducers	Substrates	Inhibitors	Inducers	Substrates
Isoenzyme 1A2			**Isoenzyme 3A4**		
cimetidine	carbamazepine	theophylline	amiodarone	carbamazepine	alprazolam
ciprofloxacin	phenobarbital		Azole antifungals	dexamethasone	atorvastatin
clarithromycin	phenytoin	tricyclic antidepressants	clarithromycin	ethosuximide	calcium channel blockers
enoxacin	rifampin	benzodiazepines	erythromycin	phenobarbital	carbamazepine
erythromycin	ritonavir	warfarin	fluoxetine	phenytoin	clindamycin
norfloxacin	smoking		fluvoxamine	rifabutin	clomipramine
oral contraceptives	polycyclic		imidazole	rifampin	clonazepam
SSRIs	aromatic		nefazodone		cyclosporine
zileuton	hydrocarbons		norfloxacin		dapsone
			protease inhibitors		dexamethasone
Isoenzyme 2C (primarily 2C9, 2C19)			quinine		dextromethorphan
amiodarone	carbamazepine	amitriptyline	telithromycin		disopyramide
cimetidine	phenobarbital	clomipramine	verapamil		erythromycin
fluconazole	phenytoin	diazepam	zafirlukast		oral contraceptives (estrogens)
fluoxetine	rifampin	imipramine			
fluvastatin		losartan			ethosuximide
fluvoxamine		omeprazole			fexofenadine
isoniazid		phenytoin			imipramine
metronidazole		tricyclic antidepressants			ketoconazole
omeprazole		warfarin			lidocaine
sertraline					lovastatin
zafirlukast					miconazole
					midazolam
Isoenzyme 2D6					nefazodone
amiodarone	carbamazepine				ondansetron
					oxycodone
cimetidine	phenobarbital				pravastatin
clomipramine	phenytoin				prednisone
codeine	rifampin				protease inhibitors
desipramine					quinidine
haloperidol					quinine
perphenazine					rifampin
propafenone					sertraline
quinidine					tacrolimus
SSRIs					tamoxifen
thioridazine					temazepam
venlafaxine					triazolam
					verapamil
Isoenzyme 2E1					warfarin
disulfiram	ethanol	acetaminophen			zileuton
ritonavir	isoniazid	chloral hydrate			
		ethanol			
		isoniazid			
		ondansetron			
		tamoxifen			

SSRIs, selective serotonin reuptake inhibitors.

Some of the more common enzyme inducers are rifampin, phenobarbital, phenytoin, and carbamazepine. Enzyme induction, like enzyme inhibition, is substrate dependent. Therefore, any drug that is a potent inducer of a cytochrome P450 system increases the metabolism of most drugs metabolized by that enzyme. Also, in a manner similar to that of enzyme inhibitors, inducers may affect more than one cytochrome P450 isoform; for example, phenobarbital is a potent inducer of the CYP3A4, CYP1A2, and CYP2C isoforms (Michalets, 1998).

Some enzyme inducers, such as carbamazepine, also increase their own metabolism. Over time, carbamazepine stimulates its own metabolism, thereby decreasing its half-life and frequently resulting in an increased dose requirement to maintain the same therapeutic drug level (Hussar, 1995). This process is termed *autoinduction*.

The onset and duration/cessation of enzyme induction depend on both the half-life of the inducer and the half-life of the isoenzyme that is being stimulated. For example, rifampin (t½ = 3 to 4 hours) results in enzyme induction within 24 hours, whereas the enzyme induction capacity of phenobarbital (t½ = 53 to 140 hours) is not evident for approximately 7 days (Michalets, 1998; Spinler, et al., 1995). The level of induction remains constant while the drugs are being administered. However, on discontinuation of the respective inducers, the inducing action of rifampin ends more rapidly because of its shorter half-life. This occurs because rifampin is removed from the body at a faster rate than phenobarbital and therefore is not available to inhibit hepatic enzymes for as long.

The initiation and duration of enzyme induction also depend on the half-life of the induced isoenzyme. It takes anywhere from 1 to 6 days for a cytochrome P450 enzyme to be degraded or produced (Cupp & Tracy, 1997). Therefore, even if a drug achieves a high enough concentration to produce induction of liver enzymes, the increase in metabolism of an object drug may not be evident until more liver enzymes have formed. The effect of rifampin on warfarin metabolism is a good example of this. Although induction begins within 24 hours of rifampin administration, its effect on warfarin metabolism is not evident for approximately 4 days (Harder & Thurmann, 1996). On discontinuation of rifampin, the remaining drug is metabolized to negligible levels before the effect on warfarin metabolism dissipates. This occurs because the half-life of the liver enzymes is greater than the half-life of rifampin, and therefore the enzymes remain to metabolize warfarin after rifampin is eliminated from the body.

These concepts are important to remember when monitoring laboratory values that demonstrate the effectiveness of the object medication. For example, the international normalized ratio (INR), which is a surrogate marker of warfarin levels, fluctuates significantly within a couple of days of the initiation or discontinuation of rifampin. However, no change in the INR is evident for approximately 1 week after administration of phenobarbital. This is also true when measuring levels of certain antibiotics and other agents that may be affected by

inducers. **Table 3.3** lists several enzyme inducers and the drugs they affect.

Excretion

Although most drugs are metabolized by the liver, the primary modes of elimination from the body are biliary and renal excretion. Drugs are removed from the bloodstream by the kidneys by filtration or by urinary secretion. However, reabsorption from the urine into the bloodstream may also occur.

Changes in these processes become important when they affect drugs that are unchanged or still active. Excretion of drug molecules can be affected in a number of ways; these include, but are not limited to, acidification or alkalinization of the urine and alteration of secretory or active transport pathways. Although they are not discussed here for various reasons, there are a select number of other mechanisms of renal drug interactions.

The ionization state of drug molecules plays a key role in the excretion process. The urine pH determines the ionization state of the excreted molecule. Because lipophilic membranes are less permeable to ionized molecules (hydrophilic), ionized molecules become "trapped" in the urine and are subsequently excreted. Drugs that are non-ionized in the urine may be reabsorbed and then recirculated, effectively decreasing their elimination and increasing their half-lives.

Acidic drugs remain in their non-ionized state in an acidic urine and become ionized in an alkaline urine. The opposite is true for basic drug molecules, which remain non-ionized in an alkaline urine and are ionized in an acidic urine. When a drug is administered that alters the urine pH, it may promote an increased reabsorption or excretion of another drug. For example, the administration of bicarbonate can potentially increase the urine pH. This leads to the increased excretion of acidic drugs (e.g., aspirin) and the increased reabsorption of basic drugs (e.g., pseudoephedrine).

Although most drugs cross the membrane of the renal tubule by simple diffusion, some drugs are also secreted into the urine through active transport pathways. These pathways, however, have a limited capacity and can accommodate only a set amount of drug molecules. Therefore, if two different drugs using the same pathway are coadministered, the transport pathway may become saturated. This causes a "traffic jam" and the excretion of one or both of the drugs is inhibited.

These interactions can be beneficial or detrimental, depending on the agents that are administered. For example, when probenecid and penicillin are given together, they compete for secretion through an organic acid pathway in the renal tubule. The probenecid blocks the secretion of the penicillin, thereby increasing the therapeutic concentration of penicillin in the bloodstream. This is a prime example of drug interactions benefiting the patient. In contrast, digoxin and verapamil also share an active transport pathway. When they are administered concomitantly, their interaction leads to an increase in digoxin levels resulting in potential cardiotoxicity (e.g., arrhythmia). **Table 3.4** lists some other clinically important excretion interactions.

TABLE 3.4	Drugs Affecting Excretion		
Renal Elimination	**Mechanism**	**Object Drug**	**Results**
acetazolamide	Increases urine pH	salicylates	Increased elimination
losartan	Unknown	lithium	Decreased elimination
salicylates	Unknown	acetazolamide	Decreased elimination
acetazolamide	Increases urine pH	quinidine	Decreased elimination
triamterene	Unknown	amantadine	Decreased elimination
amiodarone	Unknown	digoxin	Decreased elimination
	Unknown	procainamide	Decreased renal and hepatic elimination
antacids	Increases urine pH	dextroamphet-amine, quinidine, pseudoephedrine	Decreased elimination
diuretics	Inhibit sodium reabsorption with subsequent renal tubular reabsorption of lithium	lithium	Decreased elimination
salicylates	Inhibit renal tubular secretion of metho-trexate	methotrexate	Decreased elimination

The other common pathway of excretion, the biliary tract, allows for the elimination of drugs and their metabolites into the feces. This route of excretion is involved in interactions with drugs that undergo enterohepatic recirculation. Drugs subject to this process are excreted into the GI tract through the biliary ducts and have the potential to be reabsorbed through the intestinal wall into the bloodstream. Some of these drugs depend on enterohepatic recirculation to achieve therapeutic concentrations. An example of a drug class that undergoes enterohepatic recirculation is the oral contraceptive. As previously described, antibiotics can adversely affect reabsorption of the estrogen components of oral contraceptives, potentially rendering them ineffective. In addition, drugs that undergo enterohepatic recirculation may also be affected by binding agents. An example of this is warfarin in combination with the bile acid sequestrants cholestipol or cholestyramine. Warfarin undergoes enterohepatic recirculation. Once warfarin has been excreted in the bile, the bile acid sequestrant binds with warfarin, preventing its reabsorption and increasing its clearance, decreasing its efficacy. This has been shown to occur even when warfarin is administerd intravenously (Jahnchen, et al., 1978). Therefore, it is not only important to administer warfarin 2 hours before or 6 hours after cholestyramine, but consistency in the administration time of these agents is important as well (Mancano, 2005).

Pharmacokinetic interactions make up a large part of the interactions that practitioners must contend with every day. These interactions are the most studied because they have an objective measurable outcome (e.g., drug concentrations, enzyme concentrations). However, a drug's pharmacodynamic profile must also be considered when it is administered with other agents.

P-Glycoprotein Interactions

Inhibition or induction of P-glycoprotein (P-gp), an energy-dependent efflux transporter, can result in interactions involving absorption or excretion (biliary or renal). P-gp pumps drug molecules out of cells and is found in the epithelial cells of the intestine (enterocytes), liver, and kidney. As a drug passes through the enterocyte in the intestine to be absorbed into the systemic circulation, P-gp can pick up the molecule and carry it back to the intestinal lumen, preventing absorption. P-gp in the liver and kidney act to increase the excretion of drugs by transporting the molecules into the bile and urine, respectively (Horn & Hansten, 2004).

If P-gp is inhibited, more drug will be absorbed through the enterocytes. This will result in an increase in plasma concentrations of the object drug. An example of this interaction is when quinidine is administered with digoxin. Quinidine inhibits intestinal P-gp, which results in increased absorption of digoxin. In addition, quinidine inhibition of renal P-gp results in reduced elimination of digoxin by the kidney. The end result is increased concentrations of serum digoxin (Horn & Hansten, 2004).

If P-gp is induced, less drug will be absorbed through the enterocytes. An example of an induction interaction of P-gp is when rifampin is given with digoxin. Rifampin induces intestinal P-gp, resulting in reduced absorption and reduced serum digoxin concentrations (Horn & Hansten, 2004).

Table 3.5 provides examples of common substrates, inhibitors, and inducers of P-gp (Horn & Hansten, 2004; Kim, 2002).

Pharmacodynamic Interactions

The responses or effects produced by a drug's actions are referred to as the drug's *pharmacodynamic profile*. Although drugs are administered to elicit a specific response or change in

TABLE 3.5	Examples of Substrates, Inhibitors, and Inducers of P-Glycoprotein*	
Substrates	**Inhibitors**	**Inducers**
aldosterone	amiodarone	indinavir
aimetidine	atorvastatin	morphine
colchicine	clarithromycin	nelfinavir
cyclosporine	cyclosporine	phenothiazine
digoxin	diltiazem	rifampin
diltiazem	erythromycin	ritonavir
erythromycin	felodipine	saquinavir
fexofenadine	indinavir	St. John's wort
indinavir	itraconazole	
itraconazole	ketoconazole	
morphine	methadone	
nelfinavir	nelfinavir	
quinidine	nicardipine	
ranitidine	quinidine	
saquinavir	ritonavir	
tetracycline	sirolimus	
verapamil	tacrolimus	
	verapamil	

*Data from Horn, J. R., & Hansten, P. D. (2004). Drug interactions with digoxin: The role of P-glycoprotein. *Pharmacy Times* (October), available at: http://www.hanstenandhorn.com/hh-article10-04.pdf and Kim, R. B. (2002). Drugs as P-glycoprotein substrates, inhibitors, and inducers. *Drug Metabolism Reviews, 34*, 47–54.

dynamics, an agent usually causes several changes in the body. When one or more drugs are coadministered, the entire pharmacodynamic profile of each drug must be considered because of the potential for their effects to interact. Drugs that have a similar characteristic in their pharmacodynamic profile may produce an exaggerated response. For example, when a benzodiazepine (e.g., alprazolam) is administered with a muscle relaxant (e.g., cyclobenzaprine), the sedative effects of both drugs combine to produce excessive drowsiness. A less obvious pharmacodynamic interaction occurs with the coadministration of angiotensin-converting enzyme (ACE) inhibitors (e.g., enalapril) and potassium-sparing diuretics (e.g., triamterene). These agents individually can both produce an increase in the potassium (K^+) level. Unless the prescriber is aware of the pharmacodynamic profile of both drugs, the potential for an excessive increase in the potassium level may go unnoticed and arrhythmia may ensue.

In contrast, drugs may also produce opposing pharmacodynamic effects. This type of interaction may cause the expected drug response to be diminished or even abolished. Unfortunately, these interactions are often overlooked. Instead of the lack of response being interpreted as a pharmacodynamic drug interaction, it is suspected to be due to an ineffective dose or drug. This often leads to an increase in the amount of drug administered and consequent unwanted side effects or interactions. This type of interaction is illustrated by the concomitant administration of an antihypertensive agent (e.g., a diuretic) and a nonsteroidal anti-inflammatory drug

(NSAID). Thiazide diuretics produce their hypotensive effects by blocking sodium reabsorption in the distal tubule of the kidney, which leads to increased sodium and water excretion. If NSAIDs are administered concomitantly, the sodium and water retention effects of the NSAIDs may reduce or nullify the hypotensive action of the diuretic.

DRUG–FOOD INTERACTIONS

The interaction between food and drugs can affect both pharmacokinetic and pharmacodynamic parameters. The mechanism of these pharmacokinetic interactions is mediated by alteration of drug bioavailability, distribution, metabolism, or excretion, as seen with drug–drug interactions. The potential for pharmacodynamic drug–food interactions warrants concern about proper diet for patients on certain drugs. Although practicing clinicians often overlook drug–food interactions, these interactions can significantly affect efficacy of drug therapy. Awareness of significant drug–food interactions can reduce the incidence of these effects and optimize drug therapy.

Effect of Food on Drug Pharmacokinetics

Absorption

Food can affect the absorption of drugs in two ways: first, by altering the extent of drug absorption, and second, by changing the rate of drug absorption. Usually, changes in the rate of drug absorption have less significance if only the rate of absorption is delayed without affecting bioavailability. The underlying mechanisms that mediate these interactions are highly variable and depend on both the content of food and the properties of the drug involved.

Food can either increase or decrease the amount (extent) of drug absorption, potentially altering the bioavailability of a drug. One mechanism, similar to drug–drug interactions, is adsorption. For example, tetracycline and fluoroquinolone antibiotics (e.g., ciprofloxacin, ofloxacin) can chelate with calcium cations found in milk or milk products, thus significantly limiting the drug's bioavailability (Deppermann & Lode, 1993).

A second type of drug–food interaction occurs when food serves as a physical barrier and prevents the absorption of orally administered drugs (Kirk, 1995). The absorptive capacity of the small intestine is related to the accessibility of a drug to the GI mucosal surfaces, the site where absorption occurs. When food is coadministered with a drug, access to the mucosa is reduced, resulting in delayed or decreased drug absorption. For example, the bioavailability of azithromycin is reduced by 43% when the drug is taken with food (Zithromax Package Insert, 2003). Similar types of interactions can be seen when erythromycin, isoniazid, penicillins, and zidovudine are given orally. To avoid such interactions, these drugs can be administered 2 hours apart from mealtime. **Box 3.1** identifies some commonly prescribed drugs that should be taken on an empty stomach. Note, however, if patients cannot tolerate these

BOX 3.1

Drugs to Be Taken on an Empty Stomach

azithromycin
captopril
erythromycin
fluoroquinolones (e.g., ciprofloxacin, ofloxacin)
griseofulvin
isoniazid
oral penicillins
sucralfate
tetracycline
theophylline, timed release (e.g., Theo-Dur Sprinkle, Theo-24, Uniphyl)
zidovudine

medications on an empty stomach (because of GI side effects like diarrhea), coadministration with food may be advisable.

In contrast, food can also increase the absorption of some drugs. For example, a high-fat meal can significantly increase the absorption of lipophilic drugs like griseofulvin (Trovato, Nuhlicek, & Midtling, 1991). In another example, the concentration of a long-acting formulation of theophylline, such as Theo-24, can increase when taken with a high-fat meal (Jonkman, 1989). Conversely, only 40% of the Theo-Dur Sprinkle formulation is absorbed when given with meals. Because considerable variation can exist in the absorption of controlled-release formulations of theophylline, the drug is recommended to be taken apart from meals (Hussar, 1995).

Metabolism

Food can also affect drug metabolism. Grapefruit juice, for example, can affect the metabolism of many drugs. Grapefruit juice specifically inhibits the 3A4 subset of intestinal cytochrome P450 enzymes and thus increases the serum concentration of drugs dependent on these enzymes for metabolism (Ameer & Weintraub, 1997; Huang et al., 2004).

The cytochrome enzymes are found in highest concentrations in the proximal two thirds of the small intestine. These enzymes are located at the distal portion of the villi that line the small intestine and are responsible for the extrahepatic metabolism of more than 20 drugs (Ameer & Weintraub, 1997; Huang et al., 2004). The component in grapefruit juice that is responsible for this interaction remains undetermined; however, the flavonoid naringin, found in high concentrations in grapefruit juice, is suspected. Increases in the bioavailability of verapamil and dihydropyridine calcium channel blockers such as felodipine, nisoldipine, nitrendipine, nifedipine, and amlodipine have been documented with the coadministration of grapefruit juice (Bailey, et al., 1991, 1992, and 1993; Rashid, et al., 1993). The bioavailability of felodipine could be

enhanced by as much as 2.8-fold by grapefruit juice (Bailey, et al., 1991). However, unlike verapamil and dihydropyridine calcium channel blockers, diltiazem does not demonstrate an increase in bioavailability with grapefruit juice.

The amount of grapefruit juice required to increase plasma concentrations can vary between agents. A single glass of grapefruit juice can increase the area under the curve and maximum concentration (Cmax) of felodipine by severalfold (Bailey, et al., 1998) while the warnings in the product labeling for some HMG CoA reductase inhibitors metabolized by CYP3A4 say to avoid quantities greater than 1 quart per day (Zocor prescribing information/Mevacor prescribing information). The extent of the increase in felodipine plasma concentrations is maximal between simultaneous and 4 hours before administration of grapefruit juice. However, higher Cmax concentrations were evident even when grapefruit juice is consumed 24 hours before felodipine. Therefore, separating doses may reduce but does not eliminate the potential for the interaction (Bailey, et al., 1998). Because grapefruit juice appears to inhibit mostly intestinal CYP3A4 and not hepatic CYP3A4 enzymes, the metabolism of drugs administered intravenously is unlikely to be altered. Further, the data suggest that only those agents given at doses higher than usual or if the patients' livers are severely damaged, result in the intestinal CYP3A4 as the primary metabolic pathway (Huang et al., 2004). **Box 3.2** identifies some drugs that may interact with grapefruit juice.

In contrast to the ability of grapefruit juice to inhibit drug metabolism, other components of food may induce drug metabolism and therefore decrease drug efficacy. For example, in the treatment of Parkinson disease, dopamine in the brain needs to be replenished. However, exogenous dopamine does not cross the blood-brain barrier, but its precursor, levodopa, does. Unfortunately, much of the levodopa is lost

BOX 3.2

Drugs That Interact with Grapefruit Juice

benzodiazepines
  midazolam
  triazolam
cyclosporine
dihydropyridine calcium channel blockers
  amlodipine
  felodipine
  nifedipine
  nisoldipine
  nitrendipine
lovastatin
simvastatin
theophylline
verapamil
17 β-estradiol

to metabolism when given orally and only approximately 1% of the administered amount enters the brain to be converted to dopamine (Trovato, et al., 1991). Concomitant administration with food containing pyridoxine (or vitamin B$_6$) can potentially further enhance the peripheral metabolism of levodopa, thus decreasing drug efficacy (Trovato, et al., 1991). Patients taking levodopa should therefore be educated about moderate intake of pyridoxine-rich foods, such as avocados, beans, bacon, beef, liver, peas, pork, sweet potatoes, and tuna. Similarly, charcoal-broiled meats can induce the activity of the CYP1A2 isoenzymes, thus increasing the metabolism of drugs such as theophylline (Kirk, 1995).

Excretion

Ingestion of certain fruit juices can alter the urinary pH and affect the elimination and reabsorption of drugs such as quinidine and amphetamine (Trovato, et al., 1991). Orange, tomato, and grapefruit juices are metabolized to an alkaline residue, which can increase the urinary pH. For drugs that are weak bases, making the urine more alkaline by raising the pH increases the proportion of non-ionized drug and enhances the reabsorption of the drug systemically. (Recall that the ionization of drugs helps promote water solubility and ultimately enhances drug elimination into the urine.)

Effect of Food on Pharmacodynamics

Food affects the pharmacodynamics of drugs either by opposing or potentiating a drug's pharmacologic action. For example, warfarin exerts its anticoagulant effects by inhibiting synthesis of vitamin K–dependent clotting factors. Vitamin K is required for activation by several protein factors of the clotting cascade, namely, factors II, VII, IX, and X. When foods rich in vitamin K are ingested, they can significantly oppose the anticoagulatory efficacy of warfarin. Leafy green vegetables, such as collard greens, kale, lettuce, spinach, mustard greens, and broccoli, are generally recognized to contain large quantities of vitamin K. Health care providers should educate patients who are taking warfarin about this interaction. More importantly, however, practitioners should stress maintaining a balanced diet without abruptly changing the intake of foods rich in vitamin K.

Another significant drug–food interaction occurs between monoamine oxidase (MAO) inhibitors and foods containing tyramine, an amino acid that is contained in many types of food. Tyramine can precipitate a hypertensive reaction in patients taking MAO inhibitors, such as phenelzine, tranylcypromine, or isocarboxazid. Monoamine oxidases are enzymes located in the GI tract that inactivate tyramine in food. When patients are taking MAO inhibitors, the breakdown of tyramine is prevented and therefore allows for more tyramine to be absorbed systemically. Because of the indirect sympathomimetic property of tyramine, this amino acid provokes the release of norepinephrine from sympathetic nerve endings and epinephrine from the adrenal glands, resulting in an excessive pressor effect. Clinically, patients may complain of diaphore-

---

BOX 3.3
Foods High in Tyramine

Bean pods
Beer (draft)
Cheese (aged)
Cured meats (i.e., salami, pepperoni, sausage)
Fruits (overripe, such as figs, avocados, prunes, and raisins)
Herring (pickled)
Liver
Sauerkraut
Soy sauce
Wine

---

sis, mydriasis, occipital or temporal headache, nuchal rigidity, palpitations, and elevated blood pressure. Examples of foods that contain tyramine are listed in **Box 3.3**.

Effect of Drugs on Food and Nutrients

Many of the aforementioned examples indicate that food can precipitate an interaction with a drug, but in some cases, a reciprocal relationship also holds true. First, some drugs can cause a depletion of nutrients or minerals found in food through various mechanisms. For example, drugs such as cholestyramine and colestipol, which were designed to bind bile acid in the GI tract, could also potentially bind to fat-soluble vitamins (i.e., vitamins A, D, E, K) and folic acid when taken with food, resulting in the decreased absorption of these vitamins. Orlistat, an over-the-counter and prescription medication used for weight loss, reduces fat absorption. In addition to reducing fat absorption, it can also decrease the absorption of fat-soluble vitamins and beta-carotene. Similarly, the chronic use of mineral oil as a laxative reduces the absorption of fat-soluble vitamins (Kirk, 1995). Careful monitoring of the INR in patients taking warfarin and drugs that affect vitamin K absorption is warranted to avoid changes in bleeding times.

Second, drug-induced malabsorption can occur in patients with pre-existing poor nutritional status. For example, long-term use of isoniazid can cause pyridoxine (vitamin B$_6$) deficiency. Pyridoxine supplementation is recommended for patients who are malnourished or predisposed to neuropathy (e.g., patients with diabetes or alcoholism) when treated with isoniazid. Metformin is associated with vitamin B$_{12}$ deficiency in about 7% of patients, which may lead to anemia. In general, the clinical significance of these interactions may depend on the baseline nutritional status of the patient. Patients with poor nutrition or inadequate dietary intake (e.g., elderly or alcoholic patients) are potentially at greater risk for drug-induced vitamin and mineral depletion.

Third, drugs can change nutrient excretion as well. Both thiazide and loop diuretics can enhance the excretion of potassium, possibly leading to hypokalemia. Digoxin, in the presence of diuretic-induced hypokalemia can lead to digoxin-induced arrhythmias. Spironolactone, an aldosterone antagonist and potassium-sparing diuretic, can increase potassium levels, especially in the presence of an ACE inhibitor or angiotensin receptor blocker. Loop diuretics can increase urinary excretion of calcium, whereas thiazide diuretics can decrease it. In addition, ascorbic acid and potassium depletion can occur with high doses of long-term aspirin therapy (Trovato, et al., 1991).

DRUG–HERB INTERACTIONS

In today's society, the search for a "natural way" to treat and prevent diseases has become commonplace. This potentially stems from the misconception that "natural" means "safer." The National Toxicology Program estimates that there are over 1,500 botanicals sold as dietary supplements (Herb Fact Sheet, 2006). It is estimated that 20% of the U.S. population takes herbal supplements (Izzo & Ernst, 2009). For the most part, these herbal supplements are not regulated by the FDA. In many cases, little research has been conducted to assess the efficacy and safety of these agents or the potential for pharmacokinetic or pharmacodynamic interactions. Some clinical trials have been conducted to evaluate the safety and efficacy of certain herbal medications; however, much of available data is based on animal studies, case reports, and the potential for interactions derived from what is known about the chemical characteristics and pharmacokinetic parameters of the herbs.

Pharmacokinetic Interactions

Absorption

As discussed earlier in the chapter, certain agents can interact with other medications in the GI tract to prevent absorption. Likewise, some herbs can prevent absorption of medications

and reduce the effectiveness of those medications. For example, acacia, marketed as a fiber supplement, has been shown to impair the absorption of amoxicillin. This may be secondary to the fiber content of acacia. Doses of acacia and amoxicillin should be separated by 4 hours. Dandelion has a high mineral content and has been shown to reduce the effectiveness of quinolones in animals (Ulbricht, et al., 2008). **Table 3.6** summarizes some of the potential herb–drug interactions that can occur in the absorptive process.

Distribution

Meadowsweet and black willow contain salicylates that have the potential to displace highly protein-bound drugs. To avoid toxicity, coadministration of these products with highly protein-bound drugs with a narrow therapeutic index, such as warfarin and carbamazepine, should be avoided (Kuhn, 2002).

Metabolism

Certain herbs can be inducers or inhibitors of the cytochrome P450 enzyme system. St. John's wort, an herbal medication often used to treat depression, has consistently been shown to induce CYP3A4, CYP2E1, and CYP2C19. In addition, St. John's wort induces intestinal P-gp and has been shown to lower plasma concentrations of common P-gp substrates such as digoxin and fexofenadine. Induction of these enzymes are secondary to hyperforin, an ingredient in St. John's wort. St. John's wort has been shown to clinically interact with a number of drugs, including immunosuppressants, hypoglycemics, anti-inflammatory agents, antimicrobial agents, anti-migraine medications, oral contraceptives, cardiovascular agents, and antiretroviral and anti-cancer drugs as well as drugs affecting the central nervous, GI, and respiratory systems (Izzo & Ernst, 2009).

In contrast, kava, used as an anxiolytic, and garlic, used to treat dyslipidemia, have both been shown in pharmacokinetic studies to inhibit the cytochrome P450 enzyme system,

TABLE 3.6	**Herb–Drug Interactions Affecting Absorption**		
Herbal Medication	**Mechanism of Action**	**Object Drug**	**Results**
Acacia	Fiber content may slow or reduce absorption of medications	Amoxicillin	Decreased absorption (separate doses by at least 4 hours)
Carob	Decreased bowel transit time	Oral medications	Decreased absorption (separate doses by several hours)
Citrus pectin	Fiber content may slow or reduce absorption of medications	Oral medications	Take 1 hour before or 2 hours after intake of other oral medications
Dandelion	High mineral content (chelation)	Ciprofloxacin and potentially other medications affected by chelation	Decreased absorption; dandelion and quinolone coadministration should be avoided
Flaxseed	Fiber content may decrease absorption of oral agents	Oral agents/vitamins/minerals	Decreased absorption; oral agents should be taken 1 hour before or 2 hours after flaxseed
Psyllium	Fiber content may decrease absorption of oral agents	Carbamazepine, digoxin, lithium	Decreased absorption

Data from Ulbricht, C., Chao, W., Costa, D., et al. (2008). Clinical evidence of herb–drug interactions: A systematic review by the Natural Standard Research Collaboration. *Current Drug Metabolism, 9,* 1063–1120.

TABLE 3.7	Drug–Herb Metabolism Interactions		
Herbal Medication	**Mechanism of Action**	**Object Drug**	**Results**
Garlic	Inhibitor of CYP2E1	Chlorzoxazone	Increased chlorzoxazone levels and potentially other 2E1 substrates
Ginkgo	Inducer of CYP2C19	Antiseizure medications, omeprazole	Decreased levels of valproic acid, phenytoin, and omeprazole possible
Goldenseal (Berberine)	Inhibitor of CYP3A4	Cyclosporine	Increase in cyclosporine levels
Kava	Inhibitor of CYP2E1	Chlorzoxazone	Increased chlorzoxazone levels and potentially other 2E1 substrates
Licorice	Inhibitor or inducer of CYP3A4	CYP3A4 substrates	Potential increase or decrease in CYP3A4 substrate levels
Red yeast rice	CYP3A4 inhibitors can increase plasma concentrations of Monacolin K	Monacolin K	Increased plasma concentrations of Monacolin K can result in muscle toxicity
Scotch broom	Haloperidol (CYP2D6 inhibitor) has been shown to increase levels of sparteine)	Sparteine	Increased levels of sparteine, which may be potentially cardiotoxic
St. John's wort	Inhibitor of CYP3A4	Alprazolam, amitriptyline, atorvastatin, ciclosporin, ertythromycin, imatinib, indinavir, irinotecan, ivabradine, methadone, midazolam, nevirapine, nifedipine, oral contraceptives, quazepam, simvastatin, tacrolimus, verapamil, warfarin	May result in decreased efficacy and/or effectiveness of the object drugs listed
	Inducer of CYP2C19	Omeprazole	Decreased levels of omeprazole possible
	Inducer of CYP2E1	Chlorzoxazone	Decreased chlorzoxazone levels and potentially other 2E1 substrates

Data from Ulbricht, C., Chao, W., Costa, D., et al. (2008). Clinical evidence of herb-drug interactions: A systematic review by the Natural Standard Research Collaboration. *Current Drug Metabolism, 9,* 1063–1120 and Izzo, A., & Ernst, E. (2009). Interactions between herbal medicines and prescribed drugs: An updated systematic review. *Drugs, 69,* 1777–1798.

specifically CYP2E1 (Izzo & Ernst, 2009). **Table 3.7** shows some common herb–drug interactions affecting metabolism.

Pharmacodynamic Interactions

Herbs may contain ingredients that potentiate the pharmacodynamic effects of certain medications, which may lead to adverse effects. The causative mechanism of these effects may not be well understood in many cases.

Several herbal medications have been shown to inhibit platelet activity and/or have an effect on increasing the INR. Case reports of increased bleeding in patients taking herbal medications with nonsteroidal anti-inflammatory agents, antiplatelet agents, and anticoagulants has been reported (Ulbricht, et al., 2008). **Box 3.4** shows herbal medications that may increase the potential for bleeding when given concomitantly with medications that inhibit platelets or alter coagulation.

Some herbal medications have been shown to potentiate the central nervous system (CNS) depressant effects of some medications. Kava, lavender, and valerian may potentiate the effects of CNS depressants, such as barbiturates, benzodiazepines, and narcotics. In addition, kava may interfere with the effects of dopamine or dopamine antagonists and

it is potentially hepatotoxic (Ulbricht, et al., 2008; Kuhn, 2002).

Aloe has been associated with hypoglycemia in patients taking glibenclamide (glyburide). Bitter orange contains MAO inhibitor substrates such as tyramine and octopamine, and concomitant use with an MAO inhibitor may increase the potential for hypertensive effects (Ulbricht, et al, 2008).

While many patients may believe herbal medications are safe because they are "natural" and are available over the counter, the potential for herb–drug interactions still exists. Clinicians must be aware of the potential for these interactions and encourage patients to disclose all medications they are taking, including herbal remedies.

DRUG–DISEASE INTERACTIONS

Certain drug–disease interactions can change drug pharmacokinetic and pharmacodynamic parameters, leading to less-than-optimal drug therapeutic outcomes and greater risk of toxicity. In addition, certain drugs can exacerbate a patient's co-existing disease.

BOX 3.4

Herbal Supplements That Potentially Increase Bleeding When Taken with Antiplatelets/ Anticoagulants*

Borage seed oil
Clove
Danshen
Devil's claw
Dong quai
Feverfew
Garlic
Ginger
Ginkgo
Ginseng
Goji
Omega-3 fatty acids
Papaya
Peony
Policosanol
Pycnogenol
Saw palmetto
Turmeric

*Data from Ulbricht C., Chao W., Costa D., et al. (2008). Clinical evidence of herb-drug interactions: A systematic review by the Natural Standard Research Collaboration. *Current Drug Metabolism, 9,* 1063–1120.

Effect of Disease on Pharmacokinetics of Drugs

Absorption

As already discussed, the absorption of drugs may be affected by the presence of other drugs and food in the GI tract. However, drug absorption also depends on the physiologic processes that maintain normal GI function. These processes can include enzyme secretion, acidity, gastric emptying, bile production, and transit time. Thus, any disease that alters the normal physiologic function of the GI system potentially alters drug absorption.

As an example, the gastric emptying rate can be reduced in patients with duodenal or pyloric ulcers and hypothyroidism (Shargel & Yu, 1993). In addition, long-term diabetes can result in diabetic gastroparesis, which delays gastric emptying. This results in later or fluctuating maximal serum concentrations and has been documented with oral hypoglycemic agents. This may become particularly important when a rapid acting drug is required. However, drugs with longer half-lives may be less likely to be affected (Jing, et al., 2009). Another example includes bowel edema and intestinal hypoperfusion

from advancing heart failure, which can delay the absorption of diuretics prescribed to control edema (Hunt, et al., 2009). Finally, diarrhea, a manifestation of many diseases, can pose a problem for oral absorption of drugs as well as food and nutrients.

Distribution

The distribution of drugs can be affected by certain disease states. Of significance are conditions that change plasma albumin levels and therefore can increase or decrease the concentration of drugs usually bound to albumin. Examples of conditions that may decrease plasma albumin levels include burns, bone fractures, acute infections, inflammatory disease, liver disease, malnutrition, and renal disease. Examples of conditions that may increase plasma albumin levels include benign tumors, gynecologic disorders, myalgia, and surgical procedures (Braun, 1997).

Metabolism

The metabolism of drugs can often be altered by diseases that affect the functions of the liver, such as liver cirrhosis. Failure of the liver (the primary organ responsible for drug metabolism) not only impairs drug metabolism, but can cause changes in liver blood flow and a reduction in albumin synthesis. Therefore, the clinical impact of liver failure includes a strong potential for interactions with drugs. Congestive heart failure is another disease that can cause direct reduction in the ability of the liver to metabolize drugs. In patients with congestive heart failure, however, decreased metabolic capacity of the liver is also caused by a decrease in blood flow to the liver owing to changes in cardiac output.

In some cases, normal liver function is needed to activate a drug rather than to inactivate it. Certain drugs like enalapril are called *prodrugs,* meaning the drug needs to be converted by the liver to its active form (enalaprilat) to achieve maximal therapeutic effect. Therefore, use of a prodrug in patients with liver dysfunction can potentially reduce the efficacy of the drug.

Excretion

Renal function can influence serum drug concentrations because most drugs are eliminated by the kidneys either as unchanged drug or as metabolites. Chronic renal diseases that compromise the function of the kidney to clear drugs can result in drug accumulation. Glomerulonephritis, interstitial nephritis, long-term and uncontrolled diabetes, and hypertension are primary causes of declining renal function. In clinical practice, once the patient's estimated creatinine clearance has declined to less than 50 mL/min, dose adjustments usually are required for drugs that are primarily renally cleared. For example, drugs such as H_2 receptor antagonists and fluoroquinolone antibiotics commonly require dose adjustments for patients with renal insufficiency. In particular, the drug regimen of elderly patients or those with an elevated serum creatinine level above 1.5 mg/dL should be evaluated to detect any ADRs from possible drug accumulation secondary to declining renal clearance.

Effects of Drugs on Co-existing Disease

Drugs used to treat one medical condition can sometimes exacerbate the status of another comorbid disease. Practitioners, therefore, should be aware of potential drug–disease interactions. This is of particular importance in elderly individuals who have multiple concomitant diseases and often take multiple medications. Detected rates of drug–disease interactions range from 6% to 30% in older adults (Lindblad, et al., 2006). A complete discussion of this topic is beyond the scope of this chapter. However, a consensus statement has been published from a multidisciplinary panel of health care providers whose members specialize in geriatric medicine. The statement identifies several drug–disease interactions that are common in older individuals and are considered to have a deleterious impact on co-existing disease in older individuals. **Table 3.8** lists these common and clinically significant drug–disease interactions in the elderly (Lindblad, et al., 2006).

TABLE 3.8	**Drug–Disease Interactions Common in the Elderly**
Disease/Condition	**Drug/Drug Class**
Benign prostatic hyperplasia	Anticholinergics
	Tricyclic antidepressants
Chronic renal failure	Nonaspirin NSAIDS
Heart failure (systolic dysfunction)	First-generation calcium channel blockers
Constipation	Anticholinergics
	Opioid analgesics
	Tricyclic antidepressants
Dementia	Anticholinergics
	Barbiturates
	Benzodiazepines
	Tricyclic antidepressants
Diabetes	Corticosteroids
Falls	Antipsychotics (thioridazine/ haloperidol)
	Benzodiazepines
	Sedative hypnotics
	Tricyclic antidepressants
Heart block	Digoxin
	Tricyclic antidepressants
Narrow-angle glaucoma	Anticholinergics
Parkinson's disease	Metoclopramide
Peptic ulcer disease	Aspirin
	Nonaspirin NSAIDs
Postural hypotension	Thioridazine
	Tricyclic antidepressants
Seizures	Bupropion
Syncope	Alpha-blockers (e.g., doxazosin, terazosin, methyldopa)

*Data from Lindblad, C. I., Hanlon, J. T., Gross, C. R., et al. (2006). Clinically important drug-disease interactions and their prevalence in older adults. *Clinical Therapeutics, 28,* 1133–1143.

PATIENT FACTORS INFLUENCING DRUG INTERACTIONS

The outcomes of drug interactions are highly variable from one person to another. Many patient factors can influence the propensity for an interaction to occur, such as genetics, diseases, environment, smoking, diet/nutrition, and alcohol (Hansten, 1998). An understanding of these factors can help to identify potential sources of drug interactions.

Heredity

As discussed previously, the cytochrome P450 system can display genetic polymorphism (Ingelman-Sundberg, 2004; Hansten, 1998). That is, the variable metabolism of drugs by cytochrome P450 enzymes from one person to another in the population can be partly explained by genetic differences. For example, approximately 8% of Americans lack the gene to form the isoenzyme CYP2D6 and therefore are at greater risk for toxicity from psychotropic drugs and, potentially, other drugs that are metabolized by these isoenzymes (Hansten, 1998). The metabolism of isoniazid also demonstrates variation among different people; some acetylate isoniazid very rapidly, whereas others acetylate it slowly (Hussar, 1995).

Disease

Another important factor that influences drug interactions is the patient's existing disease state. Any disease affecting liver or kidney function can potentially predispose the patient to drug interactions and ADRs because these organs are primary sites of drug metabolism and elimination, respectively. Significant deterioration in drug metabolism or elimination can lead to increased serum concentrations and therefore increase the likelihood for drugs to interact. Consequently, elderly patients and those with a history of liver disease or renal insufficiency should be evaluated for dose adjustments of drugs significantly cleared by the liver and kidneys.

Environment

Environmental factors, such as DDT and other pesticides, can increase the activity of liver enzymes, potentially causing an increase in drug metabolism (Hussar, 1995). Although the general significance of the effect of environmental exposure on the clinical outcome of drug therapy has not been well studied, people working in occupations with prolonged exposure to toxins and chemicals should be more closely observed.

Smoking

Studies show that smoking can increase the liver's metabolism of certain drugs, including diazepam, propoxyphene, chlorpromazine, and amitriptyline (Hussar, 1995). For example, the polycyclic aromatic hydrocarbons in cigarettes can induce CYP1A2 metabolism, resulting in decreased theophylline serum concentrations (Schein, 1995).

Diet and Nutrition

The nutritional status and dietary intake of the patient can influence the importance of a drug–nutrient interaction. Drugs can deplete valuable vitamins and minerals from food; however, these interactions are often difficult to recognize and may go undetected. Patients with poor baseline nutrition (e.g., alcoholics) may experience more pronounced effects mainly because of underlying nutritional deficiency. Practitioners should be aware of potential drug–nutrient interactions by identifying patients who have poor dietary intake and who concurrently take medications that can deplete vitamins and minerals.

Alcohol Intake

Alcohol can complicate drug therapy on many different levels. Alcohol has a variable effect on drug metabolism depending on acute or chronic intake. Acute alcohol ingestion can inhibit drug metabolism, thus increasing serum drug concentrations; it also can enhance the pharmacodynamic effect of drugs with properties of CNS depression. Patients concurrently taking narcotics, antihistamines, antidepressants, antipsychotics, and muscle relaxants with alcohol are at greatest risk for CNS depression and should be warned of this interaction (Trovato, et al., 1991). In addition, acute ingestion of alcohol can increase the potential for hypoglycemia in diabetic patients taking insulin or insulin secretagogues (e.g., sulphonylureas).

In contrast, chronic alcohol intake tends to increase the synthesis of drug-metabolizing enzymes, leading to induction (Hansten, 1998). Enzyme induction causes decreases in serum drug levels. Enzyme induction secondary to chronic alcohol use increases conversion of acetaminophen to hepatotoxic metabolites. Chronic use of alcohol in combination with high doses of acetaminophen (often from several sources) above that recommended in the labeling may result in liver damage (Jang & Harris, 2007). In addition, chronic use of alcohol in combination with NSAIDS or aspirin increases the risk of GI bleeding. Long-term abuse of alcohol leads to liver cirrhosis, which ultimately impairs drug metabolism by destruction of functional hepatocytes.

ADVERSE DRUG REACTIONS

An ADR can be defined as an undesirable clinical manifestation that is consequent to and caused by the administration of a particular drug. ADRs are basically drug-induced toxic reactions. The World Health Organization defines an ADR as "a response to a medicine which is noxious and unintended, and which occurs at doses normally used in man."

There are two general types to consider. The first type of ADR is an exaggeration of the principal pharmacologic action of the drug. The ADR is simply a more pronounced drug response than normal. These reactions usually are dose dependent and predictable. These are often referred to as type A reactions.

In the second type, type B reactions, the ADR is unrelated to the principal pharmacologic action of the drug itself (May, 1993; Plaa & Smith, 1995). These reactions are precipitated by the secondary pharmacologic actions of the drug, may be unpredictable, and may or may not be dose dependent. In either type, the ADR can result from overdosage of drug or administration of therapeutic doses to a patient hyperreactive to the drug, or as an indirect consequence of the primary action.

ADRs are sometimes referred to as side effects. A side effect is also recognized as an undesirable pharmacologic effect that accompanies the primary drug action and usually occurs within the therapeutic dosing range (Plaa & Smith, 1995). ADRs or side effects can have varying levels of intensity. For example, the dry mouth and blurred vision that occur from drugs with anticholinergic properties are considered routine side effects of that class of medication. In contrast, drug-induced liver damage would be an uncommon and severe ADR or side effect not routinely associated with that class of medication. Patients experiencing ADRs or side effects from drugs do not necessarily require discontinuation of therapy; however, proper drug selection emphasizing agents with minimal side effect profiles may help improve patient acceptance of and compliance with the drug.

Tracking Drug Interactions and Adverse Drug Reactions

The initial source of documented ADRs comes primarily from the experience gained while using a drug during clinical trials. Usually, the number of people taking the drug in clinical trials, on the order of hundreds to several thousands, is too few to detect all the possible adverse reactions from the drug. However, after a drug is approved by the FDA, it becomes readily available for public use in hundreds of thousands to millions of people. The potential for drug interactions and ADRs then becomes much greater than during clinical trials. Therefore, practitioners should have a basic understanding of drug interactions and ADRs and report these events to the FDA when they occur.

MedWatch is a medical products reporting program conducted by the FDA (**Figure 3-3**). The purpose of the MedWatch program is to enhance the effectiveness of surveillance of drugs and medical products after they are marketed and as they are used in clinical practice. The benefit to health care providers for reporting drug interactions and ADRs is to ensure that drug safety information is rapidly communicated to health care professionals, thus improving patient care. Health care providers should also be aware of programs in their own institutions that collect and report ADRs or drug interactions.

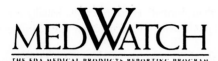

For VOLUNTARY reporting
by health professionals of adverse
events and product problems

THE FDA MEDICAL PRODUCTS REPORTING PROGRAM

Form Approved: OMB No. 0910-0291 Expires 12/31/94
See OMB statement on reverse

FDA Use Only **[DAVIS]**

Triage unit
sequence #

Page ___ of ___

PLEASE TYPE OR USE BLACK INK

A. Patient information

1. Patient identifier	2. Age at time of event: or _____ Date of birth:	3. Sex ☐ female ☐ male	4. Weight _____ lbs or _____ kgs
In confidence			

B. Adverse event or product problem

1. ☐ **Adverse event**   and/or   ☐ **Product problem** (e.g., defects/malfunctions)

2. **Outcomes attributed to adverse event**
(check all that apply)

☐ death _____
            (mo day yr)
☐ life-threatening
☐ hospitalization – initial or prolonged

☐ disability
☐ congenital anomaly
☐ required intervention to prevent permanent impairment/damage
☐ other: _____

3. Date of event (mo day yr)	4. Date of this report (mo day yr)

5. **Describe event or problem**

6. **Relevant tests/laboratory data,** including dates

7. **Other relevant history, including preexisting medical conditions** (e.g., allergies, race, pregnancy, smoking and alcohol use, hepatic/renal dysfunction, etc.)

C. Suspect medication(s)

1. **Name** (give labeled strength & mfr/labeler, if known)
#1
#2

2. **Dose, frequency & route used**	3. **Therapy dates** (if unknown, give duration) from/to (or best estimate)
#1	#1
#2	#2

4. **Diagnosis for use** (indication)	5. **Event abated after use stopped or dose reduced**
#1	#1 ☐ yes ☐ no ☐ doesn't apply
#2	#2 ☐ yes ☐ no ☐ doesn't apply

6. **Lot #** (if known)	7. **Exp. date** (if known)	8. **Event reappeared after reintroduction**
#1	#1	#1 ☐ yes ☐ no ☐ doesn't apply
#2	#2	#2 ☐ yes ☐ no ☐ doesn't apply

9. **NDC #** (for product problems only)

10. **Concomitant medical products** and therapy dates (exclude treatment of event)

D. Suspect medical device

1. **Brand name**

2. **Type of device**

3. **Manufacturer name & address**	4. **Operator of device** ☐ health professional ☐ lay user/patient ☐ other: _____
6. model # _____ catalog # _____ serial # _____ lot # _____ other # _____	5. **Expiration date** (mo day yr)
	7. **If implanted, give date** (mo day yr)
	8. **If explanted, give date** (mo day yr)

9. **Device available for evaluation?**   (Do not send to FDA)
☐ yes   ☐ no   ☐ returned to manufacturer on _____ (mo day yr)

10. **Concomitant medical products** and therapy dates (exclude treatment of event)

E. Reporter (see confidentiality section on back)

1. **Name, address & phone #**

2. **Health professional?** ☐ yes ☐ no	3. **Occupation**	4. **Also reported to** ☐ manufacturer ☐ user facility ☐ distributor

5. **If you do NOT want your identity disclosed to the manufacturer, place an " X " in this box.** ☐

FDA

Mail to: MEDWATCH
5600 Fishers Lane
Rockville, MD 20852-9787

or FAX to:
1-800-FDA-0178

FDA Form 3500 (6/93)   Submission of a report does not constitute an admission that medical personnel or the product caused or contributed to the event.

FIGURE 3–3   MedWatch form for reporting an adverse event or product problem to the U.S. FDA.

BIBLIOGRAPHY

*Starred references are cited in the text.

*Ameer, B., & Weintraub, R. A. (1997). Drug interactions with grapefruit juice. *Clinical Pharmacokinetics, 33*(2), 103–121.

*American Society of Health-System Pharmacists. (2008). *AHFS Drug Information 2008.* (1961, 3062). Bethesda, MD: Author.

*Bailey, D. C., Arnold, J. M. O., Strong, H. A., et al. (1993). Effect of grapefruit juice and naringin on nisoldipine pharmacokinetics. *Clinical Pharmacology and Therapeutics, 54,* 589–594.

*Bailey D. G., Malcolm J., Arnold O., Spence J. D. (1998). Grapefruit juice-drug interactions. *British Journal of Clinical Pharmacology, 46,* 101–110.

*Bailey, D. G., Munoz, C., Arnold, J. M. O., et al. (1992). Grapefruit juice and naringin interaction with nitrendipine [Abstract]. *Clinical Pharmacology and Therapeutics, 51,* 156.

*Bailey, D. G., Spence, J. D., Munoz, C., et al. (1991). Interaction of citrus juices with felodipine and nifedipine. *Lancet, 337,* 268–269.

*Bates, D., Spell, N., Cullen, D., et al. (1997). The costs of adverse drug events in hospitalized patients. *Journal of the American Medical Association, 277,* 307–311.

*Becker, M. L., Visser L. E., van Gelder T., et al. (2008). Increasing exposure to drug-drug interactions between 1992 and 2005 in people aged ≥55 years. *Drugs and Aging, 25,* 145–152.

*Bjerrum, L., Lopez-Valcarcel, B. G., & Petersen, G. (2008). Risk factors for potential drug interactions in general practice. *European Journal of General Practice, 14,* 23–29.

*Braun, L. D. (1997). Therapeutic drug monitoring. In L. Shargel, A. H. Mutnick, P. F. Souney, L. N. Swanson, & L. H. Black (Eds.). *Comprehensive pharmacy review* (3rd ed., pp. 586–597). Baltimore, MD: Williams & Wilkins.

*Brosen, K. (1990). Recent developments in hepatic drug oxidation: Implications for clinical pharmacokinetics. *Clinical Pharmacokinetics, 18,* 220–239.

*Classen, D. C., Pestonik, S. L., Evans, R. S., et al. (1997). Adverse drug events in hospitalized patients: Excess length of stay, extra costs, and attributable mortality. *Journal of the American Medical Association, 277,* 301–306.

*Clopidogrel (Plavix®) prescribing information. Available at: http://products. sanofi-aventis.us/PLAVIX/PLAVIX.html. Accessed July 29, 2010.

*Cupp, M., & Tracy, T. (1997). Role of the cytochrome P450 3A subfamily in drug interactions. *US Pharmacist, 22,* HS9–HS21.

*Deppermann, K. M., & Lode, H. (1993). Fluoroquinolones: Interaction profile during enteral absorption. *Drugs, 45*(Suppl. 3), 65–72.

Drew, R. H., & Gallis, H. A. (1992). Azithromycin—spectrum of activity, pharmacokinetics, and clinical applications. *Pharmacotherapy, 12,* 161–173.

*FDA Drug Safety Communication: Reduced effectiveness of Plavix (clopidogrel) in patients who are poor metabolizers of the drug. Available at: http://www.fda. gov/Drugs/DrugSafety/PostmarketDrugSafetyInformationforPatientsand Providers/ucm203888.htm. Accessed July 27, 2010.

*FDA Table of Valid Genomic Biomarkers in the Context of Approved Drug Labels. Available at: http://www.fda.gov/Drugs/ScienceResearch/ ResearchAreas/Pharmacogenetics/ucm083378.htm. Accessed July 27, 2010.

Fraser, A. G. (1997). Pharmacokinetic interactions between alcohol and other drugs. *Clinical Pharmacokinetics, 33*(2), 79–90.

*Guengerich, F. (1994). Catalytic selectivity of human cytochrome P450 enzymes: Relevance to drug metabolism and toxicity. *Toxicology Letters, 70,* 133–138.

*Hansten, P. D. (1998). Understanding drug–drug interactions. *Science and Medicine* (Jan/Feb), 16–20.

*Hansten, P. D., & Horn, J. R. (1997). *Drug interactions: Analysis and management.* Vancouver, WA: Applied Therapeutics.

*Harder, S., & Thurmann, P. (1996). Clinically important drug interactions with anticoagulants: An update. *Clinical Pharmacokinetics, 30,* 416–444.

*Herb Fact Sheet. (2006). National Toxicology Program. Available at: http:// ntp.niehs.nih.gov/ntp/Factsheets/HerbalFacts06.pdf. Accessed July 24, 2010.

*Highlights of Prescribing Information: Ziagen (abacavir sulfate) Tablets and Oral Solution. Available at: http://www.accessdata.fda.gov/drug-satfda_docs/label/2008/020977s019,020978s022lbl.pdf. Accessed July 27, 2010.

*Holmes, D. R., Dehmer, G. J., Kaul, S., et al. (2010). ACCF/AHA clopidogrel clinical alert: Approaches to the FDA "Boxed Warning": A report of the American College of Cardiology Foundation Task Force on Clinical Expert Consensus Documents and the American Heart Association. *Journal of the American College of Cardiology, 56,* 321–341.

*Horn, J.R., Hansten P.D. (2004). Drug interactions with digoxin: The role of P-glycoprotein. *Pharmacy Times* (October), available at: http://www. hanstenandhorn.com/hh-article10-04.pdf.

*Huang, S. M., Hall, S. D., Watkins P., et al. (2004). Drug interactions with herbal products and grapefruit juice: A conference report. *Clinical Pharmacology and Therapeutics, 75,* 1–12.

*Hunt, S. A., Abraham, W. T., Chin, M.H., et al. (2009). 2009 focused update incorporated into the ACC/AHA 2005 guidelines for the diagnosis and management of heart failure in adults. *Circulation, 119,* e391–e479.

*Hussar, D. A. (1995). Drug interactions. *American Journal of Pharmacy, 167,* 1–39.

*Impicciatore P., Choonara I., Clarkson A., et al. (2001). Incidence of adverse drug reactions in paediatric in/out-patients: A systematic review and meta-analysis of prospective studies. *British Journal of Clinical Pharmacology, 52,* 77–83.

*Ingelman-Sundberg, M. (2004). Pharmacogenetics of cytochromes P450 and its applications in drug therapy; the past, present and future. *Trends in Pharmacological Sciences, 25*(4), 193–200.

*Izzo, A. A., & Ernst, E. (2009). Interactions between herbal medicines and prescribed drugs: An updated systematic review. *Drugs, 69,* 1777–1798.

*Jahnchen, E., Meinertz, T., Gilfrich, H.-J., et al. (1978). Enhanced elimination of warfarin during treatment with cholestyramine. *British Journal of Clinical Pharmacology, 5,* 437–440.

*Jang, G. R., & Harris, R. Z. (2007). Drug interactions involving ethanol and alcoholic beverages. *Expert Opinion on Drug Metabolism and Toxicology, 3,* 719–731.

*Jing, M., Rayner, C. K., Jones, K. L., & Horowitz, M. (2009). Diabetic gastroparesis diagnosis and management. *Drugs, 69,* 971–986.

Johnson, K. A., Strum, D. P., & Watkins, W. D. (1995). Pharmacology and the critical care patient. In P. L. Munson, R. A. Mueller, & G. R. Breese (Eds.), *Principles of pharmacology: Basic concepts and clinical application* (pp. 1673–1688). New York, NY: Chapman & Hall.

*Jonkman, J. H. (1989). Food interactions with sustained-release theophylline preparations: A review. *Clinical Pharmacokinetics, 16,* 162–179.

*Kim, R. B. (2002). Drugs as P-glycoprotein substrates, inhibitors, and inducers. *Drug Metabolism Reviews, 34,* 47–54.

*Kirk, J. K. (1995). Significant drug-nutrient interactions. *American Family Physicians, 51*(5), 1175–1182.

*Kivisto, K., Neuvonen, P., & Koltz, U. (1994). Inhibition of terfenadine metabolism: Pharmacokinetic and pharmacodynamic consequences. *Clinical Pharmacokinetics, 27,* 1–5.

*Kuhn, M.A. (2002). Herbal remedies: Drug-herb interactions. *Critical Care Nurse, 22,* 22–32.

*Lazarou, J., Pomeranz, B., & Corey, P. (1998). Incidence of adverse drug reactions in hospitalized patients: A meta-analysis of prospective studies. *Journal of the American Medical Association, 279,* 1200–1205.

*Lindblad, C. I., Hanlon, J. T., Gross, C. R., et al. (2006). Clinically important drug-disease interactions and their prevalence in older adults. *Clinical Therapeutics, 28,* 1133–1143.

*Lovastatin (Mevacor®) prescribing information. Available at: http://www. merck.com/product/usa/pi_circulars/m/mevacor/mevacor_pi.pdf. Accessed July 30, 2010.

*Mancano, M. A. (2005). Clinically significant drug interactions with warfarin. *Pharmacy Times.* Available at: https://secure.pharmacytimes.com/ lessons/200301-01.asp. Accessed July 27, 2010.

*Mathews, D., McNutt, B., Okerholam, R., et al. (1991). Torsades de pointes occurring in association with terfenadine use. *Journal of the American Medical Association, 266,* 2375–2376.

*May, R. J. (1993). Adverse drug reactions and interactions. In J. T. DiPiro, R. L. Talbert, P. E. Hayes, et al. (Eds.), *Pharmacotherapy: A pathophysiologic approach* (2nd ed., pp. 71–83). East Norwalk, CT: Appleton & Lange.

*The Medical Letter (2009). In brief: Tamoxifen and SSRI interactions. *The Medical Letter on Drugs and Therapeutics, 51,* 45.

*Michalets, E. (1998). Update: Clinically significant cytochrome P-450 drug interactions. *Annals of Pharmacotherapy, 18,* 84–112.

*National Center for Health Statistics. (1996). *Vital and health statistics.* Series 13, No. 134 (FASTATS A to Z). [On-line; information updated 5/18/1999; retrieved 10/7/1999]. Available: http://www.cdc.gov/nch-swww/gastats/hospital.htm.

*Nebert, D., Adesnich, M., Coon, M., et al. (1987). The P450 gene superfamily: Recommended nomenclature. *DNA, 6,* 1–11.

*Olivier, P., Bertrand, L., Tubery, M., et al. (2009). Hospitalizations because of adverse drug reactions in elderly patients admitted through the emergency department: A prospective survey. *Drugs and Aging, 26,* 475–482.

*Plaa, G. L., & Smith, R. P. (1995). General principles of toxicology. In P. L. Munson, R. A. Mueller, & G. R. Breese (Eds.), *Principles of pharmacology: Basic concepts and clinical application* (pp. 1537–1543). New York, NY: Chapman & Hall.

*Rashid, J., McKinstry, C., Renwick, A. G., et al. (1993). Quercetin, an in vitro inhibitor of CYP3A, does not contribute to the interaction between nifedipine and grapefruit juice. *British Journal of Clinical Pharmacology, 36,* 460–463.

*Rolan, P. (1994). Plasma protein binding displacement interactions: Why are they still regarded as clinically important? *British Journal of Clinical Pharmacology, 37,* 125–128.

*Schein, J. R. (1995). Cigarette smoking and clinically significant drug interactions. *Annals of Pharmacotherapy, 29,* 1139–1147.

*Shargel, L., & Yu, A. B. C. (1993). *Applied biopharmaceutics and pharmacokinetics* (3rd ed.). East Norwalk, CT: Appleton & Lange.

*Shinn, A. F. (1992). Clinical relevance of cimetidine drug interactions. *Drug Safety, 7,* 245–267.

*Simvastatin (Zocor®) prescribing information. Available at: http://www.merck.com/product/usa/pi_circulars/z/zocor/zocor_pi.pdf. Accessed July 29, 2010.

*Spinler, S., Cheng, J., Kindwall, K., & Charland, S. (1995). Possible inhibition of hepatic metabolism of quinidine by erythromycin. *Clinical Pharmacology and Therapeutics, 57,* 89–94.

*Susla, G. M. (2005). Miscellaneous antibiotics. In S.C. Piscitelli, K.A. Rodvold (Eds.), *Drug interactions in infectious diseases* (2nd ed., pp. 358–359). Totowa, NJ: Humana Press, Inc.

*Tegretol (carbamazepine USP) Label. Available at: http://www.accessdata.fda.gov/drugsatfda_docs/label/2009/016608s101,018281s048lbl.pdf. Accessed July 27, 2010.

*Trovato, A., Nuhlicek, D. N., & Midtling, J. E. (1991). Drug–nutrient interactions. *American Family Practitioner, 44,* 1651–1658.

*Ulbricht, C., Chao, W., Costa, D., et al. (2008). Clinical evidence of herb-drug interactions: A systematic review by the Natural Standard Research Collaboration. *Current Drug Metabolism, 9,* 1063–1120.

*Weaver, K. & Glasier, A. (1999). Interaction between broad-spectrum antibiotics and the combined oral contraceptive pill: A literature review. *Contraception, 59,* 71–78.

*Woosley, R. (1996). Cardiac actions of antihistamines. *Annual Review of Pharmacology and Toxicology, 36,* 233–252.

*Xie, H. G., Kim, R. B., Wood, A. J., et al. (2001). Molecular basis of ethnic differences in drug disposition and response. *Annual Review of Pharmacology and Toxicology, 41,* 815–50.

CHAPTER 4

Anita Siu
Jim Thigpen

Principles of Pharmacotherapy in Pediatrics

When treating pediatric patients, many health care practitioners use the terms *infant*, *child*, or even *kid* interchangeably. However, there are currently accepted terms that define the different age categories of pediatric patients (**Table 4.1**). These terms should be used for accuracy when describing young patients and especially when determining drug dosages. Safe and effective drug therapy in pediatric patients is based on a firm understanding of three concepts:

- Ongoing maturation and development in pediatric patients and their effect on a drug's absorption, distribution, metabolism, and excretion. Interpatient variabilities may be attributed to physiologic changes throughout childhood.
- Short- and long-term effects that the prescribed drug will have on a pediatric patient's growth and development
- Effects of underlying congenital, chronic, or current diseases on the prescribed drug, and vice versa

The popular concept that the pediatric patient is merely a "little or small adult," and therefore pediatric pharmacokinetics, drug dosing, and even adverse effects can be extrapolated from the results of adult clinical drug trials is a serious misconception. Although many drugs do exhibit similarities between the adult and pediatric populations, the assumption of resemblance should not be applied to all drugs. Several tragic drug misadventures in the 1960s and 1970s illustrate this. Extrapolated data from adult responses to chloramphenicol (Chloromycetin) led to its use in neonates in the 1960s. When given chloramphenicol, these neonates developed gray baby syndrome, hypotension, and hypoxemia, leading eventually to shock and death (Haile, 1977). This occurred because neonates, unlike adults, lack the enzyme needed to metabolize chloramphenicol. Another tragedy in the 1970s involved the topical antimicrobial cleanser hexachlorophene. Used routinely and safely in adults, hexachlorophene caused vacuolar encephalopathy of the brain stem in premature neonates after they were repeatedly bathed in a 3% solution (Anonymous, 1972).

The well-grounded fears that unforeseen adverse events may affect the growth or development of or may produce fatal outcomes in pediatric study subjects, combined with the difficulties associated with obtaining informed consent or blood samples, serve as major barriers to pharmaceutical manufacturers in conducting pediatric clinical trials. In turn, the lack of clinical trials in pediatric patients prevents the U.S. Food and Drug Administration (FDA) from approving drugs for use in the pediatric population. As such, the prescribing information commonly states "Pediatric Use: Safety and effectiveness in pediatric patients has not been established."

Without FDA approval or adequate documented information, many practitioners are uncertain how to use drugs in pediatrics. This leaves prescribers little choice but to use drugs in pediatric patients in an off-label capacity, based on adult data, uncontrolled pediatric studies, or personal experience. In 1997, the FDA took the initiative to increase the quantity and quality of clinical drug trials in the pediatric population by proposing alternate ways to obtain FDA approval. The FDA would waive the need for well-controlled clinical drug trials if drug manufacturers provided other satisfactory data for drugs already approved for the same use in adults. These data could include the results of controlled or uncontrolled pediatric studies, pharmacodynamic studies, safety reports, and premarketing or postmarketing studies. Alternatively, the drug manufacturer could provide evidence demonstrating that the disease course and drug effects are sufficiently similar in adult and pediatric patients in order to support extrapolation of data from adult clinical trials. In addition, pediatric pharmacokinetic studies are necessary to provide data for an appropriate pediatric dosage recommendation, especially age-dependent dosing. An FDA regulation issued in December 1998 required manufacturers to provide additional information about the use of their drug products in pediatric patients. The nature of the studies required to support pediatric labeling will depend on the type of application, the condition being treated, and existing data about the product's safety and efficacy in pediatric patients. Manufacturers will be required to study the drug in all relevant pediatric age groups (U.S. FDA, 1998a). Over the years, the FDA has encouraged more well controlled trials on drug efficacy and safety in pediatrics. The FDA Modernization Act of 1997 and the Best Pharmaceuticals for Children Act of 2002 offered support for the pharmaceutical industries to conduct and submit pediatric clinical trials. The Pediatric Research Equity Act of 2003 mandated that drugs used in pediatrics require literature or clinical trials supporting their use. As a result, pediatric pharmacotherapy will evolve with additional clinical trials.

TABLE 4.1	Age Groups of Pediatric Population
Group	**Age**
Preterm or premature	<36 weeks gestational age
Neonate	<30 days old
Infant	Age 1 month until 1 year old
Child	Age 1 until 12 years old
Adolescent	Age 12 until 18 years old

PEDIATRIC PHARMACOKINETICS

Pediatric patients differ from adults, anatomically and physiologically. For safe use of drugs in pediatrics, prescribers and other caregivers need to recognize the potential for very different pharmacokinetics in pediatric patients as opposed to adults. The differences are based on developing body tissues and organs, which affect a drug's absorption, distribution, metabolism, and excretion.

Changes in a pediatric patient's body proportions and composition and the relative size of the liver and kidneys can alter the pharmacokinetics of a drug. During the first several years of life, a child undergoes rapid changes in growth and development, most rapid during infancy. Growth is a quantitative change in the size of the body or any of its parts, and development is a qualitative change in skills or functions. Maturation, a genetically controlled development independent of the environment, is a slower process, lasting until late childhood. **Table 4.2** summarizes pharmacokinetic differences in pediatric patients.

By the end of the first year of life, an infant's weight triples, whereas body surface area (BSA) and length double.

Accompanying these changes in growth and development are changes in body composition, intracellular and extracellular body water, fat, and protein. Approximately 75% to 80% of a full-term neonate's body weight is total body water (Friis-Hansen, 1957). By age 3 months, total body water constitutes approximately 65% of the patient's body weight. Extracellular water progressively declines and intracellular water increases faster than total body water, exceeding extracellular water (Friis-Hansen, 1957). The decreasing percentage of body weight from total body water is replaced by an increase in body fat during the first 5 months of life. In fact, the percentage of body weight from fat doubles in these 5 months. The protein percentage increases during the second year of life as fat is lost, primarily because of ambulation. The liver and kidney reach their maximum size relative to body weight by age 2, producing a "peak" in the child's metabolism and elimination. After age 2, the child's liver and kidney size/body weight ratios steadily decrease until adult liver and kidney ratios are reached by adolescence.

Oral Absorption

The extent of a drug's absorption in a pediatric patient depends on a variety of factors: gastric pH, gastric and intestinal transit time, gastrointestinal surface area, enzymes, and microorganism flora, or any combination thereof.

Gastric pH

Basal and stimulated secretion of gastric acid controls the pH of the stomach. The stomach pH is alkaline at birth (>4) because of residual amniotic fluid and the immaturity of parietal cells. As gastric acid is produced, the pH falls. By the end of the first day of life, the basal and stimulated rates are equal, although lower than the rates in adults. An increased stomach

TABLE 4.2	Age-Related Pharmacokinetic Differences in Children Compared with Adults				
	Premature Neonate	**Neonate**	**Infant**	**Child**	**Adolescent**
Absorption					
Gastric acidity	↓	↓	↓	=	=
Gastric emptying time	↓	↓	=	=	=
GI motility	↓	↓	↓	=	=
Pancreatic enzyme activity	↓↓	↓	↓	=	=
GI surface area	↑	↑	↑	↑	=
Skin permeability	↑↑	↑	=	=	=
Distribution					
Body composition					=
Blood-brain barrier	↓	↓	=	=	=
Plasma proteins	↓↓	↓	=	=	=
Metabolism					
Liver	↓	↓	↓	=/↑	=
Elimination					
Renal blood flow	↓	↓	↓	=	=
Glomerular filtration	↓	↓	↓	=	=
Tubular function	↓	↓	↓	=	=

pH (alkaline) adversely affects the absorption of weakly acidic drugs and improves the absorption of weakly basic drugs. This phenomenon results from increased ionization of the weakly acidic drug, producing more ionized (polar) drug, which moves poorly across the nonpolar gastric membrane—and vice versa for weakly basic drug. For example, the bioavailability of phenobarbital (a weak acid) is decreased in neonates, infants, and young children because their alkaline gastric pH produces more ionized phenobarbital, which crosses the gastric membrane poorly.

For weakly basic drugs, the alkaline stomach pH increases the non-ionized form of the drug, which then easily moves across the gastric membrane. By the second year of life, the child's gastric acid output on a per-kilogram body weight basis is similar to that observed in the adult (Deren, 1971). As a result, gastric pH affects the degree of drug ionization, thus changing the amount of drug absorbed.

Gastric Emptying Time and Surface Area

The gastric emptying time is delayed in both preterm and full-term neonates during the first 24 hours of life. No studies have been conducted beyond the immediate neonatal period. The combination of delayed gastric emptying time and gastroesophageal reflux can result in the regurgitation of orally administered drugs, producing irregular drug absorption. In general, gastric emptying is more prolonged in neonates and infants than in children.

The characteristics of a drug's movement through the intestines can drastically affect the rate and extent of drug absorption because most drugs are absorbed in the duodenum. Both neonates and infants have irregular peristalsis, which can lead to enhanced absorption. In addition, the type of feeding an infant receives can affect intestinal transit time. For instance, the intestinal transit time in breast-fed infants is greater than in formula-fed infants (Cavell, 1981).

The relative size of the absorptive surface area in the duodenum can significantly influence the rate and extent of drug absorption. In the young, the greater relative size of the duodenum compared with adults enhances drug absorption.

Gastrointestinal Enzymes and Microorganisms

The absorption of drugs that are fat soluble or carried in fat vehicles depends on lipase. Premature neonates have low lipase concentrations and no alpha-amylase. The reduced activity of bile acids, lipase, alpha-amylase, and protease continues until approximately age 4 months. Vitamin E absorption is decreased in neonates because of the diminished bile acid pool and biliary function; therefore, supplementation of this vitamin may be necessary.

The development of the intestinal microorganism flora depends more on diet than on age (Yaffe & Juchau, 1974), which may account for the more rapid development of flora in breast-fed infants than in formula-fed infants. The reduction of digoxin (Lanoxin) to inactive metabolites by anaerobic intestinal bacteria can be used as a marker for the development or changes in intestinal flora (Lindenbaum, et al., 1981). Digoxin metabolites are not detected in children until 16 months, and an adult-like reduction of digoxin does not occur until age 9 (Linday, et al., 1987).

Rectal Absorption

The rectal route of administration is seldom used; it usually is reserved for patients who cannot tolerate oral drugs or who lack intravenous access. In rectal administration, the drug is absorbed by the hemorrhoidal veins, which are not part of the portal circulation, therefore avoiding first-pass hepatic elimination. Unfortunately, most drugs administered by this route are erratically and incompletely absorbed. Feces in the rectum, frequent bowel movements in neonates and infants, and lack of anal sphincter muscle contribute to the poor absorption profile of drugs administered rectally.

Although rectal administration may not be appropriate for routine dosing of drugs, the rectal administration of diazepam (Valium), valproic acid (Depakote), or secobarbital (Seconal) has been used to control seizures when intravenous access could not be quickly established in infants or children with status epilepticus (Graves & Kriel, 1987).

Intramuscular and Subcutaneous Absorption

Both the characteristics of the patient and the properties of the drug influence the absorption of intramuscularly or subcutaneously administered drugs. Patient characteristics include blood flow to the muscle, muscle mass, tone, and activity. Important properties of the drug are its solubility, the pH of extracellular fluid, its ease in crossing capillary membranes, and the amount of drug administered at the injection site.

In pediatric patients, all the patient characteristics are highly variable. Neonates have decreased muscle mass, and their limited muscle activity decreases blood flow to and from the muscle. Collectively, these factors produce erratic and poor intramuscular drug absorption. On the contrary, infants possess a greater density of skeletal muscle capillaries than older children, allowing for more efficient drug absorption (Carry, et al., 1986). Some drugs, such as erythromycin, can cause pain at the injection site and should not be administered intramuscularly. However, many drugs, such as the penicillins, reach concentrations in the serum with intramuscular administration that are comparable with those achieved after intravenous administration, with minimal adverse effects.

Percutaneous Absorption

Adverse effects resulting from the inadvertent systemic absorption of percutaneously administered hexachlorophene emulsion, salicylic acid ointment, and hydrocortisone creams in neonates have limited the use of this route of drug administration. The absorption of compounds is inversely related to the thickness of the stratum corneum and directly related to hydration of the skin (Morselli, et al., 1980). Relative to body mass, the BSA is greatest in the infant and young child compared with older children and adults. The decreased thickness of the skin with increased skin surface hydration relative to body weight produces much greater percutaneous drug absorption in neonates than in adults. The percutaneous administration of drugs in neonates does pose some risks of toxic effects. Neonatal skin is structurally immature, resulting in less subcutaneous fat and a thinner stratum corneum and epidermis (Rutter, 1987). Since a greater skin surface area/body weight ratio is observed during the neonatal period, percutaneous drug absorption is also superior. Both the advantages and subsequent disadvantages of enhanced percutaneous absorption disappear after infancy, however.

Pulmonary Absorption

Aerosolized drug delivery to the lungs continues to be a favorite technique in many respiratory disorders, such as asthma. Factors affecting drug deposition in the lungs include particle size, lipid solubility, protein binding, drug metabolism in the lungs, and mucociliary transport (American Academy of Pediatrics, 1997). Aerosol particle size and lipid solubility are factors in determining whether the drug is deposited in the upper or lower airways; smaller particle size and lipid-soluble drugs are more likely to be absorbed and deposited in the lower airways (Bond, 1993).

Besides drug considerations, pediatric characteristics also affect aerosol drug delivery. Infants and children have lower tidal volumes and increased respiratory rates (especially while crying), reducing drug delivery and absorption in the lungs (Dolovich, 1999). Studies have shown that less than 2% of aerosolized drugs are deposited in young infants and toddlers (Fok, et al., 1996; Salmon, et al., 1990). Therefore, adult dosing may be necessary to counteract these effects.

Distribution

Six factors affect drug distribution in the pediatric population: vascular perfusion, body composition, tissue-binding characteristics, physicochemical properties of the drug, plasma protein binding, and route of administration (Stewart & Hampton, 1987). During the neonatal period, most of these factors are significantly different from those in the adult population, while children and adolescents are very similar to or the same as adults.

Vascular Perfusion

Changes in vascular perfusion are common in neonates. For example, in neonatal respiratory distress syndrome and post-asphyxia, a right-to-left vascular shunt may occur and divert blood from the lungs to the tissues and organs.

Body Composition

Neonates have increased total body water (75% to 80%) with decreased fat compared with adults, resulting in a higher water-to-lipid ratio. After the neonatal period, fat increases and total body water decreases steadily until puberty, especially in girls.

For instance, neonates and infants have increased total body and extracellular water, creating a larger volume of distribution and affecting the pharmacokinetics of some drugs, such as aminoglycoside. The larger volume, in turn, requires administering a larger milligram-per-kilogram dose of aminoglycoside to neonates and infants than to adults.

Tissue-Binding Characteristics

The mass of tissue available for binding can affect drug distribution. Drugs extensively bound to tissues exhibit increased "free" blood levels when the mass of tissue is reduced by disease or degeneration or immaturity, as in pediatrics.

Physicochemical Properties

The physicochemical properties of a drug include lipid solubility (ionized vs. non-ionized) and molecular configuration. These properties affect the ability of a drug to move across membranes into target cells or tissues. Drugs that display favorable properties for absorption may pose a greater risk for toxicity in neonates, who have enhanced percutaneous drug absorption.

Plasma Protein Binding

Preterm neonates have lower circulating amounts of alpha$_1$-acid glycoprotein, which binds alkaline drugs, than full-term neonates, who have lower alpha$_1$-acid glycoprotein levels than adults. Neonates also have a reduced amount of circulating albumin compared with adults. Albumin is responsible for binding acidic drugs, fatty acids, and bilirubin. While the affinity of drugs for either of these plasma proteins is harder to determine, theoretically a neonate's affinity for protein binding is reduced, resulting in the likelihood of displacing drugs or bilirubin bound to albumin and leading to increased serum concentrations. All these factors produce a larger volume of distribution and increased free drug concentrations (e.g., phenytoin [Dilantin]) in neonates than in adults.

Route of Administration

The route by which a drug is administered has a primary influence on the drug's distribution. If the drug is administered orally, the liver becomes the primary distribution site. However, if a drug is administered intravenously, the heart and lungs act as the primary distribution sites. This is important because when a drug passes through the liver before reaching its site of activity, it is subject to the first-pass effect of extensive hepatic metabolism, which typically reduces the amount of circulating active drug and thus limits its effects. Therefore, to achieve an equal effect, the dosage of a drug administered by the oral route usually needs to be higher than the dosage of a drug administered intravenously.

Metabolism

Clearance of many drugs is mainly reliant on hepatic metabolism. The two phases of drug metabolism in the liver are the oxidation, reduction, and hydrolysis reactions (phase I) and conjugation reactions (phase II). Age-related changes in

TABLE 4.3	Summary of Age-Related Changes in Metabolism		
P450 Cytochromes	**Reduced Activity Versus Adults**	**Increased Activity Versus Adults**	**Age at Which Adult Activity Is Reached**
CYP1A2	Until age 4 months	1–2 years old	End of puberty
CYP2C19			
CYP2C9	First week of life	3–4 years old	End of puberty
CYP2D6	Until age 3–5		3–5 years old
CYP2E1	Unknown	Unknown	Unknown
CYP3A4	First month of life	1–4 years ol3d	End of puberty

Based on data from Leader, J. S., & Kearns, G. L. (1997). Pharmacogenetics in pediatrics: Implications for practice. *Pediatric Clinics of North America, 44,* 55–77.

metabolism affect how drugs are broken down or transformed in pediatric patients and how certain metabolic enzymes are activated (**Table 4.3** summarizes developmental patterns in phase I oxidation reactions). Phase I and II reactions are delayed in neonates, infants, and young children, with consequential drug toxicities.

The P450 cytochrome (CYP) is the most important component of phase I drug metabolism. Cytochromes in the CYP1, CYP2, and CYP3 families have been identified as important in human drug metabolism. Additional information suggests there is substantial genetic variability in the quantity and quality of CYP in the human body (Kearns, 1995).

The metabolism of caffeine and theophylline, the prototypic substrate for CYP1A2, is reduced at birth; the drug concentration increases linearly over the first year of life and exceeds adult levels in older infants and children. To maintain therapeutic serum theophylline concentrations, smaller doses are prescribed and administered less frequently in neonates than in older infants and children.

In pediatrics, phase II reactions are less well studied than phase I reactions. In adults, acetaminophen (Tylenol) (a substrate for glucuronosyltransferase 1A6 and 1A9) is metabolized by a phase II glucuronidation reaction. In neonates and infants, however, this metabolic pathway is deficient. As a result, acetaminophen metabolism is shifted to sulfate conjugation, which results in a half-life for acetaminophen that is similar to its half-life in adults.

Elimination

Almost all drugs and their metabolites are excreted through the kidneys. The kidney eliminates drugs by glomerular filtration (passive diffusion) or tubular secretion (energy-dependent channels or pumps). The glomerular filtration rate (GFR) increases quickly during the first 2 weeks of postnatal life and does not approach adult rates until age 2 (Rubin, et al., 1949); tubular secretion and reabsorption rates do not reach adult values until age 5 to 7 months. The proximal tubules are characterized by an inability to concentrate urine or reabsorb various filtered compounds and a reduced ability to secrete organic acids. This immaturity of the renal system in neonates and infants results from restricted blood flow and a resultant decrease in cardiac

output to the kidneys, combined with incomplete glomerular and tubular development. As a result, plasma clearance of many drugs via the kidneys is altered. For example, during infancy the response to thiazide diuretics, which require a GFR greater than 30 mL/minute to be effective, is diminished. Often, a larger dosage of a thiazide diuretic or substitution by a loop diuretic is required to produce adequate diuresis. Because the elimination of aminoglycosides is directly related to the GFR, aminoglycosides have a longer half-life in neonates and infants, thus requiring a longer dosing interval than in adults. In addition, decreased tubular secretion in neonates and infants can lengthen the elimination half-life of other antibiotics, such as the penicillins and sulfonamides. Selecting the appropriate dosing regimen based on age, weight, and kidney maturation and identifying concomitant agents renally eliminated are important factors to prevent toxicity. In general, renal excretion of many drugs is directly proportional to age.

DRUG SELECTION

Various factors are considered when prescribing a drug for a pediatric patient. Among them are the benefits of the drug in relation to the risks of administration, the long-term effects, the dosage form, and the route and frequency of administration (**Figure 4-1**).

Risks and Benefits

The classic medication when discussing risks and benefits in the pediatric population is ciprofloxacin (Cipro®). Ciprofloxacin was brought to market in 1987 and carried a risk of severe degenerative arthropathy. This effect was seen in juvenile study animals during drug development. The potential for this problem led to these drugs being contraindicated in all pediatric populations. Numerous studies over the past 20 years disputing this risk has led to over 500,000 prescriptions for the drug being written annually for children younger than age 18. The American Academy of Pediatrics developed a policy statement that provides an outline for the use of ciprofloxacin/fluoroquinolones in children (American Academy of Pediatrics, 2006). The use of the drug class in children is driven more by

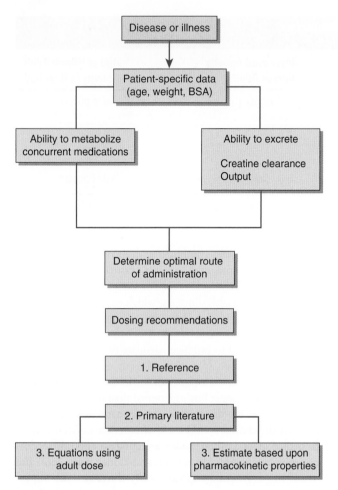

FIGURE 4–1 Approach to prescribing drug therapy for the pediatric patient.

resistance patterns in pathogens covered by the class than the potential risk of arthropathy to the patient.

Cardiovascular safety and adverse psychiatric effects are a concern with the use of psychostimulants in the treatment of attention-deficit hyperactivity disorder (ADHD). A very small number of case reports of sudden cardiac death have been reported in children prescribed psychostimulants for ADHD. The risk has been found to be greater in patients with underlying cardiac structural abnormalities. However, the risk is similar to that of strenuous exercise in this population, and the use in the general population does not necessitate additional testing beyond normal screening (Wilens, et al., 2006). There is also a small risk of psychosis and mania-type reactions in children. As a result, the FDA requires the pharmaceutical industry to provide medication guides to patients and prescribers explaining the risks of ADHD drug treatments and information on their potential side effects (Mosholder, et al., 2009).

Another widely used drug class with specific safety concerns in the pediatric population is antidepressants. There is a very slight increase in suicide risk in patients started on antidepressants, which likely reflects the current depressed state and other comorbidities (Schneeweiss, et al., 2010). The FDA has included a black box warning for increased suicidality for children and adolescents initiating all classes of antidepressants. Although this is a statistically significant increased risk compared to the normal population, the risk of suicide in untreated depressed patients is much higher.

Long-Term Effects

Drugs administered to pediatric patients may take a longer time to produce adverse effects than in adults. Certain adverse effects may not be detected until decades after treatment. For example, secondary cancers, growth retardation, hypogonadism, and sterility have all been reported as late adverse effects associated with certain antineoplastic therapies. Inhaled and intranasal corticosteroids may decrease growth velocity, which is a means of comparing growth rates among children of the same age. Studies with inhaled steroids showed approximately a 1-cm/year reduction in growth velocity. The FDA suggests that the reduction is related to dose and how long the child takes the drug (U.S. FDA, 1998b). More recently, Lone & Pederson (2000) evaluated the long-term effect on growth of inhaled or intranasal budesonide in pediatric asthma patients. At the end of this 10-year study, the researchers concluded that normal adult height was achieved in patients receiving these corticosteroids.

Potential long-term effects of medications used in children create a concern. The 5-year survival rates of most pediatric malignancies is approaching 80%. This has led to a focus on the late effects of therapy and the quality of life in this growing population of childhood cancer survivors (Shankar, et al., 2008). Nearly two-thirds of all childhood cancer survivors will experience some physical or psychological outcome that develops or persists beyond 5 years from the initial diagnosis (Shankar, et al., 2008). Other medications used in pediatrics may also carry risks for long-term effects. Unfortunately, these effects may not be seen for years after the medication is stopped, and there are likely other factors that could cause or at least contribute to the effect. Studies that evaluate the long-term effect of a medication are very difficult to perform and often yield conflicting results.

Dosage Formulation

Commercially available dosage formulations often limit the drugs that can be prescribed to children and are not always child friendly. Many drugs are available only as an oral tablet, capsule, or intravenous dilution in adult dosage strengths. Prescribing a drug as a tablet or capsule for a pediatric patient has several drawbacks. He or she may have difficulty swallowing a whole or intact tablet or capsule, and attempting to break a tablet into smaller pieces or emptying part of a capsule to provide an appropriate dose leads to questionable accuracy of the administered dose. It is important to provide a dosage form that can be administered easily, accurately, and safely to a pediatric patient. A method to improve administration is via extemporaneous formulations, especially if a product is not commercially available as an elixir, solution, suspension, or syrup. However, these oral liquid formulations also have drawbacks such as an unfavorable taste. Other alternatives to oral liquid formulations include tablet dispersion, powdered papers, and repacked capsules. Combination products are available to reduce pill burden and improve medication adherence. However, these agents contain fixed dosage forms in tablets or capsules, making it difficult for a child less than age 5 to swallow.

Ideally, a practitioner who is prescribing a dosage formulation not commercially available for a pediatric patient ought to work with a pharmacist who is willing and able to compound accurate pediatric drug dosages and formulas. Practitioners can familiarize themselves with additional drugs that can be extemporaneously compounded for use in pediatrics by a pharmacist in such publications as *Handbook on Extemporaneous Formulations* (Dice & Zenk, 1987); *Pediatric Drug Formulations* (Nahata & Hipple, 2003); *Teddy Bear Book: Pediatric Injectable Drugs* (Phelps, 2010); *Pediatric Dosage Handbook* (Taketomo, et al., 2010); *Extemporaneous Formulations for Pediatric, Geriatric, and Special Needs Patients* (Jew, et al., 2010), or *Trissel's Stability of Compounding Formulations* (Trissel, 2008). A Medline search should be conducted for drugs not contained in these publications.

Dosage

In adult drug therapy, one standard dose of a drug can be used for almost all adults, but the opposite is true in pediatric drug therapy: a pediatric drug dose changes for different illnesses or as the patient grows or develops and requires age-dependent adjustments.

When writing or assessing a pediatric medication order, the following process is recommended to ensure safe and effective pharmaceutical care.

1. Determine the patient type (i.e., neonate, pediatric, adolescent).
2. Assess the appropriateness of the drug therapy selected in this patient type, patient population, and/or disease state.
3. Establish the appropriate dose, route, formulation, and frequency based on the recommended references mentioned below.
4. If all resources have been exhausted or further information is needed regarding the pediatric dosage, contact a pharmacist. It is important to ensure that the dose is appropriate or reasonable based on his or her knowledge of pediatric pharmacokinetics and available resources.

Many drugs currently in use in pediatrics have established dosing recommendations based on body weight, BSA, concurrent drug therapy, and stage of development or physiologic function (age). Body weight–based dosing is the most common method for pediatric dosing. A total daily dose, milligrams per kilogram per day (mg/kg/day), is divided by the dosing interval to calculate each individual dose. Analgesics, antipyretics, and emergency drugs are often administered on a dose-by-dose method; as such, the recommended pediatric dose is reported as milligrams per kilogram per dose (mg/kg/dose). The starting or maximum doses for pediatric intravenous infusions are usually reported as micrograms per kilogram per minute (mcg/kg/minute) or micrograms per kilogram per hour (mcg/kg/hour). Drug dosages based on a patient's BSA are usually reserved for antineoplastic agents or critically ill patients. BSA correlates closely with many factors that influence drug elimination, including cardiac output, respiratory metabolism, blood volume, extracellular water volume, GFR, and renal blood flow. Dosages of several drugs, including docusate (Colace) and montelukast (Singulair), are based on age.

General pediatric drug references such as the *Pediatric Dosage Handbook* (Taketomo, et al., 2010) and Micromedex (DRUGDEX® System, 2010) provide comprehensive drug monographs, including dosage formulations, adverse events, pharmacology, and pharmacokinetics. *The Harriet Lane Handbook* (Custer & Rau, 2008) provides drug monographs based on the Johns Hopkins Hospital formulary and special drug topics. A specialty pediatric reference such as the *Red Book* (Pickering, et al., 2009) covers only antimicrobial agents and vaccines; *Neofax* (PDR Network, 2010) and the *Neonatal Drug Formulary Book 2002* (Bhatt, et al., 2002) provide information about drug dosing in neonates.

Obesity

Obesity, defined in children as a body mass index (BMI) at or above the 95th percentile for age, is considered a public health crisis in the United States (Ogden, et al., 2010). Since 1980, the percentage of school-age children and adolescents that are considered obese has tripled and is approximately 17% (Ogden, et al., 2010). Children with a BMI at or above the 85th percentile are considered "at risk for overweight," and nearly 32% of U.S. children ages 2 to 19 fall into this category (Ogden, et al., 2010). While it is known that there is an overall lack of information on dosing most medications in children, there is far less information on proper medication dosing in the overweight child. Obesity can affect the pharmacokinetics, dosing, half-life, and metabolism of a medication. There is a greater risk of dosing errors in overweight children, specifically for underdosing and overdosing of antimicrobials (Pediatric Pharmacy Advocacy Group, 2010). The Pediatric Pharmacy Advocacy Group recommends that weight-based dosing be utilized for all children less than age 18 and weighing less than 88 lb (40 kg). For children who weigh over 40 kg, weight-based dosing should be used, unless the patient's dose or dose/day exceeds the recommended adult dose for the specific indication (Johnson, et al., 2010).

Routes of Administration

Oral

When prescribing or administering oral drugs for pediatric patients, the caregiver needs to consider not only the drug's flavor and ease of delivery but the frequency of administration, dosage form, and "inactive" ingredients, such as alcohol and sugar. A liquid dosage form is preferred for most pediatric patients.

To ensure the accuracy of each dose administered, the drug should be measured and then administered with an oral syringe or a calibrated drug cup, with the base of the meniscus viewed at eye level. If the drug is available only in tablet form, and the tablet can be broken, the tablet may be crushed and mixed in compatible syrup. However, mixing a crushed or whole tablet with food should be done cautiously because many foods interfere with drug absorption.

If the patient is an infant, the head should be raised to prevent aspiration of the drug. Applying gentle downward pressure on the chin with a thumb helps open the patient's mouth. If a syringe is used, the tip of the syringe should be placed in the pocket between the patient's cheek and gum and the drug administered slowly and steadily to reduce the risk of aspiration.

For bottle-fed infants, the drug can be placed in a nipple and the infant allowed to suck the contents. However, a drug should never be mixed with the contents of a baby's bottle because the correct dose will not be received if the infant does not consume the full contents of the bottle. In addition, a drug–nutrient interaction may occur if a drug is mixed with formula. A classic example of a drug–nutrient interaction is the significant reduction of oral phenytoin absorption after concurrent administration with an enteral feeding formula (Sacks & Brown, 1994).

Rectal

Toddlers being toilet trained, especially children experiencing stress or difficulty, often resist the rectal administration of drugs.

Older children may perceive the procedure as an invasion of privacy and may react with embarrassment or anger and hostility. The best approach to reducing anxiety and increasing cooperation is to spend time explaining the procedure and to reassure the child that giving drugs by this route will not hurt. It may be necessary, after placing a suppository, to hold the child's buttocks together for a few minutes to prevent expulsion of the drug.

Parenteral

Establishing venous access, venipuncture for blood samples, and intramuscular injections are a great source of distress and pain for children. Several local anesthetic agents have been developed to help manage the pain and anxiety brought on by these procedures. The ideal product would have needle-free or topical administration, a rapid onset of anesthetic, and no dermal or systemic adverse effects and the product would have no impact on the success rate of the procedure. No commercially available product has all these qualities. The three general delivery methods used to bypass the stratum corneum layer include direct injection of local anesthetics, passive diffusion from topically applied gels or creams, and several needle-free methods that hasten the rate of drug passage through the skin and speed the time to onset of action. **Table 4.4** lists the methods of drug delivery, the available agents, and the advantages and disadvantages of each (Zempsky, 2008).

TABLE 4.4	Topical Anesthetics			
Method	**Product(s)**	**Medication(s)**	**Onset of Topical Anesthesia**	**Adverse Reactions**
Injection of local anesthetics	lidocaine lidocaine buffered with sodium bicarbonate	lidocaine	<1 minute	Pain associated with initial needle stick for injection of medication
Lidocaine needle-free injection	J-Tip®	lidocaine	<1 minute	"Popping noise" with administration (may frighten some children)
Passive diffusion with topical creams or gels	EMLA®, generic	lidocaine 2.5%, prilocaine 2.5%	30 minutes (minimum), 60 minutes for more complete effect	Skin blanching, rare methemoglobinemia in infants
	LMX4®	Liposomal lidocaine 4%	30 minutes	Erythema, blanching
Needle-free strategies to accelerate onset	Synera®	lidocaine/tetracaine	10 minutes	Local reactions (erythema – 71%, blanching, and edema)
Lidocaine iontophoresis	Numby Stuff®	lidocaine	10–15 minutes	Intolerable tingling, itching, burning sensation and discomfort, potential for burn
Lidocaine HCl monohydrate powder intradermal injection system	Zingo®	lidocaine HCl monohydrate	1–3 minutes	Local reactions (erythema – 62%, petechiae – 52.8%) and edema
Vapocoolant sprays	Pain Ease®	Liquid refrigerant (ethyl chloride)	Immediate (may require two providers as effect lasts <1 minute)	Some skin pigmentation changes (temporary)

TABLE 4.5	Recommended Age Groups of Aerosol Delivery Devices
Device	**Age**
Metered-dose inhaler (MDI)	• ≥5 years old • <5 years old (+ spacer or valved holding chamber)
Breath-actuated MDI	• ≥5 years old
Dry powder inhaler	• ≥4 years old
Spacer or valved holding chamber (VHC)	• ≥4 years old • <4 years old (VHC + face mask)
Nebulizer	• Any age

Pulmonary

Nebulizers, metered-dose inhalers (MDIs), and dry powder inhalers (DPIs) can be used to deliver bronchodilators, aminoglycosides, and corticosteroids in the treatment of asthma or cystic fibrosis. Nebulized drugs require connecting an air or oxygen tube to the nebulizer machine and are often used in infants and young children. MDIs require coordination between actuation and inhalation; this is difficult in any age-group, so a tube spacer is recommended for children less than age 5 (National Heart, Lung, and Blood Institute, 2007). Spacer devices have expanded the use of MDIs even to the neonatal population. A DPI such as budesonide powder (Pulmicort Turbohaler) involves coordination with the patient's inspiratory flow; therefore, the delivery mechanism is not recommended in children less than age 4. **Table 4.5** summarizes the recommended population for aerosol delivery devices (National Heart, Lung, and Blood Institute, 2007).

Topical

The topical delivery of medications is common in the pediatric population with diseases such as eczema and acne as well as other skin disorders that appear during childhood. Caution is warranted in this population due to several factors that may lead to a higher rate of drug absorption. When compared to adults, infants and children have a higher ratio of skin surface to body weight. This increases the risk of accumulating significant serum drug levels (Metry & Herbert, 2000). It is especially true in the newborn and infant because the barrier function of their skin is immature. Parents must be cautioned to follow the directions for administration of all topical medications to prevent toxic drug levels. A fatal case of diphenhydramine toxicity was reported in the literature, largely due to excessive application following a bath in a child with eczema (Turner, 2009).

Medication Adherence

The term "medication adherence" is used to describe the extent to which patients take medication as prescribed by their health care providers (Osterberg & Blaschke, 2005). Adherence (or nonadherence) to prescribed therapy is multifactorial and includes simply forgetting, busy lifestyle, complexity of the regimen, taste, education, and motivation, among others. Practitioners must consider these factors when prescribing therapy and must strive to find the balance that will help the patient and family achieve necessary adherence to the prescribed therapy. It is practical to select medications that can be administered once or twice daily because adherence falls dramatically when medications are to be administered more than twice per day (Richter, et al., 2003). Establishing a good relationship with honest communication between the prescriber and the patient/family is an important factor in medication adherence and positive outcomes. Practitioners should always look for poor adherence as a cause of less-than-optimal outcomes. Better adherence can often be achieved by additional education, simplifying the regimen, and customizing the regimen to the patient's/family's lifestyle (Osterberg & Blaschke, 2005).

BOX 4.1

Preventing Pediatric Medication Errors

American Academy of Pediatrics

- Maintain an up-to-date patient allergy profile.
- Confirm the validity of a patient's weight for medications that are dosed by body weight (or body surface area [BSA] for medications dosed by BSA).
- State specific dosage strengths or formulation.
- Do not use abbreviations for drug names or patient instructions.
- Avoid using abbreviations for dosage units.
- Use a zero before a decimal point.
- Avoid a zero after a decimal point.

The Joint Commission

- Standardize concentrations of high alert medications (i.e. heparin, insulin, or narcotics)
- Utilize oral syringes to administer liquid formulations
- Create drug order pathways for protocols
- Collaborate and educate all healthcare members involved with the patients' care
- Use technology such as automated dispensing cabinets, smart infusion pumps, bar-coding

CONCLUSION

In summary, pediatrics poses a unique challenge. The lack of medications approved by the FDA, insufficient literature resources, pharmacokinetic parameters compared to adults, individual drug dosing calculations, lack of dosage forms, and inappropriate drug delivery systems are a few examples (Levine, et al., 2001). Ensuring effective and safe delivery of drugs in pediatrics involves understanding the physiologic changes that occur throughout childhood. Since the start of the Institute for Safe Medication Practices in 1994, pediatric medication safety movements have progressed over time. In 2004, the Institute of Healthcare Improvement (IHI) introduced the 100K Lives Campaign to protect patients from medical harm. Two years later, the IHI launched the 5 Million Lives Campaign with a pediatric initiative to reduce adverse drug events and decrease harm from high alert medications (i.e., anticoagulants, sedatives, opioids, insulin) (IHI, 2006). More recently, the Joint Commission Sentinel Event Alert stated that harm caused by medication errors is three times greater in pediatric patients than adults (The Joint Commission, 2008). As a result, the Joint Commission Issue 39 recommends initiatives to prevent medication errors and suggests risk reduction strategies. **Box 4.1** gives some recommendations to assist health care professionals in reducing medication errors (The Joint Commission, 2008; American Academy of Pediatrics, 2003). In the future, pediatric pharmacotherapy will evolve with additional legislation and safety movements.

BIBLIOGRAPHY

Starred references are cited in the text.
*American Academy of Pediatrics. (1997). Alternative routes of drug administration—advantages and disadvantages (subject review). *Pediatrics, 100,* 143–152.
*American Academy of Pediatrics. (2003). Prevention of medication errors in the pediatric inpatient setting. *Pediatrics, 112,* 431–436.
*American Academy of Pediatrics. (2006). The use of systemic fluoroquinolones. *Pediatrics, 118,* 1287–1292.
*Anonymous. (1972). American Academy of Pediatrics committee on fetus and newborn: Hexachlorophene and skin care of newborn infants. *Pediatrics, 49,* 625–626.
*Bhatt, D. R., Bruggman, D. S., Thayer-Thomas, J. C., et al. (2002). *Neonatal drug formulary 2002* (5th ed.). Fontana, CA: N.D.F. Los Angeles.
*Bond, J. A. (1993). Metabolism and elimination of inhaled drugs and airborne chemicals from the lungs. *Pharmacology and Toxicology, 72,* 23–47.
*Carry, M. R., Ringel, S. P., & Starcevich, J. M. (1986). Distribution of capillaries in normal and diseased human skeletal muscle. *Muscle Nerve, 9,* 445–454.
*Cavell, B. (1981). Gastric emptying in infants fed human milk or infant formula. *Acta Paediatrica Scandinavica, 70,* 639–641.
*Custer, J. W., & Rau, R.E. (2008). *The Harriet Lane handbook* (18th ed.). St. Louis, MO: Mosby–Year Book.
*Deren, J. S. (1971). Development of structure and function of the fetal and newborn intestine. *American Journal of Clinical Nutrition, 24,* 144–159.
*Dice, J. E., & Zenk, K. E. (1987). *Handbook on extemporaneous formulations.* Bethesda, MD: American Society of Hospital Pharmacy.
*Dolovich, M. (1999). Aerosol delivery to children: What to use, how to choose. *Pediatric Pulmonology, 18*(Suppl.), 79–82.

*DRUGDEX® System (electronic version). Thomson Reuters (Healthcare) Inc., Greenwood Village, Colorado, USA. Available at: http://www.thomsonhc.com. Accessed August 16, 2010.
*Fok, T. F., Monkman, S., Dolovich, M., et al. (1996). Efficacy of aerosol medication delivery from a metered-dose inhaler versus jet nebulizer in infants with bronchopulmonary dysphasia. *Pediatric Pulmonology, 21,* 301–309.
*Friis-Hansen, B. (1957). Changes in body water compartment during growth. *Acta Paediatrica, 46*(Suppl. 110), 1–68.
*Graves, N. M., & Kriel, R. L. (1987). Rectal administration of antiepileptic drugs in children. *Pediatric Neurology, 3,* 321–326.
*Haile, C. A. (1977). Chloramphenicol toxicity. *Southern Medical Journal, 70,* 479–480.
*Institute of Healthcare Improvement. (2006). Protecting 5 million lives from harm. Available at: http://www.ihi.org/IHI/Programs/Campaign/Campaign.htm?TabId=1. Accessed August 16, 2010.
*Jew, R. K., Soo-Hoo, W., & Erush, S. C. (2010). *Extemporaneous formulations for pediatric, geriatric, and special needs patients* (2nd ed.). Bethesda, MD: American Society of Hospital Pharmacists.
*Johnson, P. N., Miller, J. L., & Boucher, E. A. (2010). Medication dosing in overweight and obese children. Available at: www.ppag.org/obesedose/. Accessed August 16, 2010.
*The Joint Commission. (2008). Preventing pediatric medication errors. Available at:http://www.jointcommission.org/sentinelevents/sentineleventalert/sea_39.htm. Accessed August 16, 2010.
*Kearns, G. L. (1995). Pharmacogenetics and development: Are infants and children at increased risk for adverse outcomes? *Current Opinion in Pediatrics, 7,* 220–233.
*Levine, S. R., Cohen, M. R., Blanchard, N. R., et al. (2001). Guidelines for preventing medication errors in pediatrics. *Journal of Pediatric Pharmacologic Therapies, 6,* 426–442.
*Linday, L., Dobkin, J. F., Wang, T. C., et al. (1987). Digoxin inactivation by the gut flora in infancy and childhood. *Pediatrics, 79,* 544–548.
*Lindenbaum, J., Rund, D. G., Butler, V. P., et al. (1981). Inactivation of digoxin by gut flora; reversal by antibiotic therapy. *New England Journal of Medicine, 305,* 789–794.
*Lone, A., & Pederson, S. (2000). Effect of long-term treatment with inhaled budesonide on adult height in children with asthma. *New England Journal of Medicine, 343,* 1064–1069.
*Metry, D. W. & Herbert A. A. (2000). Topical therapies and medications in the pediatric patient. *Pediatric Clinics of North America, 47,* 867–876.
*Morselli, P. L., Franco-Morselli, R., & Bossi, L. (1980). Clinical pharmacokinetics in newborns and infants: Age-related differences and therapeutic implications. *Clinical Pharmacokinetics, 5,* 485–527.
*Mosholder, A. D., Gelperin, K., Hammad, T. A., et al. (2009). Hallucinations and other psychotic symptoms associated with the use of attention-deficit/hyperactivity disorder drugs in children. *Pediatrics, 123,* 611–616.
*Nahata, M. C., & Hipple, T. F. (2003). *Pediatric drug formulations* (5th ed.). Cincinnati, OH: Harvey Whitney.
*National Heart, Lung, and Blood Institute. (2007). Expert panel report 3: Guidelines for the diagnosis and the management of asthma. Available at: http://www.nhlbi.nih.gov/guidelines/asthma/. Accessed August 16, 2010.
*Ogden, C. L., Carroll, M. D., Curtin, L. R., et al. (2010). Prevalence of high body mass index in U.S. children and adolescents, 2007–2008. *Journal of the American Medical Association, 303,* 242–249.
*Osterberg, L., & Blaschke, T. (2005). Adherence to medication. *New England Journal of Medicine, 353,* 487–497.
*PDR Network. (2010). *Neofax 2010* (23rd ed.). Montvale, NJ: Thomson Reuters.
*Pediatric Pharmacy Advocacy Group. (2010). Medication dosing in overweight and obese children. Available at: http://www.ppag.org/obesedose/. Accessed August 16, 2010.
*Phelps, S. J. (2010). *Teddy bear book: Pediatric injectable drugs* (9th ed.). Bethesda, MD: American Society of Hospital Pharmacists.
*Pickering, L. K., Baker, C. J., Kimberlin, D. W., & Long, S. S. (2009). *Red Book: 2009 Report of the Committee on Infectious Diseases* (28th ed). Elk Grove Village, IL: American Academy of Pediatrics.

*Richter, A., Anton, S. F., Pierce, C. (2003). A systematic review of the associations between dose regimens and medication compliance. *Clinical Therapeutics, 25,* 2307–2335.

*Rubin, M. I., Bruck, E., & Rapoport, M. J. (1949). Maturation of renal function in childhood: Clearance studies. *Journal of Clinical Investigation, 28,* 1144–1162.

*Rutter, N. (1987). Percutaneous drug absorption in the newborn: Hazards and uses. *Clinical Perinatology, 14,* 911–930.

*Sacks, G. S., & Brown, R. O. (1994). Drug-nutrient interactions in patients receiving nutritional support. *Drug Therapy, 24,* 35–42.

*Salmon, B., Wilson, N. M., & Silverman, M. (1990). How much aerosol reaches the lungs of wheezy infants and toddlers? *Archives of Disease in Childhood, 65,* 401–404.

*Schneeweiss, S., Patrick, A. R., Soloman, D. H., et al. (2010). Comparative safety of antidepressant agents for children and adolescents regarding suicidal acts. *Pediatrics, 125,* 876–888.

*Shankar, S. M., Marina N., Hudson, M. M., et al. (2008). Monitoring for cardiovascular disease in survivors of childhood cancer: Report from the cardiovascular disease task force of the children's oncology group. *Pediatrics, 121,* 387–396.

*Stewart, C. F., & Hampton, E. M. (1987). Effect of maturation on drug disposition in pediatric patients. *Clinical Pharmacy, 6,* 548–564.

*Taketomo, C. K., Hodding, J. H., & Kraus, D. M. (2010). *Pediatric dosage handbook* (17th ed.). Hudson, OH: Lexi-Comp.

*Trissel, L. (2008). *Trissel's stability of compounded formulations* (4th ed.). Washington, DC: American Pharmacist Association.

*Turner, J.W. (2009). Death of a child from topical diphenhydramine. *American Journal of Forensic Medical Pathology, 30,* 380–381.

*U.S. Food and Drug Administration. (1998a). Rules and regulations. *Federal Register, 63*(231), 66631–66672.

*U.S. Food and Drug Administration. (1998b). *FDA talk paper.* Rockville, MD: Author.

*Wilens, T. E., Prince, J. B., Spencer, T. J., et al. (2006). Stimulants and sudden death: What is a physician to do? *Pediatrics, 118,* 1215–1219.

*Yaffe, S. J., & Juchau, M. R. (1974). Perinatal pharmacology. *Annual Review of Pharmacology, 14,* 219–238.

*Zempsky, W. T. (2008). Pharmacologic approaches for reducing venous access pain in children. *Pediatrics, 122,* S140–S153.

CHAPTER 5

Stephanie A. Gaber
Andrew M. Peterson

Principles of Pharmacotherapy in Pregnancy and Lactation

Although very little is known about the effects of medications on the fetus, many women ingest drugs during their pregnancy. The World Health Organization states "there can be no doubt that at present some drugs are more widely used in pregnancy than is justified by the knowledge available." Although considerable attention has been given recently to complementary and alternative medicine use during pregnancy, the use of these ubiquitous substances continues and poses significant challenges to today's health care practitioner (Briggs, et al., 2008).

ISSUES IN MEDICATION USE DURING PREGNANCY

Studies have determined that anywhere from 35% to 80% of all pregnant women will consume at least one medication during their pregnancy (McElhatton, 2003). As the number of medications being prescribed during pregnancy increases, the practitioner needs a solid understanding of the physiologic changes that occur during pregnancy and the effects that these changes have on medication use. The practitioner must also balance the need to treat the mother against the potential risk to the fetus. Because there are few studies available discussing the pharmacokinetic changes that occur during pregnancy, appropriate dosing of medications may be difficult. Understanding these changes will assist the practitioner in making recommendations during drug therapy. The maternal and fetal response to medications ingested during pregnancy may be influenced by two factors:

- Changes in the absorption, distribution, and elimination of the drug in the mother, which are altered by physiologic changes (Yankowitz & Niebyl, 2001)
- The placental–fetal unit, which affects the amount of drug that crosses the placental membrane, the amount of drug metabolized by the placenta, and the distribution and elimination of the drug by the fetus (Loebstein, et al., 1997).

Pregnancy-Induced Maternal Physiologic Changes

Women undergo many physiologic changes during pregnancy (**Table 5.1**). These changes affect the way a medication exerts its effects on both the mother and fetus.

Absorption

Drug absorption into the maternal bloodstream can occur by different processes, including the gastrointestinal (GI) tract, skin, or lungs, or the drug may be directly placed into the bloodstream via intravenous administration.

Gastrointestinal Absorption

Pregnancy-induced maternal physiologic changes may affect GI function, and therefore the absorption of some drugs may be altered. Of the many factors that can affect GI absorption of drugs, one is the decrease in GI tract motility, especially during labor. It is believed that an increase in plasma progesterone levels causes this decrease in motility, which may delay the absorption of orally administered drugs (Fredericksen, 2001; Kraemer, et al., 1997; Loebstein, et al., 1997).

In addition, pregnant women experience a reduction in gastric acid secretions (up to 40% less than in nonpregnant women) as well as an increase in gastric mucus secretion (Fredericksen, 2001; Loebstein, et al., 1997). Together, this may lead to an increase in gastric pH and a decrease in the absorption of medications that need an acidic pH for appropriate absorption.

Another reason for decreased GI absorption may be the nausea and vomiting that is common during the first trimester of pregnancy and that is thought to be associated with increased progesterone levels. Therefore, pregnant women may be well advised to take their medications at times when nausea is minimal (Loebstein, et al., 1997).

Lung Absorption

Physiologic changes in pregnancy favor the absorption of medications administered through the inhalation route. Both cardiac and tidal volumes are increased by approximately 50% in pregnancy; this results in hyperventilation and increased pulmonary blood flow (Loebstein, et al., 1997). These alterations aid in the transfer of medications through the alveoli into the maternal bloodstream (Loebstein, et al., 1997).

Transdermal Absorption

An increase in the absorption of medications through the skin is evident during pregnancy. The increase in peripheral vasodilation and increase in blood flow to the skin (Kraemer,

TABLE 5.1	Physiologic Changes in Pregnancy
Organ System Dynamic	**Change During Pregnancy**
Cardiovascular	
Blood volume	Increased by 30%–50%
Cardiac output	Increased by 30%–50%
Systemic vascular resistance	Decreased
Gastrointestinal	
pH of intestinal secretions	Increased
Gastric emptying time	Increased
Gastric acid secretions	Decreased
Intestinal motility	Decreased
Kidney	
Renal blood flow rate	Increased
Glomerular filtration rate	Increased
Gynecologic	
Uterine blood flow	Increased

Adapted from Kraemer, K., et al. (1997). Placental transfer of drugs. *Neonatal Network, 16*(2), 65–67.

et al., 1997) enhance this increase in absorption. Because of an increase in total body water, there is increased water content in the skin, therefore favoring an increased rate and extent of absorption to water-soluble medications like lidocaine, which is used as a topical anesthetic during pregnancy (Yankowitz & Niebyl, 2001).

Distribution

Maternal blood volume increases significantly during pregnancy. The 30% to 50% increase in blood volume (Guyton & Hall, 1996; Loebstein, et al., 1997) is characteristically distributed to various organ systems serving the needs of the growing fetus. The full increase in total body water during pregnancy is 8 L, with 60% distributed to the placenta, fetus, and amniotic fluid and 40% going to maternal tissues (Loebstein, et al., 1997). It is these increases that cause the volume of distribution of medications to increase, resulting in a decrease (dilutional effect) in drug concentrations. Studies show that serum levels of water-soluble drugs decrease because of the increased volume of distribution (Simone, et al., 1994). Conversely, drug distribution is affected by an increase in maternal fat deposits. Medications that are highly lipophilic distribute to maternal fat deposits, also resulting in decreased serum drug levels. Body fat increases during pregnancy by 3 to 4 kg, and may act as a reservoir for medications that favor a fat-soluble environment (Yankowitz & Niebyl, 2001). Another factor that may affect medication distribution is the concentration of albumin in the maternal blood. The concentration of plasma albumin decreases during pregnancy (Fredericksen, 2001). This decrease is believed to be caused by a reduction in the rate of albumin in synthesis or an increase in its rate of catabolism (Fredericksen, 2001). Medications that are highly bound to plasma albumin (e.g., anticonvulsants) may have an increased drug concentration due to decreased albumin binding.

Elimination

Hormonal changes that normally occur during pregnancy can affect the elimination of various medications. The normal increase in progesterone levels can stimulate hepatic microsomal enzyme systems, thereby increasing the elimination of some hepatically eliminated medications (e.g., phenytoin [Dilantin]). Progesterone may also decrease the elimination of some medications (e.g., theophylline [Theo-Dur]) by inhibiting specific microsomal enzyme systems. Therefore, depending on the elimination pathway of a specific medication, the elimination rate cannot be predicted. The extent of these physiologic changes is difficult to quantify, and it is unknown whether changes in dosages are required.

As plasma volumes increase, so does renal blood flow (Fredericksen, 2001; Guyton & Hall, 1996; Loebstein, et al., 1997). With the increase in renal blood flow by 50% (Loebstein, et al., 1997) and increased glomerular filtration rate, drugs excreted primarily by the kidney show increased elimination. Again, the size of these increases in elimination is not known and therefore dosage adjustment may not be required.

Factors in Placental–Fetal Physiology

Until the 1960s, it was widely believed that the uterus provided a secure and protected environment for the developing fetus. Very little thought was given to the potential harm posed to the fetus from maternal drug use. After the thalidomide tragedy in the 1960s, the government required testing of drugs before human use. It is now known that by the fifth week of fetal development, virtually every drug has the ability to cross the placenta (Kraemer, et al., 1997).

The treatment of medical conditions is complicated during pregnancy by various factors that must be considered before initiating drug therapy. A key factor is whether the drug will cross the placenta and potentially cause fetal harm.

Placental Transfer of Medications

The following factors affect a drug's ability to cross the placenta:

- Lipid-soluble drugs can cross the placenta more freely than water-soluble drugs because the outer layers of most cell membranes are made up of lipids. Many antibiotics and opiate compounds are highly soluble in lipids and can therefore easily cross the placental membrane (Kraemer, et al., 1997).
- The ionization status of the drug affects placental transfer. Drugs with high lipid solubility tend to remain in a non-ionized state; therefore, placental transfer is increased. Heparin, for example, is a highly ionized drug, and therefore it does not readily cross the placental membrane (Kraemer, et al., 1997).
- The molecular weight of the drug can determine the ease of placental transfer (Kraemer, et al., 1997; Loebstein, et al., 1997). The lower the molecular weight or the smaller the drug molecule, the more readily the drug crosses the placenta (**Table 5.2**).

TABLE 5.2	Effect of Molecular Weight on Placental Transfer of Drugs	
Molecular Weight	Drug Example	Rate of Placental Transfer
<500 g/mol	acetaminophen, caffeine, cocaine, labetalol, morphine, penicillins, theophylline	Readily crosses the placenta
600–1000 g/mol	digoxin	Crosses placenta at a slower rate
>1000 g/mol	heparin, insulins	Transfer across placenta severely impeded

- Only drugs that are not bound to a protein (e.g., albumin) can cross the placenta. Albumin is the most abundant protein in the human body. During pregnancy, the concentration of albumin decreases, and therefore fewer proteins are present, allowing for more unbound or "free" drug to cross the placental membrane (Kraemer, et al., 1997).

Placental and Fetal Metabolism

Evidence exists to support the theory that the human placenta and fetus are capable of metabolizing medications. Research findings suggest that liver enzyme systems are present in fetal livers as early as 7 to 8 weeks' gestation (Juchau & Choa, 1983). Although these enzyme systems are present, they are immature and any drug elimination that occurs is a result of drug diffusing back into maternal blood.

Fetal Physiology

Not all drugs that cross the placental barrier cause fetal harm. Therefore, the practitioner needs to ask whether a specific drug will cross the placenta and cause fetal harm. Fetal factors to be considered in answering the question include the gestational age at the time of exposure to the drug, which is important because some drugs can exert their effects on the fetus throughout gestation. On the other hand, some drugs exert their effects on the fetus at different stages of gestation. For example, angiotensin-converting enzyme inhibitors, such as captopril (Capoten), quinapril (Accupril), and enalapril (Vasotec), vary in their fetal risk during pregnancy, being in category C in the second trimester and category D in the third trimester. In other words, they become less safe as the pregnancy advances.

Within the first 14 days after conception, the embryo is protected from exogenous toxicity (Kraemer, et al., 1997; Rayburn, 1997). The cells at this time are totipotential, meaning that if one cell is damaged or killed, another cell can perform the dead cell's function, and the embryo remains unharmed (Dicke, 1989). After this point, the developing fetus is susceptible to the effects of drugs. The first 3 months of gestation are the most crucial in terms of abnormalities and malformations (Briggs, et al., 2008). Some medications that may be relatively safe during the middle trimester of pregnancy may not be safe in the last trimester or during delivery. For example, aspirin use late in pregnancy is associated with increased bleeding at the time of delivery. Moreover, the effect that aspirin has on prostaglandins may delay labor.

Fetal total body water and fat deposition are associated with gestational age and they affect the absorption and distribution of drugs. As the fetus matures, total body water decreases and fat deposition increases, and the fetus is more likely to be affected by medications that are highly lipophilic (e.g., opiates) than by medications that are water soluble (e.g., ampicillin [Principen]).

Fetal circulatory patterns can alter the amount of drug distributed to the fetus. In early gestation, a disproportionately large percentage of the fetal cardiac output is presented to the brain, and consequently the concentration of drug in the fetal circulation is increased (Kraemer, et al., 1997).

Teratogenicity of Medications

The word *teratogenicity* is derived from the Greek root *teras*, meaning "monster." Teratogenicity is the ability of an exogenous agent to cause the dysgenesis of fetal organs as evidenced either structurally or functionally (Koren, et al., 1998; Kraemer, et al., 1997).

The risk of fetal abnormality depends on many factors, including not only the gestational age of the fetus at the time of exposure but the agent or medications the fetus is exposed to and the length of exposure.

The health care provider must therefore balance the risk of exposing the fetus to the drug with the benefit of treatment to the mother. If it is determined that the drug is necessary, the drug with the safest profile should be used at the lowest effective dose. The practitioner always keeps in mind that the mother is not the only recipient of the drug—the fetus is as well. It is estimated that approximately 2% or 3% of all malformations and abnormalities in the developing fetus result from drug ingestion (Oakley, 1986).

To help prevent drug-induced abnormalities in the fetus, the U.S. Food and Drug Administration (FDA) has categorized drugs according to fetal risks. The categories are based on the presence or absence of controlled studies in women to determine the level of fetal risk (**Table 5.3**). Health care providers use these categories to determine the appropriate drug therapy that will effectively treat the mother but carries the least potential for fetal harm. In pregnant women, balancing the risk–benefit ratio is of great concern for the health care provider. Any illnesses or chronic medical conditions that go untreated during pregnancy could potentially cause harm to the mother and fetus, even though treating the illness or condition may be potentially harmful to the fetus. Therefore, weighing the benefit of drug therapy to the mother with the risk of drug therapy to the fetus needs to be as balanced as possible.

TABLE 5.3	FDA Pregnancy Risk Categories	
Category	Risk Summary	Example
A	Controlled studies in women fail to demonstrate a risk to the fetus in the first trimester (and there is no evidence of a risk in later trimesters), and the possibility of fetal harm appears remote.	folic acid, thyroid hormone
B	Either animal reproduction studies have not demonstrated a fetal risk but there are no controlled studies in pregnant women, or animal reproduction studies have shown an adverse effect (other than decrease in fertility) that was not confirmed in controlled studies in women in the first trimester (and there is no evidence of a risk in later trimesters).	erythromycin, penicillin
C	Either studies in animals have revealed adverse effects on the fetus and there are no controlled studies in women, or studies in women and animals are not available. Drugs should be given only if the potential benefit justifies the potential risk.	labetalol, nifedipine, angiotensin-converting enzyme (ACE) inhibitors
D	There is positive evidence of human fetal risk, but benefits from the use in pregnancy may be acceptable despite the risk.	glyburide, diazepam, aspirin, ACE inhibitors
X	Studies in animals or human beings have demonstrated fetal abnormalities, or there is evidence of fetal risk based on human experience, or both, and the risk of the use of the drug in pregnant women clearly outweighs any possible benefit. The drug is contraindicated in women who are or may become pregnant.	oral contraceptives, lovastatin, isotretinoin

DRUG THERAPY IN THE BREAST-FEEDING MOTHER

With the number of women who choose to breast-feed their infants increasing yearly, the number of questions presented to health care practitioners concerning the safety of medication use while breast-feeding is also increasing. Recommendations to discontinue or interrupt breast-feeding while taking a medication are far too common. Health care practitioners are reluctant to recommend medication use while the mother is breast-feeding because of the potential adverse effects on the infant. Most research on lactation has been conducted in small groups or on animal models. The American Academy of Pediatrics has published lists of medications that are safe for use while breast-feeding (**Boxes 5.1** and **5.2**).

Human Breast Milk as a Drug Delivery System

Human breast milk is complex, nutrient-enriched fluid. Containing approximately 80% water, breast milk also has immunologic properties and proteins, fats, carbohydrates, minerals, and vitamins needed for normal development. The availability of the drug to be distributed into breast milk depends on many factors. For a drug to be distributed into breast milk, it must first be absorbed into the maternal circulation. The concentration or level of the drug in the mother's plasma influences the amount and degree of drug distributed into breast milk. Once drug is available for distribution into breast milk, several other factors need to be considered. These factors are similar to those determining whether a drug will cross the placental membrane, and include (Dillon, et al., 1997):

- Blood flow to the breast—the greater the blood flow to the breast, the greater the drug level in breast milk.

- Plasma pH (7.45) and milk pH (7.08)—the medication will stay in the maternal plasma if the medication favors a higher pH.
- Mammary tissue composition—high adipose or fat content of the breast tissue causes lipophilic medications to be distributed into the breast tissue and then into breast milk.
- Breast milk composition—breast milk contains proteins, fat, water, and vitamins. Any medication that has a high affinity for any component will have an increased distribution into breast milk.
- Physicochemical properties (i.e., lipophilicity, molecular weight, ionization of medication in plasma and breast milk) of the drug—drug characteristics that favor transfer of medication into breast milk are low molecular weight, low ionization in plasma, low protein binding, and high lipophilicity.
- Extent of drug protein binding in plasma and breast milk—medications that are highly protein bound in the plasma are less likely to be distributed into the breast milk.
- The rate of breast milk production—the more breast milk produced, the more diluted the medication will be in the breast milk.

When considering these factors, it can easily be appreciated that different medications distribute into breast milk at different rates and to different extents. That is one factor that makes prescribing medications to the breast-feeding woman problematic at best. Health care providers need to ask themselves many questions before selecting a drug therapy.

First, is there a need to treat the maternal condition? Many prescriptions are written for conditions that do not need to be treated. Second, what medication can be prescribed that is least likely to be secreted into the breast milk, and for which there is the greatest information about its use in breast-feeding mothers?

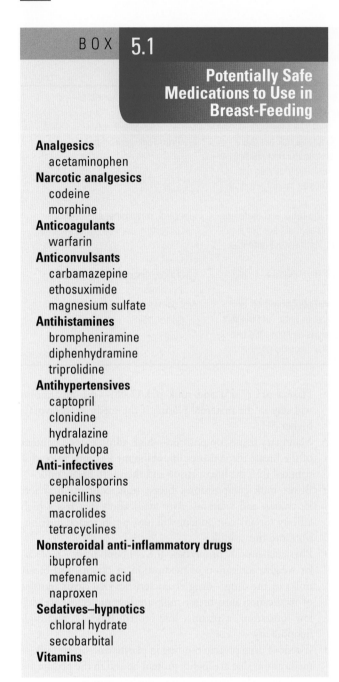

BOX 5.1

Potentially Safe Medications to Use in Breast-Feeding

Analgesics
  acetaminophen
Narcotic analgesics
  codeine
  morphine
Anticoagulants
  warfarin
Anticonvulsants
  carbamazepine
  ethosuximide
  magnesium sulfate
Antihistamines
  brompheniramine
  diphenhydramine
  triprolidine
Antihypertensives
  captopril
  clonidine
  hydralazine
  methyldopa
Anti-infectives
  cephalosporins
  penicillins
  macrolides
  tetracyclines
Nonsteroidal anti-inflammatory drugs
  ibuprofen
  mefenamic acid
  naproxen
Sedatives–hypnotics
  chloral hydrate
  secobarbital
Vitamins

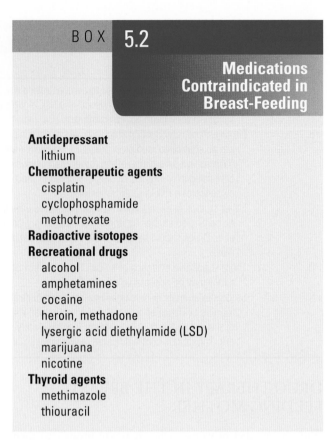

BOX 5.2

Medications Contraindicated in Breast-Feeding

Antidepressant
  lithium
Chemotherapeutic agents
  cisplatin
  cyclophosphamide
  methotrexate
Radioactive isotopes
Recreational drugs
  alcohol
  amphetamines
  cocaine
  heroin, methadone
  lysergic acid diethylamide (LSD)
  marijuana
  nicotine
Thyroid agents
  methimazole
  thiouracil

Answers to these questions are often difficult or elusive. Referring to the FDA guidelines for medication use in pregnancy and lactation is helpful. Consulting the known pharmacokinetic parameters of medications can also be helpful in prescribing medications. Selected drugs should have short half-lives, and the use of sustained-release products should be discouraged. Dosing schedules also help in minimizing the amount of drug reaching the infant. Scheduling the mother to take the medication immediately after breast-feeding minimizes the dose to the infant by circumventing peak breast milk levels (Dillon, et al., 1997).

Patients with chronic conditions, such as hypertension, epilepsy, or diabetes, need to consult their health care practitioners about continuing treatment and minimizing risk to the infant. Without other options, patients with short-term illnesses can temporarily interrupt breast-feeding for the duration of treatment and resume breast-feeding a few days after therapy is completed. By this time, no residual drug should be concentrated in the breast milk. During the interruption, however, the mother must pump the breast and discard the milk. Doing so relieves engorgement and promotes continued milk production and flow.

Balancing Benefits and Risks

Although the health benefits of breast-feeding are established, there remain a few medications that are unsafe to use during breast-feeding. As with medication use during pregnancy, the risk–benefit ratio needs to be assessed. Choice of the best medication to treat the maternal condition needs to be balanced against the risk of adverse effects to the infant.

BIBLIOGRAPHY

Starred references are cited in the text.
Anderson, G D. (2006). Using pharmacokinetics to predict the effects of pregnancy and maternal-fetal transfer of drugs during lactation. *Expert Opinion on Drug Metabolism and Toxicology, 2*(6), 947–960.
*Briggs, C. G., Freeman, R. K., & Yaffe, S. J. (2008). *Drugs in pregnancy and lactation* (8th ed.). Philadelphia, PA: Lippincott Williams & Wilkins.
Cordero, J. F., & Oakley, G. P. (1983). Drug exposure during pregnancy: Some epidemiological considerations. *Clinical Obstetrics and Gynecology, 26*, 418–428.

Dawes, M., & Chowienczyk, P. J. (2001). Drugs in pregnancy. Pharmacokinetics in pregnancy. *Best Practice and Research in Clinical Obstetrics and Gynaecology, 15*(6), 819–826.

*Dicke, J. M. (1989). Teratology: Principles and practice. *Medical Clinics of North America, 73*, 567–582.

*Dillon, A. E., et al. (1997). Drug therapy in the nursing mother. *Obstetrics and Gynecology Clinics, 24*, 676–697.

*Fredericksen, M. C. (2001). Physiologic changes in pregnancy and their effect on drug disposition. *Seminars in Perinatology, 25*(3), 120–123.

Gonsalves, L., & Scheuremeyer, I. (2009). Treating depression in pregnancy: Practical suggestions. *Cleveland Clinical Journal of Medicine 73*(12), 1098–1104.

*Guyton, A. C., & Hall, J. C. (1996). *Human physiology and mechanisms of disease* (6th ed.). Philadelphia, PA: Saunders.

*Juchau, M. R., & Choa, S. T. (1983). Drug metabolism by the human fetus. In M. Gibaldi & L. Prescott (Eds.), *Handbook of clinical pharmacokinetics* (pp. 58–78). New York, NY: Adis.

*Koren, G., et al. (1998). Drugs in pregnancy. *New England Journal of Medicine, 338*, 1128–1137.

*Kraemer, K., et al. (1997). Placental transfer of drugs. *Neonatal Network, 16*(2), 65–67.

*Loebstein, R., et al. (1997). Pharmacokinetic changes during pregnancy and their clinical relevance. *Clinical Pharmacokinetics, 33*, 328–343.

*McElhatton, P. R. (2003). General principles of drug use in pregnancy. *The Pharmaceutical Journal, 270*, 232–234.

*Oakley, G. P. (1986). Frequency of human congenital malformations. *Clinics in Perinatology, 13*, 545–554.

*Rayburn, W. F. (1997). Chronic medical disorders during pregnancy. *Journal of Reproductive Medicine, 42*, 1–24.

Scott, J. R., DiSaia, P. J., Hammond, C. B., & Spellacy, W. N. (Eds.). (1999). *Danforth's obstetrics and gynecology* (8th ed.). Philadelphia, PA: Lippincott Williams & Wilkins.

*Simone, G., Derewlany, L., & Koren, G. (1994). Drug transfer across the placenta. *Clinics in Perinatology, 21*, 463–482.

Tettenborn, B. (2006). Management of epilepsy in women of childbearing age: Practical recommendations. *CNS Drugs, 20*(5), 373–387.

Wyska, E., & Jusko W. J. (2001). Approaches top pharmacokinetic/pharmacodynamic modeling during pregnancy. *Seminars in Perinatology, 25*, 124–32.

*Yankowitz, J., & Niebyl, J. R. (2001). *Drug therapy in pregnancy* (3rd ed.). Philadelphia, PA: Lippincott Williams & Wilkins.

Principles of Pharmacotherapy in Elderly Patients

The medical and pharmacologic management of the geriatric patient presents a challenge to the practitioner that warrants an understanding of aging and its effects on the body. In prescribing drug therapy for elderly patients, the practitioner must have a sound understanding of the physiologic and social issues that are unique to older adults and that may affect the safety and efficacy of prescribing practices. As the elderly population grows, the health care community must be prepared for the challenges ahead.

Indeed, the elderly population is the fastest growing of any age group. By the year 2050, the "oldest old," those age 85 and older, will approach 19 million and 4.3% of the U.S. population (Vincent & Velhoff, 2010), with a life expectancy of 79.7 years for men and 85.6 years for women (Arias, 2004). Advances in medicine and technology have dramatically increased longevity, turning once fatal conditions, such as heart disease, into chronic illnesses (Guralnik & Havlik, 2000).

The consequences of longevity are evidenced by the rising number of older adults living with multiple chronic diseases, contributing to disability, frailty, and decline in function and presenting significant challenges for medical management (Norris, et al., 2008). Treating multiple problems with prescription as well as over-the-counter (OTC) medications can result in adverse drug reactions (ADRs) and interactions related to changes produced by aging. Problems of polypharmacy (the use of an inappropriate amount of medications to treat a host of medical conditions), improper dosing for an older adult, and a lack of understanding by patients about medications can lead to significant but preventable adverse effects, such as falls, fractures, and delirium (Pham & Dickman, 2007). This chapter discusses basic physiologic changes of aging, proper prescribing principles, and social concepts pertaining to safe medication use for the geriatric patient.

BODY CHANGES AND AGING

Every body system is affected by the aging process somewhat, although homeostasis is often maintained despite less-than-optimal functioning of organ systems. Certain systems are more vitally affected by aging and play significant roles in the pharmacokinetic and pharmacodynamic changes in drug effects. **Box 6.1** summarizes the impact of aging on the pharmacokinetics of drugs.

Absorption

With aging, physiologic changes in the gastrointestinal (GI) tract may play a role in drug absorption and availability. Stomach pH may increase, blood flow may decrease, and gastric motility may be delayed. The significance of these changes for drug metabolism is controversial. Despite these changes, it is believed that the prolonged transit time in the GI tract still allows for adequate drug absorption (Cusack & Vestel, 2000).

Distribution

Body size decreases with age. Muscle that makes up lean body tissue decreases, shifting to increased fat stores, and body water content decreases 10% to 15% by age 80. Aging results in some reduction in serum albumin (by approximately 20%), leading to an increase in free drug concentration of drugs such as warfarin (Coumadin) and phenytoin (Dilantin) (Miller, 2004).

There are two important plasma-binding proteins in drug metabolism: albumin and α-acid glycoprotein. Albumin has an affinity for acid compounds or drugs such as warfarin, whereas α_1-acid glycoprotein binds more readily with lipophilic and alkaline drugs such as propranolol (Inderal) (Semla & Rochon, 2003). The effects of chronic disease, nutritional deficits, immobility, and age-related liver changes contribute to the changes in serum proteins. The significance of decreased serum proteins is realized when highly protein-bound drugs compete for decreased protein-binding sites. The result can be greater levels of free or unbound circulating drug and, therefore, potential toxicity (Miller, 2004).

Body mass changes may lead to changes in total body content of drugs in elderly patients. A water-soluble drug (low volume of distribution $[V_d]$) is taken up more readily by lean tissue or muscle and attains higher serum concentrations in patients with less body water or lean tissue. Conversely, a lipid-soluble (high V_d) drug is retained in body fat, resulting in a higher V_d for some drugs. Coupled with a decrease or no change in total body clearance, this increase in V_d can lead to increased half-lives and drug accumulation in elderly patients.

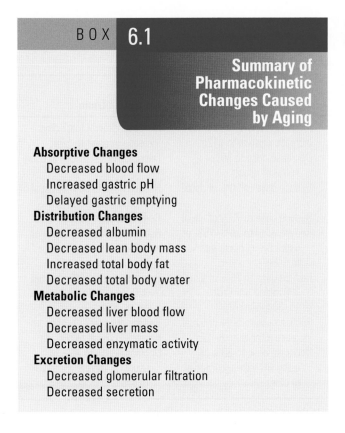

BOX 6.1

Summary of Pharmacokinetic Changes Caused by Aging

Absorptive Changes
    Decreased blood flow
    Increased gastric pH
    Delayed gastric emptying
Distribution Changes
    Decreased albumin
    Decreased lean body mass
    Increased total body fat
    Decreased total body water
Metabolic Changes
    Decreased liver blood flow
    Decreased liver mass
    Decreased enzymatic activity
Excretion Changes
    Decreased glomerular filtration
    Decreased secretion

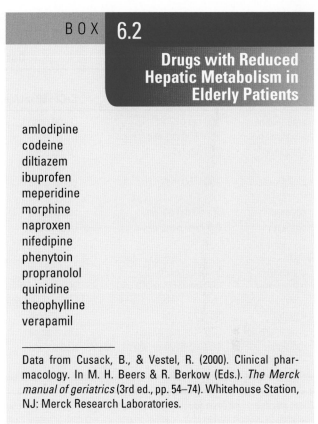

BOX 6.2

Drugs with Reduced Hepatic Metabolism in Elderly Patients

amlodipine
codeine
diltiazem
ibuprofen
meperidine
morphine
naproxen
nifedipine
phenytoin
propranolol
quinidine
theophylline
verapamil

Data from Cusack, B., & Vestel, R. (2000). Clinical pharmacology. In M. H. Beers & R. Berkow (Eds.). *The Merck manual of geriatrics* (3rd ed., pp. 54–74). Whitehouse Station, NJ: Merck Research Laboratories.

For example, diazepam (Valium) has a half-life (t½) of approximately 20 hours in a young adult, but the t½ can exceed 70 hours in the older adult. In addition, some drugs, such as tricyclic antidepressants (TCAs) and long-acting benzodiazepines, pass more readily through the blood–brain barrier, causing more pronounced central nervous system (CNS) effects (Semla & Rochon, 2003). Elderly patients who are treated for depression and anxiety may experience fatigue and confusion from drug therapy because antidepressant and antianxiety agents more readily cross their blood–brain barrier.

Elimination

The liver is the major organ of drug metabolism in the body. With aging comes a decrease in blood flow and liver size. However, in the absence of disease, function is maintained. Decreased size and hepatic blood flow may slow the clearance of certain drugs, and reduced dosages may be required. This is particularly important for drugs with high hepatic extraction ratios. Phase I metabolism, particularly oxidation, is affected by aging. The result is decreased oxidation of drugs, which in turn results in a decreased total body clearance (**Box 6.2**). The phase II metabolism of drugs by conjugation, which promotes drug elimination by breaking the drug into water-soluble components, is not affected by age (Cusack & Vestal, 2000).

After the liver, the kidneys are the most important organs for drug metabolism and excretion. After age 40, renal blood flow declines and the glomerular filtration rate (GFR) drops approximately 1% a year and accelerates with advancing age. Function is usually maintained despite decreased filtration

unless illness or disease overstresses the kidney (Kelleher & Lindeman, 2003). In elderly patients, drugs excreted primarily by the kidney are given in smaller doses, or the time between doses is extended.

A serum creatinine level alone cannot be used to estimate renal function in the aging person because reductions in lean body mass result in decreased rates of creatinine formation. This, coupled with the decreased GFR, makes the serum creatinine appear normal. It cannot be assumed that the GFR is normal from a normal serum creatinine value. The most accurate means of measuring renal function is a 24-hour urine test for creatinine clearance; however, this is not standard procedure before ordering a medication. When there is a need to determine a drug choice in the setting of a potential reduction in creatinine clearance, the Cockcroft and Gault formula (see Chapter 2) provides an estimate based on age, weight, and serum creatinine level with an adjustment for sex (Semla & Rochon, 2003). **Table 6.1** lists drugs eliminated by the kidney and recommended dosage adjustments based on estimated creatinine clearance.

PHARMACODYNAMIC CHANGES IN THE ELDERLY

Many of the changes that occur due to aging affect major organ systems and therefore affect the pharmacokinetic disposition of the drug. However, the clinician also must consider the impact drugs have on the aging body (or the

TABLE 6.1	**Examples of Dose Adjustments Based on Estimated Creatinine Clearance**			
		Dose Based on Estimated CrCl*		
Drug	**Usual Oral Dose (Nonrenally Impaired)**	**CrCl >50 mL/min**	**CrCl 10–50 mL/min**	**CrCL <10 mL/min**
amantadine	100 mg q12h	Usual dose	Increase interval to q24–72h	Increase interval to q7 days
amoxicillin	250–500 mg q8h	Usual dose	Increase interval to q12h	Increase interval to q24h
cefaclor	250 mg tid	Usual dose	Decrease dose to 50%–100% of usual	Decrease dose to 50% of usual
ciprofloxacin	250–750 mg q12h	Usual dose	Reduce dose to 50% of usual	Reduce dose to 33% of usual or extend to q24h
codeine	30–60 mg q4–6h	Usual dose	Reduce dose to 75% of usual	Reduce dose to 50% of usual
digoxin[†]	0.125–0.5 mg q24h	Usual dose	Reduce dose to 25%–75% of usual OR increase interval to q48h	Reduce dose to 10%–25% of usual
enalapril	5–10 mg q12h	Usual dose	Reduce dose to 75% of usual	Reduce dose to 50% of usual
gabapentin[†]	400 mg tid (for CrCl >60)	300 mg bid (for CrCl 30–60 mL/min)	300 mg qd (for CrCl 15–30 mL/min)	300 mg qod (for CrCl 15 mL/min)
nadolol	80–120 mg/d	Usual dose	Reduce dose to 50% of usual	Reduce dose to 25% of usual
procainamide[‡]	350–400 mg q3–4h	Usual dose	Increase interval to 6–12h	Increase interval to q8–24h
ranitidine	150 mg q12h or 300 mg qhs	Usual dose	Decrease dose to 50% of usual OR increase interval to q24h	Decrease dose to 25% of usual OR increase interval to q48h

*Dose adjustments based on actual creatinine clearance or creatinine clearance estimated by the Cockroft and Gault formula (see Chapter 2).

[†]These drugs are best monitored using actual drug levels, and dose adjustments should be made based on these results.

[‡]Based on manufacturer's information.

Data from Bennett, W. M., et al. (1991). *Drug prescribing in renal failure: Dosing guidelines for adults* (2nd ed.). Philadelphia, PA: American College of Physicians; and *Physicians desk reference* (1998). Medical Economics.

pharmacodynamic effect). Although few data are available regarding age-related pharmacodynamic changes in elderly adults, it is known that the elderly may be more sensitive to drug–receptor interactions, either because of increased sensitivity of the receptor to the drug or decreased capacity to respond to drug-induced innervation of receptors. In addition, the number or affinity of receptors may be reduced (Cusack & Vestel, 2000). Nevertheless, it is commonly accepted that the CNS effects of drugs appear to be exaggerated in the elderly patient. Particularly egregious are the agents with anticholinergic affects, such as the TCAs, antihistamines, and antispasmodics. The anticholinergic effect induced by these agents can lead to excessive dry mouth, blurred vision, constipation, and even an exacerbation of benign prostatic hyperplasia. Caution should be used if these agents are prescribed at all.

Similarly, the sedative effects of agents may be intensified in elderly patients. The benzodiazepines and potent analgesic agents are examples of drugs for which older patients are particularly susceptible to this adverse effect. Overprescribing, or typical prescribing without considering the potential for exaggerated effect, can lead to oversedation and a greater risk of falls and fractures.

The cardiovascular system also can be affected by changes due to aging. Orthostatic hypotension is more common in the elderly because of a loss of the baroreceptor reflex and changes in cerebral blood flow. Moreover, drugs that lower blood

pressure or decrease cardiac output put the elderly patient at risk for a syncopal episode.

POLYPHARMACY

Polypharmacy is a significant factor in the morbidity and mortality of elderly patients. Increasing age puts the person at risk for multiple chronic illnesses, many of which require drug therapy (**Figure 6-1**). For example, the most common chronic disease in the United States, osteoarthritis, affects 40 million people, the majority being older adults. The costs in terms of morbidity are staggering. Chronic stiffness and pain from arthritis have an impact on function, prompting the routine use of nonsteroidal anti-inflammatory drugs (NSAIDs) and aspirin products (Luggen, 2003). Long-term use of NSAIDs lowers the prostaglandin level in the GI tract, which may result in esophagitis, peptic ulcerations, GI hemorrhage, and GI perforation (Chutka, et al., 2004). In a geriatric patient, treatment with histamine-2 blockers or proton pump inhibitors to relieve the side effects of aspirin or other NSAIDs may cause additional side effects, such as confusion and mental status changes, in turn requiring more treatment. This demonstrates how easily adverse events occur and snowball in an elderly patient. ADRs account for 30% of hospital admissions for persons older than age 65; approximately 106,000 deaths are attributed

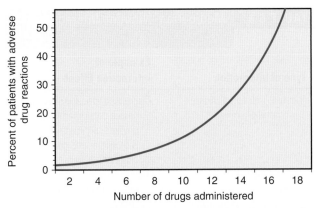

FIGURE 6–1 Relationship between probability of an adverse reaction and the number of medications taken. (Reproduced from Smith, J. W., Seidl, L. G., & Cluff, L. E. [1966]. Studies on the epidemiology of adverse drug reactions: V. Clinical factors influencing susceptibility. *Annals of Internal Medicine 65*, 629, with permission.)

to medication problems. Sadly, 15% to 65% of these events are preventable (Shiyanbola & Farris, 2010) by avoiding potentially inappropriate medications, effective communication, and patient education (Pham & Dickman, 2007).

Several factors contribute to polypharmacy. Among them are the varied symptoms and complaints associated with multiple chronic illnesses. In addition, patients often believe that a "pill will fix what ails them," and the health care provider feels pressured to "prescribe something" to satisfy the patients' expectations of a prescription for medication. When a particular medication regimen is unsuccessful, the health care provider typically prescribes another drug. Many elderly patients stockpile their discontinued medications in case they may be needed again—primarily because of the cost of prescription drugs (Rollason & Vogt, 2003).

Many providers who visit elderly patients in their homes have seen evidence of stockpiled medications. Some elderly patients keep a drawer or cabinet full of old prescription drug bottles. Some contain the same medication, differing only in brand name. Some patients may place a current medication (prescription or OTC) in a labeled prescription bottle that was used for another drug. In addition, the stockpile may reveal prescription bottles for other family members. Patients may be sharing medications or may have received medications from others who believed that the drug that helped them would help the patient (Peterson & Dragon, 1998).

Other sources of polypharmacy are "poly-providers." Many geriatric patients see multiple specialists for various chronic diseases. Medications prescribed without the provider carefully reviewing the patient's other medications can lead to drug overuse and complications. Without a primary care provider overseeing the care of the geriatric patient seeing multiple specialists, ADRs are sure to occur.

The health care provider sometimes creates a polypharmacy situation because multiple drugs are used to treat several chronic illnesses. The provider who is not astute in the principles of safe geriatric prescribing practices may create avoidable side

effects and complications. In addition, the patient, who may be a great consumer of OTC medications, often self-prescribes without knowing the consequences of mixing OTC medications with current prescription drugs.

Drug Interactions in the Elderly

Because of normal, age-related physiologic changes, the geriatric patient is at greater risk for complications from medications. Complications related to drug–disease, drug–drug, and drug–food interaction are all commonly encountered. (For more information on drug–drug interactions, see Chapter 3.)

Adverse Drug Reactions

ADRs often result in negative health outcomes, such as falls and fractures, and billions of dollars in hospital and nursing home care costs (Shiyanbola & Farris, 2010). Although age itself creates a risk for ADRs, polypharmacy and the multiplicity of drugs taken by elderly patients present the greater risk. The geriatric patient with multiple chronic illnesses and medications must be identified as a potential candidate for ADRs (Fick, et al., 2003). Older women in particular are at great risk for ADRs because they often receive more prescription drugs and have a more significant loss of muscle mass than older men.

There is a paucity of information on safety and efficacy of drugs for the elderly patient. Most research and clinical trials are performed with younger subjects. It often is difficult or impossible to predict the consequences of a medication for its intended use on an older adult because few data may be available. In an effort to better understand the effects of drugs on elderly patients, the U.S. Food and Drug Administration published guidelines in 1997 recommending older adults be included in clinical trials of drugs specifically being developed to treat prevalent diseases affecting older adults (Murray & Callahan, 2003).

Contributing Lifestyle Factors

Being unaware of potential drug interactions, elderly patients commonly take OTC medications with prescription drugs. Additional combinations of foods or nutritional supplements can slow absorption, prolonging the time for medications to reach peak levels (see Chapter 3). Fatty foods, in particular, can increase intestinal drug absorption because of the longer time required to digest a fatty meal. This, in turn, potentially leads to increased drug levels or toxicity.

Alcohol and Other Drugs

The ingestion of alcohol and other drugs can alter the metabolism of many medications in elderly patients. The combination of co-morbid conditions, physiological changes with age, and concomitant medications is often potentiated with alcohol usage (Moore, et al., 2009). CNS effects such as lethargy and confusion occur, as does hypotension, when alcohol is combined with nitrates and some cardiovascular drugs. Alcohol can be found in many OTC products such as cough and cold syrups and mouthwashes (Miller, 2004).

Alcohol abuse may be overlooked as a potential problem in the elderly, but abuse among community-dwelling (non-institutionalized) people age 65 and older has a prevalence of 14% for men and 1.5% for women. High numbers of elderly alcoholics are treated in emergency departments and medical offices or are hospitalized for medical or psychiatric admissions (Lantz, 2002). Depression, which is more prevalent in the elderly, often coexists with alcohol abuse. Moderate to heavy drinkers older than 65 are 16 times more likely to die of suicide (National Institute on Alcohol Abuse and Alcoholism, 1998). Practitioners need to be more aware of the potential for alcohol abuse in elderly patients. Although alcohol use and abuse decline with age, approximately 50% of older adults use alcohol, with between 2% and 4% meeting the *Diagnostic and Statistical Manual* (American Psychiatric Association, 1994) criteria for alcohol abuse/dependency (Oslin, 2003). The use of alcohol is anticipated to increase as Baby Boomers age. The Baby Boomer cohort has a history of greater alcohol, tobacco, and nonmedical substance usage than previous generations (Moore, et al, 2009). Life stressors such as retirement, loss of loved ones, dependency, and chronic illness are contributors to potential alcohol abuse.

Caffeine and Nicotine Use

Caffeine and nicotine are commonly used products that have the potential to interact with certain drugs, thereby altering efficacy and therapeutic drug levels. Besides its presence in coffee, tea, and some sodas, caffeine is found in many OTC drug products. The interaction of caffeine and certain medications may alter drug absorption, cause CNS effects, or decrease drug effectiveness (Miller, 2004). **Table 6.2** summarizes selected caffeine–medication interactions.

TABLE 6.2	**Medication–Caffeine Interactions**
Type of Interaction	**Example of Interaction Effect**
Caffeine-induced increase in gastric acid secretion	Decreased absorption of iron
Caffeine-induced gastrointestinal irritation	Decreased effectiveness of cimetidine; increased gastrointestinal irritation from corticosteroids, alcohol, and analgesics
Altered caffeine metabolism	Prolonged effect of caffeine when combined with ciprofloxacin, estrogen, or cimetidine
Caffeine-induced cardiac arrhythmic effect	Decreased effectiveness of antiarrhythmic medications
Caffeine-induced hypokalemia	Exacerbated hypokalemic effect of diuretics
Caffeine-induced stimulation of CNS	Increased stimulation effects from amantadine, decongestants, fluoxetine, and theophylline
Caffeine-induced increase in excretion of lithium	Decreased effectiveness of lithium

TABLE 6.3	**Medication–Nicotine Interactions**
Type of Interaction	**Example of Interaction Effect**
Nicotine-induced alteration in metabolism	Decreased efficacy of analgesics, lorazepam, theophylline, aminophylline, β blockers, and calcium channel blockers
Nicotine-induced vasoconstriction	Increased peripheral ischemic effect of β blockers
Nicotine-induced central nervous system stimulation	Decreased drowsiness from benzodiazepines and phenothiazines
Nicotine-induced stimulation of antidiuretic hormone secretion	Fluid retention, decreased effectiveness of diuretics
Nicotine-induced increase in platelet activity	Decreased anticoagulant effectiveness (heparin, warfarin); increased risk of thrombosis with estrogen use
Nicotine-induced increase in gastric acid	Decreased or negated effects of H_2 antagonists (cimetidine, famotidine, nizatidine, ranitidine)

Many elderly patients have lifelong smoking addictions and are unsuccessful in stopping. Patients and providers alike are frequently unaware of the effects of nicotine and medications. Nicotine alters the metabolism of many drugs, causes CNS effects, and interferes with platelet activity (Miller, 2004). **Table 6.3** reviews nicotine–medication effects and interactions.

ADHERENCE ISSUES

One reason elderly patients have problems with their medications is failure to adhere to the medication regimen. In many cases, prescription drugs are not taken as prescribed: up to 40% of elderly patients take their medications improperly (Cusack & Vestel, 2000). More than 40% of ambulatory adults age 65 and older take at least 5 medications per week, with 12% taking at least 10 per week (Pham & Dickman, 2007). Studies have shown that as the complexity of the medication regime increases, improper drug usage rises proportionately (Rollason & Vogt, 2003). In some cases, they may not take enough of the medication, either because they think that they will save money by making the prescription last longer or because they believe that the medicine is not needed daily. In other situations, a medication may not be taken if it interferes with the patient's lifestyle, for example, not taking a diuretic for fear of incontinence.

Cost Factors

The cost of medications today is high. Unfortunately, many elderly patients do not have health insurance plans that cover prescription medications, or they quickly reach a capitated benefit for prescription drugs under their managed care plan when treated with multiple medications for chronic illnesses. Many older adults on fixed incomes must make choices among buying food; paying rent, taxes, and utilities; or purchasing medications. In some cases, medication purchases become a low priority.

In 2003, the Medicare Modernization Act included the Medicare Part D prescription benefit option, which became effective in 2006, providing prescription coverage for Medicare enrollees in the plan. Currently, the plan has a "donut hole," which requires out-of-pocket payments for medications after the enrollee reaches $2,830. When the maximum of $4,550 is reached, coverage resumes for medication costs. This has led to much confusion on the part of enrollees, leading to stoppage or improperly taking medications (Tseng, et al., 2009). The Patient Protection and Affordable Care Act, passed in March 2010, will gradually close the donut hole by 2020 (Stefanacci & Spivack, 2010).

Side Effects

Other reasons for nonadherence to drug treatments include the unpleasant or inconvenient side effects accompanying some medications. Dry mouth, change in taste sensations, fatigue, or frequent urination are reported as reasons for stopping a medication. The form of the medication and ease of administration are reasons as well. Large tablets and capsules may be difficult to swallow. Swallowing problems may be compounded by insufficient fluid being taken with medications. Taking several oral medications at one dosing time with too little fluid may result in the medications "getting stuck," leading to chronic esophageal irritation. Presbyesophagus (the slowing of esophageal motility with advancing age) makes it difficult and frustrating to swallow multiple medications, and it can also lead to choking or aspiration.

Physical and Mental Changes

Functional deficits, especially those affecting the senses, can also challenge adherence to the medication regimen. Poor vision leads to difficulty reading labels and consequently taking the wrong pills or too many of the same pills. Arthritic hands and safety caps can make opening prescription bottles difficult and frustrating for an older adult.

The prevalence of dementia, which manifests in symptoms of cognitive impairment and poor short-term memory and recall, slowly progresses with age, affecting a substantial percentage of those residing in the community (Eslami & Espinoza, 2003). The condition may be unrecognized by the family because the patient may remain seemingly independent and functional despite mental deficits. The family may be fooled into believing the loved one is fine until the condition affects the person's ability to manage basic, daily routines. Unfortunately, the affected person is often responsible for taking his or her own medications. Poor memory results in not taking medication properly, forgetting doses, or taking too

many doses of the same drug. Approximately 30% of hospital admissions in the elderly are attributed to toxicity from medications or ADRs. Of prescription medications, almost one-third are for those age 65 and older (Feinberg & Provenzano, 2010). Improperly taking digoxin, a drug with a narrow therapeutic range, is associated with drug toxicity in the elderly (Juurlink, et al., 2003).

Self-Medication Issues

The use of OTC drugs is a significant issue. Noninstitutionalized elderly adults consume between 40% and 50% of all OTC medications sold. Of more concern is the fact that 70% of those OTC medications were consumed without the patient consulting the health care provider (Meiner, 1997). Approximately 20% of ADRs in the elderly are due to OTC medications (Chutka, et al., 2004). On average, the elderly take two OTC medications with 3.8 to 6.7 prescription drugs (Logue, 2002). Many OTC medications are taken without the medical provider's awareness in order to treat symptoms they do not want to report. Family members and friends often borrow medications believed to treat a particular ailment, again without consultation with their medical provider (Rollason & Vogt, 2003).

The use of herbal preparations contributes to ADRs, especially when taken with prescription medications. Of those over age 65 taking herbal preparations, 49% do not divulge this information to their medical providers, compounding the risk of drug interactions and toxicity (Scholz, et al., 2008).

Many OTC medications are products that were once available only by prescription. Now, despite their decreased strength, these medications that once required medical supervision and monitoring present a potential hazard for side effects.

The most common OTC medications used by the geriatric patient include analgesics, vitamins and minerals, antacids, and laxatives (Rollason & Vogt, 2003). Cough and cold products and sleeping aids such as Tylenol PM are frequently used by older adults. Combining these products may result in confusion, change in mental status, fluid and electrolyte imbalances, dysrhythmias, and nervousness. Cold medications may worsen hypertension without the patient's knowledge or worsen glucose control in a patient with diabetes.

The geriatric patient must be educated to use OTC drugs safely and to do so only after consulting with the health care provider or pharmacist. If an alternative to drug use is feasible, such as initiating sleep hygiene practices versus taking a sleeping pill, the patient should be encouraged to try these measures first.

SPECIAL CONSIDERATIONS IN LONG-TERM CARE

Advanced age coupled with years of multiple illnesses and mental decline result in frailty and disability. Placement in a long-term care facility most often occurs when the older adult requires assistance with daily functions, such as bathing and dressing, shows cognitive impairment, or becomes incontinent. The national percentage of older adults in nursing homes is about 5%, rising to 20% for age 85 and older (Kasper & Burton, 2003). With a wide array of physical, psychiatric, neurologic, and behavioral problems, the long-term care resident is the most complex of all patients (Katz & Karuza, 2003). Consequently, the complexity of prescribing medications for the nursing home resident can be challenging and frustrating.

Falls and Medication

One of the most serious problems in long-term care facilities is falls. Approximately half of nursing home residents fall annually, sustaining fractures and soft tissue and other injuries (van Doorn, et al., 2003). Among the multiple causes of falls are medications, in particular psychotropic agents (e.g., sedatives, hypnotics, antidepressants, and neuroleptics). These medications are useful for treating the depression, anxiety, and behavioral problems that are not unusual in the long-term care resident. However, their use presents an ongoing treatment challenge. Medication-related falls are often caused by orthostatic hypotension, sedation, extrapyramidal side effects, myopathy, and pupil constriction. **Table 6.4** lists drug classes leading to instability (Hile & Studenski, 2007).

The practitioner is often pressured by family members and nursing staff to "do something" when the elderly patient's behavior becomes difficult and unmanageable. At one time, psychotropics such as haloperidol (Haldol) were used to control behavior chemically. In 1987, the Omnibus Budget Reconciliation Act was enacted. Strict regulations were introduced to prevent inappropriate psychotropic drug use in long-term care, and compliance with the regulations is strictly monitored (Katz & Karuza, 2003).

TABLE 6.4	Medications That Contribute to Instability
Mechanism	**Classes of Medications**
Orthostatic hypotension	Antihypertensives, antianginals, Parkinsonian drugs, tricyclic antidepressants, antipsychotics
Sedation, decreased attention	Benzodiazepines, sedating antihistamines, narcotic analgesics, tricyclic antidepressants, selective serotonin reuptake inhibitors (SSRIs), antipsychotics, anticonvulsants, ethanol
Extrapyramidal side effects	Antipsychotics, metoclopramide, phenothiazines for nausea such as prochlorperazine, SSRIs
Myopathy	Corticosteroids; colchicine; high-dose statins, especially in combination with fibrates; ethanol; interferon
Miosis (pupil constriction)	Glaucoma medications, especially pilocarpine

Antipsychotics

Psychotropic drugs, such as the antipsychotics, are appropriately intended to treat schizophrenia, hallucinations, and violent behaviors that pose the potential for physical harm. Environmental and organic causes of aberrant behavior need to be ruled out before prescribing an antipsychotic, and all nonpharmacologic means should be explored *before therapy begins* (American Geriatric Society & American Association for Geriatric Psychiatry, 2003). Consulting with a geropsychiatrist regarding psychotropic management is recommended. In addition, monthly chart reviews are performed to evaluate side effects and the necessity of using psychotropic drugs. Long-term care facilities are subject to citation and loss of licensure for inappropriate use of psychotropic or chemical restraints.

The host of side effects of psychotropic agents makes monitoring the elderly resident receiving psychotropic therapy imperative. Extrapyramidal symptoms (EPSs), tardive dyskinesia, dystonic reactions, and anticholinergic effects can be severe. Older drugs, such as haloperidol, fluphenazine (Prolixin), and trifluoperazine (Stelazine), have a greater propensity to cause EPSs.

The newer, atypical antipsychotic agents (i.e., serotonin–dopamine antagonists) are better tolerated and are associated with fewer side effects than the older agents. Advantages include less tardive dyskinesia and fewer EPSs, although risperidone (Risperdal) has a greater dose-related response for EPSs. Increased weight gain and the potential for metabolic changes are common with the atypical antipsychotics (Jeste, et al, 2003). Studies have demonstrated an increased risk of dose-dependent sudden cardiac death with atypical antipsychotics, which is a similar risk as conventional antipsychotics (Bergman, et al., 2009). Somnolence, which usually subsides, may occur with initial titration of risperidone and olanzapine (Zyprexa). Frail elderly patients may experience more sedation with quetiapine (Seroquel). Risperidone should be avoided or used cautiously with patients who have Parkinson's disease because of their greater potential for EPSs.

One of the newer atypical antipsychotics for the treatment of psychosis in patients with Alzheimer's disease is aripiprazole (Abilify), a partial dopamine agonist. Somnolence, the most common side effect, is dose related (Jeste, et al., 2003).

For patients exhibiting hyperactivity, aggression, increased motor activity, and excitability and inability to tolerate the usual antipsychotics, the anticonvulsants divalproex (Depakote), carbamazepine (Tegretol), oxcarbazepine (Trileptal), and lamotrigine (Lamictal) are being used with greater frequency. Hyponatremia or syndrome of inappropriate antidiuretic hormone has been associated with carbamazepine and oxcarbazepine. Caution should be used with divalproex in patients with hepatic impairment (Espinoza & Eslami, 2004). Lamotrigine has been associated with serious and life-threatening rashes (toxic epidermal necrolysis or Stevens-Johnson syndrome) in 0.3% of adults, usually within 2 to 8 weeks of treatment initiation (Burdick & Goldberg, 2002; Espinoza & Eslami, 2004).

Anxiolytics

Anxiety is a problem frequently confronted in the nursing home setting. It may be precipitated by physical causes such as pain, infection, or chronic illness. Other stressors that contribute to anxiety include fatigue and change, such as a change in a daily routine or change of caregiver. An overly stimulating environment or expectations of staff members hurrying the elderly resident through daily routines may evoke anxiety. Initially, nonpharmacologic measures should be used to assess and ameliorate anxiety; prescribing a medication to relieve anxiety should be a last choice.

Several nonpharmacologic anti-anxiety treatments may be beneficial. They include establishing daily routines in a structured environment, consistently providing the same caregiver for bathing and hygiene assistance, avoiding overstimulation from activities, limiting social visits, and scheduling quiet time with rest or naps (Flint, 2001).

When anxiolytic drugs are prescribed, the benzodiazepines are often chosen for patients age 65 and older. Unfortunately, side effects are prevalent, among which are the discomforts of discontinuing the therapy. Benzodiazepines can impact cognitive function and psychomotor performance in older adults (Wetherell, et al., 2005). The patient may experience increased agitation, anxiety, and insomnia. More serious symptoms include tremors, tachycardia, diaphoresis, nausea, vomiting, and alterations in perception, anterograde amnesia, and seizures. The benzodiazepines have a propensity for dependence by accumulating in the elderly body. For this reason they should be prescribed for short courses of up to 2 weeks at most (Pontillo, et al., 2002).

The elderly patient receiving benzodiazepine therapy often experiences significant daytime sedation, dizziness, and subsequent falls. Studies indicate the "oldest old," those older than age 85, have a 15-fold increased risk of falls with benzodiazepine use. When a benzodiazepine with a long half-life is prescribed, the fall rate is 10-fold greater than when a benzodiazepine with a short to moderate half-life is prescribed (Caramel, et al., 1998). Benzodiazepines with a long half-life include diazepam and flurazepam (Dalmane); benzodiazepines with a shorter half-life include lorazepam (Ativan), alprazolam (Xanax), and oxazepam (Serax). When a benzodiazepine is prescribed, it should have a short half-life, be for short-term use, and be given in the lowest dose possible (Wetherell, et al., 2005).

The selective serotonin reuptake inhibitors (SSRIs), which treat depression, general anxiety, and panic and obsessive–compulsive disorders, are now considered the better choice for treating anxiety in the frail elderly due to their favorable side effect profile (Sheikh & Cassidy, 2003). There is often comorbid depression with anxiety, so an SSRI may treat both conditions, such as sertraline (Zoloft) for panic and depression (Pontillo, et al., 2002).

An alternative anxiolytic is buspirone (BuSpar). It is nonsedating, has minimal drug interactions, and a slow onset of action, 2 to 3 weeks. For that reason it is not indicated for acute anxiety but works well as an add-on drug (Flint, 2001). Caution must be used with buspirone in patients with Parkinson's disease because EPSs can occur. For anxiety with underlying depression and insomnia, trazodone (Desyrel) is an alternative. Because of its sedating properties, it promotes sleep and treats underlying depression that may exacerbate anxiety (Pontillo, et al., 2002).

Antidepressants

The prevalence of depression increases with age, as evidenced by 25% of those with chronic illness and a 15% to 25% rate of depression among nursing home residents (Bergman, et al., 2009). Elderly patients with late life depression exhibit more psychotic symptoms, delusions, insomnia, and somatic complaints (Attupurath, et al., 2008). In such settings, elderly patients with depression should be treated because antidepressant treatment usually improves nutrition and function and decreases symptoms of pain and insomnia (Lantz, 2001). Better choices for antidepressants include SSRIs (e.g., paroxetine, fluoxetine [Prozac], sertraline [Zoloft], citalopram [Celexa], and escitalopram [Lexapro]). SSRIs have the advantage of daily dosing and fewer side effects than TCAs, which were used frequently before the advent of SSRIs. Although the TCAs are still used, they are associated with many side effects that can lead to cognitive impairment and falls. Cardiovascular effects include hypotension, arrhythmias, and sudden death. Other troublesome side effects include sedation, dry mouth, urinary retention, and dizziness from anticholinergic properties.

Significant drug interactions and toxicity may occur with SSRI use because these drugs inhibit oxidative metabolism. Drugs that may be affected by SSRIs include warfarin, phenytoin, and class 1C antiarrhythmics (Lavretsky, 2001). Studies indicate that older adults taking SSRIs have a greater risk of falls than older adults not taking antidepressants (Leipzig, et al., 1999) and suggest higher doses of combined CNS medications, such as SSRIs, benzodiazepines, and antipsychotics, can lead to cognitive decline in older adults (Wright, et al., 2009). Common side effects of SSRIs in the elderly include headache, nausea, dry mouth, dizziness, constipation, dyspepsia, diarrhea, asthenia, insomnia, decreased appetite, tachycardia, and abnormal taste (Bergman, et al., 2009). Hyponatremia has been increasingly noted to occur in elderly patients on SSRIs. On withdrawal of the SSRI, sodium levels return to normal within days to weeks (Kirby & Ames, 2001). The prescriber needs to be aware of early signs of hyponatremia: lethargy, fatigue, muscle cramps, anorexia, and nausea.

Other Disorders and Drug Therapies

Pain medications such as narcotic analgesics should be avoided to reduce the risk of confusion, delirium, and falls. Acetaminophen (Tylenol) is often sufficient to reduce pain and discomfort.

To avoid hepatotoxicity, caution should be taken not to exceed 4000 mg in 24 hours, especially with known liver disease, alcoholism, and malnutrition. Combination pain products often contain acetaminophen, so caution must be taken to avoid going over the daily maximum dosage (Strassels, et al., 2008). Propoxyphene (Darvon) has often been used to treat mild to moderate pain in the elderly. Based on recommendations by the FDA, it was withdrawn from the U.S. market in November 2010 due to safety risks of serious heart toxicity and arrhythmias.

The chronic pain of degenerative joint disease unrelieved by acetaminophen can be treated with an NSAID. Long-term treatment with NSAIDs can result in GI bleeding, anemia, and renal insufficiency (Luggen, 2003). Caution should be taken when on highly bound drugs, such as warfarin, digoxin, and anticonvulsants, because increased bioavailability occurs due to NSAIDs being highly protein bound (Strassels, et al., 2008). The cyclooxygenase 2 (COX-2) inhibitor celecoxib (Celebrex) is a nontraditional anti-inflammatory drug developed to prevent GI bleeding by not affecting platelet aggregation and bleeding. Although the risk of bleeding with COX-2 inhibitors may be lower than traditional NSAIDs, such as naproxen or ibuprofen, it can still occur (Luggen, 2003). Cardiovascular safety issues led to the withdrawal of rofecoxib and valdecoxib from the market in the United States (Strassels, et al., 2008).

Neuropathic pain from post-herpetic neuralgia or diabetic neuropathy can be treated with mixed serotonin and norepinephrine uptake inhibitors, such as duloxetine (Cymbalta) and venlafaxine (Effexor), with a better side-effect profile than older TCAs. The anticonvulsant agents gabapentin (Neurontin) and carbamazepine (Tegretol) are also effective in treating neuropathic pain. Pregabalin (Lyrica) is indicated for diabetic peripheral neuropathy; however, it can cause somnolence and dizziness.

Topical analgesics can be effective in pain management in the long-term care setting. The 5% lidocaine patch may help with neuralgia pain, although it is often used off label for localized back pain or arthritis. A newer topical NSAID diclofenac (Flector) is indicated for chronic pain management with less systemic absorption than oral NSAIDs (AGS Panel on Pharmacological Management of Persistent Pain in Older Persons, 2009).

Other commonly encountered drug-related problems in long-term care are urinary incontinence and recurrent urinary tract infections, evidenced by confusion and mental status changes. Respiratory infections such as bronchitis and pneumonia quickly spread through a facility because of the compromised immune state of frail residents. Thus, antibiotic use is called on more frequently than for the community-residing adult. The frail elderly patient with pneumonia may not have typical signs of illness. For example, the patient may not have a cough or fever. Moreover, the frail elderly patient becomes ill more quickly and decompensates rapidly if untreated. Dehydration, sepsis, or even death may result.

Constipation is another concern, and sometimes an obsession, of elderly patients. In many instances, they think they need medications to promote bowel movements. However, alternate methods of treating this problem may be judicious, including increasing physical activity and consumption of fluids, fiber, and fruit. One or two tablespoons of a mixture of prune juice, unprocessed bran, and applesauce taken daily is an alternative to stool softeners and laxatives. When assessing constipation, a review of current medications may yield clues to drug use that contributes to the constipation. For example, anticholinergics, such as oxybutynin (Ditropan) used for urinary incontinence; antidepressants, such as the TCAs; and calcium channel blockers may all cause constipation in the frail elderly patient.

In summary, the elderly resident in long-term care is usually the frailest and at greatest risk for complications related to improper drug administration. The health care provider should attempt to keep medications at a minimum with the lowest dosage possible. A monthly or bimonthly review of all medications should be done to review medical necessity. A pharmacist from within the facility or from the company supplying the facility with medications should routinely review charts and write recommendations to decrease or stop medications. The suggestions should be evaluated by the health care provider and acted on if appropriate to reduce polypharmacy, side effects, and costs for the resident.

GUIDELINES FOR SAFE PRESCRIBING

The goal of prescribing for patients in long-term care should be to prevent adverse events, falls, and injuries that will further degrade the patient's function, both physical and mental. The provider must prescribe cautiously and keep the patient's safety in mind while promoting his or her comfort and dignity. Providers in long-term care need to familiarize themselves with the Beers criteria, a consensus-based document listing potentially inappropriate medications for use in elderly patients and guidelines for safe prescribing practices. This extensive list of medication guidelines was created by a consensus panel of nationally recognized experts in geriatrics and updated in 2002 (Fick, et al., 2003).

Exploring Alternatives to Medication

The health care provider must evaluate new problems and determine if a medication is necessary as part of the treatment plan. If there are alternatives to medications, such as diet, exercise, and weight loss for borderline hypertension, or anti-embolism stockings instead of a diuretic for pedal edema, these options should be explored. Only after nonpharmacologic treatments fail should a medication be initiated. In knowing the patient's overall situation—physically, mentally, and socially—the provider has a baseline from which to consider the risks and benefits of medication therapy. **Table 6.5** lists 20 medications that should not be prescribed to any elderly patient (General Accounting Office, 1995). All of the drugs in this table are also present in the 2002 Beers Criteria (Fick, et al., 2003) except for phenylbutazone, which is no longer marketed.

Choosing Drugs Efficiently

When deciding on a medication for an older adult, a drug that treats two coexisting conditions should be considered. For example, a calcium channel blocker might be selected for the patient with angina and hypertension. An elderly man with hyperplasia of the prostate and hypertension may benefit from an α-adrenergic blocking agent such as terazosin (Hytrin).

TABLE 6.5	Twenty Drugs to Avoid in Elderly Patients	
Prescription Drug	**Use**	**Reason for Avoiding**
amitriptyline	To treat depression	Other antidepressant medications cause fewer side effects.
carisoprodol	To relieve severe pain caused by sprains and back pain	Minimally effective while causing toxicity. Potential for toxic reaction is greater than potential benefit.
chlordiazepoxide	To tranquilize or to relieve anxiety	Shorter-acting benzodiazepines are safer alternatives.
chlorpropamide	To treat diabetes	Other oral hypoglycemic medications have shorter half-lives and do not cause inappropriate antidiuretic hormone secretion.
cyclandelate	To improve blood circulation	Effectiveness is in doubt. This drug is no longer available in the United States.
cyclobenzaprine	To relieve severe pain caused by sprains and back pain	Minimally effective while causing toxicity. Potential for toxic reaction is greater than potential benefit.
diazepam	To tranquilize or to relieve anxiety	Shorter-acting benzodiazepines are safer alternatives.
dipyridamole	To reduce blood clot formation	Effectiveness at low dosage is in doubt. Toxic reaction is high at higher dosages. Safer alternatives exist.
flurazepam	To induce sleep	Shorter-acting benzodiazepines are safer alternatives.
indomethacin	To relieve the pain and inflammation of rheumatoid arthritis	Other nonsteroidal anti-inflammatory drugs (NSAIDs) cause fewer toxic reactions.
isoxsuprine	To improve blood circulation	Effectiveness is in doubt.
meprobamate	To tranquilize	Shorter-acting benzodiazepines are safer alternatives.
methocarbamol	To relieve severe pain caused by sprains and back pain	Minimally effective while causing toxicity. Potential for toxic reaction is greater than potential benefit.
orphenadrine	To relieve severe pain caused by sprains and back pain	Minimally effective while causing toxicity. Potential for toxic reaction is greater than potential benefit.
pentazocine	To relieve moderate to severe pain	Other narcotic medications are safer and more effective.
pentobarbital	To induce sleep and reduce anxiety	Safer sedative–hypnotics are available.
phenylbutazone	To relieve the pain and inflammation of rheumatoid arthritis	Other NSAIDs cause fewer toxic reactions.
propoxyphene	To relieve mild to moderate pain	This drug is no longer available in the United States.
secobarbital	To induce sleep and reduce anxiety	Safer sedative–hypnotics are available.
trimethobenzamide	To relieve nausea and vomiting	Least effective of the available antiemetics.

Data from General Accounting Office. (1995). *Prescription drugs and the elderly: Many still receive potentially harmful drugs despite recent improvements* (HEHS-95-152). Washington, DC: Author.

Treating two conditions with one medication reduces cost, cuts down on dosing schedules, and improves adherence and patient satisfaction.

Simplifying the Regimen

Simplifying the medication plan is a key to therapeutic adherence and safety. Drugs are started at the lowest dose possible and the dosage increased as needed (Routledge, et al., 2003). Lower doses are often effective and reduce the risk of toxicity. Dosing schedules must be easy to follow and remember. If two drugs are equally suitable to treat the same condition, it is desirable to prescribe the one that requires the least frequent dosing.

Another important concern is cost of the drug, especially if the drug is for long-term use. Many elderly patients are on fixed incomes and find the cost of prescription drugs unaffordable. If the most suitable medication for the condition is expensive, this is explained to the patient before purchase to prevent "sticker shock" or the embarrassment of not having enough money to pay for the prescription. A generic drug should be prescribed whenever possible.

Educating Patients and Caregivers

Potential side effects need to be discussed in a nonthreatening way to prevent needless fear or anticipation when starting a new medication. Many older adults forgo starting a medication for fear of potential side effects that may occur. The media are powerful in alarming patients about potentially undesirable or dangerous adverse effects, proven or not. Many older patients stop taking essential medications after reading or hearing something in the media pertaining to that particular drug.

Reviewing Medications

The provider working with a geriatric population should have the patient bring in all of his or her medications to each office visit or review a current medication card if the patient carries one. The current medications taken by the patient are recorded at each office visit as part of the progress note. This review alerts the provider to improper dosing and drug administration, misunderstanding of medications, and changes made by specialists and other professionals. The specialist is not always aware of all the medications or OTC drugs the patient takes and may prescribe a drug that places the patient at risk for interactions. As part of the review, the health care provider should ask about topical creams, vitamins, eye drops, and OTC products that may interact with prescription drugs. Patients do not always view these products as medications.

The provider should review all drugs periodically to determine if the dosage can be reduced or the drug discontinued. The goal should always be to use as little medication as possible to treat the multiple illnesses that challenge the older adult.

At the end of each office visit, the provider needs to give the medication list to the patient. Doses and times to take the medications and any special instructions need to be clearly stated and communicated in writing as appropriate. New medications should be listed by brand and generic name so there is no confusion. Clear writing with large lettering should be used, particularly if the patient has common vision impairments, such as cataracts, glaucoma, or macular degeneration.

The caps of the medication bottles that the patient brings to the office can be labeled with the reason for the drug (e.g., "blood pressure," "water pill," or "diabetes"). This helps to ensure that the patient has a basic understanding of the importance of each drug. If the caregiver of an older patient is available, the provider should explain any new medication changes or special instructions, especially for the patient with cognitive impairment or other changes in mental status.

THERAPEUTIC MONITORING

When memory problems are an issue, a medication planner helps. Labeled with the days of the week and four dosing times per day, the planner is a useful device for preparing medications for a week. A patient who fails to take the medications despite visual cues and careful labeling may be sending a signal that the family or other responsible caregivers need to investigate additional interventions, home care services, or future placement in assisted living or long-term care facilities.

It is important routinely to schedule and monitor the results of laboratory tests when the patient is taking medications that may result in fluctuating drug blood levels. For example, elderly patients taking such drugs as warfarin, theophylline (Theo-Dur), digoxin, and quinidine (Quinaglute) need careful monitoring, as do patients taking anticonvulsant medications, such as phenytoin, carbamazepine (Tegretol), and valproic acid (Depakote), for seizure disorders.

Patients taking diuretics or angiotensin-converting enzyme (ACE) inhibitors require periodic evaluation with a renal profile to detect electrolyte imbalances, as well as renal insufficiency (as evidenced by rising blood urea nitrogen [BUN] and creatinine levels). Patients starting ACE inhibitor therapy should have a baseline BUN/creatinine level documented with

a follow-up test in 2 weeks to alert for renal artery stenosis (evidenced by a rise in the BUN/creatinine levels). Because of the potential for elevations in serum potassium concentration with ACE inhibitor therapy, the elderly need routine renal profiles to detect such changes, especially when drug therapy also includes diuretics and digoxin (Lanoxin). (**Box 6.3** presents guidelines for prescribing drugs safely for elderly patients.)

BOX **6.3**

Guidelines for Safe Prescribing for Elderly Patients

- Schedule routine follow-up examinations for the patient who has multiple chronic illnesses and who takes multiple medications.
- Review the risks and benefits of adding a medication. Explore nonpharmacologic options first.
- If possible, choose one medication that treats two coexisting problems.
- Always start with the lowest dose possible and titrate up slowly. "Start low; go slow."
- Choose a drug with the fewest daily required doses (i.e., daily vs. twice daily).
- Remember to consider the cost of the brand name drug and consider generic equivalents if cost issues will deter compliance.
- Reduce dosages or discontinue medications if possible to avoid polypharmacy.
- Advise patients to bring all medications (prescription or over-the-counter) to each office visit for review.
- Write down all current medications and dosages on the progress note for each office visit.
- Review medications added by other practitioners and specialists. Inform these professionals of changes made by the primary health care provider.
- Give a written list to the patient after each office visit of the medications to be taken.
- Write written medication instructions and changes in large print.
- Explain and write both the generic and brand name of the prescribed drug to avoid confusing the patient.
- Review medications and changes in the regimen with the caregivers of patients with cognitive impairments.
- Recommend or provide medication planners or weekly/daily dosage containers to improve compliance and promote safe medication administration.
- Schedule blood tests regularly to monitor levels of such medications as diuretics, ACE inhibitors, antiseizure medications, anticoagulants, antiarrhythmics, and digitalis.

BIBLIOGRAPHY

Starred references are cited in the text.

*American Geriatric Society Panel on the Pharmacological Management of Persistent Pain in Older Persons. (2009). Pharmacological management of persistent pain in older persons. *Journal of the American Geriatrics Society, 57*(8), 1331–1346.

*American Geriatric Society & American Association for Geriatric Psychiatry. (2003). Consensus statement on improving the quality of mental health care in U.S. nursing homes: Management of depression and behavioral symptoms associated with dementia. *Journal of the American Geriatric Society, 51*(9), 1287–1298.

*American Psychiatric Association. (1994). *Diagnostic and statistical manual of mental disorders* (4th ed.). Washington, DC: Author.

*Arias, E. (2004). *United States Life Tables, 2002. National Vital Statistics Reports, 53*(6). Hyattsville, MD: National Center for Health Statistics.

*Attupurath, R., Menon, R., Nair, S., et al. (2008). Late-life depression. *Annals of Long-Term Care: Clinical Care and Aging Supplement*, 21–29.

Bennett, W. M., Aranoff, G. R., Golper, T. A., et al. (1991). *Drug prescribing in renal failure: Dosing guidelines for adults* (2nd ed.). Philadelphia, PA: American College of Physicians.

*Bergman, S., Ronald, K., Gonzales, M., & Ruscin, J. (2009). Pharmacotherapy update 2009, Part 1: Cardiology, neurology, and psychiatry. *Annals of Long-Term Care, 17*(12), 30–34.

*Burdick, K., & Goldberg, J. (2002). Cognitive advantages of new anticonvulsants in treating a geriatric population. *Clinical Geriatrics, 10*(10), 25–36.

Caracci, G. (2003). The use of opioid analgesics in the elderly. *Clinical Geriatrics, 11*(11), 18–21.

*Caramel, V., Remarque, E., Knook, D., et al. (1998). Benzodiazepine users aged 85 and older fall more often. *Journal of the American Geriatric Society, 46*(9), 1178–1179.

*Chutka, D., Takahashi, P., & Hoel, R. (2004). Inappropriate medications for elderly patients. *Mayo Clinic Proceeding*s, *79*(1), 122–139.

Cooke, C., & Proveaux, W. (2003). A retrospective review of the effect of COX-2 inhibitors on blood pressure change. *American Journal of Therapeutics, 10*(5), 311–317.

*Cusack, B., & Vestel, R. (2000). Clinical pharmacology. In M. Beers & R. Berkow (Eds.), *The Merck manual of geriatrics* (3rd ed., pp. 54–74). Whitehouse Station, NJ: Merck Research Laboratories.

*Eslami, M., & Espinoza, R. (2003). Update on treatment for Alzheimer's disease—Part 1: Primary treatments. *Clinical Geriatrics, 11*(12), 42–49.

*Espinoza, R., & Eslami, M. (2004). Update on treatment for Alzheimer's disease—Part II: Management of noncognitive, psychiatric, and behavioral complications. *Clinical Geriatrics, 12*(1), 45–53.

*Feinberg, S., & Provenzano, D. (2010). *ACPA consumer guide to pain medication and treatment* (2010 ed., p. 8). Rocklin, CA: American Chronic Pain Association.

*Fick, D., Cooper, J., Wade, W., et al. (2003). Updating the Beers criteria for potentially inappropriate medication use in older adults. *Archives of Internal Medicine, 163*, 2716–2724.

*Flint, A. (2001). Anxiety disorders. *Clinical Geriatrics, 9*(11), 21–30.

*General Accounting Office. (1995). *Prescription drugs and the elderly: Many still receive potentially harmful drugs despite recent improvements* (HEHS-95-152). Washington, DC: Author.

*Guralnik, J., & Havlik, R. (2000). Demographics. In M. Beers & R. Berkow (Eds.), *The Merck manual of geriatrics* (3rd ed., pp. 9–21). Whitehouse Station, NJ: Merck Research Laboratories.

Hayes, B., Klein-Schwartz, W., & Barrueto, F. (2007). Polypharmacy and the geriatric patient. *Clinics in Geriatric Medicine, 23*(2), 2007.

*Hile, E., & Studenski, S. (2007). Instability and falls. In E. Duthie, P. Katz & M. Malone (Eds), *Practice of geriatrics* (4th ed.). Philadelphia, PA: Saunders.

Horowitz, M. (2000). Aging and the gastrointestinal tract. In M. Beers & R. Berkow (Eds.), *The Merck manual of geriatrics* (3rd ed., pp. 1000–1052). Whitehouse Station, NJ: Merck Research Laboratories.

*Jeste, D., Schneider, L., De Deyn, P., et al. (2003). Atypical antipsychotics for the management of patients with dementia and psychotic symptoms. *Clinical Geriatrics and Annals of Long-Term Care* (Suppl.).

*Juurlink, D., Mamdani, M., Kopp, A., et al. (2003). Drug-drug interactions among elderly patients hospitalized for drug toxicity. *Journal of the American Medical Association, 289*(13), 1652–1658.

*Kasper, J., & Burton, L. (2003). Demography. In E. Flaherty, T. Fulmer, & M. Mezey (Eds.), *Geriatric nursing review syllabus* (pp. 7–12). New York, NY: American Geriatric Society.

*Katz, P., & Karuza, J. (2003). Nursing-home care. In E. Flaherty, T. Fulmer, & M Mezey (Eds.), *Geriatric nursing review syllabus* (pp. 97–102). New York, NY: American Geriatric Society.

*Kelleher, C., & Lindeman, R. (2003). Renal diseases and disorders. In E. Flaherty, T. Fulmer, & M. Mezey (Eds.), *Geriatric nursing review syllabus* (pp. 357–365). New York, NY: American Geriatric Society.

*Kirby, D., & Ames, D. (2001). Hyponatremia and selective serotonin reuptake inhibitors in elderly patients. *International Journal of Geriatric Psychiatry, 16*(5), 484–493.

*Lantz, M. (2001). Depression in the elderly: Recognition and treatment. *Clinical Geriatrics, 10*(10), 18–24.

*Lantz, M. (2002). Alcohol abuse in the older adult. *Clinical Geriatrics, 10*(2), 40–42.

*Lavretsky, H. (2001). Choosing appropriate treatment for geriatric depression. *Clinical Geriatrics, 9*(5), 30–46.

*Leipzig, R., Cumming, R., & Tinetti, M. (1999). Drugs and falls in older people: A systematic review and meta-analysis: Psychotropic drugs. *Journal of the American Geriatric Society, 47*(1), 30–39.

*Logue, R. (2002). The impact of advanced practice nursing on improving medication adherence in the elderly: An educational intervention. *American Journal for Nurse Practitioners, 6*(5), 9–15.

*Luggen, A. (2003). Arthritis in older adults. *Advance for Nurse Practitioners, 11*(3), 26–35.

*Meiner, S. (1997). Polypharmacy in the elderly. *Advance for Nurse Practitioners, 5*(7), 26–34.

*Miller, C. (2004) *Nursing for wellness in older adults: Theory and practice* (4th ed., pp. 503–537). Philadelphia, PA: Lippincott Williams & Wilkins.

*Moore, A., Karno, M., Grella, C., et al. (2009). Alcohol, tobacco, and nonmedical drug use in older U.S. adults: Data from the 2001/02 national epidemiologic survey of alcohol and related conditions. *Journal of the American Geriatric Society, 57*(12), 2275–2281.

*Murray, M., & Callahan, C. (2003). Improving medication use for older adults: An integrated research agenda. *Annals of Internal Medicine, 139*(5), 425–428.

*National Institute on Alcohol Abuse and Alcoholism. (1998). Alcohol and aging. *Alcohol Alert No. 40*. Bethesda, MD: Author.

*Norris, S., High, K., Gill, T., et al. (2008). Health care for older Americans with multiple chronic conditions: A research agenda. *Journal of American Geriatric Society, 56*(1), 149–159.

*Oslin, D. (2003). Substance abuse. In E. Flaherty, T. Fulmer, & M. Mezey (Eds.), *Geriatric nursing review syllabus* (pp. 234–239). New York, NY: American Geriatric Society.

*Peterson, A. M., & Dragon, C. J. (1998). Improving medication compliance in patients receiving home care. *Home HealthCare Consultant, 5*(9), 25–27.

*Pham, C., & Dickman, R. (2007). Minimizing adverse drug events in older patients. *American Family Physician, 76*(12), 1837–1844.

Physicians desk reference (1998). Montvale, NJ: Medical Economics.

*Pontillo, D., Lang, A., & Stein, M. (2002). Management and treatment of anxiety disorders in the older patient. *Clinical Geriatrics, 10*(10), 38–49.

*Rollason, V., & Vogt, N. (2003). Reduction of polypharmacy in the elderly. *Drugs and Aging, 20*(11), 817–832.

*Routledge, P., Mahony, M., & Woodhouse, K. (2003). Adverse drug reactions in elderly patients. *British Journal of Clinical Pharmacology, 57*(2), 121–126.

*Scholz, B., Holmes, H., & Marcus, D. (2008). Use of herbal medications in elderly patients. *Annals of Long-term Care, 16*(12), 24–28.

*Semla, T., & Rochon, P. (2003). Pharmacotherapy. In E. Flaherty, T. Fulmer, & M. Mezey (Eds.), *Geriatric nursing review syllabus* (pp. 35–42). New York, NY: American Geriatric Society.

*Sheikh, J., & Cassidy, E. (2003). Anxiety disorders. In E. Flaherty, T. Fulmer, & M. Mezey (Eds), *Geriatric nursing review syllabus* (pp. 220–223). New York, NY: American Geriatric Society.

*Shiyanbola, O. & Farris, K, (2010). Concerns and beliefs about medicines and inappropriate medications: An internet-based survey on risk factors for self reported adverse drug events among older adults. *American Journal of Geriatric Pharmacotherapy, 8*(3), 245–257.

*Stefanacci, R. & Spivack, B. (2010). Impact of healthcare reform on today's Medicare beneficiaries—and on those who care for them. *Clinical Geriatrics, 18*(6), 42–48.

*Strassels, S., McNicol, E., & Suleman, R. (2008). Pharmacotherapy of pain in older adults. *Clinics in Geriatric Medicine, 24*(2), 275–298.

*Tseng, C., Dudley, R., Brook, R., et al. (2009). Elderly patients' knowledge of drug benefit caps and communication with providers about exceeding caps. *Journal of the American Geriatric Society, 57*(5), 848–854.

*van Doorn, C., Gruber-Baldini, A., Zimmerman, S., et al. (2003). Dementia as a risk factor for fall and fall injuries among nursing home residents. *Journal of the American Geriatric Society, 51*(9), 1213–1218.

*Vincent, G., & Velhoff, V. (2010). The next four decades. The older population in the United States: 2010 to 2050. Washington, DC: U.S. Census Bureau.

Wetherell L. J., Lenze, E., & Stanly, M. (2005). Evidence-based treatment of geriatric anxiety disorders. *Psychiatric Clinics of North America, 28*(4), 871–896.

*Wright, R., Roumani, Y., Boudreau, R., et al. (2009). Effect of central nervous system medication use on decline in cognition in community-dwelling older adults: Findings from the health, aging and body composition study. *Journal of the American Geriatric Society, 57*(2), 243–250.

CHAPTER 7

Maria Foy
Andrew M. Peterson

Principles of Pharmacology in Pain Management

One of the most widely encountered clinical situations is a patient in pain. Treatment of pain is one of the most difficult aspects of patient care. Pain is defined by the International Association for the Study of Pain as "an unpleasant sensory and emotional experience associated with actual or potential tissue damage, or described in terms of such damage." Pain is subjective and its intensity varies from patient to patient, day to day. The clinician has a large array of medications available to assist patients in relieving their pain. Principles of managing various types of pain will be described in this chapter and will introduce the practicing nurse to the many types and classes of drugs available for the therapeutic management of pain.

Analgesics represent one of the most frequently prescribed and administered classes of medications. Managing pain in the acutely or chronically ill patient requires both a sound comprehension of the clinical pharmacology of analgesics and a clear understanding of how pain is perceived. Clinicians caring for chronically ill patients not only find themselves assisting the patient in dealing with the physical component of pain, but often are confronted by the patient's psychological, spiritual, and social perceptions of pain and pain medication.

Age is a major consideration in assessing pain. For example, elderly patients are less likely to complain about pain and request fewer analgesics to alleviate pain, secondary to incorrect beliefs and biases. A corollary exists in pediatric patients, whose inability to adequately express suffering leads some clinicians to believe that children cannot feel pain. Clinicians, however, now realize that pediatric patients experience as much pain as adults. Because of the identified communication barrier, clinicians need to evaluate a child in pain by utilizing special pain assessment tools developed for children. Similar assessment tools are utilized for adults who may not be able to verbally communicate their pain.

TYPES OF PAIN

Pain can be categorized as nociceptive or neuropathic based on the presumed underlying cause. Nociceptive pain occurs as a result of nerve receptor stimulation following tissue injury, disease, or inflammation. Nociceptive pain can be further classified as somatic or visceral. Somatic pain is associated with injury to tissue of muscle, skin, or bone. When pain affects the visceral organs, such as pain seen in appendicitis or pancreatitis, it is referred to as visceral pain.

Neuropathic pain is caused by abnormal signal processes in the central nervous system (CNS). Pain can be peripheral or central in origin, and is often the type of pain seen long after an acute insult has healed. Neuropathic pain is often seen in metabolic diseases (i.e., diabetes), human immunodeficiency virus, tumors, neurologic diseases (i.e., multiple sclerosis), and trauma. Descriptors of neuropathic pain, such as electric-like, burning, tingling, or shooting, can differentiate this type of pain from nociceptive pain and help determine appropriate treatment.

CLASSIFICATION OF PAIN

Pain can be classified into two categories, acute and chronic, which helps identify the derivation of the pain and provides a framework for treatment. Pain can subsequently be categorized and treated based on patient-specific symptoms and whether pain is nociceptive, neuropathic, or mixed in origin.

Acute Pain

Acute pain has a sudden onset, usually subsides quickly and is characterized by sharp, localized sensations with an identifiable cause. Acute pain is a natural physiologic response to injury, useful in warning individuals of diseases or harmful situations. This process is often seen as a signal that the body is invoking critical immunologic and physiologic responses to cellular or tissue damage. Concomitant physiologic responses include excessive sympathetic nervous system activity, such as tachycardia, diaphoresis, and increased respiratory rate. Surgical intervention and trauma are common sources of acute pain.

When acute pain responses become unremitting, constant, or under-treated, the biologic responses outlive their usefulness and can lead to chronic pain. Patients with chronic pain become tolerant to the physiologic response seen in acute pain. In addition, these patients often do not appear to be suffering from pain because constant pain becomes a way of life. Undesired consequences, such as anxiety and depression, are often associated with constant, long-term pain. The goal of acute pain management is to avoid progression to a chronic pain state. Early pain control that provides comfort to the patient will often prevent the development of chronic pain.

Chronic Pain

Chronic pain is arbitrarily defined as pain lasting longer than 3 to 6 months, although some argue that chronic pain begins when pain persists after the initial injury has healed. Further classification of chronic pain is based on the taxonomy of malignancy.

Identifying and differentiating pain through careful history of the location, quality, and nature is important because treatment choices are dictated by the cause and type of pain. In any case, the primary goal of therapy in chronic pain is to decrease the pain to a tolerable level, thereby improving patient functioning and quality of life. Examples of types of chronic pain are shown in **Box 7.1**.

BOX 7.1

Classification of Chronic Pain

NOCICEPTIVE PAIN

Arthropathies (e.g., rheumatoid arthritis, osteoarthritis, gout)
Ischemic disorders
Myalgia (e.g., myofascial pain syndromes)
Nonarticular inflammatory disorders (e.g., polymyalgia rheumatica)
Skin and mucosal ulcerations
Superficial pain (sunburn, thermal burns, skin cuts)
Visceral pain (appendicitis, pancreatitis)

NEUROPATHIC PAIN

Alcoholic neuropathy
Cancer-related pain and some cancer treatments
Chronic regional pain syndrome
Human immunodeficiency virus (HIV)–related pain and some HIV treatments
Pain associated with multiple sclerosis
Painful diabetic neuropathy
Phantom limb pain
Postherpetic neuralgia
Poststroke pain (central pain)
Trigeminal neuralgia

MIXED OR UNDETERMINED PATHOPHYSIOLOGY

Chronic recurrent headaches
Painful vasculitis

Chronic Cancer Pain

Cancer pain is pain associated with malignancy and can result from the disease itself or damage to secondary tissue. Disease-induced pain includes pain secondary to direct tumor involvement of bone, nerves, viscera, or soft tissue. In addition, muscle spasm, muscle imbalance, or other body structure/function changes secondary to the tumor are considered disease induced. Pain may be associated with treatment of the disease and can be seen with biopsies, surgeries, and/or chemotherapy and radiation treatments. Pain can also be found in sites where cancer has metastasized (i.e., bone pain). Cancer and treatment interventions may activate peripheral nociceptors, causing somatic and visceral nociceptive pain. Neuropathic pain involving the sympathetic nervous system may also be seen.

Chronic Noncancer Pain

Chronic noncancer pain (CNCP) is persistent pain seen in patients not affected by cancer. Some examples of CNCP are rheumatoid arthritis, osteoarthritis, fibromyalgia, and peripheral neuropathies. Alternately, the pain may possibly be the disease itself when no cause of pain is identified, often occurring when pain persists long after an acute injury has healed. In the past, CNCP was referred to as *chronic nonmalignant pain*. The term CNCP is now preferred because pain may last for many years and is considered progressive in nature. CNCP may be nociceptive, neuropathic, or mixed in origin. (See **Box 7.1**.) Nociceptive mechanisms usually respond well to traditional approaches to pain management, including common analgesic medications and nonpharmacologic strategies. Neuropathic pain will respond to most traditional approaches including opioid therapy. However, higher doses of opioids are required to control this type of pain. Therefore, adjunctive treatment choices including anticonvulsants, antidepressants, or dual mechanism medications may be considered to replace or add to traditional treatment modalities.

Breakthrough pain

Breakthrough pain (BTP) is defined as a transitory pain seen often in chronic pain, where moderate to severe pain occurs in patients with pain otherwise well controlled. BTP is characterized as brief, lasting minutes to hours, and can interfere with functioning and quality of life. BTP has historically been associated with cancer pain. However, BTP can be seen in many other chronic pain conditions, such as neuropathic pain and chronic lower back pain. Pain may be idiopathic, due to certain activities (incident), seen during titration of medications, or when the duration of analgesia is less than the dosing interval.

PAIN PATHOPHYSIOLOGY

Several theories exist as to how information resultant from tissue damage is perceived by the brain as pain. Noxious stimuli from the point of the initial injury move through specialized nerve fibers within the spinal cord where the signal reaches consciousness and is perceived as pain. This transmission of the pain signal through the CNS is termed nociception. Once pain is perceived, pain can be lessened by activation of non-nociceptive neurons that reduce pain perception, historically explained in the "Gate Control Theory." The original Gate Control Theory proposed that "closing of the gate" to pain was accomplished primarily through the modulating actions of the CNS in response to pain. However, recent data have theorized that anxiety, fear, depression, and previous pain experiences also have an effect on pain perception. Description of nociception can be divided into four main categories: transduction, transmission, perception, and modulation (**Figure 7-1**).

Transduction

Peripheral nerves consist of many types of nerve fibers. Two fiber types, A-delta and C, are responsible for pain conduction from the area of insult to cell bodies in the CNS. Free nerve endings of the small myelinated A-delta fibers and larger unmyelinated C fibers are called nociceptors. Transduction occurs when the initial insult activates these nerve endings through the release of various chemical neurotransmitters, such as prostaglandins, substance P, histamine, bradykinins, and serotonin.

Transmission

Nociceptive information travels through the CNS via the primary afferent neurons by way of the dorsal root ganglia to the dorsal horn of the spinal cord. If the intensity of the

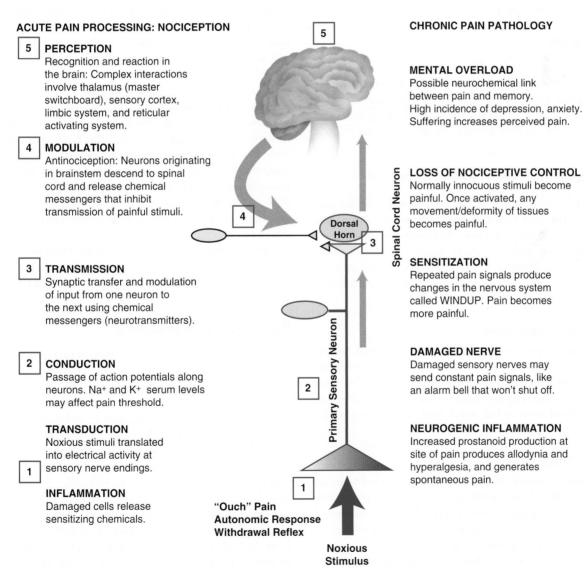

FIGURE 7–1 Acute and chronic pain pathophysiology. (From Whitten, C. E., Donovan, M., & Cristobal, K. [2005]. Treating chronic pain: New knowledge, more choices. *The Permanente Journal, 9*[4]. Retrieved from http://xnet.kp.org/permanentejournal/fall05/pain3.pdf.)

transmission is strong enough, second order neurons are stimulated and convey pain signals to the higher centers of the CNS. Neurotransmitters in the dorsal horn directly or indirectly depolarize the second order neurons, facilitating transmission of pain to the brain. Inhibitory substances are released in the dorsal horn (see section on modulation) and may decrease the number of signals reaching the brain, thereby lessening transmission.

Perception

Nociceptive information travels through different areas of the CNS, eventually reaching the cerebral cortex of the brain, where pain is perceived. Structures of both the cortical and limbic system are involved in how a person reacts to pain, explaining why pain perception is not just a manifestation of physical injury but is affected by psychosocial factors and previous experiences of pain.

Modulation

Activation of non-nociceptive neurons in the CNS inhibits nociceptive transmission along the descending pain pathways, lessening the perception of pain. Inhibitory neurotransmitters released from multiple areas of the CNS, along with other nervous system cognitive activity, can also affect pain modulation.

Peripheral and Central Sensitization

Often pain persists despite healing, and no reason for the pain can be found. Pain pathways become "broken," and pain is seen without an obvious cause. Modifications occur in the pain conduction pathways of the peripheral nervous system and CNS where hypersensitivity to pain stimulus and neuronal structural changes result in chronic pain syndromes referred to as *peripheral* and *central sensitization.*

Peripheral Sensitization

When pain receptors in the periphery are continually stimulated (i.e., untreated acute pain), the threshold for stimulation becomes lowered and increased nerve firing occurs. Increased frequency of nerve impulses result in more pain signals reaching the dorsal horn of the spinal cord, contributing to the development of central sensitization.

Central Sensitization

Central sensitization is defined as "a state of increased neuronal firing in the dorsal horn of the spinal cord." When nociceptive information repeatedly stimulates nerve fibers, increased dorsal horn neuronal activity is seen. With actual or potential nerve damage as in many cases of uncontrolled pain, the increase in firing causes increased excitability and responsiveness, termed central sensitization. The end result is a decrease of central pain inhibition, increased spontaneous neuronal activity in the dorsal horn, formation of neuromas causing an increase in receptive fields, and a decreased threshold for neuronal firing.

Sensitization of the NMDA (N-methyl-D-aspartic acid) receptor in the area of the dorsal horn also contributes to central sensitization. Allodynia (pain response to something painless), hyperalgesia (increased response to pain), persistent pain, or referred pain may result.

Central sensitization can occur in many chronic pain states, especially when associated with nerve injury or dysfunction. Alternately, inadequate treatment of acute pain may lead to sensitization of the CNS long after the acute injury has healed. Pain associated with central sensitization often responds poorly to traditional pain therapies. The addition of co-analgesics, reviewed later in the chapter, may be indicated for the treatment of chronic pain associated with central sensitization.

Chemical Mediators

Coupled with the neuronal component of pain is the release of chemical mediators initiating or continuing the stimulation of pain-conducting fibers. Peripheral chemical mediators include the neurotransmitters norepinephrine, serotonin, and histamine, and polypeptides such as bradykinin, prostaglandins (PGs), and substance P. Their role in the pain pathway is activating and sensitizing nociceptors and increasing neuronal excitability. Blocking the production of these mediators, particularly inhibiting the production of PGs with anti-inflammatory medications or similar compounds, minimizes nociceptor activation and neuronal firing, thereby lessening the transmission of pain through the CNS. Because of their role in initiating the pain pathway, these chemicals are targets for many of the medications currently available to treat pain.

Both excitatory and inhibitory neurotransmitters can be found in the dorsal horn of the spinal cord. Excitatory amino acids, glutamate, and aspartate, along with substance P, facilitate activation of second order neurons in the dorsal horn.

Pain-Modulating Receptors

Historically, pain modulation was thought to be primarily due to descending inhibitory information from the brain. Pain experts now theorize that descending inhibitory pain pathways and inhibitory neurotransmitters decrease the perception of pain. Inhibitory substances, such as endogenous opioids, norepinephrine, and GABA (gamma-aminobutyric acid) are released from the nerve fibers and attenuate the transmission of pain by modulating the pain signals in the dorsal horn. Endogenous opioid substances, primarily β-endorphins, stimulate inhibitory neuronal receptors known as the opioid receptors. Stimulation of these receptors, particularly the *mu* (μ) receptor, inhibits the transmission of pain signals to and from the higher brain centers. These receptors are stimulated by morphine-like drugs (opioids) and account for a great deal of the pain relief associated with this class of analgesics.

In contrast, neuropathic pain syndromes do not respond as well to conventional analgesic therapy. Neuropathic pain is often the result of peripheral and central sensitization.

Sensitization of the NMDA receptors by various mechanisms is primarily responsible for this type of pain and is the target for novel co-analgesics such as antidepressants, anticonvulsants, and antiarrhythmic agents.

GENERAL PRINCIPLES OF PAIN MANAGEMENT

Treatment of pain in today's society rests on two major principles: appropriate assessment of the severity and intensity of the pain and selection of the most appropriate agent to relieve pain with minimal side effects. Pain relief often requires a combination approach, using multiple agents that target different receptors and neurotransmitters in the CNS.

Pain Assessment

The individual assessment of a patient's pain is extremely important for determining proper treatments as well as monitoring effectiveness over time. According to the National Institutes of Health (NIH), self-reporting by patients is "the most reliable indicator of the existence and intensity of pain." Along with self-reporting, involving the caregiver's assessment of pain, especially in the very young or noncommunicating older patient, may be helpful. The self-report should include a description of the pain, location, intensity/severity, aggravating and relieving factors, and effect of pain on quality of life. Brief, easy-to-use assessment tools that reliably document pain intensity and pain relief and relate these to other dimensions of pain, such as a patient's mood, are recommended. One routine clinical approach to pain assessment and management is summarized by the mnemonic PQRSTU (**Box 7.2**). Assessment

tools should be used initially to obtain a baseline as well as throughout therapy to monitor progress.

Because pain is subjective and is not easily quantifiable, several tools are available to determine the quantity and quality of a patient's pain. The various pain scales can be classified as single or multidimensional and self-report or observational. Common single-dimension tools include the visual analog scale (VAS), numeric rating scale, and verbal description scale (**Figure 7-2**). The single-dimension scales evaluate the intensity of pain. Multidimensional scales consider location, pattern, and affective responses. Examples of multidimensional scales include the Brief Pain Inventory and the McGill Pain Questionnaire.

The information assessed, particularly from the numeric scale and VAS, can be used to determine appropriate treatment and drug selection. The Agency for Health Care Policy and Research (AHCPR) and the NIH have published guidelines on the appropriate evaluation and treatment of acute and chronic pain. Both organizations suggest using a 0-to-10 scale to assess a patient's current level of pain. Zero defines a pain-free state, and a 10 describes the most severe pain imaginable by the patient. Pain rated at 1 to 3 is classified as mild; 4 to 6, moderate; and 7 to 10, severe.

Subsequent assessments should evaluate the effectiveness of the treatment plan. If pain is unrelieved, determine whether the cause is related to the progression of disease, a new cause of pain, or the treatment of the disease itself. Tolerance to opioid treatments may develop in which the same amount of pain requires increasing doses of opioids. The assessment of the patient's pain and the efficacy of the treatment plan should be ongoing, and the pain reports should be documented. Continued use of the same pain scale is crucial to the continued assessment of treatment progress and communication between health care providers.

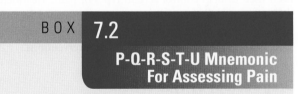

BOX 7.2

P-Q-R-S-T-U Mnemonic For Assessing Pain

P – Precipitating, palliating. What makes the pain better? What makes the pain worse?

Q – Quality of the pain. What does the pain feel like? (descriptors such as sharp, stabbing, burning)

R – Region, radiation. Where is the pain? In the area of the pain, does it stay in one place or does the pain radiate?

S – Severity. Use of pain scales (0-to-10 scale, FACES, visual analog)

T – Temporal pattern. Is the pain constant, intermittent, associated with movement?

U – How does the pain affect *you?* Quality of life indicator.

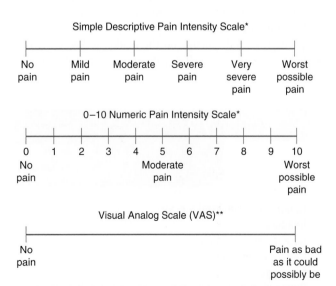

Simple Descriptive Pain Intensity Scale*

No pain / Mild pain / Moderate pain / Severe pain / Very severe pain / Worst possible pain

0–10 Numeric Pain Intensity Scale*

0 No pain ... 5 Moderate pain ... 10 Worst possible pain

Visual Analog Scale (VAS)**

No pain ... Pain as bad as it could possibly be

*If used as a graphic rating scale, a 10-cm baseline is recommended.
**A 10-cm baseline is recommended for VAS scales.

FIGURE 7–2 Visual analog scales used for ranking pain.

Pain Management

Treatment options for pain control include nonpharmacologic and pharmacologic treatment. **Box 7.3** lists treatments that complement medication management of pain. Often, a multimodal approach using a combination of treatments is necessary to reduce the pain to a tolerable level or eliminate it completely. The common goals of any type of pain therapy include relieving pain, maintaining patient function, and maximizing the patient's quality of life, while minimizing adverse effects of treatments.

An essential principle in using medications to manage chronic pain is to individualize drug regimens according to the type and severity of pain. Many routes of administration exist for the administration of pain medications. When possible, the oral route should be considered as first-line therapy because this delivery method is the least invasive.

For mild to moderate pain, acetaminophen, aspirin, or a nonsteroidal anti-inflammatory drug (NSAID) is usually considered initial therapy. Acetaminophen is used for mild pain across all age groups, mainly due to its favorable side effect profile. NSAIDs are very effective in pain associated with inflammation. However, patients may be at risk for gastrointestinal (GI) bleeding. Nonselective NSAIDS inhibit the enzyme cyclooxygenase (COX), which consists of three isoforms, COX-1, COX-2, and the recently identified COX-3. The COX-1 isoform produces PGs that regulate blood flow to the kidneys and GI tract and decrease platelet aggregation. The COX-2 isoenzyme is usually expressed in association with inflammation. First-generation NSAIDS inhibit both isoenzymes, thereby reducing inflammation but also increasing the incidence of GI adverse effects.

COX-2 inhibitors were subsequently developed in hopes of relieving pain but reducing the chance for GI toxicities. However, these agents were found to be associated with an increased risk of heart attack, stroke, and death. Only one COX-2 inhibitor, celecoxib (Celebrex), has benefits that outweigh its risks and remains on the market today. Celecoxib may be prescribed in select patients with risk factors for GI bleeding. COX-3 inhibition occurs centrally and is the proposed mechanism associated with acetaminophen's pain-relieving action.

For pain that persists or increases, combination opioids, such as oxycodone, hydrocodone, or codeine in combination with acetaminophen or ibuprofen, can be added to the regimen. These agents are indicated for the treatment of moderate to severe pain. More potent opioids, such as morphine, hydromorphone, or fentanyl, are used for the treatment of severe pain and may be used with various other co-analgesics depending on the source and type of pain. The concurrent use of co-analgesics often provides more pain control than either of the drug classes alone.

When developing a treatment plan, members of the health care team should pay particular attention to the preferences and needs of patients whose education or cultural traditions may impede effective communication. Certain cultures have strong beliefs about pain and its management. Members of these cultures may hesitate to report unrelieved pain or may have alternative methods of treating pain. Clinicians should be aware of the unique needs and circumstances of patients from different age groups or various ethnic and cultural backgrounds. In addition, many biases to opioids still exist in some patients and prescribers. Patient education may be effective in addressing cultural concerns and alleviating biases associated with pain treatments.

Pharmacologic treatment is the most common modality in pain control. However, nonpharmacologic options and therapies have been shown to be effective, especially in patients with chronic pain. Behavioral therapies, including systematic coping approaches and relaxation strategies, have been used to help control pain. Nonpharmacologic approaches include the use of physical therapies such as heat, cold, exercise, and complementary therapies such as acupuncture and massage. Transcutaneous electrical nerve stimulation therapy has also been used to help control certain types of pain. Treatment of difficult pain conditions that cannot be managed by noninvasive methods alone may require a consultation with a pain specialist to evaluate surgical options or interventions.

Drug Therapy by Type of Pain

The AHCPR suggests that mild to moderate pain be treated with step 1 drugs. Examples of step 1 drugs include acetaminophen and NSAIDs. Maximum dosages of these drugs should be used before proceeding to opioid analgesics. Aspirin has historically been used as a pain modality or as an antipyretic as well as short-term pain treatment. However, increased adverse effects limit its chronic use. Aspirin is mostly used today to prevent cardiac events and is not routinely used as first-line pain management therapy.

Step 2 drugs, such as combination opioids, ketorolac, and tramadol, are commonly used to treat moderate pain. The combination opioids contain the addition of a "non-opioid," such as acetaminophen or ibuprofen, creating a ceiling (maximum dose) of treatment. Propoxyphene, alone or in combination

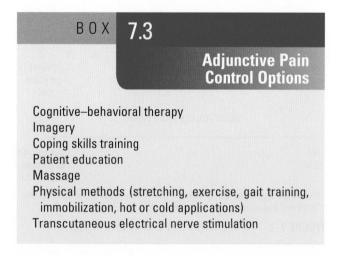

BOX **7.3**

Adjunctive Pain Control Options

Cognitive–behavioral therapy
Imagery
Coping skills training
Patient education
Massage
Physical methods (stretching, exercise, gait training, immobilization, hot or cold applications)
Transcutaneous electrical nerve stimulation

with a non-opioid, is no longer available as an agent in the treatment of pain. Propoxyphene was removed from the market by the FDA in 2010 due to increased adverse drug reactions (ADRs), especially in the elderly.

Once pain is no longer controlled by maximum doses of step 2 drugs or if ADRs occur, moving to the step 3 drugs is recommended. Severe pain is treated with step 3 drugs, of which morphine is the gold standard. When used in equivalent doses, most pure opioids (*mu* receptor agonists) are equally effective in controlling pain. Morphine, oxycodone, hydromorphone, oxymorphone, and fentanyl are opioids indicated for the treatment of severe pain. Morphine is considered the opioid of first choice unless a contraindication exists. Meperidine is another opioid that has historically been utilized for the treatment of severe pain. Use of this agent is no longer recommended because of the neurotoxicities associated with the accumulation of the active metabolite, normeperidine in the body. Accumulation is seen mostly in patients with renal insufficiency or with continual use.

In most chronic pain cases, pain medications should be administered around the clock, and as-needed medications used to treat "breakthrough" pain. This recommendation is based on the finding that regularly scheduled medications maintain a constant level of drug in the body and help prevent a recurrence of pain.

An essential principle in using medications to manage chronic pain is to individualize medication regimens according to the type and severity of pain. When at all possible, however, the oral route should be considered as first-line route of administration because this is the least invasive pain management modality. For mild to moderate pain, acetaminophen or an NSAID is usually considered initial therapy. Co-analgesics may also be used either as monotherapy or in conjunction with acetaminophen or an NSAID. For pain that persists or increases, an opioid should be added. Management for moderate to severe pain should begin first with a combination opioid, tramadol, or low doses of morphine. Severe pain is treated with higher potency opioids, such as morphine, hydromorphone, or oxycodone. Various classes of co-analgesics can also be utilized in combination with the opioids, which often provides more analgesia than either of the drug classes alone (**Table 7.1**).

Acute Pain

Acute pain is usually a response to tissue injury or trauma and is usually nociceptive in nature. Treatment includes non-opioids such as NSAIDs and acetaminophen for mild to moderate pain and opioid medications for moderate to severe pain. As acute pain increases, it becomes more difficult to manage. Therefore, it is important to treat acute pain promptly and effectively. Also, untreated acute pain is often the catalyst in the development of chronic pain conditions in which pain persists long after the injury heals.

Acetaminophen is the drug of choice for treating minor, noninflammatory pain, especially in patients at risk for GI damage. NSAIDs are also effective as monotherapy in the treatment of mild to moderate pain. Both acetaminophen and NSAIDs are available in combination with opioids in treating moderate pain. Pure or dual-mechanism opioids are used when pain is severe. The opioids as a class generally exhibit equal analgesic effects when given at equipotent doses (adjusted for route of administration and duration of action).

Various strategies are currently implemented in the control of pain. Postoperative pain is often treated with opioid medications because pain can be severe. The use of preemptive analgesia, defined as the administration of various analgesics prior to procedures, is currently being studied as a modality to decrease the development of postoperative pain. In addition, multimodal therapies using medications from more than one class may provide added benefits to better pain control while minimizing adverse effects.

Chronic Pain

Noncancer Pain

NSAIDs and salicylates are effective for chronic inflammatory conditions, such as arthritis and musculoskeletal conditions. Efficacy of NSAID treatment varies greatly among patients. Those who do not respond to one NSAID in one class may respond to an NSAID from the same or a different class. The opioids can be considered as an alternative or an addition to NSAID therapy in chronic noncancer pain if pain is moderate to severe. Administration of a lower-potency opioid in conjunction with a co-analgesic may be instituted if treatment failure of NSAIDs or acetaminophen occurs.

Historically, opioids were thought to be ineffective in chronic noncancer and neuropathic pain. It is now known that

TABLE 7.1	Recommended Order of Pain Treatment Based on Initial Pain Assessment				
Pain Rating	**Classification**	**NSAID/APAP**		**Opioids**	**Co-Analgesics**
1 to 3	Mild	√		Sometimes	√
4 to 6	Moderate	√		Usually	√
7 to 10	Severe	√		Usually	√

Supplement each level with nonpharmacologic therapy: *Psychological*—cognitive-behavioral therapy, biofeedback, relaxation, imagery, psychotherapy; *Physical Rehabilitation/Alternative Therapy*—stretching, exercise, reconditioning, thermotherapy, massage, acupuncture.

opioids will work against these types of pain but require higher doses. Utilizing co-analgesics as monotherapy or in combination with opioids may be effective in chronic pain treatment and may decrease opioid requirements.

Care should be taken when administering opioids to the elderly or in patients with respiratory diseases because of the increased chance of respiratory depression and over-sedation. Lower doses should be initiated in these patients and titrated based on response.

Physical dependence and fear of addiction should not be the overriding considerations when choosing a pain modality for patients. Often, biases exist when fear of addiction is present. Patients may "save the medication for when the pain gets bad." Patient education on the impact of untreated pain and on the differences between addiction and dependence may be needed to increase compliance to these medications.

Cancer Pain

The World Health Organization (WHO) outlines a step-wise approach to the management of cancer pain. The titration of therapy for cancer pain using this method has been effective in relieving pain for approximately 90% of patients with cancer pain (AHCPR, 1994; WHO, 1996). The WHO three-step analgesic ladder starts treatment with non-opioids ± adjuncts (co-analgesics) such as acetaminophen, aspirin, or NSAIDs. As pain persists and becomes moderate to severe, therapy should be started at the second or third step of the ladder. Step 2 medications consist of combination opioids, ketorolac, and tramadol. As pain continues to increase, substituting higher-potency opioids or dose escalation is the next consideration. As in the previous steps, the addition of non-opioids and co-analgesics is advocated as a multimodal approach. Morphine, oxycodone, hydromorphone, and fentanyl are the more common higher potency opioids used in the management of severe pain. Doses can be escalated to effect because these medications do not have an analgesic ceiling.

Methadone is a combination opioid with a dual mechanism, working by activating opioid receptors and as an NMDA receptor antagonist. Both actions help to inhibit pain. Methadone can be difficult to dose and has many drug–drug interactions and adverse reactions. Therefore, for safety reasons, methadone should be reserved for when treatment with other opioids fail. Referral to a pain professional trained in the safe dosing of methadone is recommended.

MEDICATIONS USED IN PAIN MANAGEMENT

The current pharmacotherapeutic options for pain management include non-opioid and opioid agents. Co-analgesic therapies, such as antidepressants, anticonvulsants, local anesthetics, and topical treatments, are often added especially in neuropathic and/or chronic pain conditions. Non-opioid analgesics include agents such as acetaminophen, NSAIDs, and salicylates. The opioid analgesics include oxycodone, morphine, and fentanyl.

Selection of the appropriate agent rests on an assessment of the patient's type and source of pain as well as the intensity level of the pain.

Non-Opioid Analgesics

The non-opioid analgesics are considered a first-line therapy in treating mild to moderate pain (**Table 7.2**). Pain is reduced, and a beneficial anti-inflammatory action may also be seen with some agents in this class. Onset of analgesia occurs within 1 hour of oral administration, and drug effects last anywhere from 4 to 12 hours. The agents can be classified by their mechanism of action, inhibition of PG synthesis, and anti-inflammatory activity. Aspirin, salicylates, and to a lesser extent, acetaminophen are inhibitors of PG synthesis, mediating pain through this pathway.

Acetaminophen

Acetaminophen is one of the most commonly prescribed analgesic–antipyretic medications. It is an effective alternative to aspirin. Acetaminophen's antipyretic activity comes from its direct action on the hypothalamic heat-regulating center to increase the dissipation of heat through increased vasodilation and perspiration. The analgesic activity is unknown, but may be mediated through PG inhibition in the CNS as a COX-3 inhibitor. However, lack of peripheral PG inhibition makes acetaminophen a weak anti-inflammatory agent and therefore not considered useful in treating inflammatory disorders such as rheumatoid arthritis. Acetaminophen does not adversely affect platelet aggregation or the gastric mucosa and is generally well tolerated.

Acetaminophen is almost completely absorbed from the GI tract and thus has an onset of action ranging from 30 to 45 minutes. Extensive liver metabolism to inactive substances makes acetaminophen a relatively nontoxic agent. However, a small portion (4%) of the drug is converted to a toxic metabolite, normally inactivated by glutathione pathways. Once glutathione stores are depleted, as seen in cases of chronic ingestion or acute overdosage, the toxic metabolite can cause potentially fatal liver necrosis. Generally, the maximum daily dose of acetaminophen should not exceed 4,000 mg. Lower maximum doses are recommended when two or more drinks per day are ingested or if liver disease is present.

Nonsteroidal Anti-inflammatory Drugs

NSAIDs are divided into a variety of chemical classes. Their physical and chemical properties determine their distribution in the body, leading to different therapeutic responses. NSAIDs as a class have anti-inflammatory, analgesic, and antipyretic activity because of their ability to inhibit COX, an enzyme necessary for PG synthesis. Traditional NSAIDs inhibit COX-1 and COX-2. Some NSAIDs, including aspirin, ketoprofen, and indomethacin, inhibit both enzymes but are mostly selective for COX-1. Ibuprofen and naproxen may be more selective for COX-2 inhibition and therefore less likely to cause GI toxicity. Newer agents, known as the COX-2

TABLE 7.2   Pharmacokinetic and Pharmacodynamic Properties of Non-Opioid Analgesics

Generic Name	Trade Name	Dosage Forms	Half-Life (h)	Onset (h)	Duration (h)	Route	Usual Starting Dosage	Max Dosage (24 h)
Acetaminophen	Tylenol, others	Tablet Suspension Suppository	6 to 7	0.5 to 0.75	3 to 5	PO PR	650 mg every 4 to 6 hours	4000 mg
Ibuprofen	Motrin, Advil	Tablets	1.8 to 2.4	0.25	2 to 3	PO	200 to 400 mg every 4 to 6 hours	3200 mg
	Caldolor	Suspension Injection				IV	400 to 800 mg every 6 hours	
Naproxen	Naprosyn	Tablets Suspension	12 to 15	1	8 to 12	PO	500 mg x 1, then 250 mg every 8 hours	1250 mg
Naproxen sodium	Aleve	Tablets	19	0.5	8 to 12	PO	550 mg x 1, then 275 mg every 12 hours	1375 mg
Diclofenac	Voltaren	Tablets Gel	2 1 to 2	0.5	8 to 12	PO Topical	25 mg every 12 hours	200 mg
Diclofenac Epolamine	Flector	Topical patch	12	1	12	Topical	1 patch every 12 hours	2 patches
Ketorolac	Toradol	Tablets Injection	5.5 to 7	0.5	4 to 6 5 to 6	IV, IM PO	15–30 mg IV every 6 hours 10 mg every 6 hours	120 mg 40 mg
Aspirin	Bayer, Excedrin, others	Tablet	0.25 to 0.33	0.5 to 0.75	4 to 6	PO	650 mg every 4 to 6 hours	4000 mg
Tramadol	Ultram	Tablet	6 to 7	1	5 to 7	PO	50 to 100 mg every 6 hours	400 mg
Choline magnesium trisalicylate	Trilisate	Tablet	9 to 17 (chronic dosing)	NA	NA	PO	1000 mg bid	3000 mg
Diflunisal	Dolobid	Tablet	8 to 12	1	8 to 12	PO	1 g x 1, then 500 mg every 8 to 12 hours	1500 mg

inhibitors, selectively block COX-2. COX-1 inhibition does not occur with normal doses, thereby decreasing GI side effects. However, COX-1 inhibition also decreases protective cardiovascular effects. Secondary to the platelet inhibition action of aspirin and other NSAIDs, risk of bleeding increases, especially with higher doses and/or chronic use. Other salicylates (e.g., salsalate) have minimal effects on platelet function but have been shown to be less effective pain relievers.

Lower doses of nonsteroidal therapies should be used in elderly patients to adjust for the decline in renal function. The NSAID analgesic effect is achieved within 1 hour of administration, with maximal effects within 2 or 3 hours. Anti-inflammatory effect has a longer onset, usually seen in 7 to 10 days. Decreased pain due to reduced tissue swelling is an indirect response to NSAIDs.

Long-term use of NSAIDs at high doses (anti-inflammatory doses) can cause serious adverse effects. Potentially serious ADRs are those affecting the GI tract and kidneys, such as GI bleeding and acute renal failure. Indomethacin (Indocin) is associated with more CNS and ocular adverse effects than other NSAIDs. NSAIDs should be taken with food or milk to minimize GI distress. The newer COX-2 inhibitors have less GI toxicity; however, the risk of renal adverse events is similar to traditional NSAIDs. In addition, cardiovascular toxicities, such as increased thrombotic events, heart attacks, and stroke, resulted in two of the three approved COX-2 inhibitors to be withdrawn from the market. Since that time, cardiovascular adverse effects have been shown to be a class effect. A black box warning on cardiovascular toxicities has been added to all NSAID products. Unlike NSAIDs, acetaminophen, and salsalate have minimal GI toxicity and no effect on platelet aggregation at usual doses. See Chapter 36 for more discussion of NSAIDs and acetaminophen.

Opioids

Opioids bind to opioid receptors in the CNS (*mu* (μ), *kappa* (κ), or *delta* (δ)), with analgesic effect primarily associated with μ and κ receptor binding. Full agonists include codeine, morphine, hydrocodone, oxycodone, hydromorphone, oxymorphone, fentanyl, meperidine, and propoxyphene. Meperidine and propoxyphene are associated with significant adverse effects and are no longer recommended as first-line therapy. Meperidine is metabolized to an active metabolite, normeperidine, which can accumulate and induce seizures with high doses or in patients with decreased renal function. Propoxyphene has historically been used for pain control. Due to lack of effectiveness and increased adverse reactions, propoxyphene is no longer available in the United States for treatment of pain. Pentazocine, a partial agonist–antagonist of opioid receptors, is also not recommended as a first-line pain management therapy.

Activation of the *mu* opioid receptor produces excellent analgesia as well as undesired effects, including respiratory depression, sedation, confusion, nausea/vomiting, itching, mydriasis, constipation, and urinary retention. With the exception of constipation, tolerance to these adverse effects usually develops over time. Morphine and other *mu* opioid

receptor agonists provide excellent pain relief over a broad dosage range. At equianalgesic doses and appropriate dosing intervals, there is no appreciable difference in pain relief among all of the opioid agents (**Table 7.3**). However, opioid rotation may be indicated if an allergy or an intolerable adverse reaction develops or if the maximum dosage is reached. The described potency is only a reflection of the dose needed to achieve a desired level of analgesia; the more potent the agent, the fewer milligrams needed (**Table 7.4**).

All opioids are hepatically metabolized to active and inactive metabolites, which are eliminated in the urine. Decreases in dosage and longer intervals may be needed in patients with severe liver disease. The metabolites of morphine are eliminated by the kidneys and are active. In patients with chronic renal insufficiency, morphine metabolites may accumulate and cause neurotoxicities, such as myoclonus, confusion, coma, and possible death. Therefore, morphine is relatively contraindicated in severe renal disease. Metabolites of other commonly used opioids, such as hydromorphone and oxycodone, are inactive, making them relatively safer choices to use in patients with renal failure. Fentanyl and methadone are considered the drugs of choice in the treatment of chronic pain in patients with renal disease.

The analgesic effects of oral opioids begin within 30 to 60 minutes and reach peak effect within 1 to 2 hours. Fentanyl is considered a short-acting opioid. Moderate-acting opioids, with duration of actions between 4 and 6 hours, include morphine, codeine, hydromorphone, oxycodone, and oxymorphone. Methadone, a dual-mechanism, long-acting opioid, has a variable duration of action and half life of approximately 24 to 36 hours. Steady state may take 5–7 days to be reached, therefore upward titration should not occur for at least 5 days after therapy initiation.

Morphine and Congeners

Morphine is a low-cost, readily available agent with well-characterized pharmacokinetic and pharmacodynamic properties. Morphine is absorbed erratically from the GI tract and undergoes significant first-pass hepatic metabolism when given by the oral route. Morphine is distributed throughout the body, and sufficient amounts cross the blood–brain barrier to account for most of its pharmacologic effects. Morphine has a plasma half-life of approximately 3 hours, which is due mainly to its nearly complete metabolism in the liver. Morphine crosses the placental barrier and is excreted in maternal milk.

Morphine may be administered orally, rectally, by injection, intrathecally, or intraspinally. The agent is available in short-acting, immediate-release dosage forms (tablets and liquid) and sustained-release tablets, such as MS Contin. Single-dose studies suggest that the oral dose is six times the parenteral dose, but with chronic dosing, the equivalent oral dose is three times the parenteral dose.

Morphine effectively relieves severe pain, particularly dull, chronic pain, regardless of its cause or anatomic source. Analgesia is due to the drug's effects in the CNS and spinal cord. Morphine not only alleviates pain but also alters the

TABLE 7.3 Pharmacokinetic and Pharmacodynamic Properties of Opioid Analgesics

Generic Name	Trade Name(s)	Route	Onset (min)	Half-Life (h)	Duration (h)	Usual Starting Dose
Moderate (combination opioids)						
Hydrocodone	Vicodin, Lortab, Lorcet, generic	PO	10 to 20	3.3 to 4.5	4 to 8	1 tablet (5 mg hydrocodone) every 4 hours
Oxycodone	Percocet, Percodan, generic	PO	15	2 to 3	4 to 5	1 tablet (5 mg oxycodone) every 4 hours
Moderate to severe						
Morphine immediate release	Various, generic	PO	30 to 60	2 to 3	4 to 6	10 to 15 mg every 3 to 4 hours
Sustained release	MS Contin, Kadian, Avinza	PO	15 to 60	15	8 to 12 (formulation dependent)	15 mg every 12 hours*
Injection	Various, generic	IV, SC	5 to 10	2 to 3	2 to 4	5 to 10 mg every 3 to 4 hours
Hydromorphone	Dilaudid	PO	15 to 30	1 to 3	4 to 5	2 mg every 4 hours
		IV, SC	5 to 10	1 to 3	4 to 5	0.5 mg every 4 hours
Oxycodone immediate release	Oxy IR, Roxicodone	PO	15 to 60	2 to 3	3 to 4	5 mg every 3 to 4 hours
Sustained release	Oxycontin	PO	50 to 60	5	8 to 12	10 mg PO every 12 hours*
Fentanyl	Duragesic	Transdermal patch	16 to 24	1.5 to 6	48 to 72	12 mcg patch every 72 hours*
		IV	0 to 5	2 to 4	30 to 60 minutes	
	Actiq, Fentora	Transmucosal	5 to 15	17	Related to blood level	**
Oxymorphone	Opana	PO	30	7 to 9	4 to 6	5 mg every 4 to 6 hours
	Opana ER	PO	30	10	12	5 mg every 12 hours
Levorphanol	Levo-Dromoran	PO	15	11 (up to 30)	6 to 8 (up to 15)	2 mg every 6 to 8 hours
		SC, IV	10 to 60	11 (up to 30)	6 to 8 (up to 15)	1 mg every 6 to 8 hours

(continued)

TABLE 7.3 Pharmacokinetic and Pharmacodynamic Properties of Opioid Analgesics (*Continued*)

Generic Name	Trade Name(s)	Route	Onset (min)	Half-Life (h)	Duration (h)	Usual Starting Dose
Dual Mechanism						
Methadone	Dolophine, others	PO	30 to 60	8 to 59	2 to 10 (acute) >12 (chronic)	2.5 to 5 mg every 8 to 12 hours
Tapentadol	Nucynta	IV PO	10 to 20 30 to 45	8 to 59 4	>8 (chronic) 4 to 6	1 to 2 mg every 8 hours 50 mg every 4 to 6 hours

Opioid Pearls

1. Use lower initial opioid doses in elderly and in patients with respiratory co-morbidities.
2. **Hydrocodone** for pain is only available in combination with acetaminophen or ibuprofen.
3. **Oxycodone** is available in combination with acetaminophen, aspirin, and ibuprofen.
4. **Morphine** is the opioid of choice unless contraindications exist. Morphine is relatively contraindicated in renal failure.
5. **Hydromorphone** is approximately five times the potency of morphine.
6. **Fentanyl** patch is contraindicated for acute pain and/or opioid naive.
   - Fentanyl patch may not be appropriate for patients with fever, diaphoresis, cachexia, morbid obesity, and ascites, all of which affects absorption and clinical effectiveness.
   - Patch may be appropriate for patients who cannot take long-acting oral opioids.
   - Onset of action is 12 to 24 hours after application. Utilize breakthrough pain (BTP) medications for pain control until onset of analgesia. Full effect takes 72 hours.
   - Application of external heat sources will increase the release of fentanyl from the transdermal system.
   - Titration of the patch should not occur before 3 days after the initial dose, or no more frequent than every 6 days thereafter.
7. **Methadone** has a duration of analgesia much shorter than half-life, making the drug difficult to dose.
   - Conservative dose conversions with careful titration is recommended. Use a higher conversion ratio in patients currently on high-dose opioids.
   - *Steady state not reached for at least 5 to 7 days. Use BTP medications early in the titration, as analgesic effects are shorter than the half-life of the drug. Observe for accumulation related side effects during titration (>2days treatment).
   - Consult a pain management specialist for dosing.

* Not initial therapy for opioid-naïve patients
** Cancer-related breakthrough pain only

TABLE 7.4	Basic Opioid Conversion Table	
OPIOID	**ORAL**	**PARENTERAL**
Morphine	30 mg	10 mg
Oxycodone	20 mg	–
Hydrocodone	30 mg	–
Hydromorphone	7.5 mg	1.5 mg
Oxymorphone	10 mg	1 mg
Codeine	200 mg	130 mg
Fentanyl	–	0.1 mg
Methadone	Dose dependent	2:1 oral to IV

perception of pain, so that discomfort is less distressing and/or more tolerable.

Therapeutic doses of morphine can cause respiratory depression. This effect is due both to the drug's actions on the brain's medullary respiratory control center and to the drug's ability to suppress the medulla's response to blood carbon dioxide levels. Respiratory depression is seen mainly in opioid-naïve patients or with upward dose titration. Tolerance develops relatively quickly to respiratory depressive effects. A person in whom tolerance has developed may experience only slight respiratory effects after receiving doses that could cause serious or fatal respiratory depression in a nontolerant person.

Morphine also increases smooth muscle tone in various parts of the GI tract. *Mu* receptors are located in the GI tract where receptor binding and stimulation of intestinal κ receptors result in reduced peristalsis and increased tone of the rectal sphincter. The overall resultant effect is constipation. Tolerance will not develop to opioid induced constipation; therefore, prophylactic bowel regimens consisting of a stimulant laxative and stool softener is recommended.

Hydromorphone is considered more potent and more soluble than morphine; however, it has a similar pharmacologic profile. Hydromorphone is available as an oral immediate-release tablet, a suppository, or an injectable formulation. Recently, a long acting formulation of hydromorphone was released to the U.S. market.

Oxycodone is slightly more potent than morphine. This agent may be used as monotherapy or in combination with non-opioid analgesics, such as ibuprofen or acetaminophen, for the reduction of moderate pain. Oxycodone is available as an immediate-release tablet, an oral liquid formulation, and a sustained-release tablet. No injectable form of oxycodone is currently available.

Hydrocodone, a derivative of codeine, is available in combination with non-opioid analgesics. Hydrocodone is equipotent to morphine on a milligram-to-milligram basis. However, ceiling doses of hydrocodone exist because it is only available in combination with acetaminophen or ibuprofen, thus limiting its use in more severe pain states.

Oxymorphone, the metabolite of oxycodone, is used to treat moderate to severe pain. Historically, oxymorphone was available as an injectable (Numorphan), but it is now only available as immediate-release and sustained-release tablets. Oxymorphone is approximately twice as strong as oxycodone, with 10 mg of oxymorphone equivalent to 20 mg of oxycodone. Adverse effects and mechanisms of action are similar to other opioids.

Codeine is usually administered orally either alone or in combination with non-opioid analgesics, such as acetaminophen, for mild to moderate pain. Codeine is primarily used as an antitussive agent. Other pain management modalities are more potent and better tolerated than codeine. Codeine has more of a stimulant effect on the CNS than morphine. This stimulatory effect of codeine is due to the formation of the metabolite norcodeine. The analgesic effect of codeine is due to its conversion to morphine. Approximately 10% of the population may not genetically carry the enzyme needed for this conversion, making codeine an ineffective pain therapy in these patients. Codeine has few advantages over morphine as an analgesic. At equianalgesic doses, codeine induces greater histamine release than morphine. This increases the risk of hypotension, cutaneous vasodilation, urticaria, and bronchoconstriction.

Fentanyl and Congeners

Fentanyl is an alternative to morphine and its congeners with low to no cross-allergenicity in patients with true hypersensitivity to morphine-like drugs. Fentanyl is available for acute pain as an injectable formulation only. Short-acting oral formulations are available, but its use is limited to severe breakthrough pain associated with cancer. A transdermal formulation is available for stable chronic pain and is contraindicated in opioid-naïve patients and acute pain processes. Peak systemic concentrations occur between 24 and 72 hours after initial application of the patch. Duration of action of the patch is approximately 72 hours. However, some patients may require patch changes after 48 hours.

Other agents, such as sufentanil (Sufenta) and alfentanil (Alfenta), also fall in this class but are used primarily for perioperative and postoperative pain relief and are available only in an injectable formulation.

Meperidine is a synthetic analgesic that binds strongly to both μ and κ receptors. Potency is less than that of morphine. Most of the pharmacologic effects of this drug are similar to those of morphine sulfate; however, adverse effects limit its use. High-dose meperidine may cause CNS excitation characterized by tremors and seizures due to the accumulation of its active metabolite, normeperidine. The half-life of normeperidine ranges between 15 and 20 hours and is almost completely renally eliminated. The possibility of accumulation of this metabolite leading to detrimental CNS effects has limited the use of meperidine in the treatment of pain.

Dual-Mechanism Analgesics

Tramadol is a centrally acting weak agonist of opioid receptors, inhibits norepinephrine reuptake and causes serotonin release. Tramadol is used to treat moderate to moderately severe pain and is available alone or in combination with acetaminophen. Tramadol may be useful for pain management in patients for whom an opioid is not a viable option and an NSAID may introduce undue risk (e.g., GI bleeding). In addition, tramadol may have a place in neuropathic pain management if initiated slowly and titrated to an effective dose. Tramadol may have less abuse potential when compared to other opioids. Tramadol is rapidly absorbed, and peak serum levels, which are obtained within 2 hours, persist for 4 to 6 hours. Tramadol is metabolized in the liver by the cytochrome P450 enzyme system to an active metabolite (O-dimethyl tramadol). Therefore, drug–drug interactions are common. Decreased maximum doses are recommended in the elderly and in patients with renal impairment. Increased seizure risk is seen with high doses or in patients with a history of seizure disorders.

Methadone is yet another chemical in a class historically used as an alternative to morphine-like drugs in patients with hypersensitivity. Methadone hydrochloride is effective both orally and parenterally and has an oral bioavailability exceeding 90%. It is more than 90% bound to plasma tissue proteins and is extensively metabolized in the liver to inactive products. Historically, methadone has been utilized for detoxifying opioid-dependent patients. Methadone is now being used more frequently in the treatment of chronic severe pain. Difficulty in dosing and many drug–drug interactions make methadone a second-line pain intervention recommended when conventional therapies fail. However, methadone works as both a *mu* receptor agonist and an NMDA receptor antagonist, making it effective for the treatment of severe neuropathic pain. The lack of active metabolites makes methadone a viable choice in patients with renal failure. The drug has a long half-life of nearly 40 hours in some patients, with an analgesic effect of approximately 4 to 8 hours. Early in methadone titration, pain control may not be adequate and aggressive breakthrough pain therapies are needed. Tendency to dose methadone aggressively early in titration can lead to serious adverse effects, including fatal respiratory depression and a prolonged QT interval. Patients should be monitored carefully for signs of drug accumulation or toxicity. The long biologic half-life also accounts for the mild, but prolonged, withdrawal syndrome if drug use stops abruptly.

Tapentadol is a recently approved combination opioid. Tapentadol works on opioid receptors and as a specific norepinephrine reuptake inhibitor. This medication has been shown to be effective in various pain conditions, such as osteoarthritis and postoperative pain. Currently, studies are being conducted in utilizing this medication for the treatment of neuropathic and chronic pain. Tapentadol has less affinity for the *mu* receptor than morphine, but its efficacy is comparable due to norepinephrine inhibition in addition to the *mu* receptor agonism. Tapentadol may have fewer GI-adverse effects (nausea, vomiting, constipation) when compared with other opioids due to less effect on the *mu* receptor.

Opioid Antagonist—Naloxone

Naloxone is a pure opioid antagonist that competitively binds to opioid receptors without producing an analgesic response. Naloxone is inactivated when given orally and therefore is given only by injection. Naloxone is indicated for treating opioid-induced respiratory depression (known or suspected).

The duration of naloxone's drug action is approximately 45 minutes. In most cases, this duration is shorter than the offending opioid and the overdose effect from the opioid usually returns, requiring readministration of naloxone. Care must be taken to avoid precipitation of withdrawal in opioid-tolerant patients when administering naloxone. The adverse effects of naloxone include tachycardia and hypertension, ventricular fibrillation, and cardiac arrest due to the release of neurotransmitters when naloxone is administered. Seizures have been reported, particularly in opioid-dependent patients.

Safety of Opioids

Side effects common to all opioids include sedation, confusion, respiratory depression, and GI disturbances. The GI disturbances are primarily constipation and nausea/vomiting, presumably due to stimulation of the κ opioid receptors located in the GI tract, which, when stimulated, decrease peristalsis and lead to constipation. Although considered the most dangerous side effect, severe respiratory depression is seen more often in patients with underlying pulmonary dysfunction or in cases of opioid overdose. In patients with closed head injury or recent brain surgery, opioids should be used with caution because hemodynamic effects (e.g., hypotension, orthostasis) may be exaggerated.

Bowel Regimen for the Prevention of Constipation

Tolerance usually develops within a few days to most of the adverse reactions associated with opioids except for constipation. Constipation needs to be prevented in patients receiving opioids. The general approach for patients receiving opioids is to institute a prophylactic bowel regimen consisting of a mild stimulant and a stool softener. Dose of the stimulant can be titrated to the patient's response. Initial dosing would consist of sennosides, 2 tablets daily or twice per day, and docusate sodium 100 mg twice per day. If there is no bowel movement in 48 hours, consider using an additional agent (e.g., bisacodyl suppository, lactulose) to stimulate peristalsis. If interventions continue to be ineffective, assess for impaction. If no impaction is present, utilizing an additional method (e.g., enema, mineral oil) is recommended. Once the patient has a bowel movement, titrate the dosage of senna to an effective dose. (Up to 12 tablets/day or the liquid equivalent has been used in the hospice population.) Docusate sodium should not be titrated aggressively because sodium salt may affect sodium levels.

Use of bulk-forming laxatives in patients receiving opioids is not recommended. Due to slower peristalsis in patients receiving opioids and potential inadequate fluid intake, the medication may lodge in the colon, causing bowel obstruction.

A new novel agent, methylnaltrexone, is now available to treat refractory constipation due to opioids. This agent specifically targets *mu* receptors in the GI tract and does not cross the blood–brain barrier. Therefore, reversal of analgesia does not occur.

Opioid Tolerance, Dependence, Pseudoaddiction, and Addiction

Opioid tolerance develops when chronic use of opioids causes the need for upward dose titration to maintain analgesia. Opioid dependence is defined as an emergence of withdrawal symptoms when the drug is abruptly discontinued or when the dose is rapidly decreased. Tolerance and physical dependence of opioids can develop quickly. Apparent dependence and/or tolerance in a patient with chronic pain should not impede aggressive therapy.

Patients taking opioids as briefly as 2 or 3 days may become dependent and can experience mild withdrawal symptoms upon discontinuation. These symptoms range from mild tremors to sweating and fever, and mimic flu-like symptoms. Severe withdrawal in opioid-tolerant patients may consist of increased respiratory rate, perspiration, lacrimation, mydriasis, hot and cold flashes, and anorexia.

Drug-seeking behavior may be demonstrated in patients with chronic pain and may be a result in worsening pain due to disease progression rather than drug abuse or addiction. Pseudoaddiction, defined as drug-seeking behaviors due to inadequate pain management, can be differentiated from true addiction because "pseudoaddictive" behaviors will resolve once adequate pain management is achieved.

Addiction is defined as "a primary, chronic, neurobiological disease with genetic, psychosocial and environmental factors influencing its development and manifestations. It is characterized by behaviors that include one or more of the following: impaired control over drug use, compulsive use, continued use despite harm and craving." True addiction is relatively rare in the general population, with incidence of about 10%. The concept of substance abuse with respect to opioids is an important consideration in patients with histories of substance abuse but is beyond the scope of this chapter.

Co-Analgesics

Several medications have been evaluated for use either alone or in conjunction with other analgesics to treat many persistent pain conditions. This can include many types of pain. However, the most benefit is seen in chronic pain, neuropathic pain, and postoperative pain syndromes.

Antidepressants

Antidepressants, including tricyclic antidepressants (TCAs) and selective norepinephrine reuptake inhibitors (SNRIs), exhibit analgesic effects by blocking the reuptake of primarily norepinephrine, thereby increasing pain-modulating pathway activity. TCAs have been useful in many chronic noncancer and neuropathic pain syndromes (i.e., diabetic or postherpetic neuropathy, chronic low back pain, and fibromyalgia). Several TCAs have beneficial effects in neuropathic pain, including amitriptyline, desipramine, and nortriptyline. Common side effects of urinary retention, confusion, and sedation are important to remember when considering treatment with this class of medications. Therapy with TCAs should not be initiated in the elderly due to an increased incidence of confusion and sedation due to anticholinergic activity, and may lead to falls.

Amitriptyline is the most studied TCA. The second-generation agent nortriptyline may be better tolerated than amitriptyline because there is less cholinergic and sedative effects. The SNRIs duloxetine and venlafaxine are newer agents used to treat neuropathic pain conditions. These medications are better tolerated than the TCAs because no cholinergic side effects are seen. GI disturbances, sedation, insomnia, sweating, and confusion may be seen with SNRI use. Venlafaxine has also been associated with increases in blood pressure.

Anticonvulsants

Another group of agents commonly prescribed for neuropathic pain conditions are the anticonvulsants. The most common agents used are gabapentin, pregabalin, divalproex, and carbamazepine. Gabapentin is the first-line anticonvulsant agent recommended for pain treatment. Pregabalin is structurally similar to gabapentin and has the same mechanism of action. These agents work by increasing concentration of GABA indirectly by attaching to the alpha voltage calcium channels. Gabapentin and pregabalin are generally well tolerated. Most common side effects include sedation, dizziness, fatigue, and ataxia. Gabapentin has been shown to be effective for many neuropathic pain conditions, including diabetic neuropathy, trigeminal neuralgia, restless legs syndrome, phantom limb pain, and pain after a stroke. Generally doses are started at 100 to 300 mg once daily and titrated up to 1800 to 3600 mg daily in three to four divided daily doses.

Pregabalin is better absorbed than gabapentin, and efficacy is seen in approximately 1 week, compared to 4 to 6 weeks with gabapentin. The dose should be started low and titrated. Initial doses are 50 mg two to three times daily, titrated to an effective dose. The maximum dose of pregabalin is 600 mg/day. Side effects are similar to gabapentin. Both gabapentin and pregabalin doses should be reduced in patients with renal impairment.

Carbamazepine and divalproex are additional anticonvulsants that have been used extensively in the past for neuropathic pain conditions, but side effects limit their use. Carbamazepine is primarily used for trigeminal neuralgia pain. Divalproex is currently utilized as migraine prophylaxis.

Local Anesthetics

This class of medications exerts its analgesic effects by blocking sodium channels, thereby inhibiting abnormal pain impulses. Several routes of administration exist and are chosen based on the reason for use. Topical applications help control localized pain with minimal absorption. Lidoderm patches and EMLA cream (mixture of lidocaine and prilocaine) are available for topical use. Local injections of anesthetics can be utilized as regional anesthesia, injected into tissue or the epidural space. Epidural analgesia is commonly utilized in managing obstetric or postoperative pain. Rarely, lidocaine has been administered intravenously to control refractory pain conditions in sub-anesthetic dosages. Intravenous infusions must be administered in a monitored setting because of the potential for severe ADRs.

Skeletal Muscle Relaxants

In the past, skeletal muscle relaxants have been one of the most extensively prescribed agents for short-term treatment of musculoskeletal disorders, such as low back pain, muscle sprains, fibromyalgia, or athletic injury. However, recent evidence has shown that this class of medications is no more efficacious than using NSAIDs or acetaminophen. Currently, muscle relaxants are recommended for the short-term treatment of musculoskeletal conditions when treatment failure or side effects limit NSAID and acetaminophen use. Treatment goals include increased function and reduced pain so that patients can return to work and continue their normal activities. Two categories of skeletal muscle relaxants exist: antispastic agents for central spasticity in conditions such as multiple sclerosis and cerebral palsy, and antispasmodic agents used for musculoskeletal conditions.

Antispasmodic Skeletal Muscle Relaxants

Skeletal muscle relaxants are no longer considered first-line therapy for musculoskeletal conditions. Evidence supports short-term use only (2 weeks or less) as adjunctive therapy to NSAIDs or acetaminophen, or alone if contraindications to these medications exist. These medications work on muscle tone by decreasing reflexes at a central level. Motor function is not affected.

Cyclobenzaprine (Flexeril) has been the most studied skeletal muscle relaxant and is the only agent recommended to treat the chronic pain of fibromyalgia. Choice of treatment should be individualized for other conditions, with the most benefit is usually seen within the first few days of treatment. Many of these agents have the potential for abuse and for significant toxic levels. Therefore, choice should be based on adverse effect profile, drug interaction potential, and risk of abuse.

Cyclobenzaprine is structurally related to the TCAs. As such, it is contraindicated for use in patients taking monoamine oxidase inhibitors, in the acute recovery phase of a myocardial infarction, or with arrhythmias or significant heart blockage. The onset of action of cyclobenzaprine is approximately 1 hour and its effects can last up to 12 hours. The manufacturer's recommended dose is 10 mg; however, a 5-mg dose has been shown to be effective with less toxicity. The drug is often given three times daily to ensure efficacy during the day. When the drug is considered for use in elderly patients, its anticholinergic properties also must be taken into account, particularly dry mouth, drowsiness, dizziness, and constipation. Abuse has been seen with cyclobenzaprine.

Tizanidine (Zanaflex) is a centrally acting, α_2-adrenergic agonist, putatively reducing spasticity by increasing presynaptic inhibition of motor neuron excitation. The peak effect occurs within 1 to 2 hours of oral administration and lasts 3 to 5 hours. It has an oral bioavailability of approximately 40% because of first-pass metabolism. The half-life of the agent is approximately 2.5 hours, and clearance is delayed in elderly patients. Tizanidine is very sedating and a useful adjunct in patients with sleep disturbances as a result of musculoskeletal pain.

Botulism toxin attenuates muscle spasms by inhibiting the release of substances known to increase spasms and pain (acetylcholine, substance P, and glutamate). However, use is limited because there is no oral formulation available and it is expensive.

Some of the traditional skeletal muscle relaxants produce dependence and/or respiratory depression and are no longer recommended as first-line agents. Carisoprodol and diazepam may cause physical and psychological dependence, and agents such as chlorzoxazone, methocarbamol, metaxalone, and carisoprodol may increase respiratory depression especially when combined with other agents that decrease the respiratory drive. Metaxalone may produce less dizziness and sedation than other agents in this class.

Antispastic Agents

Limited evidence exists for using antispastic agents to treat musculoskeletal conditions. Baclofen (Lioresal), dantrolene, and diazepam can reduce muscle spasticity. Baclofen is the most utilized agent in this class. Diazepam and dantrolene may also be effective in treating muscle spasticity; however, adverse effects and the risk of dependence (diazepam) limit their general use.

Baclofen is indicated for managing signs and symptoms of spasticity resulting from multiple sclerosis and for spinal cord injuries or diseases. It is available as an oral tablet. An injectable form for intrathecal administration is available for severe spasticity. Common side effects of the oral form include drowsiness, hypotension, weakness, nausea and vomiting, and headache. Intrathecal administration results in hypotension, somnolence, dizziness, constipation, and headache. Respiratory depression and difficulty with concentration or coordination are also seen with intrathecal administration. Due to possible precipitation of withdrawal with abrupt discontinuation, tapering baclofen is recommended if when discontinuing the drug.

BIBLIOGRAPHY

Starred references are cited in the text.

*Agency for Health Care Policy and Research, United States Department of Health and Human Services, Public Health Service. (1994). *Management of cancer pain.* Rockville, MD: Author.

Amadio, P., Jr., Cummings, D. M., & Amadio, P. (1993). Non-steroidal anti-inflammatory drugs: Tailoring therapy to achieve results and avoid toxicity. *Postgraduate Medicine, 93*(4), 73–76, 79–81, 85–86, 88, 93–97.

Ashburn, M., Lipman, A. G., Carr, D., & Rubingh, C. (2003). *Principles of analgesic use in the treatment of acute pain* (5th ed.). American Pain Society. Glenview, IL: Author.

Ballantyne, J. C., & Mao J. (2003). Opioid therapy for chronic pain. *New England Journal of Medicine, 349*(20), 1943–1953.

Beers, M. H., & Berkow, R. (Eds.). (1999). *Merck manual of diagnosis and therapy* (17th ed.). Whitehouse Station, NJ: Merck.

Budassi-Sheehy, S. (1992). *Emergency nursing: Principles and practice* (3rd ed.). Des Plaines, IL: Emergency Nurses Association.

Bushnell, T. G., & Justins, D. M. (1993). Choosing the right analgesic: A guide to selection. *Drugs, 46,* 394–408.

Carns, P., Stang, H., Kaye, C., et al. (2004). *Assessment and management of acute pain* (4th ed.). Bloomington, MN: Institute for Clinical Systems Improvement.

Cepeda, M.S., et al. (2003). Side effects of opioids during short-term administration: Effect of age, gender, and race. *Pharmacodynamics and Drug Action, 74*(2), 102–112.

Clive, D. M., & Stoff, J. S. (1984). Renal syndromes associated with nonsteroidal anti-inflammatory drugs. *New England Journal of Medicine, 310,* 563–572.

Cuny, C.J., et al. (1979). Pharmacokinetics of salicylate in elderly. *Gerontology, 25,* 49–55.

Ivey, K. J. (1983). Gastrointestinal effects of antipyretic analgesic. *American Journal of Medicine, 75,* 53–64.

Kane, F. J., & Pokorny, A. (1975). Mental and emotional disturbance with pentazocine (Talwin) use. *Southern Medical Journal, 68,* 808–811.

Lazarus, H., et al. (1990). A multi-investigator clinical evaluation of oral controlled-release morphine (MS Contin®) administered to cancer patients. *Hospice Journal, 6,* 1–15.

Levy, G. (1965). Pharmacokinetics of salicylate elimination in man. *Journal of Pharmaceutical Sciences, 54,* 959–967.

Lipman, A. G. (Ed.). (2004). *Pain management for primary care clinicians.* Bethesda, MD: American Society of Health-System Pharmacists, Chapter 21.

McCaffery, M., & Pasero, C. (1999). *Pain: A clinical manual.* St Louis: Mosby.

McEvoy, G. K., & Litvak, K. (Eds.). (2004). *AHFS drug information 04.* Bethesda, MD: American Society of Hospital Pharmacists.

Moreland, L. W., & St. Clair, E. W. (1999). The use of analgesics in the management of pain in rheumatic diseases. *Rheumatic Diseases Clinics of North America, 25,* 153–191.

Nikolaus, T., & Zeyfang, A. (2004). Pharmacological treatments for persistent non-malignant pain in older persons. *Drugs and Aging, 21,* 19–41.

Olin, B. R., et al. (Eds.). (2000). *Drug facts and comparisons.* St. Louis: Lippincott Williams & Wilkins.

Ortho-McNeil Pharmaceutical. (1997). *Product information: ULTRAM® (Tramadol hydrochloride tablets).* Raritan, NJ: Author.

Pasternak, G. W. (1987). Morphine 6-glucuronide, a potent mu agonist. *Life Science, 41,* 2845–2849.

Portenoy, R. K. (1996). Opioid therapy for chronic nonmalignant pain: A review of the critical issues. *Journal of Pain and Symptom Management, 11,* 203–217.

Ripamonti, C., & Dickerson, E. D. (2001). Strategies for the treatment of cancer pain in the new millennium. *Drugs, 61,* 955–977.

Vickers, M. D., et al. (1992). Tramadol: Pain relief by opioid without depression of respiration. *Anesthesia, 47,* 291–296.

Von Feldt, J. M., & Ehrlich, G. E. (1998). Pharmacologic therapies. *Physical Medicine and Rehabilitation Clinics of North America, 9,* 473–487.

Wall, R. T. (1990). Use of analgesics in the elderly. *Clinics in Geriatric Medicine, 6,* 345–364.

Wang, R. I. H., & Sandoval, R. G. (1971). The analgesic activity of propoxyphene napsylate with and without aspirin. *Journal of Clinical Pharmacology, 11,* 310–317.

Washington Department of Labor and Industries, Washington State Medical Association. (2002). *Guideline for the use of Neurontin in the management of neuropathic pain.* Seattle: Author.

Willcox, S. M., Himmelstein, D. U., & Woolhandler, S. (1994). Inappropriate drug prescribing for the community-dwelling elderly. *Journal of the American Medical Association, 272,* 292–296.

World Health Organization. (1990). Cancer pain relief and palliative care: Report of a WHO expert. *Committee Technical Report Series, No. 804.* Washington, DC: Author.

*World Health Organization. (1996). *Cancer pain relief: With a guide to opioid availability* (2nd ed.). Washington, DC: Author.

Principles of Antimicrobial Therapy

The selection of an appropriate antimicrobial agent to treat an infection is guided by a number of factors. Typically, empiric antimicrobial therapy is based on the epidemiology of the suspected infection, with therapy directed toward the most likely organisms. Laboratory studies, including Gram stain as well as culture and sensitivity testing, help to identify the pathogen and its susceptibility to a variety of antimicrobials. Although there may be several options, efficacy, toxicity, pharmacokinetic profile, and cost ultimately determine the agent of choice. The optimal dose and duration of the antimicrobial therapy are then determined by patient factors such as age, weight, and concurrent disease states as well as the site and severity of infection.

FACTORS IN SELECTING AN ANTIMICROBIAL REGIMEN

Before initiating antibiotic therapy, a systematic approach to identify the source and site of infection must be undertaken. A complete medical history and physical examination should be conducted to identify signs and symptoms consistent with the presence of infection. Identifying underlying medical or social conditions such as diabetes, immunosuppression (cancer, human immunodeficiency virus [HIV] infection), past medications, or intravenous (IV) drug use may help in identifying a predisposition toward infection or the most likely pathogen causing disease. In addition, determining where the infection was acquired (in the community versus a nursing home or hospital setting) may also help limit the list of most likely pathogens. Health care–acquired pathogens may necessitate broad-spectrum empiric therapy to cover multidrug-resistant (MDR) pathogens.

Identifying the causative pathogen is the ultimate goal because it allows for optimal antibiotic selection and patient outcome. Specimens from the most likely body sites should be properly collected and sent to the microbiology laboratory. Depending on the body site involved, specimens will be stained (e.g., Gram stain) to determine morphology and cell wall structure (gram positive versus gram negative and cocci versus bacilli) and to detect white blood cells (which indicate inflammation and infection). The gold standard of diagnosis in infectious diseases is to be able to grow the causative organism in culture and perform antibiotic susceptibility testing to determine which

agents are most likely to be effective in eradicating the pathogen. Susceptibility results often take 48 to 72 hours after cultures are obtained. Newer methods of testing can help identify specific pathogens (such as methicillin-resistant *Staphylococcus aureus* [MRSA] and *Candida*) more quickly.

Often, antibiotic therapy is initiated before culture and sensitivity testing is complete. Empiric antibiotic therapy is based on the premise of providing coverage for the most likely pathogens (**Table 8.1**). In general, the most likely organism is based on the suspected site of the infection. **Table 8.2** outlines key pathogens and spectra of activity for the most commonly prescribed antibiotics.

In most patients treated initially with a parenteral antibiotic who are clinically improving, therapy should be switched to the oral route. This does not apply to certain infections, such as osteomyelitis and endocarditis, in which parenteral antibiotics are continued to ensure adequate concentrations at the infection site. This oral conversion should be based on the following criteria:

- The patient is responding to therapy, as evidenced by a return to normal or a trend toward normal values in the patient's temperature and white blood cell count.
- The patient can take oral medications and absorb them adequately.
- An oral equivalent to the parenteral regimen exists. Not all parenteral agents are available orally. In choosing the oral equivalent, the goal is to select an agent (or agents) that provides a similar spectrum of antimicrobial activity and possesses good oral bioavailability. This may necessitate the use of oral agents that are from a different class from the parenteral agent.

The patient's response to therapy should be monitored regularly. This includes monitoring both efficacy and toxicity. If the patient responds to the prescribed antibiotic regimen, the presenting signs and symptoms of the infection should resolve. Parameters to be considered for response regardless of the site of infection include vital signs, white blood cell count, and, if the culture proved positive for bacteria, subsequent negative cultures. Other signs and symptoms are specific to the body site involved. Monitoring for adverse events is specific to the agents prescribed. (Review the drug overview sections for common adverse events.) All patients should be taught how to recognize the most common adverse events, and they should be advised

TABLE 8.1	Infection and Most Likely Infecting Organism
Body Site (Infection)	**Most Likely Organism**
Heart (Endocarditis)	
Subacute	*Streptococcus viridans*
Acute	
Injection drug user	*Staphylococcus aureus*, gram-negative aerobic bacilli, *Enterococcus* spp.
Prosthetic valve	*Staphylococcus epidermidis*
Intra-abdominal tissues	*Escherichia coli, Enterococcus* spp., anaerobes (especially *Bacteroides fragilis*), other gram-negative aerobic bacilli
Brain (Meningitis)	
Children <age 2 months	*E. coli*, group B streptococci, *Listeria monocytogenes*
Children age 2 months to 12 years	*Streptococcus pneumoniae, Neisseria meningitidis, Haemophilus influenzae*
Adults (community acquired)	*S. pneumoniae, N. meningitides*
Adults (hospital acquired)	*S. pneumoniae, N. meningitides*, gram-negative aerobic bacilli
HIV co-infected	*Cryptococcus neoformans, S. pneumoniae*
Respiratory Tract	
Upper tract, community acquired	*S. pneumoniae, H. influenzae, Moraxella catarrhalis*, group A streptococci
Lower tract, community acquired	*S. pneumoniae, H. influenzae, M. catarrhalis, Klebsiella pneumoniae* *Mycoplasma pneumoniae, C. pneumoniae*, viruses
Aspiration pneumonia	Mouth flora (anaerobic and aerobic)
Lower tract, hospital acquired	*S. aureus (including MRSA), Pseudomonas aeruginosa*, other gram-negative aerobic bacilli
HIV co-infected	*Pneumocystis jiroveci, S. pneumoniae*
Skin and Soft Tissue	
Diabetic ulcer	*Staphylococcus* spp., *Streptococcus* spp., gram-negative aerobic bacilli, anaerobes
Urinary Tract	
Community acquired	*E. coli*, other gram-negative aerobic bacilli, *Enterococcus* spp., *Staphylococcus saprophyticus*
Hospital acquired	*E. coli*, other gram-negative aerobic bacilli, *Enterococcus* spp.

to notify their health care provider if an adverse reaction occurs. The following sections highlight antimicrobials used in practice and include pharmacokinetics, pharmacodynamics, mechanism of action, spectrum of activity, common clinical uses, adverse events, drug interactions, and antimicrobial resistance.

PENICILLINS

First isolated in 1928, the penicillins were used successfully to treat streptococcal and staphylococcal infections. Since then, many synthetic penicillins have been developed to address the emerging problem of resistance. Despite resistance, the penicillins remain an important class of antimicrobials. They are classified based on their spectra of activity.

Pharmacokinetics and Pharmacodynamics

Most of the penicillins are unstable in the acid environment of the stomach and must be administered parenterally. Those that are acid stable are given orally. They are widely distributed in the body and penetrate the cerebrospinal fluid (CSF) in the presence of inflammation. Most penicillins are excreted by the kidneys, and renal impairment necessitates dosage adjustment.

The half-life of the penicillins in adults with normal renal function is 30 to 90 minutes. The penicillins are removed by hemodialysis, with the exception of nafcillin and oxacillin. The penicillins exhibit time-dependent bactericidal activity and a post-antibiotic effect against most gram-positive organisms. **Table 8.3** provides dosing information.

Mechanism of Action and Spectrum of Activity

The mechanism of action of the penicillins is the inhibition of bacterial cell growth by interference with cell wall synthesis. Penicillins bind to and inactivate the penicillin-binding proteins (PBPs).

Clinical Uses

Although the use of penicillin itself is limited due to widespread resistance, the penicillin class is effective in many infections, including those of the upper and lower respiratory tract, urinary tract, and central nervous system (CNS) as well as sexually transmitted diseases. They are the agents of choice for treating gram-positive infections such as endocarditis caused by susceptible organisms. Both the carboxypenicillins and ureidopenicillins are useful in treating infections caused by *Pseudomonas aeruginosa*.

TABLE 8.2 Sensitivity of Organisms to Specific Agents

Agent	Staphylococci and Streptococci	Enterococcus	Methicillin-Sensitive S. aureus	Methicillin-Resistant S. aureus (MRSA)	Gram-Negative Aerobes	Pseudomonas	Gram-Negative Anaerobes (Bacteroides fragilis)	Chlamydia pneumoniae, Legionella pneumophila
Penicillins								
penicillin G	+++	++	+	–	+	–	–	–
penicillin V	+++	++	+	–	+	–	–	–
ampicillin	+++	+++	+	–	+/++	–	–	–
amoxicillin	+++	+++	+	–	+/++	–	–	–
nafcillin	+++	–	+++	–	–	–	–	–
dicloxacillin	+++	–	+++	–	–	–	–	–
ticarcillin	+++	++	++	–	++	++	++	–
piperacillin	+++	+++	++	–	++	++	++	–
Beta-Lactam/Beta-Lactamase Inhibitors								
amoxicillin–clavulanic acid	+++	+++	+++	–	++	–	+++	–
piperacillin–tazobactam	+++	+++	+++	–	+++	+++	+++	–
ampicillin–sulbactam	+++	+++	+++	–	++	–	+++	–
ticarcillin–clavulanic acid	++	–	++	–	+++	++	+++	–
First-Generation Cephalosporins								
cefazolin	+++	–	+++	–	++	–	–	–
cephalexin	+++	–	+++	–	++	–	–	–
cefadroxil	++	–	+++	–	+++	–	–	–
Second-Generation Cephalosporins								
cefuroxime	+++	–	+++	–	++	–	–	–
cefoxitin	++	–	++	–	++	–	++/+++	–
cefotetan	++	–	+	–	++/+++	++	++	–
Third-Generation Cephalosporins								
ceftriaxone	+++	–	++/+++	–	+++	–	+	–
cefotaxime	+++	–	++/+++	–	+++	+	+/++	–
ceftazidime	++	–	+	–	+++	+++	–	–
Fourth-Generation Cephalosporins								
cefepime	+++	–	++	–	++/+++	++/+++	–	–
Monobactams								
aztreonam	–	–	–	–	++/+++	++/+++	–	–
Carbapenems								
ertapenem	+++	–	+++	–	+++	–	+++	–
imipenem	+++	++	+++	–	+++	++/+++	+++	–
meropenem	+++	++	+++	–	+++	++/+++	+++	–
doripenem	+++	–	++	–	+++	++	++	–
Fluoroquinolones								
ciprofloxacin	+/++	+	++	–	+++	+++	–	++
norfloxacin#	+/++	+	++	–	+++	++	–	+
levofloxacin	++/+++	+	+++	–	+++	+	+	+++
gemifloxacin	++/+++	++	++	+/++	++	+	–	+++
moxifloxacin	++/+++	++	++	+/++	+++	+	+/++	+++

Macrolides							
erythromycin	++/+++	–	++	–	+/++	–	–
clarithromycin	++/+++	–	++	–	++	–	–
azithromycin	++/+++	+	+	–	++	–	–
telithromycin	++/+++	+	++	–	++	–	–
Aminoglycosides							
gentamicin*	++	++	++	–	+++	–	–
tobramycin*	++	+	++	–	+++	–	–
amikacin*	+	–	+/+++	–	+++	–	–
Tetracyclines							
tetracycline	++/+++	+	++	+/++	+	++	+
doxycycline	++/+++	+	++	+/++	+/++	+++	++
minocycline	+++	+/+++	+/+++	+/+++	+/++	+++	++
Glycylcyclines							
tigecycline	++	++	++	++	++	–	++
Sulfonamides							
trimethoprim–sulfamethoxazole	++	–	++	+	+/+++	–	++
Glycopeptides							
vancomycin	+++	+++	++	+++	–	–	–
telavancin	+++	+++	++	+++	–	–	–
Oxazolidinones							
linezolid	+++	++	++	+++	–	–	+++
Lipopeptides							
daptomycin	+++	++	++	+++	–	–	+++
Streptogramins							
quinupristin–dalfopristin	+++	+++	+++	+++	+	–	+++
Antianaerobic Agents							
clindamycin	+++	–	+/++	+/++	–	–	–
metronidazole	–	–	–	–	–	–	–
Miscellaneous Agents							
chloramphenicol	+/++	++	++	++	++	–	+++
rifampin	++/+++	–	+++	+++	–	+	+++
nitrofurantoin#	+++	+++	++	+	+++	–	–

* Provides synergistic activity against gram-positive organisms when combined with a cell wall active agent.
# Applicable only to organisms isolated in urine.
– = No activity or no information available
+ = Poor to moderate activity; use only when known to be susceptible
++ = Good activity; resistance in some strains and geographical location may limit use
+++ = Excellent activity; generally reliable coverage for empiric therapy

TABLE 8.3	Penicillin Dosages	
Drug	**Adult Dosages**	**Pediatric Dosages**
Natural		
penicillin G	2–4 million units IV q4–6h	100,000–400,000 units/kg/d IV divided q4–6h
penicillin G benzathine	1.2–2.4 million units IM at specified intervals	300,000–2.4 million units IM at specified intervals
penicillin G procaine	0.6–4.8 million units IM in divided doses q12–24h at specified intervals	25,000–50,000 units/kg/d IM divided 1–2 times/day
penicillin VK	250–500 mg PO q6h	25–50 mg/kg/d PO divided q6–8h
Aminopenicillins		
ampicillin	1–2 g IV q4–6h	100–400 mg/kg/d IV divided 4–6h
amoxicillin–ampicillin	250–500 mg PO q8h	400–100 mg/kg/d PO divided q6–12h
	875–1000 mg PO q12h	
Carboxypenicillins		
ticarcillin sodium	3 g IV q4–6h	200–300 mg/kg/d IV divided q4–6h
Penicillinase Resistant		
cloxacillin	250–500 mg PO q6h	50–100 mg/kg/d PO divided q6h
dicloxacillin	250–500 mg PO q6h	12.5–100 mg/kg/d PO divided q6h
nafcillin	500 mg–1 g IV q4–6h	50–200 mg/kg/d IV divided q4–6h
oxacillin	500–2 g IV q4–6h	100–200 mg/kg/d IV divided q4–6h
Ureidopenicillins		
piperacillin	3–4 g IV q4–6h	200–300 mg/kg/d IV divided q4–6h

Note: Dosage adjustment of all above drugs required in patients with impaired renal function, with the exception of penicillinase-resistant penicillins.

Adverse Events

There is a low incidence of adverse reactions with penicillin administration. Hypersensitivity reactions characterized by maculopapular rash and urticaria are most common. Gastrointestinal (GI) side effects are most common with oral administration. In the presence of severe renal dysfunction, high-dose penicillins have been associated with seizures and encephalopathy. Thrombophlebitis has occurred with IV administration. The Jarisch-Herxheimer reaction, characterized by fever, chills, sweating, and flushing, may occur when penicillin is used in treating spirochetes, in particular syphilis. Release of toxic particles from the organism precipitates the reaction. In rare cases, leukopenia, thrombocytopenia, and hemolytic anemia can occur with penicillins.

Drug Interactions

Drug interactions involving penicillins are rare. Probenecid has been shown to increase the half-life of the penicillins by inhibiting tubular secretion. Both the carboxypenicillins and ureidopenicillins have been shown to inactivate the aminoglycosides, and these agents should not be mixed in the same IV solution. Also, the parenteral carboxypenicillins have a high sodium content. Caution should be used in patients with fluid or sodium restrictions.

BETA-LACTAM/BETA-LACTAMASE INHIBITOR COMBINATIONS

Resistance to penicillin develops when the drug is inactivated by the enzymes known as penicillinases or beta-lactamases produced by bacteria. After several attempts over the years to prevent penicillin degradation by this enzyme, clavulanic acid became the first beta-lactamase inhibitor introduced and combined with a beta-lactam. Two other beta-lactamase inhibitors, sulbactam and tazobactam, are also available in combination with ampicillin and piperacillin, respectively. The role of the beta-lactamase inhibitor is to prevent the breakdown of the beta-lactam by organisms that produce the enzyme, thereby enhancing antibacterial activity. These combinations are suitable alternatives for infections caused by beta-lactamase producing organisms such as *S. aureus*, *Haemophilus influenzae*, and *Bacteroides fragilis*.

Pharmacokinetics and Pharmacodynamics

The beta-lactam/beta-lactamase inhibitors diffuse into most body tissues, with the exception of the brain and CSF. The half-life of both components in each combination is approximately 1 hour. Because these drugs are eliminated by glomerular filtration, renal dysfunction necessitates dosage changes (**Table 8.4**). The compounds are removed by hemodialysis and peritoneal dialysis.

Mechanism of Action and Spectrum of Activity

The beta-lactam components of the combinations are cell wall–active agents. They interfere with bacterial cell wall synthesis by binding to and inactivating penicillin-binding proteins. The beta-lactamase inhibitors irreversibly bind to most beta-lactamase enzymes, protecting the beta-lactam from degradation and improving their antibacterial activity. The beta-lactamase inhibitors alone lack significant antibacterial activity. The spectrum of activity is similar to the penicillin derivative, with broader coverage against beta-lactamase-producing organisms.

TABLE 8.4	Beta-Lactam/Beta-Lactamase Inhibitor Dosages	
Drug	**Adult Dosages**	**Pediatric Dosages**
amoxicillin–clavulanic acid	250–500 mg PO q8h 500–875 mg PO q12h 2 g PO q12h*	20–40 mg/kg/d PO divided q8–12h 80–90 mg/kg/d PO divided q12h#
ampicillin–sulbactam	1.5–3 g IV q6h	100–400 mg/kg/d IV divided q6h
piperacillin–tazobactam	4.5 g IV q6–8h or 3.375 g IV q6h	240–300 mg/kg/d IV divided q8h
ticarcillin–clavulanic acid	3.1g IVq4–6h	200–300 mg/kg/d IV divided q4–6h

* amoxicillin-clavulanic acid (Augmentin XR®) extended release formulation
 # amoxicillin/clavulanic acid (Augmentin ES-600®) formulation
Note: Dosage adjustment required for all above drugs administered to patients with renal impairment.

Clinical Uses

Based on their broad spectrum of activity, the beta-lactam/beta-lactamase inhibitors are frequently used in treating polymicrobial infections. They are used extensively to treat intra-abdominal and gynecologic infections; and skin and soft tissue infections, including human and animal bites, as well as foot infections in diabetic patients. Respiratory tract infections, including aspiration pneumonia, sinusitis, and lung abscesses, have been successfully treated with these combinations.

Adverse Events

The addition of the beta-lactamase inhibitor to the penicillins has not resulted in any new or major adverse events. The major effects associated with the beta-lactam/beta-lactamase inhibitor combinations are hypersensitivity reactions and GI side effects such as nausea and diarrhea associated with oral administration. Elevated aminotransferase levels have been documented for all agents.

Drug Interactions

The combinations are physically incompatible with parenteral aminoglycosides. Each of the penicillins in the combinations has been associated with the inactivation of aminoglycosides in vitro. The clinical significance of this interaction is unknown.

CEPHALOSPORINS

The cephalosporins, a beta-lactam group, are structurally similar to the penicillins. Substitutions on the parent compound, 7-aminocephalosporanic acid, produce compounds with different pharmacokinetic properties and spectra of activity. The cephalosporins are divided into "generations" based on their antimicrobial spectrum of activity. The progression from first to fourth generation in general reflects an increase in gram-negative coverage and a loss of gram-positive activity.

Pharmacokinetics and Pharmacodynamics

The cephalosporins are well absorbed from the GI tract. In some cases, food enhances absorption. They penetrate well into tissues and body fluids and achieve high concentrations in the urinary tract. Non-cephamycin second-generation agents and all third- and fourth-generation agents penetrate the CSF and play a role in treating bacterial meningitis. Most of the oral and parenteral cephalosporins are excreted by the kidney, with the exception of ceftriaxone (Rocephin) and cefoperazone (not available in the United States), which are eliminated by the liver. The cephalosporins exhibit a time-dependent bactericidal effect and a prolonged post-antibiotic effect against staphylococci. **Table 8.5** provides dosing information.

Mechanism of Action and Spectrum of Activity

Like other beta-lactams, the cephalosporins interfere with bacterial cell wall synthesis by binding to and inactivating the PBPs.

Clinical Uses

The cephalosporins are used in treating many infections. In general, the first-generation cephalosporins are used in treating gram-positive skin infections, pneumococcal respiratory infections, urinary tract infections, and for surgical prophylaxis. The second-generation cephalosporins are used in treating community-acquired pneumonia, other respiratory tract infections, and skin infections. Mixed aerobic and anaerobic infections may be treated with the second-generation cephamycins (cefotetan and cefoxitin). In addition, treating community-acquired bacterial meningitis typically includes a third-generation cephalosporin such as ceftriaxone or cefotaxime (Claforan). Nosocomial infections are commonly treated with ceftazidime (Fortaz) or cefepime (Maxipime), whose broad spectrum of activity includes gram-negative organisms, especially *P. aeruginosa*. Ceftaroline fosamil (Teflaro), a new intravenous cephalosporin, has activity similar to ceftriaxone, but is the only cephalosporin that covers MRSA.

TABLE 8.5	Cephalosporin Dosages	
Drug	**Adult Dosages**	**Pediatric Dosages**
First Generation		
cefazolin	500 mg–1 g IV q8h	50–100 mg/kg/d IV divided q8h
cephalexin	250–1000 mg PO q6h	25–100 mg/kg/d PO divided q6h
cefadroxil	500 mg–1 g PO q12h	30 mg/kg/d PO divided q12h
Second Generation		
cefotetan	1–2 g IV q12h	40–80 mg/kg/d IV divided q12h
cefoxitin	1–2 g IV q6–8h	80–160 mg/kg/d IV divided q4–8h
cefuroxime	750–1.5 g IV q8h	75–150 mg/kg/d IV divided q8h
cefuroxime axetil	250–500 mg PO q12h	20–30 mg/kg/d PO divided q12h
loracarbef	200–400 mg PO q12–24h	15–30 mg/kg/d PO divided q12h
cefaclor	250–500 mg PO q8h	20–40 mg/kg/d PO divided q8–12h
Third Generation		
cefotaxime	1–2 g IV q8h	100–300 mg/kg/d IV divided q6–8h
ceftazidime	1–2 g IV q8h	90–150 mg/kg/d IV divided q8h
ceftizoxime	1–2 g IV q8h	150–200 mg/kg/d IV divided q6–8h
ceftriaxone[†]	1–2 g IV q12–24h	50–100 mg/kg/d IV divided q12–24h
ceftibuten	400 mg PO q24h	9 mg/kg/d PO divided q24h
cefpodoxime proxetil	100–400 mg PO q12h	10 mg/kg/d PO divided q12h
cefprozil	250–500 mg PO q12h	15–30 mg/kg/d PO divided q12h
cefdinir	300 mg PO q12h OR 600 mg PO q24h	7–14 mg/kg/d PO divided q12–24h
Fourth Generation		
cefepime	1–2 g IV q8–12h	50 mg/kg/d IV divided q8h

Note: Dosage adjustment necessary for all agents in patients with renal impairment except ceftriaxone.
[†]Dosage adjustment necessary in patients with liver dysfunction.

Adverse Events

The cephalosporins are a safe class of antimicrobials with a favorable toxicity profile. With a few exceptions, the adverse events are similar across the generations. Hypersensitivity reactions, not unlike those with the penicillins, are characterized by maculopapular rash and urticaria. The cross-reactivity between penicillins and cephalosporins is 3% to 10%. Patients who experience allergic reactions to penicillins (other than a type 1 allergy) can often tolerate a cephalosporin. The most common side effects with oral administration are nausea, vomiting, and diarrhea. GI effects are usually transient. Less common reactions include a positive Coombs test and rarely hemolytic reactions.

Drug Interactions

Drug interactions involving cephalosporins are rare. Probenecid has been shown to increase the half-life of some cephalosporins by inhibiting the tubular secretion.

MONOBACTAMS

The monobactams are a unique class of beta-lactams with a four-membered ring but lacking a fifth or sixth member, like other beta-lactams. Because aztreonam (Azactam) is the only agent of its class commercially available, most of the information relates specifically to that agent. With primary activity against gram-negative organisms, including *Pseudomonas*, aztreonam is considered a safer alternative to the aminoglycosides, with a similar spectrum of activity.

Pharmacokinetics and Pharmacodynamics

Aztreonam distributes well into most tissues, with a volume of distribution of 0.16 L/kg. Penetration into the CSF is increased in the presence of inflamed meninges. Aztreonam is not extensively bound to proteins. The approximate half-life is 2 hours, and dosages are typically calculated according to the severity of disease (**Table 8.6**). Aztreonam is excreted primarily

TABLE 8.6	Aztreonam Dosages	
Severity of Infection	**Adult Dosages**	**Pediatric Dosages**
Mild	500 mg IV q8–12h	90–120 mg/kg/d IV divided q6–8h
Moderate	1–2 g IV q8–12h	
Severe	2 g IV q6–8h	

Note: Dosage adjustment required in patients with impaired renal function.

unchanged by glomerular filtration, so dosage adjustments are necessary in patients with renal insufficiency. Aztreonam is cleared by hemodialysis and peritoneal dialysis.

Mechanism of Action and Spectrum of Activity

Aztreonam, like other beta-lactams, interferes with bacterial cell wall synthesis by binding to and inactivating PBPs. The principal activity of aztreonam is against most aerobic gram-negative organisms, including *P. aeruginosa, Serratia marcescens,* and *Citrobacter* species. It has virtually no activity against gram-positive organisms. Its gram-negative coverage is similar to that of the aminoglycosides and the third-generation cephalosporin ceftazidime. Aztreonam is not active against anaerobic organisms.

Clinical Uses

Aztreonam is commonly used in treating complicated and uncomplicated urinary tract and respiratory tract infections such as pneumonia and bronchitis when aerobic gram-negative coverage is necessary. To broaden coverage, it is usually used in combination with an agent exhibiting gram-positive activity. It is a reasonable substitute for the aminoglycosides in treating gram-negative infections in patients at high risk for toxicity.

Adverse Events

Aztreonam has a relatively safe toxicity profile. Most of the adverse events associated with aztreonam are local reactions and GI symptoms. Elevated aminotransferase levels have also been documented. Despite its beta-lactam structure, patients allergic to penicillins and cephalosporins usually do not manifest an allergic reaction to aztreonam. A cross-allergy specifically with ceftazidime has been reported and linked to an identical side chain on both compounds.

Drug Interactions

No clinically significant drug interactions have been documented with aztreonam.

CARBAPENEMS

The carbapenems, ertapenem (Invanz), doripenem (Doribax), imipenem (Primaxin), and meropenem (Merrem) are bicyclical beta-lactams with a common carbapenem nucleus (**Table 8.7**). Imipenem is extensively metabolized by renal dehydropeptidases, yielding only limited activity in the urine. Cilastatin, a competitive inhibitor of the dehydropeptidases, was introduced to overcome imipenem degradation and is commercially available in combination with imipenem in a one-to-one ratio. Subsequently, ertapenem, meropenem, and doripenem were developed; they maintain stability against dehydropeptidase metabolism without the addition of a cilastatin-like agent. The carbapenems are the most broad-spectrum agents commercially available.

TABLE 8.7	Carbapenem Dosages	
Drug	**Adult Dosages**	**Pediatric Dosages**
ertapenem	1 g IV/IM daily	30 mg/kg/d IV divided q12h
doripenem	500 mg IV q8h	Not recommended
imipenem	250–1000 mg IV q6h	25–100 mg/kg/d IV divided q6h
meropenem	500 mg–1000 mg IV q8h	30–120 mg/kg/d IV divided q8h

Note: Dosage adjustment required for all above drugs administered to patients with renal impairment.

Pharmacokinetics and Pharmacodynamics

Carbapenems are not absorbed after oral administration. They exhibit linear pharmacokinetics; thus, peak serum levels increase proportionately as the dose is increased. They are widely distributed into most tissues, with an approximate volume of distribution of 0.25 L/kg. With the exception of ertapenem, they are minimally bound to plasma proteins. Penetration into the CSF varies and depends on the degree of meningeal inflammation. The half-life of the carbapenems is approximately 1 hour. They are primarily eliminated by urinary excretion of unchanged drug. Imipenem, meropenem, and doripenem are removed by hemodialysis and hemofiltration.

The carbapenems, like other beta-lactams, exhibit time-dependent bactericidal effects. Unlike other beta-lactams, they exhibit a post-antibiotic effect against gram-negative aerobes lasting at least 1 to 2 hours.

Mechanism of Action and Spectrum of Activity

Similar to the penicillins and cephalosporins, the carbapenems bind to the PBPs on the cell wall and interfere with bacterial cell wall synthesis. They frequently have stability against beta-lactamases and bind to several PBPs.

Imipenem, meropenem, and doripenem possess the broadest spectrum of activity of any of the beta-lactam compounds. They have excellent activity against aerobic gram-positive organisms, including staphylococci and streptococci and gram-negative organisms such as Enterobacteriaceae, *P. aeruginosa,* and *Acinetobacter* species. They are also active against most gram-negative anaerobic organisms, including *B. fragilis.* Ertapenem has a similar spectrum of activity as the other carbapenems, with the noted exceptions of *P. aeruginosa* and *Acinetobacter* species, for which ertapenem has no clinically significant activity.

Clinical Uses

Their broad spectrum of activity and stability to many beta-lactamases make the carbapenems useful as single agents in treating polymicrobial infections. They have been used extensively in treating skin and soft tissue, bone and joint, intra-abdominal, and lower respiratory tract infections. In addition, meropenem is used in treating CNS infections because it has a lower risk than imipenem of causing seizures.

Adverse Events

Neurotoxicity, a well-known effect of the carbapenems, is characterized by seizure activity. Imipenem has been reported to lower the seizure threshold more frequently than meropenem and doripenem. Risk factors for seizures include impaired renal function, improper dosing, age, previous CNS disorder, and concomitant agents that lower the seizure threshold. Meropenem and more recently doripenem are the carbapenems of choice in patients with a seizure disorder or underlying risk factors. Such GI side effects as nausea, vomiting, and diarrhea have also been reported. Decreasing the infusion rate may lessen their severity.

Drug Interactions

Concomitant administration of probenecid and meropenem or doripenem results in decreased clearance of these agents and a substantial increase in half-life; therefore, the concurrent administration of meropenem or doripenem with probenecid is not recommended. A similar interaction with imipenem occurs, but to a lesser degree.

FLUOROQUINOLONES

Since 1990, the fluoroquinolones (FQs) have become a dominant class of antimicrobial agents. No other class of antimicrobial agents has grown so rapidly or been developed with such interest by pharmaceutical research companies. Although multiple medications in this class have been approved by the U.S. Food and Drug Administration (FDA), several FQs have been removed from the U.S. market due to the identification of post-marketing adverse events. This emphasizes the importance of post-marketing research and adverse event reporting. **Table 8.8** lists the available FQs. Ciprofloxacin, levofloxacin, and moxifloxacin are most commonly prescribed.

TABLE 8.8	Fluoroquinolone Dosages
Drug	**Adult Dosage**
ciprofloxacin	250–750 mg PO q12h; 200–400 mg IV q12h; 400 mg IV q8h (severe infections)
gemifloxacin	320 mg PO daily
levofloxacin	250–750 mg PO/IV daily
moxifloxacin	400 mg PO/IV daily
norfloxacin	400 mg PO q12h
ofloxacin	200–400 mg PO q12h

Note: With the exception of ciprofloxacin for the treatment of urinary tract infections and anthrax, these drugs are not recommended for use in children younger than age 18. Dosage adjustment required for all above drugs (except moxifloxacin) administered to patients with renal impairment.

Pharmacokinetics and Pharmacodynamics

The FQs are bactericidal antibiotics. They display a concentration-dependent killing effect. All FQs have excellent bioavailability, making it easy to transition from an IV to an oral formulation. They have a volume of distribution ranging from 1.5 to 6.1 L/kg and distribute well into most tissues and fluids except the CNS. The half-life for the FQs ranges from 4 to 12 hours, with levofloxacin, gemifloxacin, and moxifloxacin having the longest half-lives. These three agents are dosed once daily. All FQs undergo renal elimination with the exception of moxifloxacin. The FQs are removed by hemodialysis and peritoneal dialysis, with percentages varying between products. All FQs also exhibit a post-antibiotic effect, which also appears to be a concentration-dependent parameter. The newer compounds have been reported to have post-antibiotic effects of 1 to 6 hours, depending on the pathogen and drug.

Mechanism of Action and Spectrum of Activity

The quinolone antibiotics are strong inhibitors of deoxyribonucleic acid (DNA) gyrase and topoisomerase IV. These enzymes are critical to the process of supercoiling DNA. Without such enzymatic activity, bacterial DNA cannot replicate.

All FQs possess activity against aerobic gram-negative organisms. Ciprofloxacin and levofloxacin have activity against *P. aeruginosa,* representing the only oral antibiotics available to treat this pathogen. However, widespread use of the FQs since the late 1990s have led to increased resistance against gram-negative pathogens and limited use in some parts of the United States. Newer FQs, such as levofloxacin, moxifloxacin, and gemifloxacin, have activity against gram-positive organisms including *Streptococcus* species. These agents are sometimes referred to as the "antipneumococcal" or "respiratory" fluoroquinolones given their activity against *S. pneumoniae* and usefulness in treating community-acquired pneumonia. Moxifloxacin has some activity against anaerobic bacteria.

Clinical Uses

The FQs have been shown to be effective in treating many infections, including urinary tract infections (for which they are one of the agents of choice), pneumonia, sexually transmitted diseases, skin and soft tissue infections, GI infections (in combination with an agent for anaerobic coverage), traveler's diarrhea, and osteomyelitis. For hospital-acquired infections such as nosocomial pneumonia, ciprofloxacin (Cipro) or levofloxacin (Levaquin) are the preferred agents, as part of a drug combination, because they have the best activity against *P. aeruginosa.* Ciprofloxacin is also recommended for meningococcal prophylaxis as a single 500-mg oral dose.

Adverse Events

The FQs have a relatively safe side-effect profile. The most common side effects include nausea, diarrhea, dizziness, and confusion. Rare but serious side effects include QTc prolongation, tendon rupture, tendonitis, and peripheral neuropathy.

TABLE 8.9	Macrolide/Ketolide Antibiotic Dosages	
Drug	**Adult Dosage**	**Pediatric Dosages**
azithromycin	250–500 mg IV/PO daily 2000 mg (ER) PO single dose	5–12 mg/kg IV/PO daily 30 mg/kg PO single dose
clarithromycin*	250–500 mg PO q12h or 1000 mg (ER) PO daily	15 mg/kg/d PO divided ql2h
erythromycin base*	250 mg–1 g PO q6h	30–50 mg/kg/d PO divided q6–8h
ethyl succinate	400–800 mg PO q6–12h	30–50 mg/kg/d PO divided q6–8h
estolate; stearate		30–50 mg/kg/d PO divided q6–12h
injection	500–1000 mg IV q6–8h	15–50 mg/kg/d IV divided q6h
telithromycin*	800 mg PO daily	Not recommended

*Dosage adjustment necessary in patients with renal impairment.
ER = extended-release product

Drug Interactions

The FQs have several significant drug–drug interactions. Ciprofloxacin is a potent inhibitor of the cytochrome P450 (CYP) 1A2 isoenzyme and may increase the effect of other medications, including theophylline, warfarin (Coumadin), tizanidine, propranolol, and others. Antacids, sucralfate, and magnesium, calcium, or iron salts will decrease the absorption of the FQs if given concomitantly. These agents should be separated when administered orally. Due to the risk of QTc prolongation and torsades de pointes, medications that prolong the QTc interval should be used cautiously with the FQs. Prolonged administration of FQs in combination with corticosteroids increases the risk of tendonitis and tendon rupture. Hyperglycemic and hypoglycemic events have been reported with FQs when administered with insulin or other antidiabetic agents.

MACROLIDES AND KETOLIDES

Erythromycin (E-Mycin), the prototypical macrolide, has been used in treating many infections over the years. However, its use has been diminished by its GI side effects. This toxicity has even been used as a means of treating patients with diabetic gastroparesis. Newer agents (clarithromycin and azithromycin) have been developed with improved GI tolerance and longer half-lives. Telithromycin (Ketek) is the only agent in the class known as ketolides. Although separate from macrolides, telithromycin has a similar mechanism of action and antibacterial coverage.

Pharmacokinetics and Pharmacodynamics

The macrolides are usually administered orally and are absorbed from the GI tract if not inactivated by gastric acid. They have good tissue penetration, achieve high intracellular concentrations, and exhibit minimal protein binding. The macrolides are metabolized via the liver and excreted in the urine. Half-lives vary throughout the class, from 2 hours for erythromycin, 4 to 5 hours for clarithromycin (Biaxin), and 50 to 60 hours for azithromycin (Zithromax). The long half-life and high intracellular concentrations of azithromycin permit once daily dosing and short courses. Dosage adjustment in patients with renal failure is necessary with clarithromycin (Biaxin) and erythromycin (**Table 8.9**).

Telithromycin is well absorbed following oral administration and is moderately protein bound. The half-life of telithromycin is approximately 10 hours. Telithromycin is metabolized in the liver and eliminated in the urine and feces. A dosage adjustment is recommended for patients with renal failure. The macrolides and ketolides are minimally cleared via hemodialysis and peritoneal dialysis.

Mechanism of Action and Spectrum of Activity

The mechanism of action of the macrolides is inhibition of bacterial protein synthesis by binding to the 50S ribosomal subunit. The spectrum of activity of the macrolides includes gram-positive and gram-negative aerobes and atypical organisms, including chlamydia, mycoplasma, legionella, rickettsia, mycobacteria, and spirochetes. Telithromycin is classified as a ketolide and also works by binding to the 50S ribosomal subunit; however, it has a higher binding affinity compared to the macrolides. The spectrum of activity is similar to the macrolides, with coverage against most organisms isolated in respiratory tract infections, including some strains of erythromycin-resistant *S. pneumoniae*.

Clinical Uses

The macrolides are used in several settings. Their broad spectrum of activity makes them useful in treating respiratory tract, skin, and soft tissue infections, sexually transmitted diseases, HIV-related *Mycobacterium avium-intracellulare* complex infection, and other infections caused by atypical organisms such as chlamydia, rickettsiae, and legionella. Telithromycin is approved for the treatment of community-acquired pneumonia; however, its use is limited due to the risk of hepatotoxicity.

Adverse Events

The macrolides are in general considered safe agents. Particularly with erythromycin, GI effects such as abdominal pain, nausea, and vomiting are most common. The newer macrolides cause fewer GI effects. Hepatotoxicity related to the macrolides is rare but serious; it also is less frequent with the newer agents. Extremely high doses of IV erythromycin and oral clarithromycin have been associated with ototoxicity. Phlebitis may occur with IV erythromycin administration. Telithromycin has been linked to cases of acute hepatic failure and severe liver injury. Common adverse effects of telithromycin include nausea, vomiting, diarrhea, dizziness, and blurred vision.

Drug Interactions

Among the macrolides, erythromycin and clarithromycin are potent inhibitors of the CYP3A4 isoenzyme. When administered concomitantly, they have been shown to prolong the half-life of an extensive list of agents, including cyclosporine, tacrolimus, carbamazepine, theophylline, warfarin, and most HMG-CoA reductase inhibitors. Azithromycin does not undergo significant cytochrome P450 metabolism, so the possibility of similar interactions is low. Telithromycin is also a strong inhibitor of CYP3A4 and has similar interactions and precautions to erythromycin and clarithromycin. Macrolides and ketolides have the potential to increase the QTc interval, so caution should be used in patients receiving concomitant medications that can also prolong the QTc interval.

AMINOGLYCOSIDES

Despite the advent of many new antibiotics over the past several decades, the aminoglycosides remain an important therapeutic drug class. Their major drawback has been their potential for drug-related toxicities (nephrotoxicity and ototoxicity). Because of these, their use or the length of therapy has been restricted. The introduction of a modified dosing regimen that uses once-daily (or extended-interval) dosing of these agents for several infections has provided a way of maximizing their therapeutic effects while minimizing the risk of toxicity.

Pharmacokinetics and Pharmacodynamics

The aminoglycosides are poorly absorbed from the GI tract, and parenteral administration is necessary to treat systemic infections. They are weakly bound to serum proteins (10%) and freely distribute into the extracellular fluid. The approximate volume of distribution is 0.25 L/kg, which may be significantly affected in intensive care patients and in disease states such as malnutrition, obesity, and ascites. The aminoglycosides are excreted unchanged via glomerular filtration. The half-life of aminoglycosides in an adult with normal renal function is approximately 1 to 3 hours. Dosage adjustments are necessary in patients with renal impairment because substantial increases in the half-life are seen. Aminoglycosides can be removed by hemodialysis, peritoneal dialysis, and continuous hemofiltration/dialysis.

Because of a narrow range between efficacy and toxicity, renal function and serum levels are used to monitor therapy with aminoglycosides. **Table 8.10** gives dosage guidelines.

Pharmacodynamically, the bactericidal effect of the aminoglycosides depends on drug concentration. The number of organisms decreases more rapidly when a higher peak concentration is achieved. In addition, the aminoglycosides exhibit a post-antibiotic effect for both gram-positive and gram-negative organisms.

Mechanism of Action and Spectrum of Activity

The aminoglycosides are actively taken up by bacteria and subsequently bind to the smaller 30S subunit of the bacterial ribosome, thus inhibiting bacterial protein synthesis.

The principal activity of the aminoglycosides is against aerobic gram-negative bacilli such as *Escherichia coli, Klebsiella*

TABLE 8.10	Aminoglycoside Dosages	
Aminoglycoside	**Adult Dosages**	**Pediatric Dosages**
Multiple Daily Dosing		
gentamicin, tobramycin	1–1.7 mg/kg IV q8h	6–7.5 mg/kg/d IV divided q8h
netilmicin#	1.7–2 mg/kg IV q8h	
amikacin, kanamycin#	5 mg/kg IV q8h OR 7.5 mg/kg IV q12h	15–22.5 mg/kg/d IV divided q8h
streptomycin	0.5–2 g IV q24h	20–40 mg/kg/d IV divided q6-12h
*Once-Daily Dosing**		
gentamicin, tobramycin	5–7 mg/kg IV q24h	5–7.5 mg/kg IV q24h
netilmicin#	4–6 mg/kg IV q24h	
amikacin	15–20 mg/kg IV q24h	20 mg/kg IV q24h

Note: Dosage adjustment required for all above drugs administered to patients with renal impairment.
*Once-daily dosing of aminoglycosides is not recommended for enterococcal infections, during pregnancy, in instances of gram-positive synergy, or for endocarditis, meningitis, or ascites.
Not routinely available for use in the United States.

species, *Proteus mirabilis, Enterobacter* species, *Acinetobacter* species, and *P. aeruginosa.* They are also generally active against gram-positive cocci, particularly *Staphylococcus, Enterococcus,* and *Streptococcus* species, but they must be used in combination (for synergy) with a cell wall–active agent such as ampicillin, nafcillin, or vancomycin. Streptomycin is also active against *Francisella tularensis* and *Mycobacterium tuberculosis.*

Clinical Uses

The aminoglycosides are primarily used in treating gram-negative infections. They have long been used in the empiric treatment of neutropenic fever and nosocomial infections because of their broad coverage of *P. aeruginosa* and Enterobacteriaceae. They are also frequently used with cell wall–active agents such as penicillins, cephalosporins, and vancomycin to achieve synergy in treating gram-positive infections, including staphylococcal and enterococcal infections. They are routinely used in combination with other agents in treating pneumonia, bacteremia, and intra-abdominal and skin and soft tissue infections. Monotherapy usually is not recommended, with the noted exception of patients with urinary tract infections. The aminoglycosides have been used in treating tuberculosis, with streptomycin having the greatest activity against *M. tuberculosis.* Streptomycin is also the treatment of choice for tularemia, a potential agent of bioterrorism.

Adverse Events

In general, the aminoglycosides have been associated with a variety of adverse events (GI and CNS), most of which are mild and transient. They rarely produce hypersensitivity reactions and are well tolerated at the sites of administration. Nephrotoxicity and ototoxicity are also associated with aminoglycoside use.

Nephrotoxicity results from accumulation of the drug in the proximal tubule cells of the kidney, causing nonoliguric renal failure. This renal failure is usually mild and reversible and rarely progresses to the need for dialysis. Factors that increase the risk of toxicity to the kidney include increased age, renal disease, increased trough levels, dehydration, and concomitant administration of nephrotoxic agents such as amphotericin B, cyclosporine, and vancomycin. Blood urea nitrogen and serum creatinine values are monitored in addition to serum levels to ensure safe and effective therapy. **Table 8.11** provides optimal serum concentrations for aminoglycosides.

Two forms of ototoxicity—auditory and vestibular—may occur alone or simultaneously. Auditory toxicity presents as hearing loss and tinnitus; vestibular toxicity is manifested by nausea, vomiting, and vertigo. Ototoxicity may be irreversible and has been associated with high serum trough levels. The risk of ototoxicity increases when the aminoglycosides are administered in combination with high-dose loop diuretics, high-dose macrolide antibiotics, or vancomycin. Long courses of aminoglycosides warrant baseline and periodic auditory monitoring.

TABLE 8.11	Aminoglycoside Concentration Monitoring	
Aminoglycoside	**Target Peak**	**Target Trough**
Multiple Daily Dosing*		
gentamicin, tobramycin	4–10 µg/mL	<2 µg/mL
netilmicin	4–10 µg/mL	<2 µg/mL
amikacin, kanamycin	20–30 µg/mL	<8 µg/mL
streptomycin	20–30 µg/mL	<8 µg/mL
Once-Daily Dosing**#		
gentamicin, tobramycin	>15 µg/mL	<1 µg/mL
netilmicin	>15 µg/mL	<1 µg/mL
amikacin	>50 µg/mL	<5 µg/mL

* Serum concentrations based upon steady state for multiple daily dosing. Peak concentrations should be obtained 30 to 60 minutes after infusion and trough concentrations 30 minutes before next infusion.
\# Random concentrations routinely measured for once-daily dosing in lieu of peak and trough serum concentrations and dosage adjustments based upon dosing nomograms.

Drug Interactions

The aminoglycosides have the potential to cause or prolong neuromuscular blockade, although this is uncommon. It is recommended that parenteral aminoglycosides be administered over a 30-minute interval. The risk of neuromuscular blockade increases in patients receiving concurrent neuromuscular blockers, general anesthetics, or calcium channel blockers and in those with myasthenia gravis. Administration of calcium gluconate usually reverses the neuromuscular blockade.

TETRACYCLINES

The tetracyclines possess activity against gram-positive, gram-negative, and atypical organisms, including rickettsiae, chlamydia, mycobacteria, and spirochetes. They are separated into short-, intermediate-, and long-acting agents. Doxycycline and minocycline are considered long-acting and the most active of the class. The tetracyclines became the first class of antimicrobials to be labeled "broad spectrum," and they remain a frequently used class of antimicrobials.

Pharmacokinetics and Pharmacodynamics

Absorption from the GI tract along with protein binding varies among agents. The long-acting agents have the highest absorption and are bound to protein to the greatest extent. With the exception of the long-acting agents, absorption is improved with administration on an empty stomach. The tetracyclines have excellent tissue distribution. The primary route of elimination is through the kidney by glomerular filtration, with the exception of doxycycline. In general, the short-acting agents have a half-life of 8 hours; the long-acting agents, 16 to 18 hours. The

TABLE 8.12	Tetracycline Dosages*
Drug	**Adult Dosages**
demeclocycline	150 mg PO q6h
	300 mg PO q12h
doxycycline	100 mg IV/PO q12h
minocycline	100–200 mg PO q12h
tetracycline	250–500 mg PO q6h

*The tetracyclines are not recommended for use in children less than age 8 or during pregnancy and breast-feeding.
Note: Dosage adjustment for all above drugs necessary in patients with renal impairment, with the exception of doxycycline.

tetracyclines are removed to a small degree by hemodialysis. **Table 8.12** provides dosing information.

Mechanism of Action and Spectrum of Activity

The tetracyclines inhibit bacterial protein synthesis by binding to the 30S subunit of the ribosome. The tetracyclines are active against gram-positive and gram-negative bacteria and atypical organisms, including spirochetes, rickettsiae, chlamydia, mycoplasma, and legionella. They typically are bacteriostatic agents.

Clinical Uses

Because of their broad spectrum of activity, the tetracyclines are used extensively in many settings. They are typically used as alternatives when beta-lactams are not an option. They are frequently used in treating rickettsial, chlamydial, and gram-negative infections, in addition to acne vulgaris and pelvic inflammatory disease (PID). Doxycycline is the drug of choice for the treatment of early Lyme disease and used in treating community-acquired pneumonia. Doxycycline and minocycline are used as sclerosing agents for pleurodesis. Additionally, minocycline and doxycycline have gained popularity as a treatment for community-acquired MRSA infections. Though a tetracycline, demeclocycline (Declomycin) is primarily used to treat the syndrome of inappropriate antidiuretic hormone and not as an antibiotic.

Adverse Events

The most frequent side effects associated with the tetracyclines are anorexia, nausea, vomiting, and epigastric distress. These are typically lessened if the agents are administered with food. Thrombophlebitis is associated with IV administration, and it is recommended that doxycycline be administered in a large volume and infused slowly. Hepatotoxicity is a rare but potentially fatal toxicity. The risk of hepatotoxicity increases if the patient is concurrently receiving other hepatotoxic agents. Gray-brown discoloration of the teeth can be a permanent effect of the tetracyclines. It results from stable tetracycline/calcium complexes in bone and teeth and is related to dose and duration of therapy. Therefore, children younger than age 8 should not receive tetracyclines. Patients receiving tetracyclines are more sensitive to the effects of the sun because of accumulation of the drug in the skin. Minocycline has been associated with dose-related vertigo.

Drug Interactions

There are multiple drug interactions involving the tetracyclines. The absorption of the tetracyclines is affected by several agents. Tetracyclines form chelating complexes with divalent and trivalent cations, decreasing tetracycline absorption. It is recommended that the administration of tetracyclines and antacids, iron, cholestyramine, and sucralfate be separated by at least 1 hour. Likewise, food decreases the absorption of most tetracyclines, with the exception of doxycycline. Milk and dairy products also impair their absorption. Phenytoin and carbamazepine, CYP enzyme inducers, decrease the half-life of doxycycline. Concomitant administration of the tetracyclines and oral contraceptives results in decreased levels of the oral contraceptive, so an additional form of contraception is recommended. The tetracyclines also potentiate the effect of warfarin by impairing vitamin K production by intestinal flora.

GLYCYLCYCLINES

Tigecycline (Tygacil) belongs to a new class of agents known as the *glycylcyclines*. It is structurally related to the tetracycline class. Tigecycline is derived from the addition of a glycyl ring to minocycline, which significantly enhances its antimicrobial spectrum.

Pharmacokinetics and Pharmacodynamics

Tigecycline is available only in a parenteral formulation. Following IV administration, tigecycline has a half-life of 27 to 42 hours. It is moderately protein bound with a volume of distribution of 7 to 9 L/kg. Given its large volume of distribution, it does not result in prolonged serum concentrations. The dose in adults is a single 100-mg IV dose followed by 50-mg IV every 12 hours. Tigecycline is not extensively metabolized in the liver and does not require adjustments for renal insufficiency; however, the dose should be adjusted for patients with severe underlying liver disease. Tigecycline is not removed by hemodialysis.

Similar to the tetracyclines, tigecycline is bacteriostatic and has a post-antibiotic effect lasting 2 to 4 hours.

Mechanism of Action and Spectrum of Activity

Tigecycline inhibits bacterial protein synthesis by binding to the 30S subunit of the ribosome. It has a five-fold higher binding affinity to these ribosomes compared to the tetracyclines. Tigecycline is active against many gram-positive, gram-negative, and anaerobic organisms, with the exception of *Pseudomonas* and *Proteus* species. Tigecycline has activity against MRSA and vancomycin-resistant enterococci (VRE).

Clinical Uses

Tigecycline is approved by the FDA for treating complicated skin and skin structure infections, intra-abdominal infections, and community-acquired pneumonia; however, given the spectrum of activity, it is also used for gram-negative organisms resistant to alternative agents.

Adverse Events

Tigecycline is generally well tolerated, with nausea and vomiting being the most common adverse effects. Tigecycline has also been reported to cause asymptomatic hyperbilirubinemia. Given the similarity in chemical structure to minocycline, there is the potential for adverse effects seen with the tetracycline class.

Drug Interactions

Concomitant administration of tigecycline and oral contraceptives results in decreased levels of the oral contraceptive, so an additional form of contraception is recommended.

SULFONAMIDES

In 1932, the dye prontosil rubrum was found to be effective in treating streptococcal infections. Subsequent studies found that one of its by-products was sulfanilamide. Manipulation of this by-product created the class of antimicrobials known as the sulfonamides.

Pharmacokinetics and Pharmacodynamics

Oral sulfonamides are readily absorbed from the GI tract. They are distributed through all body tissues and enter the CSF, pleural fluid, and synovial fluid. They are eliminated from the body by glomerular filtration and hepatic metabolism. The half-lives of the sulfonamides vary from hours to days; sulfadoxine (Fansidar) (no longer available in the United States), at 5 to 10 days, has the longest half-life. **Table 8.13** gives dosing information.

TABLE 8.13	Sulfonamide Dosages	
Drug	**Adult Dosages**	**Pediatric Dosages**
sulfadiazine	4–8 g PO in divided doses q6–12h	100–150 mg/kg/d PO divided q6h
sulfisoxazole	4–8 g PO in divided doses q4–6h	120–150 mg/kg/d PO divided q4–6h
trimethoprim	100 mg PO q12h OR 200 mg PO q24h	4–6 mg/kg/d PO divided q12h
trimethoprim–sulfamethoxazole*	160/800 mg PO q12h 10–20 mg/kg/d IV in divided doses	6–20 mg/kg/d PO/IV divided q6–12h

Note: Dosage adjustment necessary in patients with renal impairment.
*Dosing recommendations are based on the trimethoprim component.

Mechanism of Action and Spectrum of Activity

The sulfonamides work by inhibiting the incorporation of para-aminobenzoic acid, the basic building block used by bacteria to synthesize dihydrofolic acid, the first step leading to folic acid synthesis, required for bacterial cell growth. Sulfamethoxazole (SMX) competitively inhibits the bacterial enzyme dihydropteroate synthetase.

Trimethoprim (TMP), combined with SMX, inhibits the enzyme dihydrofolate reductase, synergistically inhibiting folic acid formation at another step in the pathway. Because bacterial dihydrofolate reductase is inhibited much more than the mammalian enzyme and because humans obtain exogenous dietary folate, inhibition of folate synthesis by SMX-TMP in humans is not a major problem.

The sulfonamides are active against a wide range of gram-positive and gram-negative organisms, with the exception of *Pseudomonas* species and group A streptococci. In combination with other folate antagonists, they also demonstrate activity against *P. jiroveci* and *Toxoplasma gondii*.

Clinical Uses

The sulfonamides are frequently used in treating many infections. Sulfasalazine (Azulfidine), a sulfonamide derivative lacking significant antimicrobial activity, is poorly absorbed and is used in the management of ulcerative colitis. Because of their limited spectrum of activity and increasing resistance, the sulfonamides are typically used in combination with other agents to increase efficacy or expand coverage. Trimethoprim–sulfamethoxazole (Bactrim) is the combination of choice in treating urinary tract infections, *P. jiroveci* pneumonia (PCP), toxoplasmosis, and some resistant gram-negative infections. Mafenide (Sulfamylon) and silver sulfadiazine (Silvadene) are topical agents frequently used in treating burns.

Adverse Events

Several side effects are reported for sulfonamides. The most common are rash, fever, and GI side effects. The rash occurs within 1 to 2 weeks of initiating therapy. Severe dermatologic reactions, such as Stevens-Johnson syndrome and vasculitis, are uncommon and associated more with longer-acting preparations. Hemolytic anemia can occur in patients with glucose-6-phosphate dehydrogenase deficiency.

Drug Interactions

The sulfonamides potentiate the effects of warfarin, phenytoin, hypoglycemic agents, and methotrexate as a result of drug displacement or decreased liver metabolism.

GLYCOPEPTIDES

Vancomycin, a glycopeptide antibiotic, was first introduced in 1958. Shortly after its introduction, vancomycin became known as "Mississippi Mud" because of the color and impurities in the manufacturing process. The clinical use of vancomycin was initially limited due to its potential for drug-related toxicities, alternative available agents, and concern for the development of resistance. However, since the early 1980s vancomycin has been an important agent in treating infections. Telavancin (Vibativ), a lipoglycopeptide, was recently introduced to the market. Telavancin is a synthetic derivative of vancomycin. Both agents have a narrow spectrum of activity directed toward gram-positive organisms.

Pharmacokinetics and Pharmacodynamics

Vancomycin is poorly absorbed from the GI tract. Because of its poor bioavailability, oral administration of vancomycin provides concentrations in the stool sufficient to treat *Clostridium difficile* colitis. The volume of distribution for vancomycin and telavancin, respectively, are 0.6 to 0.9 L/kg and 0.1 L/kg. Vancomycin is minimally bound to proteins; however, telavancin is highly bound to proteins (greater than 90%). They have relatively good penetration into most body fluids and tissues. Unpredictable levels are attained in the CSF and bone. Telavancin is dosed 10 mg/kg IV once daily. Vancomycin is dosed 15 to 20 mg/kg IV with the interval based on kidney function. **Table 8.14** provides an example of a vancomycin-dosing nomogram. Monitoring renal function is important in determining proper dosing because dosage adjustments are necessary in patients with renal insufficiency. Both vancomycin and telavancin are renally excreted, primarily as unchanged drug. The vancomycin half-life in adults with normal renal function is 5 to 11 hours. The half-life of telavancin is approximately 8 hours. Neither telavancin nor vancomycin is cleared to a significant extent by hemodialysis or peritoneal dialysis.

Serum drug monitoring is used for vancomycin in patients with unpredictable kidney function or severe infections or those receiving therapy for more than 3 to 5 days. In general, the target trough concentration ranges from 15 to 20 mg/mL for pneumonia, osteomyelitis, meningitis, and endocarditis and from 10 to 15 mg/mL for other infections. Peak concentrations are generally not recommended. Serum monitoring is not required for telavancin. Both agents exhibit bactericidal activity and a post-antibiotic effect of 1 to 4 hours.

Mechanism of Action and Spectrum of Activity

Vancomycin is a cell wall–active agent that inhibits the second stage of bacterial cell wall synthesis by binding to the D-alanyl D-alanine portion of the cell wall precursor. It also alters membrane permeability and ribonucleic acid (RNA) synthesis. Telavancin inhibits bacterial cell wall synthesis by interfering with the polymerization and cross-linking of peptidoglycan. Telavancin binds to the bacterial membrane and disrupts membrane barrier function. Telavancin has more rapid bactericidal activity than vancomycin.

The principal activity of vancomycin and telavancin is limited to gram-positive aerobic and anaerobic bacteria such as methicillin-sensitive and methicillin-resistant staphylococci, streptococci, enterococci, and *Clostridium* species.

Clinical Uses

Vancomycin is used to treat many infections. It is frequently used to treat serious gram-positive infections in patients allergic to or unable to tolerate beta-lactam antibiotics, and it is the drug of choice for MRSA and other resistant gram-positive infections. Neutropenic fever, endocarditis, and meningitis are commonly treated with vancomycin. Oral vancomycin is used in treating severe cases or *C. difficile* colitis or those that have failed to respond to metronidazole. Given the limited use of telavancin, it is currently indicated only for the treatment of skin and skin structure infections. Once additional evidence becomes available, it may be used for other MRSA infections and pneumonia.

Adverse Events

The most common side effects associated with vancomycin administration are fever and chills, phlebitis, and "red man" syndrome, a histamine-mediated phenomenon associated with the rate of vancomycin infusion. The typical syndrome consists of pruritus; flushing of the head, neck, and face; and hypotension. It usually resolves when the drug is discontinued. This reaction can also occur with telavancin. Vancomycin and telavancin should be infused over at least 1 hour.

TABLE 8.14	**Vancomycin Dosages**		
Estimated Creatinine Clearance (mL/min)	**Dosing Interval**		
	40–55 kg, 500 mg*	**55–75 kg, 750 mg***	**75–100 kg, 1,000 mg***
>80	q8h	q12h	q12h
54–80	q12h	q18h	q18h
40–53	q18h	q24h	q24h
27–39	q24h	q36h	q36h
21–26	q36h	q48h	q48h
16–20	q48h		

Note: These recommendations represent one of several nomograms used in the empiric dosing of vancomycin. Some prescribers use pharmacokinetic calculations and monitor serum trough levels to evaluate the efficacy and toxicity of a particular regimen. Therapeutic trough levels are typically maintained between 10 and 20 mcg/mL.
*Patient's body weight and IV dose of vancomycin.

Nephrotoxicity as a result of vancomycin alone is uncommon. Typically, a combination of variables and risk factors precipitates renal insufficiency. Risk factors include age, pre-existing renal disease, and the use of other nephrotoxic agents such as aminoglycosides, amphotericin B, acyclovir, and cyclosporine. In clinical trials evaluating telavancin and vancomycin, an increase in serum creatinine was more common with telavancin. Vancomycin has been classified as an ototoxic agent. Although rare, ototoxicity has occurred in patients receiving high-dose therapy or concurrent ototoxic agents (e.g., aminoglycosides). Hematologic effects from vancomycin such as thrombocytopenia and neutropenia are rare. The most common reported adverse effects of telavancin are taste disturbances, nausea, vomiting, and foamy urine. Due to the risk to the fetus, telavancin is contraindicated during pregnancy.

Drug Interactions

Since neither vancomycin nor telavancin undergo significant hepatic metabolism, drug–drug interactions with these two agents are unlikely.

OXAZOLIDINONES

The oxazolidinones are a totally synthetic antibiotic class first investigated in the late 1980s as antidepressant agents. Serendipitously, these agents were discovered to have excellent antibacterial activity. The main reason for their clinical development has been the emergence and spread of resistance in gram-positive pathogens. Linezolid (Zyvox) is the only agent available in this class.

Pharmacokinetics and Pharmacodynamics

Linezolid is well absorbed from the GI tract. Peak levels are achieved within 1 to 2 hours, and levels increase linearly as the dose is increased. The absolute bioavailability is approximately 100%. The oral formulation may be administered without regard to meals. Linezolid is predominantly eliminated by nonrenal mechanisms. Its metabolism does not involve the CYP enzyme system. Two inactive metabolites are the major by-products of this conversion to more water-soluble products that are excreted by the kidney. Linezolid is removed by hemodialysis and should be dosed following hemodialysis sessions. **Table 8.15** provides dosing information.

Linezolid is considered a bacteriostatic agent. A post-antibiotic effect of 3 to 6 hours has been reported, but this has little clinical significance.

TABLE 8.15	Linezolid Dosages	
Drug	**Adult Dosages**	**Pediatric Dosages**
linezolid	400–600 mg PO/IV q12h	20 mg/kg/d PO/IV divided q12h OR 30 mg/kg/d PO/IV divided q8h

Mechanism of Action and Spectrum of Activity

Linezolid binds to the 50S ribosome at a unique binding site and disrupts bacterial protein synthesis. Antagonism has been described with chloramphenicol and clindamycin.

The principal activity of linezolid is against gram-positive aerobic organisms, including staphylococci, streptococci, and enterococci. In particular, activity against resistant pathogens, including MRSA, penicillin-resistant streptococci, and VRE is excellent.

Clinical Uses

Linezolid has FDA approval for the treatment of community and nosocomial pneumonia, skin and skin structure infections, and vancomycin-resistant *Enterococcus faecium*. Given the high cost of this agent, it is generally reserved for patients with allergies or contraindications to other agents. It is most frequently used in treating skin infections and as part of a drug combination for hospital-acquired pneumonia.

Adverse Events

In general, linezolid is well tolerated. The most common adverse events include diarrhea, nausea, taste perversion, and vomiting. As mentioned earlier, this class of agents was initially investigated for its antidepressant activity. Thrombocytopenia has been reported on average in 3% to 4% of patients in studies. Additionally, anemia, leukopenia, and pancytopenia have been reported. A complete blood count should be monitored in patients, especially if receiving linezolid for longer than 2 weeks.

Drug Interactions

Linezolid possess weak monoamine oxidase inhibitory activity. There is a potential for drug interactions with sympathomimetic agents, such as pseudoephedrine, antidepressants, some herbal products, and foods rich in tyramine.

LIPOPEPTIDES

Daptomycin is an antibacterial agent belonging to the class known as the lipopeptides. This class of agents has been studied for its antibacterial activity for several decades; however, daptomycin is the only agent available. Daptomycin is a natural product developed for the treatment of MDR gram-positive pathogens.

Pharmacokinetics and Pharmacodynamics

Daptomycin pharmacokinetics are nearly linear and time independent at doses up to 6 mg/kg administered once daily for 7 days. Its half-life is approximately 8 hours. The apparent volume of distribution in healthy adults is approximately 0.1 L/kg. Daptomycin reversibly binds human plasma proteins, primarily to serum albumin, with a mean serum protein binding of 90%. Because renal excretion is the primary route of elimination, dosage adjustments are necessary in patients with severe renal insufficiency (creatinine clearance less than 30 mL/minute). The dose for patients with normal renal function is 4 to 6 mg/kg IV administered daily. There is very limited information to support the use of daptomycin in pediatric patients. Daptomycin exhibits rapid, concentration-dependent bactericidal activity against gram-positive organisms.

Mechanism of Action and Spectrum of Activity

The mechanism of action of daptomycin is distinct from that of any other antibiotic. It binds to bacterial membranes and causes a rapid depolarization of membrane potential. The loss of membrane potential leads to bacterial cell death.

Daptomycin covers most gram-positive pathogens such as *S. aureus* (including methicillin-resistant strains), streptococcus, and enterococcus. It is active against MRSA and VRE.

Clinical Uses

Daptomycin is indicated for the treatment of complicated skin and skin structure infections and *S. aureus* bloodstream infections (bacteremia), including those with right-sided infective endocarditis, caused by methicillin-susceptible and methicillin-resistant isolates. Daptomycin is a useful alternative to other agents (linezolid, quinupristin/dalfopristin) for treating infections caused by resistant gram-positive pathogens because there are few options at present for treating these infections. For complicated skin and skin structure infections, combination therapy may be clinically indicated if the documented or presumed pathogens include gram-negative or anaerobic organisms. Daptomycin is not indicated for the treatment of pneumonia.

Adverse Events

Daptomycin may cause GI reactions such as constipation, nausea, diarrhea, and vomiting. Injection-site reactions and headache may occur. Skeletal muscle toxicity manifested as muscle pain has been reported with daptomycin. This is accompanied by an increase in creatinine phosphokinase (CPK) levels.

Drug Interactions

CPK monitoring should be done at least weekly for patients concomitantly receiving an HMG-CoA reductase inhibitor and/or those with renal insufficiency. Otherwise, daptomycin does not have any significant drug–drug interactions.

STREPTOGRAMINS

The streptogramin antibiotics are naturally occurring products that have been used clinically in Europe for more than 40 years. The semi-synthetic derivative, quinupristin/dalfopristin (Synercid), is the only streptogramin antibiotic available in the United States. It is a combination of two antibiotics.

Pharmacokinetics and Pharmacodynamics

Quinupristin/dalfopristin is not absorbed from the GI tract. After IV administration, both quinupristin and dalfopristin have a serum half-life of approximately 1 hour. Each drug is moderately protein bound; the volume of distribution is 0.45 L/kg and 0.24 L/kg for quinupristin and dalfopristin, respectively. Metabolism of both agents is through the liver. The drug is primarily excreted in the feces.

Quinupristin/dalfopristin is a bactericidal agent against most organisms, with the noted exception of vancomycin-resistant *E. faecium*. Quinupristin/dalfopristin possesses a post-antibiotic effect ranging from 8 to 18 hours. The dosage for adults and children is 7.5 mg/kg every 8 to 12 hours. It is not significantly removed by hemodialysis or peritoneal dialysis.

Mechanism of Action and Spectrum of Activity

The streptogramins inhibit protein synthesis by binding to the 50S ribosome. The interaction of quinupristin and dalfopristin is synergistic. Either compound alone is bacteriostatic, whereas the combination results in a bactericidal effect.

The principal activity of quinupristin/dalfopristin is against gram-positive aerobic organisms, including staphylococci, streptococci, and enterococci. In particular, its activity against resistant pathogens, including methicillin-resistant staphylococci, penicillin-resistant streptococci, and vancomycin-resistant *E. faecium*, is excellent. Quinupristin/dalfopristin is not active against *Enterococcus faecalis*.

Clinical Uses

Quinupristin/dalfopristin is approved by the FDA for treating skin and skin structure infections and vancomycin-resistant *E. faecium* infections. The use of this agent is limited due to adverse effects and the need for administration through a central venous line. It can be used to treat gram-positive infections caused by methicillin-resistant staphylococci, penicillin-resistant *S. pneumoniae*, and vancomycin-resistant *E. faecium* when alternative agents are contraindicated.

Adverse Events

The most common adverse reactions are infusion related. Infusion-site reactions, including pain, inflammation, edema, and thrombophlebitis, have been reported in as many as 75% of patients receiving quinupristin/dalfopristin through a peripheral IV catheter. Arthralgias and myalgias have also been reported. They may be severe and result in discontinuation of therapy. They usually occur after several days of therapy. After discontinuation of therapy, these reactions are uniformly reversible. The most common laboratory abnormality is an increased level of conjugated bilirubin.

Drug Interactions

The CYP3A4 isoenzyme (responsible for the metabolism of many drugs) is significantly inhibited by quinupristin/

dalfopristin. Close clinical or serum level monitoring of known substrates of the CYP3A4 enzyme is recommended.

ANTI-ANAEROBIC AGENTS: CLINDAMYCIN

Clindamycin (Cleocin) has been used extensively in treating gram-positive and anaerobic bacterial infections. It was first used orally to treat streptococcal and staphylococcal infections, but it soon became the drug of choice for anaerobic infections. The combination of clindamycin and gentamicin (Garamycin) is still frequently used in treating mixed aerobic and anaerobic infections.

Pharmacokinetics and Pharmacodynamics

Both the clindamycin hydrochloride and palmitate hydrochloride salts are well absorbed and converted to active forms in the blood. Clindamycin reaches most tissues and bone, but its distribution into CSF is limited. It is 93% bound to proteins. The half-life is approximately 3 hours. Clindamycin is metabolized by the liver, necessitating dosage adjustment in patients with liver impairment (**Table 8.16**). Hemodialysis and peritoneal dialysis do not remove clindamycin to a significant extent.

Mechanism of Action and Spectrum of Activity

Clindamycin binds to the 50S subunit of the bacterial ribosome and inhibits protein synthesis. It acts at the same site as chloramphenicol and the macrolides.

Clinical Uses

Clindamycin is typically included in regimens for its anaerobic coverage in mixed infections and may also be used in treating gram-positive infections, toxoplasmosis, and PCP or in combination with other agents to treat PID. In addition, it is frequently used to inhibit toxin production as part of the treatment for staphylococcal or streptococcal toxic shock.

Adverse Events

The major side effect associated with clindamycin is diarrhea and associated *C. difficile* colitis. This adverse event is unrelated to dose and may range from acute, self-limiting symptoms to life-threatening toxic megacolon. Pain at the site of IV administration may occur.

Drug Interactions

In rare cases, clindamycin use in combination with skeletal muscle relaxants has been reported to potentiate neuromuscular blockade.

ANTI-ANAEROBIC AGENTS: METRONIDAZOLE

Metronidazole (Flagyl) was first recognized for its antiprotozoal activity in treating *Trichomonas vaginalis* infections. Subsequently, its utility as an anti-anaerobic agent was used in treating *B. fragilis* infections. Metronidazole has become a treatment of choice for anaerobic infections, *C. difficile* colitis, and is part of a number of regimens to eradicate *Helicobacter pylori*–associated duodenal ulcers.

Pharmacokinetics and Pharmacodynamics

Metronidazole is completely absorbed from the GI tract after oral administration. It penetrates well into most tissues, with an apparent volume of distribution of 0.3 to 0.9 L/kg. Its binding to plasma protein is minimal. The liver metabolizes metronidazole, and dosage adjustments are necessary in patients with hepatic impairment (**Table 8.17**). The half-life is approximately 6 to 9 hours. Metronidazole is removed by hemodialysis and peritoneal dialysis.

Mechanism of Action and Spectrum of Activity

Metronidazole is reduced to a toxic product that interacts with DNA, causing strand breakage and resulting in protein synthesis inhibition. Metronidazole has excellent activity against gram-positive and gram-negative anaerobes, *H. pylori*, and protozoa such as *T. vaginalis*.

Clinical Uses

Metronidazole is typically included in regimens for its anaerobic coverage in mixed infections. In addition, metronidazole is the treatment of choice for bacterial vaginosis, trichomoniasis, and *C. difficile* diarrhea.

Adverse Events

Metronidazole is usually safe and well tolerated. GI side effects such as nausea, vomiting, abdominal pain, and a metallic

TABLE 8.16	Clindamycin Dosages	
Drug	**Adult Dosages**	**Pediatric Dosages**
clindamycin	150–450 mg PO q6–8h 600 mg IV q8h	10–30 mg/kg/d PO divided q6–8h 25–40 mg/kg/d IV divided q6–8h

Note: Dosage adjustment recommended for patients with liver dysfunction.

TABLE 8.17	Metronidazole Dosages	
Drug	**Adult Dosages**	**Pediatric Dosages**
metronidazole	250–500 mg PO q6–8h 500 mg IV q6–12h	15–35 mg/kg/d PO/ IV divided q6h

Note: Dosage adjustment recommended for patients with severe liver or kidney dysfunction.

taste are most common. More serious but rare effects include seizures, peripheral neuropathy, and pancreatitis. Seizures have been associated with high doses, whereas peripheral neuropathy has been documented in patients receiving prolonged courses of metronidazole.

Drug Interactions

Metronidazole enhances the anticoagulant effect of warfarin, resulting in a prolonged half-life of warfarin. A disulfiram-like reaction characterized by flushing, palpitations, nausea, and vomiting may occur when alcohol is consumed during metronidazole therapy. Metronidazole is an inhibitor of the CYP3A4 isoenzyme. It has the potential to interact with multiple medications. Additionally, phenobarbital, phenytoin, and rifampin increase the metabolism of metronidazole, which may result in treatment failure. A careful review of a patient's medication list for drug interactions should be done before initiating metronidazole.

MISCELLANEOUS ANTIMICROBIAL AGENTS: CHLORAMPHENICOL

Chloramphenicol has a wide spectrum of activity against gram-positive, gram-negative, and anaerobic organisms. However, its use has been limited by its toxicity profile, which includes "gray baby" syndrome, optic neuritis, and fatal aplastic anemia. Nonetheless, in selected situations, chloramphenicol remains an important agent.

Pharmacokinetics and Pharmacodynamics

Chloramphenicol is available as an IV succinate ester. The dose is based on age and indication (**Table 8.18**). The ester formulation is hydrolyzed in the body to the active drug. Chloramphenicol penetrates well into most tissues and bodily fluids, including the CSF. Chloramphenicol readily crosses the placenta in pregnant females. It is conjugated in the liver and excreted by the kidney in an inactive, nontoxic form. The serum half-life is 3 to 4 hours. Chloramphenicol is 25% to 50% bound to protein.

Serum levels are frequently monitored in high-risk patients. The therapeutic range of chloramphenicol is 5 to 20 mg/dL. Dose-related myelosuppression typically occurs at serum levels exceeding 25 mg/dL.

TABLE 8.18	Chloramphenicol Dosages
Patient Group	**Dosage**
Older children and adults	50–100 mg/kg/d IV divided q6h (max 4000 mg daily)
Older children and adults with meningitis	75–100 mg/kg/d IV divided q6h

Note: Chloramphenicol should be used with caution in patients with renal impairment, and serum concentrations should be monitored to guide dosing and prevent toxicity.

Mechanism of Action and Spectrum of Activity

Chloramphenicol reversibly binds to the larger 50S subunit of the ribosome, thereby inhibiting bacterial protein synthesis. It is variably bactericidal.

Chloramphenicol is active against gram-positive and gram-negative aerobes and anaerobes as well as atypical organisms, including mycoplasma, chlamydia, and rickettsiae. Its gram-negative activity includes *E. coli*, *Proteus* species, and *Salmonella* species, but not *P. aeruginosa*.

Clinical Uses

Newer agents have reduced the need to use chloramphenicol in treating infection. However, it can be used as an alternative in treating bacterial meningitis when a patient has a life-threatening penicillin allergy. It is also useful in treating rickettsial diseases such as Rocky Mountain spotted fever and typhus fever in patients allergic to tetracyclines or in pregnant women. Chloramphenicol may be used in treating VRE infections as well.

Adverse Events

The major adverse events associated with chloramphenicol are "gray baby" syndrome, blood dyscrasias, and optic neuritis. "Gray baby" syndrome typically occurs in neonates and is manifested by vomiting, lethargy, respiratory collapse, and death. It results from drug accumulation because neonates cannot conjugate chloramphenicol. Two forms of hematologic toxicity may occur with chloramphenicol administration. Dose-related bone marrow suppression has occurred in patients receiving doses exceeding 4 g/day and at serum levels exceeding 25 mg/dL. It may present as a combination of anemia, leukopenia, and thrombocytopenia. Aplastic anemia is an idiosyncratic effect independent of dose and may occur weeks after therapy with chloramphenicol. It is associated with a greater than 50% mortality rate and often necessitates bone marrow transplantation. Optic neuritis is a major neurologic complication and is associated with long courses of chloramphenicol. The toxicity involves red-green color changes and loss of vision. It may be reversible or permanent. GI side effects have been associated with high doses of chloramphenicol.

Drug Interactions

Chloramphenicol is metabolized by the liver and is an inhibitor of the CYP enzyme system. It prolongs the half-life of warfarin, phenytoin, and cyclosporine.

MISCELLANEOUS ANTIMICROBIAL AGENTS: RIFAMPIN

Rifampin is a macrocyclic antibiotic used in a variety of settings, and it is a first-line agent in treating tuberculosis. It is typically combined with other antibiotics such as vancomycin in treating MRSA infections.

TABLE 8.19	Rifampin Dosages	
Drug	**Adult Dosages**	**Pediatric Dosages**
rifampin	600 mg PO once daily 10–20 mg/kg IV daily	10–20 mg/kg IV generally once daily

Note: Dosage adjustment recommended for patients with liver dysfunction.

Pharmacokinetics and Pharmacodynamics

Rifampin is completely absorbed after oral administration. It distributes into most tissues and fluids, including the CSF. The half-life of rifampin is approximately 3 hours. It is metabolized by the liver and is not removed by hemodialysis or peritoneal dialysis. **Table 8.19** provides dosing information.

Mechanism of Action and Spectrum of Activity

Rifampin suppresses initiation of chain formation for RNA synthesis in susceptible bacteria by inhibiting DNA-dependent RNA polymerase. The β subunit of the enzyme appears to be the site of action.

Rifampin is extremely active against gram-positive cocci. It has moderate activity against aerobic gram-negative bacilli. *Neisseria meningitidis*, *Neisseria gonorrhoeae*, and *H. influenzae* are the most sensitive gram-negative organisms. Rifampin maintains activity against *M. tuberculosis*.

Clinical Uses

Rifampin is commonly used in combination with a cell wall–active agent to treat serious, gram-positive infections that fail to respond to other courses of therapy. This combination is used for synergistic activity and prevents rapid resistance development. It is the drug of choice for post-exposure meningitis prophylaxis against *N. meningitidis* and *H. influenzae* type B. Rifampin is a first-line agent in the treatment of *M. tuberculosis* infection, and it is used to treat nontuberculous mycobacterial infections as well.

Adverse Events

The most common side effects associated with rifampin are GI distress (nausea, vomiting, and diarrhea), headache, and fever. Rifampin changes bodily fluids such as sweat, saliva, and tears to a red-orange color. Hepatotoxicity is rare, but the risk increases when it is administered in combination with isoniazid. Liver function tests should be monitored while patients receive rifampin. Anemia or thrombocytopenia also has been reported.

Drug Interactions

Rifampin is a potent inducer of hepatic CYP drug metabolism and precipitates many drug interactions. Rifampin increases the clearance of agents such as antiarrhythmics, azole antifungals, clarithromycin, estrogens, most HMG-CoA reductase inhibitors, warfarin, and many HIV medications. A careful review of a patient's medication list for drug interactions should be done before initiating rifampin.

MISCELLANEOUS ANTIMICROBIAL AGENTS: NITROFURANTOIN

Nitrofurantoin is an antimicrobial agent used only for treating and preventing urinary tract infections. Nitrofurantoin has been used in the United States since 1953 and still remains very effective. It is a synthetic nitrofuran-compound derivative, a class that also includes furazolidone, available in Europe.

Pharmacokinetics and Pharmacodynamics

Following oral administration, nitrofurantoin is rapidly absorbed. The bioavailability of nitrofurantoin is approximately 40% to 50%. Absorption can be enhanced with food. Nitrofurantoin serum concentrations are low, with a serum half-life of less than 30 minutes. For this reason, nitrofurantoin should not be used for complicated urinary tract infections or in patients for which a concern of bacteremia exists. Nitrofurantoin undergoes renal elimination. Inadequate urinary concentrations are achieved in patients with renal insufficiency; thus, the drug is ineffective. It is contraindicated in patients with a creatinine clearance of less than 60 mL/minute. **Table 8.20** provides dosing information.

Mechanism of Action and Spectrum of Activity

The exact mechanism of nitrofurantoin is poorly understood. The drug does inhibit several bacterial enzymes, which results in impaired bacterial cell wall synthesis.

Nitrofurantoin has adequate antimicrobial coverage against common organisms that cause urinary tract infections such as *E. coli*, *Citrobacter* species, *Staphylococcus saprophyticus*, *E. faecalis*, and *E. faecium*. Nitrofurantoin frequently covers strains of VRE. Resistance has increased against some types of bacteria such as *Enterobacter* and *Klebsiella* species.

Clinical Uses

Nitrofurantoin is only used for the treatment and prophylaxis of uncomplicated urinary tract infections. As mentioned

TABLE 8.20	Nitrofurantoin Dosages	
Drug	**Adult Dosages**	**Pediatric Dosages**
nitrofurantoin	50 mg PO q6h (macrocrystal) 100 mg PO q12h (macrocrystal/ monohydrate)	5–7 mg/kg/d PO divided q6h

Note: Nitrofurantoin is contraindicated in patients with a creatinine clearance of less than 60 mL/minute.

earlier, it should not be used for complicated urinary tract infections such as pyelonephritis.

Adverse Events

The most common side effects of nitrofurantoin include nausea and vomiting. Allergic reactions are rare. Pulmonary reactions (pulmonary infiltrates, pneumonitis, pulmonary fibrosis) and hepatic effects (hepatitis, hepatic necrosis) have been reported in rare cases, usually associated with long-term use. Additionally, peripheral neuropathy has been associated with long-term use in patients with renal failure.

Drug Interactions

Nitrofurantoin is not associated with significant drug interactions.

ANTIMICROBIAL RESISTANCE

There are multiple mechanisms by which bacteria form or acquire antibiotic resistance. Some types of resistance occur naturally, while others are acquired from another strain of bacteria. Additionally, resistance can sometimes be induced during antibiotic treatment. **Table 8.21** summarizes the most common resistance mechanisms.

1. The first and most common type of resistance is bacterial enzyme production. For example, bacteria frequently produce enzymes that disrupt beta-lactam antibiotics, altering the structure so they cannot bind to the PBPs.

There are hundreds of different types of these enzymes known as *beta-lactamases*. Some enzymes have activity only against penicillins (penicillinases), whereas others, such as extended-spectrum beta-lactamases, can render almost all beta-lactam antibiotics ineffective. Separate from beta-lactamases, bacteria also produce enzymes that can alter the chemical structure or inactivate the drug. This can occur with aminoglycosides, chloramphenicol, macrolides, streptogramins, and tetracyclines.

2. Resistance can occur as the bacteria alter their own cell membranes, not permitting antibiotics to enter the bacteria. An example of this is loss of porins on the gram-negative bacterial cell outer membrane. Specifically with beta-lactam antibiotics, loss of these porins alters the ability of the antimicrobial agent to enter the cell.

3. A third, common mechanism of resistance is the activation of efflux pumps that expel antibiotics out of the intracellular space back across the cell membrane. This prevents antibiotics from acting at their intracellular target site. This is a common mechanism of resistance with classes such as tetracyclines and macrolides.

4. A fourth type of resistance is alteration of the antibiotic's target site of action. This occurs with macrolides, among other classes, when mutations alter the ribosomal binding site. The antibiotic does not bind at all or as well to the ribosome anymore. Similarly, VRE is a result of altered cell well precursors. Plasmid-mediated resistance results in a modified peptidoglycan precursor that binds vancomycin, preventing it from binding to its intended target site.

5. A fifth type of resistance is alteration of target enzymes. For example, the FQs work by inhibiting the enzymes DNA

TABLE 8.21	Antimicrobial Resistance					
Antibiotic/Antibiotic Class	**Bacterial Enzyme Production**	**Decreased Membrane Permeability**	**Promotion of Antibiotic Efflux**	**Altered Target Sites/Protection of Target Site**	**Altered Target Enzymes**	**Overproduction of Target**
Penicillins	✓	✓	✓		✓	
Cephalosporins	✓	✓	✓		✓	
Monobactams	✓	✓				
Carbapenems	✓	✓	✓			
Fluoroquinolones		✓	✓	✓	✓	
Macrolides	✓		✓	✓		
Aminoglycosides	✓			✓		
Tetracyclines	✓		✓	✓		
Sulfamethoxazole/Trimethoprim					✓	✓
Glycopeptides				✓		
Oxazolidinones				✓		
Streptogramins	✓		✓	✓		
Clindamycin	✓			✓		
Metronidazole		✓			✓	
Chloramphenicol	✓	✓				
Rifampin				✓		
Nitrofurantoin					✓	

gyrase and topoisomerase IV. Mutations to a variety of different chromosomes on these enzymes can reduce the efficacy of the FQs.

6. Last, overproduction of target enzymes can result in resistance. The best example of this is with sulfonamides and trimethoprim. Sulfamethoxazole/trimethoprim works by inhibiting folic acid synthesis by inhibiting the dihydropteroate synthetase and dihydrofolate reductase enzymes, respectively. These enzymes are required for bacterial folic acid synthesis. Excess production of these two enzymes in some strains of bacteria can render the antibiotic ineffective.

A specific area of interest in antimicrobial development is targeting the prevention or overcoming drug resistance.

ANTIMICROBIAL STEWARDSHIP

Overuse of antibiotics is well documented and has led to increased resistance to various strains of bacteria worldwide. Some examples of drug-resistant bacteria include extended-spectrum beta-lactamases against *E. coli* and *Klebsiella*, carbapenem-resistant *Klebsiella*, fluoroquinolone-resistant gonococcus, MRSA, and vancomycin intermediate *S. aureus*. Given the slow development of new antibiotics for the treatment of resistant pathogens, appropriate antibiotic use is crucial. The Infectious Diseases Society of America has developed antibiotic stewardship guidelines. These guidelines recommend a multidisciplinary approach to improving antibiotic use, particularly in the hospital setting. A few ways to improve antibiotic use include formulary restrictions, evidence-based prescribing, dose optimization, antibiotic streamlining, and de-escalation. To minimize resistance, all prescribers must make an effort to ensure appropriate antibiotic use.

BIBLIOGRAPHY

Andes, D. R., & Craig, W. A. (2005). Cephalosporins. In G. L. Mandell, J. E. Bennett, & R. Dolin (Eds.), *Principles and practice of infectious diseases* (6th ed.). Philadelphia, PA: Churchill Livingstone.

Bolon, M. K. (2009). The newer fluoroquinolones. *Infectious Diseases Clinics of North America, 23,* 1027–1051.

Calfee, D. P. (2005). Rifamycins. In G. L. Mandell, J. E. Bennett, & R. Dolin (Eds.), *Principles and practice of infectious diseases* (6th ed.). Philadelphia, PA: Churchill Livingstone.

Chambers, H. F. (2005). Penicillins. In G. L. Mandell, J. E. Bennett, & R. Dolin (Eds.), *Principles and practice of infectious diseases* (6th ed.). Philadelphia, PA: Churchill Livingstone.

Chambers, H. F. (2005). Other beta-lactam antibiotics. In G. L. Mandell, J. E. Bennett, & R. Dolin (Eds.), *Principles and practice of infectious diseases* (6th ed.). Philadelphia, PA: Churchill Livingstone.

Dellit, T. H., Owens, R. C., McGowan, J. E., et al. (2007). Infectious Diseases Society of America and the Society for Healthcare Epidemiology of America guidelines for developing an institutional program to enhance antimicrobial stewardship. *Clinical Infectious Diseases, 44,* 159–177.

Guay, D. (2007). Update on clindamycin in the management of bacterial, fungal and protozoal infections. *Expert Opinion on Pharmacotherapy, 8*(14), 2401–2444.

Hooper, D. C. (2005). Urinary tract agents: Nitrofurantoin and methenamine. In G. L. Mandell, J. E. Bennett, & R. Dolin (Eds.), *Principles and practice of infectious diseases* (6th ed.). Philadelphia, PA: Churchill Livingstone.

Kattan, J. N., Villegas, M. V., & Quinn, J. P. (2008). New developments in carbapenems. *Clinical Microbiology and Infection, 14*(12), 1102–1111.

Khardori, N. (2006). Antibiotics—Past, present, and future. *Medical Clinics of North America, 90,* 1049–1076.

Lee, S. Y., Fan, H. W., & Kuti, J. L. (2006). Update on daptomycin: The first approved lipopeptide antibiotic. *Expert Opinion on Pharmacotherapy, 7*(10), 1381–1397.

Leibovici, L., Vidal, L., & Paul, M. (2009). Aminoglycoside drugs in clinical practice: An evidence-based approach. *Journal of Antimicrobial Chemotherapy, 63,* 246–251.

Levine, D. P. (2008). Vancomycin: Understanding its past and preserving its future. *Southern Medical Journal, 101*(3), 284–291.

Matthews, S. J., & Lancaster, J. W. (2009). Doripenem monohydrate, a broad-spectrum carbapenem antibiotic. *Clinical Therapeutics, 31*(1), 42–63.

Meyers, B., & Salvatore. M. (2005). Tetracyclines and chloramphenicol. In G. L. Mandell, J. E. Bennett, & R. Dolin (Eds.), *Principles and practice of infectious diseases* (6th ed.). Philadelphia, PA: Churchill Livingstone.

Nicolau, D. P. (2008). Carbapenems: A potent class of antibiotics. *Expert Opinion on Pharmacotherapy, 9*(1), 23–37.

Opal, S. M., & Medeiros, A. A. (2005). Molecular mechanisms of antibiotic resistance in bacteria. In G. L. Mandell, J. E. Bennett, & R. Dolin (Eds.), *Principles and practice of infectious diseases* (6th ed.). Philadelphia, PA: Churchill Livingstone.

Paterson, D. L., & DePestel, D. D. (2009). Doripenem. *Clinical Infectious Diseases, 49,* 291–298.

Rice, L. B. (2009). The clinical consequences of antimicrobial resistance. *Current Opinion in Microbiology, 12*(5), 476–481.

Rose, W. E., & Rybak, M. J. (2006). Tigecycline: First of a new class of antimicrobial agents. *Pharmacotherapy, 26*(8), 1099–1110.

Rybak, M. (2006). The pharmacokinetic and pharmacodynamic properties of vancomycin. *Clinical Infectious Diseases, 42,* S35–39.

Rybak, M. J., Lomaestro, B., Rotschafer, J. C., et al. (2009). Therapeutic monitoring of vancomycin in adult patients: A consensus review of the American Society of Health-System Pharmacists, the Infectious Diseases Society of America, and the Society of Infectious Diseases Pharmacists. *American Journal of Health System Pharmacists, 66,* 82–98.

Salvatore, M., & Meyers, B. (2005). Metronidazole. In G. L. Mandell, J. E. Bennett, & R. Dolin (Eds.), *Principles and practice of infectious diseases* (6th ed.). Philadelphia, PA: Churchill Livingstone.

Saravolatz, L. D., Stein, G. E., & Johnson, L. B. (2009). Telavancin: A novel lipoglycopeptide. *Clinical Infectious Diseases, 49*(15), 1908–1914.

Stahlmann, R., & Lode, H. (2010). Safety considerations of fluoroquinolones in the elderly. *Drugs and Aging, 27*(3), 193–209.

Wilcox, M. H. (2005). Update on linezolid: The first oxazolidinone antibiotic. *Expert Opinion on Pharmacotherapy, 6*(13), 2315–2326.

Zhanel, G. G., Wiebe, R., Dilay, L., et al. (2007). Comparative review of the carbapenems. *Drugs, 67*(7), 1027–1052.

Zinner, S. H., & Mayer, K. H. (2005). Sulfonamides and trimethoprim. In G. L. Mandell, J. E. Bennett, & R. Dolin (Eds.), *Principles and practice of infectious diseases* (6th ed.). Philadelphia, PA: Churchill Livingstone.

Zuckerman, J. M., Qamar, F., Bono, B. R. (2009). Macrolides, ketolides, and glycycyclines: Azithromycin, clarithromycin, telithromycin, tigecycline. *Infectious Disease Clinics of North America, 23,* 997–1026.

Complementary and Alternative Medicine

There has been a tremendous growth in the use of complementary and alternative medicine (CAM) in the United States in recent years. *Complementary medicine* is defined as that used together with conventional medicine. *Alternative medicine* is that used in place of conventional medicine. Approximately 38% of adults and 12% of children in the United States use some form of CAM. The most frequent users of CAM are between 30 and 49 years of age with a higher education and income level. Women use CAM more frequently than men (http://nccam. nih.gov/news/camstats/2007/camsurvey_fs1.htm).

People use CAM because they want more control over their medical care, they feel an affinity for a holistic or "natural" approach, they are dissatisfied with the attitudes of their health care providers, they are discouraged with the increased cost of traditional medical care, or conventional medicine fails to meet their needs (**Box 9.1**). *Integrative medicine*, a combination of mainstream medical treatment and CAM, appears to have more scientific evidence regarding safety and efficacy. This chapter will focus on the agents that are in the mainstream of Western society, such as herbal or dietary supplements.

In 1995, the National Institute of Health's Office of Alternative Medicine defined CAM as the "broad domain of healing resources that encompasses all health systems, modalities, and practices and their accompanying theories and beliefs other than those intrinsic to the politically dominant health system of a particular society or culture in a given historical period. CAM includes all such practices and ideas self-defined by their users as preventing or treating illness or promoting health and well-being."

DOMAINS OF CAM

There are five domains of CAM (**Box 9.2**): alternative medicine system, mind/body interventions, biologically based therapy, manipulation and body-based methods, and energy therapies. Alternative medicine systems are based on complete systems of theory and practice. Mind/body interventions incorporate a variety of techniques to enhance the mind's capacity to affect bodily function; a common practice is biofeedback. Biologically based therapy is treatment with substances found in nature. Manipulation and body-based methods are based on manipulation or movement of body parts; an example is chiropractic manipulation. Energy therapies involve the use of energy fields such as magnets.

NATIONAL CENTER FOR COMPLEMENTARY AND ALTERNATIVE MEDICINE

The National Center for Complementary and Alternative Medicine (NCCAM) was established in 1998 by congressional mandate. It is dedicated to exploring complementary and alternative healing practices in the context of rigorous science. Its purpose is to train CAM researchers and disseminate authoritative information to the public and professionals. It serves as an information clearinghouse and facilitates research and training programs, which are funded by the federal government. NCCAM has four areas of focus: research, research training and career development, outreach, and integration.

NCCAM identifies CAM practitioners. It also publishes alerts and advisories for specific products and practices, lists clinical trials of CAM, and provides treatment information.

REGULATION

Over 100 million Americans use dietary supplements, which are defined as products taken orally that contain a "dietary product"

BOX	**9.1**
	Reasons to Use CAM

- Advertising
- Affinity to the natural approach
- Desire to have control over treatment
- Desperation
- Dissatisfaction with prescription drugs
- High cost of traditional medical care and drugs
- Perceived effectiveness
- Perceived safety
- Rejection of established medical practices

BOX 9.2

Domains of Complementary and Alternative Medicine

Alternative Medicine Systems — These are built upon complete systems of theory and practice and have often evolved apart from and earlier than the conventional medical approach popular in the United States. Examples are homeopathic and naturopathic medicine and traditional Chinese medicine.

Mind/Body Interventions — This incorporates a variety of techniques designed to enhance the mind's capacity to affect bodily function and symptoms. This includes biofeedback, meditation, dance therapy, and art therapy.

Biologically Based Therapy — This is treatment with substances found in nature, including dietary supplements, herbal supplements, and "natural" but scientifically unproved treatment.

Manipulation and Body-Based Methods — These are based on manipulation or movement of body parts. Examples include chiropractic manipulation and massage therapy.

Energy Therapies — This is the use of energy fields. Biofield therapy affects the energy fields that purportedly surround and penetrate the human body and includes Reiki and Therapeutic Touch. Bioelectromagnetic therapy is based on treatment involving the unconventional use of electromagnetic fields. An example is magnet therapy.

---

intended to supplement the diet. These may include vitamins, minerals, herbs, amino acids, other botanicals, or substances such as enzymes, organ tissues, and metabolites. The products may be in the form of powder, capsules, tablets, gelcaps, or liquids. The increasing use of dietary supplements reflects the increased interest in "natural" medicine, fitness, health, and disease prevention. Also, consumers want to avoid the high cost of traditional drugs and the side effects of these drugs.

More than 500 herbs are marketed in the United States; indeed, about 25% of the current pharmacopoeia is derived from botanicals. The cardiac glycoside digoxin comes from the foxglove plant. Aspirin comes from willow bark, oral contraceptives from Mexican yam, warfarin from sweet clover, and capsaicin from the red pepper plant.

BOX 9.3

Label Requirements for Herbal Preparations

- Name
- Quantity of contents
- Ingredients and amounts
- Disclaimer: "This statement has not been evaluated by the FDA. This product is not intended to diagnose, treat, cure or prevent disease."
- Supplemental facts panel
  - Serving size
  - Amount
  - Active ingredients
- Other ingredients such as herbs for which no daily values exist
- Name and address of manufacturer, packer, or distributor

In March 2003, the U.S. Food and Drug Administration (FDA) published new guidelines for dietary supplements that would prevent contamination with other herbs, pesticides, heavy metals, or prescription drugs. Manufacturers do not have to prove the supplement's quality but must meet certain FDA standards. The FDA can take action only if it finds that a product is unsafe once it is on the market. Each product must have a label accurately listing the product's ingredients. **Box 9.3** lists label requirements for herbal preparations.

Products also have a "Supplemental Facts" panel that lists the appropriate serving size. Natural remedies cannot be patented, so the manufacturer does not need to take the time and money to conduct necessary tests.

Nutrition Labeling and Education Act (NLEA)

NLEA was enacted by Congress in 1990 to provide a clear relationship of nutrition to disease. The purpose of the act was to educate consumers. Information required on the label includes nutritional information, in an easy-to-read format, with the amount of ingredient per serving, the percentage of daily values of the ingredients, and the standard serving size. The act also established that disease-related health claims could be used on labeling of nutritional products, provided there is agreement among qualified scientists that the claim is valid.

Dietary Supplement Health and Education Act (DSHEA)

DSHEA, passed in 1994, restricted the FDA's control over dietary supplements. It defined herbal products as dietary supplements, which are considered foods. Before this, products had to be proven safe by the FDA; those introduced after the act's passage had to be proven safe by the manufacturer.

The manufacturer of an herbal preparation is responsible for the truthfulness of the claims made on a label and must have evidence supporting the claims; however, there is no standard for this evidence, nor does the manufacturer need to submit it to the FDA. The manufacturer may claim that the product affects the structure or function of the body as long as there is no claim of effectiveness in the prevention or treatment of a specific disease. A disclaimer must be provided stating that the FDA has not evaluated the product. Since health claims are not pre-approved, the statement "This statement has not been evaluated by the Food and Drug Administration. This product is not intended to diagnose, treat, cure or prevent any disease" must be on the label. Information regarding therapeutic claims for herbal products can be disseminated as long as the information is not misleading or product-specific, is physically separated from the product, and has no product stickers affixed to it.

In 2000, the FDA allowed "structure and function" statements to be made. For example, cranberry products could say that the product supports urinary health but not that it treats urinary tract infections. It allowed for claims that do not relate to disease but are health maintenance claims ("maintains a healthy circulatory system"), nondisease claims ("helps you relax"), and claims for minor symptoms associated with life stages ("for common symptoms of premenstrual syndrome"). Anything that uses words such as "prevents," "treats," "cures," "mitigates," or "diagnoses disease" is subject to drug requirements. This act led to enormous growth in the dietary supplement industry, which today grosses over $18 billion annually.

RISKS

Many herbs and alternative medicines have not been studied adequately and may in fact be toxic. The fact that plants are "natural" does not make the use of agents from that plant free of risks! Adverse reactions can result from direct exposure to the component of the plant or from poor manufacturing process. The law does not require that adverse events resulting from the use of dietary supplements be reported to the FDA. Research studies of safety in people are not required because, as noted above, these agents are considered dietary supplements, not drugs. There is inappropriate dissemination of information and weak regulation in the industry. **Box 9.4** lists the dangers of herbal preparations.

One example of an adverse reaction that has brought about governmental action is ephedra. Ephedra, a common ingredient in weight-loss products, can cause an increase in blood pressure, tremors, arrhythmia, seizures, strokes, myocardial infarction, and death. In April 2004 the FDA banned its sale.

There is no check on the ingredients in preparation. Analyses of herbal supplements have found differences between what is on the label and what is actually in the bottle. There may be less or more of the supplement than the label indicates.

BOX 9.4

Dangers of Herbal Products

- Many herbs and alternative medicines have not been studied adequately and may be toxic.
- Research studies of safety in people are not required.
- Natural remedies cannot be patented, so the manufacturer does not take the time and money to conduct necessary tests.
- There is inappropriate dissemination of information and weak regulation in the industry.
- Herbal supplements can be bought by anyone.
- There can be herb–drug interactions.

Herbal medicines can be purchased and consumed by anyone. They are less expensive than prescription drugs but can still be costly.

HERB–DRUG INTERACTIONS

Interactions between dietary supplements and drugs can be pharmacokinetic or pharmacodynamic. Pharmacokinetic interactions can be a change in the amount of active compounds available and are the consequence of alteration in absorption, distribution, metabolism, or excretion. For example, senna, a common ingredient in weight-loss products, has a laxative effect that can affect drug transit time and reduce absorption. Zinc lozenges, often used to relieve cold symptoms, may chelate fluoroquinolones and tetracyclines, decreasing serum levels of these antibiotics.

Pharmacodynamic interactions occur at the site of action and may be additive or antagonistic to prescribed drugs or other herbal preparations. Vitamin E doses of greater than 1,000 units per day can increase the anticoagulant effect of warfarin. Ephedra has additive effects with caffeine and at high doses can cause death.

There can be an effect on drug metabolism. Herbal products can affect cytochrome P450 (CYP) isoenzymes. For example, St. John's wort is a potent herbal inducer of CYP3A4.

PATIENT EDUCATION

Patients must be aware that herbal preparations have pharmacologic properties. There are interactions with many prescription and over-the-counter (OTC) medications. All products should be purchased from a reliable source. The more ambitious the claim, the more suspicious the consumer should be of the product. The consumer can request professional health information from the company such as the nature of the company, testing procedures, quality control standards, and so forth.

BOX 9.5

Resources for Information About CAM

*www.naturaldatabase.com*a—subscriber-funded site.
www.herbalmedicine.com—a free database from Scripps Center for Integrative Medicine.
www.drugfacts.com—a free database to check interactions.
http://altmed.od.nih.gov—site from Office of Dietary Supplements at the National Institutes of Health.
www.nccam.nih.gov—National Center for Complementary and Alternative Medicine. Fact sheets and other publications are available. Research being conducted on CAM is also available from NCCAM. The toll-free number is 888-644-6266.
www.cfsan.fda.gov (1-888-723-3366)—provides information on safety of supplements. Adverse effects from a supplement can be reported at *www.fda.gov/medwatch* (1-800-FDA-1088).

Consumers should avoid excessive dosing. Taking higher than the recommended dosage can increase the possibility of adverse effects. All supplements should be discontinued during pregnancy and lactation and avoided in children under age 12.

Dietary supplements should not be used for serious health conditions without the advice and supervision of a qualified health professional. Most dietary supplements are meant to treat mild, short-term disorders.

Combination products should be avoided. Combining more than two or three ingredients in one product is not good because it is impossible to tell which ingredient is causing side effects if they develop. Multivitamins are the exception.

All side effects should be reported to a health professional. The side effects may be due to the dietary supplement or from interaction with a prescribed drug.

Consumers can obtain information about CAM from many websites (**Box 9.5**).

COMMONLY USED HERBS

The following section reviews some commonly used dietary supplements (herbs). **Table 9.1** lists them by use for various organ systems. People use CAM for an array of diseases and conditions. American adults are most likely to use CAM for musculoskeletal problems such as back, neck, or joint pain. The supplements most commonly used are fish oil/omega 3s, glucosamine, echinacea, flaxseed oil, gingko biloba, garlic, and coenzyme Q10 (CoQ10).

Black Cohosh

Action and Proof of Efficacy

Black cohosh has vascular and estrogenic activity. Some studies have shown that black cohosh binds to estrogen receptors.

Uses and Dosage

The action of estrogen-receptor binding is thought to mimic natural estrogen activity. Therefore, black cohosh is used for dysmenorrhea and vasomotor menopausal symptoms. The recommended dosage is 20 to 160 mg daily.

Adverse Reactions and Drug Interactions

Black cohosh can cause nausea, dizziness, increased perspiration, and bradycardia. It interacts with several classes of drugs, such as anesthetics and sedatives. It may increase the hypotensive effect of many antihypertensive agents. It also may increase the effects of estrogen supplements. Black cohosh is contraindicated in patients with estrogen-dependent tumors. Black cohosh also has salicylates.

Coenzyme Q10

Action and Proof of Efficacy

CoQ10 has antioxidant properties, is a membrane stabilizer, and is a cofactor in many metabolic pathways. It is produced by the human body and is necessary for the basic functioning of cells. CoQ10 levels are reported to decrease with age and to be low in patients with some chronic diseases such as heart conditions, muscular dystrophies, Parkinson's disease, cancer, diabetes, and human immunodeficiency virus/acquired immunodeficiency syndrome. Some prescription drugs may also lower CoQ10 levels.

Uses and Dosage

CoQ10 is used in patients with hypertension, congestive heart failure, and migraines. There are studies being conducted to determine the role of CoQ10 in many other diseases. The recommended dose is 100 to 1200 mg/day.

Adverse Reactions and Drug Interactions

Reactions may include nausea, vomiting, stomach upset, heartburn, diarrhea, loss of appetite, rash, insomnia, headache, dizziness, itching, irritability, increased light sensitivity of the eyes, fatigue, or flulike symptoms. It may reduce the effectiveness of warfarin or may add to the effects of other blood pressure-lowering drugs. It may affect thyroid hormone levels and alter the effects of thyroid drugs, such as levothyroxine, and may also interact with antiretroviral or antiviral drugs.

Echinacea

Action and Proof of Efficacy

Echinacea stimulates phagocytosis and increases respiratory cellular activity and mobility of leukocytes. A review of 19 German-controlled studies in treatment of the common cold

TABLE 9.1 Common Herbal Preparations

Suggested System	Name/Dosage	Use	Selected Adverse Events	Contraindications/Interactions	Special Considerations
Gastrointestinal (GI)	Acidophilus 10 colony-forming organisms per day	Restore normal oral, GI, and vaginal flora altered by antibiotics or *Candida* and bacterial infections	Flatulence	Warfarin—may decrease efficacy	
Health promotion	Black cohosh 40–200 PO mg/day	Relief of menstrual and menopausal symptoms	Increased perspiration, dizziness, nausea/vomiting, visual disturbances, reduced pulse	Anesthetics, antihypertensives, sedatives—may increase hypotensive effect Not for use in patients with estrogen-dependent tumors	
Respiratory disorders	Echinacea 50–1000 mg/day	Shorten duration of symptoms of URI, wound healing	Nausea, rash	Those who are immunocompromised (may suppress T cells) Human immunodeficiency virus Tuberculosis Multiple sclerosis	May increase effects of estrogen supplements
Cardiovascular disorders	Garlic 600–800 mg/day, 1 clove of garlic daily	Lower cholesterol, prevent clot formation	Dizziness, irritation of mouth and esophagus, nausea, flatulence, malodorous breath and body, sweating	Warfarin (increased risk of bleeding)	Only taken for 8 weeks
Neurologic/psycho-logical	Gingko biloba 40–80 mg/day in 2 or 3 divided doses	Peripheral vascular insufficiency, memory loss	Headache, dizziness, heart palpitations	Aspirin (increased risk of bleeding) Nifedipine (elevated nifedipine levels) Trazodone (increased sedation) Warfarin (increased risk of bleeding) Hypoglycemic agents (facilitates clearance to elevate blood sugar) Thiazide diuretics (increases blood pressure when combined)	The preparation must contain allicin, the active ingredient in garlic.
Musculoskeletal	Glucosamine 500 mg PO TID	Antiarthritic	Potential to alter blood glucose levels, heartburn, diarrhea, nausea, abdominal pain	Sulfa allergy	
Neurologic/ psychological	Kava 100 mg three times per day	Depression	Headaches, disturbance in visual accommodation	Alcohol (increases activity) Alprazolam (may induce coma) Central nervous system (CNS) depressants (additive sedative effects) Levodopa (increases parkinsonian symptoms)	

Neurologic/psychological	Melatonin 5 mg PO HS; Jet lag: 5 mg/day for 3 days before departure and ending 3 days after departure	Insomnia; Jet lag	Headache, depression, drowsiness, confusion, hypothermia	Nifedipine (interferes with antihypertensive effect); Increased anxiolytic action with benzodiazepines	Drowsiness may occur within 30 minutes, so avoid operating machinery.
Neurologic/psychological	St. John's wort 320 mg PO daily	Depression, anxiety, neuralgic pain	Dizziness, restlessness, sleep disturbances, dry mouth, constipation, GI distress, photosensitivity	Oral contraceptives (decreased efficacy); Cyclosporine (decreased levels); Digoxin (decreased levels); Nifedipine (decreased levels); Tricyclic antidepressants (decreased levels); Selective serotonin reuptake inhibitors (increased sedative effects and serotonin syndrome); Simvastatin (decreased cholesterol-lowering effect); Theophylline (decreased levels); Warfarin (decreased anticoagulant effect); Alcohol; Monoamine oxide (MAO) inhibitors	Considered an MAO inhibitor
Neurologic/psychological	Valerian 200–500 mg PO HS for insomnia; 200–300 mg PO BID for anxiety	Sleep disorders, anxiety	Excitability; Blurred vision, nausea	Additive effects with alcohol and CNS depressants	
Respiratory	Zinc	Cold symptoms, wound healing	Nausea, bad taste, diarrhea, vomiting, mouth irritation		
Genitourinary disorders	Saw palmetto 320 mg/day PO	Benign prostatic hyperplasia	GI side effects, decreased libido, headache, back pain	Warfarin (increased risk of bleeding)	
Cardiovascular disease	Omega 3s 1–6 g/day	Decrease triglyceride levels, slow growth of atherosclerotic patches	GI upset	Blood thinners, antihypertensives	

showed that there may be some effect on the immune system, but a recent study showed no effect on children ages 2 to 11.

Uses and Dosage

Echinacea is used to help heal abscesses, burns, eczema, and skin wounds and to treat the common cold. The recommended dose is 50 to 1000 mg/day.

Adverse Reactions and Drug Interactions

Echinacea may cause a rash. It should not be taken by immunocompromised patients. Long-term use may suppress T cells. There are no reported drug interactions.

Garlic

Action and Proof of Efficacy

Garlic has lipid-lowering and antithrombotic properties. Results from clinical studies are varied. Cholesterol-lowering effects, if any, have been shown to be small.

Uses and Dosage

Garlic is used to treat hyperlipidemia and to prevent clot formation. The product must contain allicin, the active ingredient in garlic. Fresh garlic is the most effective (one clove a day). The recommended dose is 600 to 800 mg/day.

Adverse Reactions and Drug Interactions

Garlic can cause dizziness, irritation of the mouth and esophagus, nausea, flatulence, malodorous breath and body odor, and sweating. Garlic increases the risk of bleeding when taking with anticoagulants. Garlic oil can reduce CYP2E1 activity by almost 40%, causing elevated serum levels of drugs whose major metabolic pathway includes CYP2E1, such as alcohol.

Gingko Biloba

Action and Proof of Efficacy

Gingko biloba promotes arterial and venous vascular changes that increase tissue perfusion and cerebral blood flow. It is also considered an antioxidant. Results from clinical trials are varied. Cholesterol-lowering effects, if any, have been shown to be small.

Uses and Dosage

Gingko biloba is used to treat peripheral vascular insufficiency and dementia. The recommended dose is 40 to 80 mg/day.

Adverse Reactions and Drug Interactions

Gingko biloba can cause headache, diarrhea, flatulence, nausea, and dermatitis. It interacts with anticoagulants and antiplatelets by affecting platelet activity. When taken with insulin and oral hypoglycemic agents, it causes increased clearance of insulin and oral hypoglycemic agents, resulting in elevated blood glucose levels. When taken with thiazide diuretics, it increases blood pressure.

Glucosamine

Action and Proof of Efficacy

Glucosamine stimulates the production of cartilage components and allow rebuilding of damaged cartilage. Studies have proven its safety and effectiveness in the treatment of osteoarthritis.

Uses and Dosage

Glucosamine is used for osteoarthritis and other joint diseases. The recommended dosage is 1500 mg/day. It may take 2 weeks to realize the positive effect.

Adverse Reactions and Drug Interactions

Glucosamine can cause drowsiness, headache, abdominal pain, constipation, diarrhea, epigastric discomfort, and nausea. There are no known drug interactions. Glucosamine contains sodium, so care needs to be used in a patient with sodium restrictions.

Kava

Action and Proof of Efficacy

Kava inhibits the limbic system, suppressing emotional excitability and mood enhancement. Randomized, controlled clinical trials of kava use with anxiety provide some reasonable support for its use, but there are no clinical comparison trials with existing anxiolytics.

Uses and Dosage

Kava has been used to treat anxiety disorders. The recommended dosage is 100 mg three times per day.

Adverse Reactions and Drug Interactions

Kava can cause headaches, dizziness, and disturbances in visual accommodation. Alcohol can increase kava's activity. Central nervous system (CNS) depressants can cause an additive sedative effect. Taken together, levodopa and kava can cause an increase in parkinsonian symptoms. Absorption of kava is increased if it is taken with food. Kava increases the effects of alcohol.

Melatonin

Action and Proof of Efficacy

Melatonin release corresponds to periods of sleep. Studies have proven melatonin to be safe and effective for the short-term prevention of jet lag.

Uses and Dosage

Melatonin is used to prevent and treat jet lag and sleeping disturbances. The recommended dosage for sleeping disturbances is 5 mg at bedtime. The recommended dosage for jet lag is 5 mg/day for 3 days before departure and ending 3 days after departure.

Adverse Reactions and Interactions

Melatonin can cause altered sleep patterns, confusion, headache, hypothermia, sedation, tachycardia, hypertension, hyperglycemia, and pruritus. Interactions include increased anxiolytic action when taken with benzodiazepines.

Omega 3s/Fish Oil

Action and Proof of Efficacy

Omega 3s promote the relaxation and contraction of muscles, blood clotting, digestion, cell division, and the growth and movement of calcium and other substances in and out of cells. It also decreases inflammation and platelet aggregation.

Uses and Dosages

Omega 3s are primarily used to decrease triglyceride levels and slow the growth of atherosclerotic plaques. There is research being done to look at the effect of omega 3s on diabetes mellitus, rheumatoid arthritis, systemic lupus erythematosus, and osteoporosis. The recommended dosage is 1 to 6 g/day.

Adverse Reactions and Interactions

Omega 3s can cause gastrointestinal (GI) upset, including diarrhea, heartburn, and abdominal bloating. In high doses, they can interfere with blood thinners and antihypertensives.

Probiotics

Action and Proof of Efficacy

Probiotics are nonpathologic bacteria that reside in the GI tract. They help maintain a healthy balance of organisms in the intestines, promote binding of enterocytes within the GI tract, and prevent harmful bacteria from attaching to these cells.

Uses and Dosage

Probiotics are commonly used to restore normal oral, GI, and vaginal flora. They treat diarrhea, urinary tract infections, vaginitis, and irritable bowel syndrome. They may be used to manage atopic dermatitis in children. They are potentially useful in patients taking antibiotics because the normal flora may be disturbed by the bactericidal or bacteriostatic activity of the drug. Further, patients with *Candida* and bacterial infections may have an imbalance of normal flora. The recommended dosage is 1 capsule of 10 colony-forming units per day.

Adverse Reactions

Adverse reactions are GI-related, primarily flatulence. Warfarin's efficacy may be reduced because acidophilus may enhance the intestinal absorption of vitamin K.

Saw Palmetto

Action and Proof of Efficacy

Saw palmetto inhibits the production of enzymes responsible for converting testosterone to more reactive dihydrotestosterone (DHT). Saw palmetto blocks the binding of DHT to prostate cells, inhibiting enlargement. Studies have shown a decrease in symptoms in patients with noncancerous enlargement of the prostate. Saw palmetto also increases urine flow and improves emptying of the bladder.

Uses and Dosage

Saw palmetto is used to treat benign prostatic hyperplasia (BPH). (See Chapter 33 for more information on BPH.) The recommended dosage is 320 mg daily.

Adverse Reactions and Drug Interactions

Adverse reactions include headache, hypertension, constipation, diarrhea, decreased libido, and back pain. There are no known drug interactions.

St. John's Wort

Actions and Proof of Efficacy

St. John's wort is a monoamine oxidase (MAO) inhibitor. It inhibits reuptake of serotonin, noradrenaline, adrenaline, and dopamine. Numerous studies of St. John's wort in patients with depressive disorders have shown that it is more effective than placebo and as effective as antidepressants; however, these studies had many flaws, and more studies need to be done.

Uses and Dosage

St. John's wort is used to treat depression, anxiety, and neuralgic pain. The recommended dosage is 100 to 500 mg daily.

Adverse Reactions and Drug Interactions

St. John's wort can cause dizziness, restlessness, sleep disturbances, dry mouth, constipation, GI distress, and photosensitivity. Drug interactions include an increase in MAO inhibition activity when taken with alcohol, MAO inhibitors, narcotics, and OTC cold and flu medicines. There is a decrease in levels of digoxin and cyclosporine. Serotonin syndrome may develop when used concurrently with amphetamines, selective serotonin reuptake inhibitors, trazodone, and tricyclic antidepressants.

Valerian

Actions and Proof of Efficacy

Valerian binds to gamma-aminobutyric acid alpha-receptor sites in the brain and CNS. It acts in a competitive action with any benzodiazepine. In nine randomized, placebo-controlled, double-blind studies in which valerian was used as a treatment for sleep disorders, some studies showed effectiveness but others showed none.

Uses and Dosage

Valerian is used for insomnia, anxiety, and stress. The recommended dosages are 200 to 500 mg at bedtime for insomnia and 200 to 300 mg two times per day for anxiety.

Adverse Reactions and Drug Interactions

Valerian can cause excitability, blurred vision, and nausea. There are additive effects with alcohol and CNS depressants.

RECOMMENDING DIETARY SUPPLEMENTS

When recommending dietary supplements, the practitioner must be aware of several key points. The patient must be educated on the use of alternative therapies. Discussions and recommendations must be documented. The provider and patient must be aware of potential interactions.

INCREASING AWARENESS

Since the use of CAM is increasing, health care providers must be aware of the different modalities. At each visit, the patient should be asked about the use of OTC medications, vitamins, and supplements. The health care provider should check whether there are any interactions between medications and supplements.

Patients who choose to use CAM can be directed to reliable providers and reliable dietary supplements. NCCAM is an excellent source of information for both the patient and provider and can be accessed on the Internet (*www.nccam.nih.gov*) or by phone (1-888-644-6226).

BIBLIOGRAPHY

Starred references are cited in the text.

DerMarderosian, A., Liberti, L., Beutler, J. A., et al. (Eds.) (2008). *The review of natural products* (5th ed.). St. Louis, MO: Wolters Kluwer Health.

Guerrea, M. (2007). Complementary and alternative medicine: A new dimension of integrative care. In R. Rakel (Ed.), *Textbook of family medicine* (7th ed.). Philadelphia, PA: Saunders Elsevier.

Loverr, E., & Ganta, N. (2010). Herbs and nutraceuticals: Tips for primary care providers. *Primary Care: Clinics in Office Practice, 37*(1), 13–30.

National Center for Complementary and Alternative Medicine. National Institutes of Health. [on-line: retrieved July 17, 2010]. http://nccam.nih.gov/.

*National Center for Complementary and Alternative Medicine. National Institutes of Health. [on-line: retrieved July 14, 2010]. http://nccam.nih.gov/news/camstats/2007/camsurvey_fs1.htm.

Straus, S. (2008). Complementary and alternative medicine. In L. Goldman & D. Ausiello (Eds.), *Cecil textbook of medicine* (23rd ed.). Philadelphia, PA: Saunders Elsevier.

Pharmacogenomics

PHARMACOGENOMICS AND PERSONALIZED MEDICINE

Clinicians have always understood that **genes** are a significant component to **personalized medicine**, as evidenced by the routine use of family history and prior drug therapy response as a guide to diagnosing and treating diseases. Personalized medicine is "a form of medicine that uses information about a person's genes, proteins, and environment to prevent, diagnose, and treat disease" (National Cancer Institute, 2010). The concept of using **deoxyribonucleic acid (DNA)**-based genetic information as a means of tailoring medicine stemmed out of the **genome** mapping project. There is a language associated with pharmacogenomics, and many of the definitions can be found in **Box 10.1**. **Pharmacogenetics**—the study of inherited differences (variation) in drug metabolism and response—focuses on how genes influence an individual's response to drug therapy, and **pharmacogenomics**—the general study of all of the many different genes that determine drug behavior—are only small components of personalized medicine. However, many supporters of personalized medicine believe that pharmacogenomics has significant promise in improving the care of patients with chronic disease.

Promises and Pitfalls

The promises of pharmacogenomics center around the clinician's ability to use genetic information to aid in the prevention of diseases, improve the sensitivity and specificity of diagnostic tests, and identify specific treatments with the best chance of success and the least chance of adverse effects. In addition to the inherent scientific challenges with linking genetic information to drug response, there are commercial and political challenges and pitfalls that need to be overcome.

Genetic testing for the presence or absence of specific markers will benefit pharmaceutical companies as they continue to develop new drugs for specific diseases. The ability to apply genetic screens for patients entering a clinical trial will streamline the inclusions/exclusion criteria and create a more homogenous group of subjects. This in turn will improve the ability to determine the efficacy and safety of a drug more rapidly and with greater precision. This pre-clinical trial screening should allow for the trials to be smaller, be completed faster, and, ultimately, be less expensive, thus reducing overall development costs. However, designing clinical trials using genetic information is complicated and requires additional time and resources with an unknown payoff. Genetically designed drugs, specific to only thousands of patients, presents a business model in stark contrast to the current pharmaceutical industry model of developing "blockbuster" drugs used by millions of patients. The return on investment from the genetically designed drugs will likely be smaller unless the cost of the drug is extraordinarily higher. It is unclear if public and private insurers will be willing to bear the additional cost without substantial evidence that pharmacogenomics will deliver on its promise of reduced costs through improved efficacy and reduced toxicity. Convincing the insurance companies to pay for these more expensive agents for smaller numbers of people poses a significant market force change that is both a commercial and a policy challenge.

In addition to the policy challenge associated with the cost and access to genetically targeted drugs, political challenges include protecting the patient's genetic information from misuse. Specifically, there is concern that patients may be denied health insurance due to a genetic indication that he or she may be at risk for contracting a disease in the future (Goldman, 2005). Current regulations, such as the Health Insurance Portability and Accountability Act, prevent insurance companies from using genetic information to exclude a patient from coverage in the absence of a medical diagnosis. However, the fear and hype still exist as a major challenge to patient participation in genetic testing, even for personal benefit.

These are only a few of the challenges facing the field of pharmacogenomics, with more pitfalls emerging as more challenges are resolved. There are several examples in which pharmacogenomics have transformed the treatment of patients with diseases such as cancer, cardiovascular disease, human immunodeficiency virus disease, and even asthma. Pharmacogenomics, as a component of personalized medicine, is a fast-growing field that has already altered how clinicians treat patients.

Adenine (A)–One of the four nucleotide bases. Pairs with thymine.

Alleles–Multiple versions of a gene. Each person typically inherits two alleles of each gene, one from the mother and one from the father.

Biomarkers–Molecules that indicate the status of a biological process.

Chromosome–The organized structure of DNA and proteins, the "double-helix." It contains genes and nucleotide sequences.

Cytosine (C)–One of the four nucleotide bases. Pairs with guanine.

DNA–Deoxyribonucleic acid–a nucleic acid that contains genetic information and/or instructions used in the function of living organisms.

Gene–A sequence of DNA that codes for a type of protein or RNA, serving a particular function in a cell.

Genome–All of the genetic material in chromosomes of an organism.

Genotype–The genetic makeup of a cell.

Guanine (G)–One of the four nucleotide bases. Pairs with cytosine.

Haplotype–A combination of alleles. A haplotype may be a single locus of alleles, multiple loci, or even an entire chromosome.

Nucleotide–Molecules that make up the structural units of DNA and RNA. The four DNA nucleotides are adenine, cytosine, guanine, and thymine. For RNA, uracil is substituted for thymine.

Personalized medicine–A form of medicine that uses information about a person's genes, proteins, and environment to prevent, diagnose, and treat disease.

Pharmacogenetics–Refers to the study of inherited differences (variation) in drug metabolism and response.

Pharmacogenomics–Refers to the general study of all of the many different genes that determine drug behavior.

Phenotype–The expressed traits of an organism based on the genotype.

Polymorphism–DNA sequence variation.

RNA–Ribonucleic acid–a nucleic acid that carries genetic information and produces proteins used in the function of living organisms.

SNPs–Single-nucleotide polymorphism–A DNA sequence variation occurring when a single nucleotide differs between members of a species.

Thymine (T)–One of the four nucleotide bases. Pairs with adenine.

BASIC CONCEPTS

The human genome is the underpinning to every human's individuality. With the exception of identical twins, the genome is different for every individual; though in the grand scheme of things, there are only small differences among people's DNA that make us unique. The human genome consists of approximately three billion base pairs, 99.9% of which are the same among all humans with only 0.1% variation among individuals. The variations that occur with DNA (**polymorphisms**), along with environmental and dietary factors, create a patient's individuality, susceptibility to disease, and response to treatments. Included in this individuality is a person's ability to absorb, distribute, metabolize, and excrete drugs. Understanding the genetic components affecting these pharmacokinetic processes can help the clinician tailor treatment for a patient.

Each human has 23 pairs of **chromosomes**—22 are autosomal and look the same in males and females, and 1 pair is the sex chromosome, in which females have two X chromosomes and males have an X and a Y chromosome (**Figure 10-1**). These chromosomes reside in the nucleus of a cell (**Figure 10-2**). Each chromosome is composed of DNA, which carries the genetic information for the individual. Each chromosome can have hundreds or thousands of genes; it is estimated that there are more than 25,000 genes on the human genome. However, genes only make up about 1% of the total DNA found in humans.

Genes function to produce proteins involved in the millions of biological processes that support the function of the body every day. Genes that mutate or malfunction can have profound effects on the body. In the case in which a single gene mutates or malfunctions, the result is a monogenic disease, such as sickle-cell anemia or cystic fibrosis. In most cases, however, there are multiple genes involved in the disease process. These are referred to as *polygenic disorders*.

Polygenic disorders may appear as a single clinical disorder but at the molecular level have multiple "**biomarkers.**" Biomarkers are molecules that indicate the status of a biological process. Examples of biomarkers include prostate-specific antigen for prostate cancer or blood glucose level for diabetes. Genetic biomarkers, specific DNA sequences, are also being discovered.

The building blocks of DNA are the four **nucleotide** bases, including the two purines—**adenine** (A) and **guanine** (G)—and the two pyrimidines—**thymine** (T) and **cytosine** (C). DNA strands are linked through base-pairing of the pyrimidines with the purines (A with T; G with C), conceptually forming the well-known double helix. (See **Figure 10-2**.) The arrangement of these base pairs along each chromosome is called the *DNA sequence*. Variations in the base pairings range from **single nucleotide polymorphisms** (SNPs), insertions or deletions of a nucleotide base, to changes in the number of copies of genes. These variations can alter the production or function of proteins, thus creating the variation in the expression of a disease or the response to drug therapy.

from different individuals: AAG**C**TA and AAG**T**TA. Note the only difference between these sequences is the substitution of thymidine (T) for cytosine (C). In this case, there are two versions (or **alleles**) of this gene. Each person typically inherits two alleles of each gene: one from the mother and one from the father. There can be up to 10 million SNPs in humans, but only those SNPs on coding regions of the gene or the area of the DNA responsible for turning genes on or off have an affect on humans. This concept of SNPs and differing alleles is important in the study of pharmacogenomics, as many of the genes responsible for drug activity and metabolism (e.g., cytochrome P450 [CYP]) have different alleles on the same gene, producing different metabolic effects.

Genetic Biomarkers

Genetic biomarkers are identified through microarrays (biochips). While the technology is still primarily a lab-based tool, there are examples of biochips that are useful in the clinical environment. Biomarkers, genetic or not, assist clinicians in diagnosing, treating, and monitoring patient progress. Moving the genetic screening to the marketplace, specifically the clinician's office, should also improve the drug use process. Currently, there are several companies marketing DNA tests. Roche Diagnostics offers a series of pharmacogenomic screening tests

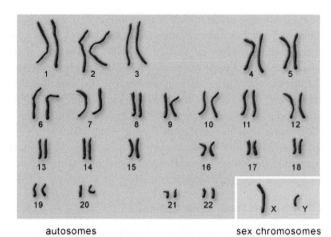

autosomes   sex chromosomes

U.S. National Library of Medicine

FIGURE 10–1   Human chromosomes. (Source: Genetics Home Reference [Internet] National Library of Medicine 2010. http://ghr.nlm.nih.gov/handbook/basics/howmanychromosomes. Cited December 30, 2010.)

Single Nucleotide Polymorphisms

An SNP is a variation in the DNA sequence that differs between members of a species or paired chromosomes in an individual. For example, the following are two sequenced DNA fragments

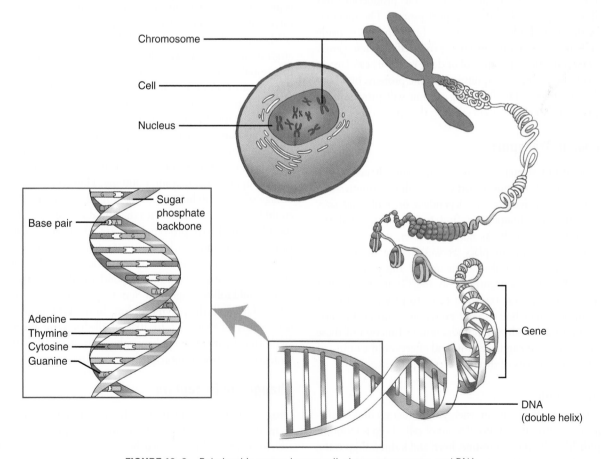

FIGURE 10–2   Relationship among human cell, chromosome, genes, and DNA.

for CYP enzymes and pathways, and AmpliChip was the first test to become available in the United States in 2005. Using microarray chip technology, AmpliChip determines which CYP2D6 and CYP2C19 variations are present and whether the patient is a poor, intermediate, extensive, or ultrarapid metabolizer of each enzyme's substrates. While this test is not used routinely in office practice, it can be used to help target the reason for a patient demonstrating irregular responses to drugs or, when planning long-term therapy, can be used prior to the prescribing to determine the patient's metabolic status and thus help select the best drug.

Another example test is for the enzyme thiopurine methyltransferase (TPMT), which catalyzes the methylation of thiopurine drugs, such as azathioprine and 6-mercaptopurine. Alterations in the TPMT enzyme lead to decreased inactivation of 6-mercaptopurine, leading to increased bone marrow toxicity.

PHARMACOGENOMICS—SPECIFIC EFFECTS

The study of pharmacogenomics remains in the early stages of development, but current research efforts are focusing on how the human gene affects drug pharmacokinetic and pharmacodynamic profiles. The drug transport mechanisms, described earlier in Chapter 2, are governed by the production and breakdown of proteins in the transport process. The metabolism of the drug, both as it enters the body and once inside the body, is controlled by enzymes produced by these genes. Also, the production and control of drug receptors can largely be affected by the genes responsible for the proteins of which they are composed. The following section will provide brief examples of how genomics affects drug therapy.

Changes in Transport

As discussed in Chapter 2, there is significant reliance on the theory that the absorption of drugs from the gastrointestinal (GI) tract is a passive process, dependent on molecular size, polarity/ionization, lipophilicity and hydrophilicity, and the pH of the GI tract itself. As noted, however, there are active transport mechanisms in place as well. These mechanisms use protein transport molecules to import and export drugs through cell walls. Concentrated in the GI tract and liver and renal systems, these transport proteins play a key role in the absorption, metabolism, and excretion of drugs. Genetic polymorphisms that alter the production or function of these transporter proteins can have profound effects on the utility of a specific drug or class of drugs in certain patients.

P-Glycoprotein

P-glycoprotein (P-gp) is an energy-dependent efflux transporter that pumps drug molecules out of cells. P-gp is found in the epithelial cells of the intestine, liver, and kidney. P-gp is the product of the gene ABCB1, also known as the *MDR1 (multidrug resistance) gene*. This gene is a member of the superfamily of ATP-binding cassette (ABC) transporters that are responsible for transporting various molecules across extra- and intracellular membranes. So far, 28 SNP variants have been identified as variants of the human ABCB1 gene; however, the significance of this number of variations is still controversial, but several reports show that this polymorphism has had an effect on patients taking cyclosporin, tacrolimus, and digoxin. Nonetheless, the importance of P-gp in drug transport is well known. When the genomics behind protein production is more well understood, so will the predictability of these polymorphisms on drug transport.

Changes in Drug Metabolism

As noted in Chapter 3, there are many drugs that have an increased interest in genetic testing to identify strategies to reduce the risk of adverse drug reactions and optimize therapy for individuals. In fact, about 10% of the labels for approved drugs contain pharmacogenomic information in an effort to identify responders and non-responders, avoid toxicity, and adjust doses of medications to optimize efficacy and ensure safety (U.S. Food and Drug Administration, 2011). Primarily, the enzymes CYP1, CYP2, and CYP3 are generally polymorphic and responsible for 70% to 80% of phase I metabolism. Mutations in these produce enzymes with reduced or increased activity. These polymorphisms form the four primary **phenotypes** with respect to metabolism: poor metabolizers (PMs), intermediate metabolizers (IMs), extensive metabolizers (EMs), and ultra metabolizers (UMs). PMs lack a functional enzyme, while IMs carry a defective allele, and EMs carry two functional alleles. UMs carry multiple copies of the gene and thus produce more enzyme than a single gene copy would. (See Chapter 3 for more information.)

To see how this is applicable in clinical practice, note the following example. Tricyclic antidepressants, such as nortriptyline, are metabolized by the CYP2D6 system. The usual starting dose of nortriptyline is 150 mg daily and can be titrated up, usually to around 300 mg. However, for PMs, the dosage of nortriptyline would be around 50 mg; for UMs, it could be high as 500 mg. With the initial start dose of 150 mg, the PM would have profound adverse effects and most likely stop the agent and conclude drug intolerance. In contrast, the UM would have little effect therapeutically or adversely and would likely be labeled a non-responder and alternative treatment would follow (Ingleman-Sundberg & Rodriguez-Antona, 2005). Given all the polymorphisms in the CYP gene system, it is estimated that 15% to 20% of all drugs are affected. In fact, often a patient has polymorphisms in more than one system, affecting two or more of the treatments.

Changes in Receptors

Drugs typically exert their effect by interacting with receptors or modulating the activity of enzymes. Receptor and enzyme activity is primarily governed by protein synthesis; therefore, genetic polymorphisms affecting protein synthesis can have an effect on receptor and enzyme production and activity.

Specifically, genetic polymorphisms that reduce or increase the production of proteins necessary to create receptors or enzymes directly impact the drug concentration necessary to elicit a therapeutic or toxic response. Further, polymorphisms that alter a receptor or enzyme configuration, disabling its ability to function, clearly alter the intent of the drug administered. Currently, the number of documented pharmacokinetic alterations outweighs the number of documented pharmacodynamic alterations, but both types are important to understand.

An example of a pharmacodynamic response is the vitamin K epoxide reductase complex subunit 1 gene polymorphisms (*VKORC1*) and warfarin response. *VKORC1* encodes vitamin K epoxide reductase, which is responsible for the carboxylation of vitamin K–dependent factors II, VII, IX, and X and anticoagulation proteins C and S. Warfarin inhibits this enzyme, thus decreasing the coagulation effects of these factors and proteins. It has been found that two **haplotypes** (A and B) formed by five noncoding *VKORC1* SNPs have been associated with differences in mean daily warfarin. That is, patients with the A haplotype appear to produce smaller amounts of *VKORC1* than do patients with the B haplotype, thus decreasing the need for warfarin in haplotype A patients. In clinical practice, this appears to be true, since most Asian patients are haplotype A and typically require lesser amounts of warfarin than other ethnicities (Limdi, et al., 2010).

β$_2$ Adrenoreceptor

The β$_2$ adrenoreceptor (ADBR2) interacts with endogenous catecholamines such as epinephrine and norepinephrine and medications such as albuterol and propranolol. Genetic polymorphism of this receptor can lead to alterations in target drug response. Several SNPs are associated with receptor down-regulation or change in expression. For example, studies have shown that there is a higher forced expiratory volume in 1-second response to oral albuterol in patients with amino acid changes from glycine to arginine. Further, this alteration leads to a desensitization of the ADBR2 receptor in patients expressing this phenotype.

CONCLUSION

This chapter provided just a small glimpse into the burgeoning area of study called *pharmacogenomics*. There are untold potential research and clinical applications—from improved diagnosis of disease to selection and monitoring of drug therapy—that today's clinician can incorporate into daily practice. As the area of study evolves, so will the opportunities for improved clinical practice and better patient care through personalized medicine.

BIBLIOGRAPHY

Starred references are cited in the text.

Catania, M. G. (2006). *An A-Z guide to pharmacogenomics*. Washington, DC: American Association for Clinical Chemistry, Inc.

Court, M. H. (2007). A pharmacogenomics primer. *Journal of Clinical Pharmacology, 47,* 1087–1103.

Genetics home reference. [Internet] National Library of Medicine 2010. http://ghr.nlm.nih.gov/handbook/basics/howmanychromosomes. Accessed December 30, 2010.

*Goldman, B. R. (2005). Pharmacogenomics: Privacy in the era of personalized medicine. *Northwestern Journal of Technology and Intellectual Property, 4,* 83. http://www.law.northwestern.edu/journals/njtip/v4/n1/4. Accessed January 3, 2011.

Holmes, D. R., Dehmer, G. J., Kaul, S., et al. (2010). ACCF/AHA clopidogrel clinical alert: Approaches to the FDA "Boxed Warning": A report of the American College of Cardiology Foundation Task Force on Clinical Expert Consensus Documents and the American Heart Association. *Journal of the American College of Cardiology, 56,* 321–341.

Horn, J. R., & Hansten, P. D. (2004). Drug interactions with digoxin: The role of P-glycoprotein. *Pharmacy Times* (October), available at http://www.hanstenandhorn.com/hh-article10-04.pdf.

Ingelman-Sundberg, M., (2004). Pharmacogenetics of cytochromes P450 and its applications in drug therapy: The past, present and future. *Trends in Pharmacological Sciences, 25*(4), 193–200.

*Ingelman-Sundberg, M., & Rodriguez-Antona C. (2005). Pharmacogenetics of drug-metabolizing enzymes: Implications for a safer and more effective drug therapy. *Philosophical Transactions of the Royal Society B: Biological Sciences, 360,* 1563–1570.

Kalow, W., Mayer, U. B., & Tyndale, R. F. (Eds.). (2005). *Pharmacogenomics* (2nd ed.). Boca Raton, FL: Taylor & Francis Group.

*Limdi, N. A., Wadelius, M., Cavallari, L., et al. on behalf of the International Warfarin Pharmacogenetics Consortium. (2010). Warfarin pharmacogenetics: A single VKORC1 polymorphism is predictive of dose across 3 racial groups. *Blood, 115,* 3827–3834.

*National Cancer Institute. (2010). Dictionary. http://www.cancer.gov/dictionary. Viewed December 10, 2010.

Shin, J., Keyser, S. R., & Langaee, T. Y. (2009). Pharmacogenetics: From discovery to patient care. *American Journal of Health-System Pharmacy, 66,* 625–637.

*U.S. Food and Drug Administration. (2011). Table of valid genomic biomarkers in the context of approved drug labels. Available at: http://www.fda.gov/Drugs/ScienceResearch/ResearchAreas/Pharmacogenetics/ucm083378.htm. Accessed February 17, 2011.

Pharmacotherapy for Skin Disorders

Contact Dermatitis

Dermatitis is an alteration in skin reactivity caused by exposure to an external agent. It is a combination of genetic and environmental factors. It can occur after a single exposure or multiple exposures to an agent or in response to an allergen. The resulting dermatitis usually appears as an inflammatory process. According to the American Academy of Dermatology, contact dermatitis is a common problem and results in approximately 5.7 million visits to health care providers each year. Almost any substance can be a potential irritant. Diaper dermatitis (sometimes called *diaper rash*) is the most common form of irritant contact dermatitis in childhood.

CAUSES

Two types of contact dermatitis are irritant and allergic dermatitis. *Irritant* contact dermatitis (ICD) results from exposure to any agent that has a toxic effect on the skin. *Allergic* contact dermatitis (ACD) results from exposure to an antigen that causes an immunologic response. Atopic dermatitis (eczema), a form of allergic dermatitis characterized as a pruritic, chronic inflammatory condition, affects between 5% and 10% of the population in the United States (Goodheart, 2008). It most often begins in childhood.

PATHOPHYSIOLOGY

Irritant contact dermatitis is not an allergic response. It is a result of damage to the water–protein–lipid matrix of the outer layer of skin. It appears as an erythematous, scaly eruption resulting from friction, exposure to a chemical, or a thermal injury. The severity of the reaction depends on the condition of the skin, the concentration and the toxicity of the irritant, and the length of exposure. The reaction appears only in the area exposed to the irritant.

Allergic contact dermatitis (e.g., poison ivy) is an immunologically mediated response to an allergen (antigen). During the initial sensitization phase, the host is immunized to the allergen. After re-exposure, a more rapid and potent secondary immune response occurs. The second phase manifests in ACD, and T cells are key mediators of the reaction. On activation, T cells release cytokines, chemokines, and cytotoxins, causing stimulation of local blood vessels; recruitment of immune

cells, such as macrophages and eosinophils; and subsequent amplification of the sensitization response. Within 5 to 7 days after sensitization, there is visual evidence of the response. On subsequent exposures, however, dermatitis may develop within 6 to 18 hours. Hypersensitivity can occur after one exposure or after years of repeated exposures. Contact dermatitis may spread extensively beyond the area of contact.

In atopic dermatitis, there are high concentrations of serum immunoglobulin (Ig) E, decreased numbers of immunoregulatory T cells, defective antibody-dependent cellular cytotoxicity, and decreased cell-mediated immunity. The pathogenesis of atopic dermatitis involves genetic factors, skin barrier defects, and immune dysregulation. The genetics of atopic dermatitis is an area of intense research and plays a significant role in IgE production and allergic sensitization. More recently, the association of atopic dermatitis with filaggrin (FLG) gene mutations suggests the role of skin barrier defects in the pathogenesis of atopic dermatitis. FLG is a protein essential to the normal barrier function of the skin. Deficiency in FLG may contribute to the physical barrier defects in atopic dermatitis and predispose patients to increased transepidermal water loss, infection, and inflammation associated with the exposure of cutaneous immune cells to allergens.

PHARMACOGENOMICS

A genetic basis for atopic dermatitis has long been recognized with a family history of disease as a risk factor. Before characterization of the human genome, heritability studies combined with family-based linkage studies supported the definition of atopic dermatitis as a complex trait in which interactions between genes and environmental factors and the interplay between multiple genes contribute to disease manifestation. The gene encoding FLG has been most consistently replicated as associated with atopic dermatitis. Most gene studies to date have focused on adaptive and innate immune response genes, but there is increasing interest in skin barrier dysfunction genes (Barnes, 2010).

DIAGNOSTIC CRITERIA

Irritant contact dermatitis and allergic contact dermatitis appear as linear streaks of papules, vesicles, and blisters that are very pruritic. In irritant contact dermatitis, the lesions are found only in the area of exposure to the irritant. In allergic contact dermatitis, the lesions are usually more diffuse, and they may present over an underlying area of edema.

Lesions in atopic dermatitis include papules, erythema, excoriations, and lichenification. In infants, the face, chest, legs, and arms are the most commonly involved areas; lesions are scaly and red and may be crusted patches and plaques. In children, the most common sites are the antecubital and popliteal fossae, the neck, wrists, ankles, eyelids, scalp, and behind the ears. Lesions are usually lichenified because of constant scratching. In adults, the neck, antecubital and popliteal fossae, face, wrist, and forearms are the most commonly involved areas. Lesions may appear as poorly defined, pruritic, erythematous papules and plaques. This may present specific therapeutic opportunities; however, at this time, maintaining a normal epidermal barrier is key.

INITIATING DRUG THERAPY

The most effective form of treatment for contact dermatitis is prevention. The patient must become aware of the causes or triggers and plan ways to avoid them. Before initiating therapy, the practitioner first needs to determine the severity of the problem. If the symptoms are mild, cool compresses may offer relief, and baths with colloidal oatmeal may offer relief from pruritus. Compresses of Burow's solution are effective for drying the vesicles and bullae that may be associated with contact dermatitis. If these treatments fail or if the dermatitis is more extensive, drug therapy is initiated.

Before initiating drug therapy, delivery of the drug to the skin, protection/barrier function, and cosmetic acceptability must be considered. Ointment and gels offer the best delivery and protection barrier. Creams are less greasy but less effective. Lotions are dilute creams. Solutions are alcohol-based liquids and are useful for treating the scalp because they do not coat the hair.

Moisturizers used generously and frequently increase skin hydration, and their lipid component improves the damaged skin barrier. Lipid-rich moisturizers both prevent and treat ICD.

Barrier creams containing dimethicone or perfluoropolyethers, cotton liners, and softened fabrics help to prevent ICD.

Goals of Drug Therapy

The goals of drug therapy for dermatitis are

- restoration of a normal epidermal barrier;
- treatment of inflammation of skin; and
- control of itching.

The mainstays of therapy for contact dermatitis are topical corticosteroids. There are also topical immunosuppressives available. Systemic corticosteroids are recommended for widespread symptoms, and antihistamines are used for relieving intense pruritus.

For mild or moderate localized dermatitis, topical corticosteroids applied twice daily are usually effective within a few days and should be continued for 2 weeks. Lower-potency agents should be applied to the face and intertriginous areas, and higher-potency steroids should be reserved for the extremities and torso. Topical calcineurin inhibitors (e.g., tacrolimus or pimecrolimus) may be used as an alternative to low-potency topical corticosteroids in chronic ICD.

Emollients or occlusive dressings may improve barrier repair in dry, lichenified skin. Traditional petrolatum-based emollients are accessible and inexpensive, and they have been shown to be as effective as an emollient containing skin-related lipids. To relieve pruritus, a lotion of camphor, menthol, and hydrocortisone (Sarnol HC) is soothing, drying, and antipruritic. Pramoxine, a topical anesthetic in a lotion base (Prax), can also relieve pruritus.

Topical Corticosteroids

Topical steroidal therapy is safer than systemic steroidal therapy. Steroidal agents are effective for smaller outbreaks. Because of their anti-inflammatory and antimitotic actions, they reduce inflammation and the buildup of scale.

Topical corticosteroids are classified according to potency (**Table 11.1**), with the fluorinated agents being more potent. Ideally, the least potent topical corticosteroid should be used for the shortest possible time in treating dermatitis. Topical corticosteroids should be avoided if there are additional bacterial, viral, or fungal skin infections, and they are not recommended for prophylaxis.

Dosage

Treatment may be initiated with an intermediate- or high-potency topical corticosteroid. A lower-potency corticosteroid may be used after the symptoms subside. As a rule, short-term therapy with more potent topical corticosteroids is preferred to longer-term therapy with less potent corticosteroids. Low-potency corticosteroids should be used in the facial and intertriginous regions because fluorinated and high-potency corticosteroids applied to the face may cause atrophy of the tissue or trigger steroidal rosacea. If it is necessary to use either type of agent, use should be limited to a very brief time. The maximum recommended length of treatment with topical corticosteroids is 2 weeks for adults and 1 week for children.

Preparations

Topical corticosteroids are available in creams, ointments, lotions, gels, solutions, or sprays. Creams are the most desirable because they are not as obvious when applied. They are, however, water based, which causes more skin drying. Ointments and gels are the most potent and the most lubricating, and they have occlusive properties. In areas with large amounts of hair or widespread dermatitis, lotions, gels, spray products, and solutions are easiest to apply. Occlusion by a dressing of an area of a topical corticosteroid application increases hydration and hence penetration, thereby enhancing efficacy.

Table 11.1	Classification of Topical Corticosteroids by Potency		
Low Potency	**Intermediate Potency**	**High Potency**	**Very High Potency**
alclometasone dipropionate 0.05% (Aclovate—c, o)	betamethasone valerate 0.12% (Luxiq-foam)	amcinonide 0.1% (Cyclocort—c, l, o)	betamethasone dipropionate augmented 0.05% (Diprolene—o, g)
fluocinolone acetonide 0.01% (Synalar—s)	desonide 0.05% (DesOwen—c, l, o Tridesilon—c, o)	betamethasone dipropionate augmented 0.05% (Diprolene AF—emollient cream Diprolene—lotion)	clobetasol propionate 0.05% (Temovate—c, g, o, scalp preparation Temovate-E—emollient cream, Clobex, Cormax, Olux)
hydrocortisone base or acetate 0.5% (Cortisporin—c Mantadil—c)	desoximetasone 0.05% (Topicort LP—emollient cream)	desoximetasone 0.05% (Topicort—g)	diflorasone diacetate 0.05% (Psorcon—o)
hydrocortisone base or acetate 1% (Cortisporin—o Hytone [1% or 2.5%]—c, l, o Proctocort—c Vytone—c)	fluocinolone acetonide 0.025% (Synalar—c, o)	desoximetasone 0.25% (Topicort—emollient cream, o)	fluocinonide 0.1% (Vanos – c)
triamcinolone acetonide 0.025% (Aristocort—c Aristocort A—c Kenalog—c, l, o)	flurandrenolide 0.025% or 0.05% (Cordran-SP—c Cordran—o)	diflorasone diacetate 0.05% (Florone—o Psorcon—c)	flurandrenolide 4mcg/sq c (Cordran tape)
	fluticasone propionate 0.005% or 0.05% (Cutivate—o 0.005%, c 0.05%)	fluocinonide 0.05% (Lidex—c, g, o, s Lidex-E—emollient cream)	halobetasol propionate 0.05% (Ultravate—c, o)
	hydrocortisone buteprate 0.1% (Pandel—c)	halcinonide 0.1% (Halog—c, o, s Halog-E—emollient cream)	
	hydrocortisone butyrate 0.1% (Locoid—c, o, s)	triamcinolone acetonide 0.5% (Aristocort—c, o Aristocort A—c Kenalog—c)	
	hydrocortisone valerate 0.2% (Westcort—c, o)		
	mometasone furoate 0.1% (Elocon—c, o, l)		
	prednicarbate 0.1% (Dermatop—emollient cream)		
	triamcinolone acetonide 0.1% (Aristocort—c, o Aristocort A—c, o Kenalog—c, o)		
	triamcinolone acetonide 0.2% (Kenalog—aerosol)		

c, cream; l, lotion; o, ointment; g, gel; s, solution.

Correct Usage

Tolerance to a topical corticosteroid is common. To prevent this, chronic use is not recommended. Using the topical corticosteroid preparation only in the case of recurrence of contact dermatitis, and not prophylactically, or prescribing intermittent dosing (e.g., every 4 days) may be effective methods of controlling tolerance.

Application

Penetration of a topical corticosteroid is enhanced when the skin is hydrated. This can be accomplished by moistening the skin before application or by using an occlusive dressing constructed from a material such as a plastic shower cap (for the scalp), gloves (for hands), or plastic wrap or a sock (on other extremities).

Adverse Events

Although topical corticosteroids are relatively safe to use, some adverse events may occur (**Table 11.2**). The prolonged use of fluorinated corticosteroids on the face can cause atrophy and acne-like eruptions. This usually is seen after therapy stops, and may last for several months. With prolonged use, ecchymoses may develop on the arms in elderly patients. Moreover, epidermal atrophy, manifested by striae, shiny, thin skin, or telangiectases, can occur with prolonged use, or a hypersensitivity reaction may occur, usually in response to the vehicle in which the medication is delivered. Frequent and prolonged use of topical corticosteroids in fold areas can cause atrophy, telangiectasia, or striae, and their use on the face can also cause steroid rosacea. Topical corticosteroids can potentiate or cause cataract formation or glaucoma when used around the eyes for prolonged periods.

Systemic Corticosteroids

If the dermatitis is widespread or resistant to treatment with topical steroidal preparations, oral corticosteroids may be used. Systemic corticosteroids inhibit cytokine and mediator release, attenuate mucus secretion, upregulate beta-adrenergic receptors, inhibit IgE synthesis, decrease microvascular permeability, and suppress the influx of inflammatory cells and the inflammatory process.

Table 11.2	Topical Corticosteroids Used for Contact Dermatitis: Selected Adverse Events and Special Considerations		
	Selected Adverse Events	**Special Considerations**	
See Table 11.1 for listing of topical corticosteroids by potency.	Skin irritation Acneiform lesions Striae Skin atrophy Burning Irritation Pruritus Erythema Folliculitis	Applying to moist skin and covering with occlusive dressing increases efficacy except with very high-potency topical corticosteroids. Can cause or intensify cataracts or glaucoma if used near eyes. Use lowest potency on thin/atrophic skin and children. Pregnancy category C	
Topical Immunosuppressants pimecrolimus (Elidel) 1% tacrolimus (Protopic) 0.03%, 0.1% 　Apply a light layer BID 　For use in children age 2 years and older	Skin burning Pruritus Flu-like symptoms Erythema	Do not use with occlusive dressing. Apply for 1 week after clearing. Pregnancy category C Not recommended for children under age 2	

Systemic corticosteroids are prescribed in a tapering dose schedule. The starting dose of 1 mg/kg is decreased by 5 mg every 2 days for 2 to 3 weeks. The entire dose of steroids can be taken at the same time in the morning. This will minimize sleep disturbances. Taking the corticosteroids for less than 2 weeks may cause rebound dermatitis, especially with poison ivy. If dermatitis flares up during the tapering, the dosage can be increased and tapered again.

Although these medications are readily absorbed when taken orally, peak plasma concentrations are not achieved for 1 to 2 hours. For more information about systemic corticosteroids, refer to Chapter 25.

Contraindications

Because they suppress the immune response, systemic corticosteroids are contraindicated in patients with systemic mycoses and in patients receiving a vaccination. These drugs also should be used cautiously in people with tuberculosis, hypothyroidism, cirrhosis, renal insufficiency, hypertension, osteoporosis, and diabetes mellitus.

Adverse Events

Systemic corticosteroids mask infection. In short-term use, they may cause gastrointestinal upset. Mood changes (hyperactivity, anxiety, depression) may be evident and sleep disturbances may occur, especially if medication is taken late in the day. The effects of systemic corticosteroids may be decreased if they are administered with barbiturates, hydantoins, or rifampin.

Topical Immunosuppressives

Topical immunosuppressives act on T cells by suppressing cytokine transcription. These agents are used in patients with moderate to severe atopic dermatitis who cannot tolerate topical steroids or are not responsive to other treatments, or where there is a concern for topical steroid-induced atrophy. Because they do not cause skin atrophy, these medications are especially useful for the treatment of atopic dermatitis involving the face, including the periocular and perioral areas.

Tacrolimus and pimecrolimus are the preparations currently available. They are applied twice a day until the lesions clear and then for an additional 7 days. The skin is dried before application.

Contraindications

Care should be used when administering these drugs with drugs in the CYP3A family. The drugs should not be used under occlusive dressings.

Adverse Effects

There can be transient burning and pruritus, which disappear with continued use. The concomitant ingestion of alcohol can cause redness and flushing. Sun protection is recommended.

Antihistamines

Antihistamines are used to relieve pruritus associated with contact dermatitis. The best time to use them is before bed to promote sleep because the main side effect is drowsiness. Antihistamines are discussed in Chapter 47.

Selecting the Most Appropriate Agent

In contact and atopic dermatitis, topical corticosteroids are the first line of therapy (see **Table 11.1**). These agents are for

Table 11.3	Recommended Order of Treatment for Contact Dermatitis	
Order	**Agent**	**Comments**
First line	Apply low-potency topical corticosteroid two times a day. Take oral antihistamine for relief of symptoms.	Occlusive dressing is helpful. Apply to moist skin surface. Use only for 14 d in adult and 7 d in child.
Second line	Increase potency of topical corticosteroid.	Avoid using moderate- or high-potency topical corticosteroid on face or intertriginous areas.
Third line	Prescribe oral corticosteroid on tapered-dosage regimen.	Common dosage: 1 mg/kg decreased by 5 mg every 2 d. Continue therapy for at least 2 wk. Consider increasing dose if dermatitis flares up; then taper as above.

short-term use. The recommended treatment order is listed in **Table 11.3.**

First-Line Therapy

A topical corticosteroid preparation with low to intermediate potency applied twice a day is the appropriate first-line therapy. If improvement does not occur, a higher-potency topical corticosteroid may be tried rather than increasing the time of administration of the lower-potency agent. Occlusive dressings and application to moist skin may be efficacious in treating the acute phase. Low-potency topical corticosteroids are used on the face and intertriginous areas. Oral antihistamines are used to relieve pruritus and reduce the response to the cause.

Second-Line Therapy

Second-line therapy calls for a more potent topical corticosteroid. Topical immunosuppressants are another consideration for second-line therapy.

Third-Line Therapy

Systemic corticosteroids are useful for treating widespread dermatitis. They are given on a tapered-dose schedule. The recommended dose is 1 mg/kg, with the dose decreased every 2 days for at least 2 weeks and up to 3 weeks. If a flare-up occurs during the tapering, the dosage can be increased again. When treating severe poison ivy, for example, oral corticosteroids are continued for 2 to 3 weeks to prevent rebound dermatitis, which may occur if therapy is discontinued before that time.

Figure 11-1 provides an algorithm of contact dermatitis treatment.

Special Populations

Pediatric

Topical corticosteroids should be used for only 7 days in children younger than age 6 and at the lowest potency. Topical corticosteroids can cause atrophy of the skin. Topical immunosuppressants are considered only for patients age 2 and older. Topical immunosuppressants will not cause atrophy of the skin.

Geriatric

The most common causes of contact dermatitis in elderly patients are topical medications (e.g., neomycin [Myciguent]) and the bases of other topical medications. The adhesives on adhesive patches may also cause contact dermatitis. The rash of contact dermatitis does not present

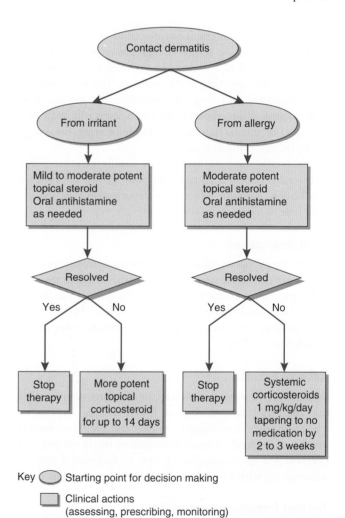

FIGURE 11–1 Treatment algorithm for contact dermatitis.

in a classic pattern in the elderly. Instead of vesicles or inflammation, the area exposed to the irritant may simply become scaly. Topical corticosteroids can cause atrophy of the skin in elderly people, which is a problem because their skin is already friable.

MONITORING PATIENT RESPONSE

The response to therapy is monitored by visual examination of the affected parts of the anatomy and the reported resolution of symptoms. The patient should return for follow-up evaluation within 2 or 3 days of initiation of therapy. If a bacterial infection recurs secondary to contact dermatitis, it may be treated as discussed in Chapter 14.

PATIENT EDUCATION

Drug Information

Education includes teaching patients to avoid the causative substance. Using mild soaps without perfume is an important preventive measure. As appropriate, the practitioner can demonstrate how to apply topical preparations to moist skin and apply an occlusive dressing to increase the efficacy of topical corticosteroids. Penetration of topical steroids is enhanced 10- to 100-fold by hydrating (moistening) the area before applying the medication. An easy-to-make occlusive dressing consists of plastic wrap applied over the medicated area and held in place by a sock or tape. On the hands, a glove can act as an occlusive dressing. On the head area, a shower cap can be used.

Occlusive dressings should not be used with topical immunosuppressants. The patient should avoid alcohol and should use sunscreen.

Most patients with atopic dermatitis require hydration though the liberal use of bland emollients, which serve to hydrate the stratum corneum and maintain the lipid barrier. Sufficient emollients applied liberally several times a day may be enough to significantly reduce the disease activity of atopic dermatitis. Parents of infants and toddlers should apply a bland emollient to the entire body with each diaper change. Older children should apply bland emollients in the morning, after school, and at bedtime. Bathing should be limited to brief, cool showers once daily. Soap, which dries and irritates the skin, should be avoided, but gentle lipid-free cleansers are beneficial.

Skin hydration is best accomplished through daily soaking baths for 10 to 20 minutes. It is important to remind patients and caregivers to apply a topical medication or moisturizer immediately after bathing. This is to seal in the water that has been absorbed into the skin and to prevent evaporation that can lead to further drying of the skin.

Complementary and Alternative Medicine

Some supplements are thought to be helpful in atopic dermatitis. Gingko biloba antagonizes platelet-aggregating factors, a key chemical mediator in atopic dermatitis. Zinc can be used at a dosage of 50 mg/day until the condition clears. Use of fish oil supplements incorporates omega-3 fatty acids into the membrane phospholipid pools.

Recommendations for supplements are as follows:

- Vitamin A 50,000 international units daily
- Vitamin E 400 international units daily
- Zinc 50 mg daily, to be decreased as the condition clears
- EPA 540 mg and DHA 360 mg daily or flaxseed oil 10 g daily
- Evening primrose oil 3,000 mg daily

Case Study

J . F., a 15-year-old boy who weighs 110 pounds, is seeking treatment for a very itchy rash consisting of linear streaks of papules, vesicles, and blisters on his arms, legs, and face. He tells you he was hiking in the woods 2 days ago along trails lined with patches of shiny weeds with three leaves. He tried using calamine lotion and over-the-counter hydrocortisone cream but has had no relief from the itching.

DIAGNOSIS: CONTACT DERMATITIS (POISON IVY)

1. List specific goals of treatment for J. F.
2. What drug therapy would you prescribe? Why?

3. What are the parameters for monitoring the success of the therapy?
4. Discuss specific patient education based on the prescribed therapy.
5. List one or two adverse reactions for the selected agent that would cause you to change therapy.
6. What would be the choice for second-line therapy?
7. What over-the-counter and alternative medications would be appropriate for J. F.?
8. What lifestyle changes would you recommend to J. F.?
9. Describe one or two drug–drug or drug–food interactions for the selected agent.

BIBLIOGRAPHY

Starred references are cited in the text.

*Barnes, K. (2010). Update on genetics of atopic dermatitis: Scratching the surface in 2009. *Journal of Allergy and Clinical Immunology, 125*(1), 16–29.

Fyhrquist-Vanni, N., Alenius, H., & Lauerma, A. (2007). Contact dermatitis. *Dermatology Clinics, 25*(4), 613–623.

*Goodheart, H. P. (2008). *A photoguide of common skin disorders: Diagnosis and management* (3rd ed.). Philadelphia: Lippincott Williams & Wilkins.

Habif, T. (2009). *Clinical dermatology* (3rd ed.). Philadelphia: Mosby Elsevier.

Jung, T., & Stingl, G. (2008). Atopic dermatitis: Therapeutic concepts evolving from new pathophysiological insights. *Journal of Allergy and Clinical Immunology, 122*(6), 1074–1081.

Kockentiet, B., & Adams, B. (2007). Contact dermatitis in athletes. *Journal of the American Academy of Dermatology, 56*(6), 1048–1055.

Lee, J., & Bielory, A. (2010). Complementary and alternative interventions in atopic dermatitis. *Immunology and Allergy Clinics of North America, 30*(3), 411–424.

Ong, P., & Baguniewicz, M. (2008). Atopic dermatitis. *Primary Care: Clinics in Office Practice, 35*(1), 105–107.

Peroni, A., Colato, C., Schena, D., & Girolmoni, G. (2010). Urticarial lesions: If not urticarial what else? The differential diagnosis of urticaria. *Journal of the American Academy of Dermatology, 62*(4), 541–555.

Piliang, M. (2009). Atopic dermatitis. In W. Carey (Ed.), *Cleveland Clinics: Current clinical medicine.* Philadelphia: Saunders Elsevier.

Scalf, L. (2007). Contact dermatitis: Diagnosing and treating skin conditions in the elderly. *Geriatrics, 62*(6), 14–19.

Taylor, J., & Amado, A. (2009). Contact dermatitis and related conditions. In W. Carey (Ed.), *Cleveland Clinics: Current clinical medicine.* Philadelphia: Saunders Elsevier.

Fungal Infections of the Skin

Fungi live in the dead, horny outer layer of the skin. The organisms penetrate only the stratum corneum—the surface layer of the skin—and infect the skin, hair, and nails. They cause tinea, tinea versicolor, and candidiasis.

TINEA

Dermatophytes are a group of fungi that infect nonviable keratinized cutaneous tissues. Dermatophytosis, more commonly called *tinea*, is a condition caused by dermatophytes. Tinea is further classified by the location of the infection (**Box 12.1**).

Tinea capitis primarily affects children ages 3 to 9. This age group may also be infected with tinea corporis. *Tinea pedis* most commonly affects the adolescent population and young adults. Immunocompromised patients have an increased incidence and more intractable dermatophytosis. *Tinea unguium*, infection of the nails, is also called *onychomycosis*. It is caused by various yeast, fungi, and molds.

CAUSES

General factors that predispose to fungal infections include warm, moist, occluded environments, family history, and a compromised immune system. Infection is spread from person to person by animals, especially cats and dogs, and by inanimate objects.

PATHOPHYSIOLOGY

Dermatophytes grow only on or within keratinized structures. Most infections result from five specific species of fungus: *Trichophyton rubrum, Trichophyton tonsurans, Trichophyton mentagrophytes, Microsporum canis,* and *Epidermophyton floccosum*. These can be found on humans, animals, and in the soil. They produce enzymes (keratinases) that allow them to digest keratin, causing epidermal scale; thickened, crumbly nails; or hair loss.

DIAGNOSTIC CRITERIA

General symptoms of fungal infections in hair and skin include pruritus, burning, and stinging of the scalp or skin. An inflammatory dermal reaction may cause erythema and vesicles. Diagnosis is confirmed by several mechanisms. One mechanism is microscopic evaluation of the stratum corneum with 10% potassium hydroxide (KOH) preparation. At the margin of the lesion, scale is scraped with a No. 15 knife blade and placed on a slide. KOH is then added and the slide inspected under the microscope. Fungi appear as rod-shaped filaments with branching.

Another mechanism for diagnosis is the fungal culture. A specimen of infected tissue is applied to a dermatophyte test medium on an agar plate. If the infecting organism is a fungus, the plate will change color—from yellow to pink or red—in approximately 2 weeks.

A third diagnostic method involves using a Wood's lamp, which produces a bright green fluorescence in the presence of a tinea infection caused by *Microsporum* species. A major disadvantage of this test is that other fungal infections may be undiagnosed because the Wood's lamp test identifies only *Microsporum*.

Tinea Capitis

Presentation of tinea capitis varies widely. There may be generalized, diffuse seborrheic dermatitis-like scalp scaling, although more common signs and symptoms include impetigo-like lesions with crusting and redness, areas of hair loss with broken hairs, and possibly inflammatory nodules. Although often impressive, cervical lymphadenitis does not correlate with the extent of scalp inflammation. Finally, approximately 15% of patients have a cross-infection with tinea corporis. Most cases of tinea capitis are found in prepubertal children, with a disproportionate amount in African Americans. It is very contagious.

Most cases (90%) are caused by *T. tonsurans. Microsporum audouinii*, spread from human to human, and *M. canis*, spread from animals, are other organisms.

Tinea capitis presents in several ways:

- inflamed, scaly, alopecic patches, especially in infants;
- diffuse scaling with multiple round areas with alopecia secondary to broken hair shafts, leaving residual black stumps;
- "gray patch" type with round, scaly plaques of alopecia in which the hair shaft is broken off close to the surface; or
- tender, pustular nodules.

Tinea Corporis

Tinea corporis is called "ringworm" when it affects the face, limbs, or trunk, but not the groin, hands, or feet. The typical

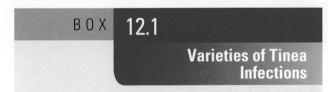

BOX **12.1**

Varieties of Tinea Infections

Tinea infections are identified by their location on the body as follows:

- Head: tinea capitis
- Body: tinea corporis
- Hand: tinea manus
- Foot: tinea pedis
- Groin: tinea cruris
- Nails: tinea unguium (onychomycosis)

presentation of tinea corporis is a ring-shaped lesion with well-demarcated margins, central clearing, and a scaly, erythematous border. It is caused by contact with infected animals, human-to-human transmission, and from infected mats in wrestling. The organisms responsible are *M. canis, T. rubrum,* and *T. mentagrophytes.*

Tinea Cruris

Tinea cruris is often referred to as *jock itch.* A fungal infection of the groin and inguinal folds, tinea cruris spares the scrotum. The most common causes are *T. rubrum* or *E. floccosum.* Typically, the lesion borders are well demarcated and peripherally spreading. The lesions are large, erythematous, and macular, with a central clearing. A hallmark of tinea cruris is pruritus or a burning sensation. There is often an accompanying fungal infection of the feet.

Tinea Pedis

Interdigital tinea pedis, commonly called *athlete's foot,* is characterized by scaling and itching in the web spaces between the toes and sometimes denudation and sodden maceration of the skin. Another variation is inflammatory tinea pedis, which presents with vesicles involving the toes or instep. A third variety is the moccasin style, which presents with itching, chronic noninflammatory scaling, and thickness and cracking of the epidermis on the sole, heel, and often up the side of the foot. This is a common problem in young men.

Most cases are caused by *T. rubrum,* which evokes a minimal inflammatory response. The *T. mentagrophytes* organism produces vesicles and bullae.

There are three types of tinea pedis:

- interdigital, which presents as scaling, maceration, and fissures between the toes;
- plantar, which presents as diffuse scaling of the soles, usually on the entire plantar surface; and
- acute vesicular, which presents as vesicles and bullae on the sole of the foot, the great toe, and the instep.

Tinea Manus

Tinea manus is a dermatophyte infection of the hand. This is always associated with tinea pedis and is usually unilateral. The lesions are marked by mild, diffuse scaling of the palmar skin, and vesicles may be grouped on the palms or fingernails involved.

Tinea Unguium

Tinea unguium (onychomycosis) is a fungal infection of the nail. Typically affected are the toenails, which become thick and scaly with subungual debris. Onycholysis, a separation of the nail from the nail bed, may be seen. The infection usually begins distally at the tip of the toe and moves proximally and through the nail plate, producing a yellowish discoloration and striations in the actual nail. Under the nail, a hyperkeratotic substance accumulates that lifts the nail up. If untreated, the nail thickens and turns yellowish brown. Onychomycosis is usually asymptomatic but can act as a portal of entry for a more serious bacterial infection.

Organisms causing onychomycosis include dermatophytes, *E. floccosum, T. rubrum, T. mentagrophytes, Candida albicans, Aspergillus, Fusarium,* and *Scopulariopsis.*

Some health insurance plans refuse to reimburse for drug therapy without confirmation of the diagnosis. Tests that verify the diagnosis include the KOH test and culture.

INITIATING DRUG THERAPY

Fungal infections can be prevented by applying powder containing miconazole (Monistat) or tolnaftate (Tinactin) to areas prone to fungal infections after bathing. The areas can be dried completely with a hair dryer on low heat.

Goals of Drug Therapy

Pharmacologic therapy is directed against the offending fungus and the site of infection. Therapy is topical or systemic, depending on the location of the lesion. Topical therapy is used for most skin infections. The exceptions are tinea capitis and tinea unguium (onychomycosis).

Topical Azole Antifungals

Topical azoles (**Table 12.1**) impair the synthesis of ergosterol, the main sterol of fungal cell membranes. This allows for increased permeability and leakage of cellular components and results in cell death. Topical azoles are fungicides that are effective against tinea corporis, tinea cruris, and tinea pedis as well as cutaneous candidiasis. They should be applied once or twice a day for 2 to 4 weeks. Therapy should continue for 1 week after the lesions clear. However, therapy is not recommended during pregnancy or lactation and is administered cautiously in hepatocellular failure. Ketoconazole (Nizoral), in particular, should be avoided in patients with sulfite sensitivity. Adverse effects include pruritus, irritation, and stinging.

TABLE 12.1	**Overview of Antifungal Medications**		
Generic (Trade) Name and Dosage	**Selected Adverse Events**	**Contraindications**	**Special Considerations**
Topical Agents			
clotrimazole ointment (Lotrimin), powder (Desenex) Gently massage ointment into affected and surrounding skin areas bid × 4 wk; powder as needed	Erythema, irritation, stinging, pruritus	Pregnancy or lactation Use cautiously in patients with hepato-cellular failure	May be purchased OTC
miconazole (Micatin, Monostat Derm) Cover affected areas with cream lotion, or powder bid for 2–4 wk	Irritation, maceration	Pregnancy or lactation	Avoid applying near eyes.
ketoconazole (Nizoral) Apply to affected and surrounding areas once daily for 2–4 wk	Irritation, stinging, pruritus	Asthma Not administered to people who are sensitive to sulfites Pregnancy or lactation	Not recommended in children
oxiconazole (Oxistat) Apply to affected and surrounding areas 1–2 times daily for 2–4 wk	Pruritus, burning	Pregnancy or lactation	Avoid applying near eyes or mucous membranes.
sulconazole (Exelderm) Apply to affected and surrounding areas bid × 4 wk	Pruritus, burning sensation, erythema	Pregnancy or lactation	Not recommended in children Avoid contact with eyes.
ciclopirox (Loprox) Apply to affected area bid × 4 wk	Pruritus, burning sensation		Not recommended in children younger than age 10 Lotion formulation good for nails Avoid occlusive dressing.
naftitine (Naftin) Apply to affected area once daily × 4 wk	Burning, stinging, dryness, erythema, itching		Not recommended in children Avoid occlusive dressings. Avoid contact with mucous membranes.
terbinafine (Lamisil) Apply to affected area bid × 4 wk	Burning, irritation, skin exfoliation, dryness		Not recommended in children Avoid occlusive dressings. Avoid contact with mucous membranes.
tolnaftate (Tinactin) Apply small amount bid × 4 wk	Stinging, burning, irritation		Not recommended in children younger than age 2
selenium sulfide (Selsun)1% (OTC); 2.5% Massage into affected area, rest 15 min, rinse thoroughly	Irritation, hair loss		
nystatin (Mycostatin) 100,000 units/mL Infants: 1 mL each side of mouth Adults: 2–3 mL each side of mouth	GI upset, oral irritation		Continue use for at least 48 h after clinical cure. Keep in mouth as long as possible before swallowing.
Oral Agents			
griseofulvin (Grifulvin V) Microsize: Adult 500–1000 mg Child 10–15 mg/kg/d Ultramicrosize: Adult 330–660 mg Child 10 g/kg/d	Headaches, nausea, vomiting, diarrhea, photosensitivity	Pregnancy Patients with porphyria or hepatic failure	Ultramicrosize particle increases absorption. Prescribe with caution to patients who are sensitive to penicillin. Drug is most effective when taken with a high-fat meal. Drug is well tolerated in young children. Monitor complete blood count and LFT with long-term use.

(continued)

TABLE 12.1 Overview of Antifungal Medications (*Continued*)

Generic (Trade) Name and Dosage	Selected Adverse Events	Contraindications	Special Considerations
			Drug use may aggravate lupus erythematosus. Use with alcohol produces Antabuse-like effects. Drug interactions: antagonizes oral contraceptives and warfarin, and is antagonized by barbiturates.
ketoconazole (Nizoral) 200 mg/d	Nausea, vomiting, abdominal pain, urticaria, pruritus	Do not use with other drugs metabolized by CYP3A	Not recommended in children
itraconazole (Sporanox) 200 mg/d	GI upset, rash, fatigue, headache, dizziness, edema	Do not use with other drugs metabolized by CYP3A	Not recommended in children May use pulse dosing Remains in nails for 4–5 mo Ingestion of food increases absorption.
terbinafine (Lamisil) 62.5–250 mg/d	GI disturbance, LFT abnormalities, urticaria, pruritus	Liver or renal disease	Not recommended in children
fluconazole (Diflucan) Adults: 100–200 mg/d Children: 3–6 mg/kg/d	GI disturbance, headache, rash, hepatotoxicity		Decrease dose if creatinine clearance < 50 mL/min. Drug interactions: potentiates warfarin, theophylline, oral hypoglycemics. May increase serum levels of phenytoin, cyclosporine. Thiazides increase fluconazole levels. May decrease effect of oral contraceptives.

CYP3A, cytochrome P450 enzyme 3A; GI, gastrointestinal; LFT, liver function tests; OTC, over the counter.

Topical Allylamine Antifungals

These agents are effective against dermatophyte infections but have limited effectiveness against yeast. Patients treated with these agents may undergo a shorter treatment period with less likelihood of relapse. Topical allylamines are applied twice daily. Potential side effects include burning and irritation.

Griseofulvin

Mechanism of Action

Griseofulvin in a fungistatic that deposits in keratin precursor cells, increasing new keratin resistance to fungal invasion.

Adverse Events

Adverse effects include nausea, vomiting, diarrhea, headache, or photosensitivity. Evaluation of renal, hepatic, and hematopoietic systems is recommended before initiating therapy, particularly because this drug may aggravate lupus erythematosus.

Interactions

Griseofulvin increases levels of warfarin (Coumadin) and decreases levels of barbiturates and cyclosporine (Sandimmune). It may decrease the efficacy of oral contraceptives and may cause a serious and unpleasant reaction with alcohol. Patients should be advised not to drink beverages or any other preparation containing alcohol while taking the drug.

Systemic Allylamine Antifungals

Terbinafine (Lamisil) is a synthetic allylamine derivative that inhibits squalene epoxidase, a key enzyme in fungal biosynthesis. This causes a deficiency of ergosterol causing fungal cell death. It is used in the treatment of onychomycosis.

Dosage

For fingernail onychomycosis the dose is 250 mg/day for 6 weeks; toenail onychomycosis requires 250 mg/day for 12 weeks.

Adverse Events

Adverse events include diarrhea, dyspepsia, rash, increase in liver enzymes, and headache. Evaluation of alanine aminotransferase (ALT) and aspartate aminotransferase (AST) levels is recommended before starting therapy and at 6 to 8 weeks into therapy if it is long-term because it can cause liver failure, although this is rare.

Interactions

Terbinafine is potentiated by cimetidine (Tagamet) and antagonized by rifampin (Rifadin). Cyclosporine levels should be monitored when the patient is taking both cyclosporine and terbinafine.

Systemic Azole Antifungals

Systemic azoles inhibit cytochrome P450 (CYP) enzymes and fungal 14-α-demethylase, inhibiting synthesis of ergosterol. Systemic therapy is required for tinea capitis and tinea unguium. Itraconazole (Sporanox), a systemic azole, has a high affinity for keratin and is lipophilic, which causes high levels to accumulate in the hair and nail. It has a long half-life, so pulse dosing, in which periods of drug therapy are alternated with periods without therapy, is feasible.

Dosage

The dosage of itraconazole is 200 mg once daily for 12 weeks for toenail infection. For fingernail infection, the dose is 200 mg twice daily for 1 week, then 3 weeks off, and repeat dosing with 200 mg twice daily for 1 week. The drug is not recommended for children, and ingestion of food increases absorption.

The dosage of fluconazole is usually 200 mg on the first day, then 100 mg each day for at least 2 weeks. For children it is 6 mg/kg/day on day 1, then 3 mg/kg/day.

Contraindications

A systemic azole should not be given with drugs metabolized by the CYP3A enzyme, including β-hydroxy-β-methylglutaryl coenzyme A (HMG-CoA) reductase inhibitors such as quinidine (Quinidex) or others. The azole antifungals should not be used in pregnancy.

Adverse Events

Adverse effects associated with systemic azole therapy include gastrointestinal upset, rash, fatigue, hepatic dysfunction, edema, and hypokalemia.

Interactions

Severe hypoglycemia may occur with hypoglycemic drugs. In addition, systemic azole therapy may potentiate triazolam (Halcion), midazolam (Versed), and warfarin. Fluconazole (Diflucan) levels are increased with use of hydrochlorothiazide (HydroDIURIL). Anticholinergics, histamine-2 blockers, and antacids should be avoided within 2 hours of taking an oral azole so that absorption is not compromised.

Selecting the Most Appropriate Agent

Topical agents work well for most tineas but not for tinea capitis and tinea unguium. If tinea capitis is especially severe and painful in a child, prednisone (Deltasone) 1 mg/kg/day can be given for 3 to 4 days as adjunct therapy. To be effective, all therapy must be adequate in dose and duration. If a pet carries the fungus, the pet must be treated. For more information, see **Figure 12-1.**

When selecting an oral agent to treat onychomycosis, consideration must be given to cost of the agent, patient motivation and compliance, the age and health of the patient, and drug interactions and side effects of the medications.

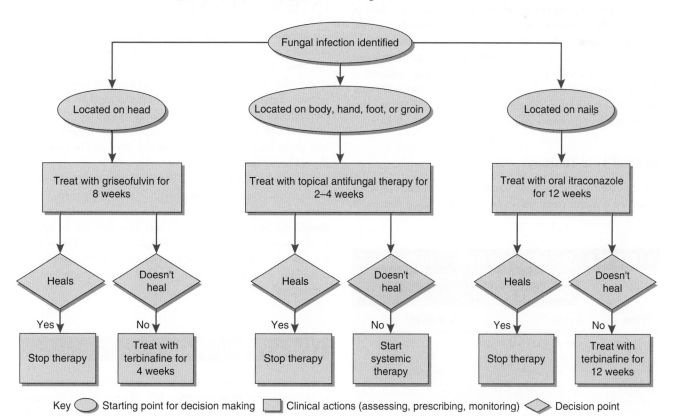

FIGURE 12–1 Treatment options for fungal skin infections.

TABLE 12.2	Recommended Order of Treatment for Tinea Capitis	
Order	**Agent**	**Comments**
First line	griseofulvin (Grifulvin V)	Treatment lasts a minimum of 8 wk. Take medication with a high-fat meal.
Second line	terbinafine (Lamisil) or itraconazole (Sporanox)	Treatment lasts 4 wk.

First-Line Therapy

Topical therapy is recommended for cases of tinea corporis, pedis, cruris, or manus when the infection affects a limited area. The topical antifungal is applied 3 cm beyond the margin of the lesion. Therapy should continue for at least 2 weeks and for 1 week after the lesion clears (**Table 12.2**).

First-line therapy for tinea capitis is microsize griseofulvin (**Table 12.3**) administered with milk or food to promote absorption. Treatment is for 8 weeks. The adult dose is 500 mg daily, and the pediatric dose ranges between 10 and 20 mg/kg/day. Children may attend school during therapy.

First-line therapy for tinea unguium (onychomycosis) consists of systemic agents. Topical preparations are not effective because they penetrate the nails poorly. Itraconazole is given by pulse dosing, 200 mg twice daily with a full meal for 7 days of each month. Treatment for fingernails lasts 3 months and for toenails, 4 months. Also effective for toenails is 200 mg itraconazole per day for 12 weeks (**Table 12.4**). Pulse dosing has less impact on the liver and is more popular than continuous dosing. Fluconazole can be given at a dose of 150 to 400 mg/day for 1 to 4 weeks or 150 mg once a week for 9 to 10 months. Treatment for onychomycosis is only 40% to 50% effective.

Second-Line Therapy

Second-line therapy for tinea corporis, pedis, cruris, or manus is needed if the infection fails to respond to topical therapy, if

TABLE 12.3	Recommended Order of Treatment for Tinea Corporis, Tinea Cruris, and Tinea Pedis	
Order	**Agent**	**Comments**
First line	Topical azole antifungals for 2–4 wk (1 wk past clinical cure)	Use medications for 2 wk even after the rash is gone.
Second line	Systemic therapy: terbinafine (Lamisil) or fluconazole (Diflucan)	

TABLE 12.4	Recommended Order of Treatment for Onychomycosis	
Order	**Agent**	**Comments**
First line	itraconazole (Sporanox) or terbinafine (Lamisil)	Take with food. Treatment lasts 12 wk. Not recommended for children

there are multiple lesions or if treatment areas are repeatedly shaved. Second-line therapy consists of terbinafine 250 mg/day for 2 to 6 weeks or fluconazole 150 mg/week for 2 to 4 weeks.

Second-line therapy for tinea capitis involves using itraconazole, terbinafine, or fluconazole if treatment failure occurs with griseofulvin despite adequate dosage and time.

MONITORING PATIENT RESPONSE

When patients use terbinafine or itraconazole, the AST/ALT levels and white blood cell counts need to be monitored at 6 to 8 weeks. Follow-up evaluations need to monitor both the effectiveness of the therapy and results of liver, kidney, and hematopoietic diagnostic studies. If tests disclose elevated liver function or if creatinine clearance exceeds 40 mL/minute, drug therapy should be discontinued.

PATIENT EDUCATION

An important role of the practitioner is to teach the patient about hygiene and ways to avoid transferring fungal infection to others. Patients should be instructed to complete the full course of treatment and not to stop treatment when symptoms subside. Parents and other caregivers also need to know that children can attend school while being treated.

Patients may dry areas susceptible to fungus with a hair dryer after bathing to ensure full drying. The hair dryer should be set to cool or low to avoid burns.

Vinegar soaks and Vicks VapoRub may be used for onychomycosis. Vinegar is mixed with 1 part vinegar to 2 parts warm water. Feet are soaked for 15 to 20 minutes daily. It should not be used long-term. Vicks VapoRub can be applied to the toenails and socks put over the feet. Neither of these remedies have been thoroughly researched. Areas with fungal infections should be carefully dried. Antifungal powders and sprays can be used for prophylaxis.

TINEA VERSICOLOR

Tinea versicolor, also called pityriasis versicolor, is an opportunistic superficial yeast infection. It is a chronic, asymptomatic infection characterized by well-demarcated, scaling patches of varied coloration, from whitish to pink, tan, or brown.

CAUSES

An overgrowth of the hyphal form of *Pityrosporum ovale* causes tinea versicolor, which is most common in young adults (older than age 15). The fungal infection occurs mostly in subtropical and tropical areas. In temperate zones, it is more common in the summer months but is seen in physically active people year round. Moist skin surfaces predispose to tinea versicolor. The infection rarely causes symptoms other than discoloration, and patients usually seek treatment for cosmetic purposes.

PATHOPHYSIOLOGY

P. ovale has an enzyme that oxidizes fatty acids in the skin surface lipids, forming dicarboxylic acids, which inhibit tyrosinase in epidermal melanocytes and cause hypomelanosis (loss of pigmentation).

DIAGNOSTIC CRITERIA

Skin lesions of tinea versicolor are well-defined, round or oval macules with an overlay of scales that may coalesce to form larger patches. They most often form on the trunk, upper arms, and neck. There may be mild itching. The diagnosis is confirmed by positive KOH test findings, which reveal budding yeast and hyphae.

INITIATING DRUG THERAPY

Topical agents for treating tinea versicolor include selenium sulfide lotion or shampoo and azole creams. The treatment may be repeated in 3 to 4 weeks and before the next warm season or travel to a tropical area. For widespread or stubborn disease, systemic itraconazole or fluconazole may be prescribed for 7 to 10 days.

Goals of Therapy

The goal of therapy for tinea versicolor is resolution of lesions. Therapy lasts for 3 to 4 weeks. Because the lesions may recur in warm weather, prophylaxis consists of applying selenium sulfide lotion or shampoo twice a month.

Selenium Sulfide

Selenium sulfide, the drug of choice for tinea versicolor, has antifungal properties (**Table 12.5**). It is applied once a day to the affected skin for 15 minutes and then rinsed off. Contraindicated during pregnancy and lactation, it can be used with caution in instances of acute inflammation or exudation. Skin folds and genitalia are carefully rinsed. Selenium sulfide must be kept away from eyes. Potential adverse effects include irritation and increased hair loss.

TABLE 12.5	Recommended Order of Treatment for Tinea Versicolor	
Order	**Agent**	**Comments**
First line	selenium sulfide solution 1% or 2.5% topical azole cream or spray	Topical therapy is used for localized lesions. Use if lesions are resistant or widespread.
Second line	itraconazole (Sporanox)	

Selecting the Most Appropriate Agent

Lesions may reappear because the infection is a result of microorganisms that normally inhabit the skin, so twice-monthly application of selenium sulfide is suggested as prophylaxis.

First-Line Therapy

Selenium sulfide solution (2.5%) as a lotion or shampoo (Selsun) is applied once a day. Pyrithione zinc (Head and Shoulders shampoo) can also be used. An antifungal topical agent is used. Choices include terbinafine cream or spray, ketoconazole, or sulconazole (Exelderm) nitrate for 3 to 4 weeks. The treatment can be repeated before the next warm season.

Second-Line Therapy

For resistant or widespread tinea versicolor, systemic therapy with itraconazole (200 mg for 5 days) may be prescribed.

PATIENT EDUCATION

It may take several months for the discoloration to disappear. Prophylactic application of ketoconazole cream or shampoo 1 to 2 times a week can prevent recurrence. The treatment can be repeated before the next exposure to warm weather.

CANDIDIASIS

Cutaneous candidiasis is a superficial fungal infection of the skin and mucous membranes. It is commonly found in the diaper area, oral cavity, intertriginous areas, nails, vagina, and male genitalia. It can occur at any age and in both sexes. It is classified by its location on the body (**Box 12.2**).

CAUSES

Cutaneous candidiasis, which is caused by *C. albicans*, a yeast-like fungus, occurs on moist cutaneous sites. Predisposing factors include infection, diabetes, use of systemic and topical

> BOX 12.2
>
> ## Varieties of Candidiasis
>
> Candidal infections are identified by their location on the body as follows:
>
> - Axillae, under pendulous breasts, groin, intergluteal folds: intertrigo
> - Glans penis: balanitis
> - Follicular pustules: candidal folliculitis
> - Nail folds: candidal paronychia
> - Mouth and tongue: oral candidiasis (thrush)
> - Area included under diaper: diaper dermatitis

corticosteroids, and immunosuppression. It is commonly found in people who immerse their hands in water. It thrives in occluded sites.

PATHOPHYSIOLOGY

Normally found on the skin and mucous membranes, *C. albicans* invades the epidermis when warm, moist conditions prevail or when there is a break in the skin that allows overgrowth.

DIAGNOSTIC CRITERIA

Candidiasis has several classifications. Intertrigo presents as red, moist papules or pustules. It is found in the axillae, inframammary areas, groin, and between fingers and toes.

Diaper dermatitis presents as erythema and edema with papular and pustular lesions, erosion, and oozing. Scaling may be evident at the margin of the lesions.

Interdigital candidiasis is an erythematous eroded area with surrounding maceration between the fingers and toes, whereas balanitis presents as multiple discrete pustules on the glans penis and preputial sac. Balanitis that involves the scrotum can be painful. It is most common in uncircumcised men.

Paronychia and onychia present as redness and swelling of the nail folds. Swelling lifts the wall from the nail plate, causing purulent infection.

Follicular candidiasis appears as small, discrete pustules in the ostia of hair follicles, and oral candidiasis (thrush) presents as white plaques on an erythematous base. It is found mostly in infants and immunocompromised patients. The tongue is usually involved.

INITIATING DRUG THERAPY

Candidiasis can be prevented by keeping intertriginous areas dry when possible. Also, washing with benzoyl peroxide and applying powder containing miconazole may be beneficial.

Goals of Therapy

The goal of therapy is restoration of the mucous membranes to normal.

Nystatin

Nystatin (Mycostatin) is a fungicide that binds to sterols in the cell membrane of the fungus, causing a change in the membrane's permeability. This allows intracellular components to leak, thereby causing cell death.

Used to treat thrush in infants and adults, nystatin is placed in each side of the mouth 3 times daily. (See **Table 12.1.**) The solution is kept in the mouth as long as possible, then swallowed. Therapy continues for 10 to 14 days and at least 48 hours after clinical clearing. Adverse effects include GI upset and oral irritation.

Selecting the Most Appropriate Agent

First-Line Therapy

For cutaneous candidiasis, cool wet soaks with Burow's solution can be applied 2 to 3 times daily in macerated areas. Intertriginous areas are kept dry by powdering (e.g., with Zeasorb A-F Powder), exposing them to air, or by drying with a hair dryer after bathing. Antifungal creams (clotrimazole [Lotrimin], ketoconazole) can be applied once or twice a day for 10 days (**Table 12.6**).

TABLE 12.6	Recommended Order of Treatment for Candidiasis		
Order	**Cutaneous Agent**	**Oral Agent**	**Comments**
First line	Cool soaks with Burow's solution Topical azole	oral nystatin (Mycostatin)	Burow's solution is used in macerated areas. Topical azole is used for 10 days. Systemic therapy is used if no response to topical therapy.
Second line	itraconazole (Sporanox) or fluconazole (Diflucan)	itraconazole or fluconazole	NA

For oral candidiasis, oral nystatin is used for 10 to 14 days, or one clotrimazole troche is given orally 5 times a day for 2 weeks.

Second-Line Therapy

For failure to respond to treatment, patients have the option of second-line therapy. Systemic itraconazole may be prescribed to adults only for cutaneous or oral candidiasis. For children and adults, oral fluconazole may be prescribed.

MONITORING PATIENT RESPONSE

Response to therapy should be evaluated in 2 weeks. Follow-up for patients receiving long-term systemic therapy (2 weeks; not necessary for pulse therapy) is recommended every month to monitor liver function. Patients undergoing pulse therapy do not need monitoring as regularly. Human immunodeficiency virus infection and diabetes mellitus should be ruled out in patients who have recurring problems with candidiasis.

Case Study

M. B. is a 42-year-old diabetic woman who presents with thickened, yellow toenails that are painful when she wears dress shoes. Her blood sugar level is well controlled. She is taking the following medications: metformin 500 mg tid, cimetidine 300 mg qid, Accupril 10 mg daily. A toenail culture comes back positive for fungus.

1. List specific goals of treatment for M. B.
2. What drug therapy would you prescribe? Why?
3. What are the parameters for monitoring success of the therapy?
4. Discuss specific patient education based on the prescribed therapy.
5. List one or two adverse reactions for the selected agent that would cause you to change therapy.
6. What would be the choice for second-line therapy?
7. What over-the-counter and/or alternative medications would be appropriate for M. B.?
8. What lifestyle changes would you recommend to M. B.?
9. Describe one or two drug–drug or drug–food interactions for the selected agent.

BIBLIOGRAPHY

Andrews, R., McCarthy, J., Carapetis, J., & Currie, B. (2009). Skin disorders, including pyoderma, scabies and tinea infections. *Pediatric Clinics of North America, 56*(6), 1421–1440.

Goodheart, H. P. (2008). *A photoguide of common skin disorders: Diagnosis and management* (3rd ed.). Philadelphia: Lippincott Williams & Wilkins.
Habif, T. (2009). *Clinical dermatology* (5th ed.). Philadelphia: Mosby Elsevier.
Pleacher, M., & Dexter, W. (2007). Cutaneous fungal and viral infections in athletes. *Clinics in Sports Medicine, 26*(3), 397–411.

Viral Infections of the Skin

Viruses producing skin lesions may be categorized into three groups: herpes viruses, papilloma viruses, and pox viruses. Herpes and papilloma viruses each affect approximately 20% of the adult population in the United States, with an even distribution between the sexes.

Viruses are further classified by family—either the ribonucleic acid family or the deoxyribonucleic acid (DNA) family. Herpes viruses, papilloma viruses, and pox viruses are members of the DNA family.

Viruses are obligate intracellular parasites that consist of a nucleic acid core surrounded by one or more proteins. A host cell is required for viral replication. Several mechanisms exist for viral replication, and different DNA viruses replicate by their own specific mechanism. Pox viruses replicate entirely in the cytoplasm. Herpes viruses replicate their own polymerase, along with several of their own enzymes. Papilloma virus proteins contribute to the initiation of DNA replication.

HERPES VIRUS INFECTIONS

CAUSES

Seven types of herpes viruses are associated with human illness: herpes simplex type 1 (HSV-1), herpes simplex type 2 (HSV-2), varicella-zoster virus (VZV), Epstein-Barr virus, cytomegalovirus, human herpes virus type 6 (HHV-6), and human herpes virus type 8 (HHV-8).

HSV-1 infection usually involves the face and skin above the waist. HSV-2 is most commonly associated with the genitalia and the skin below the waist. A life-threatening neonatal infection is associated with HSV-2 in a baby whose mother is infected with the virus; the infection is transmitted during vaginal birth. Herpes zoster (shingles) and varicella (chickenpox) are the result of VZV infection. The overall incidence of herpes zoster is 3.2 per 1000 (Htwe, et al., 2007). Risk factors include aging, female gender, recent transplant, human immunodeficiency virus (HIV) infection, and cancer. Infectious mononucleosis is a result of Epstein-Barr virus infection. HHV-6 is associated with a mild childhood illness called roseola. HHV-8 is associated with Kaposi's sarcoma, especially in patients with HIV infection. HSV-1 and VZV are discussed in this chapter; HSV-2 is discussed in Chapter 35.

PATHOPHYSIOLOGY

Herpes viruses replicate their own polymerase along with several of their own enzymes. HSV is highly contagious. It is spread by direct contact with skin or mucous membrane. After the primary infection, the virus retreats to the dorsal root ganglion, where it remains latent until it is reactivated by triggers such as stress, viral infections, or sunlight.

Those who have had varicella virus infection are most prone to herpes zoster. After the primary infection resolves, the virus retreats to the dorsal root ganglion, where it remains dormant. Herpes zoster is caused by reactivation of the virus, most often with no apparent cause. There is a migration of virions through the axon to the skin of one or several adjacent axons. In immunocompetent patients, recurrent episodes are uncommon.

DIAGNOSTIC CRITERIA

Infection with HSV-1 and HSV-2 causes vesicular eruptions that are painful and often recurrent. The common incubation period of 4 to 10 days is followed by the eruption of clustered vesicles on an erythematous base. Distribution of the virus into autonomic and sensory nerve endings allows the virus to remain latent.

Typically, HSV-1 causes oral or facial infections, with the most common sites being the mouth, pharynx, lips, or face. Primary occurrences usually have intense symptoms. Prodromal symptoms include burning, tingling, or itching; these symptoms may accompany recurrent infection as well. Recurrence of the infection is thought to be precipitated by fatigue, stress, trauma, fever, or ultraviolet radiation. The lesion presents as a single vesicle or group of vesicles that overlie an erythematous base. They become pustules and become crusted or erode. Lesions recur at the site innervated by the dorsal root ganglion inhabited by the virus.

The two different diseases caused by VZV (chickenpox and shingles) have similar symptoms. After an incubation period of 10 to 20 days, chickenpox (primary varicella) manifests with fever and malaise followed by the outbreak of itchy, vesicular lesions on an erythematous base. The outbreak usually begins on the trunk and progresses to the extremities and face. Primary varicella occurs most often in children. Adults infected with primary varicella tend to have more systemic effects, especially if they have pre-existing medical conditions.

A reactivation of VZV in the nerve root ganglion is referred to as herpes zoster, or shingles. The infection characteristically begins with neuralgia in the affected dermatome, followed by an outbreak of grouped vesicles on an erythematous base, clustered in a unilateral pattern of the dermatome. In two thirds of infections, the lesions are on the trunk. Additional symptoms include fever, myalgia, and increasing localized pain. The most common presentation of herpes virus infection in the elderly is VZV in the form of herpes zoster. Three fourths of all cases of shingles occur in patients older than age 50. A significant complication of herpes zoster is postherpetic neuralgia, pain in the dermatome site that lasts longer than 6 weeks after resolution of the infection.

INITIATING DRUG THERAPY

Although nonpharmacologic interventions, such as soaks with Burow's solution, help to relieve symptoms, HSV-1 infection is treated primarily with other topical agents. In the case of severe infection in an immunocompromised patient, treatment may be with systemic drug therapy, which shortens the duration of symptoms; however, there is no treatment to prevent recurrence.

For oral HSV-1 infections (oral herpes), symptoms may or may not respond to viscous lidocaine (Xylocaine) 2% applied to the lesion. A solution of diphenhydramine (Benadryl) elixir and aluminum hydroxide/magnesium hydroxide (Maalox) mixed in a 1:1 proportion can be used as an oral rinse four times a day. Sucking on popsicles also can provide temporary relief.

For primary VZV infections that manifest as chickenpox, systemic therapy is used only in special cases and is not recommended for uncomplicated disease. For VZV infections that manifest as herpes zoster, antiviral agents may help relieve symptoms. Patients should be treated if the rash has been present for fewer than 72 hours or if new lesions are still developing. If therapy starts within 72 hours of the appearance of the lesion, systemic therapy decreases the duration of the rash and the acute pain associated with herpes zoster. In addition, any patient older than age 50 who is immunocompromised should be treated with antiviral agents. The use of antiviral therapy in herpes zoster decreases the symptoms of postherpetic neuralgia from 62 days with placebo to 20 days with acyclovir. Antiviral agents used are acyclovir, famciclovir, and valacyclovir. All antiviral agents have shown to shorten the duration of postherpetic neuralgia, but none prevent it.

Goals of Drug Therapy

In herpes virus infections, the goal of therapy is to reduce the duration of symptoms and suppress pain.

Topical Antiviral Agents

Two topical agents—acyclovir 5% and penciclovir (Denavir)—are available to treat herpes infections. These agents work by inhibiting viral DNA synthesis (**Table 13.1**). They may decrease healing time.

Patients usually apply topical acyclovir every 3 hours, six times per day, for 7 days. Penciclovir is applied every 2 hours, during waking hours, for 4 days. Adverse effects include mild skin irritation and pruritus.

Systemic Antiviral Agents

The three first-line systemic agents are acyclovir (Zovirax), famciclovir (Famvir), and valacyclovir (Valtrex), although famciclovir and valacyclovir are more bioavailable than acyclovir. Systemic antivirals are highly effective against herpes virus. In general, antiviral therapy is recommended for adolescents, adults, and high-risk patients, but not usually for healthy children younger than age 12. (See **Table 13.1.**)

Contraindications

Caution should be used in patients with renal disease because antivirals are excreted by the renal system. They are also contraindicated in patients with congestive heart failure and in lactation. Dosage adjustments are made for patients with a creatinine clearance rate less than 25 mL/minute.

Adverse Events

Adverse effects include headaches, vertigo, depression, and tremors. Patients may also experience gastrointestinal symptoms and rashes.

Interactions

The effect of antiviral agents is increased in patients taking probenecid, and patients taking zidovudine (Retrovir) may experience drowsiness.

Acyclovir

The prototypical antiviral agent acyclovir acts by inhibiting viral DNA replication. The drug works only in cells infected by HSV. A disadvantage of oral acyclovir is its low bioavailability of 10% to 20%.

The recommended acyclovir dosage for an initial episode of HSV disease in an immunocompetent host is 200 mg orally five times per day for 7 to 10 days. (See **Table 13.1.**) The recommended dosage for recurrent episodes is 200 mg five times per day for 5 days. For patients with recurrent infections, treatment prophylaxis is recommended with 400 mg twice daily. For an immunocompromised patient, the recommended treatment is 400 mg five times per day for 7 to 10 days. For suppression therapy, 400 mg twice a day is the dosage. The children's dosage of acyclovir is 5 mg/kg/day in five divided doses for 7 days.

The recommended dosage for treating VZV infections in children is 20 mg/kg four times per day for 5 days. Adult dosing is 800 mg five times per day for 7 to 10 days.

Famciclovir

Famciclovir is the diacetyl ester prodrug of penciclovir. It is an acyclic guanosine analog. After first-pass metabolism, it is well absorbed and converted to penciclovir. The oral bioavailability of famciclovir ranges from 5% to 75%.

The dosage of famciclovir is 250 mg three times per day for 7 to 10 days for an initial episode of illness; for recurrent episodes, the dose is 1000 mg twice daily for 1 day and 250 mg twice a day for suppression therapy.

TABLE 13.1	Overview of Antiviral Agents for Herpes Virus Infections		
Generic (Trade) Name and Dosage	**Selected Adverse Events**	**Contraindications**	**Special Considerations**
Topical Therapy			

acyclovir 5% (Zovirax)
    Apply every 3 h, six times per day for
        7 d
	Pruritus, pain on application	Do not use on mucous
		    membranes or near
		    eyes.
			Must use glove or finger cot for
			    application

penciclovir 1% (Denavir)
    Apply every 2 h for 4 d while awake
	Headache, mild skin irritation	Renal impairment	Begin using drug at earliest sign or
			    symptom.

Systemic Therapy			

acyclovir (Zovirax)
    For HSV-1
        200 mg five times per day for 10 d
            for initial outbreak; 200 mg five
            times a day for 5 d for recurrence
    For VZV infection
        Children: 20 mg/kg qid for 5 d
        Adults: 800 mg five times a day
            for 7 d
	Nausea, vomiting, headache,
	    CNS disturbance, rash,
	    malaise
		Renal impairment	Do not exceed maximum dose.
			Least effective antiviral
			Reserved for use in children

famciclovir (Famvir)
    For HSV-1
        250 mg tid for 10 d for initial out-
            break; 125 mg tid for recurrence
            or 1000 mg bid for 1 day
    For VZV infection
        500 mg tid for 7 d
	Headache, GI disturbance,
	    paresthesias
		Renal dysfunction	May be affected by drugs
			    metabolized by aldehyde oxi-
			    dase

valacyclovir (Valtrex)
    For HSV-1
        1 g bid for 10 d
    For VZV infection
        1 g tid for 7 d
    For recurrent HSV
        2000 mg bid for 1 d
	GI upset, headache, dizzi-
	    ness, abdominal pain
		Renal impairment
		HIV
			Be alert for renal or CNS toxicity
			    with nephrotoxic drugs.

HSV, herpes simplex virus; VZV, varicella-zoster virus.

Valacyclovir

Valacyclovir is a prodrug of acyclovir and is converted rapidly. First-pass metabolism converts valacyclovir to acyclovir with 50% bioavailability.

The dosage of valacyclovir is 1000 mg three times a day for 7 to 10 days for initial infection, 2000 mg two times a day for 1 day for recurrent infections, and 1000 mg daily for suppression therapy.

Selecting the Most Appropriate Agent

Of the various antiviral agents available, which is most effective for which disorder? Which agents are used when the first choice fails?

First-Line Therapy: Herpes Simplex Virus Type 1

First-line therapy for HSV-1 is topical acyclovir 5% every 3 hours six times a day for 7 days or penciclovir cream 1% every 2 hours during waking hours for 4 days in immunocompetent patients. Acyclovir is usually the first choice because it is less expensive than valacyclovir or famciclovir. Immunocompromised patients may need oral acyclovir 200 mg five times a day for 7 days, valacyclovir 500 mg twice a day for 5 days, or famciclovir 500 mg twice a day for 7 days (**Figure 13-1** and **Table 13.2**).

First-Line Therapy: Varicella-Zoster Virus

Systemic therapy is used only in patients with complicated disease or in children with pulmonary disease or taking steroids, and not for uncomplicated disease. It is prescribed only if the rash has been present for less than 24 hours. Acyclovir is used at a dosage of 20 mg/kg four times a day for 5 days (**Figure 13-2** and **Table 13.3**).

First-Line Therapy: Herpes Zoster

Systemic antiviral therapy can be started if the herpes zoster outbreak is less than 72 hours in duration or longer than

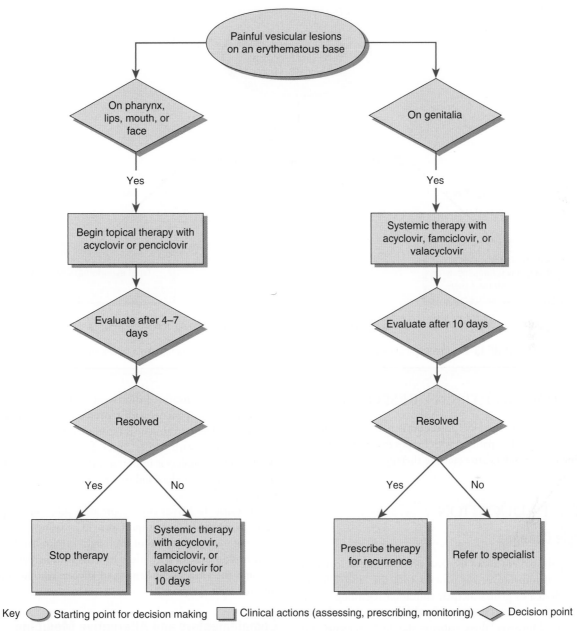

FIGURE 13–1   Treatment recommendations (left) for outbreaks of herpes simplex virus type 1 (HSV-1) and (right) for HSV-2.

TABLE 13.2	Recommended Order of Treatment for HSV-1 Infection	
Order	**Agent**	**Comments**
First line	Topical therapy with acyclovir 5% (Zovirax) or penciclovir 1% (Denavir)	Begin treatment at earliest sign of outbreak.
Second line	Systemic therapy with acyclovir (Zovirax), famciclovir (Famvir), or valacyclovir (Valtrex)	

72 hours but with new lesions appearing, the patient is older than age 50, or the patient is immunosuppressed. Therapy consists of valacyclovir 1 g three times a day or famciclovir 500 mg three times a day for 7 days (**Figure 13-3**). Cost is a driving force in prescribing valacyclovir before famciclovir because it is less expensive.

Oral analgesics, such as acetaminophen, aspirin, and nonsteroidal anti-inflammatory drugs, are helpful in pain control.

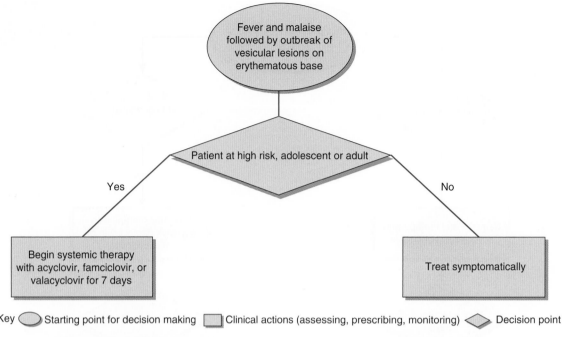

FIGURE 13–2   Treatment algorithm for the varicella-zoster virus infection manifested as chickenpox.

MONITORING PATIENT RESPONSE

Follow-up evaluation of HSV infection is not required if the symptoms resolve. For patients with herpes zoster, follow-up is recommended at 3 days after starting therapy, then at 1 week.

PATIENT EDUCATION

Lifestyle Changes

Educating the patient about hygiene, precipitating factors, and prevention is imperative. For patients with the HSV-2 infection manifested as genital herpes, education regarding sexual activity, recurrence, and the unpredictable course of the disease is necessary. Moreover, these patients should be screened for other sexually transmitted diseases. (See Chapter 35 for more information.) In patients with more than five recurrences per year, prophylactic treatment is recommended.

In patients with herpes zoster, follow-up monitoring for postherpetic neuralgia is important. Patients with postherpetic neuralgia should understand that pain management is the goal of therapy.

Because the herpes virus is spread by skin contact, patients need to recognize the importance of wearing gloves when applying medications and of thorough, careful hand washing. Skin-to-skin contact is avoided. Patients with herpes zoster can transmit the virus as chickenpox to anyone who has not been infected with the virus.

Complementary and Alternative Medicine

Capsaicin is used for pain control in herpes zoster. It is most effective when applied three or four times a day. Tea tree oil has reported antiseptic properties and is used in herpes simplex.

Special Populations

VZV infections occur occasionally during pregnancy. A primary VZV infection (varicella) may result in severe fetal abnormalities, but herpes zoster does not appear to harm the fetus.

Prevention

A vaccine, Zostavax, is now available. It is approved for everyone older than age 60 who has had chickenpox. It reduces the risk of developing herpes zoster and results in less frequent, less painful, and shorter courses of postherpetic neuralgia.

TABLE 13.3	**Recommended Order of Treatment for Varicella-Zoster Virus Infection**	
Order	**Agents**	**Comments**
First line	acyclovir (Zovirax), famciclovir (Famvir), valacyclovir (Valtrex)	For children the maximum dose is 800 mg qid. Acyclovir is the only approved agent for primary varicella. Antiviral therapy for primary varicella is recommended for adolescents, adults, and high-risk patients, but not for healthy children.

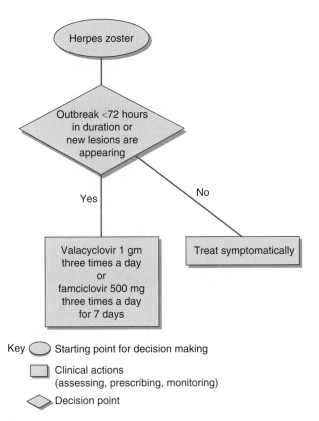

Key ⬭ Starting point for decision making

◻ Clinical actions
(assessing, prescribing, monitoring)

◇ Decision point

FIGURE 13–3 Treatment algorithm for the varicella-zoster virus infection manifested as shingles.

WARTS (VERRUCAE)

Warts are caused by the human papillomavirus (HPV). There are more than 80 types of HPV. They are transferred by skin-to-skin contact. The common viruses can be classified as those causing anogenital infections and non-anogenital infections. Anogenital infections are discussed in Chapter 35. The most common non-anogenital infections present as warts. These are very common, especially in children: at some time in their life, approximately 20% of school-age children have one or more warts, which usually regress spontaneously. Categories of warts include plantar, filiform, flat, and common.

CAUSES

Plantar warts result from HPV-1 and commonly occur on the soles of the feet and the palms of the hands. Verruca vulgaris—common warts—is an infection with HPV-2. These present on the fingers or toes or at sites of trauma. They are flesh-colored to brown, hyperkeratotic papules. HPV-3 produces flat warts, which are located on the face, neck, and chest or flexor regions of the forearms and legs.

Factors that predispose to HPV include the following:

- infection with HIV;
- intake of drugs that decrease cell-mediated immunity (prednisone, cyclosporin);
- chemotherapeutic agents;
- pregnancy (may cause proliferation); and
- handling raw meat, fish, or other animal matter.

PATHOPHYSIOLOGY

HPV proteins contribute to the initiation of DNA replication. Plantar warts are most commonly caused by HPV-1, HPV-2, HPV-4, HPV-31, and HPV-32. The virus enters through skin abrasions and infects the cells of the basal layers of the skin. There is no diffusion to the deep tissues. Viral replication is slow and is closely dependent on the differentiation of the host cells. Viral DNA is present in the basal cells, but the viral antigens and the infecting virus are produced only when the cells start to become squamous and keratinized once they reach the surface. The incubation period is usually 4 to 6 months, with transmission by direct contact or by fomite.

DIAGNOSTIC CRITERIA

Warts are papillomatous, corrugated, hyperkeratotic growths found only on the epidermis, especially in areas subjected to repeated trauma. They can be solitary, multiple, or clustered. Warts are named based on their clinical appearance, location, or both.

Filiform warts are found primarily on the face and neck and present as tan, finger-like projections. Plantar warts (verruca plantaris) are found on the metatarsal areas, heels, and toes. Common warts (verruca vulgaris) occur most often on the hands and fingers, knees, and elbows and have an asymmetric distribution. Flat warts (verruca plana) are found mostly on the forehead, chin, cheeks, arms, and dorsa of the hands. They are flat and well defined and may be flesh-colored or darker brown. Flat warts can be spread by shaving and are found in the beard area in men and on the legs in women. These HPV infections are rarely associated with malignancy. Typically, the incubation period is 2 to 6 months.

INITIATING DRUG THERAPY

The natural history of cutaneous HPV infection is spontaneous resolution in months or a few years, so aggressive therapy may not be needed unless the patient reports pain. If treatment is initiated, the choice of medication depends on age of the patient, whether pain is involved, and the location of the wart. Filiform and flat warts are removed by a dermatologist. Topical treatment with salicylic acid (DuoFilm) is usually the starting point for all other warts. It is easier to treat small verrucae rather than waiting until they are large.

Goals of Therapy

The goal of therapy is eradication of the virus and lesion, although there is no way to actually kill HPV.

Salicylic Acid

Salicylic acid is a keratolytic (peeling) agent. It is available in a variety of strengths for specific types or sites of verrucae. It comes in liquid, gel, and patches. Usually, 17% salicylic acid is used to treat small lesions. Mediplast is a patch product that is 40% salicylic acid plaster; it is useful for large lesions and can be cut to fit the wart.

Dosage

The solution is left on overnight. The patch is applied and left on for 5 to 6 days. Treatment continues for up to 12 weeks. The patient is instructed to soak the area in water for 5 minutes and dry the area before applying the topical preparation.

Contraindications

Topical therapy is contraindicated in patients with diabetes mellitus or impaired circulation and on moles, birthmarks, or unusual warts with hair growth. The most common adverse effect is skin irritation.

Selecting the Most Appropriate Agent

Since the immune system seems to play the most important role in HPV, treatment stimulates the immune system to deal more effectively with the virus. Most warts cure themselves over time, especially in the immunocompetent host.

First-Line Therapy

Filiform or flat warts are removed by a dermatologist. For common warts, topical salicylic acid in a 17% concentration is used; it is applied at bedtime for approximately 8 weeks or until the wart is gone. For plantar warts, a 40% salicylic acid preparation is used in plaster or patch form that is cut to the size of the wart and applied at bedtime. The preparation remains in place for 24 to 48 hours. When removed, the area is rubbed with a pumice stone to remove dead white keratin. This is repeated for approximately 8 weeks or until the wart is gone (**Figure 13-4** and **Table 13.4**).

Second-Line Therapy

If patient-applied therapy fails, cryosurgery, electrotherapy, or carbon dioxide laser surgery can be performed.

MONITORING PATIENT RESPONSE

In non-anogenital HPV infections, multiple treatments may be necessary. Patients should understand the importance of

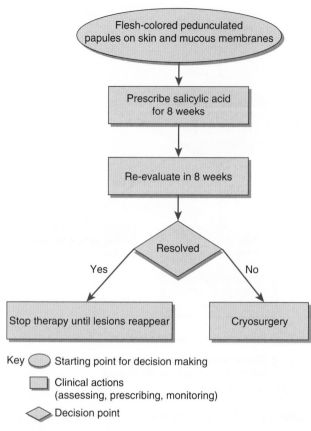

FIGURE 13–4 Treatment algorithm for non-anogenital human papillomavirus infection.

follow-up beyond the initial wart removal, because the virus may remain. Patients may need weekly treatment until the wart is eradicated.

PATIENT EDUCATION

Patients need to be informed that viral warts may recur.

TABLE 13.4	Recommended Order of Treatment for Non-Anogenital Infection with Human Papillomavirus	
Order	**Agent**	**Comments**
First line	Salicylic acid	Used as first-line agent to treat all types of verrucae
Second line	Cryosurgery, electrosurgery, or carbon dioxide laser surgery	Refer patient to specialist.

Case Study

B. H. is a 72-year-old man who presents for evaluation of several painful red bumps on his left side. The pain radiates around to his chest. The rash resembles blisters that are just forming. He noticed them yesterday, and more are forming. His wife is receiving chemotherapy for breast cancer. His laboratory results are all normal, and his creatinine is 1.2.

DIAGNOSIS: HERPES ZOSTER

1. List specific treatment goals for B. H.
2. What, if any, drug therapy would you prescribe? Why?
3. What are the parameters for monitoring the success of the therapy?
4. Discuss specific patient education based on his history and the therapy.
5. List one or two adverse effects he may get from the prescribed therapy.
6. What over-the-counter medications and/or alternative therapy might you recommend?
7. What lifestyle changes might you recommend for B. H.?
8. Describe one or two drug–drug or drug–food interactions for the selected agent.

BIBLIOGRAPHY

Starred references are cited in the text.

Decker, C. (2010). Skin and soft tissue infections in athletes. *Disease-a-Month, 56*(7), 414–421.

Elston, D. (2009). Update on cutaneous manifestations of infectious diseases. *Medical Clinics of North America, 93*(6), 1283–1290.

Goodheart, H. P. (2008). *A photoguide of common skin disorders: Diagnosis and management* (3rd ed.). Philadelphia: Lippincott Williams & Wilkins.

Habif, T. (2009). *Clinical dermatology* (3rd ed.). Philadelphia: Mosby Elsevier.

*Htwe, T. Mushtag, A. Robinson, S., et al. (2007). Infections in the elderly. *Infectious Disease Clinics of North America, 21*(3), 711–743.

Plesacher, M., & Dexter, W. (2007). Cutaneous fungal and viral infections in athletes. *Medical Clinics of North America, 93*(6), 1283–1290.

Ruocco, E., Donnarumma, G., Barone, A., & Tufano, M. (2007). Bacterial and viral skin diseases. *Dermatology Clinics, 25*(4), 663–676.

CHAPTER 14

Jason J. Schafer
Maria Foy

Bacterial Infections of the Skin

Bacterial skin infections range from those that are minor and heal without consequence to those that are more severe and may be disfiguring or even life-threatening. Minor infections are quite common and are often self-treated by patients without formal medical care. The majority of wounds seen in health care practice are easily managed with appropriate wound care and antibiotic therapy, if indicated.

Common primary skin infections resulting from bacteria include impetigo, bullous impetigo, folliculitis, felons, paronychias, and cellulitis. (See **Box 14.1** for information about associated problems.) These are discussed in this chapter, along with the less common infections erysipelas, ecthyma, furuncles, and carbuncles. This chapter also contains a brief discussion of necrotizing fasciitis, a very serious infection treated in an inpatient setting by specialists. See the accompanying color plates for an illustration of some of these infections.

CAUSES

The bacterial organisms most commonly responsible for causing skin infections are *Streptococcus pyogenes* (group A *Streptococcus*, or GAS) and *Staphylococcus aureus* (**Tables 14.1** and **14.2**).

Impetigo and Ecthyma

In the past, superficial skin infections, such as impetigo, a common infection characterized by scattered vesicular lesions, were caused by GAS. However, a shift in normal skin flora has occurred in the United States, and now impetigo is due primarily to *S. aureus* alone or less commonly in combination with GAS. Bullous impetigo, a variation of impetigo, is caused primarily by *S. aureus*.

Ecthyma is a chronic form of impetigo that affects deeper layers of the skin. Usually the causes are the same as those of impetigo; however, gram-negative organisms, such as *Pseudomonas aeruginosa*, or fungal organisms may also play a role. This is especially true in diabetic or immunocompromised patients. Ecthyma can develop from minor wounds, scabies, insect bites, or any condition that causes itching, scratching, and excoriation.

Impetigo is more common in children but can also be seen in adults. It is most often diagnosed during hot, humid weather when bacterial colonization of the skin occurs more easily. Both impetigo and ecthyma are communicable and can be transmitted through person-to-person contact, often in schools or day care centers. Poor hygiene and crowded living conditions are other factors that can contribute to the development of these infections (Gorbach, 2004).

Cellulitis and Erysipelas

Cellulitis is an infection involving the skin and subcutaneous layers. It has the potential to spread systemically and cause serious illness. It can develop in any type of wound, ranging from a minor break in the skin to more serious laceration, puncture, or burn. Other common precipitants include stasis dermatitis, stasis ulcers, edema of the lower extremity, venous insufficiency, and obesity (Odell, 2003). In intravenous (IV) drug users, cellulitis typically develops at injection sites. The characteristics of infection depend on many factors, including the type of wound, the organisms involved, and the patient.

Most cases of cellulitis are caused by GAS or *S. aureus*. Patients with predisposing factors, however, may be at risk for infections caused by other organisms, including *Escherichia coli*, *P. aeruginosa*, and *Klebsiella* species (**Table 14.2**). *Pasteurella multocida* is the primary cause of cellulitis from animal bites and scratches, although *S. aureus* and GAS may also be present. **Table 14.2** lists additional causes.

S. aureus organisms that are resistant to commonly used antibiotics have recently emerged as a major cause of community-acquired skin infections. These organisms are resistant to all penicillins and cephalosporin agents and are referred to as community-associated methicillin-resistant *S. aureus* (CA-MRSA) (DeLeo, et al., 2010). Infections resulting from these organisms can be particularly challenging to manage because of their resistance to commonly used antibiotics. Also, as opposed to other skin infections, CA-MRSA infections may occur in otherwise healthy individuals but are most common among patients with close contact with others colonized or infected with CA-MRSA. Transmission of this pathogen appears to occur most commonly when there are crowded living conditions (e.g., military bases, prisons) or close physical contact between individuals, particularly when injury to the skin is common (e.g., athletes).

Erysipelas, predominantly caused by *S. pyogenes*, is a superficial form of cellulitis and is seen more often in children, especially infants, and the elderly. Also known as *St. Anthony's fire*, it is an acute condition that can spread rapidly through the skin and lymphatics, causing significant mortality (up to 5%) if left untreated.

Danger: Bites and Other Puncture Wounds

Human and animal bites and puncture wounds of other sorts are infections waiting to develop. Because these wounds are associated with such a high risk for infection, antibiotic prophylaxis with a broad-spectrum penicillin or quinolone usually begins with the patient's request for health care. Tetanus is also an important consideration in puncture wounds and bites, and patients should be immunized as needed.

If the wound was created by a clean object and is in an area that is well vascularized, treatment, in addition to antibiotic prophylaxis, may consist simply of washing thoroughly; soaking in warm, soapy water several times a day; and observing the site for a few days.

If the wound was made by an object contaminated with fecal material, soil, or other debris, or if the patient is diabetic or has a compromised circulation, broad-spectrum antibiotic prophylaxis is required with amoxicillin-clavulanate potassium or ciprofloxacin based on the probable causative organism.

Care for bite wounds depends on several factors, including whether the biter was a human or an animal, the location of the wound, and whether the wound is primarily a puncture or a laceration. All bite wounds should be cleaned thoroughly with soap and water. Puncture bites should be irrigated with normal saline solution. Extensive

wounds may require surgical debridement, tendon repair, or suturing. If the bite is located on an extremity, elevation of the extremity will help prevent swelling.

All human bites that break the skin should be treated with broad-spectrum antibiotic prophylaxis. Appropriate choices include amoxicillin-clavulanate, or ampicillin–sulbactam of intravenous treatment. Oral doxycycline can be used for patients who are allergic to penicillin. Treatment should be given for a full 7 to 10 days.

Minor animal bites may not require antibiotic prophylaxis unless the wound is on the hand, foot, or face. However, the infection rate in animal bites can range from 2% to 20%, and it may be prudent to treat the wound with a course of antibiotic prophylaxis. The possibility of rabies must also be addressed. The same agents used for human bites are also appropriate for animal bites.

Although most puncture wounds heal without incident, patients should be instructed to observe for signs of infection, including inflammation, persistent pain, swelling, or purulent drainage. If a puncture wound becomes infected, further systemic antibiotic therapy is required and should be based on culture and Gram stain results. A follow-up visit should be scheduled within days to ensure that the wound is healing without further infection.

Pustular Infections

Pustular infections include folliculitis, furunculosis, and carbunculosis. Folliculitis is a superficial infection of the hair follicle commonly caused by *S. aureus*. Patients who have been taking prolonged antibiotic therapy for acne, however, may acquire folliculitis from gram-negative organisms such as *Klebsiella*, *Enterobacter*, or *Proteus* species. Lesions

associated with folliculitis are usually found on the cheek or chin, under the nose, or on the central facial areas (Trent, et al., 2001). *P. aeruginosa* can also cause folliculitis, particularly in those who frequently use hot tubs, as a result of inadequate chlorination.

Furunculosis (furuncles) and carbunculosis (carbuncles) are also pustular infections usually caused by *S. aureus*. Both

TABLE 14.1 Selected Organisms That Cause Skin Infections

	Impetigo and Ecthyma	Bullous Impetigo	Erysipelas	Folliculitis, Furuncles, and Carbuncles	Paronychias
Gram-Positive Organisms					
Staphylococcus aureus	X	X	X (very few)	X	X
Group A *Streptococcus*	X		X		X
Group B *Streptococcus*	X (newborn impetigo)		X (newborn)		
Gram-Negative Organisms					
Proteus				X (facial) (folliculitis)	
Pseudomonas	X (occasionally ecthyma)			X (hot tub folliculitis)	X
Klebsiella				X (folliculitis)	
Enterobacter				X (occasionally folliculitis)	

TABLE 14.2 Organisms That Cause Cellulitis

Organism	Condition
Staphylococcus aureus	Common
Group A *Streptococcus*	Common
Haemophilus influenzae B	Children (periorbital cellulitis*)
Pneumococcus	Children
Escherichia coli	Opportunistic in compromised patients
Pseudomonas	Folliculitis from underchlorinated hot tubs
Klebsiella	Opportunistic in compromised patients
Enterobacter	Opportunistic in compromised patients
Pasteurella multocida	Animal bites and scratches
Anaerobic organisms	Diabetes, ulcers, trauma, crush wounds
Erysipelothrix rhusiopathiae	Fish handlers, usually on the hand
Aeromonas hydrophila	Fresh water–related injury, immunosuppressed patients
Vibrio species	Sea water–related injuries

*Uncommon now because of the use of HIB vaccine.

conditions involve deeper areas of the skin and can develop from unresolved cases of folliculitis.

Irritation from shaving, plucking, and waxing of hair may contribute to folliculitis. Other predisposing factors include humid conditions, tight clothing, diabetes, occlusion of the hair follicles from cosmetics or sunscreens, poor hygiene, and occupational exposure to heavy grease or solvents.

Other common skin infections, such as paronychia (an infection surrounding a nail bed) and a felon (an infection affecting the tip of a digit), are usually caused by *S. aureus, S. pyogenes,* or *Pseudomonas* species and occasionally other gram-negative bacilli.

Necrotizing Fasciitis

Necrotizing fasciitis, an extremely serious infection of the sub-cutaneous tissues, is life-threatening if not diagnosed early and treated appropriately. It is most likely to occur in middle-aged, elderly, or seriously debilitated patients (Sadick, 1997). The mortality rate is typically 20% to 30% but can approach up to 50% in patients with underlying vascular disease. Often, the initial lesion is minor, such as an insect bite or boil; it is rarely associated with Bartholin's gland or perianal abscesses (Gorbach, 2004). However, 20% of cases have no visible lesions (Gorbach, 2004). Patients with diabetes and alcoholism may have no evidence of trauma (Odell, 2003).

Necrotizing fasciitis is often monomicrobial and can be caused by *S. pyogenes, S. aureus,* or anaerobic streptococcus species. Infections can also be polymicrobial and involve up to 15 different organisms. Varicella infection is often considered

a risk factor for invasive skin infections, including necrotizing fasciitis (Wilhelm, et al., 2001).

Patients with necrotizing fasciitis are very ill and require intensive care. Surgical debridement of infected areas and IV antibiotic therapy are also commonly indicated. Patients who are elderly or debilitated or who have predisposing medical conditions, such as diabetes, advanced atherosclerotic disease, and lesions starting in an extremity and progressing into the back, chest wall, or buttock muscles, have a poor prognosis (Gorbach, 2004).

PATHOPHYSIOLOGY

The skin is composed of three layers. The outer layer is the epidermis, the first line of defense against infection. Nail tissue is part of the epidermis. Underneath is the dermis, which contains connective tissue, blood vessels, nerves, hair follicles, sweat glands, and sebaceous glands. The innermost layer is composed of subcutaneous tissue. Skin infections may be classified according to the depth of penetration and the layer and skin structure affected.

Under normal circumstances, bacteria present on the skin as normal flora cause no harm. However, a break in the skin can allow these organisms to penetrate and proliferate, resulting in a skin infection. Some people are persistent carriers of *S. aureus* in the nasal, perineal, or axillary areas. These individuals may be more prone to development of skin infections and more likely to experience recurrences.

Patients with predisposing medical conditions (**Box 14.2**), such as diabetes, immune system disorders, and malnutrition from alcoholism or other causes, are more prone to skin infection because of poor wound healing. Also at a higher risk for skin infection are those with circulatory compromise of the arterial, venous, or lymphatic systems. Wound infections in

BOX 14.2

Predisposing Factors in Skin Infections

Chronic carriers of *Staphylococcus aureus*
Diabetes mellitus
Peripheral vascular disease
Venous stasis
Alcoholism (malnutrition)
Immune deficiency
Corticosteroid therapy
Obesity
Trauma or burns
Poor hygiene
Warm, humid conditions
Topical irritants
Tight clothing

patients with these conditions have the potential to become more serious and invasive, requiring IV antibiotic therapy, hospitalization, or referral to a specialist. Wound infections can also become more serious when treatment is delayed. The practitioner must be alert for these situations and act promptly.

In addition, many organisms aside from GAS or *S. aureus* may cause infections in patients with chronic conditions. These organisms include *E. coli, Klebsiella* species, and *P. aeruginosa*. Infections in these patients are often more difficult to manage clinically and have the tendency to become chronic. Furthermore, those whose infections do resolve with appropriate therapy have a high risk of recurrence.

DIAGNOSTIC CRITERIA

Impetigo and Ecthyma

Impetigo, a highly contagious, common primary skin infection in children, is most frequently found on the face, scalp, or extremities. It begins as scattered, discrete macules that itch and are spread by scratching. These macules then develop into vesicles and pustules on an erythematous base that eventually rupture, oozing a purulent liquid. Once dried, the lesions appear thick, with a characteristic honey-colored crust on the surface. Once healed, scarring is rare. Regional lymphadenopathy may be present and lesions may itch; however, fever or other systemic complaints are uncommon. The infection is diagnosed clinically by the appearance of hallmark honey-colored crusts. A Gram stain of the vesicular fluid can confirm the diagnosis if there is clinical uncertainty.

Impetigo may also present with bullous lesions and can be referred to as bullous impetigo. Found on the face, scalp, extremities, trunk, and intertriginous areas, it affects primarily newborns and children ages 3 to 5 (Wilhelm, et al., 2001). Bullous impetigo is characterized by the formation of superficial, flaccid bullae on the skin. The brownish-gray lesions are sometimes crusted or have an erythematous halo. They also appear to be smooth and shiny, as if they were coated with lacquer.

In the most severe form of bullous impetigo, exfoliation of large areas of the skin can occur in what is called "scalded skin" syndrome. This presentation is most common in infants but can also occur in those who are immunosuppressed. It is thought to occur more often in patients who are sensitive to toxins produced by staphylococcal organisms (Barg, et al., 1998). Such cases carry a greater risk for more invasive infection because of the loss of large amounts of the skin, which is the body's protective barrier.

Ecthyma occurs when a case of impetigo worsens and spreads deeply to the dermis. Much less common than impetigo, ecthyma usually affects debilitated individuals and the elderly (Odell, 2003). Signs of ecthyma are usually found on the lower extremities, beginning with the formation of vesicles that then develop into shallow ulcerations. The ulcerations enlarge over several days and are surrounded by an erythematous halo. Because the infection affects the deeper layers of the skin, scarring is often seen after ulcerations heal (Wilhelm, et al., 2001). Lesions are usually painful and may persist for weeks to months.

Cellulitis and Erysipelas

Cellulitis is a potentially serious infection involving the skin and subcutaneous tissue. In adults, it most commonly affects the lower extremities and begins with a skin break resulting from a localized trauma that may not be apparent. In children, cellulitis usually results from an insect bite or a wound. The disease can spread through the superficial layers of skin and cause painful erythema, with the affected area warm and tender to the touch. Pitting edema can also be present, and the skin may be shiny and have an "orange peel" appearance. The margins of cellulitis are diffuse, not sharply demarcated, and the affected area is flat and usually edematous. In open wounds, purulent drainage and necrosis may be present. Red streaks may develop proximal to the area of infection, indicating lymphatic spread. Crepitus may be present, suggesting involvement of anaerobic organisms. Systemic symptoms of fever, chills, and malaise and regional adenitis are also common and can indicate bacteremia. In fact, these symptoms may be present before cellulitis is clearly evident.

Cellulitis due to CA-MRSA may be accompanied by the presence of an abscess or a furuncle that contains a necrotic center (DeLeo, et al., 2010). These infections may progress rapidly and cause local tissue destruction, possibly leading to systemic infection. In addition to painful erythema, the abscess present may spontaneously drain but often will require an incision and drainage procedure for proper management.

Erysipelas, a type of cellulitis limited to the superficial layers of the skin, is most common in children, especially infants and the elderly, but it can occur in healthy individuals who have sustained only minor wounds. Other patients who are at risk include those with venous insufficiency or underlying skin ulcers, diabetics, alcoholics, or those with nephritic syndrome. Erysipelas is most commonly found on the lower extremities but can also be present on the face and scalp. Erysipelas begins as an area of sharply demarcated erythema that spreads rapidly over a period of minutes to hours. The affected area is slightly raised, firm, warm, and tender to the touch. Erythema spreads along local lymphatic channels, which gives the skin a typical "orange peel" appearance due to lymphatic obstruction.

Common systemic symptoms include pain, malaise, chills, and fever. In more serious cases, patients may appear seriously ill. Erysipelas occurring on the face often follows a respiratory infection; this presentation can be particularly serious due to the potential occurrence of cavernous sinus thrombosis (Odell, 2003). Erysipelas can recur, usually in the same area as a previous infection, especially in patients with venous insufficiency or lymphedema (Wilhelm, et al., 2001).

Pustular Infections

Folliculitis is usually superficial and occurs on hairy areas of the skin, especially the bearded parts of the face and the intertriginous areas. Early lesions appear as erythematous papules that turn into small pustules within approximately 48 hours. As a result, it is common to see various lesions at different stages of development. These lesions may itch initially and then rupture and form crusts. Folliculitis is often recurrent and can represent over months or even years.

A furuncle, which develops from folliculitis, is a painful, pus-filled nodule that encircles a hair follicle. The condition is most commonly found in adolescents or in those with predisposing conditions such as diabetes, immunodeficiency, or poor hygiene. A carbuncle is a confluence of several furuncles that form deep within the dermis. They are often found on the upper back or the thick skin at the back of the neck, especially in men over age 40.

Furuncles and carbuncles are found in hairy areas or in areas of friction. Common sites are the neck, face, axillae, forearms, upper back, groin, buttocks, and thighs. A lesion begins with pruritus and tenderness. It becomes fluctuant in several days as the collection of pus enlarges. Ranging in size from 0.5 to 3 cm, it appears as a pointed, yellow lesion on the skin. As the lesion enlarges, tenderness increases and the lesion often ruptures spontaneously. Systemic manifestations are not usually seen with furuncles, but carbuncles are frequently accompanied by systemic signs such as fever, malaise, and headache.

A paronychia is infection of the tissue surrounding a nail bed. It is associated with nail biting, hangnails, or finger sucking; it may occur in people who have their hands in water frequently. Diabetic patients are also at a higher risk. A paronychia involving the toenail most often results from an ingrown nail. The infected area appears red and swollen and is painful. Pus, which may accumulate, may sometimes be expressed with gentle pressure; this usually relieves the discomfort. Systemic symptoms are uncommon.

A felon, which may follow a fingertip wound, is an infection that involves the pulp space in the tip of a digit. It is potentially more serious than a paronychia because it is confined in a closed space. The affected digit is erythematous, edematous, and exquisitely tender. The edema has the potential to compromise the arterial supply of the digit. If left untreated, abscess and tissue necrosis can occur. An additional danger is the possibility of bony or joint involvement, which can lead to loss of function.

Necrotizing Fasciitis

Patients with necrotizing fasciitis are extremely ill, requiring intensive care and treatment by specialists. The infection may initially appear similar to cellulitis, although severe pain, erythema, and edema are commonly present. Necrotizing fasciitis may be differentiated from cellulitis by its rapid spread, tissue destruction, and lack of response to usual antibiotic therapy. The subcutaneous tissue will have a wooden-hard feel, as compared to cellulitis and erysipelas, where this tissue is usually yielding and can be palpated. Other symptoms that distinguish necrotizing fasciitis from cellulitis are high fever (102° to 105°F [38.9° to 40.6°C]), intense pain and tenderness at

the site, and swelling of the affected extremity. Drainage is also usually present and is described as "dishwater pus" (Sadick, 1997). As this infection progresses and tissue destruction spreads, pain may be replaced by anesthesia, and patients may show signs of sepsis, including hemodynamic instability and multi-organ dysfunction.

INITIATING DRUG THERAPY

An increasing challenge in treating skin infections is the problem of antibiotic-resistant organisms. Choosing the appropriate agent is not as simple as it once was, and prescribers must be aware of this fact, as well as of regional variations in infecting organisms.

Because warm, humid conditions and poor hygiene may play a role in skin infections, especially impetigo, treatment begins with good hygiene (**Box 14.3**), avoidance of irritants, and meticulous wound care as appropriate. For some very minor infections, these measures along with a topical agent may be sufficient. Adjunctive treatment for most skin infections (bullous impetigo and erysipelas, for example) includes warm soaks and elevation of the affected area if it involves an extremity. However, most bacterial skin infections require treatment with systemic antibiotics.

The majority of infections are treated in the outpatient setting with oral antibiotic agents. Patients with more serious infections, however, may require hospitalization and IV medications or referral to a specialist. Treatment decisions are based on the practitioner's knowledge of the patient's predisposing conditions, the patient's present state of health, and the type and stage of the infection.

In many cases, systemic antibiotic therapy (**Table 14.3**) is prescribed empirically based on knowledge of the organisms commonly responsible for specific skin infections, such as *S. aureus* and GAS. With potentially serious infections such as a felon or cellulitis, a specimen of wound drainage should be

---

BOX   14.3

Strategies to Prevent Skin Infections

Wash hands frequently to prevent spread of infecting organisms.

Clean skin twice daily with soap and water or antibacterial soap (e.g., Hibiclens, Lever 2000).

Avoid scratching.

Use warm soaks to promote drainage of pustular matter.

Avoid irritants, including tight clothing, shaving, sunscreens, and occlusive cosmetics and deodorants.

BIBLIOGRAPHY

Starred references are cited in the text.

Bowe, W., Joshi, S., & Shalita, A. (2010). Diet and acne. *Journal of the American Academy of Dermatology, 63*(1), 124–147.

DelRossi, J., & Kim, G. (2009). Optimizing the use of oral antibiotics in acne vulgaris. *Dermatology Clinics, 27*(1), 33–42.

Goldgar, C., Keahey, D., & Houchens, J. (2009). Treatment options for acne rosacea. *American Family Physician, 80*(5), 461–468.

Leyden, J., DelRossi, J, & Webster, G. (2009). Clinical considerations in the treatment of acne vulgaris and other inflammatory skin disorders. *Dermatology Clinics, 27*(1), 1–15.

*Mechcatie, E. (2004). Pregnancies lead to more isotretinoin restrictions. *Pediatric News, 56*(4), 651–663.

*Roche Laboratories. (2002). Accutane (isotretinoin) capsules complete product information. Nutley, NJ: Author.

Strauss, J., Krowchuk, D., Leyden, J., et al. (2007). Guidelines of care for acne vulgaris management. *Journal of the American Academy of Dermatology, 56,* 651–663.

*U.S. Food and Drug Administration. (2002). MedWatch 2002 Safety Alert–Accutane (isotretinoin) Dear Accutane Prescriber letter. Rockville, MD: Author [on-line: retrieved September 6, 2004]. Available: http://www.fda.gov/medwatch/SAFETY/2002/accutane_deardoe_10-2002.htm.

Webster, G. (2009). Rosacea. *Medical Clinics of North America, 93*(6), 1183–1194.

Pharmacotherapy for Eye and Ear Disorders

CHAPTER 17

Joshua J. Spooner

Ophthalmic Disorders

There are many conditions and disorders of the eye, but only a few, such as blepharitis and conjunctivitis, should be treated by a primary care provider. The remaining conditions are usually treated by eye care specialists. Nonetheless, prescribers should be familiar with drug therapy for the more common ophthalmic conditions (glaucoma, keratoconjunctivitis sicca) because they may encounter patients being treated for these disorders.

EYELID MARGIN INFECTIONS: BLEPHARITIS

The eye is well protected externally by the eyebrow, eyelashes, and eyelids. If these protective mechanisms are compromised, the eye becomes predisposed to disease. Externally, the eyelid structures are composed of skin with a high degree of elasticity, muscles that elevate the upper eyelid and close the eyelids, and the tarsal plate, which contains the meibomian glands. Through frequent blinking, the eyelids maintain an even flow of tears over the cornea. Internally, the eyelid structure is lined by the palpebral conjunctiva, which folds upon itself and then covers the sclera of the eyeball up to the corneoscleral junction. Located at the lid margins are the openings to the long sebaceous meibomian glands; these glands secrete the oily film that prevents tears from evaporating. At the base of the eyelash hair follicles are the superficial modified sebaceous glands of Zeiss and the sweat glands of Moll. Any of these glands may become functionally disrupted.

Blepharitis is an inflammation of the eyelid margin. Although it is a common eye disorder in the United States, epidemiologic information on its incidence or prevalence is lacking.

CAUSES

Blepharitis can be caused by a bacterial infection (staphylococcal blepharitis), inflammation or hypersecretion of the sebaceous glands (seborrheic blepharitis), meibomian gland dysfunction (MGD blepharitis), or a combination of these (American Academy of Ophthalmology [AAO], 2008a). Staphylococcal and seborrheic blepharitis involve the anterior eyelid; both have been referred to as anterior blepharitis.

PATHOPHYSIOLOGY

Although the gram-positive organisms *Staphylococcus epidermidis* and *Staphylococcus aureus* are found on the eyelids of a high proportion of healthy subjects, *S. aureus* is observed more frequently among patients with staphylococcal blepharitis. While *S. epidermidis* and *S. aureus* are thought to play a role in the development of staphylococcal blepharitis, their role in disease production remains unclear. Toxin production, immunologic mechanisms, and antigen-induced inflammatory reactions have all been reported with blepharitis (AAO, 2008a; Song, et al., 2001).

Seborrheic blepharitis typically occurs as part of the more comprehensive condition of seborrheic dermatitis, with dandruff of the scalp, eyebrows, eyelashes, nasolabial folds, and external ears. Seborrheic blepharitis is more commonly found in the geriatric population because of its association with rosacea.

Manifestations of MGD include thickening of the eyelid margin, plugging of the meibomian orifices, prominent blood vessels crossing the mucocutaneous junction, and formation of chalazia (painless firm lumps on the eyelid). These changes may lead to atrophy of the meibomian glands (AAO, 2008a). Compared to healthy patients, meibomian gland secretions are more turbid among patients with MGD blepharitis. These secretions block the gland orifices and become a growth medium for bacteria. Patients with MGD blepharitis frequently have coexisting rosacea or seborrheic dermatitis.

DIAGNOSTIC CRITERIA

There are no specific diagnostic tests for blepharitis; the diagnosis is often based upon patient history and characteristic symptoms. Patients with blepharitis frequently present with irritated red eyes and report a burning sensation. Increases in tearing, blinking, and photophobia are frequently reported, as is eyelid sticking and contact lens intolerance. Upon close inspection, the eyelid margins appear red, greasy, and crusted, with eyelid deposits that cling to the eyelashes. The eyelid margins may be ulcerated and thickened, and eyelashes may be missing.

Although the clinical features of staphylococcal, seborrheic, and MGD blepharitis are similar, there are differences that can aid in the differential diagnosis of these conditions. Eyelash loss and eyelash misdirection frequently occur in staphylococcal blepharitis but are rare in seborrheic blepharitis. The eyelid deposits are matted and scaly in staphylococcal blepharitis, oily or greasy in seborrheic blepharitis, and fatty and possibly foamy in MGD blepharitis. Chalazia are most likely to occur in MGD blepharitis.

INITIATING DRUG THERAPY

The underlying cause of the blepharitis must be treated, particularly if it is due to seborrheic dermatitis or rosacea. Treatment for all types of blepharitis includes strict eyelid hygiene and warm compresses. The use of warm compresses with a clean washcloth can soften adherent encrustations; once-daily use of compresses is generally sufficient, although some patients report benefit from using warm compresses two to four times a day (AAO, 2008a). Patients with MGD blepharitis often benefit from eyelid massage following warm compress use to remove excess oil. Following warm compress use, eyelid cleaning is performed by having the patient rub the base of the eyelashes with a commercially available eyelid cleaner (EyeScrub, OCuSOFT) or a 1:1 mixture of baby shampoo (e.g., Johnson & Johnson) and water on a cotton swab, cotton ball, or gauze pad (Shields, 2000). Performing eyelid hygiene daily or several times a week often blunts the symptoms of chronic blepharitis. Patients should be advised that eyelid hygiene may be required for life because symptoms frequently recur if eyelid hygiene is discontinued.

Patients suspected of having a new case of seborrheic or MGD blepharitis should be referred to an eye care specialist for a workup. Patients with staphylococcal blepharitis need a topical antibiotic.

Goals of Drug Therapy

The goals of drug therapy are to eradicate the pathogens causing the blepharitis and to reduce the signs and symptoms of blepharitis.

Topical Ophthalmic Antimicrobials

Topical ophthalmic antimicrobials are used for the treatment of and prophylaxis against external bacterial infections (**Table 17.1**). They kill the offending pathogen and other susceptible organisms.

Selecting the Most Appropriate Agent

Topical antimicrobials that are effective against staphylococci are listed in **Table 17.2**.

First-Line Therapy

Topical antibiotics such as bacitracin ointment or erythromycin 0.5% ophthalmic ointment are used. Therapy selection is based on allergies and patient preference for ointment or solution (drops). Ointments tend to cause a greater degree of blurry vision than the solutions; if a patient prefers a solution,

a fluoroquinolone (besifloxacin, gatifloxacin, levofloxacin, or moxifloxacin) would be suitable. The AAO (2008a) recommends that the frequency and duration of treatment should be guided by the severity of the blepharitis and the response to treatment.

Second-Line Therapy

If the blepharitis fails to respond to the first-line therapy after several weeks or the condition appears to worsen at any time (including any vision loss or corneal involvement), the patient should be referred to an ophthalmologist for a complete evaluation.

PATIENT EDUCATION

Patients should be educated about the chronic nature of blepharitis. While chronic blepharitis can rarely be eliminated, improved eyelid hygiene, warm massages, and occasional antibiotic use (for staphylococcal blepharitis) can improve symptoms. Contact lens wearers should refrain from wearing contact lenses during an acute case of blepharitis, especially if antibiotic therapy has been initiated. Contact lens wearers with chronic blepharitis should consult with their eye care professional to determine whether contact lens use is safe.

EXTERNAL SURFACE OCULAR INFECTIONS: CONJUNCTIVITIS

Conjunctivitis is the most common cause of a red, painful eye in the United States (Horton, 2008). Conjunctivitis is an inflammation of the bulbar or palpebral conjunctiva, the clear membrane that covers the white part of the eye and lines the inner surfaces of the eyelids. Conjunctivitis is commonly referred to as *pink eye*.

CAUSES

The most common organisms seen in acute bacterial conjunctivitis are the gram-positive *Staphylococcus* and *Streptococcus* species and the gram-negative *Moraxella* and *Haemophilus* species; less common organisms include *Neisseria gonorrhoeae* and *Chlamydia trachomatis* (Trattler, 2009). In children, up to 50% of conjunctivitis cases are of bacterial origin. The most common pathogens in neonates are *N. gonorrhoeae* and *C. trachomatis*, while *S. aureus*, *Haemophilus influenzae*, *Streptococcus pneumoniae*, and *Pseudomonas aeruginosa* are the most commonly isolated organisms in children with bacterial conjunctivitis (Sethuraman & Kamat, 2009).

Viruses account for the majority of conjunctivitis cases in adults. The most common viral etiology is adenovirus infection (Horton, 2008); conjunctivitis due to an adenovirus is highly contagious. Other viruses associated with conjunctivitis include the herpes simplex virus, the varicella-zoster virus, and molluscum contagiosum (AAO, 2008b).

| TABLE 17.1 | Overview of Antimicrobial Ophthalmic Agents | | |

Generic (Trade) Name and Dosage	Selected Adverse Events	Contraindications	Special Considerations
Single-Agent Products			
sulfacetamide sodium 10% solution (Bleph-10) Dosing Solution: 1–2 drops every 2–3 h initially according to the severity of infection Dosing may be tapered as the condition responds. Usual duration of therapy is 7–10 d.	Local irritation, itching, stinging, burning, periorbital edema	Allergy to sulfa drugs Do not use in infants < age 2.	A significant percentage of *Staphylococcus* species are resistant to sulfa drugs. Do not use in patients with purulent exudates.
bacitracin 500 units/g ointment	Blurred vision, redness, burning, eyelid edema		Ointments may blur vision and retard corneal wound healing.
erythromycin 0.5% ointment	Redness, ocular irritation		Ointments may blur vision and retard corneal wound healing.
gentamicin 0.3% solution or ointment (Gentak) Dosing Solution: 1–2 drops in the affected eye(s) every 4 h Ointment: ½ inch to the affected eye 2 or 3 times a day	Ocular burning and irritation, nonspecific conjunctivitis, conjunctival epithelial defects, conjunctival hyperemia, bacterial and fungal corneal ulcers		In severe infections, dosage of the solution may be increased to as much as 2 drops every 2 h. Ointments may blur vision and retard corneal wound healing.
tobramycin 0.3% solution or ointment (Tobrex) Dosing Solution: 1–2 drops into the infected eye every 4 h Ointment: ½ inch every 8–12 h	Lid itching, lid swelling, conjunctival hyperemia, nonspecific conjunctivitis, bacterial and fungal corneal ulcers		Ointments may blur vision and retard corneal wound healing. For more severe infections, the initial dose may be increased to 2 drops every 30–60 min initially (solution) or 1 inch every 3–4 h (ointment).
besifloxacin 0.6% suspension (Besivance) Dosing: 1 drop in the affected eye(s) three times a day for 7 d	Conjunctival redness, blurred vision, eye irritation, eye pain, pruritus		
ciprofloxacin 0.3% solution or ointment (Ciloxan) Dosing Solution: 1–2 drops every 2 hours while awake for 2 d, then 1–2 drops every 4 hours while awake for 5 d Ointment: ½ inch three times a day for 2 days, then ½ inch twice a day for 5 d	Local burning and discomfort, white crystalline precipitate formation, conjunctival hyperemia, altered taste		Ointments may blur vision and retard corneal wound healing. This is the only ophthalmic fluoroquinolone available as an ointment.

TABLE 17.1	**Overview of Antimicrobial Ophthalmic Agents (*Continued*)**			
Generic (Trade) Name and Dosage	**Selected Adverse Events**	**Contraindications**	**Special Considerations**	
gatifloxacin 0.3% solution (Zymar, Zymaxid) Dosing Zymar: One drop in the affected eye every 2 h while awake for 2 d, then 1 drop in the affected eye up to 4 times daily while awake for 5 d Zymaxid: One drop in the affected eye every 2 h while awake for 1 d, then 1 drop in the affected eye up to 4 times daily while awake for 6 d	Conjunctival irritation, tearing, papillary conjunctivitis, eyelid edema, ocular itching, dry eye			
levofloxacin 0.5% solution (Quixin) Dosing: One drop in the affected eye every 2 h while awake for 2 d, then 1 drop in the affected eye up to 4 times daily while awake for 5 d	Temporarily decreased or blurred vision, eye irritation, itching, dry eye		A higher-dose levofloxacin product is available (Iquix) for use in bacterial corneal ulcer.	
moxifloxacin 0.5% solution (Vigamox) Dosing: One drop in the affected eye 3 times a day for 7 d	Decreased visual acuity, dry eye, ocular itching and discomfort, ocular hyperemia			
ofloxacin 0.3% solution (Ocuflox) Dosing: 1–2 drops in the affected eye every 2–4 h for 2 d, then 1–2 drops 4 times a day	Ocular burning and stinging, itching, redness, edema, blurred vision, photophobia		Rare reports of dizziness and nausea with use	
azithromycin 1% solution (AzaSite) Dosing: One drop in affected eye(s) twice daily for 2 d, then 1 drop once daily for 5 d	Eye irritation, dry eye, ocular discharge			
Combination Products				
polymyxin B sulfate, bacitracin ointment Dosing: Apply every 3–4 h for 7–10 days, depending upon the severity of infection.	Local irritation (burning, stinging, itching, redness), lid edema, tearing, rash		Ointments may blur vision and retard corneal wound healing.	
polymyxin B sulfate, trimethoprim sulfate solution (Polytrim) Dosing: 1 drop in the affected eye(s) every 3 h (maximum 6 doses a day) for 7–10 d	Local irritation (burning, stinging, itching, redness), lid edema, tearing, rash			
polymyxin B sulfate, gramicidin, neomycin solution (Neosporin) Dosing: 1–2 drops into the affected eye(s) every 4 hours for 7–10 d	Itching, swelling, conjunctival erythema, local irritation		Dosage of the solution may be increased to as much as 2 drops every hour for severe infections.	
polymyxin B sulfate, bacitracin zinc, and neomycin ointment Dosage: Apply every 3–4 h for 7–10 d, depending upon the severity of infection	Itching, swelling, conjunctival erythema, local irritation		Ointments may blur vision and retard corneal wound healing.	

TABLE 17.2	Recommended Order of Treatment for Blepharitis	
Order	**Agent**	**Comments**
First line	Erythromycin 0.5% ophthalmic ointment	Ointments tend to cause a greater degree of blurry vision than solutions.
	or	
	Bacitracin 500 units/g ointment	Erythromycin and bacitracin are available as inexpensive generic products.
	or	
	An ophthalmic fluoroquinolone solution (besifloxacin, gatifloxacin, levofloxacin, or moxifloxacin)	The remaining ophthalmic fluoroquinolones do not provide good staphylococcal coverage.
Second line	Referral to an ophthalmologist	

Allergic conjunctivitis is fairly common and is frequently mistaken for bacterial conjunctivitis. There are three types of allergic conjunctivitis: seasonal (hay fever) conjunctivitis, due to seasonal release of plant allergens; vernal conjunctivitis, which is of unknown origin but is thought to be due to seasonal airborne antigens; and atopic conjunctivitis, which occurs in people with atopic dermatitis or asthma.

Conjunctivitis can also be caused by mechanical or chemical irritants. A foreign body on the eye (typically a contact lens) can lead to giant papillary conjunctivitis.

PATHOPHYSIOLOGY

General mechanisms of infection are at work in bacterial and viral conjunctivitis. In bacterial conjunctivitis, the infecting organism is obtained via contact with an infected individual and transmitted to the eye by fingertips. Neonates with conjunctivitis may have become inoculated during childbirth by their infected mother. Transmission of viral conjunctivitis is usually through direct contact with infected persons, contact with contaminated medical instruments, or contaminated swimming pool water (Cronau, et al., 2010). In both bacterial and viral conjunctivitis, the infectious agent causes the inflammation of the conjunctiva. Mechanical and chemical irritants that cause conjunctivitis operate in the same manner.

In allergic conjunctivitis, symptoms are caused by the immunoglobulin (Ig)E-mediated release of mast cells in the conjunctiva (Bielory, 2008).

DIAGNOSTIC CRITERIA

In addition to the hallmark red or pink eye, classic patient complaints that occur in conjunctivitis include itching or burning sensations of the eyes, ocular discharge ("leaky eye"), eyelids that are stuck together in the morning, and a sensation that a foreign body is lodged in the eye. Patients may also report a feeling of fullness around the eye. Moderate to severe pain and light sensitivity are not typical features of a primary conjunctival inflammatory process (Cronau, et al., 2010). If these symptoms are present, or if the patient reports blurred vision that does not improve with blinking, the patient should be referred to an eye care professional, as a more serious ocular disease process (such as a corneal abrasion or keratoconjunctivitis) may be occurring. Neonates with signs of conjunctivitis should be referred to an eye care professional for immediate examination, as bacterial conjunctivitis due to *C. trachomatis* or *N. gonorrhoeae* can lead to serious eye damage.

Although many symptoms of conjunctivitis are nonspecific (tearing, irritation, stinging, burning, and conjunctival swelling), inspection and patient history can help determine the cause of illness. Patients who report that their eyelids were stuck together upon awakening most likely have bacterial conjunctivitis (Bielory, 2007); this sticking is caused by a purulent ocular discharge. Because gonococcal conjunctivitis produces a copiously purulent discharge, the cause of any copiously purulent conjunctivitis should be suspected as *N. gonorrhoeae* until Gram-stain testing proves otherwise. Bacterial conjunctivitis usually starts in one eye and can become bilateral a few days later.

Viral conjunctivitis produces a profuse watery discharge. Similar to bacterial conjunctivitis, viral conjunctivitis usually starts in one eye and can become bilateral within a few days. While unlikely, photophobia and a foreign-body sensation may be reported. Examination may reveal a tender preauricular node.

In allergic conjunctivitis, itching is the hallmark symptom; it can be mild to severe and may manifest as excessive blinking. A history of recurrent itching or a personal or family history of hay fever, asthma, atopic dermatitis, or allergic rhinitis is suggestive of allergic conjunctivitis. In general, a patient with conjunctivitis who does not report an itchy eye does not have allergic conjunctivitis. Unlike bacterial or viral conjunctivitis, allergic conjunctivitis usually presents with bilateral symptoms. An ocular discharge may or may not be present; if present, it may be watery or mucoid. Aggressive forms of allergic conjunctivitis are vernal conjunctivitis in children and atopic conjunctivitis in adults. Atopic and vernal conjunctivitis are associated with shield corneal ulcers and perilimbal accumulation of eosinophils (Horner-Trantas dots) (Bielory, 2007). Atopic conjunctivitis is associated with eyelid thickening and scarring, blepharitis, and corneal scarring (AAO, 2008b).

Giant papillary conjunctivitis occurs mainly in contact lens wearers. These patients report excessive itching, mucus production and discharge, and increasing intolerance to contact lens use. Upon examination, the upper tarsal conjunctiva may show inflammation and papillae greater than 0.3 mm (Donshik, et al., 2008).

INITIATING DRUG THERAPY

Before drug therapy is prescribed, both the patient and the practitioner should be aware that bacterial and viral conjunctivitis are highly contagious and are spread by contact. Therefore, good hand-washing and instrument-cleansing techniques are imperative. The etiology of illness should be determined, as treatment is different for bacterial, viral, and allergic conjunctivitis.

Goals of Drug Therapy

The goals of drug therapy are to eradicate the offending organism (for bacterial conjunctivitis) and to relieve symptoms (for all types of conjunctivitis). A patient with bacterial conjunctivitis should experience improvement in symptoms a few days after the start of antibiotic therapy; the organisms remain active (and contagious) for 24 to 48 hours after therapy begins. With viral conjunctivitis, the disease is contagious for at least 7 days after symptoms appear; it may be contagious for up to 14 days.

Antibiotics

Although bacterial conjunctivitis caused by typical pathogens (*Staphylococcus*, *Streptococcus*, *Pneumococcus*, *Moraxella*, and *Haemophilus* species) is usually self-limiting, antibiotic therapy is justified because it can shorten the course of the disease, which reduces person-to-person spread, and lowers the risk of sight-threatening complications. The choice of antibiotic is usually empirical. Five to 7 days of therapy with agents such as erythromycin ointment or bacitracin-polymyxin B ointment or solution is usually effective. While well tolerated, sulfacetamide has weak to moderate activity against many gram-positive and gram-negative organisms. The aminoglycosides have good gram-negative coverage but incomplete coverage of *Streptococcus* and *Staphylococcus* species and a relatively high incidence of corneal toxicity. The fluoroquinolones also have good gram-negative coverage; the older fluoroquinolones (ciprofloxacin, norfloxacin, and ofloxacin) have poor coverage of *Streptococcus* species, while the newer fluoroquinolones (besifloxacin, gatifloxacin, levofloxacin, and moxifloxacin) offer improved gram-positive coverage.

Because gonococcal infection is serious, immediate treatment of conjunctivitis due to *N. gonorrhoeae* with a 1-g intramuscular (IM) injection of ceftriaxone (Rocephin) or 400 mg of oral cefixime (Suprax) is recommended for adults and children who weigh at least 45 kg. For cephalosporin-allergic patients, alternatives include single doses of oral azithromycin 2 g or IM spectinomycin 2 g. Children who weigh less than 45 kg should receive a single 125-mg IM injection of ceftriaxone, while 25 to 50 mg/kg of ceftriaxone intravenous or IM (not to exceed 125 mg) is the appropriate dose for neonates.

Topical antibiotic therapy is not necessary but is often initiated to prevent secondary infection (AAO, 2008b).

As *C. trachomatis* is now the most common cause of conjunctivitis in neonates in the United States, the long-time standard prophylactic agent for neonates, topical 1% silver nitrate solution, is no longer recommended or commercially available in America. Topical treatment of neonatal chlamydial conjunctivitis is ineffective and unnecessary (American Academy of Pediatrics, 2009). In adults and children at least 8 years old, *C. trachomatis* infection is treated with a single 1-g dose of azithromycin or 7 days of therapy with doxycycline 100 mg twice daily. Children who weigh at least 45 kg but are less than 8 years old should receive the single dose of azithromycin 1 g. Neonates and children who weigh less than 45 kg should receive 50 mg/kg/day of erythromycin base or erythromycin ethylsuccinate, divided into four doses a day for 10 to 14 days (AAO, 2008b). Identification of either *Chlamydia* or *N. gonorrhoeae* conjunctivitis requires that the patient's sexual partner also be treated.

Antihistamines

The ophthalmic antihistamine emedastine prevents the histamine response in blood vessels by preventing histamine from binding with its receptor site and is useful in reducing the symptoms of allergic conjunctivitis. Ocular adverse events include transient stinging or burning upon instillation, dry eyes, red eyes, and blurred vision. Oral antihistamines can also help to relieve symptoms in many patients. (See **Table 17.3**.)

Mast Cell Stabilizers

The mast cell stabilizers (bepotastine, cromolyn, lodoxamide, nedocromil, and pemirolast) inhibit hypersensitivity reactions and prevent the increase in cutaneous vascular permeability that accompanies allergic reactions. These agents may be helpful for patients with allergic conjunctivitis. Ocular adverse events include transient burning, stinging or discomfort, pruritus, blurred vision, dry eyes, taste alteration, and foreign body sensation. (See **Table 17.3**.)

Antihistamine/Mast Cell Stabilizer

Several products (azelastine, epinastine, ketotifen, and olopatadine) have the combined properties of an antihistamine and a mast cell stabilizer, providing immediate relief of itching and long-term suppression of histamine release. Ketotifen is available without a prescription. These agents are given two or three times a day and have a side effect profile similar to the antihistamines and mast cell stabilizers. (See **Table 17.3**.)

Nonsteroidal Anti-Inflammatory Ophthalmic Drugs

The ophthalmic nonsteroidal anti-inflammatory (NSAID) ketorolac may be useful for treating the itch associated with allergic conjunctivitis. The NSAIDs inhibit the biosynthesis of prostaglandin by decreasing the activity of the enzyme cyclooxygenase. Ketorolac is administered 1 drop four times a day into the affected eye. It should be used with caution in patients with aspirin sensitivities and patients who have bleeding

TABLE 17.3 **Overview of Antiallergy Ophthalmic Agents**

Generic (Trade) Name and Dosage	Selected Adverse Events	Contraindications	Special Considerations
Antihistamines			
emedastine 0.05% solution (Emadine) Dosing: 1 drop in the affected eye up to 4 times a day	Blurred vision, burning and stinging, dry eyes, foreign body sensation, hyperemia, itching		Labeling: Wait 10 min following administration before inserting contact lenses.
Mast Cell Stabilizers			
bepotastine 1.5% solution (Bepreve) Dosing: 1 drop into the affected eye(s) twice daily	Mild taste following instillation, eye irritation		Labeling: Refrain from contact lens use while exhibiting signs and symptoms of allergic conjunctivitis. Labeling: Wait 10 min following administration before inserting contact lenses.
cromolyn 4% solution (Crolom) Dosing: 1–2 drops in each eye 4–6 times a day at regular intervals	Burning and stinging, conjunctival injection, watery eyes, itching, dry eye, styes		Labeling: Refrain from contact lens use while under treatment.
lodoxamide 0.1% solution (Alomide) Dosing: 1–2 drops in each eye 4 times a day	Burning and stinging, ocular itching, blurred vision, dry eye, tearing, hyperemia, foreign body sensation		Labeling: Refrain from contact lens use while under treatment.
nedocromil 2% solution (Alocril) Dosing: 1–2 drops in each eye twice a day	Ocular burning and stinging, unpleasant taste, redness, photophobia		Labeling: Refrain from contact lens use while exhibiting the signs and symptoms of allergic conjunctivitis.
pemirolast 0.1% solution (Alamast) Dosing: 1–2 drops in each affected eye 4 times daily	Burning, dry eye, foreign body sensation, ocular discomfort		Pemirolast contains lauralkonium chloride, not benzalkonium chloride. Labeling: Wait 10 min following administration before inserting contact lenses.
Antihistamine/Mast Cell Stabilizer			
azelastine 0.05% solution (Optivar) Dosing: One drop into each affected eye twice daily	Ocular burning and stinging, headache, bitter taste, eye pain, blurred vision		Labeling: Wait 10 min following administration before inserting contact lenses.
epinastine 0.05% solution (Elestat) Dosing: One drop in each eye twice a day	Burning sensation, folliculosis (hair follicle inflammation), hyperemia, itching		Labeling: Wait 10 min following administration before inserting contact lenses.
ketotifen 0.025% solution (Zaditor, Claritin Eye, Zyrtec Itchy Eye) Dosing: 1 drop in the affected eye(s) every 8–12 h	Conjunctival injection, burning and stinging, conjunctivitis, dry eye, itching, photophobia		Labeling: Wait 10 min following administration before inserting contact lenses.
olopatadine 0.1% (Patanol) or 0.2% (Pataday) solution Dosing 0.1%: 1–2 drops in each affected eye twice daily 0.2%: 1 drop in the affected eye(s) once daily	Ocular burning and stinging, dry eye, foreign body sensation, hyperemia, lid edema, itching		Labeling: Wait 10 min following administration before inserting contact lenses.

TABLE 17.3   Overview of Antiallergy Ophthalmic Agents (*Continued*)

Generic (Trade) Name and Dosage	Selected Adverse Events	Contraindications	Special Considerations
Nonsteroidal Anti-Inflammatory Drugs			
ketorolac 0.5% solution (Acular) Dosing: 1 drop 4 times a day	Stinging and burning, corneal edema, iritis, ocular irritation or inflammation		Use with caution in patients with aspirin sensitivities and patients with bleeding disorders or those receiving anticoagulant therapy. Labeling: Do not administer while wearing contact lenses.
Decongestants			
naphazoline 0.012% or 0.03% solutions (Clear Eyes, Naphcon), and 0.1% solution (AK-Con) Dosing: 1–2 drops in the affected eye(s) every 3–4 h, up to 4 times a day	Stinging, blurred vision, mydriasis, redness, punctate keratitis, increased IOP	Narrow-angle glaucoma Narrow-angle without glaucoma	Use should be limited to 72 h. Contains benzalkonium chloride; use with contact lenses not addressed in labeling
oxymetazoline 0.025% solution (Visine L.R.) Dosing: 1–2 drops in the affected eye(s) every 6 h	Stinging, blurred vision, mydriasis, redness, punctate keratitis, increased IOP	Narrow-angle glaucoma Narrow-angle without glaucoma	Use should be limited to 72 h. Contains benzalkonium chloride; use with contact lenses not addressed in labeling
phenylephrine 0.12% solution (Refresh Redness Relief) Dosing: 1–2 drops up to 4 times a day as needed	Stinging, blurred vision, mydriasis, redness, punctate keratitis, increased IOP	Narrow-angle glaucoma Narrow-angle without glaucoma	May cause rebound miosis and decreased mydriatic response in older persons Use should be limited to 72 h. Contains benzalkonium chloride; use with contact lenses not addressed in labeling 2.5% and 10% solutions are available for pupil dilation for diagnostic procedures.
tetrahydrozoline 0.05% solution (Visine, Murine Plus, Optigene 3, Opti-Clear) Dosing: 1–2 drops up to 4 times a day	Stinging, blurred vision, mydriasis, redness, punctate keratitis, increased IOP	Narrow-angle glaucoma Narrow-angle without glaucoma	Use should be limited to 72 h. Contains benzalkonium chloride; use with contact lenses not addressed in labeling
Topical Corticosteroids			
fluorometholone 0.1% ointment or suspension or 0.25% suspension Dosing Ointment: ½ inch ribbon one to three times daily; during initial 24–48 h, dosing may be increased to every 4 h Suspension: 1 drop two to four times daily; during initial 24–48 h, dosing may be increased to every 4 h	IOP elevation, glaucoma, posterior subcapsular cataract formation, delayed wound healing	Dendritic keratitis Vaccinia and varicella Fungal disease Viral disease of the cornea and conjunctiva Mycobacterial eye infection	
prednisolone 0.12% or 1% suspension (Pred Mild, Omnipred, Pred Forte) or 1% solution Dosing Solution: 2 drops four times a day Suspension: 1–2 drops 2–4 times a day; dose may be increased during the initial 24–48 h	IOP elevation, cataract formation, delayed wound healing, secondary ocular infection, acute uveitis, globe perforation, stinging and burning, conjunctivitis	Dendritic keratitis Fungal disease Viral disease of the cornea and conjunctiva Mycobacterial eye infection Acute, purulent, untreated eye infections	Labeling: Wait 15 min following administration before inserting contact lenses.

(continued)

TABLE 17.3	Overview of Antiallergy Ophthalmic Agents (*Continued*)		
Generic (Trade) Name and Dosage	**Selected Adverse Events**	**Contraindications**	**Special Considerations**
dexamethasone 0.1% solution (AK-Dex, Decadron) or 0.1% suspension (Maxidex) or 0.05% ointment (Decadron) Dosing Solution: 1–2 drops every hour during the day and every 2 h at night initially, reduced to 1 drop every 4 h with favorable response Suspension: 1–2 drops <4–6 times a day in mild disease; hourly in severe disease Ointment: Apply a thin coating of ointment 3 or 4 times a day	IOP elevation, loss of visual acuity, cataract formation, secondary ocular infection, globe perforation, stinging and burning	Dendritic keratitis Fungal disease Viral disease of the cornea and conjunctiva Mycobacterial eye infection	Labeling: Wait 15 min following administration before inserting contact lenses.
loteprednol 0.2% or 0.5% suspension (Alrex, Lotemax) Dosing 0.2% solution: 1 drop in the affected eye(s) 4 times a day 0.5% solution: 1–2 drops in the affected eye(s) 4 times a day	IOP elevation, loss of visual acuity, cataract formation, secondary ocular infection, globe perforation, stinging and burning, dry eye, itching, photophobia	Dendritic keratitis Fungal disease Viral disease of the cornea and conjunctiva Mycobacterial eye infection	If needed, dosing of the 0.5% solution can be increased to 1 drop every hour during the first week of therapy. Labeling: Wait 10 min following administration before inserting contact lenses.

disorders or are receiving anticoagulant therapy because ophthalmic NSAIDs are absorbed systemically. Adverse events include transient stinging and burning, irritation and inflammation, corneal edema, and iritis. (See **Table 17.3**.)

Vasoconstrictors

Vasoconstrictor eye drops (naphazoline, oxymetazoline, phenylephrine, and tetrahydrozoline) may offer relief to patients with allergic conjunctivitis. With the exception of the higher-strength (0.1%) naphazoline solution, these agents are available without a prescription. Side effects include stinging, blurred vision, mydriasis, and increased redness; punctate keratitis and increased intraocular pressure (IOP) may also occur. These agents are contraindicated in patients with narrow-angle glaucoma or a narrow angle without glaucoma. Rebound congestion may occur with frequent or extended use of these agents; use should be limited to a maximum of 72 hours. (See **Table 17.3**.)

Topical Corticosteroids

Topical corticosteroids have been shown to reduce inflammation in allergic conjunctivitis. Low-dose corticosteroid therapy can be used at infrequent intervals for short-term periods (1 to 2 weeks) (AAO, 2008b). If a topical corticosteroid fails to improve inflammation or pain within 48 hours, therapy should be discontinued. Long-term use of topical corticosteroids is associated with severe side effects, including ocular hypertension, cataract formation, glaucoma, and infection (Calonge, 2001). (See **Table 17.3**.)

Selecting the Most Appropriate Agent

Treatment of bacterial conjunctivitis is aimed at eradicating the offending organism. Cultures are not indicated unless the infection does not resolve with first-line therapy (**Table 17.4** and **Figure 17-1**).

There is conflicting information about the use of soft contact lenses while taking ophthalmic medications that contain the preservative benzalkonium chloride. This preservative, which is in many of the ophthalmic antihistamines, mast cell stabilizers, NSAIDs, vasoconstrictors, and topical steroids reviewed in this section, may be absorbed by contact lenses. While no products identify contact lens use as an absolute contraindication to therapy, some (e.g., cromolyn, lodoxamide, and nedocromil) have warnings advising against the use of contact lenses during therapy; others advise patients to wait 10 to 15 minutes after administering the medication before reinserting contact lenses. (See **Table 17.3**.) Regardless of the etiology, contact lens wearers should refrain from wearing contact lenses during an acute case of conjunctivitis.

Bacterial Conjunctivitis

The treatment of bacterial conjunctivitis is aimed at the organisms *S. aureus*, *S. pneumoniae*, and *H. influenzae*. First-line treatments include 7 to 10 days of therapy with erythromycin ointment (two or three times a day) or polymyxin B–trimethoprim solution (1 drop every 3 to 4 hours). Therapy selection can be based on patient preference for ointment or solution. If bacterial conjunctivitis does not resolve with

TABLE 17.4   Recommended Order of Treatment for Conjunctivitis

Order	Agent	Comments
Bacterial Conjunctivitis (nongonococcal, nonchlamydial)		
First line	Erythromycin ointment *or* Bacitracin-polymyxin B ointment or solution	Ointments tend to cause a greater degree of blurry vision than solutions.
Second line	Ophthalmic fluoroquinolones (besifloxacin, gatifloxacin, levofloxacin, or moxifloxacin)	The remaining ophthalmic fluoroquinolones do not provide good staphylococcal coverage.
Seasonal (Hay Fever) Conjunctivitis		
First line	Emedastine	Minimization of exposure to the offending allergen, cool compresses, and artificial tears may also be helpful.
Second line	Addition of a brief course of low-potency topical corticosteroid to the first-line agent *or* For recurrent or persistent disease: a product with antihistamine/mast cell stabilizer properties	Use of the topical corticosteroids should not exceed 2 wk.
Third line	Ophthalmic ketorolac	
Vernal/Atopic Conjunctivitis		
First line	Emedastine or oral antihistamine or mast cell stabilizer *or*	Minimization of exposure to the offending allergen, cool compresses, and artificial tears may also be helpful.
Second line	For acute exacerbations: Addition of a brief course of low-potency topical corticosteroid to the first-line agent	
Viral Conjunctivitis		
First line	Topical antihistamines *or* Artificial tears *or* Cold compresses	There is no effective treatment for viral conjunctivitis; treatment is for symptom mitigation.
Second line	In severe cases: A low-potency topical corticosteroid	Use of the topical corticosteroids should not exceed 2 wk.
Giant Papillary Conjunctivitis		
Mild disease	One or more of the following: Replace contact lenses more frequently, decrease contact lens wearing time, increase the frequency of enzyme treatment, use preservative-free lens care systems, switch to disposable lenses, administer mast cell stabilizer, change the contact lens polymer	
Moderate or severe disease	Same as mild disease *and* Discontinuation of contact lens wear for several weeks or a brief course of topical corticosteroid treatment	

first-line therapy, the patient should be referred to an eye care professional so that cultures may be taken to rule out *C. trachomatis*. The ophthalmic fluoroquinolones with improved gram-positive organism coverage (besifloxacin, gatifloxacin, levofloxacin, or moxifloxacin) can be used as second-line therapy.

Gonococcal infection requires immediate treatment. Ceftriaxone or cefixime is recommended for adults and children who weigh at least 45 kg; alternatives include azithromycin and spectinomycin. Children who weigh less than 45 kg and neonates should receive a reduced dose of ceftriaxone. In adults and children at least 8 years old, *C. trachomatis* infection is treated with azithromycin or doxycycline. Azithromycin should be used in children who weigh at least 45 kg but are less than 8 years old, while neonates and children who weigh less than 45 kg should receive erythromycin base or erythromycin ethylsuccinate.

Seasonal (Hay Fever) Conjunctivitis

Steps should be taken to minimize exposure to the offending allergen. The ophthalmic antihistamine emedastine can be used as first-line therapy for mild seasonal conjunctivitis. If

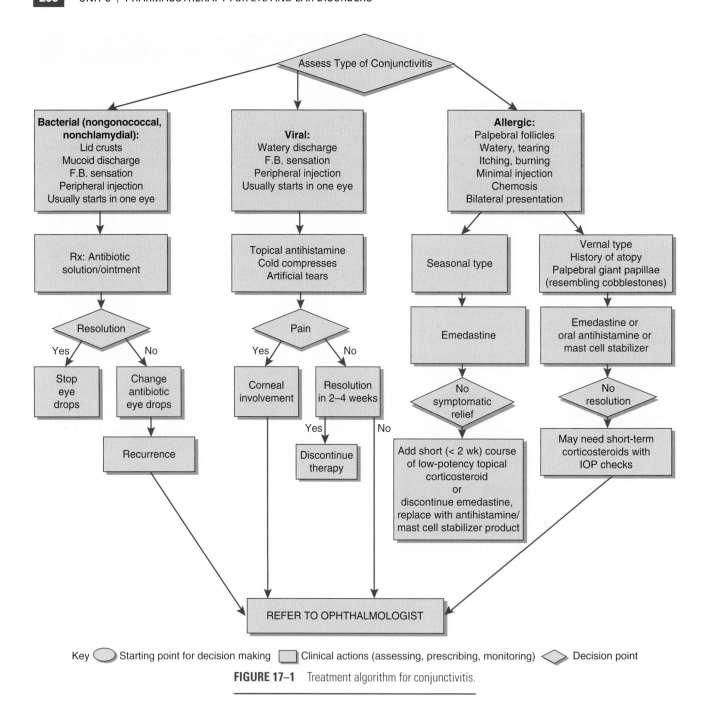

FIGURE 17–1   Treatment algorithm for conjunctivitis.

symptom control is inadequate, a brief course (1 to 2 weeks) of a low-potency topical corticosteroid can be added to the regimen. If the condition is persistent, a mast cell stabilizer or, preferably, an agent with antihistamine and mast cell stabilizer properties (azelastine, epinastine, ketotifen, or olopatadine) can be used. The ophthalmic NSAID ketorolac should be reserved for third-line therapy. Patients may also benefit from the use of cool compresses and artificial tears (which dilute allergens and help manage co-existing tear deficiency).

Vernal/Atopic Conjunctivitis

Similar to seasonal conjunctivitis, general treatment measures for vernal/atopic conjunctivitis include minimizing exposure to the offending allergen and use of cool compresses and artificial

tears. The topical antihistamine emedastine, oral antihistamines, or mast cell stabilizers (bepotastine, cromolyn, lodoxamide, nedocromil, or pemirolast) can be used as first-line agents for the treatment of vernal or atopic conjunctivitis. For patients with acute exacerbations, a topical corticosteroid can be added to the first-line agent for control of severe symptoms.

Viral Conjunctivitis

There is no effective treatment for viral conjunctivitis; patients should be informed of the risk of spreading the infection to the other eye (in unilateral infection) or to other people. Topical antihistamines, artificial tears, or cool compresses can be used to relieve symptoms. In severe cases of adenoviral keratoconjunctivitis with marked chemosis or lid swelling, epithelial sloughing, or membranous conjunctivitis, topical corticosteroids can be helpful in reducing symptoms and preventing scarring.

Giant Papillary Conjunctivitis

Treatment of giant papillary conjunctivitis centers around modifying the causative entity. Treatment of mild giant papillary conjunctivitis due to contact lens use can consist of one or more of the following: more frequent replacement of contact lenses, decrease in contact lens wearing time, increase in the frequency of enzyme treatment, use of preservative-free lens care systems, switching to disposable lenses, administration of a mast cell stabilizer, and change of the contact lens polymer. In moderate or severe giant papillary conjunctivitis due to contact lens use, discontinuation of contact lens use for several weeks or a brief course of topical corticosteroid therapy may be necessary.

MONITORING PATIENT RESPONSE

If symptoms begin to improve within 48 hours, no follow-up is needed. If there is no improvement, the patient should be referred to an eye care professional for evaluation.

PATIENT EDUCATION

It is important to instruct patients with bacterial or viral conjunctivitis to wash their hands carefully to prevent spreading infection. Organisms in bacterial conjunctivitis remain active (and contagious) for 24 to 48 hours after therapy begins, while patients with viral conjunctivitis can remain contagious for up to 14 days. Patients should be taught how to apply the medication in the inner aspect of the lower eyelid. The tip of the container should not touch the eyelashes, as it may contaminate the medication and result in therapy failure or reinfection. Patients should not share eye medications because this can spread the infection. To improve the effectiveness of an ophthalmic antibiotic, crusted eyelids should be gently cleansed before instilling medication. Regardless of the etiology, contact lens wearers should refrain from wearing contact lenses during an acute case of conjunctivitis.

DRY EYE SYNDROME: KERATOCONJUNCTIVITIS SICCA

Keratoconjunctivitis sicca, commonly referred to as dry eye syndrome (DES), is a common ophthalmologic abnormality involving bilateral disruption of tear film on the ocular surface. Estimates of the prevalence of dry eye in the United States range from 10% to 30% (Foster, et al., 2004). The prevalence of DES increases with age: 14.4% of Americans over age 48 have symptoms of DES, with the prevalence of DES doubling for patients ages 60 and above (Moss, et al., 2000). DES can occur intermittently or as a chronic condition that becomes a self-perpetuating syndrome. While the majority of patients with DES experience non-sight-threatening ocular irritation and intermittently blurred vision, patients with severe DES are at risk for severe vision loss due to ocular surface keratinization, corneal scarring, and corneal ulceration (AAO, 2008c).

CAUSES

DES is a multifactorial disease. It can be the result of decreased tear production, increased tear evaporation, or a combination of these factors (Lemp, 2007). In addition, decreased tear secretion and clearance initiate an inflammatory response on the ocular surface, and research suggests that this inflammation plays a role in the pathogenesis of DES (Pflugfelder, 2004).

Risk factors for DES include advanced age, female gender, and a history of LASIK surgery. Individuals with concomitant inflammatory conditions (allergies, asthma, or rheumatoid arthritis), infectious diseases (hepatitis C, human immunodeficiency virus/acquired immunodeficiency syndrome, or Epstein-Barr virus), or conditions such as Sjögren's syndrome, Parkinson's disease, or Bell's palsy are also at increased risk for DES. Symptoms caused by dry eye may be exacerbated by environmental factors such as wind, reduced humidity, cigarette smoke, and air conditioning. Systemic medications such as antihistamines, diuretics, anticholinergics, antidepressants, beta blockers, antipsychotics, and isotretinoin can also exacerbate dry eye symptoms (AAO, 2008c).

PATHOPHYSIOLOGY

Tears are composed of three layers: a mucus layer that coats the cornea, allowing the tear to adhere to the eye; a middle aqueous layer, which provides moisture and supplies oxygen and nutrients to the cornea; and an outer lipid film layer that seals the tear film on the eye and prevents evaporation. The outer lipid film layer is replenished by eyelid blinking, which relubricates and redistributes the lipid layer across the ocular surface. The ocular surface and tear-secreting glands function as an integrated unit to maintain the tear supply and to clear used tears. Aging, ocular surface diseases (such as herpes simplex virus keratitis) or surgeries that disrupt the trigeminal afferent sensory nerves, systemic inflammatory diseases, and systemic diseases and medications that disrupt the efferent cholinergic nerves that stimulate tear secretion can disrupt this functional unit and result in an unstable and poorly maintained tear film (Stern, et al., 1998; AAO, 2008c). Decreased tear secretion and clearance initiates an inflammatory response on the ocular surface, which is believed to play a role in DES.

DIAGNOSTIC CRITERIA

Family physicians should always refer patients reporting dry eye to an ophthalmologist if there is moderate to severe pain, vision loss, corneal infiltration or ulceration, or no response to therapy (AAO, 2008c). Making the diagnosis of DES, particularly the mild form, can be difficult because of the inconsistent correlation between reported symptoms and clinical signs, and the relatively poor sensitivity/specificity of existing diagnostic tests (AAO, 2008c). Because most dry eye conditions are chronic, repeat observation will allow a more accurate clinical diagnosis of DES.

Signs and symptoms of DES include a dry eye sensation, ocular irritation, redness, burning, and stinging, a foreign body or gritty sensation, blurred vision, contact lens intolerance, an increased frequency of blinking, and, paradoxically, increased tearing (AAO, 2008c; National Eye Institute [NEI], 2010). The inability to cry under emotional distress has also been reported among DES patients (NEI, 2010). DES symptoms tend to worsen in dry climates, in the wind, during air travel, with prolonged visual efforts, and toward the end of the day (AAO, 2008c).

A physical examination (including a test of visual acuity, an external examination, and slit-lamp biomicroscopy) should be performed to document the signs of DES and to rule out other causes of ocular irritation (AAO, 2008c). Additional tests can be used to lend some objectivity to the diagnosis. Tear break-up time testing or ocular surface dye staining (rose bengal, fluorescein, or lissamine green) can be useful for patients with mild symptoms. For patients with moderate to severe aqueous tear deficiency, the diagnosis can be made with one or more of the following tests (performed in this sequence): tear break-up time, ocular surface dye staining, or the Schirmer wetting test (AAO, 2008c).

INITIATING DRUG THERAPY

Before starting drug therapy, the patient should try nonpharmacologic interventions such as environmental control (increasing air humidity, avoiding drafts and cigarette smoke) and scheduling regular breaks during computer use and reading. Unfortunately, these interventions result in limited effectiveness and produce few lasting improvements in DES symptoms. Exogenous medical factors that can cause DES (e.g., blepharitis) should be addressed, and prescription medications that can exacerbate DES symptoms should be discontinued when possible.

If the nonpharmacologic interventions fail to eliminate DES symptoms, drug therapy is appropriate. **Table 17.5** gives information about the drugs used to treat DES.

Goals of Drug Therapy

The goals of drug therapy in DES are to relieve discomfort and prevent complications (vision loss, infection, and structural damage) (AAO, 2008c). Therapy should attempt to normalize tear volume and composition so that the eye tissues are properly lubricated, nourished, and protected, resulting in improved patient satisfaction and clinical outcomes (Wilson, 2003).

Artificial Tears and Lubricants

Artificial tears and lubricants can be used as palliative therapies to relieve DES symptoms. Designed to mimic the composition of natural tears, artificial tears contain lipids, water with dissolved salts and proteins, and mucin. Artificial tears and lubricants are over-the-counter products, available in a variety of formulations (solutions, gels, ointments). Ointments and gels may make the eyelids sticky and blur vision, and are often used only at bedtime.

For patients with mild DES, use of artificial tears four times daily plus a lubricating ointment at bedtime may be useful. As the severity of dry eye increases, administration of artificial tears can increase to hourly. Preservative-free preparations should be used if the patient applies tears more than four times a day (AAO, 2008c).

Cholinergic Agonists

The cholinergic agonists pilocarpine and cevimeline are indicated for the treatment of dry mouth in patients with Sjögren's syndrome. These agents bind to muscarinic receptors, stimulating secretion of the salivary and sweat glands and improving tear function. The main adverse event with these agents is excessive sweating, reported in 18% to 40% of patients. The use of these agents is contraindicated in patients with uncontrolled asthma and when miosis is undesirable (acute iritis, narrow-angle glaucoma).

Topical Cyclosporine

Cyclosporine ophthalmic emulsion has been reported to increase aqueous tear production and decrease ocular irritation symptoms in patients with DES. It prevents T cells from activating and releasing cytokines that incite the inflammatory component of dry eye. Side effects include ocular burning, conjunctival hyperemia, discharge, itching, and blurred vision. It is contraindicated in patients with active ocular infections.

Topical Corticosteroids

Topical corticosteroids have been shown to reduce inflammation in DES by reducing cytokine levels in the conjunctival epithelium. Low-dose corticosteroid therapy can be used at infrequent intervals for short-term (2 weeks) suppression of irritation secondary to inflammation (AAO, 2008c). Long-term use of topical corticosteroids is associated with severe side effects, including ocular hypertension, cataract formation, glaucoma, and infection (Calonge, 2001).

Selecting the Most Appropriate Agent

Agent selection is determined by the severity of DES and the underlying pathophysiology (**Table 17.6**).

First-Line Therapy

For patients with mild DES, the use of a tear substitute four times a day is appropriate. For moderate or severe DES, artificial tears can be used as often as hourly, although administration that frequently may be cumbersome. Preservative-free preparations should be used if the patient uses tears more than four times a day. A lubricating ointment applied at bedtime may also be useful.

A patient with DES and underlying Sjögren's syndrome may benefit from therapy with oral pilocarpine 5 mg four times daily or oral cevimeline 30 mg three times daily.

Second-Line Therapy

Patients with moderate to severe DES who fail to experience any improvement in symptoms with artificial tears may benefit from

TABLE 17.5	Overview of Dry Eye Syndrome Agents			
Generic (Trade) Name and Dosage	**Selected Adverse Events**	**Contraindications**	**Special Considerations**	
Artificial Tear Substitutes				
Solutions containing preservatives: 20/20, Akwa Tears, Blink Tears, Clear Eyes, Comfort Tears, Dry Eyes, GenTeal, Isopto Tears, Murine, Murocel, Nu-Tears, Optive, OptiZen, Puralube Tears, Refresh Tears, Soothe XP, Systane, Tears Plus, Tears Naturale, Visine Tears	Stinging, blurred vision		Should not be used more than 4–6 times per day; if use in excess of 4 times a day is necessary, use a preservative-free preparation	
Preservative-free solutions: AquaSite, Bion Tears, Blink Tears PF, Celluvisc, Refresh Classic, Refresh Plus, Tears Naturale Free, TheraTears, Viva-Drops	Stinging, blurred vision			
Ocular Lubricants				
Ointments containing preservatives: GenTeal PM, Stye, Tears Again, Lacri-Lube S.O.P.	Blurred vision			
Preservative-free ointments: Dry Eyes, Duratears Naturale, HypoTears, Tears Renewed, Lacri-Lube NP, LubriFresh PM, Refresh PM, Systane Nighttime, Tears Naturale PM	Blurred vision			
Cholinergic				
pilocarpine 5-mg tablets (Salagen) Dosing: 1 tablet 4 times a day	Excessive sweating, headache, urinary frequency, nausea, flushing, dyspepsia	Uncontrolled asthma Acute iritis Narrow-angle glaucoma	Dehydration may develop from excessive sweating. Visual disturbances may impair the ability to drive, especially at night.	
cevimeline 30-mg tablets (Evoxac) Dosing: 1 tablet 3 times a day	Excessive sweating, nausea, rhinitis, excessive salivation, asthenia	Uncontrolled asthma Acute iritis Narrow-angle glaucoma	Dehydration may develop from excessive sweating. Visual disturbances may impair the ability to drive, especially at night.	
Anti-inflammatory				
cyclosporine 0.05% emulsion (Restasis) Dosing: 1 drop in each eye twice a day, approximately 12 hours apart	Ocular burning, blurred vision, conjunctival hyperemia, discharge, eye pain, foreign body sensation, pruritus, stinging	Active ocular infection	Use the emulsion from a single-use vial immediately after opening; discard the remaining contents.	

therapy with 0.05% cyclosporine ophthalmic emulsion 1 drop in each eye twice a day. Due to the side effect profile, corticosteroid therapy is limited to second-line therapy for short-term (2 weeks) suppression of irritation secondary to inflammation.

Third-Line Therapy

Patients with severe DES that fails to respond to drug therapy are candidates for punctate occlusion or tarsorrhaphy.

TABLE 17.6	Recommended Order of Treatment for Dry Eye	
Order	**Agent**	**Comments**
First line	Mild DES: artificial tear substitute 4 times a day *or* Moderate to severe DES: preservative-free artificial tear substitute, administered up to hourly	If the patient has underlying Sjögren's syndrome, administer pilocarpine tablets 5 mg four times a day or cevimeline tablets 30 mg three times a day.
Second line	Cyclosporine 0.05% ophthalmic emulsion twice a day	Ophthalmic corticosteroid therapy may be useful for the short-term (2-wk) suppression of irritation secondary to inflammation.

MONITORING PATIENT RESPONSE

The frequency and extent of follow-up will depend upon the severity of DES and the therapeutic approach selected. Patients with mild DES can be seen once or twice per year for follow-up if symptoms are controlled by therapy. Patients with sterile corneal ulceration associated with DES require careful, sometime daily, monitoring (AAO, 2008c).

PATIENT EDUCATION

Patients with DES should be educated about the chronic nature of the disease and given specific instructions about their therapeutic regimens.

GLAUCOMA (PRIMARY OPEN-ANGLE GLAUCOMA)

Glaucoma is a group of eye diseases involving optic neuropathy characterized by irreversible damage to the optic nerve and retinal ganglion cells. Over time, this deterioration results in the loss of visual sensitivity and field, which frequently goes unnoticed until a significant amount of damage has occurred. Glaucoma is the leading cause of irreversible blindness in the world (Resnikoff, et al., 2004). There are numerous types of glaucoma, including primary open-angle glaucoma (POAG), acute closed-angle glaucoma, normal-tension glaucoma, and narrow-angle glaucoma. POAG accounts for up to 70% of glaucoma cases in the United States and afflicts 2.2 million Americans (Friedman, et al., 2004); as such, this section will specifically review POAG.

CAUSES

Several studies have shown that the prevalence of POAG increases with increasing IOP (Leske, et al., 2003; Gordon, et al., 2002). The median IOP in large populations is 15.5 ± 2.5 mm Hg. Previously, it was thought that increased IOP was the sole cause of POAG, but it is now recognized that IOP is one of several factors associated with the development of POAG, and an increased IOP is not required for the diagnosis of POAG.

Additional risk factors for the development of POAG include increasing age, black race (four times greater than whites), a family history of glaucoma, and a thin central cornea (AAO, 2005).

PATHOPHYSIOLOGY

The pathophysiology of glaucoma-induced vision loss is not well understood. Aqueous humor is produced by the ciliary body and secreted into the posterior chamber of the eye. A pressure gradient in the posterior chamber forces the aqueous humor between the iris and lens and through the pupil into the anterior chamber. Aqueous humor in the anterior chamber leaves the eye through two methods: filtration through the trabecular meshwork to Schlemm's canal (80% to 85%), or traversal of the anterior face of the iris and absorption into iris blood vessels (uveoscleral outflow). In POAG, the increase in IOP is a result of degenerative changes in the trabecular meshwork and Schlemm's canal that result in a decrease in the outflow of the aqueous humor (Abel & Sorensen, 2009).

DIAGNOSTIC CRITERIA

Symptoms of POAG do not manifest until substantial damage has already occurred. The diagnosis of any glaucoma should be made by an eye care professional. Any patients reporting visual field loss should be referred to an eye care professional for prompt evaluation.

During the physical examination, IOP is measured in each eye, preferably with a Goldmann-type applanation tonometer, before gonioscopy or dilation of the pupil (AAO, 2005). Unfortunately, the measurement of IOP is not an effective method for screening populations for glaucoma. At an IOP cutoff of 21 mm Hg, the sensitivity for the diagnosis of POAG by tonometry was 47.1% (Tielsch, et al., 1991), and half of all individuals with POAG are measured with an IOP of less than 22 mm Hg at a single screening (Leske, et al., 2003). As such, the AAO recommends, in addition to the measurement of IOP, that a physical examination include the following elements: patient history, test of pupil reactivity, slit-lamp biomicroscopy of the anterior segment, determination of central corneal thickness, gonioscopy, evaluation of the optic nerve head and retinal nerve fiber layer, documentation of the optic nerve head appearance, evaluation of the fundus, and evaluation of the visual field (AAO, 2005).

INITIATING DRUG THERAPY

The goals of therapy for POAG are to control IOP, stabilize the status of the optic nerve and retinal fiber layer, and to stabilize the visual field (AAO, 2005). Most cases of glaucoma can be controlled and vision loss prevented with early detection and treatment. Treatment of POAG entails decreasing aqueous humor production, increasing aqueous outflow, or a combination of both.

Over the past 15 years, glaucoma management has changed significantly, primarily due to the introduction of pharmaceutical agents that have shown clinical effectiveness (**Table 17.7**). These agents have been associated with a significant reduction in surgery rates among glaucoma patients (Fraser & Wormald, 2006).

Once a target IOP has been determined, treatment may include drug therapy, laser surgery, filtering surgery, or cyclodestructive surgery. Topical medication is, in most cases, indicated as first-line therapy. Several trials have clearly shown that reducing IOP by treatment with ocular hypotensive medication can prevent or reduce the risk of progression of glaucoma. Further, the more IOP is reduced, the risk of glaucomatous eye damage decreases.

TABLE 17.7   Overview of Glaucoma Agents

Generic (Trade) Name and Dosage	Selected Adverse Events	Contraindications	Special Considerations
Beta Blockers			
betaxolol 0.25% suspension or 0.5% solution (Betoptic S) Dosing: 1–2 drops in the affected eye(s) twice daily	Discomfort on instillation, tearing, allergic reactions, decreased corneal sensitivity, edema, bradycardia, hypotension, dizziness	Cardiogenic shock Second- or third-degree AV block Sinus bradycardia Overt cardiac failure	A cardioselective (beta-1) blocker, it has fewer effects on pulmonary and cardiovascular parameters.
carteolol 1% solution Dosing: 1 drop in the affected eye(s) twice daily	Transient eye irritation, burning, tearing, conjunctival hyperemia, edema, bradycardia, hypotension, arrhythmia, palpitations	Bronchial asthma or severe COPD Sinus bradycardia Second- or third-degree AV block Overt cardiac failure Cardiogenic shock	May be absorbed systemically; the same adverse reactions seen with oral beta blockers may occur May mask the symptoms of acute hypoglycemia or hyperthyroidism
levobunolol 0.25% or 0.5% solution (Betagan) Dosing: 1–2 drops in the affected eye(s) once daily (0.5%) or twice daily (0.25%).	Burning and stinging, blepharoconjunctivitis, urticaria, ataxia, bradycardia, arrhythmia, hypotension, syncope, heart block	Bronchial asthma or severe COPD Sinus bradycardia Second- or third-degree AV block Overt cardiac failure Cardiogenic shock	May be absorbed systemically; the same adverse reactions seen with oral beta blockers may occur May mask the symptoms of acute hypoglycemia or hyperthyroidism
metipranolol 0.3% solution (OptiPranolol) Dosing: 1 drop in the affected eye(s) twice a day	Transient local discomfort, conjunctivitis, eyelid dermatitis, blepharitis, blurred vision, headache, asthenia, angina, palpitation, bradycardia	Bronchial asthma or severe COPD Symptomatic sinus bradycardia Second- or third-degree AV block Overt cardiac failure Cardiogenic shock	May be absorbed systemically; the same adverse reactions seen with oral beta blockers may occur May mask the symptoms of acute hypoglycemia or hyperthyroidism
timolol 0.25% or 0.5% solution (Timoptic, Betimol, Istalol) or gel-forming solution (Timoptic-XE) Dosing: Solution: 1 drop in the affected eye(s) twice daily Gel-forming solution: 1 drop in the affected eye(s) once daily	Ocular irritation, decreased corneal sensitivity, visual disturbances, conjunctivitis, tearing, headache, dizziness, bradycardia, arrhythmia	Bronchial asthma or severe COPD Sinus bradycardia Second- or third-degree AV block Overt cardiac failure Cardiogenic shock	May be absorbed systemically; the same adverse reactions seen with oral beta blockers may occur May mask the symptoms of acute hypoglycemia or hyperthyroidism. Other ophthalmic medications should be administered 10 minutes before the gel-forming solution.
Carbonic Anhydrase Inhibitors			
dorzolamide 1% solution (Trusopt) Dosing: 1 drop in the affected eye(s) 3 times a day	Ocular burning and stinging, bitter taste, keratitis, ocular allergy, blurred vision, tearing, photophobia	Sulfa allergy	
brinzolamide 1% suspension (Azopt) Dosing: 1 drop in the affected eye(s) 3 times a day	Blurred vision, bitter taste, blepharitis, dermatitis, dry eye, headache, hyperemia ocular pain, pruritus	Sulfa allergy	
Prostaglandins			
latanoprost 0.005% solution (Xalatan) Dosing: 1 drop in the affected eye(s) once daily in the evening	Iris discoloration, blurred vision, burning and stinging, conjunctival hyperemia, itching, eyelash changes, eyelid skin darkening		Iris discoloration is irreversible. Requires refrigeration until dispensed

(continued)

TABLE 17.7	Overview of Glaucoma Agents (*Continued*)		
Generic (Trade) Name and Dosage	**Selected Adverse Events**	**Contraindications**	**Special Considerations**
travoprost 0.004% solution (Travatan Z) Dosing: 1 drop in the affected eye(s) once daily in the evening	Ocular hyperemia, decreased visual acuity, eye discomfort, foreign body sensation, eye pain, pruritus		Iris discoloration is irreversible. May interfere in pregnancy; should not be used during pregnancy or by those attempting to become pregnant
bimatoprost 0.03% solution (Lumigan) Dosing: 1 drop in the affected eye(s) once daily in the evening	Conjunctival hyperemia, growth of eyelashes, ocular pruritus, dry eye, iris discoloration, visual disturbance, eye pain, pigmentation of the periocular skin, foreign body sensation		Iris discoloration is irreversible; incidence less than with latanoprost.
Adrenergic Agonists			
brimonidine 0.1%, 0.15%, or 0.2% solution (Alphagan P) Dosing: 1 drop in the affected eye(s) 3 times a day, approximately 8 h apart	Ocular hyperemia, ocular pruritus, visual disturbance, somnolence, headache, fatigue, drowsiness, dry mouth	Patients receiving MAO inhibitors	Not recommended in children < age 2
apraclonidine 0.5% solution (Iopidine) Dosing: 1–2 drops in the affected eye(s) 3 times a day	Hyperemia, tearing, pruritus, lid edema, dry mouth, foreign body sensation, eyelid retraction	Hypersensitivity to clonidine Patients receiving MAO inhibitors	For short-term use only A 1% solution is available for prevention of postsurgical elevations in IOP.
Cholinergic Blocking Agents			
pilocarpine 1%, 2%, 3%, 4%, or 6% solution (Isopto Carpine) or 4% gel (Pilopine HS) Dosing: Solution: 1–2 drops 3 or 4 times a day Gel: ½-inch ribbon in the lower conjunctival sac of affected eye(s) once daily at bedtime	Stinging and burning, tearing, ciliary spasm, blurred vision, brow ache, hypertension, tachycardia, bronchospasm, salivation	Acute iritis or other conditions where papillary constriction is undesirable	A weekly pilocarpine ocular insert (Ocusert) is available.
Combination Products			
Brimonidine and timolol 0.2%–0.5% solution (Combigan) Dosing: 1 drop in the affected eye(s) every 12 h	See individual components.	See individual components.	Combined effect results in greater IOP lowering than either agent alone, but not as great as brimonidine 3 times a day and timolol 2 times a day administered concomitantly.
dorzolamide and timolol 2%–0.5% solution (Cosopt) Dosing: 1 drop into the affected eye(s) 2 times a day	See individual components.	See individual components.	Combined effect results in greater IOP lowering than either agent alone, but not as great as dorzolamide 3 times a day and timolol 2 times a day administered concomitantly.

AV, atrioventricular mode; COPD, chronic obstructive pulmonary disease; MAO, monoamine oxidase.

Goals of Drug Therapy

The goals of drug therapy for POAG are to reduce IOP to a target level and to prevent or slow the progression of vision loss. In patients with POAG, the initial IOP target should be at least 20% lower than baseline. Additional IOP lowering may be justified, based upon the severity of the existing optic nerve damage, the height of the measured IOP and the speed at which the damage occurred, and the presence of other risk factors such as family history and race (AAO, 2005). Visual fields and optic nerve status should be monitored for signs of change; if progression is detected, the IOP target should be lowered.

Beta Blockers

Beta blockers are the benchmark against which other IOP-lowering medications are measured. Beta blockers reduce adenylyl cyclase activity, which in turn reduces the production of aqueous humor in the ciliary body. Beta blockers lower IOP an average of 20% to 30%. There are five ophthalmic beta blockers available in the United States: timolol, levobunolol, carteolol, and metipranolol are nonselective beta blockers, while betaxolol is a beta$_1$-selective agent. Although nonselective beta blockers may be more efficacious in lowering IOP, selective beta blockers appear to be better tolerated systemically, particularly in patients with chronic obstructive pulmonary disease.

The ophthalmic beta blockers are typically applied twice daily. Timolol is available in a solution that forms a gel upon application, allowing once-daily dosing. Side effects include stinging, burning, dry eye, and blurred vision. Topical beta blockers can be absorbed systemically and may cause bradycardia, reduced blood pressure, aggravation of congestive heart failure, heart block, bronchospasm in asthma patients, and central nervous system (CNS) side effects such as hallucinations and depression. Betaxolol is less likely to cause these systemic side effects, but a risk still exists. All of the ophthalmic beta blockers are contraindicated in patients with sinus bradycardia, second- or third-degree atrioventricular node block, overt cardiac failure, and cardiogenic shock, and all except betaxolol are contraindicated in patients with bronchial asthma or severe chronic obstructive pulmonary disease.

Prostaglandins

The prostaglandin F$_{2\alpha}$ analogs bimatoprost, latanoprost, and travoprost reduce IOP by improving the uveoscleral outflow of aqueous humor. Given once a day, the prostaglandin F$_{2\alpha}$ analogs reduce IOP by 25% to 35%. Studies of bimatoprost, latanoprost, and travoprost found no statistical difference in IOP lowering between agents (Yildirim, et al., 2008; Parrish, et al., 2003).

These agents are more effective when given at bedtime rather than in the morning. Further, dosing in excess of once a day may decrease the IOP-lowering effect. Latanoprost requires refrigeration until dispensed; latanoprost and travoprost should be discarded within 6 weeks of the time the package is opened. Side effects of the prostaglandins include ocular hyperemia, blurred vision, pruritus, dry eye, lengthening and thickening of the eyelashes, and conjunctival hyperemia. These agents are also associated with irreversible iris discoloration, most often affecting patients with mixed-color irises. Iris discoloration is reported by 7% to 12% of latanoprost users, with discoloration starting between 18 and 26 weeks after commencement of therapy. Compared to latanoprost, the incidence of iris discoloration is lower for bimatoprost and travoprost. In addition, darkening of the eyelid skin can occur with these agents.

Carbonic Anhydrase Inhibitors

The topical carbonic anhydrase inhibitors (CAIs) brinzolamide and dorzolamide work through the reversible and competitive binding of carbonic anhydrase. Carbonic anhydrase acts as a catalyst for the reversible hydration of carbonic acid, which plays a role in fluid transport in various cell systems. By decreasing bicarbonate formation, the movement of bicarbonate, sodium, and fluid into the posterior chamber of the eye declines and less aqueous fluid is generated, reducing IOP (Abel & Sorensen, 2009). While the topical CAIs reduce IOP to a lesser extent (15% to 26%) than beta blockers, prostaglandins, or systemic CAIs, they are rarely associated with systemic side effects.

The topical CAIs are given three times a day. Side effects include ocular burning and stinging, bitter taste, blurred vision, itching, tearing, and keratitis. The topical CAIs are contraindicated in patients with hypersensitivity to sulfonamides, and are not recommended for use in patients with severe renal impairment, respiratory acidosis, and electrolyte disorders.

The systemic CAIs (acetazolamide, methazolamide, and dichlorphenamide) are the most potent agents for reducing IOP, producing a 25% to 40% decrease in IOP. However, these agents produce severe side effects such as paresthesias, gastrointestinal disturbances (anorexia, nausea, and weight loss), metallic taste, CNS effects (lethargy, malaise, and depression), electrolyte disturbances, and renal calculi, which limit their use in the elderly population (Kanner & Tsai, 2006).

Adrenergic Agonists

The adrenergic agonists apraclonidine and brimonidine activate the presynaptic alpha-2 receptors, inhibiting the release of norepinephrine. As less norepinephrine is available for activation of postsynaptic beta receptors on the ciliary epithelium, the formation of aqueous humor is reduced.

Apraclonidine and brimonidine reduce IOP by 18% to 27%. Brimonidine is a highly selective alpha-2 agonist, causing little or no alpha-1 activity. In addition to decreasing aqueous humor, it increases uveoscleral outflow. Side effects include dry mouth, fatigue, ocular hyperemia, somnolence, and headache. Apraclonidine is a relatively selective alpha-2 agonist; it is associated with some alpha-1 activity, which can lead to mydriasis, conjunctival bleeding, and eyelid retraction. Apraclonidine is primarily indicated for short-term adjunctive therapy, as the efficacy of apraclonidine diminishes over time; the benefit for most patients lasts less than 1 to 2 months. Both agents are contraindicated in patients taking monoamine oxidase inhibitors. In addition, brimonidine has been associated with respiratory and cardiac depression in infants, and should be used with caution in children under age 2.

The nonselective ophthalmic adrenergic agonists epinephrine and dipivefrin (epinephrine prodrug) are no longer available in the United States. These agents provided lackluster IOP control and were associated with adverse reactions such as stinging and tearing, brow ache, and the formation of black conjunctival spots and conjunctival deposits.

Cholinergic Blocking Agents

Pilocarpine is a direct-acting cholinergic blocking agent. Pilocarpine stimulates the parasympathetic muscarinic receptor site to increase aqueous outflow through the trabecular meshwork. While effective in lowering IOP by 20% to 30%, pilocarpine usually needs to be given four times a day. Side effects include eye pain, brow ache, blurred vision, and accommodative spasms. It can also provoke miotic responses such as papillary constriction, which can decrease night vision. The intense dosing regimen and the side effect profile make adherence difficult. A once-daily pilocarpine gel may be helpful when therapy adherence is an issue.

Combination Products

Combination products simplify administration and can promote adherence to therapy. Solutions of timolol 0.5% in combination with dorzolamide 2% or brimonidine 0.2% are available; the combined effect results in additional IOP reduction compared to either agent alone, but the result is less than each agent administered separately.

Selecting the Most Appropriate Agent

The AAO does not recommend a specific agent as first-line therapy. When the first-line agent drug fails to reduce IOP, the AAO recommends that it be discontinued in favor of another therapy before the original agent is supplanted by other medications. If a first-line agent lowers IOP but fails to lower IOP to the target level, combination therapy or discontinuation of therapy in favor of another agent are appropriate options. When selecting the first-line therapy for glaucoma, factors such as efficacy, side effects, cost, and dosing frequency should all be considered. **Table 17.8** lists the recommended order of treatment for these agents.

First-Line Therapy

The prostaglandins have been recommended as first-line therapy for POAG because they possess the best balance between efficacy, safety, and ease of dosing regimen (Schwartz & Budenz, 2004).

Second-Line Therapy

If the prostaglandin fails to decrease IOP to a significant extent, the patient should be switched to a different class of medicine. Beta blockers are recommended because of their efficacy, tolerability, and ease of dosing (Schwartz & Budenz, 2004). If the IOP decreases with a prostaglandin but fails to reach the target IOP, a beta blocker should be added.

Third-Line Therapy

If a patient fails to reach the target IOP with the first-line and second-line therapies, a topical CAI (usually the fixed combination of timolol and dorzolamide to keep the dosing regimen simple) can be added. If this fails, dorzolamide should be discontinued in favor of brimonidine (Schwartz & Budenz, 2004).

TABLE 17.8	Recommended Order of Treatment for Glaucoma	
Order	**Agent**	**Comments**
First line	Prostaglandin ophthalmic solution (bimatoprost, latanoprost, or travoprost)	An ophthalmic beta blocker may be substituted if the patient cannot afford the prostaglandins.
Second line	Substitution of an ophthalmic beta blocker (if failure to decrease IOP to a significant extent) *or* Addition of an ophthalmic beta blocker (if IOP is significantly decreased but not to goal)	
Third line	Addition of an ophthalmic carbonic anhydrase inhibitor *or* Addition of brimonidine	Dorzolamide is available in a combination product with timolol.

MONITORING PATIENT RESPONSE

Patients with POAG should receive follow-up evaluations and care from their eye care professional to determine the effectiveness of therapy. In addition to a recent history, a physical examination including a slit-lamp biomicroscopy and tests of visual acuity and IOP in each eye should be performed (AAO, 2005). The practitioner must distinguish between the impact of a prescribed agent on IOP and ordinary background fluctuations of IOP.

PATIENT EDUCATION

Patients should wash their hands before administering glaucoma medications. Patients should be taught how to apply the medication in the inner aspect of the lower eyelid. The tip of the container should not touch the eyelashes or any part of the eye because this may contaminate the medication. Contact lenses should be removed prior to administration, and patients should separate administration of different glaucoma medications by at least 10 minutes.

Case Study

V. S., age 7, presents with a feeling that there is sand in his eye. He had a cold a week ago and woke up this morning with his left eye crusted with yellowish drainage. On physical examination, he has injected conjunctiva on the left side, no adenopathy, and no vision changes. His vision is 20/20. Fluorescein staining reveals no abrasion. He is allergic to sulfa.

DIAGNOSIS: CONJUNCTIVITIS

1. List specific goals of treatment for V. S.
2. What drug therapy would you prescribe? Why?
3. What are the parameters for monitoring the success of the therapy?
4. List one or two adverse reactions for the selected agent that would cause you to change therapy.
5. What would be the choice for second-line therapy?
6. Describe one or two drug–drug or drug–food interactions for the selected agent.
7. Discuss the education you would give to the parents regarding drug therapy.
8. What over-the-counter or alternative medications would be appropriate for V. S.?
9. What dietary and lifestyle changes should be recommended for V. S.?

BIBLIOGRAPHY

Starred references are cited in the text.

*Abel, S. R., & Sorensen, S. J. (2009). Eye disorders. In M. A. Koda-Kimble, et al. (Eds.), *Applied therapeutics: The clinical use of drugs* (9th ed., pp. 51–61). Philadelphia: Wolters Kluwer.

Agarwal, R., Gupta, S. K., Agarwal, P., et al. (2009). Current concepts in the pathophysiology of glaucoma. *Indian Journal of Ophthalmology, 57*, 257–266.

*American Academy of Ophthalmology Cornea/External Disease Panel, Preferred Practice Guidelines Committee. (2005). *Primary open-angle glaucoma.* San Francisco: AAO.

*American Academy of Ophthalmology Cornea/External Disease Panel, Preferred Practice Guidelines Committee. (2008a). *Blepharitis.* San Francisco: AAO.

*American Academy of Ophthalmology Cornea/External Disease Panel, Preferred Practice Guidelines Committee. (2008b). *Conjunctivitis.* San Francisco: AAO.

*American Academy of Ophthalmology Cornea/External Disease Panel, Preferred Practice Guidelines Committee. (2008c). *Dry eye syndrome.* San Francisco: AAO.

*American Academy of Pediatrics. (2009). Chlamydia trachomatis. In L. K. Pickering (Ed.), *Red book: Report of the Committee on Infectious Diseases* (28th ed., pp. 255–259). Elk Grove Village, IL: American Academy of Pediatrics.

*Bielory, L. (2007). Differential diagnoses of conjunctivitis for clinical allergist-immunologists. *Annals of Allergy, Asthma, and Immunology, 98*, 105–115.

*Bielory, L. (2008). Ocular allergy overview. *Immunology and Allergy Clinics of North America, 28*, 1–23.

*Calonge, M. (2001). The treatment of dry eye. *Survey of Ophthalmology, 45*(Suppl. 2), S227–S239.

*Cronau, H., Kankanala, R. R., & Mauger, T. (2010). Diagnosis and management of red eye in primary care. *American Family Physician, 81*, 137–144.

Dalzell, M. D. (2002). Glaucoma: Prevalence, utilization, and economic implications. *Pharmacy and Therapeutics, 27*(Suppl. 11), 10–15.

Dalzell, M. D. (2003). Dry eye: Prevalence, utilization, and economic implications. *Managed Care, 12*(Suppl. 12), 9–13.

*Donshik, P. C., Ehlers, W. H., & Ballow, M. (2008). Giant papillary conjunctivitis. *Immunology and Allergy Clinics of North America, 28*, 83–103.

*Fraser, S. G., & Wormald, R. L. P. (2006). Hospital episode statistics and changing trends in glaucoma surgery. *Eye, 22*, 3–7.

*Friedman, D. S., Wolfs, R. C., O'Colmain, B. J., et al. (2004). Prevalence of open-angle glaucoma among adults in the United States. *Archives of Ophthalmology, 122*, 532–538.

*Foster, C. S., Yuskel, E., Anzaar, F., & Ekong, A. S. (2004). Dry eye syndrome. E-medicine: http://emedicine.medscape.com/article/1210417-overview. Accessed September 5, 2010.

*Gordon, M. O., Beiser, J. A., Brandt, J. D., et al. (2002). The Ocular Hypertension Treatment Study: Baseline factors that predict the onset of primary open-angle glaucoma. *Archives of Ophthalmology, 120*, 714–720.

*Horton, J. C. (2008). Disorders of the eye. In A. S. Fauci (Ed.), *Harrison's principles of internal medicine* (17th ed.). New York: McGraw-Hill.

*Kanner, E., & Tsai, J. C. (2006). Glaucoma medications: Use and safety in the elderly population. *Drugs and Aging, 23*, 321–332.

Lemp, M. A. (2003). Contact lenses and associated anterior segment disorders: Dry eye, blepharitis, and allergy. *Ophthalmology Clinics of North America, 16*(3), 463–469.

*Lemp, M. A. (2007). The definition and classification of dry eye disease: Report of the Definition and Classification Subcommittee of the International Dry Eye Workshop. *Ocular Surface, 5*, 77.

*Leske, M. C., Heijl, A., Hussein, M., et al. (2003). Factors for glaucoma progression and the effect of treatment: The Early Manifest Glaucoma Trial. *Archives of Ophthalmology, 121*, 48–56.

McCulley, J. P., Uchiyama, E., Aranowicz, J. D., & Butovich, I. A. (2006). Impact of evaporation on aqueous tear loss. *Transactions of the American Ophthalmological Society, 104*, 121–128.

*Moss, S. E., Klein, R., & Klein, B. E. (2000). Prevalence and risk factors for dry eye syndrome. *Archives of Ophthalmology, 118*, 1264–1268.

*National Eye Institute. (2010). Facts about dry eye. Bethesda, MD: Author.

*Parrish, R. K., Palmberg, P., Sheu, W. P., et al. (2003). A comparison of latanoprost, bimatoprost, and travoprost in patients with open-angle glaucoma or ocular hypertension: A 12-week, randomized, masked-evaluator multicenter study. *American Journal of Ophthalmology, 135*, 688–703.

Petrone, D., Condemi, J. J., Fife, R., et al. (2002). A double-blind, randomized, placebo-controlled study of cevimeline in Sjögren's syndrome patients with xerostomia and keratoconjunctivitis sicca. *Arthritis & Rheumatism, 46*, 748–754.

*Pflugfelder, S. C. (2004). Anti-inflammatory therapy for dry eye. *American Journal of Ophthalmology, 137*, 337–342.

Redmond, N., & While, A. (2008). Dry eye syndrome and watering eyes. *British Journal of Community Nursing, 13,* 471–479.

*Resnikoff, S., Pascolini, D., Etya'ale, D., et al. (2004). Global data on visual impairment in the year 2002. *Bulletin of the World Health Organization, 82,* 844–851.

*Schwartz, K., & Budenz, D. (2004). Current management of glaucoma. *Current Opinion in Ophthalmology, 15,* 119–126.

*Sethuraman, U., & Kamat, D. (2009). The red eye: Evaluation and management. *Clinical Pediatrics, 48,* 588–600.

Sheppard, J. D. (2003). Dry eye moves beyond palliative care. *Managed Care, 12*(Suppl. 12), 6–8.

*Shields, S. R. (2000). Managing eye disease in primary care. *Postgraduate Medicine, 108*(5), 83–96.

Silverman, M. A., & Bessman, E. (2010). Conjunctivitis. E-medicine: http://www.emedicine.com/emerg/topic110.htm. Accessed September 2, 2010.

*Song, P. I., Abraham, T. A., Park, Y., et al. (2001). The expression of functional LPS receptor proteins CD14 and toll-like receptor 4 in human corneal cells. *Investigative Ophthalmology & Visual Science, 42,* 2867–2877.

*Stern, M. E., Beuerman, R. W., Fox, R. I., et al. (1998). The pathology of dry eye: The interaction between the ocular surface and lacrimal glands. *Cornea, 17,* 584–589.

*Tielsch, J. M., Katz, J., Singh, K., et al. (1991). A population-based evaluation of glaucoma screening: The Baltimore Eye Survey. *American Journal of Epidemiology, 134,* 1102–1110.

*Trattler, W. B. (2009). Bacterial conjunctivitis. *Refractive Eyecare.*

Vivino, F. B., Al-Hashima, I., Khan, Z., et al. (1999). Pilocarpine tablets for the treatment of dry mouth and dry eye symptoms in patients with Sjögren syndrome. *Archives of Internal Medicine, 159,* 174–181.

*Wilson, S. E. (2003). Inflammation: A unifying theory for the origin of dry eye syndrome. *Managed Care, 12*(Suppl. 12), 14–19.

Wong, T. Y., & Hyman, L. (2008). Population-based studies in ophthalmology. *American Journal of Ophthalmology, 146,* 656–663.

*Yildirim, N., Sahin, A., & Gultekin, S. (2008). The effect of latanoprost, bimatoprost, and travoprost on circadian variation of intraocular pressure in patients with open-angle glaucoma. *Journal of Glaucoma, 17,* 36–39.

CHAPTER 18

Laura L. Bio
Jomy M. George

Otitis Media and Otitis Externa

Infections of the ear are a common problem in children, but they can also affect adults. Acute otitis media (AOM), otitis media with effusion (OME), and otitis externa (OE; also known as *swimmer's ear*) are the most common ear infections.

Antibiotics and vaccination programs have decreased the frequency of complications. However, serious complications may still occur. Identification, diagnosis, and management of these infections is essential to prevent permanent hearing loss, chronic or recurrent ear infections, mastoiditis, meningitis, and speech or language delay.

OTITIS MEDIA AND OTITIS EXTERNA

Otitis media may manifest as AOM or chronic OME (Lieberthal, et al., 2004). AOM has historically posed a major social and economic burden, occurring at an alarming rate of 19 million cases per year. It continues to impact antibiotic expenditures because it is the most common infection for which antibiotics are prescribed for children. In 1990, more than 25 million physician visits were attributed to otitis media, resulting in 809 antibacterial prescriptions per 1,000 visits (Lieberthal, et al., 2004). By the year 2000, the number of office visits decreased to 16 million, yet the number of prescriptions remained relatively the same, at 802 per 1,000 visits.

AOM is defined as an acute onset of signs and symptoms of a middle ear infection, presence of middle ear effusion, and signs and symptoms consistent with middle ear inflammation (**Table 18.1**). It is the most common bacterial respiratory tract infection in children and is a result of bacteria traveling to the middle ear from the eustachian tube. AOM is most common in infants and children age 6 months to 2 years, but the infection may occur at any age. Otitis media occurs in 60% to 70% of all children by the end of the first year of life and in more than 90% by age 7 (Hoberman, et al., 2002).

Chronic OME is distinct from AOM in that middle ear fluid persists in the absence of signs and symptoms of an acute infection (Lieberthal, et al., 2004). As of 2004, it is estimated that approximately 2.2 million episodes are diagnosed annually in the United States. It is most common in children age 6 months to 4 years (Tos, 1984). In fact, it is estimated that up to 50% of children will have OME by the first year of life and up to 60% by age 2 (Paradise, et al., 1997).

OE may also present in acute and chronic forms. OE is defined as an infection of the outer ear and ear canal. Acute OE roughly affects 1 in every 1,000 persons in the United States (Osguthorpe & Nielsen, 2006). It is most common in children ages 7 to 12, but can also occur in adults, in whom the incidence declines after age 50. OE is most often associated with swimming, local trauma, use of hearing aids, and high and humid temperatures (**Table 18.1**). Unlike AOM, in which the mainstay of treatment is systemic antibiotics, topical antibiotic therapy is usually adequate for the treatment of OE. Oral antibiotics are generally recommended for patients with compromised immunity such as patients with diabetes, those on systemic corticosteroids, or those with chronic dermatitis (Sander, 2001). Systemic antibiotics should also be considered for patients with recurrent episodes of OE and clinical signs of malignant OE. A serious and potentially life-threatening complication of OE is malignant or necrotizing OE in which the infection extends to the mastoid or temporal bone. Mortality rates as high as 53% have been reported secondary to malignant OE. Immunocompromised patients, including the elderly with diabetes and human immunodeficiency virus, are at the highest risk.

CAUSES

Acute Otitis Media and Otitis Media with Effusion

The bacterial etiology of AOM in children has remained consistent over several years (Klein, 2009). The bacteria most frequently isolated from middle ear fluid are *Streptococcus pneumoniae* (38% of infections), *Haemophilus influenzae* (27% of infections), and *Moraxella catarrhalis* (10% of infections). Infections caused by Group A *Streptococcus* and *Staphylococcus aureus* are less common and have a mean incidence of 3% and 2%, respectively.

S. pneumoniae is the most common pathogen associated with these infections. It is also the most common etiology for which antibiotics are prescribed. In fact, only up to 20% of AOM cases caused by *S. pneumoniae* resolve spontaneously. The most common serotypes responsible for AOM include, in the order of decreasing frequency, 19, 23, 6, 14, 3, and 18.

TABLE 18.1	Comparing Types of Otitis		
Type of Otitis	**Etiology**	**Symptoms**	**Clinical Findings**
Acute otitis media	*Streptococcus pneumoniae* *Haemophilus influenzae* *Moraxella catarrhalis* *Mycoplasma pneumoniae* associated with bullous myringitis	Otalgia Ear pulling Upper respiratory infection symptoms Fever Vertigo Otorrhea Decreased hearing	Diffuse redness and bulging of the tympanic membrane Decreased movement of the tympanic membrane Possibly perforation of the tympanic membrane Reddish-purple blister on the tympanic membrane or at the junction of the membrane and the canal (bullous myringitis)
Otitis media with effusion	Eustachian tube obstruction causing sterile effusion in the middle ear	Hearing loss that may be manifested by delayed language development in young children or decreased school performance in older children Feeling of ear fullness Popping sensation with swallowing, yawning, or blowing the nose	Clear, yellowish, or bluish-gray fluid behind the tympanic membrane, with or without air bubbles The tympanic membrane may be retracted with decreased movement.
Otitis externa	Infectious: *Pseudomonas aeruginosa, Staphylococcus aureus, Streptococcus* species Malignant: *P. aeruginosa*	Infectious: Erythema and swelling of the external canal with otalgia and itching, muffled hearing, watery or thick discharge from the ear Malignant: Persistent foul-smelling discharge, deep ear pain	Infectious: Pain with movement of tragus, raised area of induration on the tragus, swollen external auditory canal, red pustular lesions Malignant: Progressive cranial nerve palsies, granulations in the external ear canal

Infections caused by *H. influenzae* have a spontaneous resolution rate of 50%. Cases of otitis media in older children, adolescents, and adults are often caused by non-typable strains and can present with other serious infections such as bacteremia or meningitis. About 10% of cases are caused by type B and may be prevented by immunization.

Although many cases are caused by bacterial pathogens, viruses play a significant role in the pathogenesis and course of treatment. Viral pathogens, such as respiratory syncytial virus, influenza A and B, parainfluenza, enterovirus, and rhinovirus, have all been isolated in AOM cases. The presence of viral pathogens may prolong the symptoms associated with AOM regardless of the completion of an antibiotic regimen. Patients should be closely monitored for these reasons.

Otitis Externa

Ninety percent of cases are caused by bacteria while the remaining 10% may be caused by fungal pathogens (Osguthorpe & Nielsen, 2006; Klein, 2009). The etiology of OE is different than that found in otitis media because the flora of the external auditory canal is similar to that of the skin including *Staphylococcus epidermidis, S. aureus, Corynebacteria* species, and *Propionibacterium acnes*. Gram-negative bacilli, namely *Pseudomonas aeruginosa*, may also play a role in invasive infections such as malignant OE as

well as in situations in which the skin is constantly exposed to warm, moist environments (i.e., swimming). These infections may also be caused by fungal pathogens especially in excessive humidity. Fungal infections may also occur in cases in which prolonged antibiotic courses are given for bacterial OE, causing an alteration in ear canal skin flora. Up to 90% of these fungal infections are caused by *Aspergillus* species and to a lesser extent by *Candida* species.

PATHOPHYSIOLOGY

Otitis Media

AOM frequently follows an upper respiratory infection (URI) (usually a viral etiology) in which the eustachian tube closes secondary to inflamed mucous membranes (Lieberthal, et al., 2004). The pathophysiology of AOM is multifactorial but is mainly the result of eustachian tube dysfunction. The eustachian tube protects the middle ear from nasopharyngeal secretions, provides drainage of secretions produced in the middle ear into the nasopharynx, and permits equilibration of air pressure to atmospheric pressure in the middle ear. The structure of a child's eustachian tube differs from that of an adult's. The adult eustachian tube lies at 45 degrees to the horizontal plane and allows for secretions to drain from the middle ear to the nasopharynx. The child's eustachian tube, however, is short and horizontal. When a child develops mild inflammation or edema of the eustachian tube, the ear has difficulty clearing secretions due to the almost horizontal placement of the eustachian tube. Persistent secretions, incomplete drainage, and the absence of aeration breed an environment for bacterial growth within the middle ear (Pelton, 2008; Hoberman, et al., 2002). The result is the inflammation known as AOM. The incidence of AOM is highest during winter months, which coincide with the seasonal peak of URIs (Pelton, 2008). Risk factors for AOM include congenital defects such as cleft palate and Down syndrome, young age (highest incidence in children below age 2), family history, and children who attend day care or are relatives of children in day care. The following risk factors have also been associated, however inconsistently, with an increased risk of AOM: male sex, exposure to second-hand smoke, allergies, and lack of breast feeding (Hoberman, et al., 2002).

OME is thought to result from prolonged blockage of the eustachian tube, which in turn causes negative pressure within the middle ear that allows fluid to accumulate (Pelton, 2008). These effusions may persist for several months and may result in conductive hearing loss. The presence of effusion does not always correlate to the presence of an infection. In fact, bacterial pathogens are reported in only 20% to 30% of middle ear effusions (Pelton, 2008).

Otitis Externa

OE is a result of inflammation with or without infection that occurs in the ear canal (Osguthorpe & Nielsen, 2006). Children, adolescents, and adults are all at risk for developing this infection. This condition may occur as a result of many different factors. When the skin in the ear canal is constantly exposed to wet or humid climates, the pH may vary, compromising local immune defenses and allowing bacteria and other pathogens to harbor infection. Factors such as excessive itching, using cotton balls (local trauma), swimming, eczema, use of hearing aids, chronic ottorhea, and immunocompromise states such as diabetes all increase the risk of OE.

Resistance

The increasing rates of antimicrobial resistance are a major cause of treatment failure of AOM and OE (Hoberman, et al., 2002; Pelton, 2008). The increasing incidence warrants the judicious use of antibiotics. Mechanisms of resistance include alteration of drug binding sites and the production of antibiotic inactivating enzymes called beta-lactamases. Organisms such as *H. influenzae* and *M. catarrhalis* can produce these enzymes, which essentially render many beta-lactam antibiotics useless. It is for this reason antibiotics that remain stable in the presence of beta-lactamase producing enzymes must be chosen to ensure treatment success. Beta-lactam antibiotics commonly used in the treatment of AOM include penicillin and its derivatives as well as cephalosporins.

For infections for which beta-lactamase producing organisms are suspected, combination beta-lactam/beta-lactamase inhibitors, such as amoxicillin/clavulanic acid, should be used. A detailed discussion of treatment options is discussed in the management section of this chapter.

Drug-resistant *S. pneumoniae* (DRSP) remains a threat in the treatment of AOM and OE. Penicillin, historically, has been the mainstay of treatment against *S. pneumoniae*. However, the increasing prevalence of penicillin-intermediate and -resistant strains has discouraged the use of penicillin. Furthermore, penicillin-resistant strains may also confer resistance to other antibiotics such as macrolides, trimethoprim-sulfamethoxazole, and clindamycin. The mechanism of penicillin-resistant *S. pneumoniae* is the alteration of the penicillin-binding site. This may be overcome by administering high-dose amoxicillin. It should be noted that infections caused by penicillin-resistant *S. pneumoniae* have mostly been reported in children younger than age 2.

Beta-lactamase production is the mechanism by which organisms such as *H. influenzae* and *M. cattarhalis* develop resistance. If these organisms are suspected, specifically in the setting of treatment failure or recurrent infection, combination products such as amoxicillin/clavulanic acid and cephalosporins (i.e., cefixime, cefpodoxime), which remain stable in the presence of beta-lactamase, should be recommended for treatment.

DIAGNOSTIC CRITERIA AND CLINICAL PRESENTATION

Acute Otitis Media

The presentation of AOM includes symptoms such as fever, otalgia, irritability, tugging on the affected ear; the tympanic membrane appears bulging, erythematous, and immobile to pneumatic otoscopy upon inspection. The diagnosis of AOM requires the abrupt onset of symptoms, presence of middle ear effusion, and signs or symptoms of middle ear inflammation (**Table 18.2**). Middle ear effusion is confirmed by pneumatic otoscopy. Upon examination by pneumatic otoscopy, the tympanic membrane appears erythematous; bulging may be visualized due to air or fluid behind the membrane, leading to limited or absent motility of the membrane. Signs or symptoms of middle ear inflammation include erythema of the tympanic membrane, hearing loss, and otalgia. Severe illness is defined by the American Academy of Pediatrics (AAP) as severe otalgia and fever of 102.2°F (39°C) or more (Lieberthal, et al., 2004).

The absence of all three elements listed above presumes a diagnosis of OME. Patients with OME are usually asymptomatic, but may complain of a full sensation in the ear. Upon examination, the tympanic membrane may not appear bulging, but air-fluid levels may be apparent. AOM and OME require differentiation because OME is not treated with antibiotics because of a probable viral etiology or as the result of AOM resolution.

TABLE 18.2	**Diagnostic Criteria for Acute Otitis Media**

1. History of acute onset of signs/symptoms
2. Presence of middle ear effusion (indicated by one of the following)
   a. Bulging of tympanic membrane
   b. Limited or absent tympanic membrane mobility
   c. Otorrhea
   d. Air-fluid level behind tympanic membrane
3. Signs and symptoms of middle ear inflammation
   a. Erythema of tympanic membrane
   b. Otalgia

Data from Hoberman, A., Marchant, C. D., Kaplan, S., et al. (2002). Treatment of acute otitis media consensus recommendations. *Clinical Pediatrics, 41,* 373–390.

Tympanocentesis, the process by which fluid is drained from the middle ear, is recommended for recurrent treatment failure to ensure proper diagnosis of the causative organism and determine the presence of bacterial resistance. This process relieves pressure in the middle ear cavity and promotes drainage, but it is reserved for treatment failures because of the potential risk of permanent hearing loss and facial paralysis.

INITIATING DRUG THERAPY

Goals of Drug Therapy

The goals of therapy for AOM include symptomatic pain relief, appropriate use of antibiotics to prevent complications, and judicious use of antibiotics to prevent future antimicrobial resistance. Symptomatic pain relief can be achieved with the use of acetaminophen or a nonsteroidal anti-inflammatory drug (NSAID) such as ibuprofen. Antibiotics are utilized to eradicate the infecting organism and prevent complications such as mastoiditis and hearing impairment. Antibiotic use is not without limitations, such as resistance and adverse effects. For these reasons, clinicians should avoid unnecessary use of antibiotics.

Over-the-Counter Therapy

Acetaminophen and NSAIDs should be offered early to relieve pain regardless of antibiotic use, unless hypersensitivity exists. Local topical anesthetics such as the combination of antipyrine and benzocaine (Allergen) may be used to control otalgia.

Observational Therapy

The decision to manage AOM with antibiotics is based on patient-specific characteristics such as age, certainty of diagnosis, and severity of illness. All patients with suspected AOM who are younger than age 6 months should receive antibiotics. For patients with an uncertain diagnosis who are older than age 6 months, the role of antibiotics is unclear and the decision to provide symptomatic care with close observation can be made. The decision to observe and withhold antibiotics is based on the high rate of spontaneous resolution (~80%) and overlap of nonspecific AOM symptoms with viral URIs. The certainty of diagnosis is based on the presence of the three elements mentioned before. If less than three elements are present, the diagnosis is uncertain.

Observation is recommended for patients older than age 2 with an uncertain diagnosis or nonsevere illness. Patients age 6 months to 2 years with an uncertain diagnosis should receive antibacterial therapy if the criteria for severe illness are present, while patients with an uncertain diagnosis and nonsevere illness should be observed. The observation period for all ages is 48 to 72 hours. If the patient remains symptomatic after the observational period, antibiotic therapy should be considered. The technique for observational therapy is controversial; observe with or without a prescription with instructions to fill after 2 to 3 days if symptoms persist. This decision should be based on the prescriber's assessment to whether the caregiver is likely to adhere to the plan (Chao, et al., 2008).

Antibiotic Therapy

Beta-Lactams

Patients younger than age 6 months and patients older than age 6 months with a certain diagnosis of AOM require antibiotic therapy (**Figure 18-1**). First-line therapy for nonsevere illness is high-dose amoxicillin for adequate middle ear penetration and to overcome intermediate-resistant *S. pneumoniae* (Pichichero, 2005). Amoxicillin, a derivative of penicillin, does not possess reliable activity against beta-lactamase producing pathogens, including *S. pneumoniae and H. influenzae* (**Table 18.3**).

If the presence of a penicillin allergy is elicited from the patient or caregiver, the type of reaction must be assessed. In a non-type I hypersensitivity reaction to penicillin (rash), cephalosporins may be recommended due to the low cross-reactivity between penicillins and cephalosporins (Pichichero, 2005). The cepholosporins recommended by the AAP guidelines for the treatment of nonsevere AOM are oral formulations of cefdinir and cefpodoxime, which are third-generation cephalosporins and cefuroxime, which is a second-generation cephalosporin (**Table 18.3**).

Patients with severe illness (as defined above) should receive amoxicillin-clavulanate, which is a beta-lactam antibiotic and beta-lactamase inhibitor. Amoxicillin-clavulanate is active against more than 90% of strains of the three major pathogens that cause AOM (including certain isolates of DRSP). Amoxicillin-clavulanate is commercially available in the United States in various concentrations of the oral suspension, chewables, tablets, and extended-release tablets. The major difference among these formulations is the ratio of clavulanate to amoxicillin. It should be noted that these formulations may not be interchanged due to the differing ratios of clavulanate to amoxicillin. The most common adverse effect of amoxicillin-clavulanate is diarrhea, which is dependent on the dosage of clavulanate (Block, et al., 2006). Due to the high

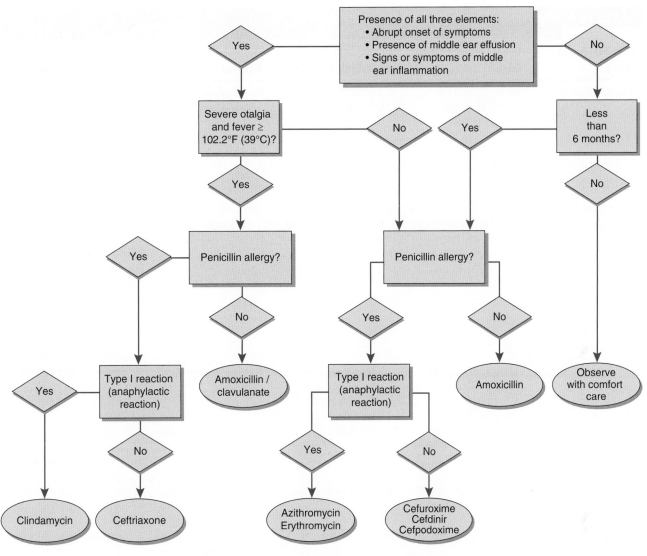

FIGURE 18–1 Treatment algorithm for acute otitis media.

amount of clavulanate administered with the high dose of amoxicillin based on the standard ratio (clavulanate to amoxicillin 1:7), the ES formulation for suspension (ratio 1:14) and XR formulation for tablets (ratio 1:16) should be recommended to limit excess exposure to clavulanate and therefore reduce the incidence of diarrhea.

If a patient with severe AOM has a history of a non-type I hypersensitivity reaction to penicillin or its derivatives, the patient should receive a single intramuscular (IM) injection of ceftriaxone. This is also an option for patients who are intolerant to oral medications or if compliance is a concern (Wang, et al., 2004).

Macrolides

Patients with a history of type 1 hypersensitivity reactions, such as anaphylaxis or hives, should avoid penicillins and its derivatives, including cephalosporins. Instead, the recommendation

by the AAP is to use a macrolide antibiotic: a 5-day course of azithromycin or a 10-day course of clarithromycin (**Table 18.3**). Macrolides are not first-line therapy due to the increased risk of treatment failure and therefore are reserved for patients with a contraindication to amoxicillin (Courter, et al., 2010).

Clindamycin

Patients who have a type I reaction to penicillin or its derivatives should receive clindamycin for treatment of severe AOM (**Table 18.3**). The limitation of clindamycin is that it lacks activity against common pathogens such as *H. influenzae* or *M. catarrhalis*.

Time Frame for Response

The standard duration of therapy is 10 days for patients younger than age 6 or to manage severe AOM, and 5 to 7 days for patients age 6 and older or treatment of mild AOM

TABLE 18.3	Overview of Antibiotics for Acute Otitis Media			
Generic (Trade) Name	**Usual Pediatric Daily Dose**	**Usual Adult Daily Dose**	**Adverse Effects**	**Dosage Formulations**
amoxicillin (various)	80–90 mg/kg/d PO divided into two doses per day	2–3 g/day PO divided into two to three doses per day	Abnormal taste, diarrhea, headache, skin rash	Suspension, oral: 125 mg/5 mL, 250 mg/5 mL, 400 mg/mL Chewable, oral: 125 mg, 200 mg, 250 mg, 400 mg Tablet, oral: 500 mg, 875 mg Capsule: 250 mg, 500 mg
amoxicillin/clavulanate (Augmentin)	80–90 mg/kg/d based on amoxicillin component PO divided into two doses per day	250–500 mg PO every 8 hours; or 875 mg PO every 12 hours	Abnormal taste, diarrhea, headache	Suspension, oral: amoxicillin[a] 200 mg/5 mL, 250 mg/5 mL, 400 mg/5 mL; Augmentin ES-600[b]: 600 mg/5 mL Chewable, oral:[a] amoxicillin 200 mg, 400 mg Tablet, oral:[c] 250 mg, 500 mg, 875 mg Augmentin XR[d] 1000 mg
azithromycin (Zithromax)	10 mg/kg PO load on day 1 followed by 5 mg/kg/d PO for 4 more days	500 mg PO load on day 1 followed by 250 mg PO for 4 more days *or* 500 mg/day PO for 3 days	Diarrhea, nausea, rash, vomiting	Suspension, oral: 100 mg/5 mL, 200 mg/5 mL Tablets, oral: 250 mg, 500 mg
ceftriaxone (Rocephin)	50 mg/kg/d IV or IM once daily for 3 days	1–2 g IV once daily	Skin rash, injection site reactions	IV: max 40 mg/mL concentration IM: 250–350 mg/mL with lidocaine
cefdinir (Omnicef)	7 mg/kg/day PO divided into two doses per day	300 mg PO twice a day	Skin rash and GI upset but otherwise generally well tolerated	Suspension, oral: 125 mg/5 mL, 250 mg/5 mL Capsule, oral: 300 mg
cefpodoxime (Vantin)	10 mg/kg/d PO once daily	200 mg PO twice a day	Skin rash and GI upset but otherwise generally well tolerated	Suspension, oral: 50 mg/5 mL, 100 mg/5 mL Tablet, oral: 100 mg, 200 mg
cefuroxime (Ceftin)	30 mg/kg/d PO divided into two doses per day	250–500 mg PO twice a day	Skin rash and GI upset but otherwise generally well tolerated	Suspension, oral: 125 mg/5 mL, 250 mg/5 mL Tablet, oral: 250 mg, 500 mg
clindamycin (various)	30 mg/kg/d PO divided into three doses per day	300–450 mg PO every 6–8 hours	Diarrhea, *C. difficile*–associated diarrhea, rash	Suspension, oral: 75 mg/5 mL Capsule, oral: 75 mg, 150 mg, 300 mg

[a]Standard ratio of clavulanate to amoxicillin of 1:7; [b] ES ratio of clavulanate to amoxicillin of 1:14; [c] Standard 125 mg of clavulanate per tablet; [d] XR ratio of clavulanate to amoxicillin of 1:16

(Lieberthal, et al., 2004). It should be noted that the duration of azithromycin is only 5 days if indicated. Symptoms of AOM should improve within 2 to 3 days, and the patient should achieve complete resolution of symptoms after 7 days. The patient or caregiver must be counseled to continue antibiotic therapy even if symptoms resolve before completion of the entire therapy course.

Treatment Failure

Despite antibiotic therapy, treatment failure may still occur. Treatment failure may be due to the presence of a resistant organism to initial therapy, a viral infection that is unresponsive to antibiotic therapy, inadequate concentration of antibiotic in the middle ear, or noncompliance with the prescribed regimen. Early failure is defined as symptom persistence for up to 72 hours after therapy initiation, and is most likely attributed to viral etiology, beta-lactamase producing organisms, or DRSP. Late failure is the presence of symptoms for more than 3 days after starting therapy, which is most likely due to re-infection with a new causative organism. Late failures can also be a result of a persistent resistant organism or new colonization of a resistant organism. Treatment failure requires escalation to the next step in management and is highly dependent on the initial therapy. For example, if a patient fails observation, the patient should be prescribed amoxicillin (unless an allergy is present; follow the algorithm in **Figure 18-1**). Patients who fail amoxicillin-clavulanate should receive a 3-day course of intravenous ceftriaxone (Khaliq, et al., 2008). Tympanocentesis is a last option for patients who have failed alternative therapy. This procedure provides symptomatic relief by releasing middle ear effusion and identifies the causative organism when the effusion is cultured. Definitive therapy should be selected based on the susceptibility data reported for the identified organism.

RECURRENT ACUTE OTITIS MEDIA

Recurrent AOM is defined as more than three episodes within 6 months or four episodes within 12 months. Recurrence is most commonly due to relapse (infection with the same organism) or reinfection (infection with a different organism). Recurrent AOM can be managed either by the placement of tympanostomy tubes or antibiotic prophylaxis. Specific indications for tympanostomy tube placement are the presence of middle ear effusion for 3 months or longer, permanent conductive-sensorineural hearing loss, vertigo or tinnitus, severe atelectasis, or changes in the middle ear (adhesive otitis or ossicular involvement). Myringotomy and insertion of tympanostomy tubes improves AOM symptoms by allowing drainage of the effusion. These tubes maintain a disease-free state typically in the first 6 months after insertion; however, the benefit thereafter is unknown (McDonald, et al., 2008). Complications of tube placement include otorrhea, myringosclerosis, perforation, and tissue granulation as seen on otoscopic examination (Vlastarakos, et al., 2007).

Prophylaxis and/or Prevention

Patients with recurrent AOM (as defined previously) may benefit from antibiotic prophylaxis, but this concept remains controversial because of a lack of supporting evidence. If the perceived benefit of prophylaxis outweighs the risk of resistance and drug-related adverse effects, the antibiotic should be initiated during winter and early spring and continued for 3 months or until therapy fails. Amoxicillin and trimethoprim-sulfamethoxazole are the most commonly used antibiotics for AOM prophylaxis. The dose of these antibiotics is approximately half of the treatment dose (refer to the dosing reference).

The Centers for Disease Control and Prevention's (CDC) recommended schedule for vaccines should be followed to reduce preventable diseases. The vaccines pertinent to the prevention of AOM are the pneumococcal, *H. influenzae* Type B, and influenza. Please refer to the prevention section of this chapter for a detailed discussion on target vaccine groups and current recommendations.

OTITIS EXTERNA

DIAGNOSTIC CRITERIA AND CLINICAL PRESENTATION

OE commonly presents with pain on movement of the auricle or tragus and a painful, erythematous auditory canal with occasional otorrhea. Hearing is usually unaffected unless pressure and fullness in the ear exist, producing occasional conductive or sensorineural hearing loss. Examination includes the ear canal, tympanic membrane, auricle, and cervical nodes. Cerumen or debris blocking the ear canal should be cleared to verify tympanic integrity. Debris usually can be cleared with a small Frazier suction tip (5 or 7 French) or an ear curette or spoon (Osguthorpe & Nielsen, 2006). To rule out otitis media, the tympanic membrane must be visualized and move normally during pneumatic otoscopy in patients with OE. If the tympanic membrane is bulging or erythematous, the patient should be worked up for otitis media. Malignant OE is osteomyelitis of the ear canal that typically presents with fever, excruciating pain, foul discharge, granulation tissue in the ear canal, and cranial nerve palsies.

INITIATING DRUG THERAPY

Goals of Drug Therapy

The goals of OE treatment are similar to otitis media, which are eradicating the causative organisms and decreasing the accompanying pain. This can be accomplished by re-establishing an acidic environment in the external auditory canal or through direct antimicrobial activity.

First-line management of OE is to clear any obstructing debris or excess cerumen from the canal and to check the integrity of the tympanic membrane and if manifestations of the infection have spread beyond the ear canal. OE treatment consists of topical, otic drops (i.e., astringents, antiseptics, antibiotics, steroids, or combination treatments). Mild, uncomplicated OE resulting from prolonged exposure to water or humidity is treated topically with an antiseptic such as acetic acid or boric acid applied to the external canal. Acute OE warrants the use of an antimicrobial ototopical agent.

Antibiotic Therapy

If edema prevents application of the drops, cotton gauze saturated with antibiotic drops can be placed into the ear. The medication should be applied to the cotton wick as often as possible. After 24 to 48 hours, the cotton can be removed and the medication applied directly into the canal. Malignant OE is usually treated with prolonged antipseudomonal antibiotic therapy (**Table 18.4**).

TABLE 18.4 **Overview of Treatment for Otitis Externa**

Generic (Trade) Name and Dosage	Selected Adverse Events	Contraindications	Special Considerations
polymyxin B sulfate, neomycin, and hydrocortisone Children: 3 drops into ear canal 3–4 times daily for maximum of 10 d Adults: 4 drops into ear canal 3–4 times daily for maximum of 10 d	Superinfection, contact dermatitis, ototoxicity with prolonged use	Herpes simplex, fungal, tubercular, or viral otic infections Perforated eardrum Prescribe with caution in pregnancy (category C drug) and in breast-feeding patients.	Use otic drops for a maximum of 10 d.
ofloxacin (Floxin) Children 1–12 y: 5 drops into ear canal bid for 10 days Children >12 y and adults: 10 drops bid for 10 d	Pruritus, site reaction, dizziness, earache, vertigo, taste perversion, paresthesia, rash	Not recommended for patients <1 y, perforated eardrum Prescribe with caution in pregnancy (category C drug) and in breast-feeding patients.	Use otic drops for a maximum of 10 d.
acetic acid, propylene glycol diacetate, and hydrocortisone (Vosol) Children >3 y: 3–5 drops into ear canal 3–4 times daily Adults: 5 drops into ear canal 3–4 times daily	Contact dermatitis, transient stinging	Perforated eardrum, viral otic infections	
acetic acid in aluminum sulfate (Otic Domeboro) Adults and children: 4–6 drops into ear canal every 2–3 h	Ear discomfort	Perforated eardrum	Discontinue in presence of excessive irritation.

Fluoroquinolones

The fluoroquinolone antibiotics, ciprofloxacin and ofloxacin, are often used to treat infections associated with OE, which have ideal antipseudomonal activity. These agents are comparable in efficacy to the gold standard, neomycin/polymyxin B, with a clinical cure rate ranging from 84% to 96% (Dohar, 2003). In addition, these agents may be more tolerable compared to neomycin/polymyxin B due to less adverse effects (i.e., stinging).

The dosage of ciprofloxacin 0.3%/dexamethasone 0.1% (Ciprodex) is four drops into the affected ear twice daily for 7 days. This regimen should show a response within 3 to 4 days of initiation. Typical adverse events include ear discomfort or pain, ear pruritus, and irritability. Ofloxacin (Floxin Otic) is administered as 5 drops once daily (children age 6 months to 13 years) or 10 drops once daily (children older than age 13 and adults).

The addition of a corticosteroid to the antibiotic formulation is controversial. The anti-inflammatory effects potentially include reduced pain, swelling, and itching. Dohar (2003) reported on a controlled study suggesting that the addition of hydrocortisone decreases the duration of pain by about 1 day. However, additional studies should be conducted to confirm this point. The risk of local immunosuppression and potential hypersensitivity reactions should be studied in light of potential benefits. The Floxin Otic preparation does not contain a corticosteroid.

Aminoglycoside Antibiotics

The combination product neomycin sulfate/polymyxin B/hydrocortisone acetate (Cortisporin) has historically been used for OE. The combination of the gram-positive coverage of the aminoglycoside neomycin and the antipseudomonal activity of polymyxin has made this combination the gold standard of treatment. The same controversy regarding the addition of a corticosteroid exists with this combination. Treatment consists of instilling 4 drops in the affected ear three or four times a day for a maximum of 10 days. The clinical cure rate of this regimen is 83% to 96% (Beers & Abramo, 2004; Dohar, 2003). However, the side effect profile, particularly the hypersensitivity reactions related to neomycin (and possibly the preservative), is high (Dohar, 2003). Further, ototoxicity with neomycin has been reported, although the number of reports is low and the data are speculative, particularly when the patient's tympanic membrane is intact.

TABLE 18.5	Recommended Order of Treatment for Otitis Externa	
Order	**Agents**	**Comments**
First line	Fluoroquinolone drops	Floxin is not recommended for patients <1 y. Use all otic drops for a maximum of 10 d. All drops are contraindicated in cases of perforated eardrum.
Second line	Combination neomycin/polymyxin B drops	Vosol is not recommended for patients <3 y. All drops are contraindicated in cases of perforated eardrum.

Selecting the Most Appropriate Agent

First-Line Therapy

OE is treated initially with a fluoroquinolone antibiotic. The selection of ciprofloxacin versus ofloxacin depends on the formulary status of the agents as well as the clinician's experience with added corticosteroids (**Table 18.5**).

Second-Line Therapy

Neomycin/polymyxin B combinations are considered second-line agents, primarily due to their side effect profile. The lower cost of these agents, however, warrants consideration, particularly in patients without insurance or other means of paying for the more expensive fluoroquinolones.

Third-Line Therapy

OE is treated with antibacterial–antifungal and astringent and solvent agents (Domeboro and Vosol) when a third-line medication is needed.

Special Population Considerations

Acetic acid 2% solution is not recommended for children younger than age 3. The concern related to the use of systemic fluoroquinolones in children is not relevant due to the minimal systemic absorption with an intact tympanic membrane.

MONITORING PATIENT RESPONSE

A gallium scan should be performed to ensure reduction in the inflammatory process. Cleaning the local affected area is needed, but extensive debridement can be reserved until the initial antibiotic therapy is completed.

PREVENTION

Prevention is the key and plays a significant role in reducing the overall burden of illness (i.e., office visits, antibiotic expenditures, severity of illness). Vaccination programs have been shown to have a favorable outcome on decreasing the overall incidence of these infections, namely those caused by *S. pneumoniae*, influenza, and *H. influenzae*.

The introduction of the heptavalent pneumococcal polysaccharide conjugate vaccine (Prevnar; serotypes 4, 6B, 9V, 14, 18C, 19F, and 23F) decreased the overall incidence of invasive pneumococcal disease by 69% in children younger than age 2 from 1998 to 1999 and 2001 (Lieberthal, et al., 2004). Reductions in otitis media office visits and severity of illness have been observed since the introduction of the vaccine (Black, et al., 2000). The serotypes in the 7-valent vaccine when brought to the market in 2000 represented approximately 70% of the serotypes found in AOM. The pneumococcal vaccine is available in two formulations: conjugated (PCV) and polysaccharide (PPSV) for infants younger than age 2 and children older than age 2 with comorbidities, respectively. The conjugate vaccine containing seven serotypes demonstrated a reduction in invasive infection/disease, but few penicillin-resistant strains are included in the vaccine (Hoberman, et al., 2002). Thus, the new conjugate vaccine containing 13 pneumococcal serotypes was approved by the U.S. Food and Drug Administration in 2010 and recommended by the Advisory Committee on Immunization Practices to replace the 7-valent PCV for routine vaccination for all children ages 6 weeks to 5 years (Advisory Committee on Immunization Practices [ACIP], 2011). This vaccine contains the aforementioned seven serotypes in addition to serotypes 1, 3, 5, 6A, 7F, and 19A (Prevnar, 2007). The polysaccharide vaccine contains 23 pneumococcal serotypes indicated for children age 2 and older with chronic disease and not indicated in infants younger than age 2 due to poor immunogenicity.

Administration of the influenza and HiB vaccines are also routinely recommended in children to decrease potential infections caused by them. The HiB vaccine is a polysaccharide, conjugated protein carrier indicated for infants age 6 weeks and older. The influenza vaccine is recommended for all children ages 6 months to 18 years, but the selection of the correct formulation is dependent on the age of the patient. The two formulations are a trivalent inactivated vaccine as an IM injection and live attenuated vaccine as an intranasal administration, which is indicated in infants older than age 6 months and children older than age 2 who are not immunocompromised, pregnant, or have exacerbative pulmonary diseases, respectively.

For up-to-date ACIP vaccine administration schedules, check the CDC website at www.cdc.gov/vaccines (*MMWR*, 2011).

PATIENT EDUCATION

Drug Information

To instill drops, the patient should lie with the affected ear upward and remain in this position for about 5 minutes to help the solution penetrate into the ear canal. Ototopicals should be warmed to body temperature before instillation to avoid dizziness. To warm the otic solution, the patient should hold or roll the bottle in the hand for 1 to 2 minutes. Counsel the patient to lie on his or her side while another person places the drops in the ear rather than the patient as a result of wide variability in self-administered dosing of eardrops. The patient should lie with the affected ear up for a few minutes after the administration of eardrops to aid passage to the medial canal. A cotton ball temporarily placed in the ear before the patient resumes an erect position will absorb excess liquid.

Nutrition/Lifestyle Changes

The use of hypoallergenic ear canal molds when swimming or showering is controversial for the prevention of OE. Drying the ears with a cool hair dryer to aid removal of fluid after swimming may be beneficial. The patient should avoid trying to remove ear wax mechanically with cotton-tipped swabs. If the ear is very swollen, the patient can insert a wick of cotton into the ear and apply the antibiotic to the wick. It is important for the patient to avoid water in the ear until the infection clears (usually 5 to 7 days) and for 4 to 6 weeks afterward. To accomplish this, hair can be washed in a sink instead of a shower or tub, and the patient can use a shower cap when bathing.

Complementary and Alternative Medications

If the patient is susceptible to recurrent OE, instillation of a few drops of a 1:1 solution of white vinegar and rubbing alcohol before and after contact with water is good prophylaxis.

Case Study

C. J., age 17, is on his high school swim team. He presents with sudden onset of right ear pain that worsens at night. He says that the pain intensifies when he touches his ear and that he has a feeling of fullness in the ear. On examination, the auditory canal is edematous and erythematous, with yellow crusting. His temperature is 97.8°F and his tympanic membranes are pearly gray with landmarks intact.

DIAGNOSIS: OTITIS EXTERNA

1. List two specific treatment goals for C. J.
2. What drug therapy would you prescribe? Why?

3. Would you recommend a complementary or alternative medication? If so, what?
4. What would indicate that treatment is successful?
5. What would you tell C. J. about the medication?
6. What adverse reactions should you be concerned about?
7. What lifestyle changes would you recommend to prevent this from happening again?
8. If C. J. returns in 2 weeks with the same symptoms, what would you prescribe?

BIBLIOGRAPHY

Starred references are cited in the text.

* Advisory Committee on Immunization Practices (ACIP). (2010). Licensure of a 13-valent pneumococcal conjugate vaccine (PCV13) and recommendations for use among children. *Morbidity and Mortality Weekly Report (MMWR), 59*(09), 258–261. Available at: http://www.cdc.gov/mmwr/preview/mmwrhtml/mm5909a2.htm. Accessed August 18, 2010.

*Beers, S. L., & Abramo, T. J. (2004). Otitis externa review. *Pediatric Emergency Care, 20*(4), 250–256.

*Black, S., Shinefield, H., Fireman, B., et al. (2000). Efficacy, safety and immunogenicity of heptavalent pneumococcal conjugate vaccine in children. Northern California Kaiser Permanente Vaccine Study Center Group. *Pediatric Infectious Disease Journal, 19,* 187–195.

*Block, S. L., Schmier, J. K., Notario, G. F., et al. (2006). Efficacy, tolerability, and parent-reported outcomes for cefdinir vs. high-dose amoxicillin/clavulanate oral suspension for acute otitis media in young children. *Current Medical Research and Opinion, 22*(9), 1839–1847.

*Chao, J. H., Kunkov, S., Reyes, L. B., et al. (2008). Comparison of two approaches to observation therapy for acute otitis media in the emergency department. *Pediatrics, 121*(5), e1352–e1356.

*Courter, J. D., Baker, W. L., Nowak, K. S., et al. (2010). Increased clinical failures when treating acute otitis media with macrolides: A meta-analysis. *Annals of Pharmacotherapy, 44*(3), 471–478.

*Dohar, J. E. (2003). Evolution of management approaches for otitis externa. *Pediatric Infectious Disease Journal, 22*(4), 299–308.

Foster, S. L. (2007). Immunization. In *The APhA complete review for pharmacy* (4th ed.). American Pharmacists Association. New York: Castle Connolly Graduate Medical Publishing.

Hendley, J. O. (2002). Otitis media. *New England Journal of Medicine, 347*(15), 1169–1174.

*Hoberman, A., Marchant, C. D., Kaplan, S., et al. (2002). Treatment of acute otitis media consensus recommendations. *Clinical Pediatrics, 41,* 373–390.

Kaushik, V., Malik, T., & Saeed, S. R. (2010). Interventions for acute otitis externa. *Cochrane Database Syst Rev, 1,* CD004740. DOI:10.1002/14651858.CD004740.pub2.

*Khaliq, Y., Forgie, S., & Zhanel, G. (2008). Upper respiratory tract infections. In J. T. Dipiro & R. L. Talbert (Eds.), *Pharmacotherapy: A pathophysiologic approach* (7th ed.). New York: McGraw-Hill.

*Klein, J. (2009). Otitis media. In G. Mandell (Ed.), *Principles and practices of infectious diseases* (7th ed.). Maryland Heights: Churchill-Livingstone.

*Lieberthal, A. S., Ganiats, T., Cox, E. O., et al. (2004). AAP/AAFP clinical practice guideline: Diagnosis and management of acute otitis media: Subcommittee on Management of Acute Otitis Media. *Pediatrics, 113*(5), 1451–1465.

*McDonald, S., Langton Hewer, C. D., & Nunez, D. A. (2008). Grommets (ventilation tubes) for recurrent acute otitis media in children. *Cochrane Database Syst Rev,* 4, CD004741.

**Morbidity and Mortality Weekly Report* (MMWR). (2011). Recommended immunization schedules for persons aged 0–18 years-United States. Available at: http://www.cdc.gov/vaccines/recs/schedules/child-schedule. htm. Accessed February 24, 2011.

*Osguthorpe, D. J., & Nielsen, D.R. (2006). Otitis externa: Review and clinical updates. *American Family Physician, 74,* 1510–1516.

*Paradise, J. L., Rockette, H. E., Colborn, D. K., et al. (1997). Otitis media in 2253 Pittsburgh area infants: Prevalence and risk factors during the first two years of life. *Pediatrics, 99,* 318–333.

*Pelton, S. (2008). Otitis media. In S. Long (Ed.), *Principles and practices of pediatric infectious diseases* (3rd ed.). Maryland Heights: Churchill-Livingstone.

*Pichichero, M. E. (2005). A review of evidence supporting the AAP recommendation for prescribing cephalosporin antibiotics for penicillin-allergic patients. *Pediatrics, 115,* 1048–1057.

Pneumovax. (2007). Pneumococcal Vaccine Polyvalent package insert. Whitehouse Station, NJ: Merck.

*Prevnar. (2011). Pneumococcal 13-valent Conjugate Vaccine package insert. Philadelphia, PA: Wyeth Pharmaceuticals.

Rosenfeld, R. M., Vertess, J. E., & Carr, J. (1994). Clinical efficacy of antimicrobial drugs for acute otitis media: Meta-analysis of 540 children from 33 randomized trials. *Journal of Pediatrics, 124,* 355–367.

*Sander, R. (2001). Otitis externa: A practical guide to treatment and prevention. *American Family Physician, 65*(5), 927–936.

*Tos, M. (1984). Epidemiology and natural history of secretory otitis. *American Journal of Otolaryngology, 5,* 459–462.

*Vlastarakos, P. V., Nikolopoulos, T. P., Korres, S., et al. (2007). Grommets in otitis media with effusion: The most frequent operation in children. But is it associated with significant complications? *European Journal of Pediatrics, 166*(5), 385–391.

*Wang, C. Y., Lu, C. Y., Hsieh, Y. C., et al. (2004). Intramuscular ceftriaxone in comparison with oral amoxicillin-clavulanate for the treatment of acute otitis media in infants and children. *Journal of Microbiology, Immunology and Infection, 37*(1), 57–62.

Pharmacotherapy for Cardiovascular Disorders

Hypertension

Hypertension is a chronic disease that affects one out of three adults in the United States. Many people are unaware that they have hypertension because the disease rarely causes symptoms; hence, the disease is appropriately nicknamed "the silent killer." High blood pressure (BP) is a major risk factor for heart disease, stroke, congestive heart failure, and kidney disease. As the prevalence of obesity and diabetes is growing, it is expected that high-risk hypertension will continue to increase. Epidemiological studies suggest that 60% to 70% of hypertension may be directly attributable to excess adiposity, both in women and in men.

Hypertension increases with age and affects all ethnic groups. However, African-Americans suffer disproportionately from hypertension and its effects, leading to high rates of cardiovascular morbidity and mortality. Hypertension in African-Americans occurs at an earlier age, is more severe, and results in organ damage such as coronary heart disease, stroke, and end-stage renal disease more often than it does in whites.

CAUSES

Hypertension is classified as primary, essential, or idiopathic when there is no identifiable cause for elevation in BP. Between 80% and 95% of hypertensive patients are diagnosed with essential hypertension. The lifestyle of a patient with documented hypertension should be evaluated to reveal identifiable causes of hypertension. Several factors may contribute to primary hypertension: environmental factors (e.g., obesity, dietary sodium, alcohol, cigarette smoking), hyperinsulinemia, defective natriuresis, abnormal neural and peripheral autoregulation, and defects in the renin-angiotensin-aldosterone system (RAAS).

When a cause for elevated BP is identified, hypertension is classified as secondary hypertension. Identifiable causes include renal disease, renal vascular hypertension, Cushing syndrome, pheochromocytoma, primary hyperaldosteronism, endocrine disorders, sleep apnea, coarctation of the aorta, and renovascular disease, to name a few (**Box 19.1**).

Medications that may increase BP include oral contraceptives, steroids, appetite suppressants, tricyclic antidepressants, the antidepressant venlafaxine (Effexor), cyclosporine (Sandimmune), nonsteroidal antiinflammatory drugs (NSAIDs), and some nasal decongestants. Herbal products that affect BP include capsicum, goldenseal, licorice root, ma huang (ephedra), scotch broom, witch hazel, and yohimbine.

PATHOPHYSIOLOGY

Role of the Nervous System

The central and autonomic nervous systems play a key role in regulating BP. Centrally located beta receptors stimulate the release of norepinephrine, whereas alpha-2 receptors inhibit norepinephrine release, which produces vasodilation and therefore reduces BP.

Receptors located in the periphery also regulate BP. These receptors are located on effector cells that are innervated by sympathetic neurons. Alpha-1 receptors located on arterioles and venules cause vasoconstriction, while the beta-2 receptors on these vessels produce vasodilation. Beta-1 receptors, which are located on the heart and kidneys, regulate heart rate and contractility, which ultimately has an effect on cardiac output. Because BP is the product of cardiac output and peripheral resistance, any reduction in cardiac output results in a decrease in BP. Blockade of beta-1 receptors decreases cardiac output, peripheral resistance, and BP. When stimulated, beta-2 receptors located in the venules and arterioles cause vasodilation.

Baroreceptors, which are nerve endings located in large arteries such as the aortic arch and carotids, play a significant role in regulating BP. These receptors are sensitive to changes in BP. When BP drops drastically, the baroreceptors send an impulse to the brain stem that results in vasoconstriction and increased heart rate and contractility. In contrast, elevation in BP increases baroreceptor firing, which results in vasodilation and decreased heart rate and contractility. Any disturbance in this system can result in elevated BP.

Peripheral autoregulatory components also play a role in controlling BP. Normally, rises in BP result in sodium and water being eliminated by the kidney. In turn, plasma volume, cardiac output, and BP decrease. Any defect in this mechanism, however, could raise plasma volume and BP.

Role of the Renal System

The RAAS regulates sodium, potassium, and fluid balance in the body. Renin, an enzyme secreted by the juxtaglomerular

BOX 19.1

Identifiable Causes of Hypertension

Adrenal steroids
Chronic kidney disease
Chronic steroid therapy and Cushing syndrome
Coarctation of the aorta
Cocaine, amphetamines, other illicit drugs
Cyclosporine and tacrolimus
Drug-induced or drug-related
Erythropoietin
Inadequate doses
Inappropriate combinations
Licorice (including some chewing tobacco)
Nonadherence
Nonsteroidal anti-inflammatory drugs; cyclo-oxygenase-2 inhibitors
Oral contraceptives
Pheochromocytoma
Primary aldosteronism
Renovascular disease
Selected over-the-counter dietary supplements and medicines (e.g., ephedra, ma huang, bitter orange)
Sleep apnea
Sympathomimetics (decongestants, anorectics)
Thyroid or parathyroid disease

cells of the afferent arterioles of the kidney, is released in response to changes in BP resulting from reduced renal perfusion, decreased intravascular volume, or increased circulation of catecholamines. Renin catalyzes the conversion of angiotensinogen to angiotensin I. Angiotensin I is converted to the potent vasoconstrictor angiotensin II by angiotensin-converting enzyme (ACE). Angiotensin II causes direct vasoconstriction and stimulation of the sympathetic nervous system. Angiotensin II also stimulates release of aldosterone from the adrenal gland, which results in the retention of sodium and water. In normotensive patients, angiotensin II directly inhibits further release of renin through a negative feedback system. If the negative feedback system fails, BP rises.

Hyperinsulinemia may contribute to hypertension by causing sodium retention and stimulating the sympathetic nervous system.

DIAGNOSTIC CRITERIA

Hypertension is generally defined as an elevation in systolic and/or diastolic BP. The following definitions were suggested by the seventh report of the Joint National Committee (JNC VII) in 2003 (**Table 19.1**):

- Normal blood pressure: systolic less than 120 mm Hg and diastolic <80 mm Hg
- Prehypertension: systolic 120 to 139 mm Hg or diastolic 80 to 89 mm Hg.
- Hypertension:

TABLE 19.1   Classification and Management of Blood Pressure for Adults*

BP Classification	SBP* (mm Hg)	DBP* (mm Hg)	Lifestyle Modification	Initial Drug Therapy Without Compelling Indications	Initial Drug Therapy With Compelling Indications
Normal	<120	and <80	Encourage		
Prehypertension	120–139	or 80–89	Yes	No antihypertensive drug indicated	Drug(s) for compelling indications[‡]
Stage 1 Hypertension	140–159	or 90–99	Yes	Thiazide-type diuretics for most. May consider ACEI, ARB, BB, CCB, or combination.	Drug(s) for the compelling indications.[‡] Other antihypertensive drugs (diuretics, ACEI, ARB, BB, CCB) as needed.
Stage 2 Hypertension	≥160	or ≥100	Yes	Two-drug combination for most[†] (usually thiazide-type diuretic and ACEI or ARB or BB or CCB)	

DBP, diastolic blood pressure; SBP, systolic blood pressure
ACEI, angiotensin-converting enzyme inhibitor; ARB, angiotensin receptor blocker; BB, beta blocker; CCB, calcium channel blocker
*Treatment determined by highest BP category.
[†]Initial combined therapy should be used cautiously in those at risk for orthostatic hypotension.
[‡]Treat patients with chronic kidney disease or diabetes to BP goal of less than 130/80 mm Hg.

– Stage 1: systolic 140 to 159 mm Hg or diastolic 90 to 99 mm Hg

– Stage 2: systolic greater than 160 mm Hg or diastolic greater than 100 mm Hg

Similar definitions were suggested in the 2007 European Societies of Hypertension and Cardiology guidelines for the management of arterial hypertension. Cardiovascular morbidity and mortality bear a continuous relationship with both systolic and diastolic BPs.

Hypertension is not diagnosed on an initial reading; rather, it is confirmed after three readings at least 1 week apart. BP measurements should be obtained after the patient has had time to relax for at least 5 minutes. Patients should be seated in a chair rather than on an examination table, with feet on the floor and arm supported at heart level. Patients should avoid smoking cigarettes 30 minutes before the reading, should not drink coffee during the hour preceding the reading, and should avoid adrenergic stimulants, such as phenylephrine, or eyedrops for pupillary dilation. For an accurate reading, the appropriate-size sphygmomanometer cuff should be used. The cuff should encompass 80% of the arm, and the width of the cuff should be at least 40% of the length of the upper arm (Screening for high blood pressure, 2007).

Ambulatory BP monitoring (ABPM) is recommended for patients with suspected "white coat hypertension," episodic hypertension, hypertension resistant to increasing medication, hypotensive symptoms while taking antihypertensive medications, and autonomic dysfunction. Patients with "white coat hypertension" have a persistently elevated BP in the doctor's office but a persistently normal BP at other times. ABPM readings correlate better with target-organ damage than clinical measurements. ABPM also identifies patients in whom BP does not drop significantly during sleep. More aggressive treatment may be necessary for these patients, who are known to be at higher cardiovascular risk. An elevated systolic BP is a more potent cardiovascular risk factor than an elevated diastolic BP.

Physical Examination

A thorough examination should be performed, including a history of personal and family risk factors (**Box 19.2**) and a history of prescription medications, over-the-counter medications, and herbal products. For patients with documented hypertension, lifestyle should be evaluated and other cardiovascular risk factors or concomitant disorders should be identified to determine the extent of target organ damage and to assess the patient's overall cardiovascular risk status.

Physical examination includes two or more measured seated BP readings with verification in the contralateral arm; body mass index (BMI; calculated as weight in kilograms divided by the square of height in meters); distribution of body fat; muscle strength; funduscopy exam; auscultation for carotid, abdominal, and femoral bruits; palpation of the thyroid gland; thorough examination of the heart and lungs; examination of the abdomen for enlarged kidneys, masses, and

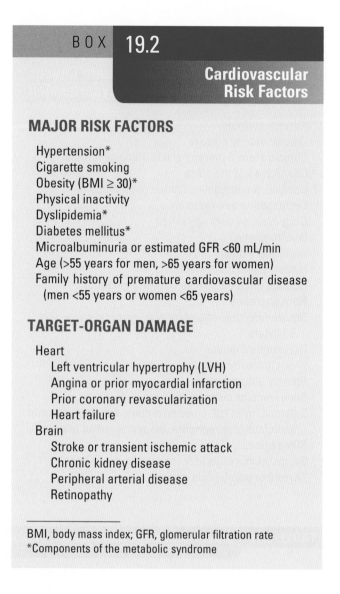

BOX 19.2

Cardiovascular Risk Factors

MAJOR RISK FACTORS

Hypertension*
Cigarette smoking
Obesity (BMI ≥ 30)*
Physical inactivity
Dyslipidemia*
Diabetes mellitus*
Microalbuminuria or estimated GFR <60 mL/min
Age (>55 years for men, >65 years for women)
Family history of premature cardiovascular disease (men <55 years or women <65 years)

TARGET-ORGAN DAMAGE

Heart
    Left ventricular hypertrophy (LVH)
    Angina or prior myocardial infarction
    Prior coronary revascularization
    Heart failure
Brain
    Stroke or transient ischemic attack
    Chronic kidney disease
    Peripheral arterial disease
    Retinopathy

BMI, body mass index; GFR, glomerular filtration rate
*Components of the metabolic syndrome

abnormal aortic pulsation; palpation of the lower extremities for edema and pulses; and neurologic assessment.

Diagnostic Tests

The following laboratory tests should be routinely performed: electrocardiogram, blood glucose, hemoglobin, hematocrit, complete urinalysis, serum potassium, creatinine, estimated glomerular filtration rate, liver function tests, calcium and magnesium, glycosylated hemoglobin (hemoglobin A1c), and fasting lipid panel (9- to 12-hour fast), which includes low-density lipoprotein (LDL) cholesterol, high-density lipoprotein cholesterol, and triglycerides. Further testing should be performed based on clinical findings.

INITIATING THERAPY

Initial therapy is determined by categorizing the patient's BP as prehypertension or stage 1 or stage 2 hypertension, and assessing for the presence of target organ damage and cardiovascular disease. **Table 19.1** and **Figure 19-1** show the current recommendations for initiating therapy.

All patients diagnosed with hypertension should be counseled about the benefits of lifestyle modifications (**Box 19.3**).

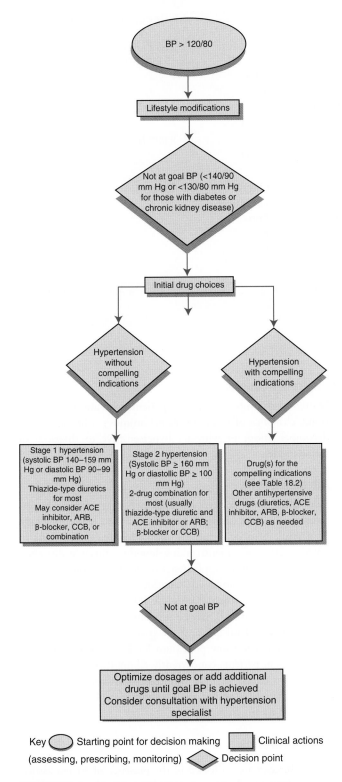

FIGURE 19–1   Modified JNC VII treatment for hypertension.

Patients are encouraged to maintain appropriate body weight (BMI of 19.5 to 24.9) and adopt the Dietary Approaches to Stop Hypertension (DASH) diet. The DASH diet is rich in fruits, vegetables, and low-fat dairy products, with a reduced content of saturated and total fat; dietary sodium is restricted to less than 100 mmol/d (2.4 g sodium or 6 g sodium chloride daily); and physical activity is encouraged, while reducing alcohol consumption. Since patients with prehypertension are at increased risk for progression to hypertension, preventive measures such as the dietary considerations mentioned above should be taken. However, if the prehypertensive patient has a concomitant disease that should also be treated, then an appropriate antihypertensive agent should be selected. If the patient progresses to stage 1 hypertension, then drug therapy is initiated.

Antihypertensive medication is initiated for patients with stage 1 hypertension. The JNC VII recommends one of the thiazide-type diuretics as initial therapy. If the goal BP is not achieved, a second drug should be added to the regimen. The diuretic should be continued and a second drug can be selected from among the ACE inhibitors, angiotensin receptor II blockers (ARBs), beta blockers, or calcium channel blockers (CCBs).

For stage 2 hypertension, the JNC VII guidelines strongly suggest starting drug therapy with two medications, usually a thiazide-type diuretic plus an ACE inhibitor, ARB, beta blocker, or CCB. Care should be taken to avoid orthostatic hypotension. Combination drug products, such as ACE inhibitors and diuretics and ARBs and diuretics, often make adhering to therapy easier for the patient.

Patients with a compelling indication (see **Table 19.3**) should be started on the indicated medication, regardless of the stage of hypertension.

Goals of Drug Therapy

The goal of antihypertensive therapy is to reduce cardiovascular and renal morbidity and mortality. Reducing BP to less than 140/90 mm Hg is associated with a decrease in the risk of cardiovascular disease (CVD). Beginning at 115/75 mm Hg, the risk of CVD doubles with each 20-mm Hg increment above systolic BP or 10-mm Hg increment above diastolic BP. Individuals who are normotensive at age 55 have a 90% lifetime risk of developing hypertension.

In patients with hypertension and comorbidities (diabetes or renal disease), the BP goal is less than 130/80 mm Hg. This goal is endorsed by the JNC VII as well as the American Diabetes Association, the National Kidney Foundation, and the Canadian Hypertensive Society. The American College of Physicians' goal for systolic BP is slightly higher, at 135 mm Hg.

Diuretics

There are five classes of diuretics: carbonic anhydrase inhibitors (which are not used for hypertension because of their weak antihypertensive effects), thiazides, thiazide-like diuretics, loop

BOX 19.3

Lifestyle Modifications to Manage Hypertension*

Modification	Recommendation	Approximate Systolic BP Reduction, Range
Weight reduction	Maintain normal body weight (BMI, 18.5–24.9).	5–20 mm Hg/10-kg weight loss
Adopt DASH eating plan	Consume a diet rich in fruits, vegetables, and low-fat dairy products with a reduced content of saturated and total fat.	8–14 mm Hg
Dietary sodium reduction	Reduce dietary sodium intake to no more than 100 mEq/L (2.4 g sodium or 6 g sodium chloride).	2–8 mm Hg
Physical activity	Engage in regular aerobic physical activity such as brisk walking (at least 30 minutes per day, most days of the week).	4–9 mm Hg
Moderation of alcohol consumption	Limit consumption to no more than 2 drinks per day (1 oz or 30 mL ethanol [e.g., 24 oz beer, 10 oz wine, or 3 oz 80-proof whiskey]) in most men and no more than 1 drink per day in women and lighter-weight persons.	2–4 mm Hg

*For overall cardiovascular risk reduction, stop smoking. The effects of implementing these modifications are dose and time dependent and could be higher for some individuals.

diuretics, and potassium-sparing diuretics. Diuretics decrease BP by causing diuresis, which results in decreased plasma volume, stroke volume, and cardiac output (**Table 19.2**). During chronic therapy their major hemodynamic effect is reduction of peripheral vascular resistance. As a result of drug-induced diuresis, hypokalemia and hypomagnesemia may lead to cardiac arrhythmias. Patients at greatest risk are those receiving digitalis therapy, those with LVH, and those with ischemic heart disease.

Thiazide Diuretics

Mechanism of Action

Thiazide diuretics work by increasing the urinary excretion of sodium and chloride in equal amounts. (See **Table 19.2.**) They inhibit the reabsorption of sodium and chloride in the thick ascending limb of the loop of Henle and the early distal tubules. Thiazide diuretics also increase potassium and bicarbonate excretion and decrease calcium excretion and uric acid retention. The thiazide diuretics are the preferred agents to reduce BP unless there are compelling or specific indications for another drug. The antihypertensive action requires several days to produce effects. The duration of action of the thiazides requires a single daily dose to control BP. Caution should be used in patients with a history of gout or hyponatremia. Diuretic-induced hyperuricemia may produce gouty arthritis or uric acid stones.

Contraindications

Diuretics are contraindicated in patients who are anuric (creatinine clearance of less than 30 mL/minute), who have renal decompensation, or who are hypersensitive to thiazides or sulfonamides.

Adverse Events

Side effects include hypokalemia, hypomagnesemia, hypercalcemia, hyperuricemia, hyperglycemia, and hyperlipidemia. As a result of drug-induced diuresis, hypokalemia occurs in 15% to 20% of patients taking low-dose thiazide diuretics; therefore, potassium supplements are needed by some patients. Combination therapy with thiazide and potassium-sparing diuretics (e.g., hydrochlorothiazide [HydroDIURIL] and triamterene [Dyrenium]) may be prudent when potassium levels are less than 4.0 mEq/L and the patient is taking a thiazide diuretic or when a low potassium level may potentiate drug toxicity, as in patients concurrently taking digoxin (Lanoxin). Other side effects include tinnitus, paresthesias, abdominal cramps, nausea, vomiting, diarrhea, muscle cramps, weakness, and sexual dysfunction.

Loop Diuretics

Loop diuretics are indicated in the presence of edema associated with congestive heart failure, hepatic cirrhosis, and renal disease. (See **Table 19.2.**) This class of drug is useful when

TABLE 19.2 Overview of Selected Antihypertensive Agents

Generic (Trade) Name and Dosage	Selected Adverse Events	Contraindications	Special Considerations
Selected Diuretics			
THIAZIDE AND THIAZIDE-LIKE			
chlorthalidone (Hygroton) 12.5–100 mg qd	Hyperuricemia, hypokalemia, hypomagnesemia, hyperglycemia, hyponatremia, hypercalcemia, hypercholesterolemia, hypertriglyceridemia, pancreatitis, rashes and other allergic reactions	High doses are relatively contraindicated in patients with hyperlipidemia, gout, and diabetes.	Preferred in patients with creatinine clearance >30 mL/min
hydrochlorothiazide (HydroDIURIL, Microzide) 12.5–25 mg qd	Same as chlorthalidone	Same as chlorthalidone	Same as chlorthalidone
indapamide (Lozol) 1.25–5 mg qd	Same as chlorthalidone	Same as chlorthalidone	Same as chlorthalidone
metolazone (Zaroxolyn) 2.5–5 mg qd	Less or no hypercholesterolemia	Same as chlorthalidone	Same as chlorthalidone
LOOP DIURETICS			
bumetanide (Bumex) 0.5–5 mg bid-tid	Dehydration, circulatory collapse, hypokalemia, hyponatremia, hypomagnesemia, hyperglycemia, metabolic alkalosis, hyperuricemia (short duration of action, no hypercalcemia)	High doses are relatively contraindicated in patients with hyperlipidemia, gout, and diabetes.	Effective in patients with creatinine clearance <30 mL/min
ethacrynic acid (Edecrin) 25–100 mg bid-tid	Same as bumetanide (only nonsulfonamide diuretic, ototoxicity)	Same as bumetanide	Same as bumetanide
furosemide (Lasix) 20–320 mg qd	Same as bumetanide	Same as bumetanide	Same as bumetanide
torsemide (Demadex) 5–20 mg qd	Short duration of action, no hypercalcemia	Same as bumetanide	Same as bumetanide
POTASSIUM-SPARING DIURETICS			
amiloride (Midamor) 5–10 mg qd-bid	Hyperkalemia, GI disturbances, rash	High doses are relatively contraindicated in patients with hyperlipidemia, gout, and diabetes.	Same as bumetanide
spironolactone (Aldactone) 12.5–100 mg qd-bid	Hyperkalemia, GI disturbances, rash, gynecomastia	Same as amiloride	Ideal in patients with heart failure
triamterene (Dyrenium) 50–150 mg qd-bid	Hyperkalemia, GI disturbances, nephrolithiasis	Same as amiloride	Same as bumetanide
Beta-Adrenergic Blocking Agents			
SELECTED BETA BLOCKERS			
atenolol (Tenormin) 25–100 mg qd	Fatigue, depression, bradycardia, decreased exercise tolerance, congestive heart failure, aggravates peripheral arterial insufficiency, bronchospasm; masks symptoms of and delays recovery from hypoglycemia, Raynaud's phenomenon, insomnia, vivid dreams or hallucinations, acute mental disorder, impotence; increased serum triglycerides, decreased high-density lipoprotein cholesterol; sudden withdrawal can lead to exacerbation of angina and myocardial infarction	Contraindicated in first trimester of pregnancy; heart failure (except carvedilol and metoprolol); relatively contraindicated in patients with asthma, diabetes; hyperlipidemia	Abrupt cessation should be avoided; taper the dose of beta blocker over a 2-wk period. Advantageous in patients with angina, tachycardia, acute myocardial infarction; hypertensive patients with left ventricular hypertrophy

(continued)

TABLE 19.2   Overview of Selected Antihypertensive Agents (Continued)

Generic (Trade) Name and Dosage	Selected Adverse Events	Contraindications	Special Considerations
betaxolol (Kerlone) 5–20 mg qd	Same as atenolol	Same as atenolol	Same as atenolol
bisoprolol (Zebeta) 2.5–10 mg qd	Same as atenolol	Same as atenolol	Same as atenolol
timolol (Blocadren) 10–60 mg bid	Same as atenolol	Same as atenolol	Same as atenolol
metoprolol tartrate (Lopressor) 50–100 qd-bid	Same as atenolol	Same as atenolol	Same as atenolol
nadolol (Corgard) 40–120 mg qd	Same as atenolol	Same as atenolol	Same as atenolol
propranolol (Inderal, Inderal LA) 40–160 mg bid 60–180 mg bid	Same as atenolol	Same as atenolol	Same as atenolol
metoprolol succinate (Lopressor, Toprol-XL) 50–100 mg qd-bid	Same as atenolol	Same as atenolol	Same as atenolol
pindolol (Visken) 10–40 mg bid	Same as atenolol, but with less resting bradycardia and lipid changes	Same as atenolol	Same as atenolol
penbutolol sulfate (Levatol) 10–40 mg qd	Same as atenolol, but with less resting bradycardia and lipid changes	Same as atenolol	Same as atenolol
acebutolol (Sectral) 200–600 mg bid	Same as atenolol, but with less resting bradycardia and lipid changes; positive antinuclear antibody test and occasional drug-induced lupus	Same as atenolol	Same as atenolol
carteolol (Cartrol) 2.5–10 mg qd	Same as atenolol, but with less resting bradycardia and lipid changes	Same as atenolol	Same as atenolol
COMBINED BLOCKERS			
carvedilol (Coreg) 12.5–50 mg bid	Similar to atenolol but more postural hypotension, bronchospasm	Same as atenolol	Same as atenolol
labetalol (Normodyne, Trandate) 200–800 mg bid	Hepatotoxicity	Same as atenolol	Same as atenolol; does not affect serum lipids
Direct Renin Inhibitor			
aliskiren (Tekturna) 150–300 mg daily		Contraindicated in pregnancy	
Selected Angiotensin-Converting Enzyme Inhibitors			
benazepril (Lotensin) 10–40 mg qd-bid	Common: cough; hypotension, particularly with a diuretic or volume depletion; hyperkalemia, rash, loss of taste, leukopenia, angioedema, neutropenia, and agranulocytosis in <1% of patients	Contraindicated in pregnancy; avoid in patients with bilateral renal artery stenosis or unilateral stenosis	First line in hypertensive diabetic patients with proteinuria; congestive heart failure patients with systolic dysfunction. Check potassium levels within 1 mo of initiating therapy. May decrease excretion of lithium
captopril (Capoten) 25–100 mg bid-tid	Same as benazepril; rash in 10% of patients; loss of taste	Same as benazepril	Same as benazepril
enalapril maleate (Vasotec) 2.5–40 mg qd-bid	Same as benazepril	Same as benazepril	Same as benazepril

Drug (dose)	Side effects	Precautions/Contraindications	Nursing considerations
fosinopril (Monopril) 10–40 mg qd			Same as benazepril
lisinopril (Prinivil, Zestril) 10–40 mg qd			Same as benazepril
moexipril (Univasc) 7.5–30 mg qd			Same as benazepril
quinapril (Accupril) 10–80 mg qd			Same as benazepril
ramipril (Altace) 2.5–20 mg qd			Same as benazepril
trandolapril (Mavik) 1–4 mg qd			Same as benazepril
Angiotensin II Receptor Blockers			
losartan (Cozaar) 25–100 mg qd-bid	Similar to ACE inhibitors but does not cause cough; angioedema (very rare), hyperkalemia		
valsartan (Diovan) 80–320 mg qd			
candesartan cilexetil (Atacand) 8–32 mg qd			
irbesartan (Avapro) 150–300 mg qd			
telmisartan (Micardis) 20–80 mg qd			
eprosartan (Teveten) 400–800 mg qd-bid			
olmesartan (Benicar) 20–40 mg qd			
Calcium Channel Blocking Agents			
NONDIHYDROPYRIDINES			
diltiazem HC1 (Cardizem SR, Cardizem CD) (Dilacor XR) (Tiazac) 180–420 mg qd (Diltia XT) 120–480 mg qd Cardizemla 120–540 mg qd	Dizziness, headache, edema, constipation (especially verapamil); lupus-like rash with diltiazem; conduction defects, worsening of systolic dysfunction, gingival hyperplasia (nausea, headache)	Avoid in patients with atrioventricular node dysfunction (second- or third-degree heart block), or left ventricular (systolic) dysfunction.	Swallow whole; do not chew, divide, or crush. Hypertensive diabetic patients with proteinuria. Increased cyclosporine levels may occur with concomitant use.
verapamil HC1 (Isoptin SR, Calan SR, Verelan) 120–480 mg qd (Covera HS) 180–480 mg qd	Constipation	Same as diltiazem	Swallow whole; do not chew, divide, or crush. Hypertensive diabetic patients with proteinuria
DIHYDROPYRIDINES			
amlodipine (Norvasc) 2.5–10 mg qd	Dizziness, headache, rash, peripheral edema, flushing, headache, gingival hypertrophy		Swallow whole; do not chew, divide, or crush. Elderly patients with isolated systolic hypertension
felodipine (Plendil) 2.5–20 mg qd	Same as amlodipine		Swallow whole; do not chew, divide, or crush.
isradipine (DynaCirc) 2.5–10 mg bid (DynaCirc CR) 5–10 mg bid	Same as amlodipine		Swallow whole; do not chew, divide, or crush.
nicardipine (Cardene SR) 60–120 mg bid	Same as amlodipine		Swallow whole; do not chew, divide, or crush.
nifedipine (Procardia XL, Adalat CC) 30–60 mg qd	Same as amlodipine		Swallow whole; do not chew, divide, or crush. Do not use sublingually.

(continued)

TABLE 19.2 Overview of Selected Antihypertensive Agents (Continued)

Generic (Trade) Name and Dosage	Selected Adverse Events	Contraindications	Special Considerations
nisoldipine (Sular) 10–40 mg qd	Same as amlodipine		Swallow whole; do not chew, divide, or crush.
Other			
ALPHA BLOCKERS			
doxazosin (Cardura) 1–16 mg qd	First-dose phenomenon, postural hypotension, lassitude, vivid dreams, depression, headache, palpitations, fluid retention, weakness, priapism, drowsiness		Administer initially at bedtime; start with low dose and titrate slowly. Ideal for hypertensive patients with benign prostatic hypertrophy
prazosin (Minipress) 2–20 mg bid-tid	Same as doxazosin		Same as doxazosin
terazosin (Hytrin) 1–20 mg qd-bid	Same as doxazosin		Same as doxazosin
CENTRAL AGONISTS			
clonidine (Catapres) 0.1–0.8 mg bid-tid	Sedation, dry mouth, bradycardia, withdrawal hypertension, bradycardia, heart block	Avoid prescribing for noncompliant patients.	Do not stop therapy abruptly without consulting health care provider first.
Transdermal (Catapres TTS) one patch weekly (0.1–0.3 mg/d)			
guanabenz (Wytensin) 4–64 mg bid	Similar to clonidine	Similar to clonidine	Tolerance of alcohol may decrease.
guanfacine (Tenex) 0.5–2.0 mg qd	Similar to clonidine	Similar to clonidine	Take at bedtime. Tolerance of alcohol may decrease.
methyldopa (Aldomet) 250–1000 mg bid	Drowsiness, sedation, fatigue, depression, dry mouth, orthostatic hypotension, bradycardia, heart block, autoimmune disorders, including colitis; hepatitis, hemolytic anemia <1% of patients		Urine may darken after voiding when exposed to air.
DIRECT VASODILATORS			
hydralazine (Apresoline) 25–100 mg bid	Tachycardia, aggravation of angina, headache, dizziness, fluid retention, nasal congestion, lupus-like syndrome, dermatitis, drug fever, hepatitis, peripheral neuropathy		May precipitate angina in patients with coronary artery disease
minoxidil (Loniten) 2.5–80 mg qd-bid	Tachycardia, aggravation of angina, dizziness, fluid retention, hypertrichosis	Avoid in patients taking nitrates.	Restrict to patients with refractory hypertension.
ADRENERGIC ANTAGONISTS			
guanadrel (Hylorel) 10–75 mg bid	Postural hypotension, exercise hypotension, diarrhea, weight gain, syncope, retrograde ejaculation		Restrict to patients with refractory hypertension.
guanethidine (Ismelin) 10–50 mg qd	Similar to guanadrel, but greater incidence of diarrhea		Maximal effect not seen for 2–4 wk. Avoid doses above 0.25 mg daily in patients with depression.
reserpine (Serpasil) 0.5–0.25–0.1 mg qd	Nasal stuffiness, drowsiness, GI disturbances, bradycardia, nightmares with high doses, fluid retention, depression, activation of peptic ulcer	Relatively contraindicated in depression	

greater diuretic potential is desired. In general, loop diuretics should be reserved for hypertensive patients with chronic renal insufficiency.

Furosemide and ethacrynic acid inhibit the reabsorption of sodium and chloride, not only in proximal and distal tubules but also in the loop of Henle. In contrast, bumetanide is more chloruretic than natriuretic and may have an additional action in the proximal tubule.

Contraindications

Loop diuretics are contraindicated in patients who are anuric, in patients hypersensitive to these compounds or to sulfonylureas, and in patients with hepatic coma or in states of severe electrolyte depletion. Ethacrynic acid is contraindicated in infants.

Adverse Events

Loop diuretics may cause the same side effects as thiazides, although the effects on serum lipids and glucose are not as significant, and hypocalcemia may occur instead. The metabolic abnormalities, such as hyperlipidemia and hyperglycemia, usually occur with high doses of diuretics and can be avoided by using low doses of the drug. Loop diuretics may lead to electrolyte and volume depletion more readily than thiazides; they have a short duration of action, but the thiazide diuretics are more effective than loop diuretics in reducing BP in patients with normal renal function. Therefore, loop diuretics should be reserved for hypertensive patients with renal dysfunction (serum creatinine of more than 2.5).

Potassium-Sparing Diuretics

In the kidney, potassium is filtered at the glomerulus and then absorbed parallel to sodium throughout the proximal tubule and thick ascending limb of the loop of Henle, so that only minor amounts reach the distal convoluted tubule. As a result, potassium appearing in urine is secreted at the distal tubule and collecting duct. The potassium-sparing diuretics interfere with sodium reabsorption at the distal tubule, thus decreasing potassium secretion. (See **Table 19.2.**)

The Randomized Spironolactone Evaluation Study (RALES) showed the benefits of low-dose spironolactone (Aldactone) to improve morbidity and mortality rates in patients with severe heart failure. Potassium-sparing diuretics have the potential for causing hyperkalemia and hyponatremia, especially in patients with renal insufficiency or diabetes and in patients receiving concurrent treatment with an ACE inhibitor, NSAIDs, or potassium supplements.

Contraindications

Contraindications are the same as for the diuretic class. Additionally, aldosterone antagonists and potassium-sparing diuretics can cause hyperkalemia and hyponatremia and should be avoided in patents with serum potassium levels of more than 5 mEq/L.

Adverse Events

Side effects of spironolactone include gynecomastia, hirsutism, and menstrual irregularities.

Beta-Adrenergic Blockers

Mechanism of Action

Beta-1 receptors, located predominantly in the heart and kidney, regulate heart rate, renin release, and cardiac contractility. (See **Table 19.2.**) Beta-2 receptors, located in the lungs, liver, pancreas, and arteriolar smooth muscle, regulate bronchodilation and vasodilation. Beta blockers reduce BP by blocking central and peripheral beta receptors, which results in decreased cardiac output and sympathetic outflow. Blockade of beta-1 receptors on the surface of juxtaglomerular cells located on the afferent arteriole of the kidney results in reduced renin release and decreased stimulation of the RAAS.

Despite several pharmacologic differences in the available beta blockers, they are all effective in treating hypertension. Beta blockers that bind specifically to beta-1 receptors are referred to as *cardioselective* because they do not block beta-2 receptors and therefore do not stimulate bronchoconstriction. These agents, which include metoprolol (Lopressor), betaxolol (Kerlone), atenolol (Tenormin), acebutolol (Sectral), and bisoprolol (Zebeta), may be safer than nonselective beta blockers for patients with asthma, chronic obstructive pulmonary disease, and peripheral vascular disease. At higher doses, selective beta blockers lose cardioselectivity and may aggravate a preexisting condition.

Some beta blockers possess intrinsic sympathomimetic activity (ISA); these agents are partial beta-receptor agonists that reduce heart rate and contractility during excessive sympathetic outflow. In resting states, heart rate and contractility are maintained. Typical medications include pindolol (Visken), penbutolol (Levatol), carteolol (Cartrol), and acebutolol.

Studies suggest that beta blockers may decrease sympathetic activity involved with the progression of heart failure. For example, carvedilol (Coreg) decreased mortality rates in patients with heart failure. Moreover, carvedilol and metoprolol decreased ventricular remodeling (which results in LVH). Beta blockers should be used only in patients with stable congestive heart failure. Practitioners should refer any patient with heart failure to a cardiologist for evaluation of therapy.

Patients should be cautioned not to discontinue therapy abruptly. The dose of beta blockers should be tapered gradually over 14 days to prevent withdrawal symptoms, which include unstable angina, myocardial infarction (MI), or even death in patients with underlying cardiovascular disease. Patients without coronary artery disease may experience sinus tachycardia, palpations, increased sweating, and fatigue.

Contraindications

Beta blockers should be avoided in patients who have sinus bradycardia, asthma, chronic obstructive pulmonary disease, second- or third-degree heart block, or overt cardiac failure. Non-ISA beta blockers are the preferred agents for treating hypertension in patients with coexisting coronary artery disease, and especially in patients after MI. Beta blockers should be used cautiously in patients with resting ischemia or severe claudication secondary to peripheral vascular disease, reactive airway disease, systolic congestive heart failure, diabetes mellitus, or depression.

Adverse Events

The most common side effects of beta blockers are fatigue, drowsiness, dizziness, bronchospasm, nausea, and vomiting. Serious side effects include bradycardia, atrioventricular conduction abnormalities, and the development of congestive heart failure.

Renin Inhibitors

Mechanism of Action

Renin inhibitors block the conversion of angiotensinogen to angiotensin I. Angiotensin I suppression decreases the formation of angiotensin II. Angiotensin II functions within the RAAS as a negative inhibitory feedback mediator within the renal parenchyma to suppresses the further release of renin. The reduction in angiotensin II levels suppresses this feedback loop, leading to further increased plasma renin concentrations and subsequent low plasma renin activity. The first effective oral direct renin inhibitor, aliskiren (Tekturna), was approved by the U.S. Food and Drug Administration in March 2007. Aliskiren lowers BP to a degree comparable to most other agents. There is no clinical trial data of aliskiren on outcomes in hypertension, diabetes, or CVD.

Contraindications

There are no contraindications listed in the manufacturer's labeling. However, this medication should be avoided during pregnancy because drugs that act directly on the renin-angiotensin system can cause fetal and neonatal morbidity.

Adverse Events

Significant adverse events include diarrhea and, infrequently, angioedema.

ACE Inhibitors

Mechanism of Action

ACE inhibitors such as captopril, enalapril, and lisinopril exert an antihypertensive effect by inhibiting ACE, which is responsible for converting angiotensin I to angiotensin II, a potent vasoconstrictor. (See **Table 19.2.**) ACE inhibitors also inhibit the degradation of bradykinin and increase the synthesis of vasodilating prostaglandins. This class of antihypertensive agents is indicated as first-line therapy in hypertensive diabetic patients who have proteinuria. ACE inhibitors decrease morbidity and mortality rates in patients with congestive heart failure and systolic dysfunction.

Contraindications

ACE inhibitors should be avoided in patients with bilateral renal artery stenosis or unilateral stenosis because of the risk of acute renal failure. They are also contraindicated in patients who have experienced angioedema and during pregnancy because of their teratogenic effects.

Adverse Events

The most common side effects associated with ACE inhibitors include chronic dry cough, rashes (most common with captopril [Capoten]), and dizziness. Hyperkalemia can occur in patients with renal disease or diabetes. Angioedema is a rare but dangerous side effect that occurs most frequently in African-Americans; it is reversible on discontinuation of the agent (Brown, et al., 1996; Burkhart, et al., 1996; He, et al., 1999). Laryngeal edema, another rare adverse effect, is life-threatening and requires immediate medical attention.

Angiotensin II Receptor Blockers

ARBs block the vasoconstriction and aldosterone-secreting effects of angiotensin II by selectively blocking the binding of angiotensin II to the angiotensin II receptor found in many tissues. (See **Table 19.2.**) They are indicated for patients with hypertension, nephropathy in type 2 diabetes, and heart failure and those who cannot tolerate the side effects associated with ACE inhibitors.

The results of the Losartan Intervention for Endpoint reduction in hypertension study (LIFE) suggest that losartan is more effective than atenolol in reducing cardiovascular morbidity and mortality in diabetic patients with hypertension and left ventricular hypertrophy. Available ARBs are losartan (Cozaar), valsartan (Diovan), candesartan (Atacand), telmisartan (Micardis), eprosartan (Teveten), olmesartan (Benicar), and irbesartan (Avapro). The incidence of cough and hyperkalemia associated with this class of drugs is lower than with ACE inhibitors.

Contraindications

Caution should be used in patients with renal and hepatic function impairment. Angioedema can also be seen with ARB therapy, but with much less frequency than with ACE inhibitors. There should be some justification (heart failure or proteinuric nephropathic) for the use of ARBs in patients having experienced ACE inhibitor–related angioedema.

Adverse Events

Adverse reactions include dizziness, upper respiratory tract infections, cough, viral infection, fatigue, diarrhea, pain, sinusitis, pharyngitis, and rhinitis. Like ACE inhibitors, ARBs are contraindicated in pregnancy.

Calcium Channel Blockers

CCBs share the ability to inhibit the movement of calcium ions across the cell membrane. (See **Table 19.2.**) The effects on the cardiovascular system include depression of mechanical contraction of myocardial and smooth muscle and depression of both impulse formation and conduction velocity. The result is muscle relaxation and vasodilation. Common CCBs, such as verapamil (Calan) and diltiazem (Cardizem), decrease heart rate and slow cardiac conduction at the atrioventricular node. The dihydropyridines (amlodipine [Norvasc], felodipine [Plendil], nifedipine [Procardia XL], nicardipine [Cardene SR], nisoldipine [Sular], and isradipine [DynaCirc]) are potent vasodilators. CCBs are effective as monotherapy and are especially effective in African-American patients. CCBs are indicated for treating hypertension associated with ischemic heart disease. The long-acting dihydropyridines are second-line therapy for elderly patients with isolated systolic hypertension. CCBs are similar in antihypertensive effectiveness but differ in other pharmacodynamic effects.

Contraindications

First-generation CCBs such as verapamil and diltiazem may accelerate the progression of congestive heart failure in a patient with cardiac dysfunction. Therefore, these agents should be avoided unless they are being used to treat angina, hypertension, or arrhythmia. Two trials with amlodipine in patients with severe heart failure showed that this agent is safe (Tierney, et al., 2004).

Diltiazem and verapamil should also be avoided in patients with atrioventricular node dysfunction (second- or third-degree heart block) or left ventricular (systolic) dysfunction when the ejection fraction measures less than 45%. Short-acting nifedipine should not be used for treating essential hypertension or hypertensive emergencies because of its association with erratic fluctuations in BP and reflex tachycardia.

Adverse Events

The most common side effects of CCBs are headache, peripheral edema, and bradycardia. The dihydropyridine agents (nifedipine, nicardipine, isradipine, felodipine, nisoldipine, and amlodipine) produce symptoms of vasodilation, such as headache, flushing, palpations, and peripheral edema. Other side effects of nifedipine include dizziness, gingival hyperplasia, mood changes, and various gastrointestinal (GI) complaints. Nifedipine may cause reflex tachycardia as a result of stimulating the baroreceptors in response to an acute drop in BP.

Diltiazem and verapamil can cause GI upset, peripheral edema, and hypotension. Rare side effects include bradycardia, atrioventricular block, and congestive heart failure. Verapamil can cause constipation in the elderly.

Peripheral Alpha-1 Receptor Blockers

Doxazosin (Cardura), prazosin (Minipress), and terazosin (Hytrin) are selective alpha-1 receptor blockers that are effective in patients with benign prostatic hypertrophy. (See **Table 19.2.**) Peripheral alpha-1 receptor blockers act peripherally by dilating both arterioles and veins, causing relaxation of smooth muscle. In clinical studies, this class of antihypertensive agents is associated with a small decrease in LDL and cholesterol.

Contraindications

In the presence of cardiovascular disease, alpha-1 receptor blockers should be avoided, as the ALLHAT study showed that these patients had an increase in mortality. The use of tadalafil (Cialis) and vardenafil (Levitra) is contraindicated with the use of alpha-1 receptor blockers. Sildenafil (Viagra) should be avoided within 4 hours of administration of alpha-1 receptor blockers due to an increased risk of symptomatic hypotension.

Adverse Events

The most common side effect associated with this class of antihypertensive medications is the first-dose phenomenon, which consists of dizziness or faintness, palpitations, or syncope. These agents should be administered initially at bedtime and the dosage should be adjusted slowly. With chronic administration, even at low doses, fluid and sodium accumulate, requiring concurrent diuretic therapy. Other side effects include vivid dreams and depression.

Central Alpha-2 Receptor Agonists

Central alpha-2 agonists stimulate alpha-2-adrenergic receptors in the brain, resulting in decreased sympathetic outflow, cardiac output, and peripheral resistance. (See **Table 19.2.**) These agents may cause fluid retention and in most cases should be used in combination with a diuretic. Clonidine (Catapres), methyldopa (Aldomet), guanabenz (Wytensin), and guanfacine (Tenex) should not be used as initial monotherapy. Abrupt cessation of alpha-2 agonist therapy may result in a compensatory increase in the norepinephrine level, which in turn raises BP. This effect is commonly referred to as rebound hypertension (JNC VI, 1997).

Adverse Events

These agents may cause fluid retention, sedation, and dry mouth. Also, the first-dose effect of dizziness and syncope are possible.

Direct Vasodilators

The direct vasodilators hydralazine (Apresoline) and minoxidil (Loniten) cause arteriolar smooth muscle relaxation, resulting in reduced BP. (See **Table 19.2.**) Direct vasodilators should be reserved for patients with essential or severe hypertension.

Both hydralazine and minoxidil may cause fluid retention and reflex tachycardia. Their use should be combined with a diuretic and a beta blocker or other agent (clonidine, diltiazem, or verapamil) that slows the heart rate.

Contraindications

Hydralazine is contraindicated in patients with coronary artery disease and mitral valvular rheumatic heart disease. Minoxidil is contraindicated in patients with pheochromocytoma, acute MI, and dissecting aortic aneurysm.

Adverse Events

Hydralazine is associated with a lupus-like syndrome that is dose-related at dosages greater than 300 mg/day. Other adverse reactions include dermatitis, drug fever, and peripheral neuropathy. Minoxidil may cause a drug-induced hirsutism, which is unacceptable to most female patients.

Adrenergic Antagonists

Reserpine (Serpasil), guanethidine (Ismelin), and guanadrel (Hylorel) inhibit the sympathetic system by depleting norepinephrine stores in the central nervous system. (See **Table 19.2.**) This results in a decrease in peripheral vascular resistance and a reduction in BP. In patients who use these agents, depression may result from decreased catecholamine and serotonin levels in the central nervous system. Reserpine's use is limited because of its side effect profile, which includes depression, impotence, diarrhea, bradycardia, drowsiness, and nasal stuffiness.

Guanadrel and guanethidine also produce numerous adverse effects, such as diarrhea, impotence, orthostatic hypotension, and syncope. They should be used with caution.

SELECTING THE MOST APPROPRIATE AGENT

First-Line Therapy

First-line therapy with diuretics is preferred in most cases of stage 1 hypertension. (See **Figure 19-1.**) The National Heart, Lung, and Blood Institute and the JNC VII endorsed the result of ALLHAT using diuretics as monotherapy in preference of other antihypertensive agents. BP was brought under control in 60% of the participants in the ALLHAT trail. ACE inhibitors, ARBs, beta blockers, CCBs, or combinations may be considered if the BP goal is not reached. However, patients with concomitant diseases may be treated with other agents as the first line, depending on the compelling indication (**Table 19.3**). The following discussion addresses some of the more common compelling indications.

Ischemic Heart Disease

Ischemic heart disease is the most common form of target organ damage associated with hypertension. For patients who also have stable angina, the first choice agent is a beta blocker followed by a long-acting CCB. In patients with acute coronary syndrome, a beta blocker and an ACE inhibitor are the initial therapy. Patients recovering from a MI are candidates for treatment with ACE inhibitors, beta blockers, and/or aldosterone antagonists. Aggressive therapy with lipid management and aspirin is also indicated in these patients.

Heart Failure

Heart failure (systolic or diastolic ventricular dysfunction) results from systolic hypertension and ischemic heart disease. Preventive measures for those at high risk include BP and cholesterol control. ACE inhibitors and beta blockers are recommended in asymptomatic individuals. For patients with symptomatic ventricular dysfunction of end-stage heart disease, ACE inhibitors, beta blockers, ARBs, and aldosterone blockers are recommended, along with loop diuretics (JNC VII, 2003).

The Metoprolol CR/XL Randomized Intervention Trial in Heart Failure (MERIT-HF) and the Carvedilol Prospective Randomized Cumulative Survival (COPERNICUS) trial showed favorable results using beta blockers to treat heart failure. Chapter 22 gives more detail.

Diabetes Mellitus

In patients with diabetic hypertension, the targeted BP goal is 130/80; achieving this goal usually requires a combination of two or more drugs. Thiazide diuretics, beta blockers, ACE inhibitors, ARBs, and CCBs are beneficial in reducing the incidence of cardiovascular disease and stroke. Studies have shown favorable effects of ACE inhibitors and ARBs on the progression of diabetic nephropathy and cardiovascular disease and in the reduction of albuminuria. Chapter 50 gives more detail.

Chronic Kidney Disease

Chronic kidney disease is defined by either reduced excretory function with an estimated glomerular filtration rate of 60 mL/min per 1.73 m^2 (creatinine of above 1.5 mg/dL in men or above 1.3 mg/dL in women) or the presence of albuminuria (above 300 mg/d or 200 mg albumin per gram of creatinine). Aggressive BP management with three or more drugs is required to reach a target BP goal of less than 130/80 mm Hg and to slow the deterioration of renal function. ACE inhibitors and ARBs offer the best renal protection, as recommended by JNC VII, the National Kidney Foundation, and the American Diabetes Association.

Cerebrovascular Disease

The rate of recurrent stroke is lowered by the combination of an ACE inhibitor and a thiazide-type diuretic. The HOPE Study and the Perindopril Protection Against Recurrent Stroke Study (PROGRESS) provided compelling evidence that treatment with an ACE inhibitor or an ACE inhibitor and a diuretic can further reduce the risk of stroke.

Obesity and the Metabolic Syndrome

Obesity is a risk factor for the development of hypertension and cardiovascular disease. The Adult Treatment Panel III guidelines for cholesterol management define metabolic syndrome as abdominal obesity (more than 40 inches in men, more than 35 inches in women), glucose intolerance (fasting glucose of above 110), BP of at least 130/85 mm Hg, triglyceride level of more than 150, and a low level of high-density lipoprotein cholesterol (<40 mg/dL in men or <50 mg/dL in women). Aggressive lifestyle modification should be pursued in all patients with the metabolic syndrome, and appropriate drug therapy should be instituted for each of its components.

Left Ventricular Hypertrophy

LVH increases the risk of subsequent cardiovascular disease. Aggressive BP management as well as weight loss and sodium

TABLE 19.3 Compelling Indications

High-Risk Conditions with Compelling Indication	Recommended Drugs					
	Diuretic	Beta Blocker	ACE Inhibitor	ARB	CCB	Aldosterone Antagonist
Heart failure	•	•	•	•		•
Post–myocardial infarction		•	•			•
High coronary disease risk	•	•	•		•	
Diabetes	•	•	•	•	•	
Chronic kidney disease			•	•		
Recurrent stroke prevention	•		•			
Atrial fibrillation		•			•	

restriction can slow the regression of LVH. Treatment with all classes of antihypertensive agents is acceptable except for direct vasodilators such as hydralazine or minoxidil.

Peripheral Arterial Disease

Peripheral arterial disease is equivalent in risk to ischemic heart disease. Treatment can include any class of antihypertensive drugs. Aspirin should be used and other risk factors should be treated aggressively.

Benign Prostatic Hypertrophy (BPH)

BPH can be treated with an alpha antagonist (doxazosin, prazosin, terazosin). The preferred drug for BPH is tamsulosin (Flomax). The ALLHAT study found alpha blockers increased the mortality rate in cardiovascular disease.

Second-Line Therapy

When the patient's systolic BP exceeds 160 mm Hg (stage 2 hypertension), antihypertensive treatment begins with combination therapy. Combination therapy can include a diuretic with an ACE inhibitor, ARB, CCB, or beta blocker, or any other combination. The second agent should be a drug from another class; typically, a diuretic is one of the two agents, unless other reasons prohibit its use or a compelling indication exists. Low-dose combination therapy has gained wide support due to its efficacy, ease of administration, compliance rate, and decreased risk of side effects. If the patient's BP remains elevated, dosages should be adjusted and additional drugs included until the goal BP is achieved.

Special Population Considerations

Pediatric

Treatment of hypertension in children can be approached in the same manner as for adults, with the appropriate agent selected for specific indications. Dosages of antihypertensive medication should be adjusted for children.

Geriatric

The Trial of Nonpharmacological Interventions in the Elderly (TONE) showed that in older patients with hypertension, BP can be reduced by low-sodium diets and weight loss. In some instances, patients could discontinue their antihypertensive medications or reduce the number of medications required to remain normotensive (Sander, 2002).

Elderly patients are very sensitive to medications that cause sympathetic inhibition and are at greater risk of becoming volume depleted than their younger counterparts. Decreased renal and hepatic function increases the risk of adverse events in this population. Antihypertensive medications should be started at half the recommended starting dose to decrease the risk of adverse effects.

Diuretics and beta blockers are effective in elderly patients because they have been shown to reduce morbidity and mortality rates. Patients with isolated systolic hypertension should start hypertensive therapy with a diuretic unless there is a compelling reason to avoid its use. The long-acting dihydropyridine CCBs are also effective and are an alternative in these patients.

Clinical trials have demonstrated that in older patients with isolated systolic hypertension, low diastolic BP was associated with a higher mortality rate for any given level of systolic BP.

Women

There are no significant differences in BP response between the sexes. Women taking oral contraceptives may have an increase in BP, and the risk of hypertension may increase with the duration of oral contraceptive use. If hypertension develops as a result of oral contraceptive use, an alternate contraception method should be used. Because of the risk of stroke associated with oral contraceptive use and cigarette smoking, women taking oral contraceptives should be encouraged not to smoke cigarettes, and women older than age 35 should not take oral contraceptives if they continue to smoke.

Women diagnosed with hypertension before pregnancy can continue taking antihypertensive agents throughout pregnancy. Most but not all antihypertensive agents are safe for use during pregnancy. ACE inhibitors and ARBs should be avoided during pregnancy because they are teratogenic. Beta blockers should also be avoided during early pregnancy because of the risk of fetal growth retardation, but beta blockers may be used during the second or third trimester. Methyldopa is recommended for women who are diagnosed with hypertension during pregnancy.

African-Americans

The incidence of hypertension and hypertension-related complications is believed to be higher in African-Americans than in any ethnic group. Some African-Americans experience hypertension before age 10. This is attributed to two major risk factors: obesity and inactivity. Other risk factors include a diet high in sodium and low in potassium. This has resulted in the greatest incidence of stroke, end-stage renal disease, cardiovascular disease, and death in this population. African-Americans who are diagnosed and treated have a lower incidence of complications.

African-Americans have physiologic characteristics that contribute to this risk, including low circulating renin levels with excessive levels of angiotensin II; endothelial dysfunction as a result of reduced bradykinin and nitric oxide; abnormal sympathetic nervous system activation; and higher levels of intracellular calcium stores. African-Americans are more responsive to monotherapy with diuretics. Results from the ALLHAT found that chlorthalidone and amlodipine were superior to ACE inhibitors in treating African-Americans (Papademetriou, et al., 2003). Alpha blockers should not be used as initial monotherapy. ACE inhibitors may induce angioedema, which occurs two to four times more frequently in African-Americans.

Diabetic Patients

Diuretics are underprescribed in patients with diabetes mellitus and hyperlipidemia because of the risk of increasing insulin resistance. However, the SHEP trial showed that morbidity and mortality rates were reduced in diabetic patients treated with low-dose diuretics (Moser, 1998; SHEP Cooperative Research Group, 1991). The goal BP in diabetic patients with hypertension is 130/85 mm Hg.

HYPERTENSIVE EMERGENCY

Hypertensive emergency or malignant hypertension is defined as a severe elevation in diastolic BP, usually higher than 120 mm Hg, in the presence of target-organ damage. Immediate treatment with an intravenous antihypertensive agent is needed to salvage viable tissue. The marked elevation in BP results in arteriolar fibrinoid necrosis, endothelial damage, platelet and fibrin deposition in the media of smooth muscle, and loss of autoregulatory function. This results in end-organ ischemia such as encephalopathy, MI, unstable angina, pulmonary edema, eclampsia, stroke, intracranial hemorrhage, life-threatening arterial bleeding, or aortic dissection. These patients require hospitalization and parenteral drug therapy. How rapidly BP should be lowered, and to what level, remains controversial.

The drug of choice to treat hypertensive emergencies depends on the clinical situation. Commonly used medications include nitroprusside, intravenous nitroglycerine, diazoxide, trimethaphan, labetalol, and hydralazine.

In cases of hypertensive urgency without evidence of target-organ damage, the BP can be reduced over 24 hours. Fast-acting oral agents, such as captopril and clonidine (**Table 19.4**), are commonly used. Most patients with hypertensive urgency are those who are newly diagnosed or who do not adhere to the therapeutic regimen. After BP is lowered, the patient's drug regimen is assessed to determine possible causes of nonadherence, such as adverse effects that interfere with the patient's lifestyle or a complex regimen that could be simplified.

MONITORING PATIENT RESPONSE

Follow-Up and Monitoring

Patients should be followed at 1-month intervals after the initiation of treatment until the goal BP is attained. Patients with a higher BP may need more frequent visits until the target BP is achieved. Patients with complicated conditions should be seen more often. Once the desired BP is attained, patients should return for visits at 3- to 6-month intervals. The patients' efforts and lifestyle modifications should be discussed at each visit. Serum creatinine and potassium levels should be monitored once or twice a year in patients taking antihypertensive medications.

Patients with stage 1 or stage 2 hypertension should be scheduled for a follow-up visit 2 to 4 weeks after initiation of

TABLE 19.4	**Oral Drugs Commonly Used to Treat Hypertensive Urgencies**				
Drug	**Dose/Route**	**Onset of Action**	**Duration of Action**	**Major Side Effects**	**Mechanism of Action**
captopril	25–50 mg PO	15 min	4–6 h	Rash, pruritus, proteinuria, loss of taste, hypotension	ACE inhibitor
clonidine	0.2 mg PO initially, then 0.1 mg/h up to 0.8 mg total	0.5–2 h	6–8 h	Sedation, dry mouth, dizziness, constipation	Alpha-2 antagonist
labetalol	200–400 mg PO 2–3 h	0.5–2 h	4 h	Orthostatic hypertension, nausea and vomiting	Alpha- and beta-adrenergic blocker
minoxidil	5–20 mg PO	0.5–1 h (max: 2–4 h)	12–16 h	Tachycardia, fluid retention	Vasodilator

drug therapy or a change in the drug regimen. Patients with stage 3 hypertension and hypertensive urgency should be seen within 2 weeks. Once BP returns to a normal range, the patient should be monitored every 3 to 6 months.

The importance of adhering to the drug regimen cannot be overemphasized. The practitioner needs to be alert for signs of nonadherence and should ask patients about their experiences or problems with adhering to the drug regimen. Side effects should be discussed, and changes in medications may or may not be considered at each visit.

PATIENT EDUCATION

Patient education is a vital part of hypertension treatment. Because most patients are free of symptoms, they must be educated about the disease, the importance of adhering to therapy, and the consequences of uncontrolled hypertension. Patient education booklets available from most pharmaceutical companies may be used to reinforce the information provided by the practitioner.

Because each antihypertensive medication has some side effects, the patient needs to be informed about what they are, what actions to take to relieve minor side effects, and what to do about intolerable or dangerous side effects. Because the objective of drug therapy is to lower BP without intolerable effects, the patient needs to know which adverse reactions should be reported to the practitioner and which ones may be relieved by switching to an alternative drug in a different class. The patient also needs to know that several different agents may be tried before finding the one that best controls his or her BP with minimal or no side effects. Other important teaching involves information about lifestyle changes and the consequences of uncontrolled hypertension.

Nutrition/Lifestyle Changes

Hypertensive adults should lose weight and increase their physical activity levels as needed. Patients should maintain an appropriate body weight, follow the DASH eating plan, and restrict sodium and alcohol consumption.

Complementary and Alternative Medications

To date, there is no evidence that alternative medications reduce BP.

Case Study

R. S., a 65-year-old African-American man, was referred to the hypertension clinic for evaluation of high BP noted on an initial screening. He reports having headaches and nocturia. He states that he has gained 8 pounds over the last year.

Past medical history
  Appendectomy 30 years ago
  Peptic ulcer disease 10 years ago
  Type 2 diabetes mellitus for 10 years
Family history
  Father had hypertension; died of myocardial infarction at age 55
  Mother had diabetes mellitus and hypertension; died of cerebrovascular accident at age 60
Physical examination
  Height 69 in, weight 108 kg
  BP: 140/89 mm Hg (left arm), 138/82 mm Hg (right arm)
  Pulse: 84 beats/min, regular
  Funduscopic examination: mild arterial narrowing, sharp discs, no exudates or hemorrhages
Laboratory findings
  Blood urea nitrogen: 24 mg/dL
  Serum creatinine: 1.5 mg/dL
  Glucose: 95 mg/dL
  Potassium: 4.0 mEq/L
  Total cholesterol: 201 mg/dL
  High-density lipoprotein cholesterol: 30 mg/dL
  Triglycerides: 167 mg/dL
  Urinalysis: 1+ proteinuria

Electrocardiogram and chest radiograph: mild left ventricular hypertrophy
Social history
  Tobacco: 35 pack years
  Alcohol: pint of vodka/week
  Coffee: 2 cups/day

DIAGNOSIS: STAGE 1 HYPERTENSION

1. List specific goals for treating R. S.'s hypertension.
2. What would you consider as first-line therapy for R. S., and why?
3. What dietary and lifestyle changes would you consider recommending for R. S.?
4. What over-the-counter and/or alternative medications would be appropriate for R. S.?
5. Beside BP, what else will you monitor to determine whether your therapy is successful? When would you monitor these?
6. Describe one or two drug–drug or drug–food interactions that you would be wary of when prescribing your selected first-line agent.
7. List one or two adverse reactions for the selected agent that would cause you to change therapy.
8. If your first-line agent was unsuccessful or a significant adverse drug event occurred, what would be your second-line agent for R. S., and why?
9. Discuss specific patient education based on both your first- and second-line choices.

BIBLIOGRAPHY

Starred references are cited in the text.

Basile, J. (2010). One size does not fit all: The role of vasodilating β-blockers in controlling hypertension as a means of reducing cardiovascular and stroke risk. *The American Journal of Medicine, 123,* S9–S15.

Bloch, M. J. (2003). The diagnosis and management of renovascular disease: A primary care perspective. *Journal of Clinical Hypertension, 5,* 210–218.

*Brown, N. J., Ray, W. A., Snowden, M., & Griffin, M. R. (1996). Black Americans have an increased rate of angiotensin-converting enzyme inhibition associated angioedema. *Clinical Pharmacology and Therapeutics, 60,* 8–13.

*Burkhart, G. A., Brown, N. J., Griffin, M. R., et al. (1996). Angiotensin-converting enzyme inhibitor-associated angioedema: Higher risk in blacks than whites. *Pharmacoepidemiology and Drug Safety, 5,* 149–154.

CAPRICORN Investigators. (2001). Effects of carvedilol on outcome after myocardial infarction in patients with left-ventricular dysfunction: The CAPRICORN randomised trial. *Lancet, 357,* 1385–1390.

Chobanian, A. (2008). Does it matter how hypertension is controlled? *New England Journal of Medicine, 359,* 2485–2488.

Escobar, C., & Barrios, V. (2009). Combined therapy in the treatment of hypertension. *Fundamental & Clinical Pharmacology, 24,* 3–8.

Forman, J., & Brenner, B. (2006). Hypertension and microalbuminuria: The bell tolls for thee. *Kidney International, 69,* 22–28.

Garcia-Donaire, J., & Ruilope, L. (2009). Multiple action fixed combinations. Present or future? *Fundamental & Clinical Pharmacology, 24,* 37–42.

Hawkins, D. W., Bussey, H. I., & Prisant, L. M. (1999). Hypertension. In J. T. Dipiro, R. L. Talbert, G. C. Yee, G. R. Matzke, B. G. Wells, & L. M. Posey (Eds.), *Pharmacotherapy: A pathophysiologic approach* (4th ed., pp. 131–152). Stamford, CT: Appleton & Lange.

*He, J., Klag, M. J., Appek, L. J., et al. (1999). The renin-angiotensin system and BP: Differences between blacks and whites. *American Journal of Hypertension, 12*(6), 555–562.

*Joint National Committee on Prevention, Detection, Evaluation, and Treatment of High BP. (1997). Sixth report of the Joint National Committee on Prevention, Detection, Evaluation, and Treatment of High BP (JNC VI). *Archives of Internal Medicine, 157,* 2413–2446.

*Joint National Committee on Prevention, Detection, Evaluation, and Treatment of High BP. (2003). Seventh report of the Joint National Committee on Prevention, Detection, Evaluation, and Treatment of High BP (JNC VII). *Journal of the American Medical Association,, 289,* 2560–2572.

Jordan, J., & Grassi, G. (2010). Belly fat and resistant hypertension. *Journal of Hypertension, 28,* 1131–1133.

*Mancia, G., De Backer, G., Dominiczak, A., et al. (2007). 2007 guidelines for the management of arterial hypertension: The task force for the management of arterial hypertension of the European Society of Hypertension (ESH) and of the European Society of Cardiology (ESC). *Journal of Hypertension, 25,* 1105–1187.

*Moser, M. (1998). Why are physicians not prescribing diuretics more frequently in the management of hypertension? *Journal of the American Medical Association, 279,* 1813–1816.

National High Blood Pressure Education Program [NHBPEP] Working Group. (1994). National High Blood Pressure Education Program Working Group report on hypertension in diabetes. *Hypertension, 23,* 145–158.

Ong, K., Cheung, B., Man, Y., et al. (2006). Prevalence, awareness, treatment, and control of hypertension among United States adults. *The Journal of Clinical Hypertension, 49,* 69–75.

Ostchega, Y., Dillon, C., & Hughes, J. (2007). Trends in hypertension prevalence, awareness, treatment, and control in older U.S. adults: Data from the national health and nutrition examination survey 1988 to 2004. *The American Geriatrics Society, 55,* 1056–1065.

*Papademetriou, V., Piller, L., Ford, C., et al. (2003). Characteristics and lipid distribution of a large, high-risk, hypertension population: The lipid-lowering component of the antihypertensive and lipid-lowering treatment to prevent heart attack trail (ALLHAT). *Journal of Clinical Hypertension, 5,* 377–385.

Poole-Wilson, P., Swedberg, K., Cleland, J., et al. (2003). Comparison of carvedilol and metoprolol on clinical outcomes in patients with chronic heart failure in the Carvedilol Or Metoprolol European Trial (COMET): Randomised controlled trial. *Lancet, 362,* 7–13.

*Sander, G. (2002). High blood pressure in the geriatric population: Treatment considerations. *American Journal of Geriatric Cardiology, 11,* 223–232.

Screening for high blood pressure: U.S. preventive services task force reaffirmation recommendation statement. (2007). *Annals of Internal Medicine, 147,* 783–787.

*SHEP Cooperative Research Group. (1991). Prevention of stroke by antihypertensive drug treatment in older persons with isolated systolic hypertension. *Journal of the American Medical Association, 265,* 3255–3264.

Sica, D. (2002). ACE inhibitors and stroke: New considerations. *Journal of Clinical Hypertension, 4,* 126–129.

Sica, D., & Black, H. (2002). ACE inhibitor-related angioedema: Can angiotensin-receptor blockers be safely used? *Journal of Clinical Hypertension, 4*(5), 375–380.

Taylor, A., & Bakris, G. (2010). The role of vasodilating B-blockers in patients with hypertension and the cardiometabolic syndrome. *The American Journal of Medicine, 123,* S21–S26.

*Tierney, L., McPhee, S., & Papadakis, M. (2004). *Current medical diagnosis and treatment.* New York: McGraw-Hill.

Ungar, A., Pepe, G., Lambertucci, L., et al. (2009). Low diastolic ambulatory blood pressure is associated with greater all-cause mortality in older patients with hypertension. *Journal of the American Geriatric Society, 57,* 291–296.

Yancy, C., Fowler M., Colucci, W., et al. (2001). Race and the response to adrenergic blockade with carvedilol in patients with chronic heart failure. *New England Journal of Medicine, 344,* 1358–1365.

Wright, J., Jamerson, K., & Ferdinand, K. (2007). The management of hypertension in African Americans. *The Journal of Clinical Hypertension, 9,* 468–475.

20

John Barron

Hyperlipidemia

Hyperlipidemia is a blood disorder characterized by elevations in blood cholesterol levels. The term is often used synonymously with *dyslipidemia* and *hypercholesterolemia*. Hyperlipidemia is one of the major contributing risk factors in the development of coronary heart disease (CHD). It is estimated that approximately 17.6 million people in the United States have CHD, with approximately 425,000 deaths each year (American Heart Association, 2010). In addition, approximately $177 billion is spent each year on direct and indirect costs from CHD.

Informed estimates indicate that approximately 102 million adults age 20 and older had total cholesterol levels above 200 mg/dL in 2006, representing approximately 47% of adults in the United States (American Heart Association, 2010). However, data from the National Health and Nutrition Examination Survey (NHANES) suggest the percentage of patients with elevated cholesterol may be decreasing.

Numerous large studies have shown that reducing elevated cholesterol levels reduces morbidity and mortality rates in patients with and without existing CHD (Downs, et al., 1998; Frick, et al., 1987; Heart Protection Study Collaborative Group, 2002; Lewis, et al., 1998; Long-Term Intervention With Pravastatin in Ischaemic Disease [LIPID] Study Group, 1998; Scandinavian Simvastatin Survival Study Group, 1994; Shepherd, et al., 1995; Ridker, et al., 2008). Although these and other trials have clearly shown the benefits of treating high cholesterol levels and other preventive measures, including the use of aspirin, beta blockers, and angiotensin-converting enzyme inhibitors in the treatment of patients with coronary artery disease, long-term use of these medications across the population are far from optimal (Newby, et al., 2006).

CAUSES

In hyperlipidemia, serum cholesterol levels may be elevated as a result of an increased level of any of the lipoproteins. (See the section on Pathophysiology: Lipoproteins and Lipid Metabolism.) The mechanisms for hyperlipidemia appear to be genetic (primary) and environmental (secondary). In fact, the most common cause of hyperlipidemia (95% of all those with hyperlipidemia) is a combination of genetic and environmental factors.

Some individuals are genetically predisposed to elevated cholesterol levels. They may inherit defective genes that lead to abnormalities in the synthesis or breakdown of cholesterol. These may include abnormalities in low-density lipoprotein (LDL) receptors and mutations in apolipoproteins that lead to increased production of cholesterol or decreased clearance of cholesterol from the bloodstream. (See the section on Pathophysiology: Lipoproteins and Lipid Metabolism.)

Secondary factors may include medications (e.g., beta blockers and oral contraceptives), concomitant disease states or other conditions (e.g., diabetes mellitus and pregnancy), diets high in fat and cholesterol, lack of exercise, obesity, and smoking (**Box 20.1**).

PATHOPHYSIOLOGY

The major plasma lipids are cholesterol, triglycerides, and phospholipids. Cholesterol is a naturally occurring substance that is required by the body to synthesize bile acids and steroid hormones and to maintain the integrity of cell membranes. Although cholesterol is found predominantly in the cells, approximately 7% circulates in the serum. It is this serum cholesterol that is implicated in atherosclerosis. Triglycerides are made up of free fatty acids and glycerol and serve as an important source of stored energy. Phospholipids are essential for cell function and lipid transport. Because these lipids are insoluble in plasma, they are surrounded by special fat-carrying proteins, called *lipoproteins*, for transport in the blood.

Lipoproteins are produced in the liver and intestines, but endogenous production of lipoproteins occurs primarily in the liver. Lipoproteins consist of a hydrophobic (water-insoluble) inner core made of cholesterol and triglycerides and a hydrophilic (water-soluble) outer surface composed of apolipoproteins and phospholipids. Apolipoproteins are specialized proteins that identify specific receptors to which the lipoprotein will bind. They are thought to play a role in the development or prevention of hyperlipidemia because they control the interaction and metabolism of the lipoproteins.

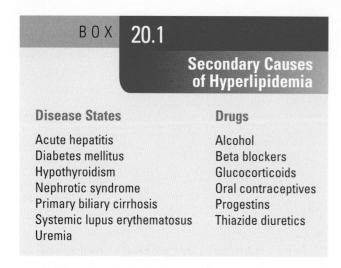

BOX 20.1

Secondary Causes of Hyperlipidemia

Disease States	Drugs
Acute hepatitis	Alcohol
Diabetes mellitus	Beta blockers
Hypothyroidism	Glucocorticoids
Nephrotic syndrome	Oral contraceptives
Primary biliary cirrhosis	Progestins
Systemic lupus erythematosus	Thiazide diuretics
Uremia	

Lipoproteins and Lipid Metabolism

The major lipoproteins are named according to their density. They include chylomicrons, very–low-density lipoproteins (VLDLs), intermediate-density lipoproteins (IDLs), LDLs, and high-density lipoproteins (HDLs).

Chylomicrons

Chylomicrons, the largest lipoproteins, are composed primarily of triglycerides. Chylomicrons are produced in the gut from dietary fat and cholesterol that has been solubilized by bile acids (exogenous pathway). Chylomicrons normally are not present in the blood after a 12- to 14-hour fast.

Very–Low-Density Lipoproteins

VLDLs are primarily composed of cholesterol and triglycerides, and are the major carrier of endogenous triglycerides. On secretion into the bloodstream, lipoprotein lipase and hepatic lipase hydrolyze the triglyceride core by a mechanism similar to that which occurs with chylomicrons. As the triglyceride content decreases, the lipoprotein becomes progressively smaller with a higher percentage of cholesterol; it is now referred to as an IDL. IDL is a short-lived lipoprotein that is converted to LDL or is taken up by LDL receptors on the liver. LDL, the final product of the metabolism of VLDL, contains the most cholesterol by weight of all the lipoproteins. It is estimated that 60% to 75% of the total cholesterol is contained in LDLs (Talbert, 1997).

Approximately 50% of LDL is taken up by the liver, and the remaining 50% is taken up by peripheral cells. Increased levels of LDL cholesterol are directly related to the probability that atherosclerosis will develop. Thus, LDL cholesterol is usually referred to as "bad" cholesterol.

High-Density Lipoproteins

HDL particles are produced in the liver and intestine. The primary function of HDL cholesterol is to remove LDL cholesterol from the peripheral cells and to remove triglycerides that result from the degradation of chylomicrons and

VLDL particles. The HDL then transports these particles to the liver for metabolism. This process is termed *reverse cholesterol transport*. For this reason, HDL is often referred to as "good" cholesterol.

Pathogenesis of Atherosclerosis

Atherosclerosis is characterized by the development of lesions resulting from accumulations of cholesterol in the blood vessel wall. Atherosclerosis primarily affects the larger arteries, including the coronary arteries.

The atherogenic process begins with the accumulation of LDL cholesterol under the endothelial lining of the innermost arterial layer, the intima. As LDLs accumulate, circulating monocytes attach to the endothelial lining and penetrate between the endothelial cells into the subendothelial space. On entry into the subendothelial space, the monocytes form into macrophages, which then ingest the LDLs. Macrophages, in particular, have a high affinity for modified (oxidized) LDL, which is believed to be more atherogenic than nonoxidized LDL. Thus, by preventing the oxidation of LDL, antioxidants such as vitamin E may be beneficial in preventing CHD, although the efficacy of antioxidants in this capacity remains unproven.

As the macrophages ingest the modified LDL, they are converted into foam cells and form the *fatty streak*, which is the initial lesion in the atherogenic process. These lesions commonly affect the coronary arteries. Formation begins in the mid-teens, and the lesions grow as the person ages.

Once the fatty streak forms, the oxidized LDL and macrophages act in other ways that promote the progression of the atherogenic lesion. Oxidized LDL appears to act as a chemotactic agent, recruiting other circulating monocytes and preventing macrophages from leaving the subendothelial space. Macrophages also produce chemotactic factors as well as growth factors. The growth factors cause proliferation of smooth muscle cells from the media into the fatty streak, leading to the formation of a fibrous plaque (Ross & Glomset, 1976). Fibrous plaques are usually raised and protrude into the lumen of the artery, thereby compromising blood flow.

As the foam cells grow, the endothelium stretches and may become damaged. This leads to platelet aggregation and clot formation. In many instances, these fissures heal and incorporate the thrombi inside the plaque. This process may occur dozens of times and eventually may produce a complicated lesion. The formation of complicated lesions is the major cause of acute cardiovascular (CV) events. However, in some instances, rupture of a small, unstable plaque may also cause the formation of a single large clot that totally occludes the vessel. The fibrous plaques that are most likely to rupture are those that have large lipid cores and a thin fibrous cap, a layer of smooth muscle cells directly over the lipid core. Large plaques with a strong fibrous cap may be more stable and less likely to rupture (Cooke & Bhatnagar, 1997; McKenney & Hawkins, 1995).

The primary symptom associated with atherosclerosis is chest pain known as *angina*. Symptoms occur when the lesion compromises blood flow in the vessel lumen. A lesion that occludes approximately 50% of the lumen usually causes symptoms when more blood flow is required (i.e., exercise-induced angina). As the lesions grow and occlude more than 70% of the vessel, anginal symptoms may occur even when the person is resting (Cooke & Bhatnagar, 1997).

RISK ASSESSMENT

The National Cholesterol Education Program's Third Report on the Detection, Evaluation and Treatment of High Cholesterol in Adults (NCEP ATP III) recommends that all adults age 20 or older should have a fasting lipoprotein panel (total cholesterol, LDL cholesterol, HDL cholesterol, and triglycerides) measured at least once every 5 years (**Table 20.1**). If the patient was not fasting, only total and HDL cholesterol are usable. In this instance, if the total cholesterol is 200 mg/dL or more or HDL cholesterol is less than 40 mg/dL, the patient should have a fasting lipoprotein profile performed. Patients should also be evaluated for CHD risk factors (**Box 20.2**) and for clinical evidence of CHD or CHD risk equivalents (**Box 20.3**).

Evaluation of patients with suspected hyperlipidemia should include a complete history and physical examination, fasting lipoprotein analysis to determine LDL and triglyceride levels, and determination of secondary causes of hyperlipidemia. For accurate results, the patient undergoing lipoprotein analysis must fast for at least 12 hours. The reason for this is that triglyceride levels can be falsely elevated in a patient who has not fasted because of circulating chylomicrons. Normal triglyceride levels are lower than 150 mg/dL. Levels of 150 to 199 mg/dL are considered borderline high. Levels of 200 to 499 mg/dL are considered high, those above 500 mg/dL are considered very high, and those above 1,000 mg/dL could lead to complications such as pancreatitis.

TABLE 20.1	Classification of LDL, Total, and HDL Cholesterol and hs-CRP	
	Result	**Initial Classification**
LDL cholesterol*	<100	Optimal
	100–129	Near or above optimal
	130–159	Borderline high
	160–189	High
	≥190	Very high
Total cholesterol*	<200	Desirable
	200–239	Borderline high
	≥240	High
HDL cholesterol*	<40	Low
	≥60	High
hs-CRP**	<1.0	Low
	1.0–3.0	Average
	>3.0	High

*mg/dL; ** mg/L

BOX 20.2

Coronary Heart Disease Risk Factors*

POSITIVE CHD RISK FACTORS

1. **Age:** Men ≥45 years old
   Women ≥55 years old
2. **Family History of Premature CHD:**
   Male first-degree relative—MI or sudden death before **55** years old
   Female first-degree relative—MI or sudden death before **65** years old
3. **Current cigarette smoking**
4. **Hypertension:**
   Blood pressure >140/90 mm Hg on several occasions or taking antihypertensive medications
5. **Low HDL cholesterol** (<40 mg/dL)

NEGATIVE CHD RISK FACTORS

1. **High HDL cholesterol** (≥60 mg/dL or 1.6 mmol/L)
Total Risk Factors = Positive risk factors minus negative risk factors

---

* Diabetes mellitus is considered a CHD risk equivalent.

BOX 20.3

Atherosclerotic Vascular Disease and CHD Risk Equivalents

Coronary Heart Disease (CHD)

Myocardial infarction
Significant myocardial ischemia (angina pectoris)
History of coronary artery bypass graft
History of coronary angioplasty
Angiographic evidence of lesions

Peripheral Vascular Disease

Claudication

Carotid Artery Disease

Thrombotic stroke
Transient ischemic attack

CHD Risk Equivalent

Diabetes mellitus

Total and HDL cholesterol values are minimally affected if a patient does not fast. However, because most laboratories calculate LDL cholesterol, the patient must be fasting because elevations in the triglyceride level may lead to falsely low LDL cholesterol levels.

The formula for calculating LDL is

$$LDL = total\ cholesterol - HDL - VLDL$$

(VLDL is equivalent to triglycerides/5.) However, as triglyceride levels approach or exceed 400 mg/dL, this formula is not accurate. In this case, the patient may require a direct LDL cholesterol level analysis. A second analysis should be performed within 1 to 8 weeks to confirm the results of the first test before a definitive diagnosis is made.

The treatment of patients who require a fasting lipoprotein analysis is primarily based on LDL cholesterol values. The LDL cholesterol goal is determined by the presence of CHD risk factors (**Box 20.2**) or by the presence of CHD or CHD risk equivalents. (See **Box 20.3**.) Patients at highest risk are those with CHD or CHD risk equivalents. These patients have a greater than 20% risk of having a coronary event within 10 years. CHD risk equivalents include patients with diabetes mellitus and patients with a 10-year risk of CHD that exceeds 20%. This includes patients with two or more risk factors and increased risk based upon the Framingham risk score. To calculate the 10-year risk for a patient, see **Table 20.2**.

Inflammatory response is a key mechanism in the pathogenesis of atherosclerosis, and a marker for inflammation within the arteries is high sensitivity C-reactive protein (hs-CRP) (Pearson, et al., 2003). Several studies have shown that hs-CRP levels may predict cardiac risk (Ridker, et al., 2000, 2008), and hs-CRP has been endorsed as the analyte of choice to associate inflammation to CV risk. A study by Harvard Women's Health Group showed that hs-CRP was more accurate than cholesterol levels in predicting risk of cardiac events (Ridker, et al., 2000). Results of hs-CRP of less than 1.0 mg/L suggest low CV risk; 1.0 to 3.0 mg/L, average risk; and over 3.0 mg/L suggest high risk (Pearson, et al., 2003). Appropriate application of hs-CRP testing in general clinical practice continues to require further investigation. However, the Canadian Cardiovascular Society recommends measurement of hs-CRP in the evaluation of healthy individuals who have a 10-year risk for CV events of 5% to 20% (Genest, et al., 2009).

INITIATING DRUG THERAPY

Management of patients with no evidence of CHD or CHD risk equivalents is termed *primary prevention*. Management of patients with CHD or CHD risk equivalents is termed *secondary prevention*. Management of patients with hyperlipidemia consists of nonpharmacologic and pharmacologic therapy. The decision to treat hyperlipidemia with drug therapy is based on LDL levels (**Table 20.3**), as is follow-up treatment (**Table 20.4**).

Lifestyle Modification

Most patients with newly diagnosed hyperlipidemia should attempt to make lifestyle modifications before beginning pharmacologic therapy. The primary lifestyle modifications include dietary therapy, exercise, weight loss, moderation of alcohol intake, and smoking cessation. Before initiating any lifestyle modifications, the patient's current lifestyle needs to be evaluated to determine what modifications would be beneficial. This evaluation should also include the patient's understanding of the disease and the importance of treating it and his or her ability to learn and follow these lifestyle modifications. Evaluation of social, cultural, and economic factors also is necessary, especially if drug therapy may be warranted.

Diet

The primary goal of dietary therapy is to reduce the intake of fat, especially saturated fat, and cholesterol and to achieve a desirable body weight. The Third National Health and Nutrition Examination Survey (NHANES III) stated that 36% or 37% of calories in the typical American diet comes from fat. All adults with hyperlipidemia should follow a "therapeutic lifestyle changes" (TLC) diet. The primary targets of the TLC diet are to reduce intake of saturated fats to less than 7% of total calories and cholesterol intake to less than 200 mg per day (**Table 20.5**). Total daily fat intake should represent 25% to 35% of total calories. The patient should follow this diet for 6 to 12 weeks before making modifications to therapy. If the LDL cholesterol goal is not met, increased intake of plant stanol/sterols and viscous fiber is recommended.

In addition to decreasing dietary fat and cholesterol, overweight patients should attempt to lose weight. The ability to lose weight depends on the amount of calories consumed and the amount of calories burned. To lose weight, most people need to reduce their caloric intake by approximately 500 calories daily and increase physical activity. The goal for overweight patients should be a realistic, gradual, and steady loss of weight. Once an ideal weight is achieved, caloric intake is adjusted to maintain that weight.

Exercise

Regular physical exercise may provide several benefits in patients with hyperlipidemia. As mentioned, it should be used along with dietary therapy to promote weight loss. Exercise may benefit the lipid profile by reducing triglycerides and raising HDL levels. Exercise may also improve control of diabetes and coronary blood flow. The most effective exercise is aerobic activity, such as walking, swimming, jogging, and tennis. The optimal schedule for aerobic exercise is at least 30 minutes a day, 5 to 7 days a week, but any exercise is beneficial.

Moderation of Alcohol Intake and Smoking Cessation

Excessive alcohol intake may elevate serum lipid levels, specifically triglyceride levels, but in moderation (no more than one drink per day for women and two drinks per day for men), alcohol may improve HDL levels and has been associated with lower CHD rates (Jackson & Beaglehole, 1993). Despite these benefits, alcohol should not be recommended for CHD prevention because the consequences associated with excessive alcohol use outweigh any benefits.

TABLE 20.2   Calculation of Estimate of 10-Year Risk

Estimate of 10-Year Risk for Men
(Framingham Point Scores)

Age	Points
20–34	–9
35–39	–4
40–44	0
45–49	3
50–54	6
55–59	8
60–64	10
65–69	11
70–74	12
75–79	13

Estimate of 10-Year Risk for Women
(Framingham Point Scores)

Age	Points
20–34	–7
35–39	–3
40–44	0
45–49	3
50–54	6
55–59	8
60–64	10
65–69	12
70–74	14
75–79	16

Men

Total Cholesterol	Points				
	Age 20–39	Age 40–49	Age 50–59	Age 60–69	Age 70–79
<160	0	0	0	0	0
160–199	4	3	2	1	0
200–239	7	5	3	1	0
240–279	9	6	4	2	1
≥280	11	8	5	3	1

Women

Total Cholesterol	Points				
	Age 20–39	Age 40–49	Age 50–59	Age 60–69	Age 70–79
<160	0	0	0	0	0
160–199	4	3	2	1	1
200–239	8	6	4	2	1
240–279	11	8	5	3	2
≥280	13	10	7	4	2

Men

	Points				
	Age 20–39	Age 40–49	Age 50–59	Age 60–69	Age 70–79
Nonsmoker	0	0	0	0	0
Smoker	8	5	3	1	1

Women

	Points				
	Age 20–39	Age 40–49	Age 50–59	Age 60–69	Age 70–79
Nonsmoker	0	0	0	0	0
Smoker	9	7	4	2	1

Men

HDL (mg/dL)	Points
≥60	–1
50–59	0
40–49	1
<40	2

Women

HDL (mg/dL)	Points
≥60	–1
50–59	0
40–49	1
<40	2

Men

Systolic BP (mm Hg)	If Untreated	If Treated
<120	0	0
120–129	0	1
130–139	1	2
140–159	1	2
≥160	2	3

Women

Systolic BP (mm Hg)	If Untreated	If Treated
<120	0	0
120–129	1	3
130–139	2	4
140–159	3	5
≥160	4	6

(continued)

TABLE 20.2 **Calculation of Estimate of 10-Year Risk (*Continued*)**

Estimate of 10-Year Risk for Men (Framingham Point Scores)		Estimate of 10-Year Risk for Women (Framingham Point Scores)	
Point Total	**10-Year Risk %**	**Point Total**	**10-Year Risk %**
<9	<1	<0	<1
9	1	0	1
10	1	1	1
11	1	2	1
12	1	3	1
13	2	4	1
14	2	5	2
15	3	6	2
16	4	7	3
17	5	8	4
18	6	9	5
19	8	10	6
20	11	11	8
21	14	12	10
22	17	13	12
23	22	14	16
24	27	15	20
≥25	≥30	16	25
		≥17	≥30

10-Year risk _____ %

10-Year risk _____ %

U.S. DEPARTMENT OF HEALTH AND HUMAN SERVICES
Public Health Service
National Institutes of Health
National Heart, Lung, and Blood Institute

NIH Publication No. 02-3305
May 2001

Cigarette smoking is an independent risk factor in the development of CHD (Hjermann, et al., 1981). Although smoking minimally affects cholesterol levels, it contributes to the development of CHD by damaging the vascular endothelium and promoting platelet aggregation, which results in increased risk of clot formation. Smoking cessation can reduce this risk and should be encouraged by all health care professionals. The risk of developing CHD decreases by approximately 50% within 1 to 2 years of smoking cessation.

Goals of Drug Therapy

Drug therapy should be used in patients who do not attain their LDL cholesterol goal with lifestyle modifications alone. As mentioned, most patients without CHD should try lifestyle changes for approximately 6 months before initiating drug therapy. Patients with very high LDL cholesterol levels who are unlikely to attain their LDL cholesterol goal with lifestyle changes alone may require drug therapy before this 6-month period. Because patients with CHD are at higher risk for future CV events, these patients should be managed more aggressively. Often, drug therapy should be considered after a trial of lifestyle modifications of 3 months or less.

The medication classes used to treat abnormal cholesterol levels are the HMG-CoA reductase inhibitors (statins), bile acid resins, nicotinic acid (niacin), cholesterol absorption inhibitors (ezetimibe), fibric acid derivatives (fenofibrate and gemfibrozil), and omega-3 fatty acids (fish oil). Statin and bile acid resins promote a decrease in LDL cholesterol and a slight increase in HDL levels, but they differ in their potency and effects on triglyceride levels. Niacin lowers LDL cholesterol (less than statins) and triglycerides, and increases HDL levels

TABLE 20.3 **LDL Cholesterol Goals Based Upon CHD Risk Factors**

Risk Factors	LDL Goal	Non-HDL Goal*
CHD and CHD risk equivalents	<100 mg/dL with desirable <70 mg/dL	<130 mg/dL
Multiple (2+) risk factors	<130 mg/dL	<160 mg/dL
0 or 1 risk factor	<160 mg/dL	<190 mg/dL

* For patients who achieve LDL cholesterol goal but have triglyceride levels >200 mg/dL.

TABLE 20.4   Treatment Decisions Based on LDL Cholesterol Levels

	LDL Goal	Initiate Dietary Therapy	Initiate Pharmacologic Therapy
0 or 1 risk factor	<160 mg/dL	≥160 mg/dL	≥190 mg/dL (160–189: drug therapy optional)
2 + risk factors			
10-year risk <10%	<130 mg/dL	≥130 mg/dL	≥160 mg/dL
10-year risk 10–20%	<130 mg/dL	≥130 mg/dL	≥130 mg/dL
Patients with CHD or CHD risk equivalents (10-year risk >20%)	<100 mg/dL or <70 mg/dL*	≥100 mg/dL	≥130 mg/dL (100–129: drug therapy optional)

* For patients with established CVD plus multiple risk factors (e.g., diabetes and continued smoking).

more than any other class. Gemfibrozil and omega-3 fatty acids are indicated for hypertriglyceridemia.

The primary goal of drug therapy in treating hyperlipidemia is to reduce cardiovascular-related morbidity and mortality without affecting quality of life. The primary surrogate marker for predicting morbidity and mortality is cholesterol levels. Patients with fewer than two risk factors and no evidence of CHD or CHD risk equivalents have an LDL cholesterol goal of less than 160 mg/dL. Patients with two or more risk factors and without evidence of CHD or CHD risk equivalents and 10-year risk of less than 20% have an LDL cholesterol goal of less than 130 mg/dL, with the ideal being less than 100 mg/dL. The intensity of LDL-lowering drug therapy for high-risk and moderately high-risk patients should be sufficient to achieve at least a 30% to 40% reduction in LDL levels, either with statins alone or a combination of lower doses of statins and other drugs, or with food products containing plant stanol/sterols. Patients with any evidence of CHD, CHD risk equivalents, or a 10-year risk of CHD that exceeds 20% are treated most aggressively and have an LDL cholesterol goal of 100 mg/dL or less, with a desired rate of below 70 mg/dL.

For patients who achieve the LDL cholesterol goal but have triglyceride levels above 200 mg/dL, a secondary goal is to achieve appropriate non-HDL cholesterol levels. Non-HDL

levels can be calculated by subtracting the HDL cholesterol result from total cholesterol. Non-HDL cholesterol goals are recommended to be 30 mg/dL higher than LDL cholesterol goals (i.e., if the LDL cholesterol goal is 130 mg/dL, then the non-HDL cholesterol goal is 160 mg/dL).

HMG-CoA Reductase Inhibitors (Statins)

The statins are the most heavily used class of lipid-lowering drugs because of their ability to lower LDL cholesterol and, more important, associated morbidity and mortality rates. These drugs are well tolerated by most patients. Lovastatin (Mevacor), the first drug in this class, became available in the United States in 1987. Since then, seven additional medications have been approved for use (**Table 20.6**). However, one of these products, cerivastatin, was removed from the market in 2001 as a result of an increased risk of rhabdomyolysis (a rapid destruction of muscle cells that can lead to kidney failure).

Mechanism of Action

The selection of a statin is based in general on its ability to lower cholesterol levels. The current guidelines from NCEP ATP III suggest that patients be treated to reach a certain LDL cholesterol goal. Trying to lower the LDL cholesterol level beyond this does not necessarily reduce morbidity and mortality. For this reason, the most potent agent may not always be necessary. Several agents in this class also lower triglyceride levels, primarily at the higher doses. (For patients who require significant lowering of triglyceride levels, niacin or fibric acid derivatives should be used.)

Primarily, the statins block the conversion of HMG-CoA to mevalonate, which is the rate-limiting step in the production of cholesterol in the liver. Blocking the production of cholesterol in the liver leads to an increase in the number of LDL cholesterol receptors on the liver. As a result, a larger amount of LDL cholesterol is taken up by the liver, thereby decreasing the amount of LDL cholesterol in the bloodstream (**Figure 20-1**).

Low-density lipoprotein receptors are also involved with the uptake of VLDL and IDL, thus leading to a decrease in triglyceride levels. In addition, modest increases in HDL

TABLE 20.5   Therapeutic Lifestyle Changes (TLC) Diet

Nutrient	Recommended Intake
Total fat	25–35% total calories
Saturated fat	<7% total calories
Polyunsaturated fat	Up to 10% of total calories
Monounsaturated fat	Up to 20% of total calories
Carbohydrates	50–60% total calories
Protein	15% total calories
Fiber	20–30 g/day
Cholesterol	<200 mg/day
Total calories	Amount to maintain desired weight/ prevent weight gain

TABLE 20.6   **Doses and Lipid-Lowering Ability of Currently Available Statins**

Generic Name (Trade Name)	Usual Daily Dose	LDL*	HDL*	Triglycerides*
lovastatin (Mevacor)	10–80 mg	↓24–48%	↑7%	↓10–14%
pravastatin (Pravachol)	10–40 mg	↓22–34%	↑2–12%	↓11–24%
simvastatin (Zocor)	20–80 mg	↓24–40%	↑7–16%	↓12–21%
fluvastatin (Lescol)	20–80 mg	↓22–36%	↑3–6%	↓12–18%
atorvastatin (Lipitor)	10–80 mg	↓39–60%	↑5–9%	↓19–37%
rosuvastatin[†] (Crestor)	5–40 mg	↓47–65%	↑2–9%	↓20%
pitavastatin (Livalo)	1–4 mg	↓32–43%	↑5–8%	↓15–18%

* Effects on lipid levels are dose dependent.
[†] Based on results from the STELLAR Study (McKenney, et al., 2003).

tend to occur. Despite having the same mechanism of action, there are differences between the agents, including their ability to lower cholesterol (**Table 20.6**). For example, fluvastatin (Lescol) can lower LDL cholesterol levels up to approximately 36% with the maximum dose, whereas atorvastatin (Lipitor) and rosuvastatin (Crestor) can lower LDL cholesterol levels up to 60% at maximum doses.

Maximum effects usually are seen after 4 to 6 weeks of therapy. For this reason, dosage adjustments should not be made more frequently than every 4 weeks.

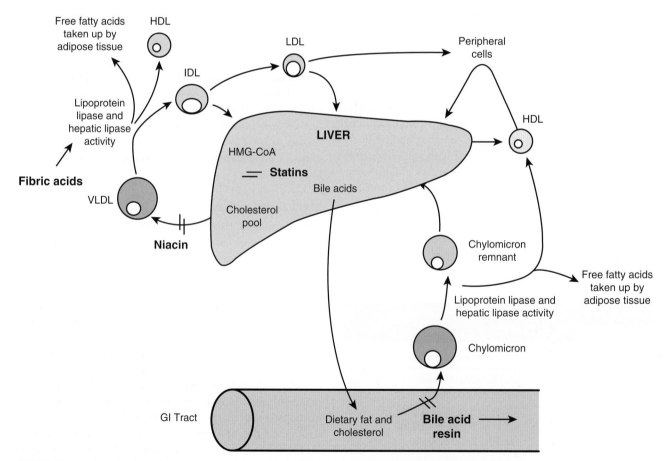

FIGURE 20–1   How lipid-lowering drugs work. The statins work in the liver by blocking the conversion of HMG–CoA to mevalonate, which is involved in producing cholesterol. The bile acid resins bind bile acid in the intestines for excretion in the feces so that lipids are not absorbed by the intestinal tract and returned to the liver. Niacin works to decrease circulating triglyceride and LDL cholesterol and fibric acid derivatives appear to lower triglyceride levels and stimulate lipoprotein lipase, which enhances the breakdown of VLDL to LDL cholesterol.

Contraindications

There are several instances when statins are contraindicated or should be used with caution. Although no studies have been conducted in pregnant women, lovastatin causes skeletal malformations in rats, so statins are contraindicated during pregnancy. These agents should be used with extreme caution in women who are breast-feeding because they may be excreted in breast milk.

Statins are also contraindicated in patients with active liver disease or with unexplained elevated aminotransferase levels. They should be used with caution in patients who consume large amounts of alcohol or have a history of liver disease.

Adverse Events

The statins are well tolerated by most patients and long-term therapy does not appear to have any serious risks. Gastrointestinal (GI) complaints and headache are the two most commonly reported adverse events, but they are usually mild and transient. The most common adverse event that occurs with the statins is asymptomatic elevations in liver function test (LFT) values. LFTs should be monitored at baseline (before starting therapy), at 6 and 12 weeks after starting or titrating therapy, and periodically thereafter. Several agents, including atorvastatin (Lipitor), pravastatin (Pravachol), and simvastatin (Zocor), do not require LFTs to be performed at 6 weeks after initiation or titration of therapy when used as monotherapy. Therapy should be discontinued if two consecutive tests disclose values that are two to three times above upper normal limits.

Other adverse effects include muscle pain and weakness, which may be a sign of myopathy. If myopathy is suspected, the patient's creatinine phosphokinase level should be checked and drug therapy discontinued if levels exceed 10 times the upper normal limits. In rare cases, patients may develop rhabdomyolysis, which is a severe breakdown of muscle cells that leak into the urine and can result in renal failure.

Interactions

The risk of myopathy is most common when using statins at high doses or in combination with drugs that can also cause myopathy (including other lipid-lowering agents) or that can affect the metabolism of the statins (e.g., cyclosporine, erythromycin, azole antifungals). Moreover, myopathy may occur at any time during therapy. Patients should be instructed to report any unusual muscle pain or weakness during therapy.

The practitioner should encourage the patient to take the statins in the evening or at bedtime because a significant amount of cholesterol production seems to occur during sleep. By taking the medication before bedtime, peak concentrations of medication occur during sleep. Exceptions are lovastatin, which has an increased bioavailability when taken with food and is usually taken with the evening meal, and atorvastatin and rosuvastatin, which can be taken at any time during the day because of their long half-lives.

Bile Acid Resins

Bile acid resins decrease cholesterol absorption through the exogenous pathway. These agents are not absorbed from the GI tract. They act to bind bile acids in the intestines, forming an insoluble complex that is excreted in the feces. This decreases the return of cholesterol to the liver. The body responds to this by increasing LDL receptors on the liver, which in turn increases the amount of LDL cholesterol taken up by the liver and thus decreases LDL cholesterol levels in the bloodstream. (See **Figure 20-1.**) Unfortunately, this process also leads to increased production of VLDL particles. As a result, triglyceride levels rise, especially in patients with elevated baseline triglyceride levels. Bile acid resins can decrease LDL cholesterol levels by 15% to 30%, increase HDL levels by approximately 3%, and increase triglyceride levels by up to 15% (**Table 20.7**). As with the statins, these effects are dose related.

Maximum effects of cholesterol lowering are seen in approximately 3 weeks. Bile acid resins are indicated as adjunct therapy for patients who do not respond to dietary therapy alone. Because of their safety with long-term use, they are extremely useful in young adult men and premenopausal women who are at relatively low CV risk. These agents are contraindicated in patients with biliary obstruction or chronic constipation.

Adverse Events

Bile acid resins are not absorbed, and therefore systemic adverse events are minimal. Monitoring for abnormal LFT values is not required. The most common adverse events are GI-related and include flatulence, bloating, abdominal pain, heartburn, and constipation. For these reasons, some patients, such as elderly patients, may not be good candidates for bile acid resins.

TABLE 20.7	Doses and Lipid-Lowering Ability of Currently Available Bile Acid Resins				
Generic Name (Trade Name)		Usual Daily Dose	LDL*	HDL*	Triglycerides*
cholestyramine (Questran, Questran Light, Prevalite)		4–16 g	↓13–32%	↑3–5%	↑0–15%
colesevelam (Welchol)		3.75 g	↓15–18%	↑3%	↑9–10%

* Effects on lipid levels are dose dependent.

Interactions

Because bile acid resins block the absorption of cholesterol from the GI tract, they should be taken with meals to maximize effectiveness. These agents are usually administered once or twice daily but can be taken up to four times a day. If taken once a day, a bile acid resin should be taken with the largest meal. The two major agents in this class are cholestyramine (Questran, Questran Light, Prevalite) and colesevelam (Welchol).

Cholestyramine is available as a powder and colestipol is available as granules or tablets. The powder and granules should be mixed with water, noncarbonated beverages, soups, or pulpy fruits such as applesauce. The tablets should be swallowed whole with water or other fluids. These agents should not be taken dry because they can cause esophageal distress. Patients should avoid taking these agents with carbonated beverages because it may result in increased GI discomfort. Medications taken concomitantly, such as thyroid hormones, antibiotics, and fat-soluble vitamins, should be taken at least 1 hour before or 4 hours after the bile acid resin because of the bile acid resin's potential to bind to other medications and decrease their bioavailability.

Niacin

Niacin (nicotinic acid) is a naturally occurring B vitamin that can improve cholesterol levels when used at doses 100 to 300 times the recommended daily allowance as a vitamin. Niacin's mechanism of action is uncertain, but the substance appears to decrease VLDL synthesis in the liver, inhibit lipolysis in adipose tissue, and increase lipoprotein lipase activity. This results in decreased triglyceride and LDL cholesterol levels in the bloodstream. (See **Figure 20-1.**) LDL cholesterol levels can be decreased by 15% to 25% and triglycerides by up to 50%, whereas HDL cholesterol levels may be increased by up to 35%. (See **Table 20.6.**) Although niacin is one of the most effective agents in improving cholesterol levels, most patients cannot tolerate the adverse events associated with its use. (See Adverse Events.)

Dosage

Doses of at least 1.5 g niacin daily are usually required to achieve beneficial effects on lipid levels. However, to minimize adverse events, dosages need to be titrated gradually. The usual starting dose is 50 to 100 mg two or three times a day. The dose can be increased every 1 to 2 weeks until a dosage of 1.0 to 1.5 g daily is reached; this should take approximately 4 to 5 weeks. This dosage range provides significant increases (15% to 30%) in HDL cholesterol levels and decreases (20% to 30%) in triglyceride levels. However, for maximal LDL cholesterol lowering, dosages of 3 g/day or more may be necessary. Niacin is available in both immediate-release and sustained-release formulations. Maximum effects usually are seen after 4 to 6 weeks of therapy on the aforementioned dosages.

Contraindications

Niacin is contraindicated in patients with hepatic dysfunction, severe hypotension, or active peptic ulcers. In addition, niacin can elevate uric acid levels and worsen glucose control.

Therefore, niacin is not a first-line treatment agent in patients with gout or diabetes mellitus, and it should be used cautiously in this population.

Adverse Events

Niacin use has been limited primarily because of its extensive adverse events. Although it is one of the most effective agents for improving lipid profiles, most patients cannot tolerate the adverse events. The most common adverse events are attributed to an increase in prostaglandin activity and include pruritus and flushing of the face and neck. A dose of aspirin, 325 mg, taken 30 minutes before the niacin dose may decrease the severity. As mentioned earlier, niacin can also increase uric acid levels and worsen glucose control and should be used cautiously, if at all, in patients with a history of gout or diabetes mellitus. Baseline glucose and uric acid levels should be checked in all patients starting niacin therapy.

Other adverse events include GI side effects (it is contraindicated in patients with an active peptic ulcer), rash, hepatotoxicity, and, rarely, acanthosis nigricans (hyperpigmentation of the skin, usually in the axilla, neck, or groin). As with the statins, LFTs should be monitored at 6 and 12 weeks after initiating or titrating therapy and periodically thereafter.

Cholesterol Absorption Inhibitors

Currently, there is only one cholesterol absorption inhibitor on the market, ezetimibe (Zetia). Ezetimibe appears to act at the brush border of the small intestine and inhibits the absorption of cholesterol, leading to a decrease in the delivery of intestinal cholesterol to the liver. This causes a reduction of hepatic cholesterol stores and an increase in clearance of cholesterol from the blood; this distinct mechanism is complementary to that of HMG-CoA reductase inhibitors.

Zetia, introduced in April 2003, is indicated for use as monotherapy or as combination therapy with a statin. LDL cholesterol levels are reduced by up to 18% with monotherapy and up to an additional 25% when added to ongoing statin therapy. Together with a statin, LDL cholesterol reductions of more than 50% have been noted. The recommended dosage of ezetimibe is 10 mg daily. If taken with a bile acid sequestrant, ezetimibe should be taken 2 hours before or 4 hours after the bile acid (**Table 20.8**).

The Ezetimibe and Simvastatin Hypercholesterolemia Enhances Atherosclerosis Regression (ENHANCE) trial, which evaluated the impact of adding ezetimibe to simvastatin, found no significant change in carotid artery inima-media thickness (a marker for atherosclerosis progression) despite significant decreases in LDL cholesterol and CRP levels (Kastelein, et al., 2008). Because there are no studies showing a decrease in CV events with the use of ezetimibe, the findings from this study question the benefits of using ezetimibe for treatment at this time.

Contraindications

Ezetimibe is contraindicated in patients who have a hypersensitivity to any component of the medication. The combination

TABLE 20.8   Doses and Lipid-Lowering Ability of Other Available Agents

Class	Generic Name (Trade Name)	Usual Daily Dose	LDL*	HDL*	Triglycerides*
Cholesterol absorption inhibitors	ezetimibe (Zetia)‡	10 mg	↓16–19% ↓33–60%	↑3–4% ↑8–11%	↓5% ↓19–40%
Niacin†	niacin (various)	1.5–3.0 g	↓12–21%	↑18–30%	↓15–44%
Fibric acid derivatives	gemfibrozil (Lopid)	600 mg BID	0	↑6%	↓31%
	fenofibrate (various)	48–200 mg QD	↓20%	↑11%	↓38%
Combination products	lovastatin/niacin	20/500 to 40/2000 mg	↓30–42%	↑20–30%	↓32–44%
	simvastatin/ezetimibe	10/10 to 80/10 mg	↓45–60%	↑6–10%	↓23–31%

*Effects on lipid levels are dose dependent.
†Dose must be titrated slowly (usually weekly) to avoid side effects.
‡Results in first line are those seen when used as monotherapy (Bays, et al., 2001). Second results are those seen when used with statin therapy (Kerzner, et al., 2003 [lovastatin]; Davidson, et al., 2002 [simvastatin]; Ballantyne, et al., 2003 [atorvastatin]).

of ezetimibe with an HMG-CoA reductase inhibitor is contraindicated in patients with active liver disease or unexplained persistent elevations in serum transaminases. There are no adequate, controlled studies of ezetimibe in pregnant women, so use during pregnancy is indicated only if the potential benefit outweighs any potential risk to the fetus.

Adverse Events

Adverse events with ezetimibe are minimal. Adverse events noted in clinical trials include headache, diarrhea, and abdominal pain. In addition, myopathy and rhabdomyolysis have been noted when given in combination with statins. The incidence of elevated liver enzymes was similar to placebo.

Fibric Acid Derivatives

Fibric acid derivatives are not considered a major class of lipid-lowering drugs because they have minimal effects on LDL cholesterol levels. The exact mechanism of action of fibric acid derivatives is unclear, but the principal effect of triglyceride lowering appears to result from the stimulation of lipoprotein lipase, which enhances the breakdown of VLDL to LDL cholesterol. (See **Figure 20-1**.)

These agents may also inhibit hepatic VLDL production, and they lower triglyceride levels up to 60% and increase HDL cholesterol by up to 30%. Although gemfibrozil and clofibrate (Atromid-S) have minimal effects on LDL cholesterol lowering, fenofibrate (TriCor) has been shown to decrease LDL cholesterol by up to 20%. Fibric acid derivatives are primarily indicated in patients who have severely elevated triglyceride levels and who have not responded to dietary therapy. (See **Table 20.8.**)

Gemfibrozil, clofibrate, and fenofibrate are the currently available fibric acid derivatives.

Dosage

Gemfibrozil is given in 600-mg doses twice daily with breakfast and dinner. A total of 2 g of clofibrate is taken in divided doses two or four times a day without regard to meals. No titration of dose is necessary for either agent, although some patients may respond at lower doses. Fenofibrate therapy is initiated at

43 to 67 mg/d (depending upon formulation). The dosage can be increased to a maximum of 200 mg/d. Because its absorption is increased when taken with food, fenofibrate should be taken with meals. Clofibrate is not commonly used because of a lack of studies showing its benefit in reducing the risk for atherosclerosis. Maximum effects usually are seen after 4 to 6 weeks of therapy.

Contraindications

Fibric acid derivatives are contraindicated in patients with a history of gallstones and in those with severe hepatic or renal dysfunction. No studies have been conducted in pregnant women, so therefore these agents should be used only if the benefits clearly outweigh any risks to the fetus.

Adverse Events

The fibric acid derivatives usually are well tolerated. The most common adverse events are GI-related and include epigastric pain, nausea and vomiting, dyspepsia, flatulence, and constipation. Myopathy can occur and is diagnosed by a creatinine phosphokinase level 10 times above the upper normal limits. The incidence of myopathy is increased when fibric acid derivatives are used with lovastatin and, to a lesser degree, other statins and niacin. As with the other systemic lipid-lowering agents, hepatotoxicity can occur, and LFTs should be monitored at 6 and 12 weeks and periodically thereafter. If LFT values increase to more than two or three times the upper normal limits, the fibric acid derivative should be discontinued. Other adverse events include rhabdomyolysis, cholestatic jaundice, gallstones, and, rarely, leukopenia, anemia, and thrombocytopenia.

Interactions

As mentioned previously, the incidence of myopathy is increased when fibric acids are used in combination with lovastatin and, to a lesser degree, other statins and niacin. Fenofibrate should be used with caution in patients taking anticoagulant therapy because it can increase the effects of the anticoagulant. Doses of the anticoagulant should be lowered and levels monitored closely if fenofibrate therapy is initiated. (See **Table 20.8.**)

Omega-3 Fatty Acids

Similar to fibric acids, omega-3 fatty acids are not considered a major class of lipid-lowering drugs due to a lack of LDL cholesterol lowering. In some cases, omega-3 fatty acids may increase LDL cholesterol levels. Additionally, there have been no studies showing reduced CV morbidity and mortality. There are numerous over-the-counter dietary supplements that contain omega-3 fatty acids; however, there is only one product available via prescription (omega-3-acid ethyl esters [Lovaza®]), which is indicated as an adjunct to diet for the treatment of severe hypertriglyceridemia. Patients should be on a lipid-lowering diet before Lovaza is initiated.

Dosage

Lovaza is given as a once- or twice-daily dose. Patients can either take 4 g (4 capsules) daily, or 2 g (2 capsules) twice daily. There is no dose titration.

Contraindications

Lovaza is contraindicated in patients with a known hypersensitivity to the drug. To date, there is no evidence to suggest that patients who have fish allergies are at an increased risk for an allergic reaction with Lovaza. There are no studies that have included pregnant women, so it should only be used if the benefits outweigh any potential risks to the fetus.

Adverse Events

Omega-3 fatty acids are generally well tolerated. Some of the side effects noted in clinical trials include flulike symptoms, belching, taste changes, upset stomach, and back pain.

Interactions

There has been some evidence to suggest that omega-3 fatty acids prolong bleeding time, but no studies have been performed to determine if there is an interaction with concomitant use of anticoagulants.

Combination Therapy

Some patients may require combination lipid-lowering therapy to achieve desired cholesterol goals, particularly those with severe hypertriglyceridemia or severely elevated LDL cholesterol levels. Combination therapy may also allow the patient to take lower doses of each of the individual drugs. Statins and niacin have been used together for patients with severely elevated LDL cholesterol, low HDL cholesterol, and hypertriglyceridemia. Currently, there are two products available that include a statin and niacin in a single formulation: lovastatin/niacin (Advicor) and simvastatin/niacin (Simcor). To date, there have been no studies showing an increased benefit in reducing CV morbidity and mortality from these combinations.

Bile acid resins can be used safely and effectively with statins, niacin, and fibric acid derivatives to enhance LDL cholesterol lowering. The only concern with using bile acid resins in combination is ensuring that the concomitant medications are taken at least 1 hour before or 4 hours after the resin to ensure adequate GI absorption. Combining statins with a cholesterol absorption inhibitor has shown added benefits in reducing LDL cholesterol.

Other combination therapies are associated with a higher risk of adverse actions, but most can still be used with close monitoring. In general, combining lovastatin with gemfibrozil should be avoided because of the high incidence of myopathy with this combination. However, other agents, such as fluvastatin, have been used successfully with gemfibrozil with close monitoring. Patients with severe hypertriglyceridemia may require the combination of a fibric acid derivative with niacin, with close monitoring for hepatotoxicity. In any case, combination therapy should be used only if the risk–benefit ratio is favorable.

Alternative Therapy

Antioxidant therapy has been a major focus of studies on preventing CHD, but its preventive benefits have yet to be determined. In theory, antioxidants block the conversion of LDL cholesterol to a modified (oxidized) LDL in the vascular endothelium. As mentioned previously, modified LDL cholesterol appears to be more atherogenic than nonoxidized LDL cholesterol. Thus, blocking the production of oxidized LDL cholesterol may slow the atherogenic process. The major antioxidants that have been studied include vitamin E, vitamin C, and beta carotene, a precursor of vitamin A. Most of the beneficial evidence has been seen with the use of vitamin E, but there is no strong evidence to support vitamin E use.

Other alternatives include garlic, vinegar, and fish oils. Although some evidence suggests that these are beneficial, no conclusive evidence exists to support their use.

Selecting the Most Appropriate Agent

Choosing which drugs to use in which order is individualized and based on the patient's clinical status, the amount of cholesterol lowering that is required, and an assessment of potential patient compliance. Factors that affect compliance include side effects, cost of therapy, health beliefs supporting the need to lower high cholesterol levels, and the understanding that this is lifelong treatment. It is estimated that 15% to 46% of patients who start lipid-lowering therapy discontinue their medication within 1 year (Andrade, et al., 1995).

Table 20.9 and **Figure 20-2** give more information. Because of its favorable effects on all lipoproteins, niacin is especially useful in patients with mixed hyperlipidemia, although severe adverse effects may lead to discontinuation of therapy. The kind of hyperlipidemia the patient has is another factor in selecting the most effective drug therapy:

- Patients who have polygenic hyperlipidemia and desired triglyceride and HDL levels are usually treated with bile acid resins, niacin, statins, or cholesterol absorption inhibitors.
- Patients with polygenic hyperlipidemia and isolated low HDL levels may benefit from niacin, a statin, or a combination of a statin and niacin.

TABLE 20.9	Selecting the Most Appropriate Agent	
	Agents	**Comments**
First line	Statins	Most experts agree that the benefits of treatment with statins are a class-wide effect. Choice of an agent depends upon the amount of LDL lowering required to reach goal.
Second line	Niacin, bile acid resins	Niacin has beneficial effects on each of the lipoproteins, but most patients cannot tolerate the side effects of the drug.
		Bile acids are not systemically absorbed and can be used in patients who cannot tolerate the effects of statins or in combination with statins for patients who are unable to reach LDL goal on a statin alone.
Third line	Fibric acid derivatives	Fibric acid derivatives are reserved for patients with very high triglyceride levels (>1,000 mg/dL) who do not respond to dietary interventions or in combination with other agents for patients with elevated triglyceride levels that cannot be controlled with other agents.
	Cholesterol absorption inhibitors	Cholesterol absorption inhibitors can be used alone or in combination with statins. When used in combination, LDL cholesterol lowering of approximately 60% has been shown.

- Patients who have familial hyperlipidemia and desired triglyceride and HDL levels may receive a statin, bile acid resin, cholesterol absorption inhibitor, or niacin.
- Nondiabetic patients with mixed hyperlipidemia may benefit from niacin, a statin, or a fibric acid derivative, such as gemfibrozil, or a combination of niacin–statin, statin–gemfibrozil, niacin–bile acid resin, or niacin–gemfibrozil.
- Diabetic patients with mixed hyperlipidemia may need a statin or fibric acid derivative, such as gemfibrozil, or combination therapy with statin–gemfibrozil, statin–cholesterol absorption inhibitor, statin–bile acid resin, or gemfibrozil–bile acid resin.

Special Population Considerations

Pediatric

Pharmacologic therapy may be considered in children older than age 10 if lifestyle modifications cannot adequately lower cholesterol levels. Use in children younger than age 10 usually is not recommended because atherosclerotic lesions are not thought to develop before this age. A consultation with a lipid specialist is recommended for any child with elevated cholesterol levels.

Geriatric

The age limit at which lipid-lowering therapy should or should not be initiated is a highly debatable issue. A subanalysis from the Cholesterol and Recurrent Events (CARE) trial showed that patients ages 65 to 75 with a previous CV event benefit from lipid-lowering drugs, specifically the statins (Lewis, et al., 1998). There is no strong evidence to support initiating these agents in patients older than age 75.

Women

Lipid-lowering therapy should usually be avoided in women who are pregnant unless the benefits outweigh the risks of use. Statins are classified as category X by the U.S. Food and Drug Administration and should not be used by pregnant women because of the potential for fetal abnormalities. Most other agents are classified as category C, meaning that tests have not been performed in humans.

MONITORING PATIENT RESPONSE

Monitoring for the beneficial effects of lipid-lowering therapy is done by a fasting lipid panel analysis. A fasting lipid panel identifies total cholesterol, HDL cholesterol, triglycerides, and a calculated LDL cholesterol level. Because the LDL cholesterol is a calculated value, inaccurate results can occur in patients with triglyceride levels approaching or exceeding 400 mg/dL. These patients may require a separate test to measure LDL cholesterol directly.

Because maximal effects are seen by 4 to 6 weeks after starting drug therapy, fasting lipid panel results should be reviewed approximately 6 weeks after starting or titrating drug therapy. If no changes are made in therapy, a fasting lipid panel test should be repeated at 3 and 6 months and yearly thereafter if the patient has achieved the LDL cholesterol goal.

PATIENT EDUCATION

Patient education consists of a thorough explanation of the value of modifying habits and making lifestyle changes (diet, exercise) to avoid or enhance drug therapy in reducing lipid levels. Equally important is thorough teaching about the need for regular laboratory tests to evaluate the effect of drug therapy on body systems and organs, such as the liver. Such education will encourage the patient to cooperate with the therapeutic plan.

Two websites that provide useful information for patients are www.americanheart.org (American Heart Association) and www.nhlbi.nih.gov (Department of Health and Human Services, National Institute of Health, National Heart, Lung and Blood Institute). On the latter site, the patient can calculate his or her 10-year risk of having a heart attack.

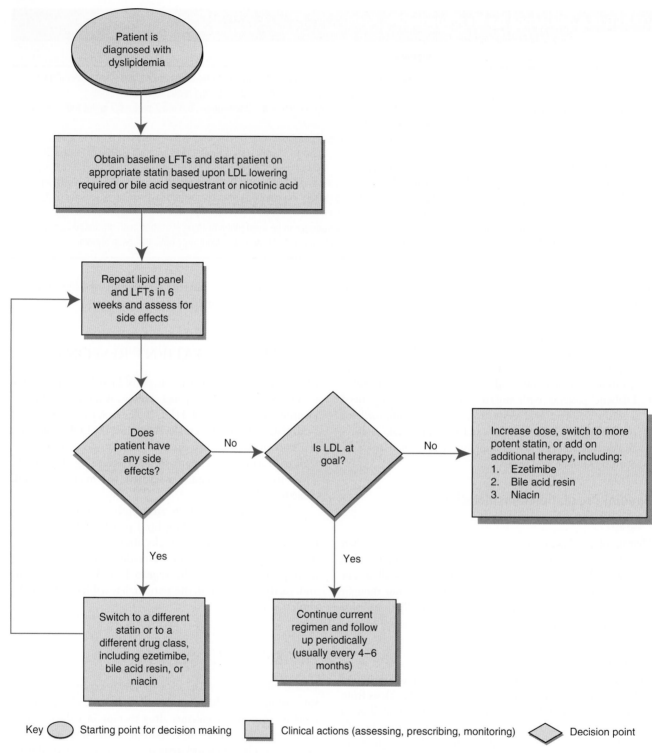

Key ⬭ Starting point for decision making   ▭ Clinical actions (assessing, prescribing, monitoring)   ◇ Decision point

FIGURE 20–2   Treatment algorithm for initiating cholesterol-lowering therapy.

Cholesterol screening should begin at age 20 and should be done every 5 years if it is normal unless there has been a significant lifestyle change, such as significant weight gain. Children should be screened if their parents have a cholesterol level greater than 240 or they have grandparents age 55 or younger with overt CHD.

Drug Information

Grapefruit juice may increase the potency of all statins except pravastatin. It may be taken occasionally with other statins, but not on a daily basis. Patients taking statins should report any new muscle pain, since these drugs can cause myopathy and, rarely, rhabdomyolysis.

Nutrition

The patient should eat a diet low in saturated fats and cholesterol. The diet can include up to 35% daily fats, but no more than 7% saturated fats. Cholesterol intake should be less than 200 mg/d.

Complementary and Alternative Medications

Dietary supplements thought to lower cholesterol include flax seed, garlic, oil of evening primrose, and wine (in moderation), but there are no good clinical studies that provide supportive evidence.

Case Study

J. J., age 55, has come in for his annual physical. He is healthy except for hypertension, which is controlled with enalapril 10 mg daily. His father died at age 55 of a myocardial infarction, and his brother, age 57, just underwent angioplasty. J. J. eats fast food at least 5 times a week because of his work schedule. He weighs 245 lb and stands 5-foot-11. His blood pressure is 134/80. His total cholesterol is 272 (LDL, 162; HDL, 32; triglycerides, 154).

1. List the specific goals of therapy for J. J. What are his ideal values for total cholesterol, LDL, HDL, and triglycerides?
2. What drug therapy would you prescribe, and why?
3. What are the parameters for monitoring the success of the therapy for lowering J. J.'s cholesterol level?
4. Discuss the specific patient education that you would provide to J. J.
5. List one or two adverse reactions for the drug therapy that you prescribed for J. J. that would cause you to change therapy.
6. When rechecked, J. J.'s total cholesterol is 234 (LDL, 135; HDL, 35). What would be your second line of therapy?
7. What over-the-counter or dietary supplements would you recommend to J. J.?
8. What dietary and lifestyle changes would you recommend for J. J.?
9. Describe one or two drug–drug or drug–food interactions for the selected agent.

BIBLIOGRAPHY

Starred references are cited in the text.

*American Heart Association. (2010). *Heart disease and stroke statistics.* www.americanheart.org.

*Andrade, S. E., Walker, A. M., Gottlieb, L. K., et al. (1995). Discontinuation of antihyperlipidemic drugs: Do rates reported in clinical trials reflect rates in primary care settings? *New England Journal of Medicine, 332,* 1125–1131.

*Ballantyne, C. M., Houri, J., Notarbartolo, A., et al. (2003). Effect of ezetimibe coadministered with atorvastatin in 628 patients with primary hypercholesterolemia: A prospective, randomized, double-blind trial. *Circulation, 107*(19), 2409–2415.

*Bays, H. E., Moore, P. B., Drehobl, M. A., et al. (2001). Effectiveness and tolerability of ezetimibe in patients with primary hypercholesterolemia: Pooled analysis of two phase II studies. *Clinical Therapy, 23*(8), 1209–1230.

*Cooke, J. P., & Bhatnagar, R. (1997). Pathophysiology of atherosclerotic vascular disease. *Disease Management and Health Outcomes, 2*(Suppl. 1), 1–8.

*Davidson, M. H., McGarry, T., Bettis, R., et al. (2002). Ezetimibe coadministered with simvastatin in patients with primary hypercholesterolemia. *Journal of the American College of Cardiology, 40*(12), 2125–2134.

*Downs, J. R., Clearfield, M., Weis, S., et al. (1998). Primary prevention of acute coronary events with lovastatin in men and women with average cholesterol levels: Results of AFCAPS/TexCAPS. *Journal of the American Medical Association, 279,* 1615–1622.

Expert Panel, National Cholesterol Education Program. (2001). Executive summary of the third report of the National Cholesterol Education Program (NCEP) Expert Panel on Detection, Evaluation and Treatment of High Blood Cholesterol in Adults (Adult Treatment Panel III). *Journal of the American Medical Association, 285,* 2486–2497.

*Frick, H., Elo, O., Kaapa, K., et al. (1987). Helsinki Heart Study: Primary prevention trial with gemfibrozil in middle-aged men with dyslipidemia. *New England Journal of Medicine, 257,* 3233–3240.

*Genest, J., McPherson, R., Frohlich, J., et al. (2009). Canadian Cardiovascular Society/Canadian guidelines for the diagnosis and treatment of dyslipidemia and prevention of cardiovascular disease in the adult—2009 recommendations. *Canadian Journal of Cardiology, 25,* 567–579.

Grundy, S. M., Cleeman, J. I., Merz, N. B., et al. (2004). NCEP report. *Circulation, 110,* 227–239.

*Heart Protection Study Collaborative Group. (2002). MRC/BHF Heart Protection Study of cholesterol lowering with simvastatin in 20,536 high-risk individuals: A randomised placebo-controlled trial. *Lancet, 360,* 7–22.

*Hjermann, I., Byre, K. V., Holme, I., & Leren, P. (1981). Effect of diet and smoking intervention on the incidence of coronary heart disease: Report from the Oslo Study Group of a randomized trial in healthy men. *Lancet, 2,* 1303–1310.

*Jackson, R., & Beaglehole, R. (1993). The relationship between alcohol and coronary heart disease: Is there a protective effect? *Current Opinion in Lipidology, 4,* 21–26.

*Kastelein, J. J., Akdim, F., Stroes, E. S., et al. for the ENHANCE Investigators. (2008). Simvastatin with or without ezetimibe in familial hypercholesterolemia. *New England Journal of Medicine, 358,* 1431–1443.

*Kerzner, B., Corbelli, J., Sharp, S., et al. (2003). Efficacy and safety of ezetimibe coadministered with lovastatin in primary hypercholesterolemia. *American Journal of Cardiology, 91*(4), 418–424.

*Lewis, S. J., Moye, L. A., Sacks, F. M., et al. (1998). Effect of pravastatin on cardiovascular events in older patients with myocardial infarction and cholesterol levels in the average range: Results of the Cholesterol and Recurrent Events (CARE) Trial. *Annals of Internal Medicine, 129,* 681–689.

*Long-Term Intervention With Pravastatin in Ischaemic Disease (LIPID) Study Group. (1998). Prevention of cardiovascular events and death with pravastatin in patients with coronary heart disease and a broad range of initial cholesterol levels. *New England Journal of Medicine, 339,* 1349–1357.

*McKenney, J. M., & Hawkins, D. W. (1995). *Handbook on the management of lipid disorders*. National Pharmacy Cholesterol Council. Springfield, NJ: Scientific Therapeutics Information, Inc.

*McKenney, J. M., Jones, P. H., Adamczyk, M. A., et al. (2003). Comparison of efficacy of rosuvastatin vs. atorvastatin, simvastatin and pravastatin in achieving lipid goals. Results from STELLAR trial. *Current Medical Research, 19*(8), 689–698.

*National Heart, Lung and Blood Institute. (2002). *Morbidity and mortality: 2002 chartbook on cardiovascular, lung and blood disease*. Bethesda, MD: U.S. Department of Health and Human Services, Public Health Service.

*Newby, L. K., LaPointe, N. M., Chen, A. Y., et al. (2006). Long-term adherence to evidence-base secondary prevention therapies in coronary artery disease. *Circulation, 113,* 203–212.

*Pearson, T. A., Mensah, G. A., Alexander, R. W., et al. (2003). Markers of inflammation and cardiovascular disease: Application to clinical and public health practice: A statement for healthcare professionals from the centers for disease control and prevention and the American Heart Association. *Circulation, 107,* 499–511.

*Ridker, P. M., Danielson, E., Fonseca, F. A., et al. (2008). Rosuvastatin to prevent vascular events in men and women with elevated C-reactive protein. *New England Journal of Medicine, 359,* 2195–2207.

*Ridker, P. M., Hennekens, C. H., Buring, J. E., & Rifai, N. (2000). C-reactive protein and other markers of inflammation in the prediction of cardiovascular disease in women. *New England Journal of Medicine, 342,* 836–884.

*Ross, R., & Glomset, J. A. (1976). The pathogenesis of atherosclerosis (first of two parts). *New England Journal of Medicine, 295,* 369–377.

Rubins, H. B., Robins, S. J., Collins, D., et al. (1999). Gemfibrozil for the secondary prevention of coronary heart disease in men with low levels of high-density lipoprotein cholesterol. *New England Journal of Medicine, 341,* 410–418.

Sacks, F. M., Pfeffer, M. A., Moye, L. A., et al. (1996). The effect of pravastatin on coronary events after myocardial infarction in patients with average cholesterol levels: The Cholesterol and Recurrent Events Trial. *New England Journal of Medicine, 335,* 1001–1009.

*Scandinavian Simvastatin Survival Study Group. (1994). Randomized trial of cholesterol lowering in 4,444 patients with coronary heart disease: The Scandinavian Simvastatin Survival Study (4S). *Lancet, 344,* 1383–1389.

*Shepherd, J., Cobb, S. M., Ford, I., et al. (1995). Prevention of coronary heart disease with pravastatin in men with hypercholesterolemia: The West of Scotland Coronary Prevention Study. *New England Journal of Medicine, 333,* 1301–1307.

*Talbert, R. L. (1997). Hyperlipidemia. In J. T. Dipiro, R. L. Talbert, G. C. Yee, G. R. Matzke, B. G. Wells, & L. M. Posey (Eds.), *Pharmacotherapy: A pathophysiologic approach* (3rd ed., pp. 459–489). Stamford, CT: Appleton & Lange.

CHAPTER 21

Alicia M. Reese
Andrew M. Peterson

Chronic Stable Angina

Cardiovascular disease was responsible for nearly 35% of deaths recorded in 2006, making it the leading cause of death in the United States (American Heart Association, 2010). Angina is a clinical syndrome caused by coronary heart disease (CHD) and affects nearly 10.2 million Americans. In 2004, the cost of cardiovascular disease was estimated to be nearly $240 billion, with CHD accounting for over $133 billion (American Heart Association, 2004).

Fortunately, the overall mortality rate from CHD has been declining. The reason for this decline is the improved treatments for cardiovascular disease, including angina. Despite this hopeful note, angina remains a significant challenge for primary care management. Successful management depends on an in-depth understanding of the pathologic process, diagnosis, and treatment of this symptom complex.

Angina is a syndrome—a constellation of symptoms—that results from myocardial oxygen demand being greater than the oxygen supply (myocardial ischemia). By definition, angina is associated with reversible ischemia, so it does not result in permanent myocardial damage. Myocardial infarction (MI) is the result of irreversible ischemia when myocardial tissue is permanently damaged.

Patients with angina may report chest pain, discomfort, heaviness, or pressure, and the sensation may radiate to the back, neck, jaw, and throat or arms. Usually these sensations last 1 to 15 minutes. Patients may also experience shortness of breath or fatigue. It is important to note, however, that not all patients present with "angina" in a typical fashion. For example, dyspnea on exertion may be the only presenting symptom. If a patient presents with unique symptoms, his or her group of symptoms associated with identified ischemia is called that patient's "anginal equivalent." **Box 21.1** lists common and unique terms used to describe angina.

Angina is called *stable* when the paroxysmal chest pain or discomfort is provoked by physical exertion or emotional stress and is relieved by rest and/or nitroglycerin (NTG). Stable angina exists when the stimulating factors or activities and the degree and duration of discomfort have not changed for the past 60 days.

Anginal episodes that increase in frequency, duration, or severity are referred to as *unstable*. Unstable angina is experienced when the patient is at rest or if the episode is prolonged or progressive. Unstable angina has also been called *preinfarction angina, crescendo angina,* or *intermittent coronary syndrome.*

It is differentiated from stable angina by the fact that symptoms may be triggered by minimal physical exertion or may be present at rest. Patients who experience unstable angina are at high risk for developing an MI.

Other types of angina include variant angina, nocturnal angina, angina decubitus, and postinfarction angina. Stable angina is most commonly managed in the primary care setting and is the focus of this chapter.

CAUSES

The development of angina is directly related to the risk factors that have been identified for CHD. Nonmodifiable risk factors for CHD cannot be altered or improved by the patient; they include age, family history, and gender. Modifiable risk factors may be controlled or treated by lifestyle modifications or pharmacologic therapy to reduce the risk of morbidity or mortality from CHD. Modifiable risk factors include cigarette smoking, hypertension, dyslipidemia, diabetes, obesity, and physical inactivity. **Box 21.2** lists the risk factors for chronic stable angina.

Nonmodifiable Risk Factors

Age

It is uncommon for men younger than age 40 and premenopausal women to have symptomatic CHD, but the incidence increases with age and is increased in women after menopause.

BOX 21.1

Words Patients Use to Describe Angina

Ache, toothache-like, dull
Burning, heartburn, soreness, bursting, searing indigestion
Choking, strangling, compressing, constricting, tightness, viselike
Discomfort, fullness, swelling, heaviness, pressure, weight, uncomfortable

BOX 21.2

Risk Factors for Chronic Stable Angina

NONMODIFIABLE RISK FACTORS

Age
Heredity
Gender

MODIFIABLE RISK FACTORS

Cigarette smoking
Hypertension
Dyslipidemia
Diabetes
Obesity
Physical inactivity

More than 80% of patients who die of CHD are over age 65 (American Heart Association, 2010). This increasing incidence of CHD with age is likely linked to age-related changes in the vasculature and the higher prevalence of other CHD risk factors among older persons.

Heredity

A family history of premature CHD in a first-degree relative (i.e., mother, father, sister, or brother) is a strong predictor for CHD in an individual. Premature CHD is defined as occurring in a man younger than age 55 or in a woman younger than age 65. The strong association between family history and the development of CHD has been consistently demonstrated in several studies. Furthermore, race has been shown to be a factor. Data show that 32% of African-Americans have high blood pressure versus 23% of Whites, thus increasing their risk of a cardiovascular event. Therefore, individuals with a family history of CHD should be carefully screened for other CHD risk factors and managed appropriately.

Gender

In general, the risk of CHD is higher for men than women. Male gender is considered a nonmodifiable risk factor for CHD. Differences for CHD susceptibility diminish, however, when comparing postmenopausal women and older men. In fact, after age 65, the incidence of CHD increases in women, but it does not reach that of men.

Modifiable Risk Factors

Cigarette Smoking

Cigarette smoking increases the risk of CHD by at least two- to threefold. Smoking increases the incidence of atherosclerosis by a mechanism that is not clearly understood. It is thought to increase the release of catecholamines, which leads to elevated blood pressure due to an increased workload of the heart caused by an increase in the heart rate and peripheral vascular constriction. Catecholamines also increase the release of free fatty acids, which increases the amount of lipids in the blood. Smoking lowers high-density lipoprotein (HDL) levels and increases low-density lipoprotein (LDL) levels, and is thought to enhance platelet adhesiveness, which increases the risk of clot formation in the arteries. All patients with CHD risk factors or established disease should be instructed to stop smoking. See Chapter 52 for a more detailed discussion of smoking cessation.

Hypertension

It is estimated that over 74 million Americans have elevated blood pressure (American Heart Association, 2010). Hypertension is a major risk factor for CHD and can lead to vascular complications that increase morbidity and mortality. Additionally, the higher the blood pressure, the higher the risk of MI and other cardiovascular events.

Atherosclerotic changes in the vasculature are exacerbated by increased pressure. Increased blood pressure alone also causes injury to the inner lining of the arteries, resulting in atherosclerotic changes and thrombus formation. As the arteries become stiff and narrow, the blood flow that normally increases during physical activity is restricted to a greater degree, resulting in ischemic symptoms. Chapter 19 provides further discussion of drug therapy for hypertension.

Dyslipidemia

Nearly half of the American population has high cholesterol (American Heart Association, 2010). Cholesterol plays a substantial role in the pathophysiology of atherosclerosis and CHD. High levels of LDL cholesterol and low levels of HDL cholesterol are associated with an increased risk of cardiovascular disease and occurrence of MI or other poor cardiovascular outcomes. Treatment of dyslipidemia in patients with CHD using pharmacologic and nonpharmacologic means has been shown in multiple large-scale studies to reduce the risk of cardiovascular death. See Chapter 20 for more detailed information on the treatment of dyslipidemia.

Diabetes

Cardiovascular disease is the most common cause of death in patients with diabetes. In fact, patients with diabetes have the same risk of having an MI as a patient who already has a history of an MI. Although data have not shown a clear or conclusive link between glucose control and cardiovascular risk reduction, an effort should be made to prevent or treat diabetes in these patients. For a complete discussion of diabetes treatment, see Chapter 45.

Obesity

In the United States, nearly two-thirds of the population is considered overweight or obese. The increasing incidence of obesity has been attributed to poorer nutrition and a more sedentary lifestyle.

Obesity is a risk factor for CHD in both men and women. Hypertension, dyslipidemia, and diabetes are more common in patients who are obese, but obesity also increases cardiovascular risk independent of these other risk factors by a mechanism that is not well understood. Even modest weight loss can improve blood pressure, hypertension, and insulin resistance and reduce cardiovascular risk. Weight loss is discussed in Chapter 54.

Physical Inactivity

A sedentary lifestyle predisposes patients to CHD. Regular physical exercise reduces blood pressure, maintains a healthy weight, and improves dyslipidemia, but it also reduces the risk of CHD independent of these changes. Patients should be carefully screened and counseled before beginning an exercise program. Exercise may include walking, running, cycling, or formalized aerobic exercise routines. It is recommended that patients get 30 to 60 minutes of aerobic exercise every day at least 5 days per week. Resistance training on 2 d/wk may also be of benefit.

PATHOPHYSIOLOGY

Angina is a symptomatic manifestation of reversible myocardial ischemia, which occurs when demand for oxygen in the myocardium exceeds available supply. This imbalance between oxygen supply and demand is caused by limited blood supply due to narrowing of the blood vessels that supply the heart muscle. The most common cause of this narrowing of the coronary arteries is atherosclerotic disease. Rarely, vasospasm of the coronary arteries narrows the arteries, thereby limiting the blood supply to the heart muscle. Other even more uncommon sources of anginal symptoms are thrombosis, aortic stenosis, primary pulmonary hypertension, and severe hypertension.

Atherosclerotic Disease

The pathophysiology of angina involves atherosclerosis, a disorder of lipid metabolism resulting in the deposit of cholesterol in the blood vessel. Over time, this causes a reactive endothelial injury that eventually results in a narrowing of the vessels by episodes of acute thrombosis. The narrow arteries impair the ability of oxygen and nutrients to reach the myocardium. This reduction in blood supply, or ischemia, impairs myocardial metabolism. The myocardial cells remain alive but cannot function normally. Once the blood supply is restored, cardiac function returns to normal. If the ischemia is caused by complete occlusion of the coronary artery, an MI (cell death) occurs.

Regardless of the risk factors that cause the development of atherosclerosis and resulting restriction of coronary blood supply, the pathophysiologic process is essentially the same. The three layers of the arterial wall—intima, media, and adventitia—are affected by structural changes that lead to CHD. The intima is a single layer of endothelial cells, comprising the innermost surface of the artery. It is impermeable to the substances in the blood. The media is the middle layer of the artery and is made up almost entirely of smooth muscle. The outer layer, or adventitia, consists mainly of smooth muscle cells, fibroblasts (which are normally only in this layer), and loose connective tissue. Atherosclerotic changes in the artery occur in stages. Normally, the intima is thin and contains only an occasional muscle cell. As a person ages, the intima slowly increases in thickness and muscle cells proliferate.

Atherosclerosis primarily affects the intima of the arterial wall. It normally takes years to develop and clinical manifestations do not occur until the disorder is well advanced. CHD progresses through three developments—the fatty streak, the fibrous plaque, and the complicated lesion.

The Fatty Streak

Thought to begin in childhood, the fatty streak is caused by the development of fatty, lipid-rich lesions that result from macrophages adhering to the intact endothelial surface. The macrophages take in lipids, which leads to a thickening of the intimal layer. Smooth muscle cells migrate to the intima and become lipid laden. The lesions at this stage do not obstruct the artery. However, on examination, fatty streaks appear in the coronary arteries as early as age 15. They continue to enlarge through the third decade of life and appear to be a precursor to plaque formation, although the process is not clearly understood.

The Fibrous Plaque

The raised fibrous plaque is a white, elevated area on the surface of the artery. It signals the beginning of progressive changes in the arterial wall, including protrusion of the lesion into the lumen of the artery. These more advanced lesions begin to develop at approximately age 30 in most patients. The major change in the arterial intima during this phase is the migration and proliferation of smooth muscle cells and the formation of a fibrous cap over a deeper deposit of extracellular lipid and cell debris. The lipid accumulation directly or indirectly reduces the blood supply. The decrease in blood supply is permanent and results in cell necrosis and cell debris.

The Complicated Lesion

A complicated lesion contains a fibrous plaque, calcium deposits, and a thrombus formed by hemorrhage into the plaque. The complicated lesion results from continuing cell degeneration. As the complicated lesion, with its lipid, necrotic center, becomes larger, it calcifies. The intimal surface may develop open or ruptured areas that degenerate into an ulcer. The damage is most likely to occur in areas where blood flow creates the greatest amount of stress in the vessel, such as at branches and bifurcations. The damaged surface allows blood from the artery lumen to enter the lipid core. Then platelets adhere and thrombus formation begins. The thrombus expands and distorts the plaque, which becomes larger and begins to block the lumen of the artery. The blockage impedes the blood flow needed to supply extra oxygen and nutrients to meet the increased workload of the heart. The result is cardiac ischemia and anginal symptoms. These symptoms are relieved when either the workload of the heart is decreased or administration of vasodilating drugs increases blood flow to the myocardium. Complete blockage can cause permanent myocardial death because the cells are entirely deprived of oxygen and blood flow cannot be restored in time to revive the cardiac cells, resulting in an MI.

Coronary Artery Vasospasm

A less common cause of restricted coronary blood supply may be coronary vasospasm, a narrowing of the coronary artery lumen. This narrowing is produced by an arterial muscle spasm and limits the blood supply to the myocardium. The exact cause is unknown, but it is thought to occur when the smooth muscles of the coronary arteries contract in response to neurogenic stimulation. Cigarette smoking and hyperlipidemia appear to play a role in this type of angina because they interfere with normal neurogenic control of the arterial intima.

Spasm is suspected of playing a role in acute MI, as well as in triggering anginal episodes. Coronary artery spasm also can occur with abrupt nitrate withdrawal, cocaine use, and direct mechanical irritation from cardiac catheterization. However, the exact mechanisms leading to spasm are still unclear.

Activation of Ischemic Episodes

Regardless of the existing pathophysiologic process, ischemic episodes that result in anginal pain are usually activated by two situations occurring simultaneously or independently: (1) ambient factors that increase myocardial oxygen demand, and (2) circumstances that decrease oxygen supply. For example, the person with atherosclerosis (noncompliant arteries) climbs a flight of stairs. The activity increases the workload of the heart and the myocardium needs more oxygen. The damaged arteries are unable to meet this demand. In some situations, the arteries may be so constricted that they are unable to deliver an adequate amount of oxygen even if the person is in a resting state. Therapy is directed at resolution or control of these situations so that the heart can receive the oxygen it needs to meet the physical demands of the body. Control of the blood flow to the heart by increasing it when necessary prevents the pathophysiologic process responsible for the myocardial ischemia.

DIAGNOSTIC CRITERIA

Health History

The health history is an important part of the diagnosis and management of angina. The chief complaint for most patients is usually chest pain or discomfort, but other symptoms may predominate, such as neck or jaw pain or shortness of breath. The patient should be asked to describe the duration, quality, location, severity, and radiation of the pain. Additionally, the practitioner should inquire about potential triggers of the pain and any accompanying symptoms, such as dyspnea, diaphoresis, nausea, or palpitations. The practitioner also should explore what interventions relieved the patient's pain or symptoms, such as rest or NTG.

For all patients with angina, an assessment of CHD risk factors should be performed to determine an individual patient's risk for CHD and to better target pharmacologic and nonpharmacologic management. Practitioners should ask patients about both nonmodifiable and modifiable risk factors, including family history, cigarette smoking, hypertension, dyslipidemia, diabetes, and physical inactivity. A past history of cerebrovascular disease or the presence of peripheral vascular disease also increases a patient's risk of CHD.

Physical Findings

Most commonly, practitioners will not have the opportunity to examine a patient during an acute anginal episode. In that case, the physical examination should focus on the assessment of risk factors and the cardiovascular system as a whole. For example, the practitioner should assess a patient for obesity during the physical examination. Additionally, the vasculature may be evaluated by looking for funduscopic changes or decreased peripheral pulses. Hypertension may be evident from taking the patient's blood pressure, and clinical signs and symptoms of heart failure may include murmurs, changes in the heart sounds, edema, rales, or organomegaly. Patients with dyslipidemia may exhibit xanthomas or cholesterol nodules.

If a physical exam is performed during an episode of anginal pain, a variety of findings may be present. These may include extra heart sounds, mild hypertension, tachycardia, or tachypnea. A paradoxical split of S_2 may indicate altered left ventricular (LV) heart function associated with the ischemic discomfort.

Diagnostic Tests

Before therapy for angina can be properly prescribed, diagnostic testing is necessary to identify a cardiac cause of the patient's chest pain. Diagnostic testing includes electrocardiography, echocardiography, exercise tolerance testing, radioisotope imaging, and coronary artery angiography.

Patients with new, current, or recent chest pain should have an electrocardiogram (ECG) to detect signs of cardiac ischemia. During an acute anginal episode, ST segment depressions with symmetric T-wave inversions may be noted in the leads that correspond to the myocardium affected. During pain-free intervals, however, the ECG reverts to baseline. ECG changes that may be present in the patient with chronic CHD include evidence of a prior MI, LV hypertrophy, and repolarization abnormalities.

Echocardiography is recommended if valvular disease or heart failure is suspected, if the patient has a history of MI, or if the patient experiences ventricular arrhythmias. All patients with intermittent episodes of chest pain should undergo an exercise tolerance test with ECG monitoring (also called a *stress test*) to evaluate the risk of future cardiac events. Those suspected of having coronary ischemia based on the presence of anginal symptoms should undergo testing within 72 hours of symptoms. Further testing with radioisotope perfusion testing or coronary artery angiography may be indicated for subgroups of patients. If diagnostic testing confirms cardiac ischemia as the cause of anginal symptoms, drug therapy is warranted.

INITIATING DRUG THERAPY

The treatment goals for the management of angina include relieving the acute anginal episode, preventing additional anginal episodes, preventing progression of CHD, reducing the risk of MI, improving functional capacity, and prolonging survival. These goals should be accomplished while maintaining the patient's quality of life and avoiding adverse events associated with therapy.

Nonpharmacologic therapy is the cornerstone of treatment for patients with angina. The clinician must assess the patient's modifiable risk factors and work with him or her to reduce the risk for CHD. Practitioners should counsel patients on smoking cessation at each clinic visit and provide support and access to pharmacologic treatment if necessary. Patients should be instructed to maintain a normal weight by consuming a low-fat, low-cholesterol diet, and practitioners should provide dietary counseling and refer interested patients to dietitians for further support. Finally, practitioners should encourage patients to engage in regular aerobic exercise. Further details on these lifestyle modifications are provided in Chapters 19, 20, 45, and 54.

The practitioner should emphasize to the patient that nonpharmacologic therapy and lifestyle modifications supplement drug therapy and should continue indefinitely.

Goals of Drug Therapy

After the patient has been properly instructed on nonpharmacologic therapy for angina, appropriate drug therapy may be initiated. A summary of selected agents is provided in **Table 21.1.** Several classes of medications are used to treat angina, including angiotensin-converting enzyme (ACE) inhibitors, nitrates, beta-blockers, calcium channel blockers, and antiplatelet agents.

Angiotensin-Converting Enzyme (ACE) Inhibitors and Angiotensin Receptor Blockers (ARBs)

The 2007 Chronic Angina Focused Update recommends that patients with ejection fractions of less than 40% or those with hypertension, diabetes, or kidney disease be placed on an ACE inhibitor unless contraindicated. When patients cannot take an ACE inhibitor, an angiotensin receptor blocker (ARB) may be used (Fraker & Fihn, 2007). ACE inhibitors include captopril (Capoten), ramipril (Altace), enalapril (Vasotec), quinapril (Accupril), benazepril (Lotensin), perindopril (Aceon), and lisinopril (Prinivil, Zestril). ARBs include losartan (Cozaar), valsartan (Diovan), candesartan (Atacand), telmisartan (Micardis), eprosartan (Teveten), olmesartan (Benicar), and irbesartan (Avapro).

Mechanism of Action

ACE inhibitors affect the enzyme responsible for the conversion of angiotensin I to angiotensin II. ARBs block the vasoconstriction and aldosterone-secreting effects of angiotensin II by selectively blocking angiotensin II from binding to angiotensin II receptors found in many tissues. Angiotensin II is a potent vasoconstrictor and also stimulates aldosterone secretion. Blocking the production of angiotensin II results in reduced vasoconstriction and sodium and water retention, thus reducing preload, afterload, and ejection fraction. These benefits are helpful in chronic stable angina, heart failure (Chapter 22), and hypertension (Chapter 19).

Dosage

ACE inhibitors and ARBs should be initiated at low doses and followed by gradual dosage increases if the lower doses are well tolerated. Renal function and serum potassium should be assessed within 1 to 2 weeks of starting therapy and periodically thereafter, especially in patients with preexisting diabetes or those receiving potassium supplementation. **Table 21.1** shows the doses of some common ACE inhibitors and ARBs when used to treat chronic stable angina.

Contraindications

ACE inhibitors are contraindicated in pregnancy and should be avoided in patients with bilateral renal artery stenosis or unilateral stenosis.

Adverse Effects

Side effects of ACE inhibitors are uncommon but may include an irritating cough and excessive drops in blood pressure, particularly in hypovolemic patients or those already on diuretics. Hyperkalemia may also occur; however, the incidence is less with ARBs than with ACE inhibitors. A serious adverse effect with ACE inhibitors is angioedema, which usually occurs early in treatment. Angioedema secondary to an ACE inhibitor is a contraindication to further ACE inhibitor use, but an ARB may be used in its place. Other adverse effects include rash, loss of taste, neutropenia, and agranulocytosis.

Interactions

Due to the effects on angiotensin II and aldosterone, ACE inhibitors contribute to potassium retention as sodium is preferentially excreted. This raises the possibility of a hyperkalemic state for the patient and must be monitored routinely. Similarly, patients taking lithium are at increased risk for lithium toxicity due to its decreased renal excretion. Other important ACE inhibitor interactions can be found in Chapter 22, **Table 22.3.**

Nitrates

The nitrates are one of the original medications used for controlling angina, and they are still commonly used to halt an acute anginal attack, to prevent predictable episodes, and for chronic treatment to prevent anginal episodes.

Mechanism of Action

Nitrates and their analogs are potent agents and have profound effects on vascular smooth muscle. The nitrates cause dilation throughout the vasculature—in the peripheral arteries and

TABLE 21.1 Overview of Agents Used to Treat Chronic Stable Angina

Generic (Trade) Name and Dosage	Selected Adverse Events	Contraindications	Special Considerations
Selected Angiotensin-Converting Enzyme Inhibitors			
captopril (Capoten) Start: 6.25 mg or 12.5 mg tid Therapeutic range: 25–100 mg tid	Common: cough; hypotension, particularly with a diuretic or volume depletion; hyperkalemia, loss of taste, leukopenia; angioedema, neutropenia, and agranulocytosis in <1% of patients; rash in >10% of patients	Contraindicated in pregnancy; avoid in patients with bilateral renal artery stenosis or unilateral stenosis	Renal impairment related to ACE inhibitors is seen as an increase in serum creatinine and azotemia, usually in the beginning of therapy. Monitor BUN, creatinine, and K levels when starting.
enalapril (Vasotec) Start: 2.5 mg qd or bid Range: 5–20 mg qd or bid daily	Same as above	Same as above	Same as above Use only 2.5 mg/d in patient with impaired renal function or hyponatremia.
fosinopril (Monopril) Start: 10 mg qd Range: 10–40 mg qd	Same as above	Same as above	Same as above Use only 5 mg/d in patient with impaired renal function or hyponatremia.
lisinopril (Zestril, Prinivil) Start: 5 mg qd Range: 5–20 mg qd	Same as above	Same as above	Same as above Use only 2.5 mg/d in patient with impaired renal function or hyponatremia.
quinapril (Accupril) Start: 5 mg bid Range: 20–40 bid	Same as above	Same as above	Same as above Use only 2.5 mg/d in patient with impaired renal function or hyponatremia.
ramipril (Altace) Start: 1.25 mg twice daily Range: 1.25–5 mg twice daily	Same as above	Same as above	Same as above
Selected Angiotensin Receptor Blockers (ARBs)			
losartan (Cozaar) Start: 12.5 mg/day Range: 50–100 mg/day	Dyspnea, hypotension, hyperkalemia	Angioedema secondary to ACE inhibition	May be used in patients experiencing cough due to ACE inhibitor
valsartan (Diovan) Start: 80 mg/day Range: 80–160 mg twice daily	Same as above	Same as above	Same as above
Short-Acting Nitrates			
nitroglycerin (Nitrostat, NitroQuick) 0.4 mg SL prn	Headache, dizziness, tachycardia, hypotension, edema	Combination with phosphodiesterase-5 inhibitors (e.g., sildenafil, vardenafil, and tadalafil)	For acute treatment of anginal episodes
isosorbide dinitrate (ISDN; Isordil, Sorbitrate) 5 mg SL prn	Above notes also apply	Above notes also apply	Above notes also apply
Long-Acting Nitrates			
nitroglycerin Topical ointment (Nitro-bid) ½–1 in bid-tid	Above notes also apply	Above notes also apply	For chronic prevention of anginal episodes Use nitrate-free interval to reduce risk of nitrate tolerance. Potential hypotensive effect with vasodilators Tapering is recommended after long-term use.
Transdermal patch (Minitran, Nitro-Dur, Nitrol, Transderm-Nitro) 0.2–0.8 mg/hr	Local irritation and erythema with topical application		Onset of action with transdermal application is approximately 60 minutes.

Medication and Dose	Adverse Effects	Contraindications/Precautions	Comments
isosorbide mononitrate (ISMN) Immediate release (Ismo, Monoket) 5–20 mg bid Extended release (Imdur) 30–120 mg bid	Above notes also apply	Above notes also apply	Above notes also apply Extended-release formulations should be swallowed whole.
Beta Blockers			
propranolol Immediate release (Inderal) 40–160 mg bid Extended release (Inderal LA) 80–240 mg qd	Fatigue, dizziness, decreased exercise tolerance, bradycardia, hypotension, dyspnea	Use with caution in patients with reactive airway disease. Bradycardia (heart rate <45 beats per minute) Acutely decompensated heart failure	Abrupt cessation of beta-blocker therapy should be avoided. Extended-release formulations should be swallowed whole.
atenolol (Tenormin) 25–100 mg qd	Above notes also apply	Above notes also apply	Above notes also apply
metoprolol Immediate release (metoprolol tartrate, Lopressor) 25–200 mg tid Extended release (metoprolol succinate, Toprol XL) 50–100 mg qd	Above notes also apply	Above notes also apply	Toprol XL tablets may be split, but should not be chewed or crushed.
Calcium Channel Blockers			
amlodipine (Norvasc) 2.5–10 mg qd	Headache, dizziness, flushing, edema, gingival hyperplasia	Severe conduction abnormalities Use with caution in patients with pre-existing bradycardia or CHF.	Useful for patients with isolated systolic hypertension
nifedipine (extended release, Adalat CC, Procardia XL) 30–60 mg qd	Above notes also apply	Above notes also apply	Should be swallowed whole
diltiazem (extended release, Cardizem CD, Dilacor XR, Tiazac) 180–420 mg qd	Headache, nausea, conduction abnormalities, gingival hyperplasia	Above notes also apply	Should be swallowed whole
verapamil Immediate release (Calan, Isoptin) 80–320 mg bid Extended release (Calan SR, Isoptin SR) 120–480 mg qd	Above notes also apply Constipation	Above notes also apply	Extended-release formulations should be swallowed whole.
Antiplatelet Agents			
aspirin 81–325 mg qd	Nausea, dyspepsia	Allergy to aspirin Bleeding disorders	For primary and secondary prevention of cardiovascular events
clopidogrel (Plavix) 75 mg qd	Nausea	Allergy to clopidogrel Bleeding disorders	Alternative antiplatelet agent for aspirin-intolerant patients
Ranolazine			
ranolazine (Ranexa) 500–1000 mg qd	Dizziness, nausea, constipation	Patients taking strong inhibitors of CYP3A4 and/or severe hepatic impairment	Should be swallowed whole

veins as well as the coronary arteries. When dilated, the veins return less blood to the heart, thereby reducing LV filling volume and pressure (preload). This decreases the workload of the heart. Another primary effect of the nitrates is coronary arterial dilation, which results in increased blood flow and oxygen supply to the myocardium. Nitrates do not directly influence the chronotropic or inotropic actions of the heart, so their administration does not affect or alter cardiac function, but rather decreases the work of the heart and increases myocardial oxygenation. Nitrates are moderately effective in lessening coronary vasospasm.

Rapid-Acting Nitrates

The sublingual forms of NTG are rapid acting. (See **Table 21.1.**) These medications are used for acute attacks of angina. Short-acting nitrates are also used for prophylaxis of angina in situations when an anginal episode can be reasonably predicted by the patient, such as during walking, climbing stairs, or sexual activity. To be effective, NTG must be administered sublingually to avoid hepatic first-pass metabolism, which would inactivate the medication.

Sublingual NTG (Nitrol, Isordil, others) remains the first-line therapy for managing acute angina episodes. NTG may be adequate treatment for patients who experience angina no more frequently than once a week. NTG usually relieves anginal symptoms within 1 to 5 minutes and provides short-term (up to 30 minutes) relief. NTG tablets or spray (0.3 to 0.6 mg) is used sublingually for immediate symptomatic treatment of anginal episodes. The practitioner instructs the patient to rest at the time of pain, take a single dose, repeat the dose if the pain does not resolve within 5 minutes, and to call emergency medical services if the pain is not relieved with 3 doses.

Patients should be instructed to mark the date they open a bottle of NTG tablets or first use an NTG spray canister. Tablets in an opened glass bottle of NTG retain efficacy for only 1 year and should be discarded after that time period. NTG canisters retain their efficacy for up to 3 years.

The main advantage of rapid-acting nitrates is their ability to halt an episode of angina once it has begun. Generally, the adverse effects of short-acting nitrates are related to their vasodilatory effects; however, patients may also experience burning under the tongue with sublingual preparations.

Long-Acting Nitrates

Due to their short duration of action, short-acting nitrates such as sublingual NTG are not suitable for maintenance therapy; long-acting nitrates must be used for chronic prophylaxis of anginal episodes. Long-acting nitrates act to maintain vasodilation, thereby continuously decreasing the workload of the heart and maintaining blood flow to the heart. The most prescribed long-acting nitrates are isosorbide dinitrate (ISDN; oral [Cedocard SR, Isordil, others]), isosorbide mononitrate (ISMN; oral [Imdur, Ismo, Monoket, others]), and long-acting NTG preparations (transdermal [Minitran, Nitro-Dur, Transderm-Nitro, others], topical [Nitro-Bid, others]).

Isosorbide Dinitrate (Oral)

Single oral doses of 20 to 40 mg significantly improve hemodynamic parameters and exercise tolerance, and the effect continues for several hours. The starting dose should be low (e.g., ISDN 5 mg three times a day) and the dosage should be advanced slowly in small increments every 1 to 2 weeks to minimize side effects. The dose is increased until control is obtained, side effects become intolerable, systolic blood pressure falls to 100 mm Hg or below, resting heart rate increases more than 10 beats per minute, or postural hypotension occurs.

Intestinal absorption with ISDN is unpredictable, especially when taken with food, so oral nitrates should be taken on an empty stomach, 1 hour before or 2 hours after food intake. A drawback to ISDN products is the short half-life (approximately 2 to 4 hours) and duration of action, which necessitates multiple doses during the day.

Isosorbide Mononitrate (Oral)

ISMN is a long-acting metabolite derivative of ISDN. Formulated in extended-release tablets, ISMN can be administered in fewer doses (Imdur, once daily; other products, twice daily). A common twice-daily starting regimen is 20 mg (immediate-release) orally at 7 AM and 3 PM, allowing for a nitrate-free period to reduce the risk of nitrate tolerance. A starting dose using extended-release ISMN (Imdur) is 30 to 60 mg orally in the morning. Like ISDN, ISMN should also be taken on an empty stomach. Extended-release formulations of ISMN must be taken whole, without crushing or chewing the tablet.

Nitroglycerin (Transdermal)

Transdermal NTG is long-acting and effective for treating and preventing anginal pain. Two percent (2%) NTG ointment may be applied to the skin as an adjunct to isosorbide therapy for nocturnal pain or, with repeated daily dosing, used alone for anginal treatment. One half to one inch of the ointment is applied to a clean, hairless area of the torso before bed. Alternatively, the ointment may be applied every 4 to 6 hours while awake, allowing for an 8- to 12-hour nitrate-free interval. Measurement guides are provided with the product to assist in dosing. The dose is increased by a half inch at a time until pain relief is achieved.

Transdermal NTG patches may also be used as a long-acting nitrate. Therapy is typically initiated with a 5-mg (0.2 mg/h) or 10-mg (0.4 mg/h) patch, which should be left in place for 12 to 14 hours and then removed to prevent nitrate tolerance. Nitrate patches should be applied to the torso intact, since cutting a patch destroys the drug delivery system. Care should be taken to ensure a previously applied patch is removed before applying a new patch.

Nitrate Tolerance

A drawback to the use of nitrates to treat angina is the potential for the development of nitrate tolerance. Nitrate tolerance refers to the loss of ability of the smooth muscles to respond to the action of the nitrates. Tolerance develops to both the peripheral and coronary vasodilator effects of nitrates. This phenomenon occurs with continuous nitrate use over prolonged periods. Tolerance is both dose- and time-dependent. Nitrate tolerance can be seen after as few as 7 to 10 days of continuous administration. Nitrate tolerance may also develop with frequent sublingual administration of nitrates, if the oral tablets are given four times daily in evenly spaced intervals, or if the transdermal patches are left on the skin for 24-hour periods.

Prevention of nitrate tolerance is based on a treatment plan that provides for rapid changes in blood nitrate levels over a given time, usually 24 hours. To prevent nitrate tolerance, one 10- to 12-hour nitrate-free interval per day is necessary. In this manner, the intervals between doses need not be equal. For example, the patch can be applied in the morning and removed in the evening. The same schedule can be developed for patients taking oral medications. The medication is given three times during the day when the patient is awake. The patient does not receive any medication during the night to minimize the risk of nitrate tolerance. Combination antianginal therapy (e.g., a beta blocker plus a long-acting nitrate) should be used for patients whose anginal symptoms are not controlled during the nitrate-free interval.

Adverse Events

The common side effects of the nitrates are related to their vasodilatory effects: headache, flushing, dizziness, weakness, and orthostatic hypotension. Additionally, since all segments of the vascular system relax in response to nitrates, reflex tachycardia often results as the heart compensates for the blood pressure drop to maintain cardiac output. Transdermal nitrate products may also cause irritation of the skin at the site of application.

Most of the side effects associated with nitrates abate or disappear with continuation of therapy. By starting therapy at a low dose and slowing titrating the dose upward, side effects are minimized and may not present at all. However, starting with a high dose can produce severe side effects (especially headache), and if side effects are intolerable, the patient may self-discontinue the medication.

If a patient has been receiving nitrate therapy long-term, it should not be abruptly discontinued because of the risk of rebound hypertension and angina. If discontinuation of nitrate therapy is required, it should be done by tapering the dose over a period of time.

Caution should be exercised when using nitrates in combination with vasodilators due to additive hypotensive effects. Concurrent use of nitrates and phosphodiesterase-5 inhibitors such as sildenafil (Viagra), vardenafil (Levitra), or tadalafil (Cialis) is contraindicated due to the potential for severe hypotension.

Beta Blockers

Beta blockers are very effective in managing angina. They reduce the workload of the heart and decrease overall myocardial oxygen demand and consumption through antagonism of adrenergic receptors. This is accomplished by a reduction in the heart rate and myocardial contractility, both at rest and during periods of normal exercise. As such, they are particularly beneficial for treating exertional angina.

Nitrates and beta blockers have complementary effects on myocardial oxygen supply and demand and therefore are often used together. Because beta blockers reduce the heart rate, they can be used to control the reflex tachycardia that sometimes occurs with the administration of nitrates. This reduction in heart rate also allows more time for myocardial perfusion during diastole.

Mechanism of Action

Beta blockers can be categorized according to their cardioselectivity, that is, the degree of preferential affinity for $beta_1$ receptors, which predominate in the heart and are the principal target of these medications. Beta antagonists that block only $beta_1$ receptors are considered *cardioselective* beta blockers. Those that block both $beta_1$ and $beta_2$ receptors are *nonselective*. There are many beta blockers available, all of which block $beta_1$ receptors. However, many agents also block $beta_2$ receptors, which predominate in the lungs.

$Beta_1$-receptor blockade is desirable in a patient with angina because it causes a slowing of the heart rate and a reduction in myocardial contractility. These effects reduce myocardial oxygen demand and therefore improve and prevent anginal symptoms.

Blockage of $beta_2$ receptors can lead to bronchoconstriction; therefore, nonselective beta blockers should be used with caution in patients with uncontrolled or unstable reactive airway disease. At low to intermediate doses, cardioselectivity is demonstrated by atenolol (Tenormin) and metoprolol (Lopressor). Propranolol (Inderal) is an example of a nonselective beta blocker. However, even cardioselective beta blockers show nonselective action at high doses.

Propranolol is a nonselective beta blocker with a short half-life (4 to 6 hours). Immediate-release formulations of propranolol must be dosed multiple times per day, but sustained-release preparations for once-daily dosing are also available. Other nonselective beta blockers include nadolol and timolol.

Atenolol and metoprolol are selective $beta_1$ antagonists. These drugs, which preferentially block $beta_1$ receptors, were developed to eliminate the unwanted bronchoconstriction effect of the agents that also block $beta_2$ receptors. These agents may be a better choice for patients with severe or uncontrolled asthma or chronic obstructive pulmonary disease (COPD). However, when these agents are prescribed at high dosage levels, they lose their cardioselective properties. Atenolol has a long duration of action, and therefore may be dosed once daily. Immediate-release metoprolol tartrate (Lopressor) must be given two to three times daily, but extended-release metoprolol succinate (Toprol XL) is given only once daily. Both atenolol and metoprolol tartrate are available in generic forms and are relatively inexpensive.

Pindolol and acebutolol are beta blockers that also possess some agonist activity. They are not completely blockers in that they have the ability also to stimulate weakly both beta$_1$ and beta$_2$ receptors, possessing so-called *intrinsic sympathomimetic activity* (ISA). Drugs possessing ISA can stimulate the beta receptor to which they are bound, yet as antagonists they block the activation of the receptor by the more potent endogenous catecholamines, epinephrine and norepinephrine. Because of the agonist action, there is a diminished effect on cardiac rate and cardiac output. Patients who cannot tolerate the other beta blockers because of pre-existing bradycardia or heart block may tolerate these agents.

Contraindications

Beta blockers are contraindicated and therefore should not be used in patients with pre-existing bradycardia because beta blockade may lower the heart rate further. Additionally, beta blockers should not be used if a patient is experiencing an acute episode of decompensated heart failure. The addition of a beta blocker in this situation has the potential to negatively impact the patient by further reducing heart rate and contractility. Finally, as discussed above, beta blockers should be used with caution in patients with reactive airway disease. In patients with stable or controlled asthma or COPD, a selective beta blocker may be a better choice to minimize the risk of bronchospasm.

Adverse Events

Beta blockers have the potential to adversely affect cardiac function. These effects include slowing the sinoatrial node and atrioventricular (AV) conduction, leading to symptomatic bradycardia and heart block. Sinus arrest is possible. If the patient has pre-existing cardiac conduction system disease, a preparation with some intrinsic beta-agonist activity may be chosen to minimize these adverse events. These patients require close and frequent monitoring to ensure that early conduction system disease is managed promptly. Beta blockers should not be given to patients with a slow heart rate at baseline due to the potential for severe bradycardia.

Since beta blockers attenuate the "fight or flight" response, the clinical manifestations of hypoglycemia may be masked. Therefore, patients with diabetes should be instructed to more closely monitor their serum glucose to avoid severe hypoglycemic reactions. Typical symptoms of hypoglycemia, including tachycardia, tremor, or sweating, may be decreased or absent when these patients are taking a beta blocker.

Abrupt withdrawal of beta blockers can precipitate tachycardia, hypertensive crises, angina exacerbation, acute coronary insufficiency, or even MI (Goroll et al., 1998). For this reason, beta blocker therapy should always be tapered. Withdrawal is of particular concern in the anginal patient on large doses of beta blockers who is faced with an emergency situation that makes it impossible to continue taking the prescribed beta blocker for more than 48 hours.

Beta blockers may also cause adverse central nervous system effects, including drowsiness and depression. These effects may occur more frequently in the elderly or in patients with pre-existing depression or psychiatric disorders. In these patients, careful monitoring of mood, sleep pattern, and sexual and cognitive functioning is necessary.

Calcium Channel Blockers

Calcium channel blockers are effective in managing angina because they exert vasodilatory effects on the coronary and peripheral vessels. Depending on the specific agent, they have the potential to depress cardiac contractility, heart rate, and conduction, which may mediate their antianginal effects. These drugs are effective in relieving coronary constriction associated with vasospastic angina.

Mechanism of Action

Calcium plays a major role in the electrical excitation and contraction of cardiac and vascular smooth muscle cells. The calcium channel blockers inhibit the entrance of calcium into smooth muscle cells of the coronary and systemic arterial vessels, which inhibits muscular contraction and therefore causes vasodilation. These vasodilatory effects are more pronounced on arteries than veins because of the relatively large amount of smooth muscle found in the arteries. Because calcium channel blockers do not cause substantial venous dilation, they do not reduce preload. Calcium channel blockers reduce heart rate by slowing conduction through the sinoatrial and atrioventricular nodes, and they depress cardiac contractility.

Two major groups of calcium channel blockers are available: the dihydropyridines and the nondihydropyridines.

Dihydropyridines

The dihydropyridine calcium channel blockers are potent dilators of the coronary and peripheral arteries. Due to the vasodilatory effect of these agents, they may cause reflex tachycardia due to a reduction in systemic blood pressure. Since dihydropyridines do not alter conduction, they do not slow the sinus rate.

There are many dihydropyridine calcium channel blockers available. Nifedipine is an example of a first-generation dihydropyridine; nicardipine, felodipine, isradipine, and amlodipine are second-generation dihydropyridines. In general, the second-generation agents are better tolerated than the first-generation agents.

All of these agents are administered orally, and they have relatively short half-lives. Doses should be titrated upward slowly to minimize orthostasis or other adverse events. Several dihydropyridines (e.g., nifedipine, nicardipine) must be administered as multiple daily doses unless the sustained formulations are used. Amlodipine is administered once daily.

Nondihydropyridines

Although diltiazem and verapamil are both nondihydropyridine calcium channel blockers, they display different effects on the cardiovascular system. Verapamil has a pronounced effect on cardiac conduction, reducing the rate of electrical conduction through the AV node. Verapamil also exerts negative inotropic and chronotropic effects, suppressing contractility, reducing heart rate, and therefore causing a reduction in oxygen demand. However, due to this effect, verapamil should be used with caution in those patients with depressed cardiac function or AV conduction abnormalities. Immediate-release formulations of verapamil must be administered as divided doses, but sustained-release products are administered once daily.

Like verapamil, diltiazem reduces the heart rate but to a lesser extent. Diltiazem also has a less potent effect than verapamil on conduction and contractility, but it is a more potent vasodilator. Diltiazem has immediate- and sustained-release formulations. The immediate-release formulation usually is taken four times a day before meals; the sustained-release formulation is taken daily on an empty stomach.

Contraindications

Before a calcium channel blocker can be selected for treating angina, a careful assessment must be done to determine a patient's LV and conduction system function. Calcium channel blockers with negative inotropic properties may worsen pre-existing LV dysfunction. Patients with conduction system disease are poor candidates for calcium channel blocker therapy because of the risk of bradyarrhythmias.

The nondihydropyridine calcium channel blockers are contraindicated in patients with heart block because of the significant depression of AV node conduction. Additionally, calcium channel blockers should be used with caution in patients with sick sinus syndrome and hypotension.

Adverse Events

In general, adverse events accompanying the dihydropyridine calcium channel blockers are more common with the first-generation than the second-generation agents. Leg edema, a common problem, results from vasodilation, which causes fluid to pool in the legs. In some cases, the edema may be so severe that new-onset heart failure may be suspected. In this situation, dosage reduction or drug discontinuation may be considered. Other common side effects of the calcium channel blockers include fatigue, dizziness, headache, flushing, and gingival hyperplasia. Verapamil is associated with constipation much more often than the other calcium channel blockers.

Antiplatelet Therapy

Antiplatelet drugs inhibit platelet aggregation through a variety of mechanisms. Aspirin inhibits platelet activation through irreversible enzyme antagonism to block prostaglandin synthesis, and clopidogrel reduces ADP-induced platelet activation. Aggregation is a normal process that causes disease when the platelets adhere to vessel walls, causing thrombus formation. Antiplatelet therapy limits the formation of the thrombus, thereby decreasing the risk of progressive CHD. When antiplatelet medications are used to treat patients with angina, the chances of having an MI are reduced.

In patients with stable angina, the risk of MI can be lowered with daily aspirin therapy. Aspirin acts by blocking prostaglandin synthesis, which prevents formation of the platelet-aggregating substance thromboxane A_2. Current angina recommendations suggest that all patients with acute or chronic ischemic heart disease receive aspirin as primary or secondary prevention of cardiovascular disease (Fraker & Fihn, 2007).

The usual dosage of aspirin for antiplatelet therapy is 75 to 162 mg taken once daily. Adverse events associated with aspirin use include dyspepsia, bruising, and bleeding. Enteric-coated aspirin may be prescribed to minimize gastrointestinal symptoms. Aspirin is contraindicated in patients with a known aspirin hypersensitivity.

Clopidogrel is another antiplatelet agent that may be used in patients with angina. It reduces ADP-induced platelet activation by antagonizing the platelet ADP receptors. Clopidogrel is recommended for prevention of MI in angina patients who have contraindications to aspirin. Like aspirin, clopidogrel has been shown to reduce the incidence of morbidity and mortality in patients with established cardiovascular disease.

The dose of clopidogrel is 75 mg daily. Since it is only commercially available as a branded product, clopidogrel is more expensive than aspirin for most patients. Bleeding events associated with clopidogrel are similar to aspirin, although it typically exhibits better gastrointestinal tolerance. However, clopidogrel is metabolized to its active component, in part by the CYP2C19 system, which in certain patients shows significant genetic variation. Data have shown that this genetic variation may play a role in the effectiveness of this agent, particularly in those who have a slow metabolism. For further discussion of antiplatelet agents, refer to Chapter 49.

Ranolazine

Ranolazine (Ranexa) is a unique antianginal agent that can be used alone or in combination with nitrates, beta blockers, calcium channel blockers, or ACE inhibitors. Currently, its primary role is as an adjunctive agent for patients who are not achieving adequate symptom relief with other agents.

Mechanism of Action

The mechanism of action of ranolazine is not well understood, but it is thought to block late-phase sodium channels, which often remain open during hypoxic or ischemic events. An increase in intracellular sodium during late-phase affects sodium-dependent calcium channels, thus increasing the amount of calcium entering the cell and causing a calcium overload. This overload can lead to further or continued contraction of the myocardium, increasing oxygen demand. By blocking late-phase sodium channels, ranolazine decreases calcium overload and breaks the cycle of ischemia.

Dosage

Ranolazine is taken orally at 500 mg twice daily and can be titrated up to a maximum of 1,000 mg twice daily. Ranexa® tablets should be swallowed whole, not crushed or split. There may need to be a dose reduction in patients taking CYP3A4 inhibitors, such as diltiazem and verapamil.

Contraindications

Ranolazine is contraindicated in patients taking ketoconazole, itraconazole, clarithromycin, and other strong CYP3A4 inhibitors.

Adverse Events

Ranolazine prolongs the QTc interval in a dose-related manner; however, in long-term studies, there has been no association with an increased risk of proarrhythmia or sudden death. Regardless, caution should still be used because there is little experience with doses greater than 1,000 mg twice daily. Dose-related dizziness, headache, constipation, and nausea are common adverse effects. Other adverse events include palpitations, vertigo, dry mouth, peripheral edema, hypotension and, less commonly, angioedema and renal failure.

Interactions

As noted earlier, patients taking potent CYP3A4 inhibitors should not take ranolazine, and less potent inhibitors warrant monitoring. Conversely, agents that induce the CYP3A4 system, such as rifampin, carbamazepine, phenytoin, and St. John's wort, may decrease plasma concentrations of ranolazine. Ranolazine, through the P-glycoprotein system, may increase digoxin levels.

Selecting the Most Appropriate Antianginal Therapy

Choosing the appropriate medications for treating a patient with angina can be challenging. The primary goal is to design a regimen that will reduce the frequency and severity of anginal episodes. Subsequent adjustments are made empirically based on the patient's response to treatment, disease progression, risk factor modification, and patient satisfaction and adherence (**Figure 21-1**).

Acute Treatment of Anginal Episodes

All patients with angina should be provided a short-acting nitrate for acute treatment of anginal episodes. Additionally, patients with infrequent episodes of angina can be managed effectively with short-acting nitrates alone. They are a good choice for the patient who has infrequent attacks or predictable pain on exertion.

Chronic Prevention of Anginal Episodes

Patients with repeated episodes of angina should receive long-acting therapy for chronic prophylaxis. All patients should be receiving aspirin. In addition, there are three classes of agents that may be used for chronic antianginal therapy: beta blockers, calcium channel blockers, and long-acting nitrates. The initial choice of an antianginal agent should be based on the patient's specific characteristics, such as physical exam findings and coexisting medical conditions. Treatment with a single agent is generally used for initial antianginal therapy, whereas combination therapy is instituted for patients who fail monotherapy.

First-Line Therapy

In the absence of contraindications, beta blockers are the agents of choice for prevention of acute anginal episodes in patients with or without a history of MI. Beta blockers reduce the frequency and likelihood of anginal episodes and reduce CHD-related morbidity and mortality. Additionally, beta blockers are useful as antihypertensive and antiarrhythmic agents. Beta blockers are particularly useful in patients whose anginal symptoms are related to physical exertion.

For patients whose anginal symptoms have been linked to coronary vasospasm, a calcium channel blocker may be considered for initial treatment. See **Table 21.2** for more information.

Second-Line Therapy

For patients who do not respond sufficiently to therapy with a single antianginal agent, combination therapy should be attempted. When initial treatment with a beta blocker is not successful, either a calcium channel blocker or a long-acting nitrate may be added to beta blocker therapy.

A long-acting nitrate/beta blocker program is safe, effective, and low in cost. Nitrates and beta blockers are well tolerated, and their effects are complementary. Reflex tachycardia caused by nitrates is blunted by a beta blocker. The control of reflex tachycardia is beneficial because a decrease in heart rate lowers myocardial oxygen demand. The combination of nitrates and beta blockers is an accepted treatment of angina, and they are often used together.

A beta blocker plus a calcium channel blocker is another typical combination. Patients who have anginal symptoms that cannot be controlled by beta blocker or calcium channel blocker monotherapy often respond to a combination of the two. However, a beta blocker plus calcium channel blocker combination should be used with caution. When drugs from these two classes are given together, the additive effect is the potent suppression of AV conduction, which may be problematic in patients with pre-existing cardiac conduction abnormalities. It is best to start with low doses of each drug and monitor each dosage increase so that side effects can be identified early.

Nitrates are often combined with a nondihydropyridine calcium channel blocker, such as diltiazem or verapamil, or a second-generation dihydropyridine calcium channel blocker, such as amlodipine. Since nitrates and first-generation dihydropyridine calcium channel blockers are potent vasodilators, they should be used together with extreme caution and only if no other treatment option is available.

Third-Line Therapy

In patients who are refractory to a two-drug regimen, a three-drug regimen of a calcium channel blocker, beta blocker, and a long-acting nitrate may be used. In general, patients whose anginal symptoms do not respond to two antianginal agents should be referred to a specialist's care.

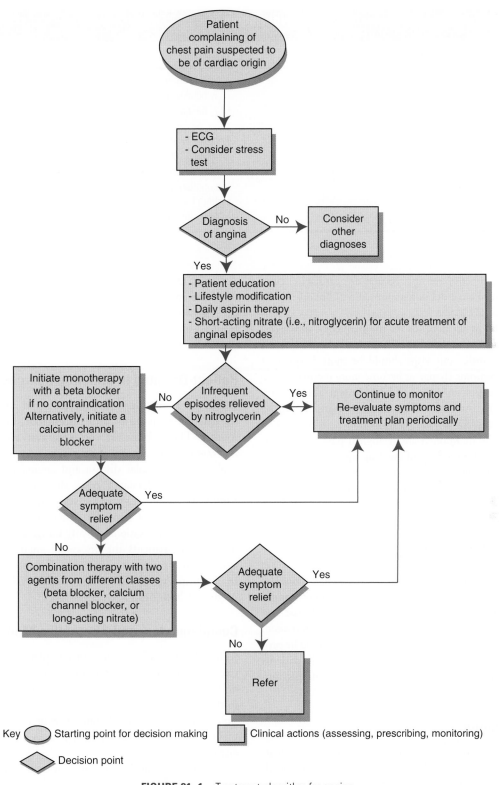

FIGURE 21–1 Treatment algorithm for angina.

MONITORING PATIENT RESPONSE

In patients with angina, monitoring is important to evaluate for progression or stability of the disease, response to therapy, and presence or absence of adverse events.

Patient monitoring begins when a stress test is performed to confirm the diagnosis of angina. Once the diagnosis is made, stress tests may be repeated if there is a change in the pattern of anginal symptoms. Additionally, patients with stable angina should have an ECG if the history or physical examination

TABLE 21.2 **Recommended Order of Treatment for Angina**

Order	Agents	Comments
For all patients	Short-acting nitrate	For acute treatment of anginal episodes
	Aspirin (if not contraindicated)	May be used to prevent predictable episodes
		May be used alone in patients with infrequent episodes
Chronic prevention of anginal episodes		
First line	Beta blocker	Reduces workload of heart by decreasing overall myocardial oxygen consumption
	Calcium channel blocker	Useful for patients who cannot tolerate a beta blocker
Second line	Combination therapy	If monotherapy fails, add another agent from a different class: beta blocker, calcium channel blocker, long-acting nitrate (e.g., beta blocker and long-acting nitrate)

changes or if the practitioner suspects new myocardial ischemia or development of a conduction abnormality (Gibbons, et al., 2003).

Routine follow-up depends on the frequency and severity of the patient's complaints. Stable patients should be seen every 2 to 6 months, but visits should be more frequent if the patient's symptoms change or become more severe or more frequent. Medication initiation and adjustment also requires more office visits. At each office visit, vital signs should be taken and a complete physical examination performed. The patient should be questioned about anginal pain and associated symptoms and side effects of the drug regimen. Additional monitoring parameters should be determined by the specific drug regimen. Ideally, a patient's antianginal regimen should make him or her symptom-free.

PATIENT EDUCATION

For optimal control of anginal symptoms, the patient should be educated on his or her disease and medications. Patients should be informed of the seriousness of coronary artery disease and the potential consequences of leaving their angina untreated. Education about lifestyle modification strategies should be provided to all patients as often as possible. Additionally, patients need to know how to recognize worsening or escalating symptoms so they know when to seek emergency care.

Drug Information

There are many sources of information relating to the treatment of angina. Several therapeutic guidelines are available to the practitioner, including those from the American College of Cardiology and American Heart Association, the American College of Chest Physicians, the European Society of Cardiology, and many other organizations. Specific questions relating to pharmacologic agents used in the treatment of angina may be addressed using the *Physician's Desk*

Reference, Drug Facts and Comparisons, Micromedex, or another drug reference. Finally, information regarding ongoing clinical trials for angina and other conditions may be obtained from a website provided by the National Institutes of Health (www.clinicaltrials.gov).

Patient-Oriented Information Sources

Practitioners may provide disease- and treatment-related information to patients with information from a variety of sources. The website for the American Heart Association (www.americanheart.org) has many resources available to explain cardiovascular disease and angina in a fashion that patients will understand. Also, the American Academy of Family Physicians (www.familydoctor.org) provides on its website a variety of resources under the heading of "Patient Ed." Finally, the National Heart, Lung, and Blood Institute describes for patients the disease of angina, its causes, and appropriate treatments under the "Diseases and Conditions Index" (http://www.nhlbi.nih.gov/health/dci/Diseases/Angina/Angina_WhatIs.html).

Complementary and Alternative Medications

Although there are a variety of complementary medications that allege to provide symptom relief for patients with angina, no herbal medication has been shown to have efficacy similar to that of the traditional agents described above. If at all possible, practitioners should counsel patients to adhere to treatment regimens that have shown efficacy in the treatment of angina.

Patients should be educated on each of the medications they are provided. They should know the importance of taking their medications as prescribed. They should be informed of each medication's indication and possible side effects, and what to do if they miss one or more doses of a scheduled medication, such as a long-acting nitrate. Additionally, practitioners should educate patients about the proper storage of all medications.

Case Study

E. H. is a 45-year-old African-American man who recently moved to the community from another state. He requests renewal of a prescription for a calcium channel blocker, prescribed by a physician in the former state. He is unemployed and lives with a woman, their son, and the woman's two children. His past medical history is remarkable for asthma and six "heart attacks" that he claims occurred because of a 25-year history of drug use (primarily cocaine). He states that he used drugs as recently as 2 weeks ago. He does not have any prior medical records with him. He claims that he has been having occasional periods of chest pain. He is unable to report the duration or pattern of the pain.

Before proceeding, explore the following questions: What further information would you need to diagnose angina (substantiate your answer)? What is the connection between cocaine use and angina? Identify at least three tests that you would order to diagnose angina.

DIAGNOSIS: ANGINA

1. List specific goals of treatment for E. H.
2. What dietary and lifestyle changes should be recommended for this patient?
3. What drug therapy would you prescribe for E. H. and why?
4. How would you monitor for success in E. H.?
5. Describe one or two drug–drug or drug–food interactions for the selected agent.
6. List one or two adverse reactions for the selected agent that would cause you to change therapy.
7. What would be the choice for the second-line therapy?
8. Discuss specific patient education based on the prescribed first-line therapy.
9. What over-the-counter and/or alternative medications would be appropriate for E. H.?

BIBLIOGRAPHY

Starred references are cited in the text.

*American Heart Association. (2004). *Heart and stroke facts: 2004 update*. Dallas, Texas: American Heart Association.

*American Heart Association. (2010). *Heart and stroke facts: 2004 update*. Dallas, Texas: American Heart Association.

Black, J., & Matassarin-Jacobs, E. (1997). *Medical-surgical nursing: Clinical management for community care* (5th ed.). Philadelphia, PA: W. B. Saunders.

Bullock, B., & Henge, R. (2000). *Focus on pathophysiology*. Philadelphia, PA: Lippincott Williams & Wilkins.

Ellsworth, A., Witt, D., Dugdale, D., & Oliver, L. (1997). *Mosby's medical drug reference*. Philadelphia, PA: Mosby–Year Book.

*Fraker, T. D., & Fihn, S. D. (2007). 2007 Chronic Angina Focused Update of the ACC/AHA 2002 Guidelines for the Management of Patients With Chronic Stable Angina: A report of the American College of Cardiology/American Heart Association Task Force on Practice Guidelines Writing Group to Develop the Focused Update of the 2002 Guidelines for the Management of Patients with Chronic Stable Angina. *Journal of the American College of Cardiology, 50*, 2264–2274.

*Gibbons, R. J., Abrams, J., Chatterjee, K., et al. (2003). ACC/AHA 2002 guideline update for the management of patients with chronic stable angina: A report of the American College of Cardiology/American Heart Association Task Force on Practice Guidelines (Committee to Update the 1999 Guidelines for the Management of Patients with Chronic Stable Angina). *Journal of the American College of Cardiology, 41*, 159–168.

*Goroll, A., May, L., & Mulley, A. (1998). Management of chronic stable angina. In *Primary care medicine*. Philadelphia, PA: Lippincott Williams & Wilkins (update on CD, Vol. 2, no. 1).

Katzung, B., & Chatterjee, M. (1998). Vasodilators and the treatment of angina pectoris. In B. Katzung (Ed.), *Basic and clinical pharmacology* (7th ed.). Stamford, CT: Appleton & Lange.

Maron, D. J., Grundy, S. M., Ridler, P. M., & Pearson, T. A. (2004). Dyslipidemia, other risk factors, and the prevention of coronary heart disease. In V. Fuster, R. W. Alexander, & R. A. O'Rourke (Eds.), *Hurst's the heart* (11th ed., pp. 1093–1122). New York, NY: McGraw-Hill.

Mycek, M., Harvey, R., & Champe, P. (1997). *Lippincott's illustrated reviews: Pharmacology*. Philadelphia: Lippincott–Raven.

O'Rourke, R. A., O'Gara, P., & Douglas, J. S. (2004). Diagnosis and management of patients with chronic ischemic heart disease. In V. Fuster, R. W. Alexander, & R. A. O'Rourke (Eds.), *Hurst's the heart* (11th ed., pp. 1465–1494). New York, NY: McGraw-Hill.

Patrano, C., Coller, B., FitzGerald, G. A., Hirsh, J., & Roth, G. (2004). Platelet-active drugs: The relationships among dose, effectiveness, and side effects: The seventh ACCP conference on antithrombotic and thrombolytic therapy. *Chest, 126*(3, Suppl.), 234S–264S.

Ross, R. (1998). Factors influencing atherogenesis. In R. Alexander, R. Schant, & V. Fuster (Eds.), *Hurst's the heart* (9th ed., pp. 1139–1160). New York, NY: McGraw-Hill.

Uphold, C., & Graham, M. (1998). *Clinical guidelines in family practice* (3rd ed.). Gainesville, FL: Barmarrae Books.

Walker, B. F. (2004). Nonatherosclerotic coronary heart disease. In V. Fuster, R. W. Alexander, & R. A. O'Rourke (Eds.), *Hurst's the heart* (11th ed., pp. 1173–1214). New York, NY: McGraw-Hill.

Heart Failure

Heart failure (HF), one of the most serious consequences of cardiovascular disease, has rapidly become one of the most important health problems in cardiovascular medicine. Nearly 5 million Americans have HF today, with an incidence approaching 10 per 1,000 among persons older than age 65 (Jessup & Brozana, 2003). At age 40, the lifetime risk of developing HF for both men and women is 1 in 5. At age 80, the remaining lifetime risk of developing new heart failure remains at 20% for men and women (American Heart Association [AHA], 2010). HF is more common in men than in women, probably because of the higher incidence of ischemic heart disease in men. Approximately 75% of all ambulatory patients with HF are age 60 or older (AHA, 1999). In people diagnosed with HF, sudden cardiac death occurs at 6 to 9 times the rate of the general population (AHA, 2010).

The economic impact of HF also is significant. The large number and often high complexity of hospitalizations for HF make this diagnosis very costly. The total cost of HF hospitalizations in the United States has been estimated at $8 billion. After hypertension, HF is the second most common indication for physician office visits. The estimated direct and indirect cost of HF in the United States for 2009 was $37.2 billion (AHA, 2010). Consequently, improved quality of life is considered a worthy health care goal, and the therapeutic approach to HF is directed toward increasing the patient's ability to maintain a positive quality of life with symptom-free activity and to enhance survival. Vasodilator therapy, especially with the angiotensin-converting enzyme (ACE) inhibitors, has made significant contributions toward achieving this goal.

CAUSES

The development of HF may be related to many etiologic variables. Coronary artery disease, hypertension, and idiopathic cardiomyopathy are the most frequently cited risk factors for HF (Braunwald, 1988; Franciosa, et al., 1983; Packer & Cohn, 1999). Acute conditions that may result in HF include acute myocardial infarction (MI), arrhythmias, pulmonary embolism, sepsis, and acute myocardial ischemia (Braunwald, 1988). Gradual development of HF may be caused by liver or renal disease, primary cardiomyopathy, cardiac valve disease, anemia, bacterial endocarditis, viral myocarditis, thyrotoxicosis, chemotherapy, excessive dietary sodium intake, and ethanol abuse.

Drugs also can worsen HF. Drugs that may cause fluid retention, such as nonsteroidal anti-inflammatory drugs (NSAIDs), steroids, hormones, antihypertensives (e.g., hydralazine [Apresoline], nifedipine [Procardia XL]), sodium-containing drugs (e.g., carbenicillin disodium [Geopen]), and lithium (Eskalith, others) may cause congestion. Beta blockers, antiarrhythmics (e.g., disopyramide [Norpace], flecainide [Tambocor], amiodarone [Cordarone], sotalol [Betapace]), tricyclic antidepressants, and certain calcium channel blockers (e.g., diltiazem [Cardizem], nifedipine, verapamil [Calan]) have negative inotropic effects and further decrease contractility in an already depressed heart. Direct cardiac toxins (e.g., amphetamines, cocaine, daunorubicin [DaunoXome], doxorubicin [Adriamycin], ethanol) also can worsen or induce HF (Covinsky & Willett, 1999).

PATHOPHYSIOLOGY

HF is a pathophysiologic state in which abnormal myocardial function inhibits the ventricles from delivering adequate quantities of blood to metabolizing tissues at rest or during activity. It results not only from a decrease in intrinsic systolic contractility of the myocardium, but also from alterations in the pulmonary and peripheral circulations (Braunwald, 1988).

When the heart fails as a pump and cardiac output (the volume of blood pumped out of the ventricle per unit of time) decreases, a complex scheme of compensatory mechanisms to raise and maintain cardiac output occurs. These compensatory mechanisms include increased preload (volume and pressure or myocardial fiber length of the ventricle prior to contraction [end of diastole]); increased afterload (vascular resistance); ventricular hypertrophy (increased muscle mass); and dilatation, activation of the sympathetic nervous system (SNS), and activation of the renin–angiotensin–aldosterone system (RAAS) (Covinsky & Willett, 1999).

Although initially beneficial for increasing cardiac output, these compensatory mechanisms are ultimately associated with further pump dysfunction. In effect, the consequence of activating the compensatory systems is worsening HF. This is often referred to as the *vicious cycle of HF* (**Figure 22-1**). Without therapeutic intervention, some of the compensatory mechanisms continue to be activated, ultimately resulting in a reduced cardiac output and a worsening of the

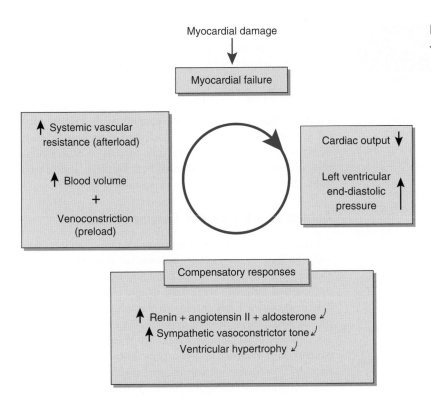

FIGURE 22–1 Vicious circle of heart failure.

patient's symptoms. An understanding of the compensatory mechanisms makes it clear why one goal in treating HF is to interrupt this vicious cycle and why various drugs are used in managing patients with HF.

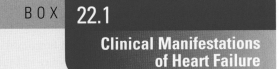

BOX 22.1

Clinical Manifestations of Heart Failure

Left Ventricular Failure–Pulmonary Congestion

Symptoms: Cough, dyspnea, dyspnea on exertion, orthopnea, paroxysmal nocturnal dyspnea, nocturia

Signs: Cardiomegaly, S_3 heart sound, bibasilar rales, signs of pulmonary edema, tachycardia, increased respiratory rate

Right Ventricular Failure–Systemic Congestion

Symptoms: Peripheral pitting edema, abdominal pain, anorexia, bloating, constipation, nausea, vomiting

Signs: Hepatomegaly, distention of the jugular veins, hepatojugular reflex, signs of portal hypertension, ascites, splenomegaly

Decreased Cardiac Output

Peripheral cyanosis, fatigue, decreased tissue perfusion, decrease in metabolism and renal elimination of drugs, decreased appetite, angina, increased risk for thromboembolism

DIAGNOSTIC CRITERIA

The signs and symptoms of HF are useful in diagnosing and assessing a patient's clinical response to therapy. The clinical manifestations of HF are in part due to pulmonary or systemic venous congestion and edema. When the left ventricle malfunctions, congestion initially occurs proximally in the lungs. When the right ventricle functions inadequately, congestion in the supplying systemic venous circulation results in peripheral edema, liver congestion, and other indicators of right HF (**Box 22.1**). Both pulmonary and systemic congestion eventually develop in most patients with left HF. In fact, the chief cause of right HF is left HF (Covinsky & Willett, 1999).

Depressed ventricular function may be confirmed by echocardiography, radionuclide ventriculography, or cardiac catheterization. Abnormalities in the electrocardiogram (ECG) are common and include arrhythmias, conduction delays, left ventricular (LV) hypertrophy and nonspecific ST-T changes, which typically reflect the underlying etiology. Laboratory findings from liver function or other tests disclose such abnormalities as elevated blood urea nitrogen (BUN) and creatinine levels, hyponatremia, and elevated serum enzymes of hepatic origin. The circumstances in which the symptoms of HF occur are also particularly important in determining the severity of disease in a particular patient.

The New York Heart Association (NYHA) classifies the functional incapacity of patients with cardiac disease into four levels depending on the degree of effort needed to elicit symptoms (**Table 22.1**):

- *Class I:* Patients may have symptoms of HF only at levels that would produce symptoms in normal people.

TABLE 22.1	New York Heart Association Functional Classification for Heart Failure
Class	**Definition**
I	No limitation of physical activity. Ordinary physical activity does not cause undue fatigue or dyspnea.
II	Slight limitation of physical activity. Comfortable at rest, but ordinary physical activity results in fatigue or dyspnea.
III	Marked limitation of physical activity. Comfortable at rest, but less than ordinary activity causes fatigue or dyspnea.
IV	Unable to carry on any physical activity without symptoms. Symptoms are present even at rest. If any physical activity is undertaken, symptoms are increased.

- *Class II:* Patients may have symptoms of HF on ordinary exertion.
- *Class III:* Patients may have symptoms of HF on less than ordinary exertion.
- *Class IV:* Patients may have symptoms of HF at rest.

INITIATING DRUG THERAPY

In the past, digitalis, glycosides, and diuretics were the mainstays of therapy for HF. However, the concept of HF has changed dramatically from a narrow focus on the weakened heart to a broadened view of the systemic pathophysiologic state, with peripheral as well as myocardial factors playing important roles. The goals of therapy are to improve the quality of life, decrease mortality, and reduce the compensatory mechanisms causing the symptoms. Three general approaches are used:

1. An underlying cause of HF is treated if possible (e.g., surgical correction of structural abnormalities or medical treatment of conditions such as infective endocarditis or hypertension).
2. Precipitating factors that produce or worsen HF are identified and minimized (e.g., fever, anemia, arrhythmias, medication noncompliance, or drugs).
3. After these two steps, drug therapy to control the HF and improve survival becomes important.

Nonpharmacologic management techniques should be used along with pharmacologic therapy in patients with HF. In the past, reduced activities and bed rest were considered a standard part of the care of patients with HF. However, it has been determined that short periods of bed rest result in reduced exercise tolerance and aerobic capacity. There is insufficient evidence to recommend a specific type of training program or the routine use of supervised rehabilitation programs. Although most patients should not participate in heavy labor or exhausting sports, aerobic activity should be encouraged (except during periods of acute decompensation). For example,

according to the Agency for Health Care Policy and Research (AHCPR), regular exercise (e.g., walking or cycling) is recommended for patients with stable class I to III disease.

Goals of Drug Therapy

Pharmacologic management of patients with HF is critical in reducing symptoms and decreasing mortality. In most cases, drug therapy is long term and consists of ACE inhibitors, diuretics, digoxin (Lanoxin), beta blockers, and others. **Table 22.2** gives an overview of drugs used to treat HF.

Angiotensin-Converting Enzyme Inhibitors

Patients who have HF resulting from LV systolic dysfunction and who have an LV ejection fraction less than 35% to 40% should be given a trial of ACE inhibitors, unless they cannot tolerate treatment with these drugs. The ACE inhibitors may be considered sole therapy in the subset of patients who present with fatigue or mild dyspnea on exertion and who do not have any other signs or symptoms of volume overload. In patients with evidence for, or a prior history of, fluid retention, ACE inhibitors are usually used together with diuretics. (See section on Selecting the Most Appropriate Agent.) ACE inhibitors are also recommended for use in patients with LV systolic dysfunction who have no symptoms of HF (Packer & Cohn, 1999). The clinical and mortality benefits of the ACE inhibitors have been shown in numerous uncontrolled and controlled, randomized clinical trials.

ACE inhibitors have a positive effect on cardiac function (i.e., reduced preload and afterload, increased cardiac index, and ejection fraction) and the signs and symptoms of HF (e.g., dyspnea, fatigue, orthopnea, and peripheral edema). As a result, exercise capacity is increased, NYHA functional classification is significantly improved, and morbidity and mortality rates in patients with HF, including those who have suffered an MI, is reduced because these drugs can attenuate ventricular dilation and remodeling.

Captopril (Capoten), enalapril (Vasotec), fosinopril (Monopril), lisinopril (Zestril), quinapril (Accupril), trandolapril (Mavik), and ramipril (Altace) are the ACE inhibitors currently indicated for treating HF. (See **Table 22.2.**) The ACE inhibitors that are approved for use in patients with LV dysfunction, and have been shown to prolong survival, are enalapril, captopril, and lisinopril. Quinapril and fosinopril are labeled for symptom reduction in HF, but data are lacking as to their effect on mortality rates.

Mechanism of Action

"Balanced" vasodilators, including the ACE inhibitors and angiotensin II receptor blockers, cause vasodilation on both the venous and arterial sides of the heart and therefore provide the hemodynamic and clinical benefits of both preload and afterload reduction.

Activation of the RAAS is an important compensatory mechanism in HF (**Figure 22-2**). ACE catalyzes the conversion of angiotensin I to angiotensin II, a potent vasoconstrictor and

TABLE 22.2   Overview of Selected Agents Used to Treat Heart Failure

Generic (Trade) Name and Dosage	Selected Adverse Events	Contraindications	Special Considerations
Selected Angiotensin-Converting Enzyme Inhibitors			
captopril (Capoten) Start: 6.25 mg or 12.5 mg tid Therapeutic range: 25–100 mg tid	Common: cough; hypotension, particularly with a diuretic or volume depletion; hyperkalemia, loss of taste, leukopenia; angioedema, neutropenia, and agranulocytosis in <1% of patients; rash in >10% of patients	Contraindicated in pregnancy Avoid in patients with bilateral renal artery stenosis or unilateral stenosis.	Renal impairment related to ACE inhibitors is seen as an increase in serum creatinine and azotemia, usually in the beginning of therapy. Monitor BUN, creatinine, and K levels when starting.
enalapril (Vasotec) Start: 2.5 mg qd or bid Range: 5–20 mg qd or bid daily	Same as above	Same as above	Same as above Use only 2.5 mg/d in patient with impaired renal function or hyponatremia.
fosinopril (Monopril) Start: 10 mg qd Range: 10–40 mg qd	Same as above	Same as above	Same as above Use only 5 mg/d in patient with impaired renal function or hyponatremia.
lisinopril (Zestril, Prinivil) Start: 5 mg qd Range: 5–20 mg qd	Same as above	Same as above	Same as above Use only 2.5 mg/d in patient with impaired renal function or hyponatremia.
quinapril (Accupril) Start: 5 mg bid Range: 20–40 bid	Same as above	Same as above	Same as above Use only 2.5 mg/d in patient with impaired renal function or hyponatremia.
ramipril (Altace) Start: 1.25 mg twice daily Range: 1.25–5 mg twice daily	Same as above	Same as above	Same as above
trandolapril (Mavik) Start: 0.5–1 mg daily Target dose: 4 mg	Same as above	Same as above	Same as above
Selected Thiazide and Thiazide-Like Diuretics			
chlorthalidone (Hygroton) 12.5–50 mg qd	Hyperuricemia, hypokalemia, hypomagnesemia, hyperglycemia, hyponatremia, hypercalcemia, hypercholesterolemia, hypertriglyceridemia, pancreatitis, rashes and other allergic reactions	High doses are relatively contraindicated in patients with hyperlipidemia, gout, and diabetes.	Thiazide diuretics preferred in patients with CrCl >30 mL/min
hydrochlorothiazide (HydroDIURIL, Microzide) 12.5–50 mg qd	Same as chlorthalidone	Same as chlorthalidone	Same as chlorthalidone
metolazone (Zaroxolyn) 2.5–10 mg qd	Less or no hypercholesterolemia	Same as chlorthalidone	Same as chlorthalidone
Loop Diuretics			
bumetanide (Bumex) 0.5–5 mg qd-bid	Dehydration, circulatory collapse, hypokalemia, hyponatremia, hypomagnesemia, hyperglycemia, metabolic alkalosis, hyperuricemia (short duration of action, no hypercalcemia)	High doses are relatively contraindicated in patients with hyperlipidemia, gout, and diabetes.	Effective in patients with CrCl <30 mL/min Monitor BUN, creatinine, and K levels when starting and with dosage changes.
ethacrynic acid (Edecrin) 25–100 mg bid-tid	Same as bumetanide (only nonsulfonamide diuretic, ototoxicity)	Same as bumetanide	Same as bumetanide

(continued)

TABLE 22.2   Overview of Selected Agents Used to Treat Heart Failure (*Continued*)

Generic (Trade) Name and Dosage	Selected Adverse Events	Contraindications	Special Considerations
furosemide (Lasix) 20–320 mg bid-tid	Same as bumetanide	Same as bumetanide	Same as bumetanide
torsemide (Demadex) 5–20 mg qd-bid	Short duration of action, no hypercalcemia	Same as bumetanide	Same as bumetanide
Potassium-Sparing Diuretics			
amiloride (Midamor) 5–20 mg qd-bid	Hyperkalemia, GI disturbances, rash	High doses are relatively contraindicated in patients with hyper-lipidemia, gout, and diabetes.	Same as bumetanide
spironolactone (Aldactone) 12.5–100 mg qd-bid	Hyperkalemia, GI disturbances, rash, gynecomastia	Same as amiloride	Spironolactone ideal in patients with heart failure
triamterene (Dyrenium) 50–150 mg qd-bid	Hyperkalemia, GI disturbances, nephro-lithiasis	Same as amiloride	Same as bumetanide
Other Agents			
digitalis/digoxin (Lanoxin) 0.25 mg qd	Ventricular tachycardia, paroxysmal atrial tachycardia, fatigue, anorexia, nausea	Allergy, ventricular tachy-cardia, ventricular fibrillation, heart block, sick sinus syndrome, idiopathic hypertrophic subaortic stenosis, acute MI, renal insuf-ficiency, electrolyte abnormalities Use with caution in preg-nancy and lactation.	Check potassium levels before starting. Check serum levels once a year.
hydralazine (Apresoline) 25–75 mg tid	Postural hypotension, tachycardia	Coronary artery disease, aortic stenosis	Advise patient to avoid rapid changes in position. Patient can be started on 10 mg tid if elderly, with severe heart failure, or hypotensive.
isosorbide dinitrate (ISDN) (Isordil) 10–40 mg tid	Headache, dizziness, tachycardia, retros-ternal discomfort, blurred vision, rash, flushing	Hypersensitivity to nitrates, closed-angle glaucoma, early MI, head trauma, pregnancy (category C)	Advise patient to avoid rapid changes in position.
Beta Blockers			
bisoprolol (Zebeta) Start: 5 mg daily Range: 5–20 mg daily	Bradycardia, congestive heart failure, atrioventricular block, postural hypotension, vertigo, fatigue, depression, bronchospasm, impotence, insomnia, decreased exercise toler-ance, impaired peripheral circulation, generalized edema, sinusitis	Sinus bradycardia, second- or third-degree heart block, asthma, liver abnormalities	Advise patient to avoid abrupt cessation of therapy. Observe for signs of dizziness for 1 h when dose is increased.
carvedilol (Coreg) 3.125–50 mg bid	Same as above	Same as above	Same as above
metoprolol Start: 6.25 mg 2–3 times daily Range: 50–100 mg 2–3 times daily	Same as above	Same as above	Same as above

TABLE 22.2 Overview of Selected Agents Used to Treat Heart Failure (Continued)

Generic (Trade) Name and Dosage	Selected Adverse Events	Contraindications	Special Considerations
Selected Angiotensin Receptor Blockers			
losartan (Cozaar) Start: 12.5 mg/d Range: 50–100 mg/d	Dyspnea, hypotension, hyperkalemia	Angioedema secondary to ACE inhibition	May be used in patients experiencing cough due to ACE inhibitor
valsartan (Diovan) Start: 80 mg/d Range: 80–160 mg twice daily	Same as above	Same as above	Same as above
Other Agents			
dobutamine (Dobutrex) 2–5 mcg/kg/min intravenously	Elevated blood pressure, increased heart rate, angina, hypotension	Idiopathic hypertrophic subaortic stenosis	May increase insulin requirements

stimulant of aldosterone secretion. ACE inhibitors are uniquely effective in managing HF by interrupting stimulation of the RAAS, inhibiting the contributions of this system to the downward spiral of HF. The pharmacodynamic properties of ACE inhibitors involve specific competitive binding to the active site of ACE.

Angiotensin II interacts with at least two known membrane receptors, type 1 and type 2 (AT_1 and AT_2). By blocking formation of angiotensin II, ACE inhibitors indirectly produce vasodilation and a decrease in systemic vascular resistance (LV afterload). In addition, because angiotensin II stimulates aldosterone secretion by the adrenal cortex and provides negative feedback for plasma renin, inhibition of angiotensin II may lead to decreased aldosterone and increased renin activity. This prevents aldosterone-mediated sodium and water retention and may produce a small increase in serum potassium levels. The reduction in volume expansion due to ACE inhibition decreases ventricular end-diastolic volume (i.e., preload). Because ACE (kininase II) is involved in the breakdown of bradykinin, a vasodilator, a decrease in kininase II activity by an ACE inhibitor could increase bradykinin as well as prostaglandin production, either of which can lead to vasodilation (Borek, et al., 1989).

ACE inhibitors produce vasodilation, inhibit fluid accumulation, and increase blood flow to vital organs, such as the brain, kidney, and heart, without precipitating reflex tachycardia. The hemodynamic effects of ACE inhibitors in HF include decreased preload, afterload, and mean arterial pressure, as well as increased cardiac output. Ejection fraction is also improved. Clinical benefits to patients with HF include improvement in exercise duration, NYHA functional class, dyspnea/fatigue focal index, and signs and symptoms of HF, as well as increased survival.

Dosage

ACE inhibitors should be initiated at low doses followed by gradual dosage increases if the lower doses have been well tolerated. Renal function and serum potassium should be assessed within 1 to 2 weeks of starting therapy and periodically thereafter, especially in patients with pre-existing hypotension, hyponatremia, diabetes, or azotemia, or if they are receiving potassium supplementation. Doses should be titrated to the target doses shown in clinical trials to decrease morbidity and mortality (e.g., at least 150 mg/day of captopril or at least 20 mg/day of enalapril or lisinopril). The doses of ACE inhibitors can be increased to these effective doses unless the patient cannot tolerate high doses. The practitioner should provide the following information to patients taking ACE inhibitors:

- Adverse effects may occur early in therapy but do not usually prevent long-term use of the drug.
- Symptomatic improvement may not be seen for several weeks or months.
- ACE inhibitors may reduce the risk of disease progression even if the patient's symptoms have not responded favorably to treatment (Packer & Cohn, 1999).

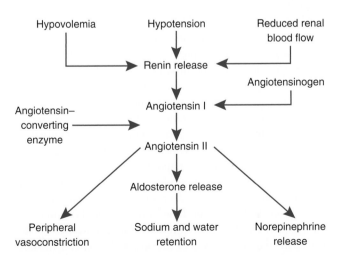

FIGURE 22–2 The renin-angiotensin-aldosterone (RAA) syndrome.

Captopril, lisinopril, ramipril, and trandolapril have been shown to reduce mortality rates in patients who have had an MI and who have HF symptoms. The indications for these

ACE inhibitors in this population vary slightly and the dosing in patients after MI differs from the dosing for patients with chronic HF. Captopril is indicated to improve survival after MI in clinically stable patients with LV dysfunction manifested as an ejection fraction of 40% or less and to reduce the incidence of overt HF and subsequent hospitalizations for HF. Captopril may be initiated as early as 3 days after an MI with a single dose of 6.25 mg. If the patient tolerates this dose, he or she should receive 12.5 mg three times a day, increasing to 25 mg three times a day over the next several days. Over the next several weeks, the dose should be increased to a target of 50 mg three times a day. Other post-MI therapies (e.g., thrombolytics, aspirin, and beta blockers) may be used concurrently.

Lisinopril has been shown to decrease mortality rates in both acute and post-MI patients. Lisinopril also is indicated for treating hemodynamically stable patients within 24 hours of an acute MI to improve survival. Patients should receive, as appropriate, the standard recommended treatments, such as thrombolytics, aspirin, and beta blockers. The first 5-mg dose of lisinopril may be given to hemodynamically stable patients within 24 hours of the onset of symptoms of acute MI, followed by 5 mg after 24 hours, 10 mg after 48 hours, and then 10 mg once daily. Dosing should be continued for 6 weeks. At that time, the patient should be assessed for signs and symptoms of HF and therapy should be continued if necessary. The dose should be decreased to 2.5 mg in patients with a low systolic blood pressure (below 120 mm Hg) when treatment is started, or during the first 3 days after the MI. If hypotension occurs (systolic blood pressure below 100 mm Hg), a daily maintenance dose of 5 mg may be given with temporary reductions to 2.5 mg if needed. If prolonged hypotension occurs (systolic blood pressure below 90 mm Hg for at least 1 hour), lisinopril therapy should be discontinued. Patients who develop symptoms of HF should receive the usual effective dose of lisinopril for HF, with a goal of 20 mg/d.

Ramipril has also been approved for stable patients who have shown clinical signs of HF within the first few days after an acute MI. It is used to decrease the risk of death (principally cardiovascular death) and to decrease the risks of failure-related hospitalization and progression to severe or resistant HF. The starting dose is 2.5 mg twice daily. A patient who becomes hypotensive at this dose may be switched to 1.25 mg twice daily, but all dosages should then be titrated, as tolerated, toward a target dose of 5 mg twice daily. In patients with a creatinine clearance less than 40 mL/minute/1.73 m² (serum creatinine level of less than 2.5 mg/dL), the dose should be decreased to 1.25 mg once daily. The dosage may be increased to 1.25 mg twice daily up to a maximum dose of 2.5 mg twice daily, depending on clinical response and tolerability.

Trandolapril also is approved for use in stable patients who have evidence of LV systolic dysfunction (identified by wall motion abnormalities) or who have symptoms of HF within the first few days after an acute MI. However, this drug is not used for chronic HF. In white patients, trandolapril decreases the risk of death (principally cardiovascular death) and of HF-related hospitalization (Kober, et al., 1995), but data regarding outcomes in other patients are insufficient. The recommended starting dose is

1 mg once daily. Dosages should be titrated, as tolerated, toward a target dose of 4 mg/day. If the 4-mg dose is not tolerated, patients can continue therapy with the highest tolerated dose.

Contraindications

Patients should not receive an ACE inhibitor if they have experienced life-threatening adverse effects (e.g., angioedema or anuric renal failure) during previous exposure, or if they are pregnant. Angioedema is a potentially fatal allergic reaction that may cause sudden difficulty in breathing, speaking, and swallowing accompanied by obvious swelling of the lips, face, and neck. Patients should receive an ACE inhibitor with caution if they have any of the following:

- Very low systemic blood pressure (systolic blood pressure less than 80 mm Hg)
- Markedly increased serum creatinine levels (above 3 mg/dL)
- Bilateral renal artery stenosis (previously considered a contraindication)
- Elevated serum potassium levels (above 5.5 mmol/L)

In addition, ACE inhibitors should not be given to hypotensive patients who are at immediate risk for cardiogenic shock and who require intravenous (IV) pressor support (e.g., dobutamine [Dobutrex] or epinephrine [Adrenalin, others]). These patients should receive treatment for their pump failure first; then, once they are stabilized, the HF should be re-evaluated (Packer & Cohn, 1999).

When taken by pregnant women during the second and third trimesters, ACE inhibitors can cause injury and even death to the fetus. When pregnancy is detected, the ACE inhibitor should be discontinued immediately.

Adverse Events

The most common adverse reactions of ACE inhibitors are dizziness, headache, fatigue, diarrhea, cough, and hypotension. Angioedema of the face, extremities, lips, tongue, glottis, or larynx also has been reported in patients treated with ACE inhibitors. Angioedema associated with throat or laryngeal edema may be fatal because of airway blockage, which causes suffocation. Patients should be advised about this possible adverse effect and told to go to an emergency department immediately if they experience any of the symptoms suggesting angioedema.

Hypotension may occur with any of the ACE inhibitors and is usually observed after the first dose. It is more common in patients who are sodium or volume depleted, such as those treated vigorously with diuretics or those on dialysis, and in patients with severe HF. Hypotension can be minimized by starting with a very low dose, then increasing it slowly (usually every 3 to 7 days based on response) to the highest clinically effective level that does not produce hypotension. The diuretic dose may also need to be decreased or discontinued before starting the ACE inhibitor. Blood pressure should be followed closely after the first dose (until the blood pressure is stabilized), for the first 2 weeks of therapy, and whenever the dose of the ACE inhibitor or diuretic is increased. Hypotension, an anticipated problem among older patients with HF because of blunted baroreceptor reflexes, is no more common in the elderly than in other age groups.

Changes in renal function may occur in susceptible patients (i.e., patients with hyponatremia; those taking high doses of diuretics; those with low cardiac output, diabetes mellitus, severe HF, or pre-existing renal impairment) because of inhibition of the RAAS. Patients with bilateral or unilateral renal artery stenosis should receive ACE inhibitors with extreme caution and should be monitored closely because renal failure may occur. The increases in serum creatinine and BUN that may occur are usually reversible by adjusting the dose of the ACE inhibitor, diuretic, or both. Furthermore, an increase in serum creatinine not exceeding 30% of the basal value is now being viewed as an indicator that the drug is working (i.e., there is adequate ACE inhibition) and not that it has caused renal failure. However, the initial dose of an ACE inhibitor should be reduced with increasing severity of HF and the titration period should be monitored carefully. Age-related declines in renal function may slow the elimination of ACE inhibitors and thus increase the level and duration of their effects. Therefore, it may be necessary to reduce the initial dose of ACE inhibitors in the elderly or in patients with a serum creatinine level of 2.5 mg/dL or more. These patients may not tolerate as high a dose as other patients with HF, but should be titrated to the highest possible dose.

Diuretic-induced potassium loss (hypokalemia) may be reduced when an ACE inhibitor is used in combination with a diuretic. However, hyperkalemia may occur in patients with renal impairment or in those receiving a potassium-sparing diuretic, a potassium supplement, or potassium-containing salt substitutes. ACE inhibitors should be administered cautiously if hypokalemia exists. Frequent monitoring of serum potassium levels should be performed.

A cough is a common adverse event associated with ACE inhibitor therapy, occurring in 5% to 15% of patients. It is thought to be due to increased production of bradykinins or substance P, both of which lower the cough reflex. The cough is described as an annoying, ticklish, dry cough that is reversible on discontinuation of the ACE inhibitor. In patients with HF, cough is rarely severe enough to require discontinuation of therapy. Patients who experience cough should be questioned to determine whether this symptom is due to the ACE inhibitor or to pulmonary edema. The ACE inhibitor should be implicated only after other causes have been excluded. The cough severity may be lessened with the use of inhaled cromolyn (Intal), although this does add another medication to an already complicated regimen. In most cases, the patient and family can be advised that if the cough is bothersome but not intolerable, the benefits of ACE inhibitor therapy outweigh this adverse effect. However, if the cough is persistent and troublesome, the clinician can suggest withdrawing the ACE inhibitor and trying alternative medications (e.g., an AT_1 receptor antagonist or a combination of hydralazine and isosorbide dinitrate [HYD/ISDN]).

Because HF is common among the elderly and increases in prevalence with age, safety and efficacy in this population is important. When ACE inhibitors first became available, many experts believed that because elderly patients tend to have low

TABLE 22.3	Drug Interactions Associated with the Angiotensin-Converting Enzyme Inhibitors
Interacting Agent	**Potential Effect**
antacids	Decrease the bioavailability of captopril; therefore, separate administration times by 2 h
aspirin	Decreases hemodynamic response of ACE inhibitor
capsaicin	Triggers or exacerbates the coughing that is associated with ACE inhibitor treatment
lithium	In combination with ACE inhibitor, causes increased serum lithium levels and symptoms of lithium toxicity
nonsteroidal anti-inflammatory drugs	In combination with ACE inhibitor, promotes sodium and water retention and diminishes control of hypertension and heart failure
potassium supplements/potassium-sparing diuretics/salt substitutes	In combination with ACE inhibitor, increases risk of hyperkalemia
rifampin	Reduces the pharmacologic effects of enalapril
tetracycline	In combination with quinapril, tetracycline undergoes decreased absorption (28% to 37%), possibly from the high magnesium content in quinapril.

plasma renin activity, these agents would be relatively ineffective. Furthermore, the physiologic consequences of aging may alter the absorption, distribution, and elimination of drugs, as well as the sensitivity of the patient to drugs. Thus, it was recognized that safety and efficacy studies should be conducted in this important patient population. A number of studies have been completed, and they document that ACE inhibitors are well tolerated and effective for elderly patients with HF. Studies have not yet identified differences in response between the elderly and younger patients. However, greater sensitivity of some older patients cannot be ruled out. Older patients receiving ACE inhibitors do not experience more adverse effects than younger patients (Giles, 1990; SOLVD Investigators, 1991, 1992).

Interactions

The ACE inhibitors have been associated with very few significant drug–drug interactions. One or all of the ACE inhibitors have been used in combination with digoxin, methyldopa (Aldomet), prazosin (Minipress), hydralazine, beta blockers, nitrates, and calcium channel blockers. The drug interactions that should be kept in mind are listed in **Table 22.3.**

Diuretics

During initial evaluation, the clinician should determine whether the patient manifests symptoms (e.g., orthopnea,

systolic dysfunction should receive a beta blocker unless they have a contraindication to its use or have shown to be unable to tolerate treatment with the drug. Beta blockers should not be used in unstable patients or in acutely ill patients ("rescue" therapy), including those who are in the intensive care unit with refractory HF requiring IV support. There are clinical trials underway that will help define the role of beta blockers in such patients. Beta blockers are recommended to improve symptoms and clinical status and to decrease the risk of death and hospitalization in patients with mild to moderate (NYHA class II) or moderate to severe (NYHA class III) HF who have an LV ejection fraction of less than 35% to 40%. Beta blockers should be added to pre-existing treatment with diuretics and an ACE inhibitor, and may be used together with digitalis or vasodilators (Packer & Cohn, 1999).

Carvedilol, a nonselective beta-adrenergic receptor blocker with vasodilating action (through alpha-adrenergic blocking action) previously approved for the management of essential hypertension, has become the first beta blocker approved in the United States for treating HF. It is intended to reduce the progression of disease as evidenced by cardiovascular death, cardiovascular hospitalization, or the need to adjust other HF medications. Similarly, the extended-release formulation of metoprolol, metoprolol succinate, was shown to be superior to placebo in decreasing mortality in HF patients. There are no trials comparing this extended-release agent to the immediate-release version (metoprolol tartrate). However, most clinicians use either of these formulations interchangeably, depending on the cost and the patient's insurance coverage. Bisoprolol (Zebeta) is also a beta blocker used in the treatment of HF that decreases mortality.

Mechanism of Action

Catecholamines can cause peripheral vasoconstriction that can exacerbate loading conditions in the failing heart and may precipitate myocardial ischemia and ventricular arrhythmias. In addition, activation of the SNS can increase heart rate, which may adversely affect the relation between myocardial supply and demand and more importantly may exacerbate the abnormal force–frequency relation that exists in HF. In addition, catecholamines activate cellular pathways that can lead to the loss of myocardial cells by a process of programmed cell death (apoptosis), which has been implicated in the progression of HF.

In experimental models of HF, pharmacologic interference with the SNS can favorably alter the natural history of the disease, similar to the manner in which antagonism of the RAAS by ACE inhibitors can modify the course of HF. Extensive research implicating the target mechanism, increased adrenergic drive, as being unfavorable to the natural history of systolic dysfunction and the HF clinical syndrome has been done. This has led to the conclusion that the primary mechanism of action of beta blockers in chronic HF is to prevent and reverse adrenergically mediated intrinsic myocardial dysfunction and remodeling. This occurs through a time-dependent, biologic effect involving inhibition of beta-adrenergic mechanisms

directly or indirectly responsible for the development of cellular contractile dysfunction and remodeling (Bristow, 1997). In addition, one of the beta blockers used in patients with HF, carvedilol, has direct antioxidant effects that may decrease the role played by apoptosis in the progression of HF (Bristow, 1993).

Studies have shown that carvedilol and metoprolol improve LV function, hemodynamic parameters, and various symptoms of HF. Carvedilol also improves submaximal exercise tolerance and NYHA classification (Krum, et al., 1995; Metra, et al., 1994). In multicenter clinical trials, carvedilol was associated with a highly significant 65% reduction in the risk of death versus placebo (all patients received conventional therapy in addition to carvedilol or placebo). This was due to a decrease in both death due to pump failure and sudden death (Packer & Cohn, 1999). In addition, carvedilol decreases the risk of hospitalization for cardiovascular causes and the combined risk of all-cause mortality and cardiovascular hospitalization.

Dosage

Adverse effects with carvedilol usually occur early in therapy and are more frequent and severe with higher doses. Because of this, the starting dose of carvedilol is 3.125 mg twice daily, and each dose titration should be done slowly over a 2-week period, doubling the dose each time. At initiation of each new dosage, the patient should be observed for 1 hour for signs of dizziness or lightheadedness. In addition, blood pressure should be monitored. The maximum recommended dosage is 25 mg twice daily in patients weighing less than 85 kg, and 50 mg twice daily in patients weighing 85 kg or greater. In addition, patients should be seen in the office during titration and evaluated for symptoms of worsening HF, vasodilation (i.e., dizziness, lightheadedness, and symptomatic hypotension), or bradycardia to determine their tolerance for carvedilol. Treatment with metoprolol starts at 6.25 mg two or three times daily and the dose is titrated slowly up to a target of 100 mg two or three times daily.

Initiation of therapy with a beta blocker may produce fluid retention, which may be severe enough to cause pulmonary or peripheral congestion and worsening symptoms of HF. Increases in body weight may occur after 3 to 5 days of starting treatment and if untreated may lead to worsening symptoms within 1 to 2 weeks. For this reason, practitioners should ask patients to weigh themselves daily. The amount of weight gain then guides the practitioner in prescribing an increase in the diuretic dosage until the patient's weight is restored to pretreatment levels. The dose of carvedilol may also have to be decreased; occasionally, the drug must be temporarily discontinued.

Excessive vasodilation may occur with initiation of therapy. It is usually asymptomatic but may be accompanied by dizziness, lightheadedness, or blurred vision. Vasodilatory adverse effects are usually seen within 24 to 48 hours of the first dose or increments in dose but usually subside with repeated dosing without any change in the dose of carvedilol or other medications. The risk of hypotension may be minimized by taking the beta blocker, ACE inhibitor, or vasodilator (if used) at different times during the day. Practitioners can work with patients to develop a regimen that is convenient and minimizes adverse effects. The practitioner may need to reduce the dose of the ACE inhibitor or vasodilator if hypotension is excessive. If the patient's heart rate decreases to less than 50 beats per minute or second- or third-degree heart block occurs, the patient should contact the practitioner, who may then decrease the dose of the beta blocker. Practitioners should evaluate the patient's concomitant medications for drug interactions that also may decrease heart rate or cause heart block (e.g., diltiazem or flecainide).

Contraindications

Beta blockers should not be used in patients with bronchospastic disease, symptomatic bradycardia, or advanced heart block (unless treated with a pacemaker). Patients should receive a beta blocker with caution if they have asymptomatic bradycardia (heart rate below 60 beats per minute). Despite concerns that beta blockade may mask some of the signs of hypoglycemia, patients with diabetes mellitus may be particularly likely to experience a reduction in morbidity and mortality with beta blocker therapy.

Adverse Events

The adverse effect profile of beta blockers in patients with HF is consistent with the pharmacology of the drug and the health status of the patient. The most common adverse effects are dizziness, fatigue, and worsening of HF. Other adverse reactions that occur less frequently include bradycardia, hypotension, generalized edema, dependent edema, sinusitis, and bronchitis (Packer, et al., 1996c). Rare cases of liver function abnormalities have been reported in patients receiving carvedilol, but no deaths due to these abnormalities have been reported. Mild hepatic injury related to carvedilol has been reversible and has occurred after short- and long-term therapy. Carvedilol should be discontinued if a patient has laboratory evidence of liver function abnormalities or jaundice.

Practitioners should advise patients receiving therapy with carvedilol or other beta blockers of the following:

- Adverse effects may occur early in therapy but usually do not prevent long-term use of the drug.
- Symptomatic improvement may not be seen for 2 to 3 months.
- Beta blockade may reduce the risk of disease progression even if the patient's symptoms have not responded favorably to treatment.

Digoxin

Digoxin can prevent clinical deterioration in patients with HF due to LV systolic dysfunction and can improve these patients' symptoms. However, it does not decrease the mortality rate. The latest large trial, the Digitalis Investigation Group (DIG) study, showed that survival was not changed by use of digoxin (0.125 to 0.5 mg) in NYHA class II and III patients with HF who were taking diuretics and ACE inhibitors. However, digoxin significantly decreased the number of hospitalizations compared with placebo. This effect seemed to be more pronounced in patients with the lowest ejection fractions and the most enlarged hearts. However, digoxin increased the risk of non-HF causes of cardiac death from presumed arrhythmia or MI (DIG, 1997).

The AHCPR guidelines state that digoxin should be used in patients with severe HF and should be added to the medical regimen of patients with mild or moderate failure who remain symptomatic after optimal management with ACE inhibitors and diuretics. The ACTION HF organization recommends digoxin to improve the clinical status of patients with HF due to LV systolic dysfunction, and recommends that it should be used in conjunction with diuretics, an ACE inhibitor, and a beta blocker. In addition, digoxin is recommended in patients with HF who have rapid atrial fibrillation, even though beta blockers may be more effective in controlling the ventricular response during exercise (Packer & Cohn, 1999). If a patient is receiving digoxin but not an ACE inhibitor or a beta blocker, treatment with digoxin should not be withdrawn, but appropriate therapy with the neurohormonal antagonists should be instituted. Patients should not receive digoxin if they have significant sinus or atrioventricular (AV) block, unless the block has been treated with a permanent pacemaker. Digoxin should be used cautiously in patients receiving other drugs that can depress sinus or AV nodal function (e.g., amiodarone or a beta blocker), although these patients usually tolerate digoxin without difficulty. In addition, digoxin is not indicated for the stabilization of patients with acutely decompensated HF (unless they have rapid atrial fibrillation). There are no data to recommend using digoxin in patients with asymptomatic LV dysfunction (NYHA class I).

Mechanism of Action

Digoxin produces a mild inotropic effect by inhibiting cell membrane sodium–potassium adenosine triphosphatase activity and thereby enhancing calcium entry into the cell. Calcium enhances contractile protein activity, allowing for a greater force and velocity of contraction.

Dosage

Loading doses of digoxin usually are not needed in patients with HF. The typical dosage of 0.25 mg daily may be initiated if there is no evidence of renal dysfunction. Patients who have reduced renal function, who have baseline conduction abnormality, or who are small or elderly should be started on 0.125 mg daily or lower and titrated to an adequate serum digoxin level. Levels of 0.9 to 1.2 ng/mL are considered therapeutic, but levels as high as 2.5 ng/mL may be tolerated. It is not clear whether the beneficial effects of digoxin are greater at higher serum levels. Although it has been suggested that serum levels may be used to guide the selection of an appropriate dose of digoxin, there is no evidence to support this approach (Packer & Cohn, 1999).

Steady state is reached in approximately 1 week in patients with normal renal function, although 2 to 3 weeks may be required in patients with renal impairment. When steady state is achieved, the patient should be evaluated for symptoms of toxicity. In addition, an ECG, serum digoxin level, serum electrolytes, BUN, and creatinine should be obtained. It is not clear whether regular serum digoxin monitoring is necessary, but levels should be checked once a year after a steady state is achieved. In addition, levels should be checked if HF status worsens, renal function deteriorates, signs of toxicity develop (e.g., confusion, nausea, anorexia, visual disturbances, arrhythmias), or additional medications are added that could affect the digoxin level (Konstam, et al., 1994).

Adverse Events

Signs of digoxin toxicity develop in approximately 20% of patients, and up to 18% of digoxin-toxic patients die from the arrhythmias that occur. Noncardiac symptoms are related to the central nervous system (CNS) and gastrointestinal (GI) tract. Anorexia is often an early manifestation, with nausea and vomiting following. The CNS adverse effects include headache, fatigue, malaise, disorientation, confusion, delirium, seizures, and visual disturbances. The noncardiac symptoms do not always precede the cardiac symptoms. Cardiac toxicity manifested by arrhythmias can take the form of almost every known rhythm disturbance (e.g., ectopic and re-entrant cardiac rhythms and heart block).

Digoxin should be discontinued (often with consideration of reinstitution at a lower dose after 2 to 3 days if the patient is benefiting from therapy) if any of the following is noted:

- Elevated digoxin level
- Substantial reduction in renal function
- Symptoms of toxicity
- Significant conduction abnormality (e.g., symptomatic bradycardia due to second- or third-degree AV block or high-degree AV block in atrial fibrillation)
- An increase in ventricular arrhythmias (Konstam, et al., 1994)

Practitioners should counsel patients about the potential adverse effects of digoxin. They also should stress the importance of taking digoxin exactly as it is prescribed to avoid toxicity or a subtherapeutic effect.

Interactions

The medications that most often cause an increase in digoxin levels are quinidine (Cardioquin, others), amiodarone, flecainide, propafenone (Rythmol), spironolactone, and verapamil. It may be necessary to decrease the dose of digoxin when treatment with these drugs is initiated (Packer & Cohn, 1999). Antibiotics may decrease gut flora and prevent bacterial inactivation of digoxin, and anticholinergic agents may decrease intestinal motility. Both of these drug classes also may increase digoxin levels. Antacids, cholestyramine (Questran), neomycin (Mycifradin Sulfate), and kaolin–pectin (Kaopectate) may

inhibit the absorption of digoxin and decrease digoxin levels. Patients should be advised to take digoxin at least 2 hours before these medications. Diuretics can enhance digoxin toxicity by decreasing renal clearance of digoxin and by causing electrolyte changes, including hypokalemia, hypomagnesemia, and hypercalcemia (thiazides). Before any new medications are added to a patient's regimen, the prescriber should determine whether the medication interacts with digoxin.

Hydralazine/Isosorbide Dinitrate

The HYD/ISDN combination of vasodilators is an appropriate alternative in patients with contraindications to or intolerance of ACE inhibitors (Konstam, et al., 1994). The combination should not be used for treating HF in patients who have not tried ACE inhibitors, and should not be substituted for ACE inhibitors in patients who are tolerating ACE inhibitors without difficulty (Packer & Cohn, 1999). No studies have specifically addressed the use of HYD/ISDN for patients who cannot take or tolerate ACE inhibitors, and the FDA has not approved HYD/ISDN for use in patients with HF. Isosorbide mononitrate also is not approved for HF and has not been studied for treating HF. HYD/ISDN is not as beneficial as the ACE inhibitor enalapril in reducing mortality rates during the first 2 years of treatment. However, this combination has been shown to achieve an absolute reduction in mortality rates compared with placebo during the first 3 years of treatment. The combination increases exercise capacity as much as enalapril, but adverse effects are a significant problem.

Mechanism of Action

Vasodilators may be classified by their mechanism of action or their site of action (venodilators, arteriolar dilators, or "balanced" vasodilators). ISDN is a venodilator that redistributes blood volume to the venous side of the heart to the systemic circulation, away from the lungs, which decreases the ventricular blood volume (preload). Hydralazine, along with prazosin and minoxidil (Loniten), which are not used for treating HF, is an arteriolar dilator. Hydralazine decreases the resistance the heart encounters during contraction (afterload), which allows for increased stroke volume (volume of blood leaving the heart) and increased cardiac output. Balanced vasodilators, including the ACE inhibitors and ARBs, cause vasodilation on both the venous and arterial sides of the heart and therefore provide the hemodynamic and clinical benefits of both preload and afterload reduction (as discussed in other sections).

Dosage

Isosorbide dinitrate usually should be initiated at 10 mg three times a day and increased weekly to 40 mg three times a day as tolerated (up to 160 mg/day). Hydralazine should be initiated at 25 mg three times a day and increased weekly to 75 mg three or four times a day (up to 300 mg/day) (Konstam, et al., 1994; Packer & Cohn, 1999). Patients with low blood pressure, severe HF, or advanced age can be started on 10 mg three times a day for both agents.

Adverse Events

Adverse events include reflex tachycardia, headache, flushing, nausea, dizziness, syncope, nitrate tolerance, and sodium and water retention. Nitrate tolerance can be avoided by providing a nitrate-free period of 10 to 14 hours.

Interactions

Other drugs that lower blood pressure, including diuretics, may cause additive hypotension, and blood pressure should be monitored.

Other Agents

Amiodarone

Amiodarone is approved in the United States for treating refractory life-threatening ventricular arrhythmias. Amiodarone has been studied in patients with HF with ventricular arrhythmias to assess whether it reduces mortality rates. Some studies demonstrated that low-dose amiodarone (300 mg/d) reduced mortality rates, whereas others found no improvement (Doval, et al., 1994; Singh, et al., 1995). A meta-analysis of 13 randomized, controlled trials of prophylactic amiodarone in patients with recent MI (8 trials) or HF (5 trials) found that amiodarone reduced the rate of arrhythmic/sudden death in high-risk patients with recent MI or HF (Amiodarone Trials Meta-Analysis Investigators, 1997).

The FDA has not approved amiodarone for treating HF. Further studies are needed to determine whether it is useful for routine prophylactic treatment of patients with ventricular arrhythmias and nonischemic HF. It may be beneficial in patients at high risk for arrhythmic/sudden death, patients with primary cardiomyopathy, or patients with both (Amiodarone Trials Meta-Analysis Investigators, 1997; Gheorghiade, et al., 1998). The recommendations suggest that some class III antiarrhythmic agents (e.g., amiodarone) do not appear to increase the risk of death in patients with chronic HF. Such drugs are preferred over class I agents when used for treating atrial fibrillation in patients with LV systolic dysfunction. Because of its known toxicity and equivocal evidence for efficacy, amiodarone is not recommended for general use to prevent death (or sudden death) in patients with HF already treated with drugs that reduce mortality rates (e.g., ACE inhibitors or beta blockers).

Mechanism of Action

Amiodarone is classified as a Vaughn-Williams class III (potassium channel blocking) antiarrhythmic drug, but it also possesses class I (sodium blocking), class II (beta blocking), and class IV (calcium channel blocking) antiarrhythmic effects. It also has vasodilatory properties (Doval, et al., 1994). The therapeutic benefit of amiodarone may be due to its beta-blocking effects and not to an antiarrhythmic effect.

Dosage

Before treatment with amiodarone starts, the practitioner should make sure the patient does not have hyperthyroidism or advanced liver disease. In addition, pulmonary function tests, chest radiography, ophthalmologic examination, and neurologic assessment are recommended before initiating therapy. The maintenance dosage should be 200 to 300 mg/d. High doses of amiodarone may cause initial cardiac decompensation with abnormal hemodynamics; therefore, use of high loading doses in patients with very severe forms of HF should be avoided (Gheorghiade, et al., 1998).

Interactions

Amiodarone interacts with warfarin (Coumadin; increases the international normalized ratio) and digoxin (increases digoxin levels).

Calcium Channel Blockers

Because vasodilator therapy with ACE inhibitors or the HYD/ISDN combination reduces symptoms and improves survival in patients with HF, it was thought that the vasodilatory effects of calcium channel blockers would be beneficial also. However, early short-term and long-term studies with calcium channel blockers have shown that these agents may actually worsen HF and increase the risk of death in patients with advanced LV dysfunction. This effect, which was found with most of the calcium channel blockers, may be due to a baroreceptor-mediated catecholamine release that is seen with short-acting dihydropyridine agents or to the negative inotropic effects of some calcium channel blockers. Thus, health care practitioners were advised to avoid calcium channel blockers in patients with HF, even if the drugs would treat coexisting angina or hypertension (Gheorghiade, et al., 1998; Konstam, et al., 1994).

It was not clear whether longer-acting dihydropyridines or more vascular-selective calcium channel blockers would have the same effect when trials with amlodipine (Norvasc) and felodipine (Plendil) extended release (ER) were conducted. A trial using amlodipine found that patients with ischemic HF had no decrease in mortality or morbidity rates with the drug. Amlodipine was safe in patients with ischemic HF, did not increase the mortality rate, and decreased anginal symptoms. In contrast, among patients with nonischemic cardiomyopathy, amlodipine significantly reduced the combined risk of fatal and nonfatal events by 31% and decreased the risk of death by 46%. The possibility that amlodipine prolongs survival in patients with nonischemic dilated cardiomyopathy requires further study. The investigators concluded that amlodipine can be used with relative safety in patients with severe HF with concomitant hypertension or angina. This is an important finding because these diseases can be difficult to treat in patients with LV dysfunction.

Felodipine ER was also studied to evaluate whether a long-acting, vascular-selective calcium channel blocker would benefit patients with HF. Felodipine significantly reduced blood pressure and, at 3 months, increased the ejection fraction. Exercise tolerance, quality of life, and the need for hospitalization did not improve. During long-term follow-up, the favorable effects on ejection fraction did not persist, but felodipine prevented worsening of exercise tolerance and quality of life. Mortality and hospitalization rates were similar between the two groups.

The researchers concluded that felodipine ER therapy was not associated with clear-cut short- or long-term clinical benefit or reduction in mortality rates, but that it can be used safely in patients with HF if used for another indication. In addition, it confirmed the results of the trial with amlodipine that long-acting dihydropyridine therapy did not cause an excess of cardiovascular events (Cohn, et al., 1997b).

In addition, despite more recent study findings and FDA approval, the ACTION HF recommendations remain consistent with the AHCPR guidelines. They do not recommend using calcium channel blockers to treat HF because of the lack of evidence supporting efficacy and because large-scale trials of newer agents have not provided evidence that long-term treatment with these drugs can improve the symptoms of HF or prolong survival. Because of concerns about safety, most calcium channel blockers should be avoided in patients with HF, even when used to treat angina or hypertension. The possibility that amlodipine might have a favorable effect on survival in patients with a nonischemic cardiomyopathy requires further study before such a finding is applied to the care of patients with HF (Packer & Cohn, 1999).

Dosage

Amlodipine and felodipine ER should be prescribed for treating hypertension or angina at a dosage of 5 to 10 mg/d.

Adverse Events

The most common adverse effects with these drugs include hypotension, dizziness, flushing, headache, and edema. Patients should be monitored for hypotension and worsening of HF.

Selecting the Most Appropriate Agent

The revised AHCPR clinical practice guidelines changed the approach to the management of patients with HF. Instead of digoxin, an ACE inhibitor is now the drug of first choice. **Table 22.4** and **Figure 22-3** summarize therapeutic regimens.

First-Line Therapy

The ACE inhibitors are now considered the first-line choice for routine use in patients with HF. According to the clinical practice guidelines, patients with systolic dysfunction should receive a trial of an ACE inhibitor unless contraindications are present. (See discussion of ACE inhibitors.) The ACE inhibitors may be considered sole therapy in HF patients who have fatigue or mild dyspnea on exertion and who do not have any other signs or symptoms of volume overload. However, if these symptoms persist after the target dose of the ACE inhibitor is reached, a diuretic should be added. (See Second-Line Therapy.) Thus, ACE inhibitor therapy is appropriate for patients in NYHA class I as a means of preventing HF and in patients in NYHA class II to IV with symptoms to decrease mortality rates. (See discussion of ACE inhibitors.) They may be used alone or in conjunction with other drugs, such as beta blockers, which some practitioners consider first-line therapy.

The AHCPR guidelines state that beta blockers should be used with caution, however, because these drugs have a negative inotropic effect. However, since the publication of the AHCPR clinical practice guidelines, a beta blocker with vasodilating action has been approved for treating HF. (See discussion of beta blockers.) Until the recent ACTION HF organization recommendations, there were no published guidelines to address the role of beta blockers in managing patients with HF (Packer & Cohn, 1999). These latest recommendations have elevated the use of beta blockers to initial therapy.

The recommendations state that all patients with stable NYHA class II or III HF due to LV systolic dysfunction should receive a beta blocker unless the drug is contraindicated or cannot be tolerated. Beta blockers should be used with diuretics and ACE inhibitors. Blockers should not be used in unstable patients or in acutely ill patients (rescue therapy), including those who are in the intensive care unit with refractory HF requiring IV support (Packer & Cohn, 1999). Studies of beta-blocker therapy in various types of patients with HF are continuing to define their role.

Second-Line Therapy

Diuretics are used to increase sodium and water excretion, correct volume overload (which manifests as dyspnea on exertion), and maintain sodium and water balance. Patients with HF and signs of significant volume overload should be started imme-

TABLE 22.4	Recommended Order of Treatment for Heart Failure	
Order	**Agents**	**Comments**
First line	ACE inhibitor, beta blocker with or without a diuretic (depends on patient)	Monitor patient's response carefully.
Second line	ACE inhibitor, with a diuretic and digoxin	In patient with mild heart failure, use a potassium-sparing diuretic when serum potassium level is <4.0 mEq/L.
Third line	ACE inhibitor, beta blocker, diuretic, and digoxin	An angiotensin II receptor antagonist can be substituted if ACE inhibitor cannot be tolerated.

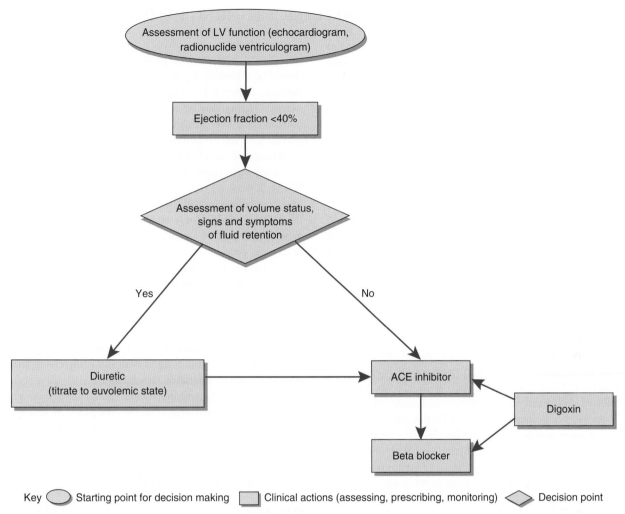

FIGURE 22–3   Treatment algorithm for chronic heart failure. (Modified from Packer, M., & Cohn, J. N. on behalf of the Steering Committee and Membership of the Advisory Council to Improve Outcomes Nationwide in Heart Failure. [1999]. Consensus recommendations for the management of chronic heart failure. *American Journal of Cardiology, 83*[2A], 1A–38A.)

diately on a diuretic in addition to an ACE inhibitor. Patients with mild HF or concomitant hypertension may be managed adequately on thiazide diuretics. However, a loop diuretic is preferred in most patients, particularly those with renal impairment or marked fluid retention. A potassium-sparing diuretic or potassium supplement should be used for patients with serum potassium concentrations less than 4.0 mEq/L. Patients with persistent volume overload despite initial medical management may require more aggressive administration of the current diuretic (e.g., IV administration), more potent diuretics, or a combination of diuretics (e.g., furosemide and metolazone, or furosemide and spironolactone) (Konstam, et al., 1994; Packer & Cohn, 1999).

Third-Line Therapy

Although digitalis preparations have been used for more than 200 years in managing chronic HF, only recently has the FDA approved digoxin for use in patients with HF who are in sinus rhythm or atrial fibrillation (AHA, 1999).

The AHCPR clinical practice guidelines state that digoxin should be used in patients with severe HF and should be added to the medical regimen of patients with mild or moderate failure who remain symptomatic after optimal management with ACE inhibitors and diuretics. The ACTION HF recommendations state that digoxin is recommended to improve the clinical status of patients with HF due to LV systolic dysfunction and should be used with diuretics, an ACE inhibitor, and a beta blocker (Packer & Cohn, 1999). Both groups suggest that digoxin may be beneficial in patients with HF when there is a second indication for digoxin therapy (e.g., a supraventricular arrhythmia for which digoxin is specifically indicated) (Konstam, et al., 1994). However, there remains a question of whether the benefits of digoxin therapy outweigh its risks.

Fourth-Line Therapy

Fourth-line therapy consists of ARBs, such as losartan, the HYD/ISDN combination of vasodilators, or an aldosterone antagonist, such as spironolactone.

According to the AHCPR guidelines and the ACTION HF recommendations, the HYD/ISDN combination is an appropriate alternative in patients with contraindications to or intolerance of ACE inhibitors (Konstam, et al., 1994; Packer & Cohn, 1999). There is little evidence to support using nitrates alone or hydralazine alone in treating HF (Packer & Cohn, 1999). The AHCPR guidelines note that nitrates and aspirin may be used to treat patients with both angina and HF (Konstam, et al., 1994).

According to the Guideline Committee for the Heart Failure Society of America (2000), spironolactone at a low dosage of 12.5 to 25 mg once daily should be considered for patients who are receiving standard therapy and who have severe HF (with recent or current NYHA class IV standing) caused by LV systolic dysfunction. Patients should have a normal serum potassium level (5.0 mmol/L) and adequate renal function (serum creatinine 2.5 mg/dL).

Special Populations

Pediatric

Children with HF usually have maturational differences in contractile function or congenital structural or genetic heart dysfunction. Drug data for children with HF are not well established. In general, treatment for class I acute HF includes IV inotropes (excluding digoxin) and IV diuretics. For class II failure, digoxin may be added, and for class III oxygen may be administered. Drug therapy in children is highly individualized according to the child's condition and setting and is usually managed by a specialist in pediatric cardiology.

Geriatric

Because of age-related reductions in renal function, elderly patients may be particularly susceptible to drug-induced decreases in blood pressure, making careful monitoring essential not only at baseline but also when dosage or drug adjustments are instituted. Blood pressure, renal function, and potassium levels should be monitored regularly. Changes in renal function may also affect the elimination of digoxin, and patients should be monitored for digoxin toxicity and educated to recognize its signs and symptoms.

An important issue in drug therapy for elderly patients with HF is therapeutic compliance. In one study, investigators identified the primary reason for hospitalization of elderly patients with HF as noncompliance with diet and medication therapy; moreover, the investigators concluded that up to 40% of readmissions could be prevented by therapeutic compliance and appropriate discharge planning, follow-up, and adequate patient and caregiver education (SOLVD Investigators, 1991).

Women

In pregnant women, ACE inhibitor therapy may pose the risk of congenital birth defects. The same is true for ARB therapy.

MONITORING PATIENT RESPONSE

A careful history and a physical examination guide outcomes and direct therapy. The patient's symptoms and activities should be explored; any worsening suggests the need to adjust therapy. Although ECG exercise testing is not recommended, repeated testing may be ordered if the patient has a new heart murmur or a new MI, or suddenly deteriorates despite compliance with the medication regimen. Serum electrolyte levels, renal function, blood pressure, and diuretic use should be monitored regularly, particularly in patients taking ACE inhibitors. Within 2 weeks of initial ACE inhibitor therapy, serum potassium, creatinine, and BUN measurements should be repeated. If values are stable, monitoring can occur at 3-month intervals or within 1 week of a change in dosage of the ACE inhibitor or diuretic drug.

Response to initial ACE inhibitor therapy should be monitored by blood pressure measurements at 1 to 2 hours (captopril) and 4 to 6 hours for long-acting drugs (enalapril or lisinopril). Blood pressure and heart rate should be monitored for 1 hour after initiating carvedilol to assess tolerance to the drug; clinical re-evaluation should occur at each increase in dose and with any worsening of symptoms (increasing fatigue, decreased exercise tolerance, weight gain).

Patients taking spironolactone should have their serum potassium level measured after the first week of therapy, at regular intervals thereafter, and after any change in dose or concomitant medications that may affect potassium balance.

PATIENT EDUCATION

Practitioners must take an active role in patient education to enhance compliance and help prevent medication errors and adverse effects. Patients taking ACE inhibitors, such as captopril and moexipril (Univasc), should take them at least 1 hour before meals. They should also be advised of potential adverse effects, particularly the effects that signal a dangerous reaction: sore throat, fever, swelling of hands or feet, irregular heartbeat, chest pains, and signs of angioedema (swelling of the face, eyes, lips, or tongue; difficulty swallowing or breathing; hoarseness). If these occur, the patient should notify the health care professional at once.

Patients taking diuretics need to know that they can take the medication with food or milk to prevent GI upset and they can schedule administration so that the need to urinate does not interrupt sleep. Because some diuretics cause photosensitivity, patients should use sunblock or avoid extensive exposure to sunlight. The practitioner can show the patient how to rise slowly from a lying or sitting position to avoid orthostatic hypotension.

Patients taking digoxin should understand that discontinuing the medication can be dangerous and that they should consult their health care provider before doing so. They should avoid taking over-the-counter medications, such as antacids, cold and allergy products, and diet drugs. Reportable signs and symptoms are loss of appetite, low stomach pain, nausea, vomiting, diarrhea, unusual fatigue or weakness, headache, blurred or yellow vision, rash or hives, or mental depression.

Women of childbearing age need to know that ARBs should be avoided if pregnancy is a possibility. Patients taking spironolactone should know the signs and symptoms to report (muscle weakness or cramps and fatigue).

Nutrition/Lifestyle Changes

Dietary sodium intake should be limited to 2 or 3 g daily. Although a 2-g daily sodium intake is preferred, patient compliance may be poor because most patients find such a diet unpalatable. Patients with mild or moderate (NYHA class II or III) HF may tolerate 3 g daily. Alcohol decreases myocardial contractility, and therefore consumption of alcoholic beverages should be discouraged or limited to one drink (i.e., a glass of beer or wine or a cocktail containing 1 ounce or less of alcohol) per day. Patients with HF should avoid excessive fluid intake, but fluid restriction is not advisable unless hyponatremia develops.

Patients should stop smoking because cigarettes cause cardiac injury. Some patients with HF experience severe limitation or repeated hospitalizations despite aggressive drug therapy. If revascularization (e.g., bypass surgery or angioplasty) is unlikely to be beneficial, consideration should be given to cardiac transplantation (Konstam, et al., 1994).

Case Study

I. W., age 62, is a white man who is new to your practice. He is reporting shortness of breath on exertion, especially after climbing steps or walking three to four blocks. His symptoms clear with rest. He also has difficulty sleeping at night (he tells you he needs two pillows to be comfortable).

He tells you that 2 years ago he suddenly became short of breath after hurrying for an airplane. He was admitted to a hospital and treated for acute pulmonary edema. Three days before the episode of pulmonary edema, he had an upper respiratory tract infection with fever and mild cough. After the episode of pulmonary edema, his blood pressure has been consistently elevated. His previous physician started him on a sustained-release preparation of diltiazem 180 mg/d. His medical history includes moderate prostatic hypertrophy for 5 years, adult-onset diabetes mellitus for 10 years, hypertension for 10 years, and degenerative joint disease for 5 years. His medication history includes hydrochlorothiazide (HydroDIURIL) 50 mg/d, atenolol (Tenormin) 100 mg/d, controlled-delivery diltiazem 180 mg/day, glyburide (DiaBeta) 5 mg/d, and indomethacin (Indocin) 25 to 50 mg three times a day as needed for pain. While reviewing his medical records, you see that his last physical examination revealed a blood pressure of 160/95 mm Hg; a pulse of 95 bpm; a respiratory rate of 18; normal peripheral pulses; mild edema bilaterally in his feet; a prominent S3 and S4; neck vein distention; and an enlarged liver.

DIAGNOSIS: HEART FAILURE

1. List specific goals of treatment for I. W.
2. What drug(s) would you prescribe? Why?
3. What are the parameters for monitoring the success of your selected therapy?
4. Discuss specific patient education based on the prescribed therapy.
5. Describe one or two drug–drug or drug–food interactions for the selected agent(s).
6. List one or two adverse reactions for the selected agent(s) that would cause you to change therapy.
7. What would be the choice for the second-line therapy?
8. What over-the-counter or alternative medications would be appropriate for this patient?
9. What dietary and lifestyle changes should be recommended for I. W.?

BIBLIOGRAPHY

*Starred references are cited in the text.

Acute Infarction Ramipril Efficacy (AIRE) Study Investigators. (1993). Effect of ramipril on mortality and morbidity of survivors of acute myocardial infarction with clinical evidence of heart failure. *Lancet, 342,* 821–828.

Ahmed, A., & Dell'Italia, L. J. (2004). Use of beta-blockers in older adults with chronic heart failure. *American Journal of the Medical Sciences, 328*(2), 100–111.

*American Heart Association. (1999). *2000 heart and stroke statistical update.* Dallas: American Heart Association.

American Heart Association. (2009). 2009 Focused update: ACCF/AHA guidelines for the diagnosis and management of heart failure in adults. A report of the American College of Cardiology Foundation/American Heart Association Task Force on practice guidelines: Developed in collaboration with the International Society for Heart and Lung Transplantation. *Circulation, 119,* 1977–2016.

*American Heart Association. (2010). Heart disease and stroke statistics 2010 update: A report from the American Heart Association. *Circulation, 121,* e46–e215.

American Society of Health-System Pharmacists. (1997). ASHP therapeutic guidelines on angiotensin-converting-enzyme inhibitors in patients with left ventricular dysfunction. *American Journal of Health-System Pharmacists, 54,* 299–313.

*Amiodarone Trials Meta-Analysis Investigators. (1997). Effect of prophylactic amiodarone on mortality after acute myocardial infarction and in congestive heart failure: Meta-analysis of individual data from 6500 patients in randomized trials. *Lancet, 350,* 1417–1424.

Australia–New Zealand Heart Failure Research Collaborative Group. (1997). Randomised, placebo-controlled trial of carvedilol in patients with congestive heart failure due to ischaemic heart disease. *Lancet, 349,* 375–380.

*Borek, M., Charlap, S., & Frishman, W. H. (1989). Angiotensin-converting enzyme inhibitors in congestive heart failure. *Medical Clinics of North America, 73,* 315–338.

*Braunwald, E. (1988). Clinical manifestations of heart failure. In E. Braunwald (Ed.), *Heart disease* (pp. 471–484). Philadelphia, PA: W.B. Saunders.

*Bristow, M. R. (1993). Pathophysiologic and pharmacologic rationales for clinical management of chronic heart failure with beta-blocking agents. *American Journal of Cardiology, 71,* 12C–22C.

*Bristow, M. R. (1997). Mechanisms of action of beta-blocking agents in heart failure. *American Journal of Cardiology, 80,* 26L–40L.

Bristow, M. R., Gilbert, E. M., Abraham, W. T., et al., for the MOCHA investigators. (1996). Carvedilol produces dose-related improvements in left ventricular function and survival in subjects with chronic heart failure. *Circulation, 94,* 2807–2816.

Brown, E. J., Chew, P. H., MacLean, A., et al. (1995). Effects of fosinopril on exercise tolerance and clinical deterioration in patients with chronic congestive heart failure not taking digitalis. *American Journal of Cardiology, 75,* 596–600.

Cohn, J. N., Fowler, M. B., Bristow, M. R., et al. (1997a). Safety and efficacy of carvedilol in severe heart failure. *Journal of Cardiac Failure, 3,* 173–199.

Cohn, J. N., Johnson, G., Ziesche, S., et al. (1986). Effect of vasodilator therapy on mortality in chronic congestive heart failure: Result of a Veterans Administration Cooperative Study. *New England Journal of Medicine, 314,* 1547–1552.

Cohn, J. N., Johnson, G., Ziesche, S., et al. (1991). A comparison of enalapril with hydralazine-isosorbide dinitrate in the treatment of chronic HF. *New England Journal of Medicine, 325,* 303–310.

*Cohn, J. N., Ziesche, S., Smith, R., et al., for the Vasodilator-Heart Failure Trial (V-HeFT) Study Group. (1997b). Effect of the calcium antagonist felodipine as supplementary vasodilator therapy in patients with chronic heart failure treated with enalapril (V-HeFT III). *Circulation, 96,* 856–863.

Colucci, W. S., Packer, M., Bristow, M. R., et al. (1996). Carvedilol inhibits progression in patients with mild symptoms of heart failure. *Circulation, 94,* 2800–2806.

CONSENSUS Trial Study Group. (1987). Effects of enalapril on mortality in severe HF: Results of the Cooperative North Scandinavian Enalapril Survival Study (CONSENSUS). *New England Journal of Medicine, 316,* 1429–1435.

*Covinsky, J. O., & Willett, M. S. (1999). Congestive heart failure. In J. T. DiPiro, R. L. Talbert, G. C. Yee, G. R. Matzke, B. G. Wells, & L. M. Posey (Eds.), *Pharmacotherapy: A pathophysiologic approach* (pp. 153–181). Stamford, CT: Appleton & Lange.

Crozier, I., Ikram, H., Awan, N., et al. (1995). Losartan in heart failure: Hemodynamic effects and tolerability. *Circulation, 91,* 691–697.

*Dickstein, K., Chang, P., Willenheimer, R., et al. (1995). Comparison of the effects of losartan and enalapril on clinical status and exercise performance in patients with moderate or severe chronic heart failure. *Journal of the American College of Cardiology, 26,* 438–445.

*Digitalis Investigation Group. (1997). The effect of digoxin on mortality and morbidity in patients with heart failure. *New England Journal of Medicine, 336,* 525–533.

*Doval, H. C., Nul, D. R., Grancelli, H. O., et al. (1994). Randomized trial of low-dose amiodarone in severe congestive heart failure. *Lancet, 344,* 493–498.

*Franciosa, J. A., Wilen, M., Ziesche, S., et al. (1983). Survival in men with severe chronic left ventricular failure due to either coronary heart disease or idiopathic dilated cardiomyopathy. *American Journal of Cardiology, 51,* 831–836.

*Gheorghiade, M., Cody, R. J., Francis, G. S., et al. (1998). Current medical therapy for advanced heart failure. *American Heart Journal, 135,* S2231–S2248.

*Giles, T. D. (1990). Clinical experience with lisinopril in congestive heart failure. Focus on the older patient. *Drugs, 39*(Suppl. 2), 17–22.

Gottlieb, S. S., Dickstein, K., Fleck, E., et al. (1993). Hemodynamic and neurohormonal effects of the angiotensin II antagonist losartan in patients with congestive heart failure. *Circulation, 88,* 1602–1609.

Gruppo Italiano per lo Studio della Sopravvivenza nell'Infarto Miocardico (GISSI-3). (1994). GISSI-3: Effects of lisinopril and transdermal glyceryl trinitrate singly and together on 6-week mortality and ventricular function after acute myocardial infarction. *Lancet, 343,* 1115–1122.

*Guideline Committee for the Heart Failure Society of America. (2000). HFSA guidelines for the management of patients with heart failure caused by left ventricular systolic dysfunction—Pharmacologic approaches. *Journal of Cardiac Failure, 5,* 357–382.

Hargreaves, M. R., & Benson, M. K. (1995). Inhaled sodium cromoglycate in angiotensin-converting enzyme inhibitor cough. *Lancet, 345,* 13–16.

Hood, W. B., Jr., Dans, A. L., Guyatt, G. H., et al. (2004). Digitalis for treatment of congestive heart failure in patients in sinus rhythm. *Cochrane Database of Systematic Reviews,* (2), 002901.

Hunt, S. A., Baker, D. W., Chin, M. H., et al. (2002). ACC/AHA guidelines for the evaluation and management of chronic heart failure in the adult: Executive summary. *Journal of Heart & Lung Transplantation, 21*(2), 189–203.

ISIS-4 (Fourth International Study of Infarct Survival) Collaborative Group. (1995). ISIS-4: A randomized factorial trial assessing early oral captopril, oral mononitrate, and intravenous magnesium sulphate in 58,050 patients with suspected acute myocardial infarction. *Lancet, 345,* 669–685.

*Jessup, M., & Brozana, S. (2003). Heart failure. *The New England Journal of Medicine, 318,* 2007–2018.

Johnston, C. I. (1995). Angiotensin receptor antagonists: Focus on losartan. *Lancet, 346,* 1403–1407.

*Kober, L., Torp-Pedersen, C., Carlsen, J. E., et al. (1995). A clinical trial of the angiotensin-converting-enzyme inhibitor trandolapril in patients with left ventricular dysfunction after myocardial infarction. *New England Journal of Medicine, 333,* 1670–1676.

*Konstam, M., Dracup, K., Baker, D., et al. (1994). *Heart failure: Evaluation and care of patients with left-ventricular systolic dysfunction.* Clinical practice guideline no. 11 (AHCPR Publication No. 94-0612). Rockville, MD: Agency for Health Care Policy and Research, Public Health Service, U.S. Department of Health and Human Services.

*Krum, H., Sackner-Bernstein, J. D., Goldsmith, R. L., et al. (1995). Double-blind, placebo-controlled study of the long-term efficacy of carvedilol in patients with severe heart failure. *Circulation, 92,* 1499–1506.

LacourciPre, Y., Brunner, H., Irwin, R., et al., for the Losartan Cough Study Group. (1994). Effects of modulators of the renin-angiotensin-aldosterone system on cough. *Journal of Hypertension, 12,* 1387–1393.

*Lang, R. M., Elkayam, U., Yellen, L. G., et al., for the Losartan Pilot Exercise Study Investigators. (1997). Comparative effects of losartan and enalapril on exercise capacity and clinical status in patients with heart failure. *Journal of the American College of Cardiology, 30,* 983–991.

LaPointe, N., Zhou, Y., Stafford, J., et al. (2009). Coronary artery disease: Association between mortality and persistent use of beta blockers and angiotensin-converting enzyme inhibitors in patients with left ventricular systolic dysfunction and coronary artery disease. *The American Journal of Cardiology, 103*(11), 1518–1524.

Massie, B. M., & Shah, N. B. (1997). Evolving trends in the epidemiologic factors of heart failure: Rationale for preventive strategies and comprehensive disease management. *American Heart Journal, 133,* 703–712.

The Medical Letter. (2009). Treatment guidelines: Drugs for the treatment of chronic heart failure. *The Medical Letter, 7*(83), 53–56.

*Metra, M., Nardi, M., Giubbini, R., et al. (1994). Effects of short- and long-term carvedilol administration on rest and exercise hemodynamic variables, exercise capacity, and clinical conditions in patients with idiopathic dilated cardiomyopathy. *Journal of the American College of Cardiology, 24,* 1678–1687.

O'Connell, J. B., & Bristow, M. R. (1994). Economic impact of heart failure in the United States: Time for a different approach. *Journal of Heart and Lung Transplantation, 13,* S107–S112.

Olsen, S. L., Gilbert, E. M., Renlund, D. G., et al. (1995). Carvedilol improves left ventricular function and symptoms in chronic heart failure: A double-blind randomized study. *Journal of the American College of Cardiology, 25,* 1225–1231.

Packer, M., Bristow, M.R., Cohn, J.N., et al., for the U.S. Carvedilol Heart Failure Study Group. (1996a). The effect of carvedilol on morbidity and mortality in patients with chronic heart failure. *New England Journal of Medicine, 334*, 1349–1355.

*Packer, M., & Cohn, J.N., on behalf of the Steering Committee and Membership of the Advisory Council to Improve Outcomes Nationwide in Heart Failure. (1999). Consensus recommendations for the management of chronic heart failure. *American Journal of Cardiology, 83*, 1A–38A.

Packer, M., Colucci, W. S., Sackner-Bernstein, J.D., et al., for the PRECISE Study Group. (1996b). Double-blind, placebo-controlled study of the effects of carvedilol in patients with moderate to severe heart failure: The PRECISE Trial. *Circulation, 94*, 2793–2799.

*Packer, M., O'Connor, C. M., Ghali, J.K., et al., for the Prospective Randomized Amlodipine Survival Evaluation Study Group. (1996c). Effect of amlodipine on morbidity and mortality in severe chronic heart failure. *New England Journal of Medicine, 335*, 1107–1114.

Parker, R., Patterson, H., & Johnson, J. (2005). Heart failure. In J. T. DiPiro, R. L. Talbert, G. C. Yee, G. R. Matzke, B. G. Wells, & L. M. Posey (Eds.). *Pharmacotherapy: A pathophysiologic approach* (6th ed., pp. 219–260). New York, NY: McGraw-Hill.

Pfeffer, M. A., Braunwald, E., Moye, L. A., et al. (1992). Effect of captopril on mortality and morbidity in patients with left ventricular dysfunction after myocardial infarction: Results of the Survival and Ventricular Enlargement Trial. *New England Journal of Medicine, 327*, 669–677.

*Pitt, B., Segal, R., Martinez, F. A., et al. (1997). Randomised trial of losartan versus captopril in patients over 65 with heart failure (Evaluation of Losartan in the Elderly Study, ELITE). *Lancet, 349*, 747–752.

*Pitt, B., Zannad, F., Remme, W. J., et al. (1999). The effect of spironolactone on morbidity and mortality in patients with severe heart failure. *New England Journal of Medicine, 341*(10), 709–717.

*Singh, S. N., Fletcher, R. D., Fischer, S. G., et al. (1995). Amiodarone in patients with congestive heart failure and symptomatic ventricular arrhythmias. *New England Journal of Medicine, 333*, 77–82.

Smith, T. W., Braunwald, E., & Kelly, R. A. (1988). The management of heart failure. In E. Braunwald (Ed.), *Heart disease* (pp. 485–543). Philadelphia, PA: W. B. Saunders.

*SOLVD Investigators. (1991). Effect of enalapril on survival in patients with reduced left ventricular ejection fractions and HF. *New England Journal of Medicine, 325*, 303–310.

*SOLVD Investigators. (1992). Effect of enalapril on mortality and the development of congestive heart failure in asymptomatic patients with reduced left ventricular ejection fractions. *New England Journal of Medicine, 327*, 685–691.

Williams, J. F., Bristow, M. R., Fowler, M. B., et al. (1995). Guidelines for the evaluation and management of heart failure: Report of the American College of Cardiology/American Heart Association Task Force on Practice Guidelines (Committee on Evaluation and Management of Heart Failure). *Journal of the American College of Cardiology, 26*, 1376–1398.

CHAPTER 23

Arrhythmias

Cynthia A. Sanoski
Andrew M. Peterson

Cardiac arrhythmias are abnormal cardiac rhythms, including tachyarrhythmias (an increase in heart rate) and bradyarrhythmias (a decrease in heart rate). Arrhythmias may be asymptomatic or symptomatic, causing palpitations, weakness, loss of consciousness, heart failure (HF), and sudden death. Searching for a reversible cause of the arrhythmia is the first step in patient care. However, in many cases, antiarrhythmic drugs (AADs) are necessary to permit stabilization until the underlying condition is normalized. Many patients require chronic drug therapy for an arrhythmia due to an underlying disease condition that makes them chronically susceptible to cardiac arrhythmias that are associated with high morbidity and mortality rates.

CAUSES

Arrhythmias may result from structural or electrical/conduction system changes in the heart that may compromise cardiac function and output. Conditions that give rise to arrhythmias include myocardial ischemia, chronic HF, hypertension, valvular heart disease, hypoxemia, hypercapnia, thyroid abnormalities, electrolyte disturbances, drug toxicity, excessive caffeine or ethanol ingestion, anxiety, and exercise. Some of these conditions are reversible, and some cause structural changes that are not reversible.

PATHOPHYSIOLOGY

Basic Electrophysiology

Electrically active myocardial cells (non–pacemaker-type cells) at rest maintain a potential difference between their intracellular fluid and the extracellular fluid. When excited, these cells manifest a characteristic sequence of transmembrane potential changes called the *action potential*. The resting membrane potential is –90 mV with respect to the extracellular fluid. The activity of the sodium-potassium pump and the permeability of the membrane to sodium, potassium, and calcium ions determine the membrane potential of a cardiac cell at any given time. Permeability is defined by the diffusion of ions across the membrane through various ion-selective channels. The phases of the action potential correspond to the excitation state of a myocardial cell (**Box 23.1**).

Arrhythmias are considered to result from disorders of impulse formation and/or impulse conduction. Several factors are believed to be involved in precipitating arrhythmias. There may be a defect in the normal mechanism of spontaneous phase 4 depolarization or an increased automaticity of pacemaker cells. In addition, ectopic pacemakers in normally quiescent tissue are responsible for arrhythmias originating from disorders of impulse formation. Impulse conduction defects occur when the impulse is slowed or blocked because of functional unidirectional block, a change in conduction velocity, or a change in the refractory period. Furthermore, simultaneous abnormalities of impulse formation and conduction may occur.

AADs are used to treat abnormal electrical activity of the heart. The drugs outlined in this chapter are used to treat, suppress, or prevent two major mechanisms of arrhythmias—an abnormality in impulse formation (i.e., increased automaticity) or an abnormality in impulse conduction (i.e., reentry).

Automaticity

Automaticity refers to the ability of the cardiac cells to depolarize spontaneously. Three factors determine automaticity: maximum diastolic depolarization, the rate of depolarization, and the level of the threshold potential. Arrhythmias resulting from abnormal automaticity include sinus tachycardia and junctional tachycardia. The sinoatrial (SA) node has the most rapid rate of depolarization during diastole and reaches threshold first. Cells of the atrioventricular (AV) node and His-Purkinje system have automaticity but a slower rate of phase 4 depolarization. The primary role of the SA node is as the pacemaker of the heart. The SA node is sensitive to alterations in autonomic nervous system output and in its biochemical surroundings. Catecholamine stimulation leads to a shorter action potential duration and increases the spontaneous rate of depolarization. Vagal stimulus and endogenous purines such as adenosine (Adenocard) increase outward potassium currents, thus inhibiting depolarization. Increased adrenergic innervation produces major changes in ionic current activity in the SA node.

Another mechanism for arrhythmias due to abnormal impulse formation is intracellular calcium overload, called *after-depolarization*. If after-depolarizations reach threshold, a new action potential is generated and propagated in adjacent cells. After-depolarizations may occur in response to hypothermia, electrolyte imbalance, catecholamine excess, or stretch. Late after-depolarizations may also be of particular importance in some of the arrhythmias caused by digoxin toxicity.

BOX 23.1

Phases of the Action Potential

- **Phase 0** is when rapid depolarization occurs due to the rapid influx of Na^+.
- **Phase 1** is a brief initial repolarization period. Inactivation of the inward Na^+ current and activation of the outward K^+ current cause this brief but rapid phase of repolarization.
- **Phase 2** is a plateau period during which there is little change in membrane potential. The outward K^+ current and the influx of Ca^{2+} through calcium channels typify the plateau period. The offsetting effect of these currents creates only a small net change in potential, thus creating a plateau.
- **Phase 3** is a period of repolarization that is characterized primarily by K^+ efflux.
- **Phase 4** is a gradual depolarization of the cell, with Na^+ gradually leaking into the intracellular space, balanced by decreasing efflux of K^+. As the cell is slowly depolarized during this phase, an increase in Na^+ permeability occurs, which again leads to phase 0.

Reentry

Reentry involves indefinite propagation of the impulse and continued activation of previously refractory tissue (Wit, et al., 1974). Reentrant foci occur if there are two pathways for impulse conduction, an area of unidirectional block (prolonged refractoriness) in one of these pathways, and slow conduction in the other pathway. A refractory period occurs when the cell cannot be activated after having already fired. Excitability determines the strength of a stimulus required to initiate a new action potential at any given point during the action potential cycle.

Types of Arrhythmias

Arrhythmias evolve either above or below the ventricles and can be regular or irregular. *Supraventricular arrhythmias* evolve above the ventricles in the atria, SA node, or AV node. These arrhythmias may present with either tachycardia or bradycardia or with regularity or irregularity. *AV nodal arrhythmias* originate at or within the AV node and are caused by delayed or absent SA node conduction to the AV node. Supraventricular and AV nodal arrhythmias are not usually life-threatening; however, they may become troublesome and lead to reduced cardiac output related to decreased ventricular filling.

Ventricular arrhythmias originate in the ventricles or the bundle of His. These types of arrhythmias may be symptomatic, causing loss of consciousness or death. Therefore, arrhythmias in this category require immediate intervention. Underlying clinical conditions that usually give rise to these arrhythmias are myocardial ischemia/infarction, dilated and hypertrophic cardiomyopathies, electrolyte disorders, hypoxia, hyperthyroidism, valvular diseases, and drug toxicity. **Box 23.2** lists arrhythmias by category.

DIAGNOSTIC CRITERIA

The practitioner must first assess the patient via a thorough and sometimes urgent history and physical examination. There may be no symptoms, or the patient may report symptoms such as chest pain, shortness of breath, decreased level of consciousness, syncope, confusion, diaphoresis, weakness, and palpitations. The practitioner should ask when the symptoms

BOX 23.2

Categories of Supraventricular, Junctional, and Ventricular Arrhythmias

Supraventricular Arrhythmias
Sinus tachycardia
Paroxysmal supraventricular tachycardia (originates above or within the AV node and conducts to the His-Purkinje system) (e.g., AV nodal reentrant tachycardia, AV reentrant tachycardia)
Sinus bradycardia
Atrial fibrillation
Atrial flutter
Atrial tachycardia
Premature atrial contractions
Wolff-Parkinson-White syndrome

Junctional Arrhythmias
Nonparoxysmal AV junctional tachycardia (heart rate > 60 beats/minute)
Junctional escape rhythm (heart rate 40–60 beats/minute)
Premature AV junctional complexes
AV dissociation
First-degree heart block
Second-degree heart block (Mobitz type I [Wenckebach], Mobitz type II)
Third-degree (complete) heart block

Ventricular Arrhythmias
Premature ventricular contractions
Ventricular tachycardia
Ventricular fibrillation
Torsades de pointes (a rapid form of polymorphic ventricular tachycardia associated with a long QT interval)

started, how long they have lasted, their frequency, and how the patient tolerated the symptoms.

It also is important to assess the patient's risk factors for development of arrhythmias, such as previous coronary artery disease, myocardial infarction (MI), dilated or hypertrophic cardiomyopathy, hypertension, valvular heart disease, alcohol or drug abuse, or prescription drug use (e.g., digoxin [Lanoxin], AADs). The practitioner should focus the physical examination on heart rate and blood pressure; presence of extra, irregular, or skipped beats; rate, rhythm, amplitude, and symmetry of peripheral pulses; and response to exercise.

Laboratory and diagnostic studies also are vital in diagnosing arrhythmias. The practitioner should examine the electrocardiogram (ECG) for evidence of myocardial ischemia; calculation of the PR interval, QRS interval, and QT interval; presence of premature atrial or ventricular contractions; characteristics of Wolff-Parkinson-White (WPW) syndrome; presence or absence of P waves; and relationship between P waves and QRS complexes. Continuous cardiac monitoring is needed for patients who have episodes of life-threatening arrhythmias so that electrical cardioversion and/or AADs can be administered as immediate interventions.

A complete blood count, chemical profile (to assess electrolyte concentrations), thyroid function tests, and a digoxin level should be performed as necessary to determine any underlying causes of the arrhythmia. In addition, an echocardiogram should be performed to assess left ventricular (LV) function. If myocardial ischemia is suspected as a cause of the arrhythmia, the patient should undergo further evaluation with measurement of cardiac enzymes, performance of cardiac stress testing and, possibly, cardiac catheterization.

INITIATING DRUG THERAPY

The past several decades have seen the introduction of numerous agents to treat arrhythmias, but there have been no "miracle cures" in terms of drug therapy. In fact, more recent studies disclose that many of these drugs are proarrhythmic. Therefore, the decision to administer AADs must be based on whether the morbidity and mortality associated with the arrhythmia outweigh the potential adverse events associated with the drugs.

Treatable conditions may cause the arrhythmia. Identification of treatable causes before administering an AAD is a priority. Conditions that may cause arrhythmias are electrolyte imbalances (e.g., hypokalemia, hypomagnesemia), drug overdose, drug interactions with other medications or herbal supplements, renal failure, thyroid disorders, metabolic acidosis, hypovolemia, MI, pulmonary embolism, cardiac tamponade, tension pneumothorax, dissecting aortic aneurysm, hypoxemia, fever, and valvular or congenital defects in the heart.

Most AADs are used to treat tachyarrhythmias; however, atropine is used to treat bradycardia. Management of these arrhythmias is focused on relieving the acute episode of the arrhythmia, establishing sinus rhythm (SR), and preventing

further episodes of the arrhythmia. Certain AADs are known to be more effective for one type of arrhythmia than another.

Nonpharmacologic therapies, such as radiofrequency catheter ablation and implantable cardioverter–defibrillators (ICDs), are also available to treat various arrhythmias. ICDs are used in the management of ventricular arrhythmias, and their benefits have been demonstrated in several clinical trials (Antiarrhythmics Versus Implantable Defibrillators [AVID] Investigators, 1997; Connolly, et al., 2000; Kuck, et al., 2000; Moss, et al., 1996; Buxton, et al., 1999; Moss, et al., 2002; Bardy, et al., 2005). Radiofrequency catheter ablation permanently terminates the arrhythmia by ablating the focal area where the arrhythmia occurs. This procedure can be used for atrial fibrillation (AF), atrial flutter, and symptomatic drug-refractory ventricular tachycardia (VT).

Goals of Antiarrhythmic Drug Therapy

The overall goals of AAD therapy are to relieve the acute episode of irregular rhythm, establish SR, and prevent further episodes of the arrhythmia. This is usually achieved through modification of the ion fluxes described previously by blocking sodium, potassium, or calcium channels and/or β-adrenergic receptors. Typical agents used to treat arrhythmias include AADs (classes I through IV), digoxin, adenosine, and atropine (**Table 23.1**).

Drug Classification

AADs are organized into four classes, I (Ia, Ib, Ic), II, III, and IV (Vaughan Williams, 1984). Although the Vaughan Williams classification system is the most widely used method for grouping AADs based on their electrophysiologic actions, using this classification system requires some points of exception to be made. This system is somewhat incomplete, and it excludes such drugs as digoxin, adenosine, and atropine. In addition, the classification is not pure, and there is some overlapping of drugs into more than one category. For instance, amiodarone and dronedarone have electrophysiologic properties of all four Vaughan Williams classes. Furthermore, this system does not take into account that the active metabolites of AADs may have different electrophysiologic effects than their parent drugs. For example, N-acetyl-procainamide (NAPA), the major active metabolite of procainamide, blocks outward potassium channels and therefore can be considered a class III AAD. Although procainamide blocks outward potassium channels, it also primarily blocks inward sodium currents, thereby making it a class Ia AAD. Therefore, the overall electrophysiologic effect produced by procainamide depends upon the relative concentrations of procainamide and NAPA that are present in the body, which can vary based on several clinical factors. The Vaughan Williams classification scheme (**Box 23.3**) identifies drugs that block sodium channels (class Ia, Ib, and Ic), those that are β-blockers (class II), those that block potassium channels (class III), and those that are nondihydropyridine calcium channel blockers (CCBs) (class IV).

TABLE 23.1 Overview of Selected Antiarrhythmic Agents

Generic (Trade) Name and Dosage	Selected Adverse Events	Contraindications	Special Considerations
adenosine (Adenocard) Adult: 6 mg IV push over 1–2 s; repeat with 12 mg IV push if sinus rhythm not obtained within 1–2 min after first dose; may repeat 12 mg dose a second time if no response in 1–2 min	Headache, chest pain, lightheadedness, dizziness, nausea, flushing, dyspnea, blurred vision	2nd- or 3rd-degree heart block or sick sinus syndrome in the absence of a pacemaker	Monitor ECG during administration. Use cautiously in patients with asthma as bronchoconstriction may occur. Instruct patient to report adverse reactions immediately or any discomfort at IV site. Each dose should be immediately followed with a 10-mL saline flush.
amiodarone (Cordarone) *Atrial Fibrillation* Adult IV: 5 mg/kg over 30 min, then continuous infusion of 1 mg/min for 6 h, then 0.5 mg/min; convert to PO therapy when hemodynamically stable and able to take PO medications Adult PO: 800–1,200 mg/d in 2 or 3 divided doses for 1 wk, until patient receives ~10 g total, then 200 mg PO daily *Pulseless VT/VF* Adult IV: 300 mg IV push/IO; can give additional 150 mg IV push/IO if persistent VT/VF; if stable rhythm achieved, can initiate continuous infusion at 1 mg/min for 6 h, then 0.5 mg/min; convert to PO therapy when hemodynamically stable and able to take PO medications (see PO dose under Stable VT) *Stable VT (with a pulse)* Adult IV: 150 mg (diluted in 100 mL of D5W or saline) over 10 min; may repeat dose every 10 min, if necessary for breakthrough VT; if	IV: hypotension, phlebitis, bradycardia, heart block PO: corneal microdeposits, optic neuritis, nausea, vomiting, anorexia, pulmonary fibrosis, bradycardia, tremor, ataxia, paresthesias, insomnia, constipation, abnormal liver function tests, hypothyroidism, hyperthyroidism, blue-gray discoloration of skin, photosensitivity	2nd- or 3rd-degree heart block or sick sinus syndrome in the absence of a pacemaker	Instruct patient to report adverse reactions immediately. Advise patient to apply sunscreen and to minimize areas of exposure to sun. Patients should have a chest x-ray performed on an annual basis. Liver function and thyroid function tests should be performed every 6 mo. Pulmonary function tests and an ophthalmologic exam should be performed if the patient becomes symptomatic. A chest x-ray, pulmonary function tests, liver function tests, and thyroid function tests should also be performed at baseline when amiodarone is initiated. An ophthalmologic exam should be performed at baseline if a patient has significant visual abnormalities.

(continued)

TABLE 23.1 **Overview of Selected Antiarrhythmic Agents (*Continued*)**

Generic (Trade) Name and Dosage	Selected Adverse Events	Contraindications	Special Considerations
stable rhythm achieved, can initiate continuous infusion at 1 mg/min for 6 h, then 0.5 mg/min; convert to PO therapy when hemodynamically stable and able to take PO medications Adult PO: 1,200–1,600 mg/d in 2 or 3 divided doses for 1 wk, until patient receives ~15 g total, then 300–400 mg PO daily			
atropine Adult: 0.5 mg IV every 3–5 min; not to exceed 3 mg total dose	Palpitations, tachycardia, dry mouth, dizziness	Acute angle-closure glaucoma, obstructive uropathy, tachycardia, obstructive disease of GI tract	Administer IV over 1 min. Monitor ECG during administration.
digoxin (Lanoxin) Adult LD (IV or PO): 0.25–0.5 mg over 2 min; may give 0.125–0.25 mg q6h for 2 more doses for a total dose of 1 mg or 10–15 mcg/kg Adult MD: 0.125–0.25 mg IV or PO daily in normal renal function	Anorexia, nausea, vomiting, diarrhea, headache, fatigue, dizziness, vertigo, visual disturbances (yellow-green halos), confusion, hallucinations, arrhythmias, AV conduction disturbances (heart block, AV junctional rhythm, bradycardia)	2nd- or 3rd-degree heart block or sick sinus syndrome in the absence of a pacemaker	Instruct patient to report adverse reactions immediately. Teach patient how to take pulse. Dose adjustment required in renal insufficiency
diltiazem (Cardizem) Adult IV: 0.25 mg/kg over 2 min; if ventricular rate remains uncontrolled after 15 min, can repeat with 0.35 mg/kg over 2 min; initiate continuous infusion of 5–15 mg/h Adult PO: Start with 30 mg 4 times daily and increase to 180–480 mg/d in divided doses (SR form can be given once daily)	Dizziness, headache, edema, heart block, bradycardia, HF exacerbation, hypotension	2nd- or 3rd-degree heart block or sick sinus syndrome in the absence of a pacemaker, LV systolic dysfunction	Teach patient how to take pulse and blood pressure. Increased levels of cyclosporine may occur with concomitant use.
disopyramide (Norpace) Adult (<50 kg): 100 mg PO q6h or SR form, 200 mg PO q12h Adult (>50 kg): 150 mg PO q6h or SR form, 300 mg PO q12h; may increase up to 800 mg/d	Hypotension, HF exacerbation, nausea, anorexia, dry mouth, urinary retention, blurred vision, constipation, TdP	2nd- or 3rd-degree heart block or sick sinus syndrome in the absence of a pacemaker, HF	Dose adjustment required in patients with renal insufficiency (CrCl ≤40 mL/min)

TABLE 23.1   Overview of Selected Antiarrhythmic Agents (*Continued*)

Generic (Trade) Name and Dosage	Selected Adverse Events	Contraindications	Special Considerations
dofetilide (Tikosyn) Adult: 125–500 mcg PO BID	Chest pain, headache, dizziness, insomnia, nausea, diarrhea, dyspnea, TdP	CrCl <20 mL/min, QT interval >440 ms, concomitant use of cimetidine, hydrochlorothiazide, ketoconazole, megestrol, prochlorperazine, QTc-prolonging drugs, trimethoprim/sulfamethoxazole, or verapamil	Specialized training and facilities are required for initiation of therapy. Dose adjustment required in patients with renal insufficiency (CrCl ≤60 mL/min) Dose must also be adjusted based on QT interval.
dronedarone (Multaq) Adult: 400 mg PO BID (with meals)	Nausea, vomiting, diarrhea, increased serum creatinine concentrations	NYHA class IV HF, NYHA class II or III HF with a recent hospitalization for decompensated HF, 2nd- or 3rd-degree heart block or sick sinus syndrome in the absence of a pacemaker, heart rate <50 bpm, concomitant use of potent CYP3A4 inhibitors or QTc-prolonging drugs, QT interval ≥500 ms, PR interval >280 ms, severe hepatic impairment	Instruct patient to report adverse reactions or any signs/symptoms of HF immediately.
esmolol (Brevibloc) Adult: 500 mcg/kg/min IV for 1 min followed by a maintenance infusion of 50 mcg/kg/min; if inadequate response, re-bolus with 500 mcg/kg/min for 1 min and increase infusion rate by 50 mcg/kg/min; repeat this process until desired response achieved or maximum infusion rate of 300 mcg/kg/min is reached	Hypotension, wheezing, bronchospasm, heart block, bradycardia, HF exacerbation	2nd- or 3rd-degree heart block in the absence of a pacemaker, decompensated HF, sinus bradycardia	Instruct patient to report adverse reactions immediately or any discomfort at IV site.
flecainide (Tambocor) Adult: 50 mg PO q12h up to a maximum of 300 mg/d	Dizziness, headache, lightheadedness, syncope, blurred vision or other visual disturbances, dyspnea, HF exacerbation, arrhythmias	2nd- or 3rd-degree heart block in the absence of a pacemaker, recent MI, ischemic heart disease, cardiogenic shock, HF	Instruct patient to report adverse reactions immediately.
ibutilide (Corvert) Adult (<60 kg): 0.01 mg/kg IV over 10 min; can repeat with another dose if atrial fibrillation/flutter does not terminate within 10 min after end of initial dose	TdP, hypotension, heart block, headache, nausea	Pre-existing hypokalemia or hypomagnesemia, QT interval >440 ms	Stop infusion if the QT interval increases or ventricular arrhythmias occur. Monitor ECG during administration. Correct any electrolyte abnormalities before administering.

(*continued*)

TABLE 23.1 **Overview of Selected Antiarrhythmic Agents (*Continued*)**

Generic (Trade) Name and Dosage	Selected Adverse Events	Contraindications	Special Considerations
Adult (≥60 kg): 1 mg IV over 10 min; can repeat with another dose if atrial fibrillation/flutter does not terminate within 10 min after end of initial dose			
lidocaine (Xylocaine) *Pulseless VT/VF* Adult: 1–1.5 mg/kg IV push/IO; may give additional 0.5–0.75 mg/kg IV push/IO every 5–10 min, if persistent VT/VF (maximum cumulative dose = 3 mg/kg); if stable rhythm achieved, can initiate continuous infusion of 1–4 mg/min *Stable VT (with a pulse)* Adult: 1–1.5 mg/kg IV push; may give additional 0.5–0.75 mg/kg IV push every 5–10 min, if persistent VT (maximum cumulative dose = 3 mg/kg); if stable rhythm achieved, can initiate continuous infusion of 1–4 mg/min	Seizures, confusion, stupor, dizziness, bradycardia, respiratory depression, slurred speech, blurred vision, muscle twitching, tinnitus	Hypersensitivity to amide local anesthetics, 2nd- or 3rd-degree heart block in the absence of a pacemaker	A lower infusion rate (1–2 mg/min) should be used in elderly patients or patients with HF or hepatic disease.
metoprolol (Lopressor) Adult IV: 2.5–5 mg over 2 min; can repeat every 5 min up to a total of 3 doses Adult PO: 25 mg BID or 50 mg daily (SR form); may increase up to 400 mg/d	Bradycardia, HF exacerbation, heart block, bronchospasm, fatigue, dizziness, hypotension	2nd- or 3rd-degree heart block in the absence of a pacemaker, decompensated HF, heart rate <45 beats/min	Use with caution in patients with severe LV systolic dysfunction or respiratory disease. Teach patient how to take pulse and blood pressure. Because sudden withdrawal can lead to exacerbation of angina and MI, instruct patient not to discontinue drug abruptly. Instruct patient to report adverse reactions immediately.
mexiletine (Mexitil) Adult: 200 mg PO q8h; may increase up to 400 mg PO q8h	Dizziness, drowsiness, paresthesias, blurred vision, tremor, seizures, confusion, arrhythmias, nausea, vomiting	2nd- or 3rd-degree heart block in the absence of a pacemaker, cardiogenic shock	Instruct patient to report adverse reactions immediately.

TABLE 23.1   Overview of Selected Antiarrhythmic Agents (*Continued*)

Generic (Trade) Name and Dosage	Selected Adverse Events	Contraindications	Special Considerations
procainamide (Pronestyl) *Supraventricular Arrhythmias or Stable VT (with a pulse)* Adult: 15–18 mg/kg IV over 60 min, then continuous infusion of 1–4 mg/min	Bradycardia, heart block, hypotension, HF exacerbation, TdP	Hypersensitivity to procaine, 2nd- or 3rd-degree heart block in the absence of a pacemaker	Use with caution, if at all, in patients with renal insufficiency.
propafenone (Rythmol) Adult: 150 mg PO q8h; up to a maximum of 300 mg PO q8h	Dizziness, drowsiness, HF exacerbation, arrhythmias, heart block, bradycardia, blurred vision, taste disturbances, bronchospasm	2nd- or 3rd-degree heart block in the absence of a pacemaker, bradycardia, cardiogenic shock, HF, bronchospastic disorders	Instruct patient to report adverse reactions immediately.
propranolol (Inderal) Adult IV: 1 mg over 1 min; may repeat every 5 min up to a total dose of 5 mg Adult PO: 10–20 mg q6–8h; can increase to 80–240 mg/d in 2–4 divided doses	Hypotension, bradycardia, heart block, HF exacerbation, fatigue, bronchospasm, depression, decreased exercise tolerance, aggravated peripheral arterial insufficiency, masking of symptoms of and delayed recovery from hypoglycemia, Raynaud's phenomenon, insomnia, vivid dreams or hallucinations, impotence, increased serum triglyceride levels, decreased high-density lipoprotein cholesterol levels	2nd- or 3rd-degree heart block or sick sinus syndrome in the absence of a pacemaker, LV systolic dysfunction Relatively contraindicated in asthma	Because sudden withdrawal can lead to exacerbation of angina and MI. Instruct patient not to discontinue drug abruptly. Teach patient how to take pulse and blood pressure, weigh self daily and report weight gain, and report any dyspnea on exertion or when lying down.
quinidine (Quinidex, Quinaglute) Adult: Quinidine sulfate, 200–400 mg PO q6h, up to a maximum of 600 mg PO q6h; quinidine gluconate, 324 mg PO q8–12h, up to a maximum of 972 mg PO q8–12h	TdP, heart block, hypotension, tinnitus, diarrhea, nausea, vomiting, fever, HF exacerbation, thrombocytopenia	Allergy or sensitivity to quinidine or cinchona derivatives, long QT syndrome (may predispose to TdP)	Instruct patient to take drug with food if GI distress occurs. Instruct patient to report adverse reactions immediately.
sotalol (Betapace, Betapace AF) *Atrial Fibrillation (Betapace AF)* Adult: 80 mg PO bid, up to a maximum of 160 mg PO bid	Bradycardia, heart block, HF exacerbation, TdP, bronchospasm	2nd- or 3rd-degree heart block in the absence of a pacemaker, bradycardia, HF, asthma, long QT syndrome (may predispose to TdP)	Dosing interval must be adjusted in patients with renal insufficiency. Instruct patient to take drug on an empty stomach. Instruct patient not to discontinue drug abruptly.

(continued)

TABLE 23.1	**Overview of Selected Antiarrhythmic Agents (*Continued*)**		
Generic (Trade) Name and Dosage	**Selected Adverse Events**	**Contraindications**	**Special Considerations**
Ventricular Arrhythmias (Betapace) Adult IV: 75 mg (given over 5 h) BID, up to a maximum of 150 mg (given over 5 h) BID Adult PO: 80 mg BID, up to a maximum of 320 mg BID			
verapamil (Calan) Adult IV: 2.5–5 mg over 2 min; if ventricular rate remains uncontrolled after 15–30 min, can double initial dose and administer over 2 min; initiate continuous infusion of 5–10 mg/h Adult PO: 240–360 mg/d in three divided doses (SR form can be given once daily)	Constipation, bradycardia, heart block, HF exacerbation, hypotension, dizziness, peripheral edema	2nd- or 3rd-degree heart block or sick sinus syndrome in the absence of a pacemaker, LV systolic dysfunction	Encourage patient to increase fluid and fiber intake to combat constipation. Teach patient how to take pulse and blood pressure.

AV, atrioventricular; BID, twice daily; CrCl; creatinine clearance; D5W, 5% dextrose in water; ECG, electrocardiogram; GI, gastrointestinal; HF, heart failure; IV, intravenous; LD, loading dose; LV, left ventricular; MD, maintenance dose; MI, myocardial infarction; NYHA, New York Heart Association; PO, oral; SR, sustained release; TdP, torsades de pointes; VF, ventricular fibrillation; VT, ventricular tachycardia.

Class I Antiarrhythmic Drugs

This class of drugs, known as the sodium channel blockers, may be subdivided into classes Ia, Ib, and Ic according to the rate of sodium channel dissociation. These agents vary in the rate at which they bind and then dissociate from the sodium channel receptor. Class Ib AADs bind to and dissociate from the sodium channel receptor quickly ("fast on-off"), while class Ic AADs slowly bind to and dissociate from this receptor ("slow on-off"). The binding kinetics of the class Ia AADs are intermediate between those of the class Ib and Ic agents. In addition, class I AADs possess rate dependence, whereby sodium channel blockade is greatest at fast heart rates (i.e., tachycardia) and least during slower heart rates (i.e., bradycardia). (See **Table 23.1**.)

Class Ia Antiarrhythmic Drugs
Quinidine

Quinidine (Quinidex, Quinaglute) is a broad-spectrum AAD that may be used to treat supraventricular and ventricular arrhythmias. This drug slows conduction velocity

(phase 0), prolongs refractoriness (phase 3), and decreases automaticity (phase 4). Quinidine widens the QRS complex, prolongs the QT interval, and slightly prolongs the PR interval on the ECG. Quinidine has been used in the management of AF, atrial flutter, AV nodal reentrant tachycardia, and VT.

Quinidine has potent anticholinergic properties that affect the SA and AV nodes. Therefore, quinidine can increase the SA nodal discharge rate and AV nodal conduction. Consequently, in patients with AF or atrial flutter, these anticholinergic effects may lead to a more rapid ventricular rate. Therefore, the AV node should be adequately inhibited with the use of an AV nodal blocking drug, such as a β-blocker, nondihydropyridine CCB (e.g., diltiazem or verapamil), or digoxin prior to administering quinidine in these patients. Quinidine also blocks α_1-receptors, which can lead to vasodilation and subsequent dose-related hypotension, especially when administered intravenously.

The most common adverse events associated with quinidine are gastrointestinal (GI) (nausea, vomiting, and diarrhea). As with other class Ia drugs, quinidine can cause proarrhythmia,

---

BOX 23.3

Classification of Antiarrhythmic Drugs

Class I—Sodium Channel Blockers
Ia (intermediate onset/offset)
   disopyramide (Norpace)
   procainamide (Pronestyl)
   quinidine (Quinidex [sulfate], Quinaglute [gluconate])
Ib (fast onset/offset)
   lidocaine (Xylocaine)
   mexiletine (Mexitil)
   phenytoin (Dilantin)
Ic (slow onset/offset)
   flecainide (Tambocor)
   propafenone (Rythmol)*

Class II—β-Blockers
atenolol (Tenormin)
esmolol (Brevibloc)
metoprolol (Lopressor)
propranolol (Inderal)

Class III—Potassium Channel Blockers
amiodarone (Cordarone)†
dofetilide (Tikosyn)
dronedarone (Multaq)†
ibutilide (Corvert)
sotalol (Betapace, Betapace AF)*

Class IV—Calcium Channel Blockers
diltiazem (Cardizem)
verapamil (Calan)

---

* Also has β-blocking properties (class II)
† Also has sodium-channel blocking (class I), β-blocking (class II), and calcium-channel blocking (class IV) properties

---

specifically torsades de pointes (TdP). Other adverse events associated with quinidine include thrombocytopenia, hepatitis, cinchonism (tinnitus, blurred vision, headache), worsening of underlying HF, and hemolytic anemia.

Quinidine is a substrate of the cytochrome P-450 (CYP) 3A4 isoenzyme and an inhibitor of the CYP2D6 isoenzyme. Therefore, quinidine can interact with any other drug that inhibits or induces CYP3A4 (e.g., inhibitors: ketoconazole, erythromycin, amiodarone, verapamil, diltiazem; inducers: rifampin, phenobarbital, phenytoin) or is a substrate of CYP2D6 (e.g., β-blockers). Quinidine can also significantly increase serum digoxin concentrations.

Procainamide

Procainamide (Pronestyl) has basically the same electrophysiologic effects as those of quinidine, except that procainamide does not have the anticholinergic activity of quinidine. Procainamide slows conduction velocity (phase 0), prolongs refractoriness (phase 3), and decreases automaticity (phase 4). Procainamide widens the QRS complex, prolongs the QT interval, and slightly prolongs the PR interval on the ECG. NAPA, the major metabolite of procainamide, blocks outward potassium currents and thereby has class III electrophysiologic properties. NAPA prolongs the QT interval. Procainamide is a broad-spectrum AAD and has been used to treat supraventricular and ventricular arrhythmias.

Procainamide is only available in the intravenous (IV) formulation; all of its oral formulations have been discontinued. Consequently, adverse events that would be most likely to occur with chronic therapy (e.g., systemic lupus erythematosus, agranulocytosis) should no longer be a concern. Most of the adverse events associated with IV administration of procainamide include bradycardia, AV block, hypotension, worsening of underlying HF, and TdP.

Procainamide and NAPA can accumulate in patients with renal insufficiency. Therefore, serum concentrations must be monitored regularly to assess for efficacy and toxicity. The therapeutic ranges of procainamide and NAPA are 4 to 10 mcg/mL and 15 to 25 mcg/mL, respectively.

Disopyramide

Disopyramide (Norpace) slows conduction velocity (phase 0), prolongs refractoriness (phase 3), and decreases automaticity (phase 4). These effects are manifested as a prolonged QT interval and a slightly prolonged QRS complex on the ECG. Disopyramide has direct and indirect effects on the heart rate similar to those of quinidine. Disopyramide is a broad-spectrum AAD and has been used to treat supraventricular and ventricular arrhythmias. However, the clinical use of this agent is limited because of its potent anticholinergic and negative inotropic effects. If disopyramide is used to treat AF or atrial flutter, the practitioner should give an AV nodal blocking agent (e.g., β-blocker, diltiazem, verapamil, or digoxin) to minimize its vagolytic effect.

The primary adverse events associated with disopyramide are precipitation of HF and anticholinergic effects (e.g., dry mouth, urine retention, constipation, blurred vision). Disopyramide is contraindicated in patients with LV systolic dysfunction (LVSD) (left ventricular ejection fraction [LVEF] of 40% or less) because of significant myocardial depression. Disopyramide can also cause TdP.

Class Ib Drugs

The class Ib AADs include lidocaine (Xylocaine), mexiletine (Mexitil), and phenytoin (Dilantin). These agents decrease automaticity and conduction velocity and shorten refractoriness. These agents primarily exert their electrophysiologic effects on the ventricular myocardium since they have little or no effect on atrial tissue.

Lidocaine

Lidocaine is categorized as a class Ib AAD; however, its electrophysiologic effects are different in that it is selective to ischemic tissue, and especially to active fast sodium channels in the bundle of His, Purkinje fibers, and ventricular myocardium. Thus, lidocaine has little effect on conduction in nonischemic tissue and the atrial myocardium. Lidocaine also has very little effect on the automaticity of the SA node. However, lidocaine does suppress the automaticity of ectopic ventricular pacemakers and Purkinje fibers. In normal tissues, the action potential duration is shortened and conduction velocity shows little change with lidocaine. However, in depolarized fibers or in fibers damaged by ischemia, lidocaine prolongs the action potential and slows conduction.

Lidocaine is primarily effective in treating ventricular arrhythmias, especially those associated with acute MI. Prophylactic administration in patients with acute MI demonstrated a decreased incidence of ventricular fibrillation (VF) but no difference in prehospital treatment outcomes of acute MI and no improvement or even higher mortality rates in hospitalized patients. Selective administration of lidocaine to patients with VF associated with MI or cardiac arrest also demonstrated no improvement in survival rates (Teo, et al., 1993; Wyse, et al., 1988). The use of lidocaine as prophylaxis against VT or VF in patients with MI is not warranted. Its use should be reserved for the treatment of ventricular arrhythmias.

Lidocaine is not effective in the treatment of supraventricular arrhythmias such as AF or atrial flutter. However, lidocaine can be used for treatment of digoxin-induced arrhythmias (atrial and ventricular) because of its selectivity for depolarized myocardium.

Lidocaine is eliminated primarily by hepatic metabolism, with the metabolic rate being proportional to hepatic blood flow. In patients with systolic HF, the volume of distribution in the central compartment is decreased and hepatic blood flow may be decreased if cardiac output is depressed. Hepatic failure slows lidocaine's clearance rate but does not affect its volume of distribution.

The principal adverse events associated with lidocaine are central nervous system (CNS) effects (i.e., dizziness, paresthesia, disorientation, tremor, agitation). At higher concentrations, seizures and respiratory arrest may occur with the use of lidocaine. Lidocaine's adverse events are more frequent in the elderly, patients with HF or hepatic disease, and during prolonged administration (more than 24 hours). Therefore, these patients should be closely monitored for signs and symptoms of lidocaine toxicity. Lidocaine concentrations should also be closely monitored in these patients. The therapeutic range of lidocaine is 1.5 to 6 mg/L. Lidocaine toxicity is most commonly observed at concentrations greater than 5 mg/L.

Mexiletine

Mexiletine is a structurally related oral analog of lidocaine and has similar electrophysiologic effects, antiarrhythmic effects, and adverse events. Mexiletine decreases conduction velocity (phase 0) preferentially in ischemic tissue.

Mexiletine is effective in the treatment of VT. However, its use as a single agent in refractory ventricular arrhythmias has not proved effective (Duff, et al., 1983). Combining mexiletine with a second AAD (class IA or III) has proven more effective for the treatment of refractory VT. However, its clinical use is limited by a high incidence of GI reactions such as nausea and vomiting. Neurologic side effects of dizziness, confusion, ataxia, and speech disturbances may lead the practitioner to discontinue treatment with this drug. Mexiletine can also cause proarrhythmia, although the incidence is lower when compared to other AADs.

Phenytoin

Phenytoin can be used to treat acute arrhythmias caused by tricyclic antidepressant and digoxin toxicity and in TdP because of its unique effect in increasing AV nodal conduction (Vukmir & Stein, 1991). It has an action similar to that of lidocaine, with decreased conduction velocity (phase 0) and automaticity (phase 4) in ischemic tissue. However, refractoriness is essentially unchanged. Adverse effects of phenytoin include hypotension caused by the phenol vehicle and occasional CNS toxicity after excessive dosing (Vukmir & Stein, 1991).

Class Ic Drugs

Flecainide

Flecainide (Tambocor) is a potent blocker of sodium channels during phase 0 of the action potential, thereby slowing conduction velocity in the Purkinje fibers and AV node and diminishing automaticity in the Purkinje fibers. Because of the slowed cardiac conduction, increases in the PR interval and QRS duration may be seen on the ECG.

Flecainide is most commonly used in clinical practice for the treatment of supraventricular arrhythmias, such as AF and atrial flutter. Although flecainide is approved by the U.S. Food and Drug Administration (FDA) for the treatment of life-threatening ventricular arrhythmias, its efficacy is rather poor and the potential for serious adverse events is rather high (Anderson, et al., 1983). In fact, flecainide has been known to cause a rapid, sustained VT that is resistant to resuscitation.

The Cardiac Arrhythmia Suppression Trial (CAST) I study (CAST Investigators, 1989) was a prospective, double-blind, randomized study that was conducted to determine if the suppression of asymptomatic or mildly symptomatic premature ventricular contractions (PVCs) with the class Ic AADs, flecainide, encainide, or moricizine would decrease the incidence of death from arrhythmia in survivors of MI. Despite adequate suppression of ventricular arrhythmias, flecainide significantly increased mortality from arrhythmia or cardiac arrest (presumably due to proarrhythmia) and significantly increased total mortality. Overall, the results of this trial demonstrated that the use of AADs to suppress asymptomatic PVCs in post-MI patients does not improve survival and is most likely detrimental. The use of flecainide should be avoided in patients with any form of structural heart disease (SHD), which includes coronary artery disease, LV dysfunction, valvular heart disease, or LV hypertrophy.

Adverse events associated with flecainide include blurred vision, dizziness, headache, tremor, nausea, vomiting, conduction disturbances, and ventricular arrhythmias (sustained VT) that can be quite resistant to cardioversion. Flecainide also has potent negative inotropic effects that may lead to worsening HF.

Propafenone

Propafenone (Rythmol) has the same ability to block sodium channels, slow conduction velocity, and diminish automaticity in the AV node and Purkinje fibers as flecainide. However, propafenone also has a mild, nonselective β-blocking effect. Although propafenone is FDA-approved for the treatment of life-threatening ventricular arrhythmias, its use in clinical practice has been limited to the management of supraventricular arrhythmias such as AF. Propafenone has been shown to be effective for restoring and maintaining SR in patients with AF (Miller, et al., 2000; Roy, et al., 2000). The use of single, oral loading doses of propafenone (450 to 600 mg) in patients with recent-onset AF has been associated with conversion rates of 72% to 76% at 8 hours (Slavik, et al., 2001). Although propafenone was not evaluated in the CAST and has not been associated with increased mortality in other trials, there still tends to be an overall negative perception of this drug's safety in patients with SHD. Until the safety of propafenone can be demonstrated conclusively in a large, randomized, prospective trial in patients with SHD, its use should be avoided in this population.

Adverse events associated with propafenone include blurred vision, dizziness, headache, nausea, vomiting, fatigue, bronchospasm, taste disturbances (metallic taste), conduction disturbances (bradycardia, heart block, QRS prolongation), and ventricular arrhythmias (sustained VT) that can be quite resistant to cardioversion. Propafenone also has potent negative inotropic effects that may lead to worsening HF.

Class II Antiarrhythmic Drugs

The β-blockers are useful in suppressing ventricular arrhythmias. They also are used for treating many supraventricular arrhythmias because of their ability to block receptor sites in the conduction system and subsequently slow AV nodal conduction and the SA nodal rate, which in turn slows the ventricular rate. Furthermore, β-blockers are helpful when used in combination with other AADs or in treating the underlying cause of some arrhythmias (ischemia, catecholamine excess). (See **Table 23.1.**)

β-blockers decrease automaticity (decrease the slope of phase 4 depolarization in the sinus node and in the Purkinje fibers) and conduction velocity (phase 0) and prolong refractoriness (phase 3). Changes in the ECG caused by β-blockers are a sinus bradycardia, consisting of a normal or slightly prolonged PR interval and occasional shortening of the QT interval. In addition to being negative chronotropic drugs (decrease AV nodal conduction), β-blockers are also negative inotropic agents (decrease cardiac contractility). Both of these properties enable β-blockers to decrease myocardial oxygen consumption, which is useful especially in patients with underlying ischemic heart disease. Exercise-related or stress-related sinus tachycardia may be treated with β-blockers. Patients with sinus node dysfunction or AV conduction system defects may have significant sinus bradycardia when a β-blocker is initiated.

In general, β-blockers lower the heart rate and blood pressure, decrease myocardial contractility, decrease oxygen consumption in the myocardium, and lower cardiac output. β-blockers have a diverse range of uses, including paroxysmal supraventricular tachycardia (PSVT), AF, atrial flutter, and arrhythmias caused by catecholamine excess, ischemia, mitral valve prolapse, hypertrophic cardiomyopathy, and MI. β-blockers also reduce complex ventricular arrhythmias, including VT (Lichstein, et al., 1983). The VF threshold is increased with the use of β-blockers in animal models, and β-blockers have been found to decrease VF in patients with acute MI. β-blockers reduce myocardial ischemia, which may reduce the likelihood of VF. In the CAST, patients receiving β-blockers had a 66% decrease in the incidence of death or cardiac arrest at 30 days, a 53% decrease at 1 year, and a 36% decrease at 2 years (Kennedy, et al., 1994). All β-blockers (without intrinsic sympathomimetic activity) are relatively similar in efficacy for the treatment of supraventricular and ventricular arrhythmias. Selection of a particular β-blocker is usually based on the safety profile of the individual agent.

The adverse events associated with β-blockers depend on their selectivity for β_1 or β_2 receptors. Bronchospasm may be seen in patients with asthma and chronic obstructive pulmonary disease; this adverse event is not eliminated by the use of selective β_1-blockers. HF, hypotension, bradycardia, and depression also are common side effects of β-blockers. In addition, patients receiving β-blockers often report fatigue and impotence.

Class III Antiarrhythmic Drugs

Class III AADs include amiodarone (Cordarone), dofetilide (Tikosyn), dronedarone (Multaq), ibutilide (Corvert), and sotalol (Betapace, Betapace AF). Ibutilide and dofetilide are used to treat AF and atrial flutter. Amiodarone and sotalol can be used to treat both supraventricular and ventricular arrhythmias. Dronedarone is FDA approved to reduce the risk of cardiovascular hospitalization in patients with paroxysmal of persistent AF or atrial flutter who experience a recent episode of this arrhythmia, have cardiovascular risk factors (age 70 or older, hypertension, diabetes, prior stroke, left atrial diameter of at least 50 mm, or LVEF of <40%), and are in or who are cardioverted to SR.

Patients receiving class III AADs should be monitored closely for ECG changes such as increased ventricular ectopy and changes in PR interval, QRS duration, and QT interval. Practitioners should avoid using class III AADs concomitantly with other drugs that can prolong the QT interval to minimize the risk of TdP. (See **Table 23.1.**)

Amiodarone

Amiodarone is a unique drug in that it possesses electrophysiologic characteristics of all four Vaughan Williams classes of AADs. While amiodarone is primarily a potassium channel blocker (blocks the rapid and slow components of the delayed rectifier potassium current), it also blocks sodium channels, has nonselective β-blocking activity, and has weak calcium-channel blocking properties. As a result, amiodarone reduces automaticity (phase 4) and conduction velocity (phase 0) and prolongs refractoriness (phase 3). Its binding characteristics to the sodium channels are similar to those of the class Ib AADs ("fast on/fast off"). When administered intravenously, amiodarone's β-blocking and calcium-channel blocking activity is more predominant. Amiodarone has minimal to no negative inotropic effects, which makes it one of the few AADs that can be safely used in patients with LVSD. Amiodarone prolongs the PR and QT intervals and widens the QRS complex. Amiodarone is used to treat both supraventricular and ventricular arrhythmias.

Since the proportion of patients with AF who have concomitant SHD appears to be increasing, amiodarone's use for this particular arrhythmia has dramatically increased because this is one of the few AADs proven to be safe in this population. Amiodarone is often given IV for the acute treatment of life-threatening ventricular arrhythmias, such as VT or VF. IV amiodarone can also be used to terminate AF acutely. Even though ICDs now play a primary role in the chronic management of ventricular arrhythmias, amiodarone is still used in patients who refuse or are not candidates for these devices. Also, amiodarone (with a β-blocker) can also be used as adjunctive therapy in these patients if frequent ICD discharges occur (Connolly, et al, 2006).

Because of amiodarone's poor oral bioavailability, large volume of distribution, and long half-life, its onset of action may not be apparent for several months. To achieve efficacy more quickly, loading doses of oral amiodarone must be initially used to saturate the myocardial stores. Once the patient is appropriately loaded with oral amiodarone, the dose should be reduced to the recommended maintenance dose to minimize the incidence of adverse events.

Because of its extremely large volume of distribution and high lipophilicity, amiodarone has the potential to accumulate and cause adverse effects in numerous organs with chronic use, with the lungs, thyroid, eyes, heart, liver, skin, GI tract, and CNS being most notably affected. Unlike other amiodarone-induced adverse effects, pulmonary toxicity can be life-threatening. Definitive diagnosis of amiodarone-induced pulmonary toxicity is difficult, since many of the subjective and objective findings are nonspecific. Patients may present with cough, dyspnea, or fever. The chest radiograph may reveal diffuse infiltrates, and pulmonary function tests may demonstrate a reduction in the diffusion capacity. If pulmonary toxicity is detected, amiodarone should be immediately discontinued. Corticosteroids may be needed to treat the pulmonary inflammation. To screen for pulmonary toxicity in patients receiving amiodarone, pulmonary function tests and a chest radiograph should be obtained at baseline. Subsequently, a chest radiograph should be obtained on an annual basis, while pulmonary function tests can be repeated if symptoms develop (Goldschlager, et al., 2007).

Because it contains approximately 38% iodine by weight, amiodarone may also cause thyroid abnormalities that can manifest as either hypothyroidism or hyperthyroidism. Hypothyroidism is the more common form of amiodarone-induced thyroid dysfunction. Although patients often report increased lethargy, the diagnosis of amiodarone-induced hypothyroidism is made upon detection of elevated levels of thyroid-stimulating hormone (TSH). Patients developing amiodarone-induced hypothyroidism can usually be treated with thyroid hormone supplementation (i.e., levothyroxine). The diagnosis of amiodarone-induced hyperthyroidism should be suspected if patients present with new or recurrent arrhythmias. Patients developing hyperthyroidism have abnormally low TSH levels and can usually be treated with antithyroid medications (i.e., methimazole, propylthiouracil). To screen for thyroid dysfunction in patients receiving amiodarone, thyroid function tests should be performed at baseline and then at 6-month intervals throughout therapy (Goldschlager, et al., 2007).

Ocular complications induced by amiodarone often manifest as corneal and lens opacities. Amiodarone-induced corneal microdeposits occur in virtually every patient. Although these opacities rarely produce visual disturbances, photophobia, halos, and blurred vision have been reported. Because of their relatively benign nature, these opacities do not require routine monitoring or discontinuation of amiodarone when they develop. Chronic amiodarone therapy has also been associated with optic neuritis and optic neuropathy. Since these ocular disturbances are vision-threatening, amiodarone must be discontinued once the diagnosis is confirmed. To screen for these complications, ophthalmologic examinations should be performed at baseline only if patients have significant visual abnormalities and then later only if symptoms develop (Goldschlager, et al., 2007).

GI adverse effects are relatively common and occur most frequently when amiodarone-loading doses are administered. Typically, patients report nausea, vomiting, loss of appetite, and abdominal pain. Constipation can also occur during long-term therapy. These GI disturbances can be minimized by dividing the total daily dose and by taking the drug with food. Liver function test abnormalities can also develop. Although elevations in aspartate aminotransferase and alanine aminotransferase levels are relatively common with amiodarone therapy, only rarely do patients develop clinical hepatitis. Liver enzyme levels usually return to baseline following reduction of the amiodarone dose or discontinuation of the drug. To screen for these hepatic abnormalities, liver function tests should be performed at baseline and then every 6 months throughout therapy (Goldschlager, et al., 2007).

Although laboratory tests cannot detect amiodarone-induced cardiovascular, neurologic, and dermatologic toxicities, patients should still be clinically evaluated on a routine basis. Compared with other AADs, amiodarone produces fewer cardiovascular adverse effects. The bradycardia and heart block that can develop merely represent an accentuation of amiodarone's pharmacologic and electrophysiologic properties. Additionally, even though amiodarone markedly prolongs the QT interval, TdP is rare. Neurologic toxicities associated with amiodarone occur frequently and may include tremors, ataxia, peripheral neuropathy, fatigue, and insomnia. The most common dermatologic reactions observed during amiodarone therapy are photosensitivity and a blue-gray skin discoloration. Photosensitivity reactions can range from extremely tanned areas to sunburned areas with erythema and edema. Blue-gray skin discoloration, which often appears on the patient's face and hands, may be related to the cumulative dose and duration of therapy. To prevent these dermatologic toxicities, patients receiving amiodarone should use opaque sunscreens such as zinc oxide while outdoors.

Patients receiving amiodarone also need to be monitored for drug interactions. Amiodarone is a substrate of the CYP3A4 isoenzyme, a potent inhibitor of the CYP3A4, 2C9, and 2D6 isoenzymes and an inhibitor of P-glycoprotein. Amiodarone significantly interacts with digoxin and warfarin, which are commonly used in patients with AF. Amiodarone potentiates the anticoagulant effects of warfarin, which results in an increased international normalized ratio (INR) and an increased risk of bleeding (Sanoski & Bauman, 2002). When amiodarone and warfarin are initiated concurrently or when warfarin is initiated in a patient already receiving amiodarone, warfarin should be started at a dose of 2.5 mg daily. When amiodarone is initiated in a patient already receiving warfarin, the warfarin dose should be empirically reduced by approximately 30% (Sanoski & Bauman, 2002). Amiodarone can also double serum digoxin concentrations. Therefore, the digoxin dose should be empirically reduced by 50% when amiodarone is initiated.

Dronedarone

Dronedarone is the first AAD in nearly a decade to be approved for the treatment of AF and atrial flutter. Like amiodarone, dronedarone is primarily considered a class III AAD, but it exhibits electrophysiological properties of all four Vaughan Williams classes. Although structurally related to amiodarone, dronedarone's structure has been modified through the addition of a methylsulfonyl group and the removal of iodine. The lack of iodine in dronedarone's structure confers several potential benefits, including less toxic effects on the thyroid and less lipophilicity, which make the drug much less likely to accumulate in tissues and to subsequently cause various organ toxicities. Dronedarone also has a considerably shorter half-life (24 hours) when compared with amiodarone (greater than 50 days), which allows for steady state to be achieved in 5 to 7 days without the need for loading doses.

Dronedarone was shown to be more effective than placebo in maintaining SR in patients with AF or atrial flutter in the European Trial in Atrial Fibrillation or Flutter Patients Receiving Dronedarone for the Maintenance of Sinus Rhythm (EURIDIS) and the American-Australian-African Trial with Dronedarone in Atrial Fibrillation or Flutter Patients for the Maintenance of Sinus Rhythm (ADONIS) (Singh, et al., 2007). In another trial (a placebo-controlled, double-blind, parallel arm trial to assess the efficacy of dronedarone 400 mg bid for the prevention of cardiovascular hospitalization or death from any cause in patients with AF/atrial flutter [ATHENA]), the use of dronedarone was associated with a significant reduction in the incidence of hospitalization due to cardiovascular events or death in patients with AF (Hohnloser, et al., 2009). The Antiarrhythmic Trial with Dronedarone in Moderate to Severe CHF Evaluating Morbidity Decrease (ANDROMEDA) evaluated the efficacy and safety of dronedarone in patients with New York Heart Association (NYHA) class III or IV HF and an LVEF of 35% or less. This trial was terminated prematurely after significantly more patients in the dronedarone group died (primarily because of worsening HF) compared with the placebo group (Køber, et al., 2008). Based on the results of this particular trial, dronedarone is contraindicated in and has received a black box warning for patients with advanced HF (NYHA class IV or NYHA class II or III with a recent hospitalization for decompensated HF).

Like amiodarone, dronedarone is a substrate of the CYP3A isoenzyme and a moderate inhibitor of the CYP3A and CYP2D6 isoenzymes. Because of the potential for significantly increasing dronedarone concentrations, concomitant use of potent CYP3A inhibitors (i.e., ketoconazole, itraconazole, voriconazole, cyclosporine, clarithromycin, nefazodone, and ritonavir) or inducers (e.g., rifampin, phenobarbital, phenytoin, carbamazepine, and St. John's wort) should be avoided. No significant interaction has been observed when dronedarone is used with warfarin. Dronedarone also inhibits P-glycoprotein and has been shown to significantly increase serum digoxin concentrations by about 2.5-fold. Therefore, when concomitantly using dronedarone with digoxin, the digoxin dose should be empirically reduced by 50%.

Unlike amiodarone, dronedarone is not associated with extensive organ toxicities. Dronedarone has been associated with diarrhea, nausea, vomiting, and increased serum creatinine concentrations. Dronedarone is believed to increase serum creatinine by inhibiting tubular secretion without having an adverse effect on glomerular filtration. Although a prolonged QT interval can occur with dronedarone, TdP is rare.

Sotalol

Sotalol is a class III AAD that also has nonselective β-blocking properties. Sotalol blocks the rapid component of the delayed rectifier potassium current, which prolongs atrial and ventricular refractoriness. Sotalol exhibits reverse-use dependence, whereby its action potential-prolonging effects are lessened at higher heart rates and increased at lower heart rates. Sotalol increases the QT interval by prolonging ventricular repolarization and may give rise to TdP. The QT interval prolongation with sotalol is a dose-dependent effect. The QT interval should be closely monitored during treatment. Sotalol should be discontinued if the QT interval exceeds 550 msec. The practitioner should avoid combining sotalol with other drugs that increase the QT interval.

Because sotalol is eliminated primarily by the kidneys, the initial dose must be based on the patient's creatinine clearance. The practitioner should routinely monitor the patient's renal function throughout therapy to determine if any dosing adjustments are necessary. Sotalol should not be used to treat AF if the patient's creatinine clearance is less than 40 mL/min. The practitioner should also routinely monitor electrolytes, especially if the patient is concomitantly receiving diuretics, since hypokalemia and hypomagnesemia can increase the risk of TdP. Because of concern about TdP when initiating therapy with sotalol, patients must be hospitalized and placed on telemetry for at least 3 days.

Most of the adverse effects associated with sotalol can be attributed to its β-blocking activity (e.g., bradycardia, fatigue, dyspnea). The β-blocking effect of sotalol may decrease cardiac contractility, so this drug should be avoided in patients with LVSD.

Sotalol is effective for the treatment of supraventricular and ventricular arrhythmias. Although sotalol is not effective for conversion of AF, it is an effective agent for maintaining SR in patients with AF (Roy, et al., 2000). In patients with an ICD, sotalol has also been shown to significantly reduce arrhythmia recurrence and discharge from the ICD (Pacifico, et al., 1999).

Dofetilide

Dofetilide acts as a selective potassium channel blocker, affecting the rapid component of the delayed rectifier potassium current. This results in a prolonged action potential and QT interval. Dofetilide affects the atria more than the ventricles. It also exhibits reverse-use dependence.

Dofetilide appears to be a pure class III AAD, with few to no hemodynamic effects. This AAD has no negative inotropic effects. Therefore, like amiodarone, dofetilide is also safe to use in patients with LVSD (Køber, et al., 2000).

Dofetilide is approved for the conversion of AF or atrial flutter to SR and for the maintenance of SR in patients with AF or atrial flutter of greater than 1 week's duration who have been converted to SR. In the Symptomatic Atrial Fibrillation Investigative Research on Dofetilide (SAFIRE-D) trial, approximately 6%, 10%, and 30% of patients receiving 125, 250, and 500 mcg of dofetilide, respectively, converted to SR. At 1 year, slightly more than 50% of patients in the group taking 500 mcg of dofetilide remained in SR (Singh, et al., 2000).

As with other AADs, the main concern with dofetilide is the dose-dependent onset of TdP and other ventricular arrhythmias. Other adverse events associated with dofetilide include headache and dizziness.

Dofetilide has a number of important drug interactions. The concomitant use of cimetidine, ketoconazole, hydrochlorothiazide, megestrol, prochlorperazine, trimethoprim–sulfamethoxazole, or verapamil with dofetilide is contraindicated since these drugs can significantly increase plasma concentrations of dofetilide. Drugs that prolong the QT interval should not be used concomitantly with dofetilide because of the increased risk of a prolonged QT interval and TdP. Since dofetilide is metabolized to a small extent by the CYP3A4 isoenzyme, drugs that are inhibitors of this isoenzyme should be used cautiously with dofetilide because they can increase dofetilide concentrations. Examples of such inhibitors include macrolide antibiotics, azole antifungals, protease inhibitors, selective serotonin reuptake inhibitors, diltiazem, grapefruit juice, nefazodone, and zafirlukast. Caution should also be exercised when using dofetilide with metformin.

The recommended dosage of dofetilide in patients with a creatinine clearance of greater than 60 mL/min is 500 mcg twice daily. The dosage of dofetilide should be decreased in patients with renal dysfunction (creatinine clearance of less than 60 mL/min). The drug should not be given to patients with a creatinine clearance of less than 20 mL/min or a QT interval greater than 440 msec at baseline. Because of concerns over TdP, the manufacturer recommends that patients be started on dofetilide in a setting where creatinine clearance testing, ECG monitoring, and cardiac resuscitation are available consistently for 3 days. Therefore, this agent is available only to facilities and prescribers who have undergone appropriate dosing and initiation training.

Ibutilide

Ibutilide is structurally related to L-sotalol, but it has no β-blocking activity. It prolongs the action potential by increasing the slow inward sodium current and blocking the rapid component of the delayed rectifier potassium current. Electrophysiologic studies have demonstrated increases in atrial and ventricular effective refractory periods and suppression of induction of arrhythmias with ibutilide (Buchanan, et al., 1993). Ibutilide is available only in IV form. It is indicated only for the acute termination of AF or atrial flutter.

Ibutilide restores SR in approximately 50% of patients with AF or atrial flutter. However, it is more effective for restoring SR in patients with atrial flutter than in those with AF (Stambler, et al., 1996; Volgman, et al., 1998). Ibutilide also appears to be effective for facilitating direct-current cardioversion (DCC) of AF (Oral, et al., 1999). The major adverse effect associated with ibutilide is TdP. Patients with LVSD or electrolyte abnormalities (e.g., hypokalemia or hypomagnesemia) are especially at risk for developing proarrhythmia with ibutilide.

Class IV Antiarrhythmic Drugs

The class IV AADs, verapamil (Calan) and diltiazem (Cardizem), are nondihydropyridine CCBs used to treat supraventricular arrhythmias, usually of reentry origin. These arrhythmias include PSVT, AF, and atrial flutter. These drugs slow conduction, prolong refractoriness, and decrease automaticity in the SA and AV nodes. In AF or atrial flutter, these drugs slow conduction through the AV node and thereby slow the ventricular rate. Their cardiac effects are vascular relaxation, a negative inotropic effect, and a negative chronotropic effect. Verapamil has more potent negative inotropic effects than diltiazem.

The primary action of these drugs is to inhibit the inward movement of calcium through calcium channels located in cell membranes. The AV node depends on the influx of calcium through voltage-dependent calcium channels or "slow" channels; therefore, supraventricular tachycardias are sensitive to treatment with nondihydropyridine CCBs. Although these drugs rarely affect normal sinus node function, they may produce sinus arrest or sinus block in patients with SA nodal disease. Use of verapamil or diltiazem in these patients may lead to severe hypotension, bradycardia, or asystole. These drugs also should not be used in patients with an accessory pathway or WPW syndrome because they can shorten the refractory period of the accessory pathway and subsequently increase the ventricular rate, which may lead to VF. (See **Table 23.1.**)

Because of their potent negative inotropic effects, both verapamil and diltiazem should be avoided in patients with LVSD because they are likely to precipitate worsening HF symptoms. The practitioner should use caution when using IV verapamil because significant hypotension can occur (Phillips, et al., 1997). It is recommended that IV verapamil be slowly administered over at least 2 minutes to minimize the risk of hypotension; its use in the elderly may require an even slower rate of administration. Bradycardia, heart block, headache, flushing, dizziness, and peripheral edema are the most common adverse effects of diltiazem and verapamil. Verapamil can also cause constipation. The practitioner should be cautious when administering these agents concomitantly with β-blockers, digoxin, or clonidine because of the increased risk of bradycardia and heart block. Since diltiazem and verapamil are substrates and inhibitors of the CYP3A4 isoenzyme, the practitioner should use caution when concomitantly administering either of these drugs with other agents that are also metabolized by this isoenzyme.

Other Antiarrhythmic Agents

Several other AADs are commonly used to treat abnormal cardiac impulse formation or conduction. Digoxin, adenosine, and atropine are used in the treatment of various cardiac arrhythmias. (See **Table 23.1.**)

Digoxin

Digoxin is a digitalis glycoside whose predominant antiarrhythmic effect is on the AV node of the conduction system. It can be used for ventricular rate control in AF and as a positive inotrope in chronic HF. Digoxin affects the autonomic nervous system by stimulating the parasympathetic division, which increases vagal tone. This vagal effect slows conduction through the AV node and prolongs the AV nodal refractory period. An increased

PR interval, a downward-sloping ST-segment depression, and a shortened QT interval are seen on the ECG.

Digoxin is commonly used to slow electrical impulse conduction through the AV node, thus slowing the ventricular rate in supraventricular arrhythmias such as AF or atrial flutter. Digoxin is not effective for converting AF or atrial flutter to SR. Although digoxin is frequently used to control the ventricular rate in patients with LVSD and concomitant AF or atrial flutter, its use tends to be limited by its relatively slow onset of action and its inability to control heart rate during exercise. Even after an appropriate loading dose is administered, digoxin's peak onset of effect is delayed for up to 6 to 8 hours. Achievement of steady-state concentrations may take up to a week in patients with normal renal function, or even longer in patients with renal dysfunction. The increased sympathetic tone generated during exercise tends to offset the vagal effects of digoxin, which limits its efficacy under these conditions. In patients with LVSD and concomitant AF or atrial flutter, digoxin can provide effective ventricular rate control without increasing the risk of worsening HF symptoms because of its additional positive inotropic effects.

Digoxin toxicity can be precipitated by declining renal function, electrolyte disturbances, and drug interactions. Because digoxin is primarily excreted unchanged by the kidneys, a decline in the creatinine clearance can predispose a patient to digoxin toxicity. Hypokalemia, hypomagnesemia, and hypercalcemia can also predispose the myocardium to the toxic effects of digoxin. Concomitant drug therapy with agents such as amiodarone, dronedarone, or verapamil can also increase serum digoxin concentrations. Potential signs and symptoms of digoxin toxicity include heart block, AV junctional tachycardia, ventricular arrhythmias, visual disturbances (e.g., blurred vision, yellow/green halos), dizziness, weakness, nausea, vomiting, diarrhea, and anorexia. Digoxin toxicity can essentially precipitate the development of virtually any type of supraventricular or ventricular arrhythmia. Digoxin has a narrow therapeutic index. The therapeutic range for digoxin in patients with AF and normal LV systolic function (LVEF >40%) is 0.8 to 2 ng/mL. Because of the potential risk of increased mortality with higher serum concentrations, the therapeutic range for digoxin in patients with AF and concomitant LVSD (LVEF of 40% or less) is 0.5 to 1 ng/mL.

Adenosine

Adenosine is an AAD used for converting PSVT to SR. It activates potassium channels and by increasing the outward potassium current, hyperpolarizes the membrane potential, decreasing spontaneous SA nodal depolarization. Adenosine may also decrease the inward calcium current by blocking adenylate cyclase, which normally increases the inward calcium current. Automaticity (phase 4) and conduction (phase 0) are inhibited in the SA and AV nodes. The most common adverse effects of adenosine include chest discomfort, dyspnea, flushing, and headache. Sinus arrest can also occur. However, because of adenosine's short half-life of 10 seconds, these adverse effects are short-lived. Adenosine is administered IV because of its short half-life.

Atropine

Atropine sulfate is a parasympatholytic drug that enhances both sinus nodal automaticity and AV nodal conduction through direct vagolytic action. Atropine blocks acetylcholine at parasympathetic neuroeffector sites. Atropine is used almost exclusively in the monitored clinical setting for the treatment of symptomatic bradycardia.

Patients who do not experience signs or symptoms of hemodynamic compromise, ischemia, or frequent ventricular ectopy do not require atropine in bradycardic events. Atropine has been reported to be harmful in some patients with AV block at the His-Purkinje level (type II AV block and third-degree AV block with a new wide QRS complex). Atropine can be used in these situations, but the practitioner must monitor the patient closely for paradoxical slowing of the heart rate.

Atropine may induce tachycardia, which may result in poor outcomes in patients with myocardial ischemia or an MI. Therefore, atropine should be used cautiously in these patients.

Selecting the Most Appropriate Agent

Determining the cause and type of the arrhythmia is essential to selecting the most appropriate drug therapy. **Figures 23-1** to **23-5,** as well as **Table 23.1,** guide the practitioner in the initial assessment of which drug to use for each patient. The practitioner should know how to manage arrhythmias in cardiovascular and cardiopulmonary conditions in which the patient is not in cardiovascular compromise or collapse. These arrhythmias could lead to life-threatening arrhythmias and cardiac arrest. This discussion presents the initial approach to arrhythmias that, unless identified and treated, may deteriorate to cardiac arrest. These arrhythmias can be categorized as serious, nonlethal arrhythmias that are either "too fast" or "too slow."

The first main question to ask when selecting drug therapy is whether the slow or fast rate of the arrhythmia makes the patient ill or symptomatic. A symptomatic patient is one with an arrhythmia characterized by low blood pressure, shock, chest pain, shortness of breath, decreased level of consciousness, pulmonary congestion, HF, or acute MI. The practitioner should not make clinical decisions or take clinical actions based only on the monitor display. For instance, AF may be a stable rhythm from a hemodynamic perspective and may not need immediate treatment. However, treatment of a new onset AF, even though the patient's heart rate is not too slow or too fast, is important. Treatment of various arrhythmias is discussed in the first-line and second-line therapy sections. **Table 23.2** consolidates the various treatment regimens.

Second, the practitioner must think of treatable conditions that might be causing the arrhythmia. Laboratory values and history are important to assess whenever patients present with arrhythmias. Some possible causes of arrhythmias are electrolyte imbalances (i.e., hypokalemia, hypomagnesemia), drug overdose/toxicity, drug interactions, renal failure, thyroid disorders (i.e., hypothyroidism, hyperthyroidism), metabolic acidosis, hypovolemia, MI, pulmonary embolism, cardiac tamponade, tension pneumothorax, dissecting aortic aneurysm, hypoxemia related to pulmonary disorders, fever, or structural

defects in the heart itself. The practitioner may have to correct the cause of the arrhythmia before initiating drug therapy, especially if the patient is asymptomatic. However, time may be a critical factor when treating symptomatic arrhythmias.

Initial vagal maneuvers may serve both a diagnostic and therapeutic purpose. For example, carotid sinus massage may make the flutter waves in atrial flutter more apparent. Appearance of flutter waves allows the practitioner to differentiate atrial flutter from AF, PSVT, or other tachycardias. Vagal maneuvers may include some of the following: unilateral carotid sinus massage, breath holding, facial immersion in ice water, coughing, nasogastric tube placement, gag reflex stimulation by tongue blade or fingers, eyeball pressure, squatting, digital sweep of the anus, and bearing down during a bowel movement. Many patients who have recurrent PSVT with disorders such as mitral valve prolapse learn how to do these maneuvers and terminate the arrhythmia themselves. It is important to note that eyeball massage should never be taught, encouraged, or performed because it may cause retinal detachment. Carotid massage (firm massage of the carotid sinus that never lasts for more than 5 to 10 seconds) should be performed only with continuous ECG monitoring and an IV line in place. The procedure should be avoided in elderly patients and should not be performed on patients with carotid bruits because it may occlude already impaired circulation to the brain. Likewise, the practitioner should avoid ice water facial immersion in patients with ischemic heart disease.

Atrial Fibrillation/Atrial Flutter

AF and atrial flutter may be stable or unstable. If the patient has hemodynamic instability (severe hypotension, syncope, HF, or angina), immediate DCC is indicated. When the patient is hemodynamically stable, the practitioner should consider acute conditions that might cause the AF or atrial flutter that may be reversible. Such conditions include acute MI, hypoxia, pulmonary embolism, electrolyte imbalance (i.e., hypokalemia, hypomagnesemia), drug toxicity (especially digoxin or sympathomimetic agents), thyrotoxicosis, and alcohol intoxication. Since new-onset AF can be due to acute MI, the practitioner should look for ischemic changes on the 12-lead ECG. If acute ischemic changes appear, admission of the patient to the hospital in a monitored bed may be needed. Obviously, correction and treatment of acute causes of AF or atrial flutter should be a priority.

If untreated, AF and atrial flutter can lead to serious hemodynamic and thromboembolic consequences. A rapid ventricular rate can induce angina in patients with ischemic heart disease or worsening signs and symptoms of HF in patients with LVSD. A persistently rapid ventricular rate may lead to the development of a tachycardia-induced cardiomyopathy. Loss of synchronized atrial contraction can lead to a significant reduction in cardiac output, which can especially affect patients with underlying HF. In addition, loss of coordinated atrial contraction can lead to the pooling of blood and subsequent thrombus formation. Therefore, these arrhythmias can lead to serious thromboembolic complications, particularly ischemic stroke. Overall, the treatment goals for AF and atrial flutter are controlling the

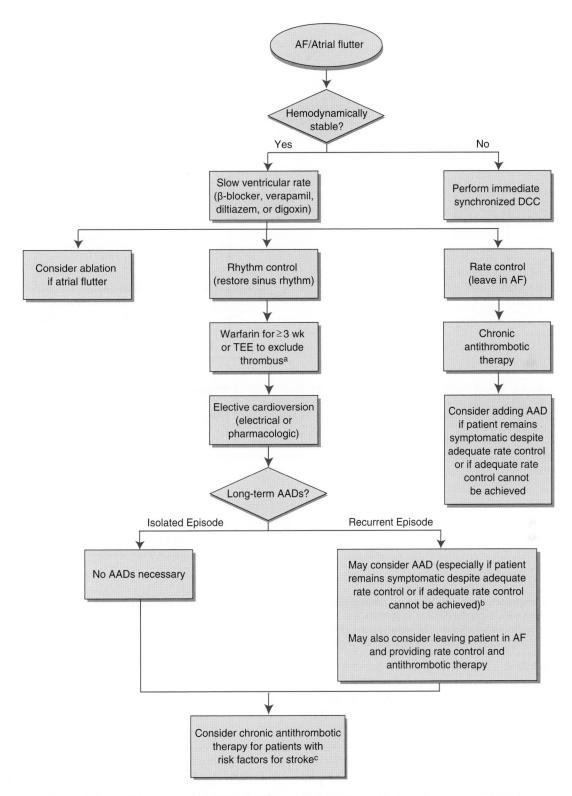

AAD, antiarrhythmic drug; AF, atrial fibrillation; DCC, direct current cardioversion; TEE, transesophageal echocardiogram
[a] If AF <48 h, anticoagulation prior to cardioversion is unnecessary; may consider TEE if patient has risk factors for stroke.
[b] Radiofrequency ablation may be considered for patients who fail or do not tolerate ≥1 AAD.
[c] Chronic antithrombotic therapy should be considered in all patients with AF and risk factors for stroke regardless of whether they remain in sinus rhythm.

FIGURE 23–1   Treatment algorithm for atrial fibrillation and atrial flutter.

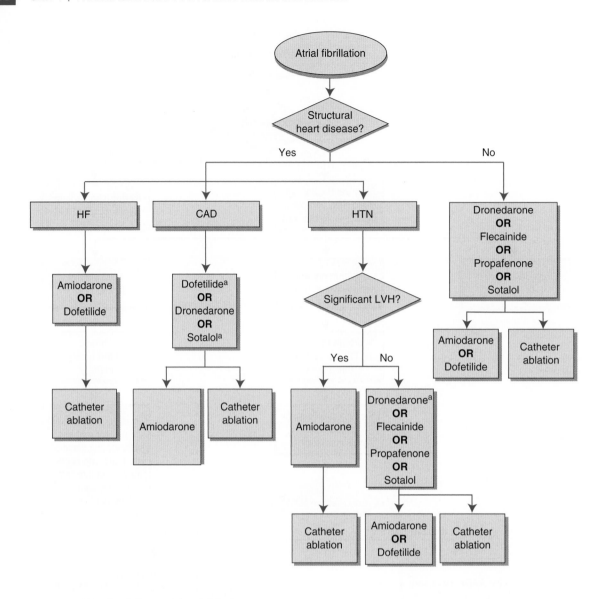

Within each of the boxes, the drugs are listed alphabetically and not in order of suggested use. However, the sequence of the boxes does imply the order of suggested use.

CAD, coronary artery disease; HF, heart failure; HTN, hypertension; LVH, left ventricular hypertrophy

[a]Should only be used if patient has normal left ventricular systolic function.

FIGURE 23–2   Treatment algorithm for selecting antiarrhythmic drug therapy for maintenance of sinus rhythm in patients with recurrent paroxysmal or persistent atrial fibrillation. (Adapted from Wann, L. S., Curtis, A. B., January, C. T., et al. [2011]. 2011 ACCF/AHA/HRS focused update on the management of patients with atrial fibrillation [updating the 2006 guidelines]: A report of the American College of Cardiology Foundation/American Heart Association Task Force on Practice Guidelines. *Circulation, 123,* 104–123.)

ventricular rate, preventing thromboembolic events, and possibly restoring and maintaining SR. **Figure 23-1** illustrates an algorithm for the management of AF and atrial flutter.

First-Line Therapy

If the patient is hemodynamically unstable (i.e., severe hypotension, syncope, HF, or angina), immediate DCC is first-line therapy. If the patient is hemodynamically stable and has a rapid ventricular rate, the first priority is to control the

ventricular rate. In the acute treatment of AF, the selection of a drug to control the ventricular rate depends on the patient's LV systolic function (Fuster, et al., 2006). In patients with normal LV systolic function (LVEF >40%), IV diltiazem, verapamil, β-blockers, or digoxin can be used. Of these options, IV diltiazem, verapamil, or a β-blocker is usually preferred because of digoxin's relatively slow onset of action. β-blockers are especially useful in high adrenergic states (i.e., postoperative patients, hyperthyroidism). The use of digoxin is limited by its

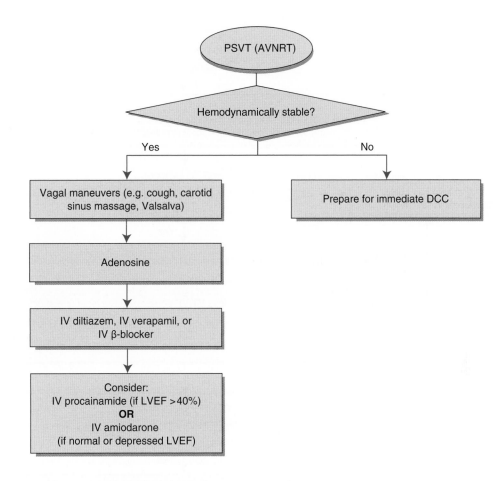

AVNRT, atrioventricular nodal reentrant tachycardia; DCC, direct current cardiversion; IV, intravenous; LVEF, left ventricular ejection fraction; PSVT, paroxysmal supraventricular tachycardia

FIGURE 23–3   Treatment algorithm for paroxysmal supraventricular tachycardia (due to atrioventricular nodal reentrant tachycardia). (Adapted from 2010 American Heart Association guidelines for cardiopulmonary resuscitation and emergency cardiovascular care. [2010]. *Circulation, 122*[Suppl 3], S729–S767.)

relatively slow onset of action and its inability to control heart rate in high adrenergic states (i.e., exercise). In patients with LVSD (LVEF of 40% or less), IV diltiazem or verapamil should be avoided because their potent negative inotropic effects may precipitate worsening HF symptoms. IV β-blockers should be used with caution in these patients and avoided in patients who are exhibiting signs and/or symptoms of decompensated HF. In those patients who are having worsening HF symptoms, IV digoxin or IV amiodarone is recommended as first-line therapy for controlling the ventricular rate. IV amiodarone can also be used in patients who are refractory to or have contraindications to β-blockers, diltiazem, verapamil, and digoxin. Since amiodarone is a class III AAD, the practitioner should be aware that the patient may convert to SR when using this agent. Patients with AF that has persisted for longer than 48 hours are at risk for thromboembolic events if conversion to SR occurs in the absence of therapeutic anticoagulation. Therefore, in these patients who have not been therapeutically anticoagulated, IV amiodarone should be avoided.

Second-Line Therapy

Once the ventricular rate is acutely controlled, patients should be evaluated for the possibility of restoring SR if AF persists. The results of six landmark clinical trials (Pharmacological Intervention in Atrial Fibrillation [PIAF], Rate Control versus Electrical Cardioversion for Persistent Atrial Fibrillation [RACE], Atrial Fibrillation Follow-up Investigation of Rhythm Management [AFFIRM], Strategies of Treatment of Atrial Fibrillation [STAF], How to Treat Chronic Atrial Fibrillation [HOT-CAFE], and Atrial Fibrillation and Congestive Heart Failure [AF-CHF]) have provided practitioners with significant insight into the comparative efficacy of rate control (controlling ventricular rate; patient remains in AF) and rhythm control (restoring and maintaining SR) treatment strategies in patients with AF (Hohnloser, et al., 2000; Van Gelder, et al., 2002; AFFIRM Investigators, 2002; Carlsson, et al., 2004; Opolski, et al., 2004; Roy, et al., 2008). The results of all of these trials essentially demonstrated that there were no significant differences in outcomes between patients who

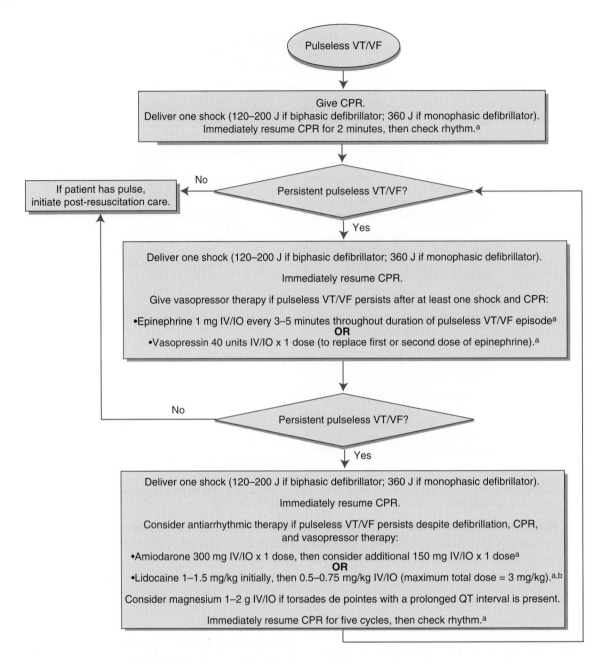

a If IV or IO access cannot be established, epinephrine, vasopressin, and lidocaine may be administered by the endotracheal route. Because of the potential risk of pulmonary toxicity, IV amiodarone should not be administered down an endotracheal tube.

b Lidocaine should be used if IV amiodarone is unavailable.

CPR = cardiopulmonary resuscitation; IO = intraosseous; IV = intravenous; J = joules; VF = ventricular fibrillation; VT = ventricular tachycardia;

FIGURE 23–4 Treatment algorithm for pulseless ventricular tachycardia/ventricular fibrillation. (Adapted from 2010 American Heart Association guidelines for cardiopulmonary resuscitation and emergency cardiovascular care. [2010]. *Circulation, 122*[Suppl 3], S729–S767.)

received a rate-control strategy and those who received a rhythm-control strategy. Therefore, based on these findings, a rate-control strategy appears to be a viable alternative to a rhythm-control strategy in patients with persistent or recurrent AF. Consequently, considering the potential toxicities of

AADs, it is reasonable to initially consider a rate-control strategy in these patients, including those with concomitant HF. However, a rhythm-control strategy should be considered for those patients who remain symptomatic despite having adequate ventricular rate control or for those in whom adequate

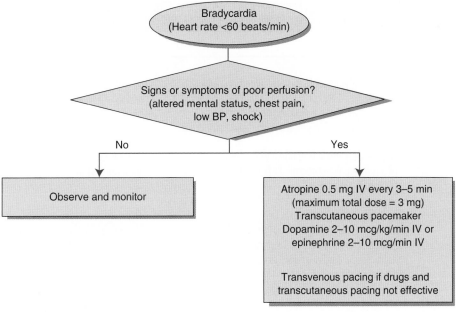

BP, blood pressure; IV, intravenous

FIGURE 23–5   Treatment algorithm for bradycardia. (Adapted from 2010 American Heart Association guidelines for cardiopulmonary resuscitation and emergency cardiovascular care. [2010]. *Circulation, 122*[Suppl 3], S729–S767.)

ventricular rate control cannot be achieved. The results of the above clinical trials do not necessarily apply to patients experiencing their first episode of AF. If these particular patients are likely to convert to and remain in SR, a rhythm-control strategy may be considered.

If the decision is made to restore SR in hemodynamically stable patients with AF, either electrical (i.e., DCC) or pharmacologic (i.e., AADs) cardioversion may be used. The decision to use either of these methods is often based on the practitioner's or patient's preference. DCC is associated with higher success rates than pharmacologic cardioversion. However, this method requires sedation or anesthesia and may be rarely associated with complications such as sinus arrest or ventricular arrhythmias. Pharmacologic cardioversion is associated with adverse effects (e.g., TdP) and drug interactions.

In those patients in whom it is decided to restore SR, it is important to note that the process of cardioverting the patient from AF to SR may place the patient at risk for a thromboembolic event. Restoration to SR may dislodge thrombi in the atria. This risk is present regardless of whether an electrical or pharmacologic method is used. In patients undergoing DCC or pharmacological cardioversion, it is imperative to determine how long the patient has been in AF because the risk of thrombus formation increases if the duration of AF exceeds 48 hours. If AF has been present for more than 48 hours or for an unknown duration, cardioversion should not be performed acutely because of the risk of thromboembolism. These patients should be therapeutically anticoagulated with warfarin (target INR 2.5; range 2.0 to 3.0) for at least 3 weeks. After that time,

the patient can then undergo DCC or pharmacologic cardioversion, which should be followed by at least another 4 weeks of therapeutic anticoagulation with warfarin. Patients with risk factors for thromboembolism should continue on warfarin for longer than 4 weeks unless it is definitive that they remain in SR. If the 3 weeks of therapeutic warfarin therapy prior to cardioversion is not feasible, there is an alternative regimen in which the patient undergoes a transesophageal echocardiogram (TEE) prior to cardioversion. If no thrombus is observed on TEE, the patient can undergo cardioversion. In these patients, anticoagulation therapy required at the time of cardioversion includes IV unfractionated heparin or having received at least 5 days of warfarin therapy (INR target range 2.0 to 3.0) at the time of cardioversion. If cardioversion is successful, therapeutic warfarin (INR target range 2.0 to 3.0) should be continued for at least 4 weeks. Again, patients with risk factors for thromboembolism should continue on warfarin therapy for longer than 4 weeks unless it is definitive that they remain in SR. If a thrombus is seen on TEE, cardioversion should not be performed, and the patient should be anticoagulated indefinitely. If cardioversion is considered in these patients at a later time, a TEE should again be performed (Singer, et al., 2008).

When the duration of AF is definitively known to be less than 48 hours, a prolonged period of anticoagulation is not necessary prior to proceeding with electrical or pharmacological cardioversion because the risk of thromboembolism is deemed to be low. In these patients, IV unfractionated heparin or a low-molecular-weight heparin (subcutaneously at treatment doses) should be initiated before cardioversion. Alternatively,

TABLE 23.2   Recommended Order of Treatment for Arrhythmias

Order	Agents	Comments
Atrial Fibrillation/Atrial Flutter		
First line	Hemodynamically unstable patient: synchronized DCC. Start with 100 J and proceed to 200, 300, and 360 J if not successful in the preceding cardioversions. Hemodynamically stable patient with rapid ventricular rate: • Normal LV systolic function (LVEF >40%): IV diltiazem, IV verapamil, IV β-blocker, or IV digoxin • LV systolic dysfunction (LVEF ≤40%): IV digoxin or IV amiodarone	Start with 50 J in patients with atrial flutter. Premedicate whenever possible when performing DCC. Avoid the use of IV amiodarone for rate control in patients with LV dysfunction if the AF/atrial flutter has been present >48 h as these patients may be at risk for thromboembolic events induced by conversion to sinus rhythm.
Second line	Patients with 1st episode of arrhythmia (if likely to convert to and remain in sinus rhythm): Electrical or pharmacologic cardioversion can be considered once ventricular rate acutely controlled. Decision of whether to proceed acutely with cardioversion depends on the duration of the arrhythmia: • <48 hrs: May proceed with cardioversion without anticoagulation. IV unfractionated heparin or a low-molecular-weight heparin (subcutaneously at treatment doses) should be initiated before cardioversion. In those patients with risk factors for thromboembolism, a TEE-guided approach can be considered. Those patients with risk factors for thromboembolism should be considered for at least 4 weeks of post-cardioversion anticoagulation therapy. For pharmacologic cardioversion, the AAD used depends on the presence of SHD. • >48 h or unknown duration: Anticoagulate with warfarin (target INR 2.5; range 2–3) for at least 3 weeks before proceeding with cardioversion. Anticoagulate with warfarin (target INR 2.5; range 2–3) for at least 4 wk following cardioversion. Patients with risk factors for thromboembolism should be continued on warfarin or dabigatran for longer than 4 weeks unless it is definitive that they remain in sinus rhythm. For patients with persistent or recurrent AF, a strategy of ventricular rate control and anticoagulation is a reasonable alternative to rhythm control. Selection of PO drug for ventricular rate control (diltiazem, verapamil, β-blocker, or digoxin) depends on patient's LV function. Warfarin therapy should be maintained at target INR of 2.5 (range 2–3).	A TEE can be performed in patients with AF (>48 h or unknown duration) to exclude the presence of thrombi and to facilitate cardioversion. IV heparin should be started in these patients. If a thrombus is detected, cardioversion should not be performed and the patient should be anticoagulated with warfarin (target INR 2.5; range 2–3) or dabigatran indefinitely. If no thrombus is detected, cardioversion can be performed within 24 h without the need for the initial 3-wk period of anticoagulation. These patients will still require anticoagulation after cardioversion for at least 4 wk. Patients with risk factors for thromboembolism should be continued on warfarin or dabigatran therapy for longer than 4 wk unless it is definitive that they remain in sinus rhythm. For AADs to be used for acute pharmacologic cardioversion, see Figure 22–2. Goal heart rate is based on patient's LV systolic function: • LVEF >40% and no or acceptable symptoms of AF: <110 beats/min (at rest) • LVEF ≤40%: <80 beats/min (at rest) PO agents for ventricular rate control: • Normal LV systolic function (LVEF >40%): diltiazem, verapamil, or β-blockers • LV systolic dysfunction (LVEF ≤40%): β-blockers or digoxin
Third line	Chronic AAD therapy can be considered for patients who remain symptomatic despite having adequate ventricular rate control or for those in whom adequate ventricular rate control cannot be achieved. The AAD used depends on patient's LV function and the type of SHD that may be present. For patients with permanent AF, a strategy of ventricular rate control and anticoagulation should be considered.	PO AADs for chronic rhythm control: • No SHD: dronedarone, flecainide, propafenone, sotalol, amiodarone, or dofetilide • LV systolic dysfunction (LVEF ≤40%): amiodarone or dofetilide • Coronary artery disease: dofetilide, dronedarone, sotalol, or amiodarone

TABLE 23.2	Recommended Order of Treatment for Arrhythmias (*Continued*)

Order	Agents	Comments
	Selection of PO drug for ventricular rate control (diltiazem, verapamil, β-blocker, or digoxin) depends on patient's LV function. Warfarin therapy should be maintained at a target INR of 2.5 (range 2–3). Radiofrequency catheter ablation may be considered in patients with symptomatic episodes of recurrent AF who fail or do not tolerate at least one class I or class III AAD.	• Significant LV hypertrophy: amiodarone Avoid flecainide and propafenone in patients with *any* form of SHD.

Paroxysmal Supraventricular Tachycardia (due to AVNRT)

Order	Agents	Comments
First line	Hemodynamically unstable patient: synchronized DCC (50–100 J, biphasic). Hemodynamically stable patient: vagal maneuvers	Premedicate whenever possible when performing DCC. Examples of vagal maneuvers include unilateral carotid sinus massage, Valsalva maneuver, facial immersion in ice water, and coughing. Carotid sinus massage should be avoided in patients with carotid bruits or history of cerebrovascular disease.
Second line	IV adenosine If persistent PSVT, use IV diltiazem, IV verapamil, or IV β-blockers; if PSVT remains persistent, can use IV procainamide (if LVEF >40%) or IV amiodarone (for normal or depressed LVEF)	
Third line	If patient continues to have frequent episodes of PSVT or infrequent episodes accompanied by severe symptoms, refer for possible radiofrequency catheter ablation. If patient is not a candidate for or refuses radiofrequency catheter ablation, PO diltiazem, verapamil, β-blocker, or digoxin can be used for chronic therapy.	If PSVT is infrequent and/or accompanied by only mild symptoms, no chronic therapy is needed.

Premature Ventricular Contractions

Order	Agents	Comments
First line	No SHD: • Asymptomatic or minimal symptoms: No drug therapy • Symptomatic: PO β-blocker SHD: • Asymptomatic or minimal symptoms: PO β-blocker (especially patients who are post-MI or those with LV systolic dysfunction [LVEF ≤40%]) • Symptomatic: PO β-blocker	Patients who are post-MI or with LV systolic dysfunction (LVEF ≤40%) should receive a β-blocker even if they have no or minimal symptoms associated with the PVCs to reduce mortality associated with these disease states.

Nonsustained Ventricular Tachycardia

Order	Agents	Comments
First line	No SHD: • Asymptomatic or minimal symptoms: No drug therapy • Symptomatic: PO β-blocker Post-MI patients: • Normal LV systolic function (LVEF >35%): PO β-blocker regardless of the presence of symptoms • LV systolic dysfunction (LVEF ≤35%): EP testing; if sustained VT/VF, ICD should be placed (once >40 days post-MI); if sustained VT/VF noninducible, PO β-blocker or amiodarone may be used.	Correct reversible causes. Post-MI patients with normal LV systolic function should receive a β-blocker even if they have no or minimal symptoms associated with the NSVT to reduce mortality associated with the MI. If frequent shocks occur in patients with an ICD, PO amiodarone and β-blocker combination therapy or sotalol monotherapy can be used.

(continued)

TABLE 23.2	Recommended Order of Treatment for Arrhythmias (*Continued*)	
Order	**Agents**	**Comments**
Sustained Ventricular Tachycardia		
First line	Hemodynamically unstable patient: synchronized DCC (100 J, biphasic). Hemodynamically stable patient: IV procainamide, IV amiodarone, or IV sotalol	Premedicate whenever possible when performing DCC. Correct reversible causes.
Second line	Hemodynamically stable patient: IV lidocaine; synchronized DCC should be considered if AAD therapy fails. Once arrhythmia acutely terminated, patient should be considered for ICD placement. If patient refuses or is not a candidate for an ICD, PO amiodarone can be considered.	If frequent shocks occur in patients with an ICD, PO amiodarone and β-blocker combination therapy or sotalol monotherapy can be used.
Pulseless Ventricular Tachycardia/Ventricular Fibrillation		
First line	Start CPR, establish an airway, and deliver one shock (biphasic defibrillator: 120–200 J; monophasic defibrillator: 360 J); immediately resume CPR for 2 min, then check rhythm.	Correct reversible causes.
Second line	If patient remains in pulseless VT/VF, deliver one shock and then immediately resume CPR; if pulseless VT/VF persists after at least one shock and CPR, give vasopressor therapy (epinephrine 1 mg IV push/IO every 3–5 min through pulseless VT/VF episode or vasopressin 40 units IV push/IO [to replace first or second dose of epinephrine]) (give drugs during CPR; do not interrupt CPR to give drugs); immediately resume CPR for 2 min, then check pulse.	
Third line	If patient remains in pulseless VT/VF, deliver one shock and then immediately resume CPR; if pulseless VT/VF persists despite defibrillation, CPR and vasopressor therapy, consider AAD therapy (IV amiodarone; lidocaine may be used if IV amiodarone unavailable) (give drugs during CPR; do not interrupt CPR to give drugs); consider IV magnesium sulfate if torsades de pointes present; immediately resume CPR for 2 min, then check pulse.	
Bradycardia		
First line	Patient with stable bradycardia: Close observation Patients with bradycardia and signs/symptoms of poor perfusion (e.g., altered mental status, chest pain, hypotension, shock): Immediately administer IV atropine (0.5 mg every 3 to 5 min, up to 3 mg total dose. If the atropine is ineffective, transcutaneous pacing or sympathomimetic continuous infusion (dopamine or epinephrine) should be initiated.	Correct reversible causes.
Second line	If drug therapy and transcutaneous pacing are ineffective, transvenous pacing should be utilized.	

AV, atrioventricular; CPR, cardiopulmonary resuscitation; DCC, direct current cardioversion; ICD, implantable cardioverter-defibrillator; INR, International Normalized Ratio; IV, intravenous; J, joules; LV, left ventricular; LVEF, left ventricular ejection fraction; MI, myocardial infarction; NSVT, nonsustained ventricular tachycardia; PO, oral; PSVT, paroxysmal supraventricular tachycardia; PVC, premature ventricular contraction; TEE, transesophageal echocardiogram; VF, ventricular fibrillation; VT, ventricular tachycardia

in those patients with risk factors for thromboembolism, a TEE-guided approach (see above) can be considered. Those patients with risk factors for thromboembolism should also be considered for at least 4 weeks of post-cardioversion anticoagulation therapy (Singer, et al., 2008).

If the practitioner decides to proceed with pharmacologic cardioversion as the initial therapy, the selection of drug should be based on the patient's LV systolic function. Pharmacologic cardioversion is most effective when initiated within 7 days of the onset of AF. The AADs with proven efficacy during this time frame include dofetilide, flecainide, ibutilide, propafenone, or amiodarone (oral or IV). The class Ia AADs, disopyramide, procainamide, and quinidine have limited efficacy or have been incompletely studied for this purpose. Sotalol is not effective for converting AF to SR. Although the use of single, oral loading doses of propafenone or flecainide is effective in restoring SR, these drugs should only be used in patients without underlying SHD. Ibutilide may also be considered in these patients. A patient's ventricular rate should be adequately controlled with AV nodal-blocking drugs prior to administering a class Ic (or class Ia) AAD for cardioversion. In patients with SHD, propafenone, flecainide, and ibutilide should be avoided because of the increased risk of proarrhythmia. Instead, amiodarone or dofetilide should be primarily used in this patient population. In patients with AF present for more than 7 days, the only AADs with proven efficacy are dofetilide, amiodarone (oral or IV), and ibutilide. The selection of AAD therapy during this time frame should again be based on the presence of SHD (Fuster, et al., 2006).

If the practitioner does not wish to proceed with cardioversion, an initial management strategy of ventricular rate control and anticoagulation is also reasonable. As previously stated, this strategy, whereby the patient is left in AF, has been shown to be an acceptable alternative to rhythm control for the chronic management of AF. The selection of an oral drug for chronic ventricular rate control is primarily based on the patient's LV systolic function. In patients with normal LV systolic function (LVEF >40%), an oral β-blocker, diltiazem, or verapamil is preferred over digoxin (Fuster, et al., 2006). Digoxin can be added if adequate ventricular rate control cannot be achieved with one of these drugs. In patients with LVSD (LVEF of 40% or less), an oral β-blocker or digoxin is preferred because these drugs can also concomitantly be used to treat chronic HF. The nondihydropyridine CCBs should be avoided in patients with LVSD because of their potent negative inotropic effects. In patients with AF and stable HF symptoms (NYHA class II or III), the β-blockers carvedilol, metoprolol succinate, or bisoprolol should be used as first-line therapy because of their documented survival benefits in patients with HF (CIBIS II Investigators and Committees, 1999; MERIT-HF Study Group, 1999; Packer, et al., 1996). Other β-blockers should be avoided in these patients because their effects on survival in HF are unknown. Digoxin should be used as first-line therapy in patients with AF and decompensated HF (NYHA class IV) because β-blocker therapy may exacerbate HF symptoms. For patients with normal or depressed

LV systolic function, oral amiodarone may also be considered if adequate ventricular rate control cannot be achieved with the use of β-blockers, nondihydropyridine CCBs, and/or digoxin (Fuster, et al., 2006). In patients with persistent AF who have no or acceptable symptoms and stable LV systolic function (LVEF greater than 40%), the goal heart rate should be less than 110 beats/minute at rest (Van Gelder, et al., 2010; Wann, et al., 2011). In patients with LVSD (LVEF of 40% or less), a stricter heart rate goal (less than 80 beats/minute) should be considered to minimize the potential harmful effects of a rapid heart rate response on ventricular function (Wann, et al., 2011).

Assessing the patient's risk of stroke becomes important for selecting the most appropriate antithrombotic regimen. The CHADS2 index is recommended for stroke risk stratification in patients with AF (Singer, et al., 2008). With this risk index, patients with AF are given 2 points if they have a history of a previous stroke or transient ischemic attack and one point each for being at least 75 years old, having hypertension, having diabetes, or having congestive HF (CHADS2 is an acronym for each of these risk factors). The points are added up, and the total score is then used to determine the most appropriate antithrombotic therapy for the patient. Patients with a CHADS2 score of at least 2 are considered to be at high risk for stroke and should receive warfarin (target INR: 2.5; range: 2.0 to 3.0). Patients with a CHADS2 score of 1 are considered to be at intermediate risk for stroke and should receive either warfarin (target INR: 2.5; range: 2.0 to 3.0) or aspirin 75–325 mg/d. However, because of its superior efficacy in preventing stroke, the use of warfarin is suggested over that of aspirin in this particular group of patients. Patients with a CHADS2 score of 0 are considered to be at low risk for stroke and should receive aspirin 75–325 mg/d. Dabigatran, an oral direct thrombin inhibitor, can also be considered as an alternative to warfarin for stroke prevention in patients with paroxysmal or persistent AF and risk factors for stroke or systemic embolism (Wann, et al., 2011). Patients with prosthetic heart valves, hemodynamically significant valvular disease, a creatinine clearance less than 15 mL/minute, or advanced liver disease are not appropriate candidates for dabigatran therapy. Please refer to Chapter 54 for a further discussion of anticoagulation in AF.

Antithrombotic therapy should be considered for all patients regardless of whether a rate-control or rhythm-control strategy is initiated. In addition, antithrombotic therapy should be continued if SR is restored because of the potential for patients to have episodes of recurrent AF.

Third-Line Therapy

For those patients who remain symptomatic despite having adequate ventricular rate control or for those patients in whom adequate ventricular rate control cannot be achieved, it is reasonable to consider AAD therapy to maintain SR once they have been converted to SR. The selection of an AAD to maintain SR is primarily based on the presence of SHD (Wann, et al., 2011). (See **Figure 23-2.**) In patients without SHD, any oral class Ia, Ic, or III AAD can be used to maintain SR.

However, dronedarone, flecainide, propafenone, or sotalol should be considered as initial therapy in these patients because of their less toxic adverse effect profiles. Amiodarone or dofetilide can be used as alternative therapy if the patient fails or does not tolerate one of these initial AADs. In patients with any type of SHD, the class Ic AADs flecainide and propafenone should be avoided. In these patients, the selection of AAD therapy is based upon the type of SHD present. In patients with LVSD (LVEF of 40% or less), either oral amiodarone or dofetilide can be used. Both dronedarone and sotalol should be avoided in patients with LVSD because of the risk of increased mortality (dronedarone) or worsening HF (sotalol). In patients with coronary artery disease, sotalol, dofetilide, or drone-darone can be used as initial therapy. In these patients, sotalol and dronedarone should only be used if their LV systolic function is normal. Amiodarone can be considered as an alternative therapy in these patients if these AADs are not tolerated. In patients with significant LV hypertrophy, amiodarone is the drug of choice.

For patients with permanent AF, a treatment strategy of ventricular rate control and anticoagulation should be used because the efficacy of AADs is extremely poor in this population. The oral drugs used for ventricular rate control are discussed in the "Second-Line Therapy" section. Patients with symptomatic episodes of recurrent AF who fail or do not tolerate at least one class I or III AAD may also be considered for radiofrequency catheter ablation (Calkins, et al., 2007).

Paroxysmal Supraventricular Tachycardia (Due to Atrioventricular Nodal Reentrant Tachycardia)

First-Line Therapy

Hemodynamically unstable PSVT requires first-line therapy of synchronized DCC to restore SR and correct hemodynamic compromise. Unless contraindicated, patients with mild to moderate symptoms can be initially managed with vagal maneuvers (e.g., unilateral carotid sinus massage, Valsalva maneuver, facial immersion in ice water, and coughing). **Figure 23-3** illustrates an algorithm for the management of PSVT due to AV nodal reentrant tachycardia.

Second-Line Therapy

If vagal maneuvers are unsuccessful or if PSVT recurs after successful vagal maneuvers, second-line therapy is AADs. The drug of choice for PSVT is adenosine (American Heart Association, 2010). Clinical studies have shown that adenosine is as effective as IV verapamil in initial conversion of PSVT. Adenosine does not produce hypotension to the degree that verapamil does, and it has a shorter half-life. If a total of 30 mg of adenosine does not successfully terminate PSVT, further doses of this agent are unlikely to be effective. Therefore, in patients with persistent PSVT, other AADs will need to be used. In these patients, IV diltiazem, verapamil, or a β-blocker can be used. If PSVT continues despite these treatment measures, the use of IV procainamide (LVEF >40%) or amiodarone (normal or depressed LVEF) can also be considered.

Third-Line Therapy

Third-line therapy focuses on the management of chronic PSVT. Chronic preventive therapy is usually necessary if the patient has either frequent episodes of PSVT that require therapeutic intervention or infrequent episodes of PSVT that are accompanied by severe symptoms. Radiofrequency catheter ablation is considered first-line therapy for most of these patients because of its effectiveness in preventing recurrence of PSVT and its relatively low complication rate. Drug therapy with oral diltiazem, verapamil, β-blockers, or digoxin can also be considered if the patient is not a candidate for or refuses to undergo radio-frequency catheter ablation.

Premature Ventricular Contractions

Occasional PVCs occur in most people and rarely compromise cardiac output or function. Correcting reversible causes such as an electrolyte imbalance sometimes eliminates these benign PVCs. Asymptomatic or minimally symptomatic PVCs in patients without associated heart disease carry little or no risk. PVCs in patients with heart disease were traditionally treated in the past. Decreasing the number and frequency of PVCs was thought to diminish the risk of sudden cardiac death. However, the results of the CAST showed that the use of AADs to suppress asymptomatic PVCs in patients after MI may increase mortality rates (CAST Investigators, 1989). Therefore, if patients with SHD have symptomatic PVCs, drug therapy should be limited to β-blockers. These agents have been associated with a reduction in mortality and sudden cardiac death in post-MI patients. These agents are also effective for suppressing symptomatic PVCs in patients without SHD. Asymptomatic PVCs do not require treatment.

Nonsustained Ventricular Tachycardia

Ventricular tachycardia that spontaneously terminates within 30 seconds is known as nonsustained VT. Given the poor survival of patients who experience cardiac arrest, it is essential to identify the most effective treatment strategies to prevent the initial episode of sustained VT or sudden cardiac death from occurring.

The presence of nonsustained VT in patients without SHD is not associated with an increased risk of sudden cardiac death. Therefore, drug therapy is not necessary in these patients if they are asymptomatic. However, if these patients do become symptomatic, β-blocker therapy can be initiated. Post-MI patients (especially those with LVSD) who develop nonsustained VT are at increased risk for sudden cardiac death. For these patients, the selection of therapy is based on the patient's LV systolic function. In post-MI patients with an LVEF greater than 35%, drug therapy is not necessary to treat the arrhythmia if they are asymptomatic. However, these patients should still chronically receive a β-blocker specifically to reduce mortality associated with the MI. β-blockers are also effective if these patients develop significant symptoms associated with the nonsustained VT. In post-MI patients with an LVEF of 35% or less, electrophysiologic testing is often performed when asymptomatic nonsustained VT occurs (Moss, et al., 1996; Buxton, et al., 1999). If sustained VT or VF is induced, an ICD is then recommended (Epstein, et al., 2008). In these patients, implantation of the ICD should be delayed until more than 40 days have elapsed since the MI occurred. If sustained VT or VF is not induced, a β-blocker or amiodarone can be initiated.

Sustained Ventricular Tachycardia

VT that persists for at least 30 seconds or that requires electrical or pharmacologic termination because of hemodynamic instability is known as sustained VT. Since sustained VT can degenerate into VF, the treatment goals are to terminate the VT acutely and then prevent recurrence of the arrhythmia.

First-Line Therapy

If the patient is hemodynamically unstable (i.e., severe hypotension, syncope, HF, or angina), immediate synchronized DCC is first-line therapy. If the patient is hemodynamically stable, IV amiodarone, IV procainamide, or IV sotalol can be considered (American Heart Association, 2010). Lidocaine can be used as alternative therapy. Synchronized DCC should be considered if AAD therapy fails.

Second-Line Therapy

Once the acute episode is terminated, measures should be taken to prevent recurrent episodes of VT. Based on the results of several trials, ICDs are clearly indicated as first-line therapy in patients with a history of sustained VT or VF (AVID Investigators, 1997; Connolly, et al., 2000; Kuck, et al., 2000, Epstein, et al., 2008). If the patient with an ICD experiences frequent discharges because of recurrent ventricular arrhythmias or new-onset supraventricular arrhythmias (e.g., AF), either amiodarone and a β-blocker or sotalol monotherapy can be used. For the patient who refuses or is not a candidate for an ICD, oral amiodarone should be used as an alternative therapy.

Pulseless Ventricular Tachycardia/ Ventricular Fibrillation

The majority of cases of sudden cardiac death can be attributed to VF. Sustained VT usually precedes VF and most commonly occurs in patients with ischemic heart disease. VF is usually not preceded by any symptoms and always results in a loss of consciousness and eventually death if not treated. Immediate treatment is essential in patients who develop VF or pulseless VT, since survival is reduced by 10% for every minute that the patient remains in the arrhythmia. It is imperative to identify and correct any potential reversible causes for the arrhythmia.

For administration of drug therapy during an episode of pulseless VT/VF, while IV access is preferred, the guidelines recommend the intraosseous (IO) route as an alternative if IV access cannot be established (American Heart Association, 2010). IO access can be used not only for administration of drugs and fluids, but also for obtaining blood for laboratory monitoring. If neither IV nor IO access can be established, the endotracheal route can then be used for the administration of only certain agents (i.e., atropine, lidocaine, epinephrine, and vasopressin). **Figure 23-4** illustrates an algorithm for the management of pulseless VT/VF.

First-Line Therapy

In patients with pulseless VT/VF, high-quality cardiopulmonary resuscitation (CPR) should be immediately initiated until a defibrillator or automated external defibrillator (AED) arrives (American Heart Association, 2010). High-quality CPR is considered to be delivery of at least 100 compressions per minute, with the depth of chest compressions being at least 2 inches. Each cycle of CPR involves delivering 30 chest compressions followed by two breaths. If a defibrillator or AED is not readily available, hands-only CPR (compressions only; no ventilations) should be provided if the bystander possesses no CPR training or is trained but lacks confidence in providing effective CPR with rescue breaths. If the bystander possesses CPR training and is confident in their ability to provide effective CPR with rescue breaths, conventional cycles of CPR (30 chest compressions followed by two breaths) should be delivered until a defibrillator or AED becomes available. Once an advanced airway (e.g., endotracheal tube) is placed, chest compressions should be delivered continuously at a rate of 100 compressions per minute without pausing for ventilation (should be provided by a separate individual at a rate of one breath every 6 to 8 seconds). Once a defibrillator or AED arrives, defibrillation should be administered immediately.

With regard to defibrillation, delivery of only one shock at a time is recommended in patients with pulseless VT/VF to minimize interruptions in chest compressions (American Heart Association, 2010). For biphasic defibrillators, the dose of the shock is device-specific (usually 120 to 200 J); the maximum dose available can be used for the initial shock if the effective dose range of the defibrillator is unknown. This dose or a higher dose can then be used for any subsequent shocks that may be needed. After delivery of the initial shock in patients with pulseless VT/VF, CPR should be immediately resumed and continued for 2 minutes, after which the patient's pulse and rhythm should be checked. Delaying pulse and rhythm checks until after this period of CPR is administered is intended to minimize interruptions in chest compressions and increase the potential for success with defibrillation. If pulseless VT/VF persists, another shock should be delivered at the appropriate dose, followed by 2 minutes of CPR. This general sequence of resuscitation and defibrillation should be followed for as long as the patient remains in pulseless VT/VF.

Second-Line Therapy

If pulseless VT/VF persists after delivery of at least one shock and CPR, vasopressor therapy with either epinephrine or vasopressin should be initiated (American Heart Association, 2010). One dose of vasopressin may be given to replace either the first or second dose of epinephrine. Vasopressin's half-life of approximately 10 to 20 minutes is considerably longer than the 3- to 5-minute half-life of epinephrine, which suggests that its vasopressor effects may be more sustained than those of epinephrine during cardiac arrest. Unlike epinephrine, vasopressin also maintains its vasoconstrictive effects under acidotic and hypoxic conditions, which suggests that this agent may continue to work during prolonged cardiac arrest situations. The recommended dosage of epinephrine for pulseless VT/VF is 1 mg given IV push/IO every 3 to 5 minutes throughout the duration of the pulseless VT/VF episode. The recommended dosage of vasopressin for pulseless VT/VF is 40 units IV push/IO for one dose only.

Third-Line Therapy

If pulseless VT/VF persists despite the use of defibrillation, CPR, and vasopressor therapy, AAD therapy can be considered. IV amiodarone is recommended as first-line AAD therapy for the treatment of pulseless VT/VF (American Heart Association, 2010). This agent has been shown to be safe and effective in the management of both in-hospital and out-of-hospital pulseless VT/VF (Dorian, et al., 2002; Kudenchuck, et al., 1999). Compared to lidocaine, IV amiodarone has been associated with a significantly higher rate of survival to hospital admission in patients with out-of-hospital cardiac arrest due to VF (Dorian, et al., 2002). Therefore, lidocaine should only be considered for the treatment of pulseless VT/VF if IV amiodarone is not available (American Heart Association, 2010). IV procainamide is no longer recommended for pulseless VT/VF. IV magnesium sulfate can be considered if TdP is present or suspected.

If the patient is resuscitated from the pulseless VT/VF episode, measures should be taken to prevent recurrent episodes of cardiac arrest. Based on the results of several trials, ICDs are clearly indicated as first-line therapy in patients with a history of sustained VT or VF (AVID Investigators, 1997; Connolly, et al., 2000; Kuck, et al., 2000; Epstein, et al., 2008). If patients with an ICD experience frequent discharges because of recurrent ventricular arrhythmias or new-onset supraventricular arrhythmias (e.g., AF), either amiodarone and a β-blocker or sotalol monotherapy can be used. For patients who refuse or are not candidates for an ICD, oral amiodarone should be used as an alternative therapy.

Bradycardia

If patients with bradycardia present with signs and symptoms of adequate perfusion, only close observation is required. If patients with bradycardia develop signs or symptoms of poor perfusion (e.g., altered mental status, chest pain, hypotension, shock), IV atropine (0.5 mg every 3 to 5 minutes, up to 3 mg total dose) should be immediately administered (American Heart Association, 2010). If atropine is not effective, either transcutaneous pacing or a continuous infusion of a sympathomimetic agent, such as dopamine (2 to 10 mcg/kg/min) or epinephrine (2 to 10 mcg/min) (i.e., dopamine or epinephrine) should be initiated. If symptomatic bradycardia persists despite any of these measures, transvenous pacing should be utilized. **Figure 23-5** illustrates an algorithm for the management of bradycardia.

Special Population Considerations

Pediatric

The epidemiology of arrhythmias is different between adults and children. Adults have arrhythmias primarily of a cardiac origin, whereas children have arrhythmias primarily of a respiratory origin.

Tachyarrhythmias occasionally compromise infants and young children. PSVT is the most common arrhythmia in young children. It typically occurs during infancy or in children with congenital heart disease. PSVT with ventricular rates exceeding 180 to 220 beats/minute can produce signs of shock. If signs of shock appear, synchronized cardioversion or administration of adenosine can be done in an emergency. Common causes of PSVT in young children and infants are congenital heart disease (preoperative) such as Ebstein's anomaly, transposition of the great arteries, or a single ventricle. Postoperative PSVT also can occur after atrial surgery for correction of congenital defects of the heart. Other common causes of PSVT in children are drugs such as sympathomimetics (cold medications, theophylline, β-agonists). WPW syndrome and hyperthyroidism also can cause PSVT. Common causes of AF and atrial flutter in children are intra-atrial surgery, Ebstein's anomaly, heart disease with dilated atria (aortic valve regurgitation), cardiomyopathy, WPW syndrome, sick sinus syndrome, and myocarditis.

Bradycardia is a common arrhythmia in seriously ill infants or children. It is usually associated with a fall in cardiac output and is an ominous sign, suggesting that cardiac arrest is imminent. The first-line therapy for this arrhythmia in infants and young children is administration of oxygen, support respiration, epinephrine and, possibly, atropine.

Pulseless VT and VF are treated much the same way as in adults; however, vasopressin is not currently recommended for children (American Heart Association, 2010). The recommended dose of epinephrine for a child with pulseless VT/VF is 0.01 mg/kg IV/IO, administered as 0.1 mL/kg of a 1:10,000 dilution. If IV/IO access cannot be established, epinephrine can be administered endotracheally (0.1 mg/kg administered as 0.1 mL/kg of a 1:1,000 dilution).

Geriatric

With aging, body fat increases, lean body tissue decreases, and hepatic and renal system changes set the stage for potential overdosage and toxicity, particularly in the case of AADs. Similarly, declining function affects the amount and dosage of the drug prescribed as well as the occurrence of adverse effects. Cardiac disease and chronic conditions such as HF exacerbate the decline in organ function. Together, these factors can increase the risk of an adverse effect from the AADs the practitioner prescribes.

For example, digoxin toxicity is relatively common in elderly patients who are not receiving a reduced dosage to accommodate for the reduced renal function. The practitioner must always assess the patient's baseline renal function (to identify abnormalities in the blood urea nitrogen and serum creatinine) and baseline hepatic function (to identify impairment in liver function). These two tests are important in prescribing the proper dosage of many of the AADs discussed in this chapter.

Signs and symptoms of adverse effects of many drugs are confusion, weakness, and lethargy. These signs and symptoms are often attributed to senility or disease. Therefore, it is important for the practitioner to take a thorough drug history and to document accurately the dosages and frequencies prescribed in the patient record. If the practitioner merely attributes confusion to old age, the patient may continue to receive the drug while actually experiencing drug toxicity. Furthermore, the practitioner may add another drug to treat the complications caused by the original AAD, compounding the issue of polypharmacy and excessive medication.

In elderly patients taking AADs, the practitioner must be particularly alert to adverse effects from diuretics, digoxin, sleeping aids, and nonprescription drugs.

AADs sometimes require accurate and timely dosing. If an elderly patient forgets to take a dose or cannot remember when he or she took the last dose, undermedication or overmedication may occur. This can be dangerous when AADs are prescribed. Many of the elderly have multiple prescriptions, even for the same medication, and therefore take an overdose of the drug. Consequently, it is essential to review medications with elderly patients and make sure they understand and can follow a safe drug therapy regimen.

MONITORING PATIENT RESPONSE

The goals of AAD therapy are to restore SR and prevent recurrences of the original arrhythmia or development of new arrhythmias. Evaluating the outcomes of AAD therapy requires the practitioner to schedule regular follow-up visits after initial treatment of the arrhythmia. The outcomes to be closely monitored include impulse generation and conduction from the SA node to the AV node, time interval for conduction, heart rate within a normal range that is age-specific, and patterns of AV and ventricular conduction.

Data to be monitored to evaluate therapeutic outcomes vary from the simple to complex. The patient may monitor some of them and needs to be taught the signs and symptoms to look for and the expectations from the therapeutic regimen. Patients with arrhythmias may be monitored on a regular or periodic basis with 12-lead ECG, 24-hour Holter monitors, electrophysiologic testing, monitoring of vital signs (blood pressure, pulse rate), echocardiograms for cardiac function, electrolytes, and serum drug levels.

In addition, the patient needs to self-monitor for symptoms such as lightheadedness, dizziness, syncopal episodes, palpitations, chest pain, shortness of breath, or weight gain. Other clinical outcomes to be monitored are those that affect quality of life, such as activity tolerance, organ perfusion, cognitive function, fear, anxiety, and depression.

PATIENT EDUCATION

Drug Information

Included in the therapeutic plan for arrhythmia is patient education. Learning outcomes can be evaluated by monitoring compliance with the medication regimen, recurrences of arrhythmia, adverse effects, weight gain, blood pressure, heart rate, and emergency department visits or hospitalizations.

AADs have narrow therapeutic windows. Toxicity is common at normal dosages. Consequently, patient education is essential for providing maximal benefits and avoiding adverse effects and accidental overdosing or underdosing.

The patient, family, and significant others should be taught the basics, such as the name of the drug (both the generic and trade name), the dose, the frequency and timing of the dose, and the reason the drug is needed. This may avoid duplicate prescribing and administration of AADs. The patient should communicate, either verbally or in writing, the names and dosages of these drugs to all other health care providers and should wear a medical identification device listing all medications. In addition, the patient should inform his or her health care provider when any new prescription, over-the-counter, or complementary or alternative medications are started so that potential drug interactions can be minimized or avoided.

The practitioner should provide written instructions for the medication regimen. Providing instructions in large print and simple language may be helpful to patients who have difficulty with memory, hearing, or vision. Instructions should include what to do when the patient misses a dose of medication, has an adverse response to the medication, or wants to stop taking the drug. If β-blockers are prescribed, the patient should be warned that abrupt discontinuation may result in rebound angina, an increased heart rate, and hypertension. The symptoms associated with these adverse effects also should be identified.

The practitioner can also teach the patient or caregiver how to take blood pressure and pulse readings, how to interpret the readings, and how to recognize and respond to signs and symptoms of hypotension, dizziness, chest pain, shortness of breath, peripheral edema, or palpitations. The patient should take his or her weight each day and call the practitioner if weight gain of over 2 pounds occurs. If the patient has difficulty learning these monitoring techniques or cannot perform them, he or she may need to schedule regular follow-up appointments for monitoring. Patients with AF or atrial flutter should know the signs and symptoms of a stroke.

In today's health care environment, the insurance plan's pharmacy provider sometimes makes substitutions with generics or less expensive brands of medications. To prevent harmful drug effects, the patient needs to be aware of this practice and should be cautioned not to change brands of the prescribed AAD or anticoagulant without the approval of the practitioner.

An important teaching point from an ethical and legal perspective is to warn the patient to avoid hazardous activities such as driving, using electrical tools, climbing ladders, or any activity that would put the patient or others in harm's way until the effects of the drug are demonstrated. Patients with an ICD should refrain from driving for at least 6 months after either implantation of the device or an appropriate discharge from the device for a ventricular arrhythmia. Documentation of patient teaching on risks, benefits, lifestyle modification, and safety issues with AAD treatment should always be entered in the patient's record. Documenting a review of this information on a follow-up visit aids health care providers who follow up on the patient's progress in the future.

Nutrition

Clear instructions should be given to avoid alcohol, excessive salt intake, and caffeine during treatment for arrhythmias. Many AADs may cause periods of hypotension resulting in dizziness, or the dose of the drug may need to be regulated, especially in the initial weeks.

Complementary and Alternative Medications

The practitioner must emphasize to the patient the importance of reporting the use of any of these agents so that interactions with AAD therapy can be minimized or avoided. While the information regarding potential interactions between AADs and specific complementary and alternative medications is relatively sparse, there are a few notable interactions of which practitioners should be aware. Patients taking AADs should avoid licorice root. Licorice has mineralocorticoid effects, which can promote hypokalemia. In patients taking digoxin, the presence of hypokalemia may predispose the patient to digoxin toxicity. In patients taking other AADs, the presence of hypokalemia may promote the development of atrial or ventricular arrhythmias. In addition, certain licorice preparations have been shown to cause a prolonged QT interval, which may be additive in patients receiving class Ia or III AADs. This interaction could lead to TdP. The use of Siberian ginseng or oleander should also be avoided in patients receiving digoxin, as digoxin toxicity may result. The use of St. John's wort may decrease digoxin concentrations; therefore, digoxin concentrations should be closely monitored when concomitant therapy is used. St. John's wort may also decrease plasma concentrations of amiodarone and dronedarone, which may predispose the patient to arrhythmia recurrence. Consequently, the use of St. John's wort in patients receiving amiodarone or dronedarone should be avoided. Patients with a history of atrial or ventricular arrhythmias should also be instructed to avoid the use of any medication containing ephedra (e.g., Ma Huang) because it can promote the development of arrhythmias.

BIBLIOGRAPHY

Starred references are cited in the text.

*2010 American Heart Association guidelines for cardiopulmonary resuscitation and emergency cardiovascular care science. (2010). *Circulation, 122*(Suppl 3), S1–S933.

*The Atrial Fibrillation Follow-up Investigation of Rhythm Management (AFFIRM) Investigators. (2002). A comparison of rate control and rhythm control in patients with atrial fibrillation. *New England Journal of Medicine, 347*, 1825–1833.

*Anderson, J. L., Lutz, J. R., & Allison, S. B. (1983). Electrophysiologic and antiarrhythmic effects of oral flecainide in patients with inducible ventricular tachycardia. *Journal of the American College of Cardiology, 2*, 105–114.

*Antiarrhythmics Versus Implantable Defibrillators (AVID) Investigators (1997). A comparison of antiarrhythmic-drug therapy with implantable defibrillators in patients resuscitated from near-fatal ventricular arrhythmias. *New England Journal of Medicine, 337*, 1576–1583.

*Bardy, G. H., Lee, K. L., Mark, D. B., et al. (2005). Amiodarone or an implantable cardioverter-defibrillator for congestive heart failure. *New England Journal of Medicine, 352*, 225–237.

*Buchanan, L. V., Turcotte, U. M., Kabell, G. G., & Gibson, J. K. (1993). Antiarrhythmic and electrophysiologic effects of ibutilide in a chronic canine model of atrial flutter. *Journal of Cardiovascular Pharmacology, 33*, 10–14.

*Buxton, A. E., Lee, K. L., Fisher, J. D., et al. (1999). A randomized study of the prevention of sudden death in patients with coronary artery disease. *New England Journal of Medicine, 341*, 1882–1890.

Cairns, J. A., Connolly, S. J., & Roberts, R. (1997). Randomized trial of outcome after myocardial infarction in patients with frequent or repetitive ventricular premature depolarizations: CAMIAT. *Lancet, 349*, 675–682.

*Calkins, H., Brugada, J., Packer, D.L., et al. (2007). HRS/EHRA/ECAS expert consensus statement on catheter and surgical ablation of atrial fibrillation: Recommendations for personnel, policy, and follow-up. *Heart Rhythm, 4*, 816–861.

*Cardiac Suppression Trial Investigators. (1989). Preliminary report: Effect of encainide and flecainide on mortality in a randomized trial of arrhythmia suppression after myocardial infarction. *New England Journal of Medicine, 321*, 406–412.

*Carlsson, J., Miketic, S., Windeler, J., et al. (2004). Randomized trial of rate-control versus rhythm-control in persistent atrial fibrillation: The Strategies of Treatment of Atrial Fibrillation (STAF) study. *Journal of the American College of Cardiology, 41*, 1690–1696.

*CIBIS II Investigators and Committees. (1999). The Cardiac Insufficiency Bisoprolol Study II (CIBIS-II): A randomised trial. *Lancet, 353*, 9–13.

*Connolly, S., Gent, M., Roberts, R. S., et al. (2000). Canadian Implantable Defibrillator Study (CIDS): A randomized trial of the implantable cardioverter defibrillator versus amiodarone. *Circulation, 101*, 1297–1302.

*Connolly, S. J., Dorian, P., Roberts, R. S., et al. (2006). Comparison of beta-blockers, amiodarone plus beta-blockers, or sotalol for prevention of shocks from implantable cardioverter defibrillators: The OPTIC study. *Journal of the American Medical Association, 295*, 165–171.

Dager, W. E., Sanoski, C. A., Wiggins, B. S., & Tisdale, J. E. (2006). Pharmacotherapy considerations in advanced cardiac life support. *Pharmacotherapy, 26*, 1703–1729.

*Dorian, P., Cass, D., Schwartz, B., et al. (2002). Amiodarone as compared with lidocaine for shock-resistant ventricular fibrillation. *New England Journal of Medicine, 346*, 884–890.

*Duff, H. J., Roden, D., & Primm, R. K. (1983). Mexiletine in the treatment of resistant ventricular arrhythmias: Enhancement of efficacy and reduction of dose-related side effects by combination with quinidine. *Circulation, 67*, 1124–1128.

*Epstein, A. E., DiMarco, J. P., Ellenbogen, K. A., et al. (2008). ACC/AHA/HRS 2008 guidelines for device-based therapy of cardiac rhythm abnormalities: A report of the American College of Cardiology/American Heart Association Task Force on Practice Guidelines (Writing Committee to Revise the ACC/AHA/NASPE 2002 Guideline Update for Implantation of Cardiac Pacemakers and Antiarrhythmia Devices). *Journal of the American College of Cardiology, 51*, e1–e62.

*Fuster, V., Rydén, L. E., Cannom, D. S., et al. (2006). ACC/AHA/ESC 2006 guidelines for the management of patients with atrial fibrillation: A report of the American College of Cardiology/American Heart Association Task Force on Practice Guidelines and the European Society of Cardiology Committee for Practice Guidelines (Writing Committee to Revise the 2001 Guidelines for the Management of Atrial Fibrillation). *Journal of the American College of Cardiology, 48*, e149–e246.

*Goldschlager, N., Epstein, A. E., Naccarelli, G., et al. (2007). A practical guide for clinicians who treat patients with amiodarone. *Heart Rhythm, 4*, 1250–1259.

*Hohnloser, S. H., Crijns, H. J., van Eickels, M., et al. (2009). Effect of dronedarone on cardiovascular events in atrial fibrillation. *New England Journal of Medicine, 360*, 668–678.

*Hohnloser, S. H., Kuck, K. H., & Lilienthal, J. (2000). Rhythm or rate control in atrial fibrillation—Pharmacological Intervention in Atrial Fibrillation (PIAF): A randomised trial. *Lancet, 356,* 1789–1794.

Julian, D. G., Camm, A. J., & Fragnin, G. (1997). Randomized trial of effect of amiodarone on mortality inpatients with left ventricular dysfunction after recent myocardial infarction: EMIAT. *Lancet, 349,* 667–674.

*Kennedy, H. L., Brooks, M. M., & Barker, A. H. (1994). Beta blocker therapy in the Cardiac Arrhythmia Suppression Trial. *American Journal of Cardiology, 74,* 674–680.

*Køber, L., Bloch-Thomsen, P. E., Møller, M., et al. (2000). Danish Investigations of Arrhythmia and Mortality on Dofetilide (DIAMOND) Study Group. Effect of dofetilide in patients with recent myocardial infarction and left-ventricular dysfunction: A randomised trial. *Lancet, 356,* 2052–2058.

*Køber, L., Torp-Pedersen, C., McMurray, J. J., et al. (2008). Increased mortality after dronedarone therapy for severe heart failure. *New England Journal of Medicine, 358,* 2678–2687.

*Kuck, K. H., Cappato, R., Siebels, J., et al. (2000). Randomized comparison of antiarrhythmic drug therapy with implantable defibrillators in patients resuscitated from cardiac arrest: The Cardiac Arrest Study Hamburg (CASH). *Circulation, 102,* 748–754.

*Kudenchuck, P. J., Cobb, L. A., Copass, M. K., et al. (1999). Amiodarone for resuscitation after out-of-hospital cardiac arrest due to ventricular fibrillation. *New England Journal of Medicine, 341,* 871–879.

*Lichstein, E., Morganroth, J., Harrist, R., & Hubble, M. S. (1983). Effect of propranolol on ventricular arrhythmia: The beta blocker heart attack trial experience. *Circulation, 67* (Suppl. I), 5–10.

*MERIT-HF Study Group (1999). Effect of metoprolol CR/XL in chronic heart failure: Metoprolol CR/XL Randomized Intervention Trial in Congestive Heart Failure (MERIT-HF). *Lancet, 353,* 2001–2007.

*Miller, M. R., McNamara, R. L., Segal, J. B., et al. (2000). Efficacy of agents for pharmacological conversion of atrial fibrillation and subsequent maintenance of sinus rhythm: A meta-analysis of clinical trials. *Journal of Family Practice, 49,* 1033–1046.

*Moss, A. J., Hall, W. J., Cannom, D. S., et al. (1996). Improved survival with an implanted defibrillator in patients with coronary disease at high risk for ventricular arrhythmia. *New England Journal of Medicine, 335,* 1933–1940.

*Moss, A. J., Zareba, W., Hall, W. J., et al. (2002). Prophylactic implantation of a defibrillator in patients with myocardial infarction and reduced ejection fraction. *New England Journal of Medicine, 346,* 877–883.

*Opolski, G., Torbicki, A., Kosior, D. A., et al. (2004). Rate control vs rhythm control in patients with nonvalvular persistent atrial fibrillation: The results of the Polish How to Treat Chronic Atrial Fibrillation (HOT CAFE) Study. *Chest, 126,* 476–486.

*Oral, H., Souza, J. J., Michaud, G. F., et al. (1999). Facilitating transthoracic cardioversion of atrial fibrillation with ibutilide pretreatment. *New England Journal of Medicine, 340,* 1849–1854.

*Pacifico, A., Hohnloser, S. H., Williams, J. H., et al. (1999). Prevention of implantable-defibrillator shocks by treatment with sotalol: Sotalol Implantable Cardioverter-Defibrillator Study Group. *New England Journal of Medicine, 340,* 1855–1862.

*Packer, M., Bristow, M. R., Cohn, J. N., et al. (1996). The effect of carvedilol on morbidity and mortality in patients with chronic heart failure. *New England Journal of Medicine, 334,* 1349–1355.

*Phillips, B. G., Gandhi, A. J., Sanoski, C. A., et al. (1997). Comparison of intravenous diltiazem and verapamil for the acute treatment of atrial fibrillation and flutter. *Pharmacotherapy, 17,* 1238–1245.

*Roy, D., Talajic, M., Dorian, P., et al. (2000). Amiodarone to prevent recurrence of atrial fibrillation. *New England Journal of Medicine, 342,* 913–920.

*Roy, D., Talajic, M., Nattel, S., et al. (2008). Rhythm control versus rate control for atrial fibrillation and heart failure. *New England Journal of Medicine, 358,* 2667–2677.

*Sanoski, C. A., & Bauman, J. L. (2002). Clinical observations with the amiodarone/warfarin interaction: Dosing relationships with long-term therapy. *Chest, 121,* 19–23.

*Singer, D. E., Albers, G. W., Dalen, J. E., et al. (2008). Antithrombotic therapy in atrial fibrillation: American College of Chest Physicians Evidence-Based Clinical Practice Guidelines (8th ed.). *Chest, 133,* 546S–592S.

*Singh, B. N., Connolly, S. J., Crijns, H. J., et al. (2007). Dronedarone for maintenance of sinus rhythm in atrial fibrillation or flutter. *New England Journal of Medicine, 357,* 987–999.

*Singh, S., Zoble, R. G., Yellen, L., et al. (2000). Efficacy and safety of oral dofetilide in converting to and maintaining sinus rhythm in patients with chronic atrial fibrillation or atrial flutter: The Symptomatic Atrial Fibrillation Investigative Research on Dofetilide (SAFIRE-D) Study. *Circulation, 102,* 2385–2390.

*Slavik, R. S., Tisdale, J. E., & Borzak, S. (2001). Pharmacological conversion of atrial fibrillation: A systematic review of available evidence. *Progress in Cardiovascular Diseases, 44,* 121–152.

*Stambler, B. S., Wood, M. A., Ellenbogen, K. A., et al. (1996). Efficacy and safety of repeated intravenous doses of ibutilide for rapid conversion of atrial flutter or fibrillation. *Circulation, 94,* 1613–1621.

Stroke Prevention in Atrial Fibrillation Investigators. (1991). Stroke prevention in atrial fibrillation study: Final report. *Circulation, 84,* 527–539.

*Teo, K. K., Yusuf, S., & Furberg, C. D. (1993). Effects of prophylactic antiarrhythmic drug therapy in acute myocardial infarction: An overview of results from randomized controlled trials. *Journal of the American Medical Association, 270,* 1589–1595.

*Van Gelder, I. C., Groenveld, H. F., Crijns H. J. G. M., et al. (2010). Lenient versus strict rate control in patients with atrial fibrillation. *New England Journal of Medicine, 362,* 1363–1373.

*Van Gelder, I. C., Hagens, V. E., Bosker, H. A., et al. (2002). The Rate Control Versus Electrical Cardioversion for Persistent Atrial Fibrillation Study Group. A comparison of rate control and rhythm control in patients with recurrent persistent atrial fibrillation. *New England Journal of Medicine, 347,* 1834–1840.

*Vaughan Williams, E. M. (1984). A classification of antiarrhythmic actions reassessed after a decade of new drugs. *Journal of Clinical Pharmacology, 24,* 129–147.

*Volgman, A. S., Winkel, E. M., Pinski, S. L., et al. (1998). Conversion efficacy and safety of intravenous ibutilide compared with intravenous procainamide in patients with atrial flutter or fibrillation. *Journal of the American College of Cardiology, 31,* 1414–1419.

*Vukmir, R. B., & Stein, K. L. (1991). Torsades de pointes therapy with phenytoin. *Annals of Emergency Medicine, 20,* 198–200.

*Wann, L. S., Curtis, A. B., Ellenbogen, K. A., et al. (2011). 2011 ACCF/AHA/HRS focused update on the management of patients with atrial fibrillation (update on dabigatran): A report of the American College of Cardiology Foundation/American Heart Association Task Force on Practice Guidelines. *Circulation, 123,* 1144–1150.

*Wann, L. S., Curtis, A. B., January, C. T., et al. (2011). 2011 ACCF/AHA/HRS focused update on the management of patients with atrial fibrillation (updating the 2006 guidelines): A report of the American College of Cardiology Foundation/American Heart Association Task Force on Practice Guidelines. *Circulation, 123,* 104–123.

*Wit, A. L., Rosen, M. R., & Hoffman, B. F. (1974). Electrophysiology and pharmacology of cardiac arrhythmias: Relationship of normal and abnormal electrical activity of cardiac fibers to the genesis of arrhythmias. *American Heart Journal, 88,* 664–670, 798–806.

*Wyse, D. G., Kellen, J., & Rademaker, A. W. (1988). Prophylactic versus selective lidocaine for early ventricular arrhythmias of myocardial infarction. *Journal of the American College of Cardiology, 12,* 507–513.

*Wyse, D. G., Waldo, A. L., DiMarco, J. P., et al. (2002). A comparison of rate control and rhythm control in patients with atrial fibrillation. *New England Journal of Medicine, 347,* 1825–1833.

Zipes, D. P., Camm, A. J., Borggrefe, M., et al. (2006). ACC/AHA/ESC 2006 guidelines for management of patients with ventricular arrhythmias and the prevention of sudden cardiac death: A report of the American College of Cardiology/American Heart Association Task Force and the European Society of Cardiology Committee for Practice Guidelines (Writing Committee to Develop Guidelines for Management of Patients with Ventricular Arrhythmias and the Prevention of Sudden Cardiac Death). *Journal of the American College of Cardiology, 48,* e247–e346.

Pharmacotherapy for Respiratory Disorders

Upper Respiratory Infections

Upper respiratory tract infections (URIs), including the common cold and sinusitis, are some of the most common problems seen in primary care. URIs are usually self-limiting, minor illnesses that account for half or more of all acute illnesses. It is difficult to differentiate the common cold from sinusitis or allergic rhinitis. (See Chapter 47.) URIs share common symptoms, such as nasal discharge, nasal congestion, tenderness over the sinuses, fever, headache, malaise, sore throat and myalgias, sneezing, a full feeling around the eyes and ears, and coughing. Symptoms may present individually or in combination, and it is difficult to determine whether the cause is viral or bacterial.

URIs can progress to acute or chronic complications. In children especially, URIs may progress to otitis media. In 5% to 10% of cases, the viral or bacterial cause may travel, causing sinusitis and bronchitis. There is an enormous economic burden associated with URIs.

COMMON COLD

Acute infectious rhinitis (coryza), or the common cold, is a viral URI. One of the most common infections, it is self-limiting. Coryza is an acute inflammation of the mucous membranes of the respiratory passages, particularly of the nose, sinuses, and throat, and is characterized by sneezing, rhinorrhea (watery nasal discharge), and coughing. The common cold has a short duration.

Approximately 100 million colds occur annually in the United States, resulting in approximately 26 million days off from school, 23 million absent days from work, 27 million visits to a primary care provider, and 250 million days of restricted activities. Nearly $1 billion is spent on cold remedies and $1.5 billion on analgesics. Adults average three colds per year. Children average six episodes per year, and the common cold is more common in children who attend day care or preschool (where they are in contact with other children and groups that may spread disease) than in those who spend more time at home and have less contact with crowds. Exposure to smoke is also a predisposing factor.

CAUSES

The pathogens most frequently associated with common colds are rhinovirus (30% to 40% of cases), especially during the

fall and spring, and coronavirus (10% to 15%), which is most prevalent during the winter. The respiratory syncytial virus, influenza virus, parainfluenza virus, and adenovirus are also responsible, but the rhinovirus is the single most pervasive cause of colds. The rhinovirus is a single-stranded ribonucleic acid virus that replicates well at 95°F (35°C) or below but poorly at 99 to 100°F (37.2 to 37.8°C), which is probably why it causes URIs and not pneumonia.

Predisposition to viral infections can be attributed to many factors, including frequent exposure to viral infectious agents; in children, the age of the child; and the inability to resist invading organisms because of allergies, malnutrition, immune deficiencies, physical abnormalities, or other comorbid conditions. Some experts propose a relationship between the host response to the virus and the production of cold symptoms. Studies show that common colds are more frequent or more severe in those under increased stress, probably as a result of stress weakening the immune system.

PATHOPHYSIOLOGY

If the protective barriers of the upper respiratory tract (i.e., cough, gag, and sneeze reflexes, lymph nodes, immunoglobulin [Ig] A antibodies, and rich vasculature) fail, viral pathogens trigger an acute inflammatory reaction with release of vasoactive mediators and increased parasympathetic stimuli. This produces congestion and rhinorrhea. Rhinoviruses grow in the upper airway, and attach and gain entry to host cells by binding to an intracellular adhesion molecule. Infection begins in the adenoidal area and spreads to the ciliated epithelium in the nose. Rhinoviruses are hardy and remain infectious for at least 3 hours after drying on hard surfaces such as telephones or countertops, but they do not last as long on porous surfaces such as tissues.

Transmission of the virus has been attributed to three methods: airborne transmission by small particles (droplets), airborne transmission by large particles, and direct contact. Large particle transmission is not efficient and requires prolonged exposure. The major means of transmission is by direct contact from a donor's nose to a donor's hand, and from there to the recipient's hand and subsequently to the nose or eye. Although conjunctival cells are not thought to harbor rhinovirus, it probably can be passed through the tear duct into the nose. Incubation of the rhinovirus is 1 to 10 days. Onset of signs and symptoms occurs 1 to 2 days after viral infection, and they peak in approximately 2 to 4 days. The virus may remain present for a week or longer after the onset of symptoms. A cough may persist after other symptoms resolve.

DIAGNOSTIC CRITERIA

Diagnostic tests have no cost/benefit effect in diagnosing the common cold. Symptoms consist primarily of clear nasal discharge, sneezing, nasal congestion, cough, low-grade fever (below 102°F [38.9°C]), scratchy or sore throat, mild aches, chills, headache, watery eyes, tenderness around the eyes, full feeling in the ears, and fatigue. In children, the presentation could also include nasal blockage, fever with seizures, anorexia, vomiting, diarrhea, and abdominal pain. Symptoms usually resolve in approximately 1 week, but they may linger for 2 weeks.

INITIATING DRUG THERAPY

Mistreatment of the common cold by clinicians is common for two reasons:

- It is difficult to determine whether the cause is viral or bacterial.

- Patients often have preconceived notions and demand antibiotics for their URI even though it is simply the common cold, which is caused by a virus.

There is no cure for the common cold. Treatment is geared toward minimizing symptoms (**Table 24.1**).

Nonpharmacologic alternatives to treating the common cold are the first line of treatment. For example, rest allows the body to gain strength and be more effective in defending itself against the pathogen. The body can then dictate the increase in activities. An alternative to decongestants and expectorants is increasing water or juice intake. This assists in liquefying tenacious secretions, making expectoration easier, soothing scratchy, sore throats, and relieving dry skin and lips. Saline gargles also are effective for soothing sore throats.

Coughing caused by chest congestion can cause a muscular chest pain. Menthol rubs can soothe this ache and open airways for some congestion relief. Menthol lozenges also have been effective in soothing scratchy throats and clearing nasal passages. Saline nasal flushes are also effective for clearing nasal passages without the rebound side effect. Petrolatum-based ointments for raw and macerated skin around the nose and upper lip ease the drying effects of dehydration and the use of multiple tissues. (See **Table 24.1**.)

Other measures, such as drinking chicken soup, taking a hot shower, or using a room humidifier, may prove helpful.

TABLE 24.1	Alternative Therapies for Cold Symptoms		
Symptoms	**Nonpharmacologic**	**Pharmacologic**	**Alternative Therapy**
Any cold symptoms	Eat proper diet, rest, drink fluids.		Echinacea (prevention) Zinc lozenges (decreased duration of symptoms)
Rhinorrhea Nasal obstruction	Use disposable paper tissues. Decrease ingestion of milk products. Inhale warm, moist heat, such as showers. Increase fluid intake.	Anticholinergic nasal spray Children: saline nose drops by bulb syringe Apply topical decongestants. If nasal obstruction is still a problem after 3 d, take oral decongestants unless contraindicated by hypertension or coronary artery disease.	Bayberry tea
Serous otitis media or sensation of fullness in ears		Decongestants (oral)	
Headache, sore throat, malaise, myalgia, fever	Gargle with salt water, drink plenty of fluids, suck on menthol lozenges.	Nonsteroidal anti-inflammatory drugs	Chaparral, aromatherapy rubs, boneset
Chest congestion	Drink fluids, have menthol rubs, and humidify room air.	Expectorants	
Sneezing and watery eyes	Humidify room air.	Two schools of thought: antihistamine of choice, but critics say antihistamines not needed in treating colds, especially in children	
Cough	Humidify room air.	Antitussives, naproxen Vicks VapoRub on the soles of feet covered by socks at bedtime	

Inhaling warm, moist heat helps raise the temperature of the nasal mucosa to at least 98.6°F (37°C), a temperature at which the virus does not replicate so readily.

Applying Vicks VapoRub on the soles of the feet and then putting on socks may help with a persistent night-time cough.

Goals of Drug Therapy

The main goals of treatment for the common cold are relief of symptoms, reduction of the risk for complications, and prevention of spread to others (**Box 24.1**). Polypharmacy is often used to treat intolerable symptoms.

Decongestants

Mechanism of Action

Decongestants are sympathomimetic agents that stimulate alpha- and beta-adrenergic receptors, causing vasoconstriction in the respiratory tract mucosa and thereby improving ventilation (**Table 24.2**). Decongestants come in topical or oral preparations. Topical decongestants in the form of nasal sprays slow ciliary motility and mucociliary clearance. Topical agents have little systemic absorption. However, topical decongestants should not be used for more than 3 days because prolonged use can cause rhinitis medicamentosa (rebound congestion), which is characterized by severe nasal edema, rebound congestion, and increased discharge due to decreased receptor sensitivity.

BOX 24.1

Preventing Upper Respiratory Infections

- Avoid touching face with hands.
- Wash hands frequently.
- Avoid people with colds or URIs.
- Avoid crowded areas during peak URI/flu season.
- Stop smoking.
- Avoid excessive intake of alcohol.
- Avoid second-hand smoke.
- Avoid excessive dry heat.
- Use disposable tissues and dispose of them properly.
- Obtain influenza vaccine, if recommended.
- Eat a nutritious diet.
- Get adequate rest and sleep.
- Avoid or reduce stress.
- Exercise regularly.
- Increase humidity in the house, especially during winter months.
- Maintain good oral hygiene.
- Avoid certain environmental irritants and allergens (dust, chemicals, smoke, and animal dander) when possible.
- Use central ventilation fans/air conditioning with microstatic air filters.

Oral decongestants are frequently used and are sold over the counter (OTC) alone or in combination with other drugs. A common example of a combination preparation is an antihistamine and a decongestant. The most common oral decongestant is pseudoephedrine (Sudafed, others). Oral decongestants have the same mode of action as topical agents but can cause more systemic responses. Decongestants assist in clearing nasal obstruction. Their use may be encouraged to prevent sinusitis and eustachian tube blockage.

Contraindications

Decongestants are contraindicated in patients with narrow-angle glaucoma, hypertension, and severe coronary artery disease. Caution is recommended in patients with hyperthyroidism, diabetes, and prostatic hypertrophy (causes difficulty with urination).

Adverse Events

Adverse events include increased blood pressure, increased heart rate, palpitations, headache, dizziness, gastrointestinal (GI) distress, and tremor. These reactions are especially seen at doses above 210 mg.

Interactions

Decongestants interact with appetite suppressants, monoamine oxidase (MAO) inhibitors (hypertensive crisis), and beta-adrenergic agents (bradycardia and hypertension). Decongestants are less effective when taken with drugs that acidify the urine and more effective when taken with drugs that alkalize the urine.

Expectorants

One of the most important nondrug considerations in treating coughs is discovering its cause, because the prolonged use of OTC expectorants or other cough products may mask symptoms of a serious underlying disorder. The drug should not be used for more than a week. If the cough persists, additional measures may be investigated.

Mechanism of Action

Expectorants, including water, increase the output of respiratory tract fluid by decreasing the adhesiveness and surface tension of the respiratory tract and by facilitating removal of viscous mucous. (See **Table 24.2**.) The effect is noted within 1 to 2 hours.

Adverse Events

Adverse events include drowsiness, headache, and GI symptoms.

Antitussives

Cough is a frequent complaint of a person with an URI. Cough can be stimulated from congestion or can occur as a result of postnasal drip. There are many cough suppressants available, but studies have shown minimal benefit with the common cold.

TABLE 24.2	Overview of Agents for Upper Respiratory Infections		
Generic (Trade) Name and Dosage	Selected Adverse Events	Contraindications	Special Considerations
Decongestants			
oxymetazoline hydrochloride (Afrin) ≥6 y: 2–3 sprays bid 2–6 y (use children's spray): 2–3 sprays bid	Palpitations, headaches		These drugs may cause rebound congestion. Use only 2 to 3 days, then switch to oral decongestants.
phenylephrine hydrochloride (Neo-Synephrine) Adults: 1 spray q3–4h as needed	Palpitations, headaches	Not recommended for children	These drugs may cause rebound congestion. Use only 2 to 3 days, then switch to oral decongestants.
pseudoephedrine (Sudafed, Benylin decongestant) Adults: short acting: 60 mg q4–6h; long acting: 120 mg q12h Children 7–12 y: short acting: 30 mg q4–6h Children 3–6 y: 15 mg q4–6h	Palpitations, headaches, increased blood pressure, dizziness, GI upset, tremor	Hypertension, coronary artery disease	Give at least 2 h before bedtime. Do not crush, break, or chew tablets.
Expectorants			
guaifenesin (Antitussin, Mucinex, Robitussin, Uni-Tussin) Adults: short acting: 200–400 mg q4h long acting: 600–1,200 mg q12h Children 7–12 y: short acting: 100–200 mg q4h long acting: 600 mg q12h Children 2–6 y: 50–100 mg q4h	GI upset, drowsiness, headache, rash, dizziness	Breast-feeding mothers, pregnancy category C	Not given for prolonged time if cough persists or accompanied by high fever Humibid sprinkles may be swallowed whole or opened and sprinkled on soft food.
Antitussives			
dextromethorphan (Benylin—15 mg/5 mL) 10 mL q6–8h (Delsym—30 mg/5 mL) Adults: 10 mL q12h Children 2–5 y: 2.5 mL q12h 6–12 y: 5 mL q12h	Drowsiness, palpitations, excitability in children	Hypertension, diabetes, asthma	None
benzonatate (Tessalon) 100–200 mg tid Not for ≤ 10 years old	Drowsiness, headache, GI upset, confusion	Pregnancy category C	
Narcotic Antitussives			
codeine phosphate 10 mg, guaifenesin 300 mg tablets and liquid (Brontex) Adults: 20 mL q4h Children 6–12 y: 10 mL q4h	Lightheadedness, dizziness, sedation, sweating, nausea, vomiting	Known addiction, cautious use in asthmatics, COPD, cardiac disease, seizure disorders, renal/hepatic impairment, BPH, head injuries, hypothyroidism, and pregnancy	Increased CNS depression if used with alcohol or other narcotics Usually used with antihistamines, expectorants, decongestants, or analgesics Controlled substance (Drug Enforcement Agency number required for prescription)
Phenergan with codeine (codeine 10 mg and promethazine 6.25 mg/5 mL) Adults: 5 mL Children: 2–5 y: 1.25–2.5 mL q4h 6–12 y: 2.5–5 mL q4h	Same as above	Same as above	Same as above

(continued)

TABLE 24.2 Overview of Agents for Upper Respiratory Infections (*Continued*)

Generic (Trade) Name and Dosage	Selected Adverse Events	Contraindications	Special Considerations
codeine 10 mg, guaifenesin 100 mg/5 mL (Robitussin AC) or codeine 10 mg, pseudoephedrine 30 mg, and guaifenesin 100 mg/5 mL (Tussar SF) Adults: 10 mL q4h to maximum of 40 mL/d	Same as above	Children: not recommended	Same as above
hydrocodone (in combination with other agents) 5 mg up to 4 qid	Same as above	Known addiction; cautious use in asthmatics, COPD, cardiac disease, seizure disorders, renal/hepatic impairment, BPH, head injuries, hypothyroidism, and pregnancy	Same as above
hydrocodone 2.5 mg, guaifenesin 100 mg, pseudoephedrine 30 mg/ 5 mL (Duratuss HD) Adults: 10 mL q4–6h Children 6–12 y: 5 mL q2–6h Maximum of 4 doses/d	Same as above	Same as above	Same as above
hydrocodone 5 mg and homatropine 1.5 mg (Hycodan tablets and syrup) Adults: 1 tablet or 5 mL q4–6h Children: 6–12 y: ½ tablet or 2.5 mL q4–6h	Same as above	Same as above	Same as above
hydrocodone 5 mg and guaifenesin 100 mg/5 mL (Hycotuss) Adults: 5 mL after meals and hs Children: 6–12 y: 2.5–5 mL after meals and hs	Same as above	Same as above	Same as above
hydrocodone 10 mg and chlorpheniramine maleate 8 mg/5 mL (Tussionex) Adults: 5 mL q12h Children: 6–12 y: 2.5 mL q12h	Same as above	Same as above	Same as above
hydrocodone 5 mg guaifenesin 100 mg per 5 mL (Vicodin Tuss) Adults: 5 mL at meals and hs Children 6–12 y: 2.5 mL at meals and hs	Same as above	Same as above	Same as above
Combination Products—Non-Narcotic			
dextromethorphan hydrobromide 10 mg, brompheniramine maleate 2 mg, pseudoephedrine 30 mg/5 mL (Bromfed-D, Dimetane-DX) Adults: 10 mL q4h Children: 2–5 y: 2.5 mL q4h 6–12 y: 5 mL q4h	Drowsiness, sedation, nausea, dizziness, palpitations, increased blood pressure, excitation in children, constipation	Asthma, lower respiratory disorders, neonates, severe hypertension, severe cardiovascular disease, within 14 d of monoamine oxidase inhibitors, nursing mothers; use cautiously in patients with history of urinary obstruction, mild hypertension, and hyperthyroidism	These drugs are combination antitussives, antihistamines, and sympathomimetics. Used for cough and congestion Pregnancy category C Not recommended for children <2 y These drugs are sold over the counter.

TABLE 24.2 Overview of Agents for Upper Respiratory Infections (*Continued*)

Generic (Trade) Name and Dosage	Selected Adverse Events	Contraindications	Special Considerations
dextromethorphan Hbr 10 mg, pseudoephedrine HCl 30 mg, guaifenesin 100 mg/5 mL (Novahistine DMX, Robitussin-DM) Adults: 10 mL q4h to maximum of 4 doses/d Children: 2–5 y: 2.5 mL q4h 6–12 y: 5 mL q4h to maximum of 4 doses/d Robitussin-DM indicated for infants in the following doses: 6–11 mo (14–17 lb): 1.25 mL 12–23 mo (18–23 lb): 2.5 mL q6–8h	Same as above	Same as above	Same as above
carbinoxamine maleate 4 mg, pseudoephedrine HCl 60 mg per tab or per 5 mL (Rondec syrup). Over 6 y: 5 mL or 1 tab qid. 18 mo–6 y: 2.5 mL qid. Comes in drops for infants and the drops should be used for children ≤18 mo pseudoephedrine HCl 60 mg/5 mL Children 1–3 mo: 0.25 mL 3–6 mo: 0.5 mL 6–9 mo: 0.75 mL 9–18 mo: 1 mL qid	Same as above	Same as above	Same as above
carbetapentane tannate 60 mg, chlorpheniramine tannate 5 mg, ephedrine tannate 10 mg, phenylephrine tannate 10 mg (Rynatuss) tablets Adults: 1–2 tablets q12h carbetapentane tannate 30 mg, chlorpheniramine tannate 5 mg, ephedrine tannate 5 mg, phenylephrine tannate 5 mg (Rynatuss Pediatric Syrup) 2–5 y: 2.5–5 mL q12h 6–12 y: 5–10 mL q12h	Same as above	Same as above	Same as above Is a prescription medication

Anti-Inflammatories and Antipyretics

naproxen sodium (Naprosyn, Aleve) Adults: 500 mg q12h or 250 mg q6–8h; maximum 1 g/d Children >2 y may take suspension form 10 mg/kg in two divided doses	Nausea, vomiting, dyspepsia	Not for children <2 y	Take on full stomach to reduce side effects of possible GI discomfort.

Anticholinergics

ipratropium bromide (Atrovent) Adults: two 36-μg inhalations qid or two sprays of 0.06% per nostril tid–qid Spray: two 0.03% sprays per nostril bid–tid	Headache, epistaxis, pharyngitis, nasal dryness	Hypersensitivity to atropine Use caution in patients with narrow-angle glaucoma, BPH, bladder neck obstruction, pregnancy, and lactation.	Protect inhalable solution from light.

Antibiotics

amoxicillin (Amoxil) Adults: 500 mg tid for 10 d Children: 20–40 mg/kg/d in divided doses	Nausea, vomiting, diarrhea, rash, allergic reactions, fungal infections, pseudomembranous colitis, Stevens-Johnson syndrome, seizures (high doses)	Hypersensitivity or allergy to penicillin or cephalosporins Use cautiously in renal impairment.	Therapy should continue for at least 10 d or 1 wk after symptoms subside.

(continued)

TABLE 24.2	Overview of Agents for Upper Respiratory Infections (*Continued*)		
Generic (Trade) Name and Dosage	**Selected Adverse Events**	**Contraindications**	**Special Considerations**

amoxicillin with clavulanic acid (Augmentin)
   Adults: 500 mg tid or 875 mg bid for 10 d
   Children: same as amoxicillin for adults
	Same as above	Same as above	Same as above
			Combination drug
			Clavulanic acid protects amoxicillin from breakdown by bacterial beta-lactamase enzymes.

cefpodoxime (Vantin)
   Adults: 200 mg q12h
   Children (>2 mo.): 5 mg/kg q12h
	GI upset, rash, abdominal pain, headache	Caution with penicillin allergy	Interacts with antacids, H2 antagonists. Avoid diuretics.

cefuroxime (Ceftin)
   Adults: 250 mg q12h
   Children (>6 mo.): 7.5–15 mg/kg q12h
	As above	As above	As above

trimethoprim-sulfamethoxazole (TMP-SMZ, Bactrim, Septra)
   Adults: 160 mg trimethoprim and 800 mg sulfamethoxazole orally q12h for up to 14 d
   Children: 8 mg/kg/d; trimethoprim in 2 doses × 10 d
	Nausea, vomiting, anorexia, megaloblastic anemia, hallucinations, depression, seizures	Megaloblastic anemia, pregnancy category C, breast-feeding, sulfa allergy	Hemolysis may develop in patients with glucose-6-phosphate dehydrogenase deficiency.
			May cause falsely elevated creatinine level
			Advise patient to increase fluid intake.

clarithromycin (Biaxin)
   Adults: 500 mg bid for 10 d
   Biaxin XL 1,000 mg qd for 7 d
	Nausea, vomiting, diarrhea, dyspepsia, abnormal taste, allergic reactions, fungal infection
	Serious: pseudomembranous colitis
		Allergy to macrolides
		Pregnancy and lactation
		Use with caution in severe hepatic or renal disease.
			Take with or without food.
			   Monitor for drug interactions with other agents that are metabolized by the cytochrome P450 3A4 isoenzyme.
			Interactants: warfarin, digoxin, carbamazepine, theophylline, cisapride

telithromycin 800 mg daily for 5 days	Diarrhea, nausea, headache, dizziness, elevated LFTs	Hypersensitivity to macrolides, visapride use, caution if hypokalemia, QT prolongation	Pregnancy category C May decrease efficacy of oral contraceptives

BPH, benign prostatic hypertrophy; COPD, chronic obstructive pulmonary disease; GI, gastrointestinal.

However, cough suppressants, such as dextromethorphan, may reduce cough frequency and help the patient sleep. There is little evidence to support the use of codeine and hydrocodone to relieve cough.

Mechanism of Action

Antitussives diminish the cough reflex by direct inhibition of the cough center in the medulla. (See **Table 24.2.**) There are narcotic antitussives and non-narcotic antitussives. Onset of action is noted within 15 to 30 minutes. Many practitioners believe that cough suppressants are ineffective in children.

Contraindications

Antitussives are contraindicated in a patient with a productive cough, a history of substance abuse, or chronic obstructive pulmonary disease.

Adverse Events

Adverse events include dizziness, nausea, drowsiness, and sedation.

Interactions

Drug–drug interactions occur with concomitant use of amiodarone (Cordarone), MAO inhibitors, quinidine (Cardioquin, others), selective serotonin reuptake inhibitors, and other antidepressants.

Anti-Inflammatories and Antipyretics

Nonsteroidal anti-inflammatory drugs (NSAIDs) inhibit prostaglandin secretions, which serves to decrease mucus secretion. Effects are noted within 1 to 2 hours.

NSAIDs alleviate constitutional symptoms such as headache, sore throat, malaise, myalgia, and fever. The NSAID naproxen (Naprosyn) is given 500 mg every 12 hours or 250 mg every 6 to 8 hours, not to exceed 1 g/day. Naproxen alleviates symptoms without increasing viral shedding. NSAIDs are contraindicated in patients with asthma, renal disease, severe hepatic disease, and ulcers. Adverse events include nausea, GI ulceration, bleeding, nephrotoxicity, and blood dyscrasias. NSAIDs may increase the action of heparin.

Aspirin (Bayer, others), a common NSAID, should not be used in children because of the secondary risk of Reye's syndrome. The patient should also refrain from taking acetaminophen (Tylenol) and nonprescription doses of ibuprofen (Motrin) because these drugs are believed to shed the virus. NSAIDs are discussed in greater detail in Chapter 38.

Anticholinergic Agents

Ipratropium bromide (Atrovent) nasal spray (0.03% and 0.06%) has been recommended for rhinorrhea associated with the common cold. It can be prescribed in both strengths for adults and in the 0.03% strength for children age 6 and older. It inhibits vagally mediated reflexes by antagonizing the action of acetylcholine at the cholinergic receptor, thereby inhibiting secretions from the serous and seromucous glands lining the nasal mucosa. The result is a decrease in nasal discharge. The dosage is two sprays per nostril three or four times a day.

Ipratropium bromide is not used in patients with a history of sensitivity to atropine or in pregnant or lactating women. It is used with caution in patients with narrow-angle glaucoma, prostatic hypertrophy, or bladder neck obstruction. Adverse events include epistaxis, dry mouth, nasal congestion, and nasal dryness.

Antihistamines

For sneezing and rhinorrhea, a combination of pseudoephedrine and a first-generation antihistamine seems to be effective. Some critics say the use of antihistamines is irrational and has no place in treatment of the common cold (Berman & Chan, 1999). They state that their drying effect might exacerbate symptoms of congestion and cause upper airway obstruction by impairing the flow of mucous. In contrast, antihistamines have been effective in controlling the symptoms of watery eyes, runny nose, and a feeling of fullness in the ears. Antihistamines are discussed further in Chapter 47.

Selecting the Most Appropriate Agent

Because symptoms of a cold are manifest individually or in combination, depending on the patient, not everyone has the same signs and symptoms. Therefore, the therapeutic approach is to treat symptoms as specifically as possible. In addition, if the cold is caused by a bacterial infection, as evidenced by throat culture results and the like, antibiotic treatment is prescribed (**Figure 24-1**).

First-Line Therapy

Initial therapy consists of symptom relief. For nasal obstruction and rhinorrhea, which are caused by secretions and increased vascular permeability with leakage of serum into the nasal mucosa, topical decongestants, such as oxymetazoline hydrochloride (Afrin) or phenylephrine hydrochloride (Neo-Synephrine), are often used for the first 3 days, when the patient feels the worst (**Table 24.3**). Topical vasoconstrictors are recommended for only 3 days because they predispose many patients to rebound congestion. Rebound congestion interferes with ciliary action and dries the nasal mucosa. If other symptoms are diminished but nasal obstruction remains a problem, the use of an oral decongestant, such as pseudoephedrine, or a combination decongestant and antihistamine, or an antihistamine alone may relieve symptoms and help prevent complications such as sinusitis and eustachian tube blockage. Antipyretics, such as acetaminophen, or anti-inflammatories, such as ibuprofen, may be recommended to relieve fever and accompanying aches and discomfort.

Second-Line Therapy

Second-line therapy may be instituted if first-line therapy fails to relieve symptoms or if complications, such as secondary infection (ear infections, sinusitis, bronchitis, or pneumonia), develop. The therapy should be specific to the disorder.

Special Population Considerations
Pediatric

In infants, using saline nose drops with a bulb syringe before feedings may be helpful. Saline nose drops may be prepared by adding one quarter of a teaspoon of salt to 8 oz of water. Children younger than age 7 should not be encouraged to blow their nose because the pressure of blowing increases the risk of ear congestion great enough to promote infection. Aspirin is not given to children because of the risk of Reye's syndrome. There is controversy over whether antitussives are effective in children.

MONITORING PATIENT RESPONSE

Patient response is monitored by the decrease of symptoms. If symptoms decrease without onset of complications, then therapy was successful. If the common cold does not improve in 8 to 10 days, a bacterial cause is suspected and antibiotic therapy is considered.

PATIENT EDUCATION

The most important aspect of patient education is to prevent contracting the virus by practicing good hygiene, such as frequent hand washing, getting adequate sleep and exercise, avoiding contact with infected people, eating a nutritious diet, and so on. Another important aspect of patient education is teaching patients to prevent spreading the virus through correct tissue disposal, hand washing, covering the mouth when coughing, and so on. (See **Box 24.1**.)

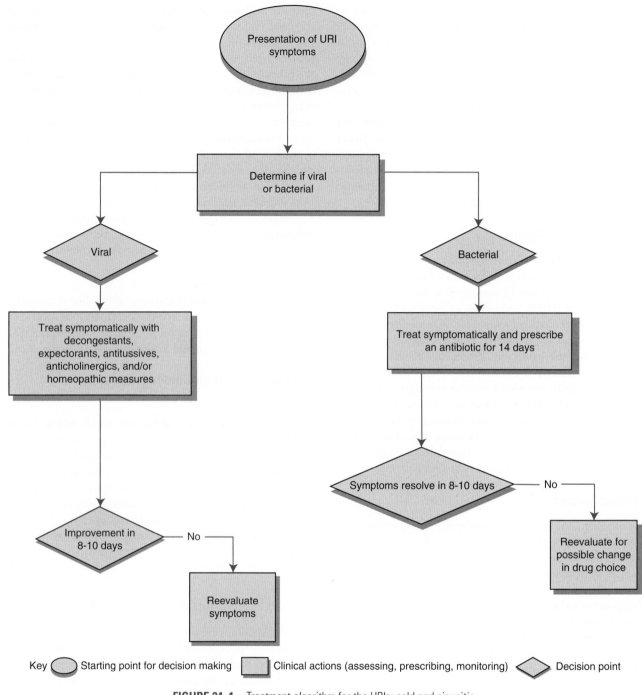

FIGURE 24–1 Treatment algorithm for the URIs: cold and sinusitis.

Alternative Therapies

There is a growing interest in alternative or complementary therapies for treating colds. The root of the bayberry bush in large doses has been used to increase the secretion of nasal mucus during head colds. Echinacea's medicinal properties inhibit microbial infections by stimulating the body's immune system. It is used for prevention. However, prolonged use can lead to immune system overstimulation and eventual suppression. (See **Table 24.1.**)

SINUSITIS

Sinusitis, also called *rhinosinusitis,* is a bacterial URI characterized by inflammation of the mucous membranes that line the paranasal sinuses. Air trapped within a blocked sinus, along with pus or other secretions, can cause pressure on the sinus wall. The result is the sometimes-intense sinus pain. Similarly, when air is prevented from entering a paranasal sinus by a swollen membrane at the opening, a vacuum can be created that also causes pain.

TABLE 24.3	Recommended Order of Treatment for the Common Cold	
Order	**Agent**	**Comments**
First line	Symptom relief with oral and topical decongestants, topical vasoconstrictors, antihistamines, expectorants or antitussives, anti-inflammatories, and antipyretics as indicated	Cold treatment is symptom specific. There is no cure. The disorder is self-limiting.
Second line	Specific drug therapy aimed at treating complications if symptoms progress to sinusitis, bronchitis, or other disorders	Patient should be advised to contact practitioner if cold symptoms do not subside in approximately 7 days.

It can be acute or chronic. Acute sinusitis often results from progression of the common cold (5% to 10% of cases) and lasts for 3 weeks or less. Chronic sinusitis is defined as episodes of prolonged inflammation or repeatedly treated acute sinus infections. Symptoms last for 3 to 8 weeks but may be present for longer than 3 months. Bacterial infections can occur from impaired drainage resulting from polyps, enlarged turbinates, a deviated septum, the common cold, anatomic abnormalities, tooth infections, exacerbation of allergic rhinitis, and so on. Health care experts estimate that 37 million Americans are affected by sinusitis every year.

CAUSES

Rhinosinusitis is a more appropriate term than either rhinitis or sinusitis to describe inflammatory disease involving the upper respiratory tract. The nasal and sinus mucosa are contiguous; sinusitis rarely occurs in the absence of rhinitis.

A preceding viral URI often is the trigger for acute sinusitis; about 0.5% to 5% of common colds become complicated by the development of acute sinusitis. Acute sinusitis is defined pathologically by transient inflammation of the mucosal lining of the paranasal sinuses lasting less than 30 days. Clinically, acute sinusitis is characterized by nasal congestion, nasal discharge, and facial pain.

Most cases of acute sinusitis start with a common cold of viral etiology that inflames the sinuses. Both the cold and the sinus inflammation usually resolve without treatment in 2 weeks. The nose reacts to an invasion by viruses that cause infections such as the common cold or flu by producing mucus and sending white blood cells to the lining of the nose, which congest and swell the nasal passages.

When this swelling involves the adjacent mucous membranes of the sinuses, air and mucus are trapped behind the narrowed openings of the sinuses. When sinus openings become too narrow, mucus cannot drain properly. This increase in mucus sets up prime conditions for bacteria to multiply.

The most common causes are the bacterial pathogens *Streptococcus pneumoniae* and *Haemophilus influenzae*, which account for 75% of cases of rhinosinusitis. *Moraxella catarrhalis* is most common in children. Other organisms that may cause sinusitis, but less frequently, are group A *Streptococcus*, *Chlamydia pneumoniae*, and *Streptococcus pyogenes*.

Most healthy persons harbor bacteria such as *S. pneumoniae* and *H. influenzae* in their upper respiratory tracts with no problems until the body's defenses are weakened or drainage from the sinuses is blocked by a cold or other viral infection. Then, bacteria that may have been living harmlessly in the nose or throat can multiply and invade the sinuses, causing an acute sinus infection.

Chronic inflammation of the nasal passages also can lead to sinusitis. Persons with allergic rhinitis or hay fever can also experience episodes of acute sinusitis. Vasomotor rhinitis, caused by humidity, cold air, alcohol, perfumes, and other environmental conditions, can also be complicated by sinus infections.

Persons with asthma may have frequent episodes of chronic sinusitis. Persons who are allergic to airborne allergens, such as dust, mold, and pollen, that trigger allergic rhinitis, may develop chronic sinusitis. Persons vulnerable to chronic sinusitis can also be affected by damp weather (especially in northern temperate climates) or pollutants in the air and in buildings. In addition, persons with nasal polyps or a severe asthmatic response to aspirin and aspirin-like medicines such as ibuprofen may develop chronic sinusitis often.

Other risks for developing sinusitis include the following: overuse of nasal decongestants, presence of deviated nasal septum, presence of a nasal foreign body, frequent swimming or diving, dental work, pregnancy, changes in altitude, exposure to air pollution and cigarette smoke, gastroesophageal reflux disease, and hospitalization.

PATHOPHYSIOLOGY

There are four paired, air-filled cavities that make up the sinuses. Small tubular openings, the sinus ostia, connect the sinus cavities and facilitate drainage of the sinuses into the nasal cavity using ciliated cells. Proper sinus functioning requires motile cilia, patent ostia, and mucus of a low viscosity that allows transport. Inflammation causes dysfunctional cilia, obstruction of the ostia, or both. Negative pressure develops in the clogged sinuses, facilitating the transport of intranasal bacteria into the sinuses. This can promote bacterial growth and inflammation and bacterial sinusitis.

DIAGNOSTIC CRITERIA

Bacterial infections (i.e., sinusitis) share the same symptoms of a viral cold with respect to nasal congestion, cough, fever, sore throat, aches, chills, headaches, tenderness around the eyes, a full feeling in the ears, and fatigue. The distinction lies with the severity and duration of symptoms with a bacterial URI. In sinusitis, there is persistent rhinitis without resolution and a cough that lasts more than 8 to 10 days after a cold. The nasal discharge increases in quantity, viscosity, and purulence. In addition, there is often malodorous breath without poor dental hygiene, and by morning periorbital swelling may be present. The patient reports facial pain on movement. Fever and malaise also may occur.

Differentiation between infectious and noninfectious disease usually can be made by history. The typical patient reports a URI that has been unusually severe and failed to resolve or improve after 7 to 10 days. The general course of the disease may be biphasic. Major symptoms include facial pain, pressure, congestion, fullness, obstruction, blockage, or discharge with a temperature greater than 100.4°F (38°C). Purulent drainage in the middle meatus may be a strong indicator of acute sinus disease; however, nasal purulence does not differentiate a viral from a bacterial infection. There may be a lack of response to decongestants. Symptoms may include headache, fatigue, dental pain, halitosis, otalgia, or cough. Other symptoms include toothache and a poor response to decongestants. There is usually edema of the mucous membranes upon examination and tenderness over the sinus areas upon percussion.

Characteristic signs are purulent, green or yellow nasal discharge and abnormal sinus illumination. Acute bacterial sinusitis is a consideration in patients who report cold symptoms lasting more than 8 days or with prolonged nasal obstruction, or a cold that seems to have gotten better but returns with more severe symptoms.

Chronic sinusitis is a persistent, low-grade infection involving the paranasal sinuses with mucosal thickening. It is diagnosed with sinus x-ray or computed tomography scan. Characteristics of chronic sinusitis include nasal discharge, nasal congestion, cough lasting more than 30 days, or a combination of all three.

INITIATING DRUG THERAPY

Initial treatment is to observe the patient with nonsevere illness (mild pain, temperature below 101°F [38.3°C]) and provide symptomatic relief. If the condition persists or worsens or if it fails to improve within 7 days, antibiotic treatment is used in addition to symptomatic treatment. Antibiotic therapy should be considered when the patient has a combination of the following: temperature above 102°F (38.9°C); pain or tenderness in the ears, sinuses, or face; purulent, colorful sputum; sore throat; dyspnea and pleuritic chest pain; and symptoms that persist with no improvement for over 10 days.

Nonpharmacologic therapies are the same as those for the common cold, particularly when the symptoms are the same. Surgical intervention is avoided in acute cases, but irrigation and surgical drainage may be necessary in recurrent chronic cases of sinusitis in which complications are present and the patient fails to respond to medical therapy.

Goals of Drug Therapy

The primary treatment goal is to restore sinuses to health; decrease the duration of symptoms to enable patients to resume daily activities more quickly; prevent severe, albeit rare, complications such as meningitis or brain abscess; and prevent the emergence of chronic disease. Other goals include reducing mucosal swelling and relieving pain. Decongestants are often prescribed to treat intolerable symptoms of acute sinusitis, and topical corticosteroids may be used to treat mucosal swelling associated with acute or chronic sinusitis.

Antibiotics

The recommended length of therapy for acute bacterial sinusitis is at least 14 days, or 7 days beyond the resolution of symptoms, whichever is longer. Amoxicillin is appropriate for the initial treatment of acute, uncomplicated, mild sinusitis in patients with no recent antibiotic use. Antimicrobial agents with more broad-spectrum activity may be indicated as initial therapy for patients who have more severe infection, comorbidity, risk factors for bacterial resistance, or who have not responded to amoxicillin therapy. These agents include amoxicillin and clavulanic acid, the newer quinolones (e.g., levofloxacin, gatifloxacin, moxifloxacin), and some second- and third-generation cephalosporins (cefdinir, cefuroxime-axetil, and cefpodoxime proxetil). Patients who are allergic to penicillin may be treated with macrolides, trimethoprim-sulfamethoxazole, tetracyclines, or clindamycin.

Many of the pathogens found in chronically inflamed sinuses are resistant to penicillin through the production of beta-lactamase. Therapy should be effective against both aerobic and anaerobic organisms in chronic sinusitis. These agents include the combination of a penicillin (e.g., amoxicillin) and a beta-lactamase inhibitor (e.g., clavulanic acid), clindamycin, the combination of metronidazole and a macrolide, or the newer quinolones (e.g., levofloxacin, gatifloxacin, moxifloxacin). If aerobic gram-negative organisms such as *Pseudomonas aeruginosa* are involved, an aminoglycoside, a fourth-generation cephalosporin (cefepime or ceftazidime), or a fluoroquinolone (only in postpubertal patients) is added. Therapy is given for at least 21 days and may be extended up to 10 weeks.

Symptomatic Therapy

Therapy is also initiated to relieve the symptoms of sinusitis. For the most part, drug choices are the same as for the common cold: aspirin or acetaminophen for fever and aches and decongestants for stuffy nose and the like, unless contraindicated. Topical corticosteroids usually are not used because they may impede the immune system's response to infection.

Selecting the Most Appropriate Agent

Due to the increasing levels of antimicrobial resistance worldwide, clinicians must re-evaluate their approaches to URIs by using evidence-based methods of diagnosis and treatment. Although clinical diagnosis is necessary for most URIs, bacterial and nonbacterial diseases are difficult to distinguish on clinical grounds. When a bacterial pathogen is suspected or diagnosed, antibiotics are not always indicated as a first-line therapy. Patients need to be educated regarding the appropriate initial treatment regimens. When prescribing antibiotics, the regimen should be tailored to the patient. If a patient is not at risk for resistant bacteria, an agent with proven efficacy, narrow spectrum, and low cost is indicated.

First-Line Therapy

Amoxicillin is the first-line antibiotic for treating sinusitis (**Table 24.4**). Amoxicillin–clavulanate (Augmentin) is also appropriate because it provides coverage for *H. influenza* and *M. catarrhalis*. For penicillin-allergic patients, TMP-SMZ, telithromycin (Ketek), erythromycin, doxycycline, and clarithromycin (Biaxin) are used. Antibiotic treatment lasts 14 days or 1 week after resolution of symptoms.

Nasal steroid sprays are indicated in sinusitis if there is mucosal swelling. Topical and systemic decongestants may be used to help relieve congestion.

Second-Line Therapy

If there is no relief of symptoms in 8 days, the antibiotic may need to be changed. A different antibiotic should also be used if the patient was treated with antibiotics in the past 4 to 6 weeks. If the organism is thought to be beta-lactamase–producing, amoxicillin–clavulanate may be prescribed. Clarithromycin (Biaxin), cefpodoxime (Vantin), and cefuroxime (Ceftin) are other choices.

Decongestants may be administered topically (oxymetazoline or phenylephrine) or orally (pseudoephedrine), and mucolytics (guaifenesin) may facilitate drainage of involved sinuses. In patients with atopy, reactive airways disease, or nasal polyposis, oral steroid therapy may help decrease mucosal inflammation and work synergistically with antibiotics in re-establishing drainage through the frontal recess and ostiomeatal complex.

MONITORING PATIENT RESPONSE

The patient who has sinusitis and who is taking an antibiotic should notice relief from symptoms in 48 to 72 hours. If there is no response, the patient should be advised to return as soon as feasible for adjustment in medication and a general assessment of the condition. If symptoms resolve, the patient can be seen for a general checkup in 10 to 14 days.

Special Population Considerations

The challenges in diagnosis and management of rhinosinusitis in children are greater than those in adults. Although the typical adult has two or three acute viral rhinosinusitis episodes annually, the typical child has six to eight episodes that must be distinguished from acute bacterial rhinosinusitis. More than half of patients are given an antibiotic prescription, even though antibiotic therapy does not hasten resolution or prevent bacterial complications of viral rhinosinusitis. Education and counseling are important components in the response to demands by parents to resolve purulent rhinorrhea, which is part of the natural course of viral rhinosinusitis. Bacterial infection is suggested when symptoms persist without improvement for more than 10 days or when they are unusually severe. Facial tenderness, transient periorbital swelling, daytime cough, or fever of 102.2°F (39°C) or higher in combination with purulent rhinorrhea is suggestive of bacterial infection.

The high frequency of acute infection in children also may lead to overdiagnosis of chronic rhinosinusitis. Although structural problems play a central role in the etiology of adults with chronic rhinosinusitis, they do not in children, so surgery plays a minor role in management. Immaturity of the immune system, evidenced by higher frequency of viral infection and atopic disease, is a significant etiologic factor in this population. Gastroesophageal reflux is also an important etiologic factor for pediatric chronic rhinosinusitis. The prevalence of reflux disease is higher in children with chronic rhinosinusitis, and treatment of reflux improves sinus symptoms.

TABLE 24.4	**Recommended Order of Treatment for Sinusitis**		
Order	**Agents**		**Comments**
First line	Antibiotic therapy (depends on suspected or confirmed bacterial organisms)		Treatment lasts for 10–14 d.
	Common selections include amoxicillin, trimethoprim–sulfamethoxazole, and symptom relief with decongestants, such as pseudoephedrine; nasal sprays, such as Neo-synephrine (no more than 3 d); and antihistamines, only if allergic process exists.		If the patient is severely penicillin allergic, clarithromycin may be substituted.
Second line	Change antibiotic therapy, for e.g., to amoxicillin with clavulanic acid.		
	Continue symptom relief.		

As in purulent otitis media, most cases of acute rhinosinusitis are caused by *S. pneumoniae*, *H. influenzae*, and *M. catarrhalis*. In addition, they can be caused by anaerobic organisms and *Staphylococcus aureus*. Resistance patterns are important in predicting response to antimicrobial therapy: *H. influenzae* and *M. catarrhalis* can be resistant to beta-lactam antibiotics such as ampicillin due to beta-lactamase production. In contrast, *S. pneumoniae* and *S. aureus* can be resistant to the penicillins and most other antibiotics by a genetic alteration in penicillin-binding proteins. This form of resistance is much more significant because it is not treated successfully by the typical "second-line" agents such as cephalosporins, macrolides, and amoxicillin–clavulanate. Oral antibiotic options include high-dose amoxicillin and clindamycin.

More than 80% of children with sinusitis have a family history of allergy, as opposed to a general population frequency of 15% to 20%. More than half of the cases of sinusitis are closely associated with asthma. Allergy can contribute to sinusitis by either nasal congestion and subsequent ostia obstruction, or direct allergic effects on sinus-lining cells. Although not IgE mediated, cow's milk protein allergy may be present in very young children with a history of rashes or colic and can be a contributing factor to rhinosinusitis in these children.

For young children with mild to moderate sinusitis, amoxicillin is recommended at the normal dose (45 mg/kg) or high dose (90 mg/kg). Patients with amoxicillin allergy should be treated with a cephalosporin such as cefdinir, cefuroxime, or cefpodoxime, whereas severely allergic patients should be treated with a macrolide such as clarithromycin or azithromycin. Children who do not respond to first-line therapy, children with more severe initial disease, and children who are considered at high risk for resistant *S. pneumoniae* (those who recently have used antibiotics or attend day care) should be treated with high-dose amoxicillin–clavulanate (90 mg/kg of amoxicillin component).

Adjuvant therapies are not necessary in the treatment of uncomplicated acute rhinosinusitis, although saline spray may make children feel better by clearing out secretions, and the newer nonsedating antihistamines may be beneficial in children where allergy is suspected as the causative factor.

PATIENT EDUCATION

The role of the practitioner is to make the patient aware not only of the importance of the therapeutic regimen but also of prevention. (See **Box 24.1**.) Education needs to begin before cold and flu season so that patients can take steps to prevent disease and to make educated decisions on whether a health care visit is needed or whether the symptoms are likely to be self-limiting.

Patients also need to know that symptoms of viral and bacterial URIs are similar, but that viral URIs and allergies are more prevalent than bacterial sinusitis. Decongestants may be used in almost all situations, unless the patient has hypertension or coronary artery disease, and they may even be helpful in preventing sinusitis in patients with recurrent symptoms.

Drug Information

Possibly the most important thing for patients to learn is to complete the full course of antibiotic therapy and not to stop taking the medication because symptoms subside in 48 to 72 hours. The patient also needs to know how to recognize and respond to adverse effects of antibiotic therapy, especially because allergic reactions are more prevalent with these drugs than other drugs. The patient should be encouraged to schedule a follow-up visit to assess the potential for chronic sinusitis or other complications, especially if he or she does not feel completely better.

Lifestyle Changes

Although sinusitis cannot be completely prevented, certain measures can reduce the number and severity of the attacks and may prevent acute sinusitis from becoming chronic. These measures include the following: use of a humidifier, particularly if the environment is heated by a dry forced-air system; use of air conditioners to help provide an even temperature; and use of electrostatic filters attached to heating and air conditioning equipment to help remove allergens from the air.

Persons prone to developing sinus disorders, especially persons with allergies, should avoid cigarette smoke and other air pollutants. If allergies inflame the nasal passages, the likelihood for a strong reaction to all irritants is increased.

Drinking alcohol also causes nasal and sinus membranes to swell. For persons prone to sinusitis, it may be uncomfortable to swim in pools treated with chlorine because it irritates the lining of the nose and sinuses. Divers often get sinus congestion and infection when water is forced into the sinuses from the nasal passages.

Air travel may pose a problem for persons with acute or chronic sinusitis. As the air pressure in a plane is reduced, pressure can build up in the head, blocking sinuses or eustachian tubes. The patient may feel discomfort in the sinus or middle ear during the plane's ascent or descent.

Case Study

M. R., a 28-year-old Asian-American, presents with complaints of a cold. He states he has been sick for 6 days and is feeling worse. He complains of a thick, green nasal discharge, congestion, and inability to breathe through his nose. He also says he has had a thick, yellow-green expectoration for 4 days, and has chills off and on. He complains of a pounding headache all over his head with sudden movement. He has pain in his neck over the submaxillary and submental nodes when touched, but he is able to swallow. He has tried "flu medicine," but it is not effective. Nothing makes it better or worse.

Objective data include the following:

Vital signs: temperature, 100.4°F; pulse rate 88; respiratory rate 18; blood pressure 120/70

Ears: tympanic membrane intact bilaterally, landmarks visible

Eyes: conjunctivae pale and moist

Nose: anterior nasal turbinates erythematous and boggy

Throat: pharynx injected without exudates

Neck: (+) tenderness and lymphadenopathy submaxillary and submental cervical nodes, (2) thyroid

Sinuses: frontal and maxillary sinuses tender on palpation; minimal transillumination

Lungs: anterior upper lobes bilaterally with scattered rhonchi—clears with coughing

Other lobes clear to auscultation; (+) thoracic expansion and thorax symmetric; resonance on percussion; no shortness of breath

Neurologic: cranial nerves 2 to 12 intact

DIAGNOSIS: ACUTE SINUSITIS

1. List specific goals for treatment for M. R.
2. What drug therapy would you prescribe? Why?
3. What are the parameters for monitoring the success of the therapy?
4. Discuss specific patient education based on the prescribed therapy.
5. List one or two adverse reactions for the selected agent that would cause you to change therapy.
6. What would be the choice for the second-line therapy?
7. What OTC or alternative medications would be appropriate for this patient?
8. What dietary and lifestyle changes should be recommended for this patient?
9. Describe one or two drug–drug or drug–food interactions for the selected agent.

BIBLIOGRAPHY

Starred references are cited in the text.

Ahmad, N., & Zacharek, M. (2008). Allergic rhinitis and rhinosinusitis. *Otolaryngology Clinics of North America, 41*(2), 267–281.

Anon, A. (2006). Upper respiratory infections. *American Journal of Medicine, 123*(4, Suppl 1), S16–S25.

*Berman, S. & Chan, K. (1999). Infections: Viral and rickettsial. In W. Hay, A. Hayward, M. Levine, & J. Sondheimer (Eds.), *Pediatric diagnosis and treatment* (pp. 406, 960–967). Stanford, CT: Appleton & Lange.

Brook, I. (2007). Acute and chronic sinusitis. *Infectious Disease Clinics of North America, 21*(2), 427–448.

Dykewicz, M., & Hamilas, D. (2010). Rhinitis and sinusitis. *Journal of Allergy and Clinical Immunology, 125*(2, Suppl 2), S103–S115.

Leung, R., & Kateal, R. (2008). Diagnosis and management of acute and chronic sinusitis. *Primary Care: Clinics in Office Practice, 35*(1), 11–24.

Morris, P. (2009). Upper respiratory infections (including otitis media). *Pediatric Clinics of North America, 56*(1), 101–117.

Pratter, M. (2006). Cough and the common cold: ACCP evidence-based practice. *Chest, 129*(1, Suppl 1), S725–S745.

Simasek, M., & Blandino, D. (2007). Treatment of the common cold. *American Family Physician, 75*(4), 515–520.

Small, C., Bachert, C., Lund, V., et al. (2007). Judicious antibiotic use and intranasal corticosteroids in acute rhinosinusitis. *American Journal of Medicine, 120*(4), 289–294.

CHAPTER 25

Virginia P. Arcangelo

Asthma

Asthma is a chronic inflammatory disease of the airways that affects approximately 8% to 10% of the U.S. population. Approximately 7 million of these people are children. It is one of the leading causes for both outpatient and hospital care, with approximately 500,000 hospitalizations and approximately 1.2 deaths per 100,000 annually (http://www.cdc.gov/nchs/fastats/asthma.htm, accessed 5/30/2010). At greatest risk for hospitalization with asthma are African-Americans and children. African-Americans are 2.5 times more likely to have emergency room visits and be hospitalized for asthma and are 5 times more likely to die from asthma and asthma-related symptoms (Bryant-Stephans, 2009). The cost for asthma-related treatment in 2007 was estimated to be $37.2 billion (Kamble & Bharma, 2009). Approximately half of all cases of asthma develop during childhood and another third before age 40. However, asthma can begin at any age, and it can affect both sexes and all cultures.

An expert panel was commissioned by the National Asthma Education and Prevention Program (NAEPP) Coordinating Committee, coordinated by the National Heart, Lung, and Blood Institute (NHLBI) of the National Institutes of Health. They developed 2007 Guidelines for the Diagnosis and Management of Asthma. These guidelines were modified from the 1997 and 2002 guidelines.

CAUSES

Childhood-onset asthma is strongly related to atopy. Approximately 80% of all people with asthma have allergies. Adult-onset asthma can be caused by factors such as coexisting sinusitis, nasal polyps, sensitivity to aspirin or nonsteroidal anti-inflammatory drugs (NSAIDs), and occupational exposure to workplace materials. Those with the greatest risk for development of asthma are children with atopy and a family history of asthma.

Several factors increase the severity of asthma. These include untreated rhinitis or sinusitis, gastroesophageal reflux disorder (GERD), aspirin sensitivity, sleep apnea, stress, depression, exposure to sulfites or beta blockers, and influenza.

PATHOPHYSIOLOGY

Asthma is a chronic inflammatory disorder of the airways characterized by airway obstruction, inflammation, and hyperresponsiveness. There is increased resistance to airflow and a decreased flow rate from airway obstruction. Hyperinflation distal to the obstruction, altered pulmonary mechanics, and increased difficulty breathing are a result of the airway obstruction. In the healthy human airway, there is normally a fine balance among immune cells, the epithelium, and the host immune response. Airway inflammation in asthma reflects a distortion of this balance and is orchestrated through complex interplay between multiple effector and target components.

There are complex interactions among inflammatory cells, mediators, and the cells and tissues in the airways. Atopic asthma causes bronchospasm, resulting from increased responsiveness of the smooth muscle in the bronchioles to external stimuli. This, in turn, promotes a release of endogenous allergic mediators from the mast cells. These mediators include histamine, leukotrienes, and eosinophil chemotactic factor. There are two phases of symptoms, the acute-phase response and the late-phase response. The acute phase occurs within a few minutes and lasts for several hours, during which there is an interaction of allergens and macrophages. Up-regulation of T cells causes the production of interleukins. The response in this phase is bronchospasm. The late-phase response occurs in 2 to 6 hours and lasts approximately 12 to 24 hours.

T-helper (Th) lymphocytes are recognized as having a central role in asthma. It is thought that individuals predisposed to allergic asthma have an imbalance favoring Th-2 cells, which produce a family of cytokines that mediate allergic inflammation rather than favoring Th-1 cells, which normally produce cytokines to fight infection. The hygiene hypothesis suggests that reduced exposure to other children, frequent antibiotic use, and reduced exposure to certain infections (e.g., tuberculosis, measles, and hepatitis A) promote the development of a Th-2 phenotype more prone to respond to environmental allergens. This gene-by-environment interaction is offered as a plausible explanation for the observed higher prevalence of asthma in Westernized countries.

Mast cells are critical in mediating the acute response in asthma. While classically, mast cell activation occurs following the binding of antigens to FcɛR1-bound, antigen-specific immunoglobulin (Ig) E, they may also be activated through other mechanisms, including stimulation of complement receptors and FcɛR1 and via Toll-like receptors (TLRs).

Basophils have a crucial role in initiating allergic inflammation through the binding of antigen-specific IgE antibodies at the FcεR1. Basophils also drive Th-2 cell differentiation of activated naive CD4+ T cells via the production of interleukin (IL)-4 and direct cell-cell contact. Murine studies show that following activation, basophils migrate in small numbers to adjacent lymph nodes. Using a basophil FcεR1-specific monoclonal antibody, it has been demonstrated that the presence of basophils but not mast cells is an absolute requirement for Th-2 cell differentiation. Basophils also increase humoral immune responses on repeat antigenic exposure in the presence of activated CD4+ cells through the release of IL-4 and IL-6, which provide support for B-cell proliferation and antibody generation.

Pulmonary dendritic cells are potent antigen-presenting cells with the capability to rapidly migrate to draining lymph nodes, suggesting an innate role in initiating immune response against airborne antigens. Hence, dendritic cells may dictate the subsequent T-cell response.

Long-lived cytokines, such as ILs, activate eosinophils, and T lymphocytes in the airways and release mediators that reproduce the acute asthma attack. Non-atopic asthma does not have an allergic cause but can be a result of exposure to drugs, such as aspirin, NSAIDs, or beta-adrenergic antagonists; chemical irritants; chronic obstructive pulmonary disease; dry air; excessive stress; and exercise. These cause stimulation of the parasympathetic reflex pathway with release of acetylcholine, which constricts bronchial smooth muscle.

In acute, severe exacerbations of asthma, there are increased eosinophils and neutrophils within the airway, with the increase in neutrophils proportionately higher than that of eosinophils. Inhaled corticosteroids reduce airway eosinophils, but increase airway neutrophils and increase the expression of the neutrophil chemoattractant IL-8, which is associated with loss of asthma control.

Increased permeability and sensitivity to inhaled allergens, irritants, and inflammatory mediators is a consequence of epithelial injury. The chronic inflammation of the airways that is characteristic of asthma can cause thickening of the basement membrane and the deposition of collagen in the bronchial wall. These changes cause the chronic small airway obstruction seen in asthma. The release of inflammatory mediators causes bronchospasm, vascular congestion, vascular permeability, edema, production of thick mucus, and impaired mucociliary function.

PHARMACOGENOMICS

Inhaled beta$_2$ agonists, such as albuterol (Proventil), are used to control acute attacks of asthma and are prescribed to be used "as needed." Several studies have shown that some patients benefit from the use of short-acting beta$_2$–adrenergic agonists (SABAs), whereas others do not. This variation in response is partly explained by the alteration in the amino acid sequence of the protein or altered transcription of the beta$_2$ receptors. Patients with the beta$_2$ receptor arginine genotype experience poor asthma control with frequent symptoms and a decrease in scores on forced expiratory volume in one second (FEV$_1$) compared with patients who have the glycine genotype. Studies show that 17% of Whites and 20% of African-Americans carry the arginine genotype. Leukotriene modifiers block the 5-lipoxygenase (5-LO) and LTC$_4$ synthase pathways, preventing leukotriene-mediated bronchoconstriction. Only a minority of patients benefit from treatment with lT receptor agonists. Polymorphism in 5-LO and LTC$_4$ synthase pathways has been identified. Approximately 5% of patients with asthma have the 5-LO polymorphism. Patients who have the 5-LO polymorphism show a greater improvement in their lung function with zafirlukast therapy compared with patients who have the normal 5-LO genotype. Similarly, polymorphisms in the LTC$_4$ synthase gene may predispose a person to asthma. Patients with the variant LTC$_4$ synthase genotype have higher levels of cysteinyl leukotrienes, which have been linked with severe asthma. The use of lT modifiers in this population may be beneficial.

Variation in the genes involved in the biologic action of inhaled corticosteroids may explain the variability in response and adverse effects to inhaled corticosteroids. Polymorphisms in corticotropin-releasing hormone receptor-1 and T-box expressed in T cells have been associated with improved response in patients with asthma. Although these findings are promising in predicting therapeutic response to asthma medication, their usefulness in clinical practice is still under investigation.

Prospective genetic testing could be beneficial for drugs in which a clear genotype-response relationship has been demonstrated.

DIAGNOSTIC CRITERIA

Key indicators for diagnosing asthma include the following:

- wheezing on exhalation
- history of cough that is worse at night, recurrent chest tightness, and recurrent shortness of breath
- reversible airflow restriction with variability during the day
- increased symptoms with exercise, viral infections, exposure to allergens, change in weather, exposure to irritants, stress, and in women during their menstrual cycle
- awakening at night with symptoms.

When the practitioner suspects asthma, further evaluation is called for by measuring pulmonary function. Obstruction of small airways is indicated if there is a reduction in FEV$_1$, in peak expiratory flow (PEF), in the ratio of FEV$_1$ to fluid volume capacity (FEV$_1$:FVC), or in the mid-expiratory flow rate. If asthma is suspected, a beta-adrenergic agonist is administered and pulmonary function tests are repeated in 15 to 30 minutes to see if there is an improvement in test values. An increase of PEF or FEV$_1$ exceeding 12% from baseline values strongly supports the diagnosis of asthma.

Normal FEV$_1$:FVC is 85% for 8- to 19-year-olds, 80% for 20- to 39-year-olds, 75% for 40- to 59-year-olds, and 70% for 60- to 80-year-olds.

| TABLE 25.1 | Classification of Asthma |

	Clinical Features Before Treatment		
	Symptoms†	**Nighttime Symptoms**	**Lung Function**
Step 4: Severe persistent*	Symptoms throughout the day SABA several times a day Very limited physical activity	Often 7× per week	FEV$_1$ ≤60% predicted FEV$_1$ / FVC 5%
Step 3: Moderate persistent	Daily symptoms Daily use of SABA Some limitation of activity	>1 time a week but not nightly	FEV$_1$ >60%–<80% predicted FEV$_1$ / FVC reduced by 5%

Step 2: Mild persistent	Symptoms >2 times a week but
	  <1 time a day
	Minor limitation of activity
	Use SABA 2 days a week but not
	  daily and not more than 1 × on
	  any day
		3–4 times a month	FEV$_1$ 80% predicted
			FEV$_1$/ FVC normal

Step 1: Mild intermittent	Symptoms ≤2 times a week
	Asymptomatic and normal PEF
	  between exacerbations
	Exacerbations brief (from a few
	  hours to a few days); intensity
	  may vary
	Use SABA ≤ 2 d/wk
	No interference with normal
	  activity
		≤2 times a month	Normal FEV$_1$ between
			  exacerbations
			FEV$_1$ 80% predicted
			FEV$_1$ / FVC normal

FEV$_1$, forced expiratory volume in 1 second; FVC, fluid volume capacity; PEF, peak expiratory flow; SABA, short-acting beta$_2$-adreneric antagonist.
*The presence of one of the features of severity is sufficient to place a patient in that category. An individual should be assigned to the most severe grade in which any feature occurs. The characteristics noted in this table are general and may overlap because asthma is highly variable. Furthermore, an individual's classification may change over time.
†Patients at any level of severity can have mild, moderate, or severe exacerbations. Some patients with intermittent asthma experience severe and life-threatening exacerbations separated by long periods of normal lung function and no symptoms.
(Data from National Asthma Education and Prevention Program, National Heart, Lung and Blood Institute, National Institutes of Health. [2007]. *Expert Panel Report III: Guidelines for the diagnosis and management of asthma: Update on selected topics.* Bethesda, MD: U.S. Department of Health and Human Services.)

Asthma is classified according to four steps, which are based on the frequency and intensity of presenting symptoms: intermittent, mild persistent, moderate persistent, and severe persistent (**Table 25.1**). There can be movement up and down the steps, depending on symptoms.

INITIATING DRUG THERAPY

Because asthma is a chronic disease, medication is needed for treatment. However, nonpharmacologic management of asthma also is an essential part of therapy. Patients must be aware of what triggers their asthma symptoms and should remove or avoid all precipitating factors. Smoke, seasonal allergies, animal dander, and cockroach droppings are strong triggers for asthma exacerbations. Stress and depression can also cause an exacerbation of asthma. Outdoor exercise and exertion also should be avoided when pollution levels are high or temperatures are extreme.

Because GERD plays a role in asthma symptoms, the clinician should evaluate the patient for GERD and treat for the problem. (See Chapter 30 for a discussion of GERD.)

Tight medication control of asthma is desired. Two categories of drugs are used in asthma: long-term medications to control symptoms and quick-relief medications (or rescue medications) to treat acute exacerbations. Long-term control medications include inhaled steroids, cromolyn sodium (Intal, others) and nedocromil (Tilade), leukotriene modifiers, and methylxanthines. Quick-relief medications are bronchodilators (beta$_2$-adrenergic agonists) and systemic (oral) corticosteroids. Medications are available in oral forms, nebulizer solutions, and metered-dose inhalers (MDIs), which deliver a predetermined amount of medication with each inhalation.

Recommendations for the initiation of therapy in neonates to children age 4 include four or more episodes of wheezing in the past year that lasted more than 1 day and that affected sleep *and* those who have risk factors for developing persistent asthma:

- EITHER one of the following: parental history of asthma, a physician diagnosis of atopic dermatitis, or evidence of sensitization to aeroallergens
- OR two of the following: evidence of sensitization to foods, 4% or more peripheral blood eosinophilia, or wheezing apart from colds.

Goals of Asthma Therapy

The goals of asthma therapy, as determined by the National Asthma Education and Prevention Program (NAEPP) (2002), include the following:

- Minimal or no symptoms
- Normal PEF rate with variations of less than 20%
- Minimal episodes of exacerbation
- No emergency visits
- Minimal need for "as needed" beta$_2$-adrenergic agonists
- No limitation of activities
- Minimal adverse effects from medications
- Decrease in or amelioration of the long-term airway remodeling, leading to irreversible lung changes
- Reduced morbidity and mortality

Inhaled Steroids

Inhaled steroids are the most effective therapy in the treatment of asthma and are indicated for long-term prevention of symptoms and the suppression, control, and reversal of inflammation (**Table 25.2**).

Mechanism of Action

Inhaled steroids are very lipophilic and quickly enter target cells of the airway and bind to cytosolic glucocorticoid receptors. Glucocorticoid receptors may directly bind certain transcription factors that are activated by cytokines. Inhaled steroids reduce the number of circulating eosinophils and the number of mast cells in the airways. In addition, they reduce airway hyperresponsiveness by reducing airway inflammation. Chronic treatment with inhaled steroids reduces responsiveness to histamine, cholinergic agonists, exercise, allergens, and irritants. They also reduce symptoms and improve pulmonary function. These drugs provide long-term prevention of symptoms and suppression, control, and reversal of inflammation when taken regularly. However, inhaled steroids are *not* effective for relieving acute episodes.

Dosage

The lowest dose required to control symptoms is recommended. The recommended dose is two to four inhalations two to four times a day. Inhaled corticosteroids now come in powder form, which is thought to deliver more of the drug to the lungs. **Table 25.3** lists comparative doses for inhaled corticosteroids.

The dose-response curve for inhaled corticosteroid treatment begins to flatten for many measures of efficacy at low to medium doses, although some data suggest that higher doses may reduce the risk of exacerbations. Most benefit is achieved with relatively low doses, whereas the risk of adverse effects increases with the dose.

Onset of Action

It takes approximately 2 weeks of continuous therapy for inhaled steroids to achieve maximum effectiveness.

Contraindications

These drugs are contraindicated for use in acute attacks and should be used cautiously in children because of the potential impact on linear growth. However, low-dose inhaled steroids can be used in children younger than age 5 with a spacer and a mask.

Adverse Events

Inhaled steroids usually are well tolerated. Side effects are minimal; the most common adverse events are oropharyngeal candidiasis, dysphonia, hoarseness, cough, and headache. Most of these effects are dose-dependent and can be minimized by using a spacer for delivery and rinsing the mouth after use. Spacers also increase the amount of the drug delivered to the airways. The potential for adverse effects on linear growth from inhaled corticosteroids appears to be dose dependent. In treatment of children who have mild or moderate persistent asthma, low- to medium-dose inhaled corticosteroid therapy may be associated with a possible, but not predictable, adverse effect on linear growth. High doses of inhaled corticosteroids have greater potential for growth suppression. Inhaled corticosteroids appear to have no serious adverse effects on bone mineral density.

Mast Cell Stabilizers

Mechanism of Action

Cromolyn sodium and nedocromil inhibit the release of mediators from mast cells, probably by preventing calcium influx across the mast cell membrane. (See **Table 25.2**.) They suppress the influx of inflammatory cells and antigen-induced bronchial hyperactivity. These drugs are especially useful in reducing bronchospasm induced by stimuli such as exercise and dry air.

These are used as first-line therapy in children because they do not have the potential for negatively affecting linear growth. These agents are not used for the immediate relief of bronchospasm but for long-term control and for exercise-induced asthma. Cromolyn is effective only as an inhaled agent.

Dosage

The recommended dosage is two to four inhalations three or four times a day.

Time Frame for Response

Plasma concentrations are seen approximately 15 minutes after inhalation; the half-life is 45 to 100 minutes. Any of the medication that is absorbed is excreted unchanged in the bile and urine. It takes 1 to 2 weeks for the medication to become effective, but it may take longer to achieve maximum benefit.

Contraindications

These agents are contraindicated in acute asthma exacerbations for immediate relief.

TABLE 25.2	**Overview of Selected Drugs Used to Treat Asthma**		
Generic (Trade) Name and Dosage	**Selected Adverse Events**	**Contraindications**	**Special Considerations**
Inhaled Corticosteroids			
beclomethasone 40 μg/inh 80 μg/inh (QVAR) >6 y: 1 inh bid Children: not for use <5 y Max. 160 mcg/d for children 320 mcg/d for adults	Hoarseness, dry mouth, oral candidiasis, dysphonia, throat irritation, coughing, headache, GI upset, dizziness	Not for primary treatment of acute attack	Early intervention with inhaled corticosteroids can improve asthma control, normalize lung function, and may prevent irreversible airway injury. They must be used on a regular basis to be effective. It is most effective when administered with a spacer. Patients should rinse their mouths after use. Monitor growth with children. High doses of inhaled corticosteroids have some potential for suppression of growth. Consider calcium supplements or hormone replacement for postmenopausal women on doses >1,000 μg/d.
flunisolide (AeroBid) 250 μg/inh Adult: 2–4 inh bid Children: not for use <6 y 6–15 y: as adult dosage	Same as above	Same as above	Same as above
fluticasone propionate (Flovent) 44, 110, 220 μg/inh 88–440 μg bid Rotadisk—50, 100, 250 μg/inh Rotadisk—100–500 μg bid Children 4–11 y: 50–100 μg bid	Same as above	Same as above	Same as above Not used for children <4 y Caution with ketoconazole
triamcinolone acetonide 100 μg/inh (Azmacort) Adults: 2 inh, tid–qid Children: 1–2 inh, tid–qid or 2–4 inh bid	Same as above	Same as above	Same as above
budesonide (Pulmicort Flexhaler) 90 & 180 μg/inh Adults: 360 mcg bid Max. 4 inh bid Children ≤6 180mcg bid (Pulmicort Respules) 0.25 mg, 0.5 mg & 1 mg/2mL 1–8 y 0.5 mg once a day	Same as above	Same as above	Inhalation powder Use once a day in intermittent or mild persistent asthma. Use nebulizer with Respules. Rinse mouth and face (if face mask used) after each use.
ciclesonide (Alvesco) 80 and 160 mcg/inh ≥12 initial dose 80 mcg bid	Same as above	Same as above	

TABLE 25.2 **Overview of Selected Drugs Used to Treat Asthma (*Continued*)**

Generic (Trade) Name and Dosage	Selected Adverse Events	Contraindications	Special Considerations
mometasone (Asmanex Twisthaler) 110 & 220 mcg/inh 4–11 years 110 mcg in pm; ≥12, 220 mcg in pm Max 440 mcg daily	Same as above	Same as above	
Mast Cell Stabilizers			
cromolyn sodium (Intal) MDI: 1 mg/inh Nebulizer solution: 20 mg/ampule Adults: MDI: 2–4 inh tid–qid Nebulizer: 1 ampule tid–qid Children: same as adult	Transient bronchospasm, coughing, dry throat, laryngeal edema, joint swelling and pain, dizziness, dysuria, nausea, headache, rash, unpleasant taste, nasal irritation	Not for treatment of acute attacks	Used for long-term control Very effective for exercise-induced asthma One dose before exposure to irritant or before exercise provides protection for 1–2 h.
nedocromil (Tilade) MDI: 1.75 mg/inh nebulizer solution Adults: 2–4 inh bid–qid Children: 1–2 inh bid–qid	Distinctive taste, dizziness, headache, nausea and vomiting	Same as above	Same as above
Leukotriene Modifiers			
zafirlukast (Accolate) 10/20 mg tablets Adults: 20 mg bid Children: >75 yrs old 10 mg bid	Headache, respiratory tract infection, GI upset, pain, fever, elevated liver enzymes (rare), dizziness	Potentiates warfarin Increases prothrombin time Potentiated by aspirin May be antagonized by erythromycin and theophylline Not for acute asthma attack	Administration with meals decreases bioavailability; take at least 1 h before meals or 2 h after meals. Not for treatment of acute attacks
montelukast sodium (Singular) 4 mg, 5 mg chewable, drug granules 10 mg tablets Children 12–23 mo 4 mg 2–5 yr 4 mg, 14 y: 5 mg in PM Adults: 10 mg in PM	Headache, asthenia/fatigue, fever, GI disturbances, laryngitis, pharyngitis		Use chewable or granules in children. Pregnancy category B Monitor closely with phenobarbital and rifampin.
Beta₂-Adrenergic Agonists			
albuterol (90 µg/inh, 0.5% and 0.83% solution for nebulizers) Adults: Inhaler: 1–2 inh q4–6h Nebulizer solu: 1.25–5 mg in 2–3 mL saline q4–6h	Tachycardia, skeletal muscle tremor, hypokalemia, hyperglycemia, increased lactic acid, dizziness	Patients with preexisting cardiovascular disease may have adverse cardiovascular reactions with inhaled therapy. Antagonized by beta blockers Use with caution in patients taking other sympathomimetics, monoamine oxidase inhibitors, tricyclics.	Very few systemic effects with inhaled therapy Drug of choice for acute bronchospasm Regularly scheduled daily use is not recommended because it does not affect asthma control. Increased use indicates poor asthma control (use of >1 canister per month).

(continued)

TABLE 25.2   **Overview of Selected Drugs Used to Treat Asthma (*Continued*)**

Generic (Trade) Name and Dosage	Selected Adverse Events	Contraindications	Special Considerations
pirbuterol (Maxair Autoinhaler) (200 μg/inh) Adults: 1–2 inh q4–6h with a max of 12 inh/d Children: not recommended	Paradoxical bronchospasms, nervousness, tremors, headache, dizziness, cough, nausea	Not to be used with other inhaled beta agonists Same as above	
terbutaline (Brethine) (0.2 mg/inh) (2.5 and 5 mg tablets and mg/mL) Adults: 2 inh q4–6h Adults: 2.5–5 mg tid 0.25 mg into deltoid; may repeat after 15–30 min with max. 0.5 mg/4 h Children 12–15 y: 2.5 mg tid, otherwise not recommended			
levalbuterol (Xopenex) 0.31 mg/3 mc, 0.63 mg/3 mc, 1.25 mg 6–11 y old 0.31 mg tid >11 y old 61.3–1.25 mg	Same as above	Same as above	May increase serum digoxin levels
Long-Acting Beta₂-Agonists			
salmeterol (Serevent Diskus) 50 mcg/blister ≥4 y old 1 inh bid	Same as above	Same as above	
formoterol (Foradil) 44, 110, and 220 mcg/inh 4–11 y old 88 mcg bid ≥12 88–220 mcg bid	Same as above	Same as above	
Combination Long-Acting Beta₂-Agonist and Inhaled Steroid			
(Advair Diskus) Fluticasone propionate and salmeterol 100/50, 250/50 and 500/50 mcg/inh 4–11 y: 100/50 one inhalation bid Adults: start at 100/50 bid and increase if symptoms persist (Advair HFA) 45/21, 115/21 & 230/21 mcg/inh ≥12 y old 45–115/21 bid budesonide and formoterol (Symbicort) 80/4.5 and 160/4.5 mcg/inh ≥2 puffs bid; max 640/18 mcg daily	URI, hoarseness, dry mouth, headache, cough, palpitations, pharyngitis, dizziness	Acute asthma attack, caution with cardiac disease	Rinse mouth after use.

TABLE 25.2 Overview of Selected Drugs Used to Treat Asthma (*Continued*)

Generic (Trade) Name and Dosage	Selected Adverse Events	Contraindications	Special Considerations
Systemic Corticosteroids methylprednisolone (Medrol) (2, 4, 8, 16, 32-mg tablets) prednisolone (5-mg tablets or 5-mg/mL, 15-mg/mL solutions) prednisone (Deltasone) (1, 2.5, 5, 10, 20, 25-mg tablets or 5-mg/mL solution) Adults: 7.5–60 mg/d Short course: 30–60 mg/d as single dose or 2 divided doses for 5–14 d Children: 0.25–2.0 mg/kg/d in single dose or qid as needed for control Short course: 1–2 mg/kg/d to a maximum of 60 mg/d	*Skin:* acne, decreased wound healing, ecchymosis, petechiae, hirsutism *Central nervous system:* depression, euphoria, headache, personality changes *Cardiovascular:* hypertension *GI:* anorexia, nausea, peptic ulcer *Endocrine:* hyperglycemia, adrenal suppression, weight gain, moon face *Hematologic:* thromboembolism *Musculoskeletal:* muscle wasting, osteoporosis, muscle pain *Fluid and electrolyte:* fluid retention, hypokalemia	Herpes, varicella, tuberculosis, hypertension, peptic ulcer, untreated infections, lactation (with chronic use)	Lowest effective dose should be used. Alternate-day or AM dosing reduces toxicity. Increased efficacy if administered at 3 PM May increase requirements of hypoglycemics Oral contraceptives may block metabolism. Increased risk of tendon rupture with fluoroquinolones Decreased effectiveness of phenytoin, phenobarbital, and rifampin

Adverse Events

Adverse events include headache, nasal irritation, transient bronchospasm, cough, an unpleasant taste, rash, and dry throat.

Leukotriene Modifiers

Leukotrienes are potent biochemical mediators—released from mast cells, eosinophils, and basophils—that contract

TABLE 25.3 Estimated Comparative Daily Dosages for Inhaled Corticosteroids

Drug	Low Daily Dose		Medium Daily Dose		High Daily Dose	
	Adult	Child*	Adult	Child*	Adult	Child*
beclomethasone CFC 42 or 84 mcg/puff	168–504 mcg	84–336 mcg	504–840 mcg	336–672 mcg	>840 mcg	>672 mcg
beclomethasone HFA 40 or 80 mcg/puff	80–240 mcg	80–160 mcg	240–480 mcg	160–320 mcg	>480 mcg	>320 mcg
budesonide DPI 200 mcg/inhalation	200–600 mcg	200–400 mcg	600–1,200 mcg	400–800 mcg	>1,200 mcg	>800 mcg
Inhalation suspension for nebulization (child dose)		0.5 mg		1.0 mg		2.0 mg
flunisolide 250 mcg/puff	500–1,000 mcg	500–750 mcg	1,000–2,000 mcg	1,000–1,250 mcg	>2,000 mcg	>1,250 mcg
fluticasone MDI: 44, 110, or 220 mcg/puff	88–264 mcg	88–176 mcg	264–660 mcg	176–440 mcg	>660 mcg	>440 mcg
DPI: 50, 100, or 250 mcg/inhalation	100–300 mcg	100–200 mcg	300–600 mcg	200–400 mcg	>600 mcg	>400 mcg
triamcinolone acetonide 100 mcg/puff	400–1,000 mcg	400–800 mcg	1,000–2,000 mcg	800–1,200 mcg	>2,000 mcg	>1,200 mcg

*Children ≤12 years of age.

National Asthma Education and Prevention Program, National Heart, Lung and Blood Institute, National Institutes of Health. (2007). *Expert Panel Report III: Guidelines for the diagnosis and management of asthma. Update on selected topics.* Bethesda, MD: U.S. Department of Health and Human Services.

airway smooth muscle, increase vascular permeability, increase mucus secretions, and attract and activate inflammatory cells in the airways of patients who have asthma. Levels of the leukotrienes, potent inflammatory mediators, are increased in asthma. Leukotriene modifiers block the 5-LO and LTC_4 synthase pathways, preventing leukotriene-mediated bronchoconstriction. They are considered an alternative, not a preferred treatment option, for mild, persistent asthma by the Expert Panel. They can also be used as adjunct therapy with inhaled corticosteroids for youths age 12 and older and adults. They are not the preferred, adjunct therapy compared to the addition of long-acting beta₂-adrenergic agonists (LABAs).

Mechanism of Action

Zafirlukast (Accolate), a receptor antagonist, and montelukast sodium (Singular) block binding of leukotrienes to the receptor. These medications reduce symptoms, improve pulmonary function, and inhibit acute asthma attacks. They are also thought to have anti-inflammatory properties because they reduce the eosinophil count.

Contraindications

The leukotriene modifiers, which dilate the bronchial pathways from the beginning of use, are contraindicated for the reversal of acute bronchospasm. Their effect on breast milk is not determined, so caution should be used in lactating women. Patients with liver impairment may require lower doses.

Adverse Events

Adverse events include headache, dizziness, weakness, gastrointestinal symptoms, elevated liver enzyme levels, back pain, myalgias, fever, and infection.

Interactions

Blood levels of zafirlukast are increased by aspirin and decreased by erythromycin (Eramycin, others) and theophylline (Theo-Dur, others). There is an increased effect of warfarin (Coumadin) when taken with zafirlukast. Food decreases the absorption of zafirlukast. Increased blood levels of theophylline, propranolol (Inderal), and warfarin are found when administered with leukotrienes. (See **Table 25.2**.)

Methylxanthines

Methylxanthines inhibit the enzyme phosphodiesterase, preventing the breakdown of cyclic adenosine monophosphate (cAMP). This relaxes bronchial smooth muscle and may prevent the release of endogenous allergens, such as histamine and leukotrienes, from mast cells. The methylxanthines are thought to antagonize prostaglandin-mediated bronchoconstriction and block receptors for adenosine. The main effects are smooth muscle relaxation, central nervous system excitation, and cardiac stimulation. They also increase cardiac output and lower venous pressure. The most common methylxanthine

is theophylline. In elderly patients, use of theophylline is considered unsafe because of concomitant disease that may alter theophylline pharmacokinetics, multiple drug interactions, and the frequent inability to tolerate the medication. These are discussed in Chapter 26.

Beta₂-Adrenergic Agonists

In asthma, SABAs are considered rescue medications that relieve bronchospasm. LABAs last for 12 hours but do not act rapidly. (See **Table 25.2**.)

SABAs are the mainstay of treatment for acute symptoms of bronchospasm, but the regular scheduled use of SABAs is not recommended. The use of more than one SABA canister per month suggests poor control.

The Expert Panel concluded that LABAs are to be used as an adjunct to inhaled corticosteroids for long-term control of symptoms but not to be used for monotherapy or for treatment of acute symptoms or exacerbations. LABAs may be used before exercise to prevent exercise-induced bronchospasm.

For the most part, beta₂-adrenergic agonists are inhaled through a nebulizer or MDI, although they come in oral form. It is important that the patient learn the proper inhalation technique to ensure optimal benefit of the medication. The patient who uses more than one canister of these drugs every month is poorly controlled.

Mechanism of Action

Beta₂-adrenergic agonists provide smooth muscle relaxation after adenylate cyclase activation and an increase in cAMP. This relieves bronchoconstriction.

Dosage

The usual dosage is two or three inhalations every 3 to 4 hours from an MDI. (See **Table 25.2** for doses of oral and nebulizer solutions.) Beta₂-adrenergic agonists work rapidly to increase airflow.

Contraindications

Caution is recommended in patients with ischemic heart disease, hypertension, cardiac arrhythmia, seizure disorder, and hyperthyroidism.

Adverse Events

Adverse events include tachycardia, skeletal muscle tremor, hypokalemia, hyperglycemia, increased lactic acid, headache, hyperglycemia, and dizziness. These drugs can interact with other sympathomimetics, tricyclic antidepressants, and monoamine oxidase inhibitors; they are antagonized by beta blockers.

Cromolyn and Nedocromil

Cromolyn and nedocromil are alternative therapies in children for step-2 therapy. They can also be used as preventive therapy before exercise or unavoidable exposure to allergens.

Mechanism of Action

Cromolyn and nedocromil block chloride channels and modulate mast cell mediator release and eosinophil recruitment.

Dosage

Recommended dosing for both is four times a day.

Contraindications

There are no contraindications.

Adverse Events

Adverse events include an unpleasant taste, sore throat, rash, and cough.

Immunomodulators

Omalizumab is the only available immunomodulator. The Expert Panel recommends that omalizumab may be considered as adjunctive therapy in step 5 or 6 care for patients who have allergies and severe persistent asthma that is inadequately controlled with the combination of high-dose inhaled corticosteroids and LABAs. It is approved for patients age 12 and older with proven sensitivity to aeroallergens. This should be prescribed and administered by a specialist.

Mechanism of Action

Omalizumab, a recombinant deoxyribonucleic acid-derived humanized monoclonal antibody to the Fc portion of the IgE antibody, binds to the portion that prevents binding of IgE to its high-affinity receptor (FcεRI) on mast cells and basophils. The decreased binding of IgE on the surface of mast cells leads to a decrease in the release of mediators in response to allergen exposure. Omalizumab also decreases FcεRI expression on basophils and airway submucosal cells.

Dosage

The dosage is 150 to 375 mg subcutaneously every 2 to 4 weeks. If more than 150 mg is given, multiple sites must be used.

Contraindications

Omalizumab is contraindicated in patients having an acute asthma attack.

Adverse Events

Anaphylaxis occurs in an estimated 0.2% of treated patients, which resulted in an U.S. Food and Drug Administration alert. Most of these reactions occurred within 2 hours of the omalizumab injection, and after the first, second, or third injections. However, reactions have occurred after many injections and after many hours. Therefore, clinicians who administer omalizumab are advised to be prepared and equipped for the identification and treatment of anaphylaxis that may occur, to observe patients for an appropriate period following each injection (the optimal length of the observation is not established), and to educate patients about the risks of anaphylaxis and how to recognize and treat it if it occurs (e.g., using prescription auto injectors for emergency self-treatment and seeking immediate medical care).

Other adverse events include injection-site pain and bruising, upper respiratory infection, and headache.

Systemic Corticosteroids

Systemic corticosteroids are effective in treating an acute asthma exacerbation. (See **Table 25.2.**) The Expert Panel recommends the use of oral systemic corticosteroids in moderate or severe exacerbations. It also recommends that multiple courses of oral systemic corticosteroids, especially more than three courses per year, should prompt a reevaluation of the asthma management plan for a patient.

Mechanism of Action

These drugs inhibit cytokine and mediator release, attenuation of mucus secretion, and upregulation of beta-adrenergic receptor numbers. They also inhibit IgE synthesis, decrease microvascular permeability, and suppress inflammatory cell influx and the inflammatory process. Airway reactivity is reduced by the suppression of airway inflammation, which in turn inhibits mucus secretion, reduces edema of the airway mucosa, and decreases denudation of airway epithelia.

Time Frame for Response

Although these medications are readily absorbed when taken orally, peak plasma concentrations are not achieved for 1 to 2 hours. Short-term (5 days to 2 weeks) therapy with systemic corticosteroids is recommended for acute exacerbations that cannot be controlled with bronchodilators. Symptoms usually improve quickly with oral corticosteroids, within 24 hours.

Dosage

Treatment is usually initiated with an oral dose of 30 to 60 mg of prednisone daily. The daily dose can be tapered or a short course of therapy (5 to 14 days) can be given without tapering. The corticosteroid therapy usually can be discontinued in 5 to 14 days. When symptoms are controlled, the patient is then maintained on inhaled corticosteroids and bronchodilators. If corticosteroids are used in the short term for treating an asthma exacerbation, there is improved efficacy when they are administered at 3 PM because the drug mimics the body's natural cortisone level. Short-term treatment should be continued until the patient achieves 80% PEF or the symptoms resolve.

If corticosteroids are prescribed for long-term therapy to maintain pulmonary function, the lowest possible dose should be used. Corticosteroids can be administered in the morning, either daily or every other day. Dosing late in the day may cause insomnia. Dosing every other day may produce less adrenal suppression.

Contraindications

Oral corticosteroids are contraindicated in untreated infections, lactation (chronic use), and known alcohol intolerance.

Adverse Events

Serious adverse events include psychosis and peptic ulcer. Less serious adverse events include nausea, vomiting, dyspepsia, edema, headache, mood swings, hypokalemia, elevated blood pressure, hyperglycemia, ecchymosis, and acne. Adverse events affecting all body systems are much more common in long-term corticosteroid therapy than in short-term therapy. (See **Table 25.2.**)

Interactions

Systemic corticosteroid therapy may increase the dosage requirements of insulin or oral hypoglycemic agents. Metabolism of corticosteroids may be blocked with oral contraceptives. Corticosteroids combined with quinolones may increase the risk of tendon rupture. The effectiveness of phenytoin (Dilantin), phenobarbital (Luminal), and rifampin (Rifadin) may be decreased when using corticosteroids.

Selecting the Most Appropriate Agent

Asthma treatment consists of a stepwise approach that corresponds to the patient's asthma classification (i.e., the features or severity of asthma; **Figures 25-1 through 25-4**). Control of asthma symptoms should be achieved as quickly as possible.

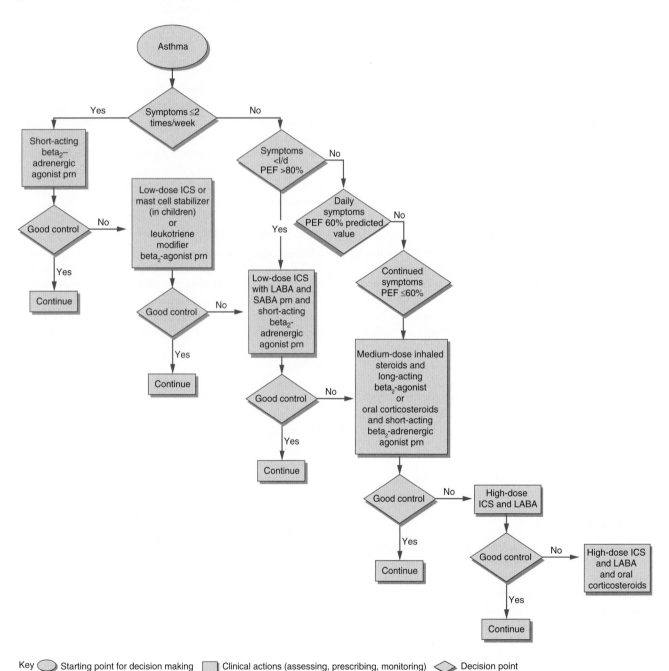

FIGURE 25–1 Treatment algorithm for asthma.

Classifying Asthma Severity and Initiating Therapy in Children

Components of Severity		Intermittent		Mild		Moderate		Severe	
		Ages 0–4	Ages 5–11	Ages 0–4	Ages 5–11	Ages 0–4	Ages 5–11	Ages 0–4	Ages 5–11
Impairment	Symptoms	≤ 2 days/week		≤ 2 days/week but not daily		Daily		Throughout the day	
	Nighttime awakenings	0	< 2x/ month	1-2x/month	3-4x/ month	3-4x/ month	>1x/week but not nightly	>1x/ week	Often 7x/week
	Short-acting beta₂-agonist use for symptom control	≤ 2 days/week		≤ 2 days/week but not daily		Daily		Several times per day	
	Interference with normal activity	None		Minor limitation		Some limitation		Extremely limited	
	Lung Function • FEV₁ (predicted) or peak flow (personal best)	Normal FEV₁ between exacerbations N/A	> 80%	N/A	> 80%	N/A	60–80%	N/A	60%
	• FEV₁/FVC		> 85%		> 85%		75-80%		75%
Risk	Exacerbations requiring oral systemic corticosteroids (consider severity and interval since last exacerbation)	0-1/year (see notes)		≥ 2 exacerbations in 6 months requiring oral systemic corticosteroids, or ≥ 4 wheezing episodes/1 year lasting >1 day AND risk factors for persistent asthma	≥ 2x/year (see notes) Relative annual risk may be related to FEV₁				
Recommended Step for Initiating Therapy (See "Stepwise Approach for Managing Asthma" for treatment steps.) The stepwise approach is meant to assist, not replace, the clinical decision-making required to meet individual patient needs.		Step 1 (for both age groups)		Step 2 (for both age groups)		Step 3 and consider short course of oral systemic cortico-steroids	Step 3: medium-dose ICS option and consider short course of oral systemic cortico-steroids	Step 3 and consider short course of oral systemic cortico-steroids	Step 3: medium-dose ICS option OR step 4 and consider short course of oral systemic cortico-steroids

In 2-6 weeks, depending on severity, evaluate level of asthma control that is achieved.
- Children 0-4 years old: If no clear benefit is observed in 4-6 weeks, stop treatment and consider alternative diagnoses or adjusting therapy.
- Children 5-11 years old: Adjust therapy accordingly.

Key: FEV₁, forced expiratory volume in 1 second; FVC, forced vital capacity; ICS, inhaled corticosteroids; ICU, intensive care unit; N/A, not applicable

Notes:
- Level of severity is determined by both impairment and risk. Assess impairment domain by caregiver's recall of pervious 2–4 weeks. Assign severity to the most severe category in which any feature occurs.
- Frequency and severity of exacerbations may fluctuate over time for patients in any severity category. At present, there are inadequate data to correspond frequencies of exsacerbations with different levels of asthma severity. In general, more frequent and severe exacerbations (e.g., requiring urgent, unscheduled care, hospitalization, or ICU admission) indicate greater underlying disease severity. For treatment purposes, patients with ≥2 exacerbations described above may be considered the same as patients who have persistent asthma, even in the absence of impairment levels consistent with persistent asthma.

FIGURE 25–2 Classification of asthma severity and initiating therapy in children.

Step up if needed (first check inhaler technique, adherence, environmental control, and comorbid conditions)

Assess control

Step down if possible (and asthma is well controlled at least 3 months)

Children 0–4 Years of Age

	Step 1	Step 2	Step 3	Step 4	Step 5	Step 6
	Intermittent Asthma	**Persistent Asthma: Daily Medication** Consult with asthma specialist if step 3 care or higher is required. Consider consultation at step 2.				
Preferred	SABA PRN	Low-dose ICS	Medium-dose ICS	Medium-dose ICS + LABA or montelukast	High-dose ICS + LABA or montelukast	High-dose ICS + LABA or montelukast + Oral cortico-steriods ICS
Alternative		Cromolyn or Montelukast				
Each Step: Patient Education and Environmental Control						
Quick-Relief Medication	• SABA as needed for symptoms. Intensity of treatment depends on severity of symptoms. • With viral respiratory symptoms: SABA q 4–6 hours up to 24 hours (longer with physician consult). Consider short course of oral systemic corticosteroids if exacerbation is severe or patient has history of previous severe exacerbations. Caution: Frequent use of SABA may indicate the need to step up treatment. See text for recommendations on initiating daily long-term-control therapy.					

Children 5–11 Years of Age

	Step 1	Step 2	Step 3	Step 4	Step 5	Step 6
	Intermittent Asthma	**Persistent Asthma: Daily Medication** Consult with asthma specialist if step 4 care or higher is required. Consider consultation at step 3.				
Preferred	SABA PRN	Low-dose ICS	Low-dose ICS + LABA, LTRA, or theophylline *OR* Medium-dose ICS	Medium-dose ICS + LABA	High-dose ICS + LABA	High-dose ICS + LABA + Oral cortico-steriods
Alternative		Cromolyn, LTRA, nedocromil, or theophylline		Medium-dose ICS + LRTA or theophylline	High-dose ICS + LRTA or theophylline	High-dose ICS + LRTA or theophylline + Oral cortico-steriods
Each Step: Patient Education, Environmental Control, and Management of Comorbidities						
	Steps 2–4: Consider subcutaneous allergen immunotherapy for patients who have persistent, allergic asthma.					
Quick-Relief Medication	• SABA as needed for symptoms. Intensity of treatment depends on severity of symptoms: up to 3 treatments at 20-minute intervals as needed. Short course of oral systemic corticosteroids may be needed. Caution: Increasing use of SABA or use >2 days a week for symptom relief (not prevention of EIB) generally indicates inadequate control and the need to step up treatment.					

Notes

• The stepwise approach is meant to assist, not replace, the clinical decision-making required to meet individual patient needs.
• If an alternative treatment is used and response is inadequate, discontinue it and use the preferred treatment before stepping up.
• If clear benefit is not observed within 4–6 weeks, and patient's/family's medication technique and adherence are satisfactory, consider adjusting therapy or an alternative diagnosis.
• Studies on children 0–4 years of age are limited. Step 2 preferred therapy is based on Evidence A. All other recommendations are based on expert opinion and extrapolation from studies in older children.
• Clinicians who administer immunotherapy should be prepared and equipped to identify and treat anaphylaxis that may occur.

Key: **Alphabetical listing is used when more than one treatment option is listed within either preferred or alternative therapy.** ICS, inhaled corticosteroid; LABA, inhaled long-acting beta$_2$-agonist; LTRA, leukotriene receptor antagonist; oral corticosteroids, oral systemic corticosteroids; SABA, inhaled short-acting beta$_2$-agonist.

• The stepwise approach is meant to assist, not replace, the clinical decision-making required to meet individual patient needs.
• If an alternative treatment is used and response is inadequate, discontinue it and use the preferred treatment before stepping up.
• Theophylline is a less desirable alternative due to the need to monitor serum concentration levels.
• Steps 1 and 2 medications are based on Evidence A. Step 3 ICS and ICS plus adjunctive therapy are based on Evidence B for efficacy of each treatment and extrapolation from comparator trials in older children and adults — comparator trials are not available for this age group; steps 4–6 are based on expert opinion and extrapolation from studies in older children and adults.
• Immunotherapy for steps 2–4 is based on Evidence B for house-dust mites, animal danders, and pollens; evidence is weak or lacking for molds and cockroaches. Evidence is strongest for immunotherapy with single allergens. The role of allergy in asthma is greater in children than adults.
• Clinicians who administer immunotherapy should be prepared and equipped to identify and treat anaphylaxis that may occur.

Key: **Alphabetical listing is used when more than one treatment option is listed within either preferred or alternative therapy.** ICS, inhaled corticosteroid; LABA, inhaled long-acting beta$_2$-agonist; LTRA, leukotriene receptor antagonist; SABA, inhaled short-acting beta$_2$-agonist.

FIGURE 25–3 Stepwise management of asthma long term in children.

Key: Alphabetical order is used when more than one treatment option is listed within either preferred or alternative therapy. ICS, inhaled corticosteroid; LABA long-acting inhaled beta₂-agonist; LTRA, leukotriene receptor antagonist; SABA, inhaled short-acting beta₂-agonist

Notes:

- The stepwise approach is meant to assist, not replace, the clinical decision-making required to meet individual patient needs.
- If alternative treatment is used and response is inadequate, discontinue it and use the preferred treatment before stepping up.
- Zileuton is a less desirable alternative due to limited studies as adjunctive therapy and the need to monitor liver function. Theophylline requires monitoring of serum concentration levels.
- In step 6, before oral corticosteroids are introduced, a trial of high-dose ICS + LABA + either LTRA, theophylline, or zileuton may be considered, although this approach has not been studied in clinical trials.
- Step 1, 2, and 3 preferred therapies are based on Evidence A; step 3 alternative therapy is based on Evidence A for LTRA, Evidence B for theophylline, and Evidence D for zileuton. Step 4 preferred therapy is based on Evidence B, and alternative therapy is based on Evidence B for LTRA and theophylline and Evidence D zileuton. Step 5 preferred therapy is based on Evidence B. Step 6 preferred therapy is based on (EPR — 2 1997) and Evidence B for omalizumab.
- Immunotherapy for steps 2–4 is based on Evidence B for house-dust mites, animal danders, and pollens; evidence is weak or lacking for molds and cockroaches. Evidence is strongest for immunotherapy with single allergens. The role of allergy in asthma is greater in children than in adults.
- Clinicians who administer immunotherapy or omalizumab should be prepared and equipped to identify and treat anaphylaxis that may occur.

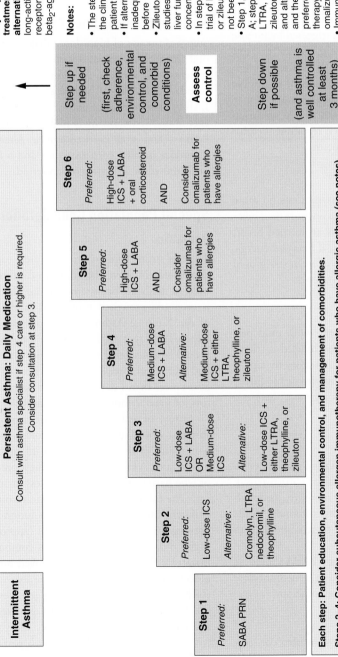

FIGURE 25–4 Stepwise management of asthma for those age 12 and up.

To gain control, treatment may be started at the step most appropriate to the severity of symptoms, or a higher level. There needs to be a step up if symptoms increase or are uncontrolled. If symptoms are controlled for more than 3 months, there can be a step down that is closely monitored.

A rescue course of systemic corticosteroids may be needed at any time and for patients diagnosed in any step for quick symptomatic relief. Acute exacerbations of asthma can be treated with inhaled, short-acting beta$_2$-adrenergic agonists. If the patient has a good response to systemic corticosteroid therapy (PEF 70% normal), it may be used to manage the condition with close follow-up. The dose of systemic corticosteroids is 1 to 2 mg/kg/d in a single dose for children and 30 to 60 mg/d for adults.

Exercise-Induced Bronchospasm

Exercise-induced bronchospasm is asthma triggered by intense physical activity. The treatment is long-term control therapy, pretreatment before exercise with SABAs, leukotriene receptor antagonists, cromolyn, or nedocromil. Frequent or chronic use of LABAs for pretreatment is discouraged because it may disguise poorly controlled persistent asthma. A warm-up period or a mask or scarf over the mouth is recommended for cold-induced, exercise-induced bronchospasm.

First-Line Therapy (Step 1)

In the patient with intermittent asthma (symptoms no more than twice a week and nighttime awakenings no more than twice a month), the recommended treatment is an inhaled SABA as needed. No daily medication is needed. If beta$_2$-adrenergic agonists are used more than twice a week, or a canister is used in a month, the patient should move up to step 2.

Second-Line Therapy (Step 2)

The treatment recommendation for patients with mild persistent asthma is step 2. This is a low-dose inhaled corticosteroid. An alternative to inhaled anti-inflammatory therapy is cromolyn, nedocromil, theophylline, or leukotriene modifiers. If symptoms are not controlled with this regimen, there is a need to move to step 3.

Third-Line Therapy (Step 3)

Step 3 treatment consists of a low-dose inhaled corticosteroid and a LABA or a medium-dose inhaled corticosteroid. Alternatives include adding a leukotriene modifier, theophylline, or zileuton to low-dose inhaled corticosteroids. If the patient is not controlled on this regimen, there is the need to move to step 4.

In children younger than age 5, either a LABA should be added to a low-dose inhaled corticosteroid or a medium-dose inhaled corticosteroid should be used as monotherapy.

Fourth-Line Therapy (Step 4)

Step 4 consists of the use of a medium-dose inhaled corticosteroid and a LABA. Oral corticosteroids are added as needed.

Alternatives include adding a leukotriene modifier, theophylline, or zileuton to medium-dose inhaled corticosteroids. If the patient is not controlled, there is the need to move to step 5.

Fifth-Line Therapy (Step 5)

Step 5 is the use of high-dose inhaled corticosteroids and a LABA and the consideration of omalizumab in patients with allergies. Uncontrolled patients should move to step 6.

For neonates up to children age 4, the recommendation is a high-dose inhaled corticosteroid and a LABA or montelukast. For children ages 5 to 11, a high-dose inhaled corticosteroid and a LABA is recommended. An alternative regimen is a high-dose inhaled corticosteroid and a leukotriene modifier or theophylline.

Sixth Line Therapy (Step 6)

Step 6 is the use of high-dose inhaled corticosteroids, LABAs, oral corticosteroids, and consideration of omalizumab in patients with allergies. In neonates to children age 4, recommended treatment is high-dose inhaled corticosteroids and LABAs or montelukast and oral corticosteroids. For children ages 5 to 11, treatment is high-dose inhaled corticosteroids, LABAs, and oral corticosteroids. Alternative treatment is high-dose inhaled corticosteroids and a leukotriene modifier or theophylline and oral corticosteroids.

Special Population Considerations

Pediatric

There is strong evidence from clinical trials that inhaled corticosteroids improve the control of asthma for children with mild to moderate persistent asthma. The lowest effective dose is used and growth is monitored carefully. It is the opinion of the National Asthma Education and Prevention Program Expert Panel that the initiation of long-term control therapies should be considered in infants and young children who have had more than three episodes of wheezing in the past year that lasted more than 1 day and affected sleep and who have risk factors for the development of asthma. Risk factors include parental history of asthma or diagnosed atopic dermatitis, allergic rhinitis, wheezing apart from colds, and peripheral blood eosinophils. This applies also to infants and young children who require symptomatic treatment more than twice per week or who have severe exacerbations less than 6 weeks apart.

The following medications are recommended for use by children: budesonide nebulizer solution (approved for children ages 1 to 8), fluticasone DPI (approved for children age 4 and older), salmeterol DPI and combination product (salmeterol + fluticasone) DPI (approved for children age 4 and older), montelukast in 4-mg chewable tablets (approved for children age 2 to 6) and in 4-mg granules (approved down to age 1), and cromolyn nebulizer (approved for children age 2 and older).

Data in children followed for 6 years suggest that low to medium doses of inhaled corticosteroids may decrease growth by about 1 cm in the first year of treatment, but this effect is not sustained in subsequent years of treatment and the final predicted height is reached. The height of any child taking corticosteroids, either oral or inhaled, should be monitored; if growth retardation is seen, the benefits of asthma control should be weighed against the possibility of growth delay.

Oral corticosteroids can cause growth retardation in young children and are used only if the exacerbation of asthma is moderate to severe. Instead of using inhalers, children age 5 and younger should use nebulizers or MDIs with a face mask to promote maximum delivery of inhaled medications. **Figures 25-2 through 25-4** summarize asthma severity and treatment for infants and children younger than age 5, from ages 5 to 11, and from age 12 and up.

It is recommended that a written asthma action plan is shared with the childcare or school setting so that treatment can be carried over into that setting.

Women

There may be a decrease in bone mineral content with inhaled corticosteroids, increasing the risk for osteoporosis. Postmenopausal women are already at risk for osteoporosis, so the practitioner should prescribe supplemental calcium, 1,000 to 1,500 mg/d, and vitamin D, 400 to 800 U/d.

Asthma management during pregnancy is similar to management in nonpregnant women, with medications that are safe and well tolerated by the mother and fetus. If oral corticosteroids are prescribed, blood glucose levels should be monitored regularly because of the drug's association with an increased risk for gestational diabetes. Asthma control should be evaluated at each prenatal visit; asthma worsens in about one-third of women and improves in about one-third of women during pregnancy. Medications should be adjusted accordingly.

There are proven negative effects from exacerbations and poor control on pregnancy outcome, whereas there are clear benefits of good control. Patient education about the importance of good asthma control is essential for improving compliance and self-monitoring.

Asthma medications are excreted in small and varying amounts into breast milk. The NAEPP found that there was no contraindication for the use of prednisone, theophylline, cromolyn, antihistamines, inhaled corticosteroids, or inhaled β agonists for breast-feeding. Patients should be instructed, and strongly encouraged, to continue their asthma medications postpartum with or without breast-feeding.

Geriatric

Because older patients with cardiovascular disease may experience tremors and tachycardia with beta$_2$-adrenergic agonists, it is helpful to use combination beta$_2$-adrenergic agonists and anticholinergics to prevent this. Because theophylline clearance is decreased in elderly patients, the build-up of theophylline may exacerbate a pre-existing heart condition, so the drug should be used cautiously in the elderly.

In elderly patients, prolonged use of systemic corticosteroids can have an adverse effect on bone metabolism by decreasing calcium deposition and enhancing calcium resorption, predisposing some patients to osteoporosis.

MONITORING PATIENT RESPONSE

After beginning therapy, the patient should be evaluated in 1 to 2 weeks. Subsequent evaluations every 1 to 6 months are necessary to determine if the asthma is well controlled. If there is good control, the patient should be moved down a treatment step; if control is poor, the patient should be moved up a treatment step. Before moving the patient up to the next step, a careful history of medication use and technique and exposure to triggers is taken. For instance, if the patient has been diagnosed with moderate persistent asthma and has been well controlled on a low-dose inhaled steroid and a LABA with a SABA as needed, he or she can be tried on a low-dose inhaled steroid with the SABA used as needed. The patient monitors his or her PEF and uses the SABA if the PEF drops below 80% of predicted value or if there is increased wheezing. If asthma is not controlled with the intervention initiated, the prescriber must assume that the patient is at the next step and initiate treatment accordingly.

The patient should be referred to a specialist if there is difficulty controlling the asthma, if a child ages 0 to 4 requires step 3 or higher, or if a child ages 5 to 11 requires step 4 or higher. Also, specialist care is recommended if a patient has required hospitalization during an exacerbation or immunotherapy or immunomodulators are indicated.

PATIENT EDUCATION

Medication

The various types of delivery systems for inhaled medications include inhalers, nebulizers, disks, and rotosystems. Each product includes information on how many inhalations are contained in the device. It is important that the patient does not run out of medications. The patient must learn the correct way to use each system and should have an extra system on hand as a backup for use at all times. These systems are described and a detailed description of their use is provided in **Box 25.1**.

Internet sites for information on asthma include www.aaaai.org (American Academy of Allergy, Asthma and Immunology), www.lungusa.org/asthma (American Lung Association), and www.nhlbl.gov/guidelines/asthma (guidelines from the National Asthma Education and Prevention Program).

The patient with asthma is prescribed a peak flow meter, which measures PEF, and is instructed to monitor and record PEF. PEF rates measure control and exacerbations of asthma. This monitoring allows the patient to determine when

BOX 25.1

Directions for Use of Delivery Devices for Asthma Medications

METERED-DOSE INHALER (MDI) (FOR USE IN ≥ 5 YEARS)

1. Remove the cap and hold the inhaler upright.
2. Shake the inhaler.
3. Tilt your head back slightly and breathe out.
4. Use the inhaler in any of these ways:
   a. Open mouth with inhaler 1 to 2 inches away
   b. Use spacer
   c. In the mouth
5. Press down on the inhaler to release the drug as you start to breathe in slowly.
6. Breathe in slowly for 3 to 5 seconds.
7. Hold your breath for 10 seconds to allow the drug to reach deeply into your lungs.
8. Repeat puffs as directed, waiting 1 minute between puffs.
9. Rinse your mouth after use if using an inhaled corticosteroid.

BREATH-ACTIVATED MDI

1. Remove the cover.
2. Breathe out to empty your lungs.
3. Make a tight seal around the mouthpiece.

DISKHALER

1. Lift the back of the lid until it points straight up and down to pierce the blister of drug.
2. Breathe out to empty your lungs.
3. With the diskhaler level, place the mouthpiece between your teeth with lips snug around it and tongue out of the way. Keeping the device horizontal prevents the powder from spilling.
4. Breathe deeply and quickly.
5. Hold your breath for 10 seconds to allow the drug to reach deeply into your lungs.
6. Repeat as directed.
7. Clean the device regularly with the brush provided.
8. Don't cover the air inlet holes at the base.
9. Rinse your mouth after use.

DISKUS

1. Open the diskus by holding the outer case in one hand and putting the thumb of the other hand on the thumb grip and push as far as it will go. Keep the diskus horizontal.
2. Slide the lever away until you hear a click.
3. Breathe out to empty your lungs.
4. Place the mouthpiece between your teeth with your lips snug around it.

5. Breathe in as deeply and as quickly as possible.
6. Hold your breath for 10 seconds to allow the drug to reach deeply into your lungs.
7. Close the diskus by sliding the thumb grip backwards as far as it will go. This automatically resets the lever to its initial position.
8. If a second dose is needed, close the diskus and repeat.
9. Rinse your mouth after use.

SPACER WITH MASK FOR CHILDREN UNDER AGE 3

1. Remove the cap from the canister.
2. Shake the canister.
3. Place the canister upside down with the mouthpiece in the rubber opening of the spacer device.
4. Place the mask of the spacer over the child's mouth and nose, making a good seal.
5. Press down on the canister, releasing a puff of medication into the spacer.
6. Hold the mask in place until the child has taken at least 6 breaths, as seen from movement of a window on the mask.
7. Rinse the mask with warm water weekly and let it dry in room air.

SPACER WITH MOUTHPIECE FOR CHILDREN OVER AGE 3

1. Remove the cap from the canister.
2. Shake the canister.
3. Place the canister upside down with the mouthpiece in the rubber opening of the spacer device.
4. Have the child take a deep breath out to empty the lungs.
5. Place the mouthpiece in the child's mouth.
6. Press down on the canister, releasing a puff of medication into the spacer.
7. Have the child breathe in deeply and slowly.
8. Have the child hold his or her breath for 10 seconds.
9. Repeat to be sure that all of the drug is used.

NEBULIZER WITH MASK OR MOUTHPIECE

1. Measure the drug into the cup below the mask or mouthpiece.
2. Put the mask over the mouth and nose or the mouthpiece between the teeth with the tongue out of the way.
3. Switch on the machine.
4. Use the nebulizer for 10 to 15 minutes until all of the drug in the cup has been used.
5. Rinse the nebulizer with warm water after each use.

TABLE 25.4	Normal Predicted Average Peak Expiratory Flow (PEF) (L/minute)

Men						Women						Adolescents		
	Height (in)						Height (in)							
Age (y)	60	65	70	75	80	Age (y)	55	60	65	70	75	Height (in)	Boys	Girls
15	511	531	548	564	578	15	423	438	451	463	473	50	249	248
20	554	575	594	611	626	20	444	460	474	486	497	51	262	261
25	580	603	622	640	656	25	455	471	485	497	509	52	276	275
30	594	617	637	655	672	30	458	475	489	502	513	53	289	288
35	599	622	643	661	677	35	458	474	488	501	512	54	303	302
40	597	620	641	659	675	40	453	469	483	496	507	55	316	315
45	591	613	633	651	668	45	446	462	476	488	499	56	329	328
50	580	602	622	640	656	50	437	453	466	478	489	57	343	342
55	566	588	608	625	640	55	427	442	455	467	477	58	356	355
60	551	572	591	607	622	60	415	430	443	454	464	59	370	369
65	533	554	572	588	603	65	403	417	430	441	451	60	383	382
70	515	535	552	568	582	70	390	404	416	427	436	61	397	395
75	496	515	532	547	560	75	377	391	402	413	422	62	410	409
												63	423	422
												64	437	436
												65	450	449
												66	464	462
												67	477	476
												68	491	489
												69	504	503
												70	517	516

NOTE: All tables are averages and are based on tests with a large number of people. The peak flow of an individual can vary widely. Individuals at altitudes above sea level should be aware that peak flow readings may be lower than those provided in the tables. (Reproduced with permission of Glaxo Wellcome Inc., Research Triangle Park, NC.)

additional intervention is warranted. The practitioner should bring the record of PEF readings for review at each office visit. Predicted PEF values are shown in **Table 25.4**, although these may vary by individual. The best personal value is determined by having the patient measure PEF rates twice a day for 2 weeks during a symptom-free period, or after maximum therapy. The patient is instructed to do three measurements and take the best of the three. Instructions on using a peak flow meter are found in **Box 25.2**.

The patient is then taught the concept of zones as they pertain to PEF monitoring. The zones are green, yellow, and red (**Box 25-3**). If the patient is in the green zone, treatment remains as usual. If he or she is in the yellow zone, an inhaled beta$_2$-adrenergic agonist should be taken right away. The red zone signals a medical emergency, and the patient should take an inhaled beta$_2$-adrenergic agonist at once and seek medical treatment.

All patients with asthma should have an action plan. The contents are outlined in **Box 25.3**. There are multiple websites for information on asthma. They are listed in **Box 25.4.**

Lifestyle Changes

Since asthma is associated with allergies and is exacerbated when the patient is exposed to allergens, the patient should be aware of triggers and avoid them. Many asthmatics are sensitive to scents and should avoid them when possible. If asthma is induced by exposure to cold, one should gradually warm up or wear protection over the nose and mouth.

BOX 25.2

How to Use Your Peak Flow Meter

A peak flow meter is a device that measures how well air moves out of your lungs. During an asthma episode, the airways of the lungs usually begin to narrow slowly. The peak flow meter may tell you if there is narrowing in the airways hours—sometimes even days—before you have any asthma symptoms.

By taking your medicine(s) early (before symptoms), you may be able to stop the episode quickly and avoid a severe asthma episode. Peak flow meters are used to check your asthma the way that blood pressure cuffs are used to check high blood pressure.

The peak flow meter also can be used to help you and your doctor:

- Learn what makes your asthma worse
- Decide if your treatment plan is working well
- Decide when to add or stop medicine
- Decide when to seek emergency care

A peak flow meter is most helpful for patients who must take asthma medicine daily. Patients age 5 and older are usually able to use a peak flow meter. Ask your doctor or nurse to show you how to use a peak flow meter.

HOW TO USE YOUR PEAK FLOW METER

- Do the following five steps with your peak flow meter:
  1. Move the indicator to the bottom of the numbered scale.
  2. Stand up.
  3. Take a deep breath, filling your lungs completely.

4. Place the mouthpiece in your mouth and close your lips around it. Do not put your tongue inside the hole.
5. Blow out as hard and fast as you can in a single blow.
- Write down the number you get. If you cough or make a mistake, don't write down the number, do it over again.
- Repeat steps 1 through 5 two more times and write down the best of the three blows in your asthma diary.

FIND YOUR PERSONAL BEST PEAK FLOW NUMBER

Your personal best peak flow number is the highest peak flow number you can achieve over a 2- to 3-week period when your asthma is under good control. Good control is when you feel good and do not have any asthma symptoms.

Each patient's asthma is different, and your best peak flow may be higher or lower than the peak flow of someone of your same height, weight, and sex. This means that it is important for you to find your own personal best peak flow number. Your treatment plan needs to be based on your own personal best peak flow number.

To find out your personal best peak flow number, take peak flow readings:

- At least twice a day for 2 to 3 weeks
- When you wake up and between noon and 2:00 PM
- Before and after you take your short-acting inhaled beta$_2$-agonist for quick relief, if you take this medicine
- As instructed

Data from National Asthma Education and Prevention Program, National Heart, Lung and Blood Institute, National Institutes of Health. (2002). *Expert Panel Report II: Guidelines for the diagnosis and management of asthma.* Bethesda, MD: U.S. Department of Health and Human Services.

BOX 25.3

Asthma Action Plan

Written asthma action plans must include two important elements:

DAILY MANAGEMENT

- What medicine to take daily, including the specific names of the medications
- What actions to take to control environmental factors that worsen asthma

HOW TO RECOGNIZE AND HANDLE WORSENING ASTHMA

- What signs, symptoms, and PEF measurements (if peak flow monitoring is used) that indicate worsening asthma
- What medications to take in response to these signs
- What symptoms and PEF measurements that indicate the need for urgent medical attention
- Emergency telephone numbers for the physician, emergency department, and person or service to transport the asthmatic for emergency care

BOX 25.4

Asthma Education Resources

American Academy of Allergy, Asthma and Immunology
1-414-272-6071
555 East Wells Street, Suite 100
Milwaukee, WI 53202-3823
www.aaaai.org
American Lung Association 1-800-586-4872
61 Broadway
New York, NY 10006
www.lungusa.org
Association of Asthma Educators 1-888-988-7747
1215 Anthony Avenue
Columbia, SC 29201
www.asthmaeducators.org

Asthma and Allergy Foundation of America
1-800-727-8462
1233 20th Street, N.W., Suite 402
Washington, DC 20036
www.aafa.org
National Heart, Lung, and Blood Institute Information Center 1-301-592-8573
P.O. Box 30105
Bethesda, MD 20824-0105
www.nhlbi.nih.gov

Case Study

M. L. is a 15-year-old boy who plays soccer for his school team. He has noticed that when running, he sometimes has trouble catching his breath. He also reports an increased runny nose and itchy eyes. He has a frequent dry cough and is awakened with coughing spells at least four times a week. His mother and father have seasonal allergies and his mother has asthma. This morning he woke up and heard "funny sounds" when he took a breath. His coughing increased when he took a deep breath. In his nose, the mucosa is pale and swollen bilaterally. His lungs have bilateral expiratory wheezing; respirations are 22 and PEF is 400. His heart shows a normal sinus rhythm, with no murmurs or gallops; pulse is 72; and there is no cyanosis.

DIAGNOSIS: MILD PERSISTENT ASTHMA

1. List specific goals of therapy for M. L.
2. What drug therapy would you prescribe?
3. What are the parameters for monitoring the success of the therapy?
4. Discuss specific patient education based on the prescribed therapy.
5. List one or two adverse reactions for the selected agent(s) that would cause you to change therapy.
6. If the patient is still having symptoms with the prescribed therapy, what would be your next course of action?
7. What lifestyle changes would you recommend for M. L.?
8. When would you instruct him to return for evaluation?
9. If upon return his symptoms have resolved, what would be your course of action?

BIBLIOGRAPHY

Starred references are cited in the text.

Belle, D. G., & Singh, H. (2008). Genetic factors in drug metabolism. *American Family Physician, 77*(11), 1553–1568.

*Bryant-Stephans, T. (2009). Asthma disparities in urban environments. *Journal of Allergy and Clinical Immunology, 123*(6), 1119–1206.

Centers for Disease Control and Prevention. (1998). Surveillance for asthma—United States, 1960–1995. *MMWR, 47*(SS1), 1–28.

*Kamble, S., & Bharma, M. (2009). Incremental direct expenditures of treating asthma in the United States. *Journal of Asthma 46*, 73–80.

*National Asthma Education and Prevention Program, National Heart, Lung and Blood Institute, National Institutes of Health. (2007). *Expert Panel Report III: Guidelines for the diagnosis and management of asthma. Update on selected topics.* Bethesda, MD: U.S. Department of Health and Human Services.

Yawn, B. (2009). New asthma guidelines. *American Family Physician, 79*(9), 727–731. http://www.cdc.gov/nchs/fastats/asthma.htm, accessed 5/30/2010.

CHAPTER 26

Virginia P. Arcangelo

Chronic Obstructive Pulmonary Disease

Chronic obstructive pulmonary disease (COPD), also called *chronic obstructive lung disease,* is a pulmonary disorder characterized by small airway obstruction and reduction in expiratory flow rate. COPD is the fourth leading cause of death in the United States and affects 10.1% of the population (Buist, et al., 2007). It accounts for 120,000 deaths a year. The cost of caring for patients with COPD in the United States exceeds $37 billion annually. By 2020, it is expected to be the third leading cause of death. COPD begins early in life, but significant symptoms do not usually appear until the middle years. The prevalence of COPD increases with age. Prevalence is also higher in men than in women and in whites compared with other racial groups. One of the biggest problems with COPD is that there are no clinical findings during the early stages of the disease process, and by the time the patient is symptomatic, the disease has progressed significantly.

The most common forms of COPD are chronic bronchitis and emphysema. Chronic bronchitis is diagnosed in patients who have a history of excessive secretion of bronchial mucus with a productive cough for 3 months or longer in at least 2 consecutive years. The lungs of patients with emphysema are characterized by an abnormal, permanent enlargement of the air spaces distal to the terminal bronchiole, with destruction of the acinar wall. The patient usually demonstrates some features of both types of COPD, but one dominates.

CAUSES

The most common cause is smoking: smokers have a 30 times greater risk of death from COPD. Other risk factors are air pollution, occupational exposure to respiratory irritants, chronic respiratory infections, and hyperresponsive airways due to asthma.

Emphysema, unlike chronic bronchitis, may also result from a genetic deficiency of the protein alpha$_1$-antitrypsin. This protein deficiency can trigger early-onset emphysema, even in nonsmokers. Both parents must carry the gene for the disease to be acquired by offspring. The genetic factor accounts for only approximately 3% of cases.

PATHOPHYSIOLOGY

Chronic bronchitis, defined as cough and sputum production for most days over 3 months for 2 consecutive years, is marked by thickened bronchial walls, hyperplastic and hypertrophied mucus glands, and mucosal inflammation in the bronchial walls and airways. Emphysema, defined as enlargement of the airways, is characterized by permanent destruction of the alveoli as a result of irreversible destruction of elastin, a protein in the lung that maintains the strength of the alveolar walls. The destruction of elastin causes enlargement of air spaces as the walls of the small airways and alveoli lose elasticity. In addition, there is a narrowing of the bronchioles, limiting airflow to the lungs. The walls of the airways thicken, closing off some of the smaller air passages and narrowing larger ones. Air enters the alveoli during expansion of the lung in inhalation but cannot escape during exhalation because the air passages collapse. Air is trapped in the lungs, causing uneven blood flow and airflow to the walls of the alveoli. In some alveoli, there is adequate blood flow but little air; in others, there is adequate air but inadequate blood flow. This results in a decreased oxygen exchange. It becomes more difficult for air to flow through narrow airways, and the patient's respiratory muscles tire. Inadequate air reaches the alveoli, causing inadequate removal of carbon dioxide from the lungs. This results in a buildup of carbon dioxide and a decreased level of oxygen in the blood. Pathological changes in COPD occur in the large (central) airways, the small (peripheral) bronchioles, and the lung parenchyma. The pathogenic mechanisms are not clear but most likely involve diverse mechanisms. The increased number of activated polymorphonuclear leukocytes and macrophages release elastases in a manner that cannot effectively be counteracted by antiproteases, resulting in lung destruction. The primary offender has been human leukocyte elastase, with a possible synergistic role suggested for proteinase 3 and macrophage-derived matrix proteinases, cysteine proteinases, and a plasminogen activator. Apoptosis or necrosis of exposed cells can be caused by increased oxidative stress caused by free radicals in cigarette smoke, the oxidants released by phagocytes, and polymorphonuclear cells. Accelerated aging and autoimmune mechanisms are also thought to have roles in the pathogenesis of COPD.

The cellular composition of the airway inflammation in COPD is predominantly mediated by the neutrophils. Cigarette smoking induces macrophages to release neutrophil chemotactic factors and elastases, thus unleashing tissue destruction. Severity of airflow obstruction has correlated with greater induced sputum neutrophilia that is also more prevalent in patients with chronic cough and sputum production and is associated with an accelerated decline in lung function. Macrophages also play an important role through macrophage-derived matrix metalloproteinases (MMPs). Cigarette smoke causes neutrophil influx and is required for the secretion of MMPs, suggesting that both neutrophils and macrophages are required for the development of emphysema. Studies have shown that T lymphocytes, particularly $CD8^+$, in addition to the macrophages, play an important role in the pathogenesis of smoking-induced airflow limitation. Evidence supports that the dysregulation of apoptosis and defective clearance of apoptotic cells by macrophages play a prominent role in airway inflammation, particularly in emphysema.

Diagnostic Criteria

The symptoms of COPD depend on whether the disease results from chronic bronchitis or pulmonary emphysema. Chronic bronchitis presents with wheezing; copious, purulent sputum production; and shortness of breath. For a diagnosis of chronic bronchitis to be made, there must be cough and sputum production on most days for more than 3 months during 2 consecutive years. Emphysema presents with dyspnea with light exertion; scant, thick sputum production; and possibly a slight cough with little sputum production. A patient presenting with symptoms of COPD usually has lost between 50% and 70% of lung tissue.

Pulmonary function studies are essential in diagnosing COPD. Forced vital capacity is the maximum volume of air that can be exhaled with force. This indicates lung size. Forced expiratory volume measures the maximum volume of air expired in 1 second (FEV_1). Lung function as measured by FEV_1 diminishes with age at a rate of approximately 25 mL/y from age 35 on. Smoking increases the rate of decline. FEV_1 and symptoms are used to stage COPD (**Table 26.1**).

INITIATING DRUG THERAPY

COPD is a progressive disease, but early intervention is beneficial in relieving symptoms and slowing disease progression. Avoidance of irritants such as allergens and smoke is essential in managing asthma and COPD. Outdoor exercise and exertion should be avoided when pollution levels are high or temperatures are extreme. The patient with COPD is taught how to conserve energy to maintain quality of life. For example, the most strenuous activity should be done in the early morning, when the patient has the most energy.

Drug therapy is initiated when the patient becomes symptomatic. Patients with COPD usually are older and are more

TABLE 26.1	**Stages of COPD**	
Stage 0	At risk	Chronic cough and sputum production Lung function normal
Stage I	Mild	Mild airflow limitation FEV_1/FVC <70% but FEV_1 ≥80% predicted value Usually chronic cough and sputum production
Stage II	Moderate	Airflow limitation FEV_1/FVC >70% 50%≤FEV_1 <80% predicted value Progression of symptoms with shortness of breath, especially on exertion
Stage III	Severe	Further worsening of airflow limitation FEV_1/FVC <70% 30%≤FEV_1 <50% predicted value Increased shortness of breath, repeated exacerbations
Stage IV	Very severe	Severe airflow limitation FEV_1/FVC <70% FEV_1 <30% predicted value plus chronic respiratory failure

FEV_1, forced expiratory volume in 1 second; FVC, forced vital capacity.

susceptible to the side effects of medications, so a stepwise approach is useful in treatment. The dose response of FEV_1 to most bronchodilators is flatter in COPD than in asthma, while the rate of adverse effects increases progressively with dosing. Thus, managing COPD is unlike managing many other chronic diseases. In hypertension, for example, it is common to start with a low dose and increase the dosing progressively to attain the target blood pressure. In COPD, combining bronchodilators of different classes is more often the strategy used to achieve a better FEV_1 response while limiting adverse effects.

Both the Global Initiative for Chronic Obstructive Lung Disease (GOLD) and the American Thoracic Society and European Respiratory Society ATS/ERS guidelines for COPD emphasize treatment based on disease severity. Somewhat confusingly, the GOLD guidelines emphasize postbronchodilatory FEV_1 in defining severity, whereas the ATS/ERS guidelines focus more on the nature of the symptoms (e.g., intermittent versus persistent).

Goals of Drug Therapy

Although COPD is not reversible, the major goals of therapy are to slow the progression of the disease, prevent acute exacerbations, maintain quality of life (i.e., minimize limitation of activities and loss of productivity), improve the symptoms associated with obstruction, improve exercise tolerance, improve sleep quality, and reduce mortality. Drug therapy relieves cough and bronchospasm and enhances airflow. Drugs used to treat COPD include beta$_2$ agonists, anticholinergics, theophylline, corticosteroids, and antibiotics for infectious processes (**Table 26.2**).

TABLE 26.2 Overview of Selected Agents Used to Treat COPD

Generic (Trade) Name and Dosage	Selected Adverse Events	Contraindications	Special Considerations
Beta$_2$ Agonists			
albuterol (Proventil) 90-μg/inhalation, 0.5% and 0.83% solution for nebulizers Inhaler: 1–2 inhalations q4–q6 Inhalable solution: 2.5 mg (0.5 mL) of 0.5% solution diluted with 3 mL normal saline solution or 3 mL of 0.083% solution	Tachycardia, skeletal muscle tremor, increased lactic acid levels, hypokalemia, hyperglycemia, dizziness	Antagonized by beta blockers in patients taking other sympathomimetic drugs, monoamine oxidase inhibitors, tricyclic antidepressants Patients with pre-existing cardiovascular disease may have adverse cardiovascular reactions with inhaled therapy.	Very few systemic effects with inhaled therapy Drug of choice for acute bronchospasm At least 1 min should elapse between inhalations.
Long-Acting Beta$_2$-Agonists			
arformoterol (Brovana) 15 mcg/2 mL solution for inhalation 15 mcg by nebulizer bid	Bronchitis, headache, nervousness, serum K changes	Concomitant with other LABAs No use within 2 weeks of MAO inhibitors	Monitor K
formoterol (Perforomist 20 mcg/2 mL; 20 mcg by nebulizer q 12 h) (Foradil Aerolizer) 12 mcg/inh; 1 inh q 12 h)	Same as above	Same as above	Same as above
salmeterol (Serevent Diskus) 50 mcg/inh 1 inh q 12 h	Same as above	Same as above	Same as above
Combination Long-Acting Beta$_2$-Agonist and Inhaled Steroid			
fluticasone propionate and salmeterol (Advair Diskus) 100/50, 250/50, and 500/50 Adults: 250/50 bid	URI, hoarseness, dry mouth, headache, cough, palpitations, pharyngitis, dizziness	Acute asthma attack, caution with cardiac disease	Rinse mouth after use.
budesonide and formoterol (Symbicort) 80/4.5 and 160/4.5 Start at 2 inh of 80/4.5 bid and increase to 2 inh of 160/4.5 bid if symptoms persist	Same as above	Same as above	Same as above

TABLE 26.2 Overview of Selected Agents Used to Treat COPD (*Continued*)

Generic (Trade) Name and Dosage	Selected Adverse Events	Contraindications	Special Considerations
Anticholinergics			
ipratropium bromide (Atrovent) 18 μg/inhalation 2 inhalations qid	Exacerbation of symptoms, cough, nervousness, dizziness, GI upset, headache, palpitations, rash, urinary retention	Allergy to atropine Allergy to peanuts Caution with BPH & narrow-angle glaucoma	Patients using this drug for the first time need to learn how to use inhaler device properly for best effect.
ipratropium bromide (18 μg) and albuterol (90 μg) (Combivent) 2 inhalations qid	Same as above Also, URI and rhinitis	Same as above	Antagonized by beta blockers
tiotropium bromide (Spiriva) 18 mcg/capsule 1 capsule inhaled daily	Same as above	Same as above	Use with HandiHaler device only.
Combination Anticholinergic and Beta₂-Agonist			
ipratropium and albuterol (DuoNeb) 0.5 mg ipratropium and 2.5 mg albuterol/3 mL 1 vial by nebulizer q 4–6 h	Pharyngitis, chest pain, UTI, leg cramps, headache, dizziness	Atropine allergy Not recommended for nursing mothers Not to be used within 2 wk of MAO inhibitors and tricyclic antidepressants	Not for primary treatment of acute attack
ipratropium and albuterol inhaler (Combivent)	Same as above	Same as above	Same as above
Methylxanthines			
theophylline (Slo-Phyllin) 200–400 mg bid or 400–800 mg at night for nocturnal symptoms	Exacerbation of symptoms, cough, nervousness, dizziness, GI upset, headache, palpitations, rash	Allergy to atropine Allergy to peanuts	Monitor theophylline levels regularly to detect potential toxicity early.

BPH, benign prostatic hyperplasia; GI, gastrointestinal; K, potassium; LABAs, long-acting beta₂ agonists; MAO, monoamine oxidase; URI, upper respiratory infection; UTI, urinary tract infection.

Inhaled Beta$_2$ Agonists

Beta$_2$ agonists relax smooth muscle, dilate airways, and improve pulmonary function. These drugs are used for symptom relief in patients with COPD. The dosage should not exceed 12 inhalations a day for short-acting preparations.

Beta$_2$ agonists are sympathomimetic agents that stimulate bronchodilation by activating adenyl cyclase to produce cyclic 3'5' adenosine monophosphate.

Dosage and Time Frame for Response

Short-acting beta$_2$ agonists (SABAs) have a 3- to 6-hour duration of action, and the duration of action of long-acting beta$_2$ agonists (LABAs) exceeds 12 hours. Because of their rapid onset of action, SABAs are effective for relieving symptoms of COPD. LABAs—salmeterol and formoterol—have been shown to significantly improve lung function, health status, and symptom reduction. Dosages vary by the drug. (See **Table 26.2.**)

The SABA albuterol (Proventil) can be used in combination with the inhaled anticholinergic agent ipratropium. If this combination therapy is used, ipratropium should be taken 2 hours before albuterol. Inhaled beta$_2$ agonists are discussed in more detail in Chapter 25.

Because of their rapid onset of action, SABAs are very effective in relieving symptoms of COPD. In addition to their bronchodilatory properties, these agents are effective in increasing mucociliary clearance.

Contraindications

Monoamine oxidase inhibitors and tricyclic antidepressants must be avoided for 14 days before starting therapy. Beta$_2$ agonists are antagonized by beta blockers.

Adverse Events

Common adverse events associated with beta$_2$ agonists include tremor, nervousness, cough, insomnia, tachycardia, and throat irritation.

Anticholinergics

Mechanism of Action

Inhaled anticholinergics relax the bronchial muscles and act as a bronchodilator. They also block the contraction of bronchial smooth muscle and decrease the mucus secretion from parasympathetic activity. Anticholinergics prevent the acetylcholine-induced release of allergenic mediators from mast cells. The most common anticholinergic is ipratropium (Atrovent). There is also a long-acting anticholinergic, tiotropium (Spiriva HandiHaler). The use of tiotropium results in improved health status, dyspnea, and exercise capacity, and reduced hyperinflation and COPD exacerbation rate in patients with moderate to severe COPD.

Dosage and Time Frame for Response

The dosage of ipratropium is two to four puffs four to six times a day. Onset of action after inhalation is 15 minutes, with a peak response of 1 to 2 hours and a duration of action of 3 to 4 hours.

The dosage of tiotropium is one capsule inhaled daily. Onset of action is within 5 minutes; it is effective for 24 hours.

Contraindications

Anticholinergics are not used in a patient with hypersensitivity to atropine. They also are not used for acute episodes of bronchospasm. Caution is used in a patient with narrow-angle glaucoma or benign prostatic hypertrophy, and in pregnancy and lactation. It should not be used in people with soy or peanut allergies.

Adverse Events

Common adverse events associated with anticholinergic use include restlessness, dizziness, headache, gastrointestinal (GI) distress, blurred vision, hoarseness, cough, palpitations, and urinary obstruction.

Methylxanthines (Theophyllines)

Theophylline is a nonselective phosphodiesterase inhibitor that acts as both a weak bronchodilator and a respiratory stimulant. Because of its potential adverse effects and narrow therapeutic index, it should only be used when symptoms persist despite optimal bronchodilator therapy.

Mechanism of Action

Methylxanthines inhibit the enzyme phosphodiesterase, preventing the breakdown of cyclic adenosine monophosphate. This relaxes bronchial smooth muscle and may prevent the release of endogenous allergens such as histamine and leukotrienes from mast cells. The methylxanthines are thought to antagonize prostaglandin-mediated bronchoconstriction and block receptors for adenosine. The main effects are smooth muscle relaxation, central nervous system excitation, and cardiac stimulation. They also increase cardiac output and lower venous pressure. The most commonly used methylxanthine is theophylline.

Dosage and Time Frame for Response

The dosage of the sustained-release preparation is 200 to 400 mg twice a day or 400 to 800 mg at night for nocturnal symptoms. The drug is usually taken at 8 PM for relief of nocturnal symptoms. Smokers may require a dose 50% higher than the recommended dose. The dosage prescribed for patients with hypoxia, congestive heart failure, or liver disease is 25% to 50% lower than the normal dose.

The half-life of theophylline is 3 to 15 hours (4 to 5 hours in smokers), with extended-release formulas having the longer half-life.

Contraindications

Theophylline is contraindicated in peptic ulcer disease, seizure disorders, arrhythmias, and severe respiratory obstruction. Theophylline is metabolized in the liver and excreted in the urine, so it is used cautiously in patients with heart failure, liver disease, and thyroid dysfunction, and theophylline levels are carefully monitored.

Adverse Events

Adverse effects include headache, irritability, and insomnia. The patient also may experience palpitations, loss of appetite, GI distress, tachypnea, urinary retention, and flushing. Toxicity can produce cardiac arrhythmias and seizures.

Interactions

Excessive caffeine intake (greater than the equivalent of six cups of coffee a day) can cause increased concentration of the drug. Theophylline interacts with many drugs, including cimetidine (Tagamet), erythromycin, quinolones, oral contraceptives, and barbiturates. Food may alter bioavailability of the sustained-release theophylline preparation; therefore, the prescriber may recommend taking the medication 1 hour before or 2 hours after a meal.

Corticosteroids

Inhaled steroids diminish airway inflammation. Inhaled corticosteroids are much less effective in COPD than in asthma, likely due to the different types of inflammation seen in each disease. Thus, they are only approved at low doses in combination with a β-agonist. They do appear to lower the exacerbation rate, although this response is seen primarily in patients with severe disease who have frequent exacerbations. It is unclear whether they have an effect on symptoms or exercise capacity.

Inhaled corticosteroids have also been shown to be more effective in improving lung function when combined with LABAs. However, the guidelines recommend that corticosteroids be reserved for patients with severe COPD with frequent exacerbations who are already on treatment with a long-acting bronchodilator. Inhaled corticosteroids should be used to reduce the frequency of COPD exacerbations, but they are not useful for symptom control.

Systemic corticosteroids suppress inflammation of the airways and inhibit prostaglandin-induced narrowing of the airways. Systemic corticosteroids are used only for severe flare-ups and are most useful in patients with chronic bronchitis. They enhance the effects of the bronchodilators. If the corticosteroids are used for long-term therapy, the lowest possible dose should be used. They can be administered either daily or every other day, in the morning or early afternoon because they may cause insomnia. Dosing every other day may produce less adrenal suppression.

High-dose oral corticosteroids may improve lung function in patients with COPD, but they have no clinically significant benefits for patient-oriented outcomes. Inhaled corticosteroids should be used instead. Corticosteroids are discussed in Chapter 24.

Antibiotics

Patients with chronic bronchitis are predisposed to repeated respiratory infections resulting from mucus stagnation due to impaired ciliary movement and plugging. Aggressive management of respiratory infections is paramount to the management of COPD. The most common bacterial causes of respiratory infection in patients with COPD are *Haemophilus influenzae*, *Streptococcus pneumoniae*, *Chlamydia pneumoniae*, and *Legionella pneumophila*. Treatment of these infections is discussed in Chapter 27.

Selecting the Most Appropriate Agent

Medications cannot alter the course of COPD, but they can control symptoms and improve quality of life. A stepwise approach to therapy is recommended, adding medications as symptoms increase (**Table 26.3** and **Figure 26-1**). GOLD and ATS/ERS have developed guidelines for diagnosis and management of COPD.

First-Line Therapy

A short-acting bronchodilator is recommended when needed for mild COPD for intermittent symptoms (GOLD I). The recommended agent is a beta$_2$ agonist such as albuterol. As a "rescue drug," albuterol has a more rapid onset and is preferred by more patients than a short-acting anticholinergic such as ipratropium.

Second-Line Therapy

Many patients with COPD do not get relief from just one medication. If the patient has persistent symptoms (GOLD II), combination therapy is recommended. This is needed when

TABLE 26.3	Recommended Order of Treatment for COPD	
Order	**Agent**	**Comments**
First line	Inhaled short-acting bronchodilator	
Second line	Inhaled beta$_2$ agonists and anticholinergics	The combination drug ipratropium and albuterol (Combivent) can be used.
Third line	Long-acting beta$_2$ agonists (LABAs) and anticholinergics and albuterol as needed	
Fourth line	LABAs and anticholinergics and albuterol as needed and inhaled corticosteroids	Combined LABAs and inhaled corticosteroids can be used.

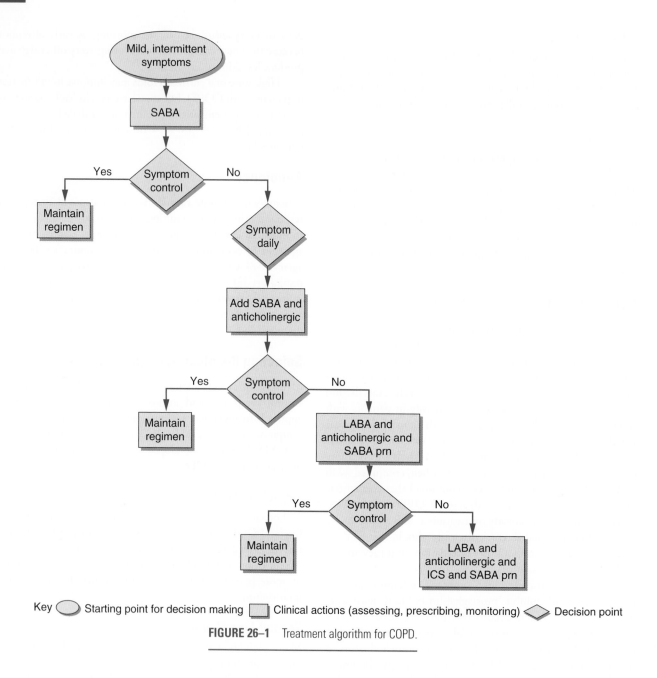

FIGURE 26–1 Treatment algorithm for COPD.

symptoms become persistent (e.g., need for rescue medication two times per week or more, breathlessness with exertion, reduced physical activity levels, nocturnal symptoms). The combinations of tiotropium and albuterol or salmeterol and ipratropium are recommended.

Third-Line Therapy

When there is increasing severity of symptoms (GOLD III), tiotropium and LABAs are recommended. Albuterol is also used as needed.

Fourth-Line Therapy

In patients with frequent exacerbations (GOLD III/IV), tiotropium and LABAs along with inhaled corticosteroids is

the recommended treatment. Physiological and clinical benefits of LABAs have been shown to be enhanced when administered in conjunction with inhaled corticosteroids. Albuterol is used as needed. See Chapter 24 for a discussion of inhaled corticosteroids.

Special Population Considerations

Geriatric

In older patients with cardiovascular disease, tremors and tachycardia may develop with beta$_2$ agonist therapy. The combination of ipratropium and albuterol may be prescribed to help prevent tremors and tachycardia. Theophylline clearance is decreased in elderly patients, and the subsequent buildup of theophylline may exacerbate a pre-existing heart condition. Therefore, this drug should be prescribed cautiously for elderly patients.

Women

Inhaled corticosteroids may promote a decrease in bone mineral content, thereby increasing the risk for osteoporosis. Postmenopausal women are already at risk for osteoporosis, so they may be advised to take 1,000 to 1,500 mg of supplemental calcium and 400 units of vitamin D daily.

MONITORING PATIENT RESPONSE

Patients taking theophylline on a regular basis need to have their blood theophylline levels monitored routinely. Safe theophylline levels in patients with COPD are 8 to 12 mg/dL. Theophylline levels are analyzed 2 weeks after initiation of therapy, then every 6 to 12 months. If theophylline levels are too low, the dose is increased by 25% and levels are rechecked after 2 weeks. If the levels are too high, the next dose is withheld if it is 20 to 25 mg/L and the dosage decreased by 10%. At 25 to 30 mg/L, the next dose is withheld and subsequent doses are decreased by 25%. Levels are rechecked in several days. If the level is greater than 30 mg/L, the next two doses are withheld and the dosage is decreased by 50% and levels are rechecked in several days. Theophylline levels should be checked 1 to 2 hours after administration of a short-acting preparation or 4 hours after administration of a long-acting preparation.

Follow-up examinations should be scheduled at 2 to 3 months. Meanwhile, the patient needs to be aware of the warning signs of respiratory infection and symptoms that suggest worsening of the condition. Pulmonary function tests are recommended every 1 to 2 years to determine the efficacy of therapy.

PATIENT EDUCATION

Drug Information

Patients with COPD are cautioned to avoid antihistamines, cough suppressants, sedatives, tranquilizers, beta blockers, and narcotics because these may further compromise the patient's already depressed respiratory state. All patients with COPD should be immunized against pneumonia and influenza.

Patient-Oriented Information Sources

The best source for patients about COPD is the National Heart, Lung and Blood Institute's website, www.nhlbi.nih.gov. Other sources are the American College of Chest Physicians (www.chest.net.org/education/patient/guide/copd) and the American Lung Association (www.lungusa.org/lungprofilers/copdlungprofiler.html).

Nutrition/Lifestyle Changes

The practitioner should explain to the patient that preventing respiratory infection is very important in COPD management. This is because serious consequences—and most deaths—result from respiratory failure caused by infection. The patient should be advised to stay away from anyone with a respiratory infection, and the practitioner should ensure that the patient can recognize the warning signs of infection, including a change in the color, consistency, and amount of sputum. If symptoms develop, treatment should be sought immediately.

The practitioner should also discuss the advantages of conserving energy to maintain activities of daily living. Activities should be attempted early in the day, when the patient has the most energy. The patient can do aerobic exercises using the arms and legs to increase endurance.

Another important aspect of management of COPD is rehabilitation: the patient should partake in at least 2 months of pulmonary rehabilitation.

Additional teaching involves showing the patient how to use inhalers, nebulizers, or spacer devices. (See Chapter 25 for more information.)

Weight loss frequently occurs in patients with COPD and is a determining factor of functional capacity, health status, and mortality. As many as one third to one half of patients with COPD are undernourished. Low body weight in patients with COPD is associated with an impaired pulmonary status, reduced diaphragmatic mass, lower exercise capacity, and a higher mortality rate than in adequately nourished individuals with COPD. Weight loss occurs because of increased energy requirements unbalanced by dietary intake. Both metabolic and mechanical inefficiency contribute to the elevated energy expenditure. An imbalance between protein synthesis and protein breakdown may cause a disproportionate depletion of fat-free mass in some patients. Patients need to eat a high-calorie diet and should be encouraged to use supplemental feedings to maintain a desirable weight.

Case Study

R. W. is a 64-year-old postal clerk who has smoked a pack of cigarettes a day for the past 35 years. He presents with progressive difficulty getting his breath while doing simple tasks. He is having difficulty doing any manual work, but he has no symptoms when working behind his desk. He also reports a cough, fatigue, and weight loss. He has been treated for three respiratory infections a year for the past 3 years and feels like another one is developing now.

On physical examination, you notice clubbing of his fingers, use of accessory muscles for respiration, wheezing in the lungs, and hyperresonance on percussion of the lungs. Pulmonary function studies show an FEV_1 of 58%.

DIAGNOSIS: CHRONIC OBSTRUCTIVE PULMONARY DISEASE

1. List specific treatment goals for R. W.
2. What drug therapy would you prescribe? Why?

3. What are the parameters for monitoring the success of the therapy?
4. Describe specific patient education based on the prescribed therapy.
5. List one or two adverse reactions for the selected agent that would cause you to change therapy.
6. What would be the choice for second-line therapy?
7. What dietary and lifestyle changes should be recommended for this patient?
8. Describe one or two drug–drug or drug–food interactions for the selected agent.

BIBLIOGRAPHY

*Starred references are cited in the text.

Barnes, P. (2008). Emerging pharmacotherapies for chronic obstructive pulmonary disease. *Chest, 134*(6). 278–286.

*Buist, A., McBurnie, M., Vollman, W., et al. (2007). International variation in the prevalence of COPD (the BOLD study): A population based prevalence study. *Lancet, 370*(9589), 741–750.

Evensen, A. (2010). Management of COPD exacerbation. *American Family Physician, 87*(5), 607–613.

*Global Initiative for Chronic Obstructive Lung Disease (GOLD). Accessed at www.goldcopd.com, August 6, 2010.

Grimes, G., Manning, J., Patel, P., & Via, R. M. (2007). Medications for COPD: A review of effectiveness. *American Family Physician, 76*(8), 1141–1148.

Gross, N., & Levin, D. (2008). Primary care of the patient with chronic obstructive disease, Part 2. *American Journal of Medicine, 121*(7 Suppl 1), S13–S24.

MacNee, W. (2007). Pathogenesis of chronic obstructive pulmonary disease. *Clinics in Chest Medicine, 28*(3), 479–453.

Radin, A., & Cote, C. (2008). Primary care of the patient with chronic obstructive pulmonary disease. *American Journal of Medicine, 121* (7 Suppl 1), S3–S17.

Stephens, M., & Yew, K. (2007). Diagnosis of chronic obstructive pulmonary disease. *American Family Physician, 78*(1), 87–92.

Wan, E., & Silverman, E. (2009). Genetics of COPD and emphysema. *Chest, 136*(3), 87–92.

Bronchitis and Pneumonia

One of the most commonly occurring upper respiratory tract infections is bronchitis, which may present as an acute or a chronic infection.

ACUTE BRONCHITIS

Acute bronchitis is a frequently diagnosed condition and is the ninth most common outpatient illness in the United States. The disease is a reversible inflammatory condition of the tracheobronchial tree that occurs in all age groups and is usually self-limiting. Typically, acute bronchitis occurs during the winter months. Predisposing factors for acute bronchitis include cold air, damp climates, fatigue, malnutrition, and inhalation of irritating substances, such as polluted air and cigarette smoke.

CAUSES

Viral infections cause 95% of acute bronchitis episodes; the most common respiratory viruses associated with acute bronchitis are rhinovirus, coronavirus, influenza virus A, parainfluenza virus, adenovirus, and respiratory syncytial virus (RSV). Bacterial infections cause 5% to 20% of acute bronchitis. The only bacterial microorganisms implicated in the pathogenesis of uncomplicated acute bronchitis are *Bordetella pertussis*, *Chlamydia pneumoniae*, and *Mycoplasma pneumoniae*. Limited evidence indicates that other common respiratory tract pathogens such as *Streptococcus pneumoniae* can contribute to acute bronchitis.

PATHOPHYSIOLOGY

Acute bronchitis is characterized by infection of the tracheobronchial tree. This infection results in hyperemic and edematous mucous membranes, yielding an increase in bronchial secretions. Destruction of the respiratory epithelial lining and reduced mucociliary function result from these changes. This process is usually transient and resolves after the infection clears.

DIAGNOSTIC CRITERIA

Signs and symptoms of acute bronchitis are preceded by manifestations of an upper respiratory tract infection such as coryza, malaise, chills, back and muscle pain, headache, and sore throat. If fever is present, it rarely exceeds 102.2°F (39°C) and lasts for 3 to 5 days. Fever is more commonly seen with adenovirus, influenza virus, and *M. pneumoniae* infection. The hallmark of acute bronchitis is a cough that is initially dry and nonproductive; however, as the production of bronchial secretions increases, the cough becomes more abundant and mucoid. The cough usually lasts for 7 to 10 days, although in some patients it can persist for weeks to months. Patients also present with phlegm, hoarseness, and wheezing.

Pulmonary examination may reveal signs of coarse, moist bilateral crackles, rhonchi, and wheezing. The chest x-ray typically reveals no active disease. The usefulness of cultures to identify the causative microorganisms is limited because most cases of acute bronchitis are viral in origin, and cultures usually are negative or grow normal nasopharyngeal flora. Laboratory tests may reveal a normal or slightly elevated white blood cell (WBC) count.

The high reported incidence of acute bronchitis can be correlated with the absence of definitive diagnostic signs or laboratory tests. Thus, the diagnosis is based purely on the patient's risk factors and signs and symptoms. In many patients an upper respiratory tract infection (sinusitis or allergic rhinitis) may be misdiagnosed as acute bronchitis.

INITIATING DRUG THERAPY

The general treatment for acute bronchitis is symptomatic and supportive (**Figure 27-1**). Patients should be encouraged to drink plenty of fluids to prevent dehydration and decrease the viscosity of bronchial secretions. Bed rest is indicated until fever subsides. Mild analgesic/antipyretic therapy is effective for relief of fever and musculoskeletal pains. Aspirin or acetaminophen (Tylenol; 650 mg in adults or 10 to 15 mg/kg per dose in children) or ibuprofen (Advil, others; 200 to 400 mg in adults or 10 mg/kg per dose in children) administered every 4 to 6 hours can be used as analgesic/antipyretic therapy. Acetaminophen is the agent of choice because aspirin should be avoided, owing to the

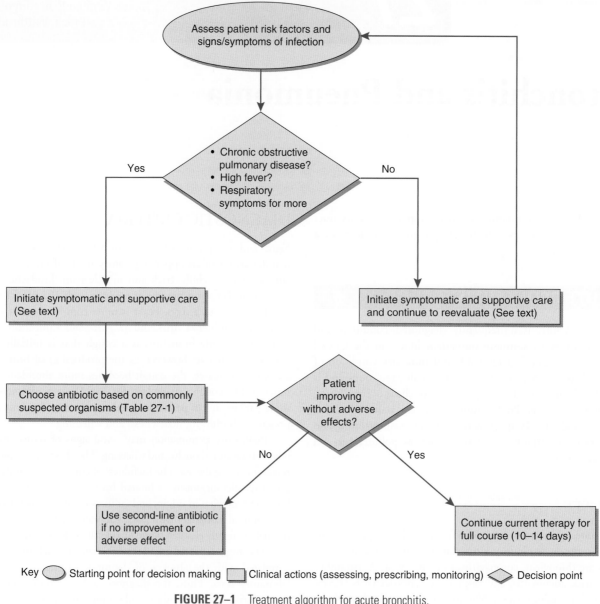

FIGURE 27–1 Treatment algorithm for acute bronchitis.

correlation of aspirin and the development of Reye syndrome in children. Aspirin and ibuprofen should also be used cautiously in elderly patients, patients with a history of peptic ulcer disease, and patients with renal insufficiency.

Nonprescription cough and cold medications (see Chapter 24) often are used by patients to help reduce the signs and symptoms of acute bronchitis. The use of nonprescription medications that contain various combinations of antihistamines, sympathomimetic agents, and antitussives can result in dehydration of bronchial secretions. This could lead to further aggravation of symptoms, which prolongs the recovery process. Cough that is associated with acute bronchitis can become bothersome for the patient. Dextromethorphan, an antitussive agent, is recommended to help treat mild, persistent cough. Severe cough may require more potent cough medications that contain codeine or similar agents.

In patients with a productive cough persisting beyond 10 to 14 days, treatment with antibiotics may be indicated to treat bacterial coinfection, especially in smokers or in patients with underlying pulmonary disease.

Goals of Drug Therapy

The goals of pharmacotherapy include providing the patient with comfort and, in severe cases, treating associated dehydration and respiratory compromise. If antibiotics are administered, minimizing side effects is also a goal.

Antibiotics

Antibiotics often are prescribed for patients with acute bronchitis; however, they offer little relief from the respiratory symptoms of the disease and do not shorten the course of the illness.

The routine use of antibiotics for acute bronchitis is discouraged. Antibiotics are indicated if the patient has concomitant chronic obstructive pulmonary disease (COPD), high fevers, purulent sputum, or respiratory symptoms for more than 4 to 6 days. Empiric antibiotic therapy should be directed against the microorganisms commonly suspected to cause acute bronchitis.

Selecting the Most Appropriate Agent

Table 27.1 lists the antibiotics that are commonly used to treat acute bronchitis caused mostly by bacteria. Aminopenicillins such as ampicillin (Omnipen) and amoxicillin (Amoxil) are effective against infections caused by pneumococci, streptococci, and *Haemophilus influenzae*.

For microorganisms that produce beta-lactamase, such as *Moraxella catarrhalis* and *H. influenzae*, aminopenicillins given in combination with a beta-lactamase inhibitor, such as clavulanate (Augmentin), should be administered.

For acute bronchitis due to atypical bacteria such as *M. pneumoniae* and *Chlamydia* species, macrolides (e.g., erythromycin [Eryc], clarithromycin [Biaxin], or azithromycin [Zithromax]) or doxycycline (Vibramycin) are usually efficacious. Doxycycline should not be used in children younger than age 8. In this population, the agent of choice is erythromycin. If *B. pertussis* is the likely microorganism, erythromycin is the drug of choice. Fluoroquinolone antibiotics (e.g., levofloxacin [Levaquin], moxifloxacin [Avelox]) are effective against typical and atypical organisms, but are usually reserved for acute bronchitis refractory to macrolides or doxycycline. Their use is not recommended for patients younger than age 18.

During epidemics caused by influenza A virus, amantadine (Symmetrel) or rimantadine (Flumadine) may be administered early in the course of the illness to minimize symptoms. Oseltamivir (Tamiflu) and zanamivir (Relenza) are also used to minimize symptoms in influenza A in adults who have been symptomatic for no longer than 2 days (See **Figure 27-1;** for more information about antibiotic/antimicrobial therapy, refer to Chapter 8.)

CHRONIC BRONCHITIS

Chronic bronchitis is a component of COPD, which is the fourth leading cause of death in the United States. (See Chapter 26 for a discussion of COPD.) The standard description/definition of chronic bronchitis is productive cough and sputum production for 3 months per year for at least 2 years, and an acute exacerbation of chronic bronchitis is defined as worsening of respiratory symptoms such as increased cough, sputum, and dyspnea. Chronic bronchitis primarily affects adults and occurs more commonly in men than in women. Between 10% and 25% of the adult population in the United States age 40 or older is afflicted with chronic bronchitis, which accounts for a large amount of health care expenditures and lost wages.

Because many infections are untreated, the exact morbidity of acute exacerbations of chronic bronchitis is unknown. Patients with chronic bronchitis are more likely to have frequent and severe episodes of acute bacterial bronchitis.

CAUSES

Several factors are implicated in the pathogenesis of chronic bronchitis; however, the precise cause of this disease is unknown. The predominant factor in chronic bronchitis is cigarette smoke, a well-known respiratory irritant, and most patients with chronic bronchitis have a history of cigarette smoking. Occupational dust, fumes, and environmental pollution also contribute to the etiology of the disease. The phrase industrial bronchitis refers to chronic bronchitis acquired from occupational and environmental exposure to pollutants. Cold, damp climates can provoke acute exacerbations of chronic bronchitis; hypersecretion of mucus in patients with asthma has also been shown to yield symptoms of chronic bronchitis. Evidence suggests that recurrent respiratory infections may predispose a person to development of chronic bronchitis, although the exact reason for this is unclear.

Colonization of the lower airways with bacteria such as *H. influenzae, M. catarrhalis,* and *S. pneumoniae* has been frequently detected in patients with chronic lung disease. Viral infections may account for nearly one third of acute exacerbations of chronic bronchitis.

PATHOPHYSIOLOGY

Several physiologic abnormalities of the bronchial mucosa may lead to chronic bronchitis. It has been suggested that patients with chronic bronchitis are predisposed to respiratory infections because of impaired mucociliary clearance due to chronic inhalation of irritating substances. Factors that can

TABLE 27.1	Acute Bronchitis: Drug Therapy for Selected Microorganisms
Microorganism	**Treatment**
H. influenzae	aminopenicillin (ampicillin or amoxicillin)
M. catarrhalis, H. influenzae (beta-lactamase producing)	aminopenicillin + clavulanic acid (Augmentin)
M. pneumoniae, Chlamydia spp.	macrolide (erythromycin, clarithromycin, or azithromycin) or doxycycline
B. pertussis	erythromycin
Methicillin-resistant *Staphylococcus aureus*	
Influenza A	amantadine or rimantadine or oseltamivir or zanamivir
Influenza B	amantadine or rimantadine or oseltamivir or zanamivir

lead to impaired mucociliary clearance are the proliferation of mucus-secreting goblet cells and the replacement of ciliated epithelium with nonciliated metaplastic cells. The latter event results in the inability of the bronchi to clear the profuse, thick, sticky secretions present in patients with chronic bronchitis.

Other changes in the bronchial mucosa of patients with chronic bronchitis that predispose them to infection are hypertrophy and dilation of the glands that produce mucus. In addition, inhalation of toxic irritants results in bronchial obstruction because of stimulation of cholinergic activity and increased bronchomotor tone.

Bacteria residing in the tracheobronchial tree also predispose patients to acute exacerbations of chronic bronchitis. *H. influenzae* and other microorganisms harbored in the bronchial epithelium act as reservoirs for infection when the patient's host defenses are compromised. Compromised host defenses include decreased phagocytosis of bacteria by polymorphonuclear neutrophils, deficient bactericidal activity, reduced numbers of macrophages, and decreased amounts of immunoglobulin A.

Diagnostic Criteria

As with acute bronchitis, cough is the hallmark of chronic bronchitis. Cough can be mild or severe (with purulent sputum) and may be stimulated by factors such as simple conversation. Many patients with chronic bronchitis expectorate a large quantity of white to yellow tenacious sputum in the morning. Because of the characteristics of sputum, many patients complain of a foul taste in the mouth.

The earliest symptom in patients with acute exacerbations of chronic bronchitis is an increase in frequency and severity of cough. Other symptoms include greater sputum production, purulent sputum, hemoptysis, chest congestion and discomfort, increased dyspnea, and wheezing. Malaise, loss of appetite, chills, and fever may also be present. True chills (rigors) and fever suggest pneumonia rather than acute exacerbations of chronic bronchitis; these findings require further diagnostic investigation (chest x-ray study, sputum culture).

Clinical assessment and the patient's medical history contribute to the diagnosis of chronic bronchitis. Other diseases such as bronchiectasis, cardiac failure, cystic fibrosis, tuberculosis, and lung carcinoma must be excluded before diagnosing a patient with chronic bronchitis. Patients with chronic bronchitis must have had a sputum-producing cough for at least 3 consecutive months each year for 2 consecutive years. An additional criterion for diagnosis is loss of wages for 3 or more weeks in a year due to cough and sputum production.

Physical examination of patients with chronic bronchitis is usually unremarkable except that chest auscultation reveals inspiratory and expiratory rales, rhonchi, and mild wheezing; normal breath sounds are diminished. As the severity of the disease progresses, an increase in the anteroposterior diameter of the thoracic cage (barrel chest appearance), hyperresonance on percussion, and limited mobility of the diaphragm are observed. Pulmonary function tests demonstrate a decrease in vital capacity and prolongation of expiratory flow. Other features of disease progression include clubbing of the fingers, cor pulmonale, hepatomegaly, and edema of the lower extremities.

To determine the need for antibiotic treatment or hospitalization during an acute exacerbation of chronic bronchitis, the severity of the patient's symptoms needs to be evaluated. A sputum culture is necessary to identify the causative microorganism. To determine the presence of infection, the following two criteria must be present: the Gram stain must exhibit a significant concentration of bacterial growth that is not present when the patient is stable, and the increased bacterial concentration seen on the Gram stain must be accompanied by a doubling of the neutrophil count in the sputum.

Culture and sensitivity findings are not needed, although these results may guide the clinician in choosing appropriate antibiotic therapy. Culture and sensitivity are recommended if any of the following is present:

- The Gram stain reveals a significant amount of *Staphylococcus* species.
- Antibiotic resistance is suspected.
- A decrease in bacteria is detected by Gram stain after 3 to 5 days of antibiotic therapy, and the infection is hospital-acquired.
- Laboratory test results reveal a normal or slightly elevated WBC count during an acute exacerbation of chronic bronchitis.

Finally, a chest x-ray should be performed in patients who have fever or crackles on auscultation to rule out pneumonia.

A proposed classification system for patients with chronic bronchitis has been developed to help clinicians identify high-risk patients and select the appropriate antimicrobial therapy according to the suspected microorganism. **Table 27.2**

TABLE 27.2	Classification of Chronic Bronchitis	
Clinical Status	**Risk Factors**	**Microorganisms**
Simple chronic bronchitis	FEV_1 >50%, increased sputum production and purulence	*H. influenzae, M. catarrhalis, S. pneumoniae* (possible beta-lactam resistance)
Complicated chronic bronchitis	FEV_1 <50%, advanced age, ≥4 exacerbations/year	*H. influenzae, M. catarrhalis, S. pneumoniae* (resistance to beta-lactam common)
Chronic bronchial infection	Complicated chronic bronchitis and continuous sputum production throughout year	The above microorganisms and enterobacteria + *P. aeruginosa*

outlines the classification system, taking into consideration the baseline clinical status, risk factors, and most likely common pathogens.

Patients with uncomplicated chronic bronchitis have little or no lung impairment. The forced expiratory volume in 1 second (FEV$_1$) of these patients is greater than 50%, and they have increased purulent sputum production. The most common pathogens include *H. influenzae, M. catarrhalis,* and beta-lactam–resistant *S. pneumoniae*. Viral infections should be considered before bacterial infections in this category of patients.

Patients with moderate to severe chronic bronchitis include those with moderate (FEV$_1$ 50% to 80% of predicted) to severe (FEV$_1$ <50% of predicted) lung impairment, those who are elderly (older than age 65), those who have frequent exacerbations (more than four episodes per year), and those who have comorbid illnesses such as congestive heart failure, diabetes mellitus, chronic renal failure, or chronic liver disease. The most common pathogens isolated in severe chronic bronchitis are *H. influenzae, S. pneumoniae,* and *M. catarrhalis*.

Patients with chronic bronchial infections have characteristics similar to those in the previous group, but they have increased sputum production, cough, and worsening dyspnea. The same microorganisms that were found in the other groups should be considered in these patients; however, gram-negative microorganisms should also be suspected.

INITIATING DRUG THERAPY

A complete assessment of the patient's occupational and environmental history should be performed to treat chronic bronchitis properly. Patients should reduce or eliminate cigarette smoking and their exposure to second-hand smoke. This can be accomplished by counseling sessions and the use of nicotine replacement therapy. Also, exposure to inhaled irritants at work or home should be reduced or eliminated.

The approach to treatment of acute exacerbations of chronic bronchitis is multifactorial (**Figure 27-2**). The therapies listed in **Box 27.1** should be initiated in combination with antibiotic therapy by the clinician. Prompt initiation of therapy with antimicrobial agents is important for the effective treatment of most acute exacerbations of chronic bronchitis.

Goals of Drug Therapy

There are two goals for the treatment of chronic bronchitis: to reduce the severity of the chronic symptoms and to ameliorate acute exacerbations with prolonged infection-free intervals.

Antimicrobial Therapy

The concentration of the antimicrobial agent in the sputum does not reflect the success of treating the invading microorganism; the penetration of the antimicrobial agent into bronchial tissues is a better indicator of clinical success. Among the antimicrobial agents used to treat chronic bronchitis

are the aminopenicillins (ampicillin), cephalosporins, and fluoroquinolones.

Ampicillin does not penetrate well into sputum; however, it is an effective agent in the treatment of certain bacterial infections that cause acute exacerbations of chronic bronchitis. Fluoroquinolones penetrate well into bronchial tissue and have demonstrated to be very effective in treating acute exacerbations of chronic bronchitis. **Table 27.3** reviews antibiotic agents used for patients with chronic bronchitis and pneumonia.

Aminopenicillins

Aminopenicillins, such as ampicillin, inhibit the final step of bacterial cell wall synthesis by binding to one or more of the penicillin-binding proteins. They are safe for use in children, adults, and pregnant women. **Table 27.3** reviews the dosages of aminopenicillins for chronic bronchitis.

Contraindications

Aminopenicillins should not be administered to patients with severe hypersensitivity reactions to these agents.

Adverse Events

Hypersensitivity reactions to aminopenicillins manifest as eosinophilia or rash (urticarial, erythematous, morbilliform). Angioedema, exfoliative dermatitis, or erythema multiforme have also been reported as hypersensitivity reactions to aminopenicillins. These reactions occur less frequently than eosinophilia or rash. Rarely, Stevens-Johnson syndrome has been reported as a hypersensitivity reaction to aminopenicillins.

Nausea, vomiting, and diarrhea, however, are the most common adverse effects that occur with aminopenicillins. Pseudomembranous colitis may occur during or after the antibiotic treatment.

Interactions

Aminopenicillins may interrupt the enterohepatic circulation of estrogen by reducing the bacterial hydrolysis of conjugated estrogen in the gastrointestinal (GI) tract. Therefore, the efficacy of oral contraceptives is decreased. Probenecid may increase the effects of aminopenicillins by competing with renal tubular secretion. An increased risk for rash occurs with the coadministration of allopurinol (Zyloprim) and aminopenicillins; the exact mechanism of this interaction has not been established.

Cephalosporins

Cephalosporins consist of several agents, including cefaclor (Ceclor), cephalexin (Keflex), cefuroxime axetil (Ceftin), and cefpodoxime (Vantin), that are frequently used for the treatment of acute exacerbations of chronic bronchitis. Like penicillins, cephalosporins inhibit bacterial cell wall synthesis by binding to one or more of the penicillin-binding proteins. These drugs are safe for use by children and adults. The dosages of cephalosporins are listed in **Table 27.3.**

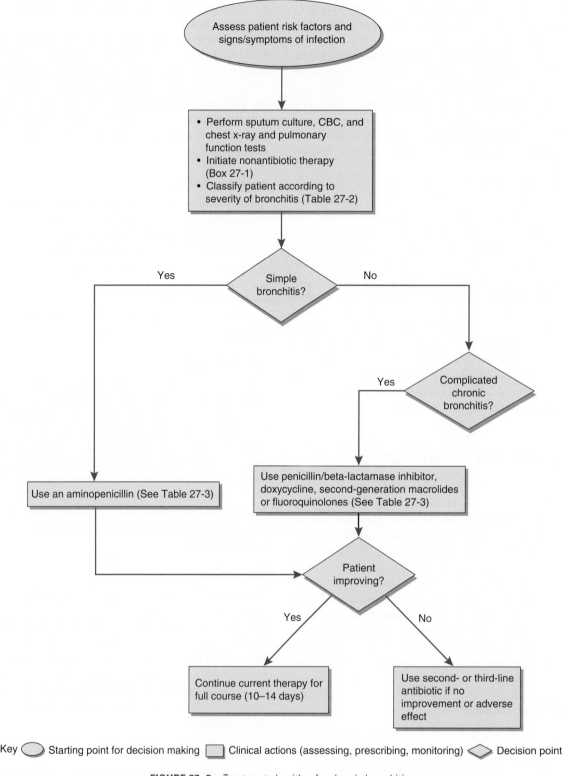

FIGURE 27–2 Treatment algorithm for chronic bronchitis.

Contraindications

Cephalosporins are contraindicated in patients who have had hypersensitivity reactions to any member of the cephalosporin class of antimicrobial agents. There is a 5% to 7% cross-sensitivity reaction between cephalosporins and penicillins, and therefore cephalosporins should be avoided in patients who have had an anaphylactic reaction to penicillins.

> ## BOX 27.1
> ### Nonantibiotic Therapy for Acute Exacerbations of Chronic Bronchitis
>
> - Stop smoking
> - Avoid inhalation of polluted air
> - Increase ingestion of fluids (nonalcoholic)
> - Humidify atmosphere
> - Use bronchodilators
> - Treat any associated asthma

Adverse Events

Nausea, diarrhea, and vomiting are common adverse effects with cephalosporins. Fungal infections and pseudomembranous colitis can also occur with the administration of cephalosporins.

Interactions

Probenecid increases the serum concentrations of cephalosporins by reducing their renal clearance.

Doxycycline

Doxycycline inhibits protein synthesis by binding with the 30S and possibly the 50S ribosomal subunits of susceptible microorganisms. The dosage of doxycycline is listed in **Table 27.3.**

Contraindications

Doxycycline is contraindicated in patients with severe hypersensitivity reactions to doxycycline or tetracycline. The drug should not be administered to children age 8 or younger; its use in infants has resulted in retardation of bone growth. Doxycycline can localize in the enamel of developing teeth, resulting in enamel hypoplasia and permanent yellow-gray to brown discoloration of the teeth. Doxycycline is a pregnancy category D drug and should not be administered to pregnant or lactating women.

Adverse Events

GI adverse effects such as nausea, vomiting, diarrhea, and bulky, loose stools commonly occur with the administration of doxycycline. Superinfection, enterocolitis, blood dyscrasias, and hepatotoxicity have also been reported to occur with the administration of doxycycline.

Interactions

The administration of antacids, iron, and bismuth subsalicylate (Pepto-Bismol), which contain divalent or trivalent cations, reduces the efficacy of doxycycline by impairing its absorption because of chelation of the cation by doxycycline. Barbiturates, phenytoin (Dilantin), and carbamazepine (Tegretol) can reduce the serum concentration of doxycycline by induction of its hepatic metabolism. The effects of warfarin (Coumadin) can be potentiated when it is administered with doxycycline.

Doxycycline can decrease vitamin K production by GI bacteria. The significance of this interaction is unknown, but patients should be monitored for signs of bleeding when anticoagulant drugs are used concomitantly with doxycycline.

Macrolides

The three macrolides—erythromycin, clarithromycin, and azithromycin—work by inhibiting ribonucleic acid–dependent protein synthesis by binding to the 50S ribosomal subunit. The dosage regimens of the macrolides are listed in **Table 27.3.**

Contraindications

Macrolides are contraindicated in patients with known hypersensitivity reactions to erythromycin, clarithromycin, or azithromycin, and these products should not be administered to patients with hepatic impairment or pre-existing liver disease. Clarithromycin and some formulations of erythromycin should not be administered to pregnant and lactating women because the safety of these agents has not been fully established.

Adverse Events

Abdominal pain, cramping, nausea, vomiting, diarrhea, and hepatic dysfunction commonly occur with the administration of macrolides. Skin rashes and pseudomembranous colitis have also been reported.

Interactions

Erythromycin and clarithromycin are inhibitors of the hepatic cytochrome P450 microsomal enzyme system. Elevations of carbamazepine, cyclosporine (Sandimmune), theophylline (Slo-Phyllin), zidovudine (Retrovir), didanosine (Videx), ritonavir (Norvir), midazolam (Versed), and warfarin can occur when these agents are administered concomitantly with erythromycin or clarithromycin. Antacids should not be administered with azithromycin because they inhibit its absorption.

Fluoroquinolones

Levofloxacin (Levaquin) and moxifloxacin (Avelox) inhibit deoxyribonucleic acid gyrase and topoisomerase intravenously in susceptible microorganisms, thereby interfering with protein synthesis. The dosing regimens of the fluoroquinolones are listed in **Table 27.3.**

Contraindications

Fluoroquinolones are contraindicated in patients with known hypersensitivity reactions to any member of the fluoroquinolone class of antimicrobial agents. Fluoroquinolones generally should not be administered to patients younger than age 18 or to pregnant or lactating women. Gatifloxacin, levofloxacin, and moxifloxacin should be used cautiously in patients with known prolongation of the QT interval, in patients with uncorrected hypokalemia, and in those receiving class IA (e.g.,

TABLE 27.3   Overview of Selected Antibiotics for Bronchitis and Pneumonia

Generic (Trade) Name and Dosage	Selected Adverse Events	Contraindications	Special Considerations
Aminopenicillins			
ampicillin (Omnipen, Principen) Adults: 250–500 mg q6h Under 20 kg: 50–100 mg/d qid	Nausea, vomiting, diarrhea, rash, hypersensitivity reactions, gastritis	Hypersensitivity reactions to penicillin Pregnancy category B	High incidence of development of rash in patients with infectious mononucleosis. Ampicillin should be used with extreme caution in this patient population.
amoxicillin (Amoxil, Trimox) 250–1000 mg tid Adults: 500 mg q8h Children: 40 mg/kg/d in divided doses	Nausea, vomiting, diarrhea, gastritis, hypersensitivity reactions	Hypersensitivity reactions to penicillin Pregnancy category B	High incidence of development of rash in patients with infectious mononucleosis. Amoxicillin should be used with extreme caution in this patient population. Take with or without food. Food may decrease GI symptoms. Interacts with warfarin and oral contraceptives; probenecid decreases renal excretion, and allopurinol increases the risk of rash. Safe for young children
amoxicillin–clavulanate Adults: (Augmentin) 500 mg/ 125 mg tid 875 mg bid Children: same as for amoxicillin	Nausea, vomiting, diarrhea, gastritis, hypersensitivity reactions, Stevens-Johnson syndrome, seizures (high doses)	Hypersensitivity reactions to penicillin, clavulanic acid Pregnancy category B	High incidence of development of rash in patients with infectious mononucleosis. Amoxicillin clavulanate should be used with extreme caution in this patient population. Take with or without food. Food may decrease GI symptoms. Interacts with warfarin and oral contraceptives; probenecid decreases renal excretion, and allopurinol increases the risk of rash. Safe for young children
Cephalosporins			
cefaclor (Ceclor) 250–500 q8h Not recommended in children <16 y	Nausea, vomiting, diarrhea, rash, hypersensitivity reactions, fungal infections Serious: pseudomembranous colitis	Hypersensitivity to cephalosporin Not recommended in children <1 mo Pregnancy category B	Cephalosporins should be avoided in patients who have had an anaphylactic hypersensitivity reaction and should be used with caution in patients with a delayed type of reaction to other beta-lactam antibiotics. Take with or without food. Food may decrease GI symptoms. Probenecid decreases renal excretion.

Drug/Dosage	Side Effects	Contraindications	Comments
cephalexin (Keflex) Adults: 500 mg qid Children: 25–50 mg/kg/d qid; max 100 mg/kg/d	Nausea, vomiting, diarrhea, rash, hypersensitivity reactions, fungal infections Serious: pseudomembranous colitis, seizures (high doses)	Hypersensitivity or allergy to cephalosporin antibiotics Not recommended in children <1 mo	Avoid cephalosporins for patients who have had an anaphylactic hypersensitivity reaction. Use with caution in patients with a delayed type of reaction to other beta-lactam antibiotics. Take with or without food. Food may decrease GI symptoms. Probenecid decreases renal excretion.
cefuroxime axetil (Ceftin) Adults: 250–500 mg bid Children: 20 mg/kg/d in 2 divided doses	Same as above	Same as above	Same as above
cefpodoxime (Vantin) Adults: 200 mg q12h Children: 85 mg/kg q12h; max 200 mg	Same as above	Same as above	Same as above
cefdinir (Omnicef) Adults: 300 mg q12h	Same as above	Same as above	Same as above
cefixime (Suprax) Adults: 400 mg daily	Same as above	Same as above	Same as above
Tetracyclines			
doxycycline (Vibramycin, Doryx, Vibra-tab, Monodox) 100 mg bid for 1 day then 100 mg qd	GI upset (nausea, vomiting, diarrhea, bulky, loose stools, anorexia), hypersensitivity reactions, photosensitivity reactions, superinfection, enterocolitis, rash, blood dyscrasias, hepatotoxicity	Hypersensitivity reactions to any tetracycline Pregnancy category D, breast-feeding Not recommended in children <8 y	Capsules or tablets should be administered with adequate amounts of fluid. Capsules or tablets should not be given to patients with esophageal obstruction or compression. Antacids containing aluminum, calcium, or magnesium should be given 1 to 2 h before. Avoid sunlight or ultraviolet light. Use of drug during tooth development may cause dental discoloration.
trimethoprim–sulfamethoxazole (Bactrim) Adults: 800 mg sulfamethoxazole/160 mg trimethoprim bid Children >2 mo: 8 mg/kg/d trimethoprim/40 mg/kg/d sulfamethoxazole		Allergy to sulfa Pregnancy	

(continued)

TABLE 27.3　Overview of Selected Antibiotics for Bronchitis and Pneumonia (Continued)

Generic (Trade) Name and Dosage	Selected Adverse Events	Contraindications	Special Considerations
Macrolides			
erythromycin (Eryc, PCE) Adults: 250–500 mg qid Children: 30–50 mg/kg qid (not to exceed 100 mg/kg/d)	Abdominal pain and cramping, nausea, vomiting, diarrhea, hepatic dysfunction, urticaria, fungal infection, skin eruptions, rash, ototoxicity	Allergy to erythromycin, hypersensitivity to macrolides, hepatic dysfunction or preexisting liver disease	Erythromycin inhibits the hepatic cytochrome P450 microsomal enzyme system. Thus, elevations of serum concentrations of the following agents can be seen: carbamazepine, cyclosporine, theophylline, zidovudine, digoxin, didanosine, ritonavir, midazolam, and warfarin. Take on empty stomach for better absorption 1 h before or 2 h after a meal.
clarithromycin (Biaxin) Adults: 500 mg bid or 1,000 mg qd Children >6 mo: 7.5 mg/kg q12h	Diarrhea, nausea, abnormal taste, dyspepsia, abdominal discomfort, fungal infection, pseudomembranous colitis, hepatic dysfunction, headache, mild urticaria, mild skin eruptions	Hypersensitivity to macrolides, hepatic dysfunction or preexisting liver or renal disease, pregnancy or breast-feeding	Clarithromycin is an inhibitor of the hepatic cytochrome P450 microsomal enzyme system. Thus, elevations of serum concentrations of the following agents can be seen: carbamazepine, cyclosporine, theophylline, zidovudine, didanosine, ritonavir, midazolam, and warfarin.
azithromycin (Zithromax) Bronchitis: Adults: 500 mg qd for 1 d then 250 qd for 4 d CAP: 500 mg for 7–10 d Children >6 mo: 10 mg/kg for 1 d then 5 mg/kd/d for 4 d	Diarrhea, loose stools, nausea, abdominal pain, dizziness, headache, rash photosensitivity, fungal infection, dizziness, fatigue, palpitations	Hypersensitivity to macrolides Use with caution in hepatic disease. Safety not established in pregnancy, lactation, or in children <2 y.	Administer the suspension 1 h before or 2 h after a meal. Use of antacids with aluminum or magnesium decreases serum levels. Interactions: warfarin, pimozide, carbamazepine
Fluoroquinolones			
levofloxacin (Levaquin) 500 mg qd Not recommended for children <18 y	Nausea, diarrhea, vomiting, abdominal pain or discomfort, photosensitivity	Same as above	Same as above
moxifloxacin (Avelox) 400 mg qd Not recommended for children <18 y	Same as above	Same as above	Same as above
gemifloxacin (Factive) 320 mg once a day	Same as above	Same as above	Should be administered 4 h before or 8 h after antacids, sucralfate, iron, or multivitamins with zinc.

quinidine [CinQuin], procainamide [Pronestyl]) or class III (e.g., amiodarone [Cordarone], sotalol [Betapace]) antiar-rhythmic agents. These agents should also be used cautiously in patients who are receiving other agents known to prolong the QT interval, such as erythromycin, antipsychotics, and tricyclic antidepressants.

Gatifloxacin and levofloxacin are eliminated through the kidneys; therefore, dosage adjustments are necessary in patients with renal impairment. Moxifloxacin, which is metabolized primarily through sulfate and glucuronide conjugation, is not recommended for use in patients with mild to severe hepatic impairment.

Adverse Events

GI adverse effects (e.g., nausea, diarrhea, vomiting, and abdom-inal pain) have commonly been reported with the adminis-tration of fluoroquinolones. Central nervous system adverse effects such as headache, agitation, confusion, and restlessness have occurred after the administration of fluoroquinolones. Photosensitivity has been reported with the administration of some fluoroquinolones.

Interactions

Fluoroquinolones should not be administered concomitantly with antacids, calcium products, sucralfate (Carafate), iron, multivitamins with zinc, and didanosine-buffered tablets or pediatric powder. These products should be spaced at least 2 to 4 hours apart from the fluoroquinolone. The manufactur-ers of moxifloxacin recommend spacing at least 4 hours before or 8 hours after the administration of iron- or zinc-containing multivitamins, magnesium, calcium, or aluminum products, sucralfate, or didanosine-buffered tablets or pediatric powder.

Selecting the Most Appropriate Agent

For simple chronic bronchitis, treatment with an amin-openicillin (ampicillin or amoxicillin) is sufficient. In patients with complicated chronic bronchitis, therapy with a second- or third-generation cephalosporin, amoxicillin–clavulanate, a macrolide, or a fluoroquinolone is effective. For chronic bron-chial infections, a fluoroquinolone is the agent of choice because gram-negative microorganisms, such as *Pseudomonas* species, need to be considered as potential pathogens. (**Table 27.4** and **Figure 27-2** provide more information about treatment choices.)

Special Population Considerations

Pediatric

Antimicrobials related to the tetracyclines (e.g., doxycycline) may discolor dental enamel in fetuses and children while teeth are developing.

Women

Women who take antibiotics, especially the aminopenicillins, may experience secondary symptoms, such as vaginitis, that require treatment.

TABLE 27.4	Recommended Order of Treatment for Chronic Bronchitis	
Order	**Agent**	**Comments**
First line	Aminopenicillin (ampicillin or amoxicillin) for 10–14 d	Therapy typically used for simple chronic bronchitis
Second line	Fluoroquinolone Penicillin plus beta-lactamase inhibitor (Augmentin), doxycycline Second- or third-generation cephalosporin Macrolide antibiotics (eryth-romycin, clarithromycin, azithromycin)	Therapy typically initiated for complicated chronic bronchitis
Third line	Fluoroquinolone	Effective for chronic bronchial infections

MONITORING PATIENT RESPONSE

Signs and symptoms of infection should improve within days of drug administration. If patients fail to improve, sputum culture and sensitivity analyses should be performed to evaluate the possibility of resistance.

The recommended duration of therapy for acute exacer-bation of chronic bronchitis is 10 to 14 days. This decreases morbidity and increases the posttherapy infection-free period in patients. Some patients may require a longer duration of therapy or hospitalization with parenteral therapy. Because patients with chronic bronchitis are predisposed to recurrent infections, antimicrobial agents that were previously successful in eradicating the infection should be readministered.

Measures to prevent exacerbations of chronic bronchi-tis should be initiated by the clinician. One such method is annual administration of an influenza vaccine. This reduces the rate and severity of infections with the influenza virus in some patients with chronic bronchitis. Patients should also receive the pneumococcal vaccine, with readministration 6 years later. Sufficient data do not exist to support the theory that the pneumococcal vaccine may reduce the frequency or severity of exacerbations in patients with chronic bronchitis. However, this vaccine may potentially reduce the frequency of pneumococcal pneumonia.

PATIENT EDUCATION

Drug Information

The patient needs to understand that the entire course of anti-microbial therapy should be finished to ensure eradication of the causative microorganisms. Moreover, the patient should be cautioned to report adverse effects, such as diarrhea, immedi-ately to the health care provider for further evaluation. Other adverse effects may include photosensitivity, and the patient needs to be advised to protect the skin from excessive exposure to sunlight or ultraviolet light, particularly when taking doxy-cycline. If sunburn-like reactions or skin eruptions occur, the patient should contact the prescriber immediately.

Additional patient counseling includes whether to take the drug with food or on an empty stomach. Absorption of ampicillin, for example, is decreased both by rate and extent when taken with food. Thus, ampicillin should be taken on an empty stomach (i.e., 1 hour before or 2 hours after a meal). Storage instructions include whether the drug needs refrigeration, as do the oral suspensions of ampicillin and amoxicillin, which are stable for only 7 days at room temperature but for 14 days under refrigeration. The reconstituted oral suspension of amoxicillin–clavulanate should be kept in the refrigerator, as should oral cephalosporin suspensions.

Patients should be encouraged to take the macrolides with food to lessen the GI adverse effects, except for the oral suspension of azithromycin, which must be taken on an empty stomach. The oral suspension of erythromycin should be refrigerated, but the oral suspension of clarithromycin should not be refrigerated because it is more palatable when taken at room temperature. The oral suspension of azithromycin can be refrigerated if the patient so desires.

Because fluoroquinolones may cause dizziness and light-headedness, patients need to be aware of this when operating an automobile or other potentially dangerous machinery or engaging in activities requiring mental alertness or coordination.

A Web source for patient information on updated information about bronchitis is www.nih.gov/medlineplus/bronchitis.html.

COMMUNITY-ACQUIRED PNEUMONIA

Pneumonia is an infection of the lungs that leads to consolidation of the usually air-filled alveoli. It occurs in all age groups and can be caused by various agents, including viruses, bacteria, mycobacteria, mycoplasma, and fungi. Systemic viral infections such as influenza A or B in adults and measles or varicella in children can also lead to bacterial pneumonia.

Pneumonia occurs in about 3 to 4 million patients per year in the United States, with approximately 1 million patients requiring hospitalization. The symptoms of pneumonia include cough, shortness of breath, sputum production, and chest pain. Physical examination includes fever in most, with crackles and bronchial breath sounds on auscultation in about 80% of cases. Pneumonia is classified by where it was acquired: community-acquired pneumonia (CAP) and health care–acquired pneumonia (sometimes called *hospital-acquired pneumonia*).

Pneumonia carries an age-adjusted mortality rate of up to 22%. CAP is an acute infection of the lower respiratory tract that is usually associated with:

- some symptoms of acute infection, and acute infiltrates detected by chest x-ray, OR
- auscultatory findings consistent with pneumonia on physical examination.

The bacteriology and antibiotic choices for CAP have changed in the last decade. The elderly and patients with other coexistent illnesses such as COPD, diabetes mellitus, renal insufficiency, congestive heart failure, and chronic liver disease are at a high risk for acquiring pneumonia compared with other patient populations. New microorganisms have been identified as possible causes for bacterial infections in these patients. More potent antibiotics have been developed to treat CAP and decrease the likelihood of resistance.

CAUSES

Although several pathogens are identified in CAP, the etiology is only established in about 40% of cases. *S. pneumoniae* is the most commonly isolated pathogen in patients with CAP. Nearly 65% of all diagnosed CAP cases can be attributed to *S. pneumoniae*. Other pathogens that have been commonly isolated in patients with CAP are *H. influenzae* (12%), *S. aureus* (2%), and gram-negative bacilli (1%). Less common pathogens that have been implicated in CAP are *M. catarrhalis, Streptococcus pyogenes, Chlamydia psittaci,* and *Neisseria meningitidis.* Atypical microorganisms, such as *Legionella* species, *M. pneumoniae,* and *C. pneumoniae,* account for 10% to 20% of cases of CAP. Between 2% and 15% of CAP cases are due to viral infections. The most common virus known to be associated with CAP is the influenza virus; however, parainfluenza virus, RSV, and adenovirus also have been isolated as CAP pathogens. Methicillin-resistant *S. aureus* (MRSA) has rapidly emerged as the most common pathogen isolated in community-acquired skin and soft-tissue infections and is increasingly recognized as a cause of CAP.

PATHOPHYSIOLOGY

Microorganisms gain access to the lower respiratory tract by inhalation as airborne particles, by way of the bloodstream to the lung from an extrapulmonary site of infection, or, most commonly, through aspiration of oropharyngeal contents. This is a common method of transmission of microorganisms into the lower respiratory tract for both healthy and ill people.

DIAGNOSTIC CRITERIA

Patients with pneumonia typically present with cough, fever, dyspnea, malaise, and/or sputum production. It is difficult to distinguish other respiratory tract infections such as bronchitis from pneumonia based on signs and symptoms (**Figure 27-3**). A chest x-ray can help differentiate pneumonia from other infections and can also indicate whether coexisting conditions, such as COPD or pleural effusions, are present.

The presence of infiltrates on chest x-ray usually indicates pneumonia, which necessitates treatment with an antibiotic. In general, chest x-rays cannot distinguish between bacterial and

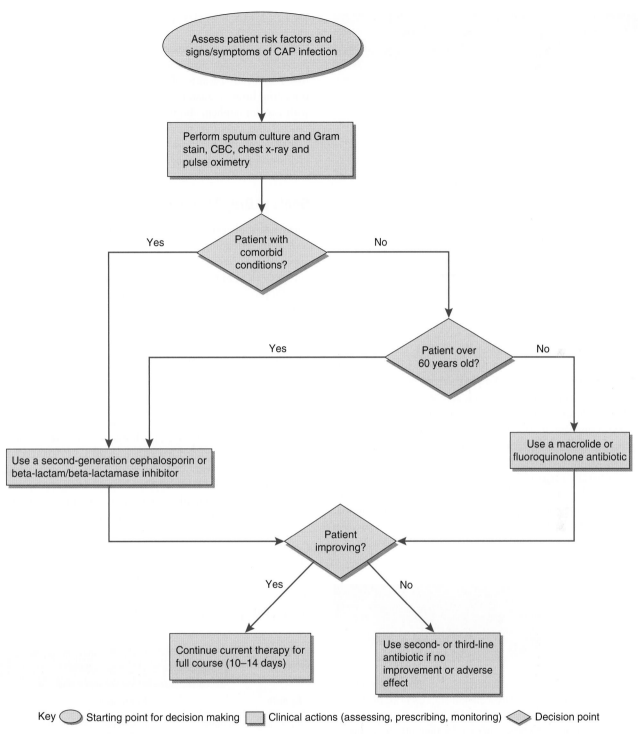

FIGURE 27–3 Treatment algorithm for outpatient treatment of community-acquired pneumonia.

nonbacterial microorganisms. However, certain findings on the chest x-ray can guide the practitioner to a diagnosis. The severity of illness can also be detected by an x-ray; multilobar involvement typically indicates severe illness. **Table 27.5** depicts common findings on chest x-rays in immunocompetent patients and suggests possible pneumonia-causing pathogens. A Gram stain of the sputum specimen is useful in the initial evaluation

of patients with pneumonia. The sensitivity and specificity of a Gram stain can vary; however, it can provide the practitioner with some clues to the causative microorganism. Bacterial cultures of sputum are useful when resistant microorganisms are suspected. Invasive diagnostic techniques such as transtracheal aspiration, bronchoscopy, bronchoalveolar lavage, and direct needle aspiration may be useful in patients with severe CAP.

TABLE 27.5	Differential Diagnosis of Pneumonia Based on Chest X-Ray in Immunocompetent Patients
X-Ray Finding	**Possible Pathogen**
Focal opacity	*S. pneumoniae*
	C. pneumoniae
	H. influenzae
	S. aureus
	Legionella
	M. pneumoniae
Interstitial/miliary involvement	Viruses
	M. pneumoniae
Hilar adenopathy ± segmental or interstitial infiltrate	*C. psittaci*
	M. pneumoniae
Cavitation	Anaerobes

Data from Bartlett, J. G. (1997). *Management of respiratory infections.* Baltimore: Williams & Wilkins.

It can be difficult to determine when an outpatient needs hospitalization for closer observation. **Box 27.2** lists the indications for hospitalization in a patient with severe CAP. However, once patients are hospitalized, several routine tests must be performed to determine the severity of the illness, possible complications, the status of underlying conditions, and the most appropriate treatment choices. A WBC count is not useful for distinguishing between the various causative microorganisms; however, a WBC count greater than 12,000 cells/mm^3 typically suggests bacterial infection. A complete blood count can determine whether a patient has anemia, which can indicate *Mycoplasma* infections or complicated pneumonia. Pulse oximetry can help reflect the severity of the disease. An arterial oxygen saturation of less than 90% on room air is a standard criterion for hospital admission.

BOX	27.2
	Indications for Hospitalization

- Severe vital sign abnormality: pulse >140/min; systolic blood pressure <90 mm Hg; respiratory rate >30/min; temperature >101°F (38.3°C)
- Altered mental status (newly diagnosed): disorientation to person, place or time; stupor or coma
- Arterial hypoxemia: PO2 <60 mm Hg on room air
- Suppurative pneumonia-related infection: empyema, septic arthritis, meningitis, endocarditis
- Severe electrolyte, hematologic, metabolic laboratory value not known to be chronic

Data from Bartlett, J. G. (1997). *Management of respiratory infections.* Baltimore, MD: Williams & Wilkins.

INITIATING DRUG THERAPY

General treatment approaches for pneumonia consist of providing adequate hydration (replacement of loss of water that may occur because of fever, poor intake, or vomiting), providing bronchodilators for dyspnea, and controlling fever with acetaminophen, ibuprofen, or aspirin. Early identification of the causative microorganism is optimal for proper management of CAP. However, diagnostic tests cannot always identify all potential pathogens, and therefore empiric therapy is often initiated by the clinician.

Goals of Drug Therapy

The goals of pharmacotherapy for pneumonia include eradication of the offending microorganism through the selection of appropriate antibiotic therapy and effecting a complete clinical cure, as well as minimizing adverse effects of medications.

Empiric antibiotic treatment for outpatients with pneumonia should always be active against *S. pneumoniae* because this pathogen is one of the most commonly identified causes of bacterial pneumonia. Aminopenicillins and cephalosporins are not recommended as agents of choice for treating pneumonia on an outpatient basis because of the increasing resistance of *S. pneumoniae* to these agents. A macrolide (i.e., erythromycin, clarithromycin, and azithromycin), or doxycycline are the agents of choice for treating pneumonia on an outpatient basis. A fluoroquinolone (e.g., gatifloxacin, levofloxacin, moxifloxacin) is recommended if a patient with CAP has received antibiotic therapy within the previous 10 to 14 days or has other comorbidities (**Table 27.6**).

A-MRSA has rapidly emerged as the most common pathogen isolated in community-acquired skin and soft-tissue infections and is increasingly recognized as a cause of CAP. CA-MRSA pneumonia typically presents as a severe, rapidly progressing pneumonia with sepsis, often in children or healthy young adults. Antimicrobial agents with consistent in vitro activity against CA-MRSA isolates include vancomycin, trimethoprim-sulfamethoxazole, daptomycin, tigecycline,

TABLE 27.6	Recommended Antimicrobial Treatment for Outpatients with CAP*
Agents	**Comments**
macrolides (erythromycin, azithromycin, clarithromycin)	Azithromycin is preferred if *H. influenzae* is the suspected cause of CAP.
fluoroquinolones	Preferred treatment if high-level penicillin-resistant *S. pneumoniae* is the suspected cause of CAP
doxycycline	Good agent to use in patients ages 17 to 40

*In CAP, the order of treatment depends on the cause of CAP. If the cause remains unknown, the prescriber recommends empiric therapy and makes adjustments if needed depending on the patient's response.

and linezolid. Although it is not necessary to provide empiric coverage of MRSA for all pneumonia cases, it should be strongly considered for patients with severe pneumonia associated with sepsis, especially persons with concurrent influenza, contact with someone infected with MRSA, or radiographic evidence of necrotizing pneumonia.

Differences among these agents were discussed previously in the chronic bronchitis section, and must be considered when choosing antimicrobial therapy for CAP. Resistance patterns also should be considered when choosing an agent. For erythromycin and clarithromycin, resistance patterns to *S. pneumoniae* and *H. influenzae* have been documented in certain regions of the United States. *S. pneumoniae* and *H. influenzae* appear to be less resistant to azithromycin than to erythromycin and clarithromycin. If a *Legionella* species is suspected, erythromycin should be added to the regimen. Ciprofloxacin should not be used for treating pneumonia because of the high level of resistance that *S. pneumoniae* exhibits to this drug. A fluoroquinolone with good *S. pneumoniae* coverage should be used, such as levofloxacin or moxifloxacin. In young adults ages 17 to 40 years, doxycycline can be helpful.

If aspiration pneumonia is suspected, then the agent of choice is amoxicillin–clavulanate. If the prescriber suspects that the CAP is caused by a high level of penicillin-resistant *S. pneumoniae* (defined as a minimum inhibitory concentration ≤2 µg/mL), a fluoroquinolone is the agent of choice.

Hospitalized patients should receive a fluoroquinolone or a combination of a macrolide (azithromycin or clarithromycin) and beta-lactam, such as cefotaxime (Claforan) or ceftriaxone (Rocephin) (**Box 27.3**). Patients hospitalized in the intensive care unit for pneumonia should receive the same therapy as other hospitalized patients, unless *Pseudomonas aeruginosa* is a concern. If the latter is true, then an antibiotic with broader gram-negative coverage (i.e., piperacillin–tazobactam, cefepime) should be added.

Selecting the Most Appropriate Agent

Identification of the likely microorganism simplifies treatment for pneumonia. The reader is referred to the comprehensive references for appropriate antimicrobial agents that are commonly used once pathogens have been identified. (See **Figure 27-3**.)

MONITORING PATIENT RESPONSE

The patient's response to therapy must be evaluated carefully. Response to treatment should be based on clinical illness, pathogen isolated, severity of illness, host, and chest x-ray findings. Subjective symptoms usually respond within 3 to 5 days of initiating therapy. Objective findings such as fever, leukocytosis, and chest x-ray abnormalities resolve at different times. Fever lasts for 2 to 4 days in most cases of CAP; however, defervescence occurs more quickly with *S. pneumoniae* infection. Leukocytosis usually resolves by the fourth day of initiation of antimicrobial therapy. Chest x-rays indicate that signs of pneumonia last longer than symptoms. Of course, this depends on many factors, such as the causative microorganism and underlying illness. The overall suggested chest x-ray follow-up is 7 to 12 weeks after initiation of therapy.

Duration of therapy for treating CAP depends on the severity of the illness and the antimicrobial agent that was used to treat the infection. Patients treated for mild episodes of CAP with azithromycin typically have a short duration of therapy. Because the half-life of azithromycin is 11 to 14 hours, it remains in the tissues longer than erythromycin or clarithromycin. Five days of azithromycin therapy is sufficient to treat mild CAP. Bacterial infection with *S. pneumoniae* is treated for 7 to 14 days. *M. pneumoniae* and *C. pneumoniae* infections usually require 10 to 14 days of therapy. Patients with Legionnaires disease who are immunocompetent typically receive 14 days of treatment.

PATIENT EDUCATION

The patient must take the full course of medication even though he or she may feel better within days of initiation of antibiotics. Early discontinuation of therapy can result in reinfection or the development of resistant microorganisms. If the patient continues to worsen despite several days of therapy, he or she should contact the prescriber immediately. The organism causing infection in the patient could be resistant to the antibiotic originally prescribed. Readers should refer to the chronic bronchitis section for further information on drug therapy.

BOX 27.3

Preferred Antimicrobial Choices for Patients Hospitalized with Pneumonia

General Inpatient
- Beta-lactam antibiotic with or without a macrolide antibiotic
- Fluoroquinolone

Alternatives include cefuroxime with or without a macrolide antibiotic or azithromycin (alone).

Intensive Care
- Antipseudomonal cephalosporin (cefotaxime, ceftriaxone) plus a macrolide or fluoroquinolone
- Beta-lactam/beta-lactamase inhibitor (e.g., ampicillin/sulbactam, ticarcillin/clavulanate, piperacillin/tazobactam)

Case Study

R. R., a 58-year-old man, presents to the clinic with complaints of increasing shortness of breath, chills, malaise, and cough productive of a yellowish-green sputum. His medical history is significant for hypertension and chronic lower back pain. He has a 35 pack-year history of cigarette smoking. Physical examination is significant for rales on auscultation of the chest. Clubbing of the fingernails is apparent. Vital signs are blood pressure, 138/88 mm Hg; pulse rate, 96 beats/min; respiration rate, 32 breaths/min; and temperature, 99.7°F. Laboratory test results and chest x-ray findings are pending.

DIAGNOSIS: PNEUMONIA

1. List specific treatment goals for R. R.
2. What drug therapy would you prescribe? Why?

3. What are the parameters for monitoring success of the therapy?
4. Describe specific patient goals based on the prescribed therapy.
5. List one or two adverse reactions for the selected agent that would cause you to change therapy.
6. What would be the choice for second-line therapy?
7. What dietary and lifestyle changes should be recommended for this patient?
8. Describe one or two drug–drug or drug–food interactions for the selected agent.

BIBLIOGRAPHY

Ewig, S., Welte, T., Chastre, J., & Torres, A. (2010). Rethinking concepts of community-acquired and health-care–acquired pneumonia. *The Lancet Infectious Diseases 10*(4), 279–283.

Fu, C., Metlay, J., Canargo, C., et al. (2010). ED antibiotic use for respiratory illness since pneumonia performance measure inception. *Chest, 28*(1), 23–31.

Mandell, L., Wunderink, R., Anzueto, A., et al. (2007). Infectious Disease Society of America/American Thoracic Society consensus guidelines on the management of community-acquired pneumonia in adults. *Clinics of Infectious Diseases, 44*(Suppl 2).

Moran, J., Talon, D., & Abrahamian, F. (2008). Diagnosis and management of pneumonia in the emergency department. *Infectious Disease Clinics of North America, 22*(1), 53–72.

Nazarian, D., Eddy, O., Lukens, T., et al. (2009). Critical issues in management of the adult patient presenting to the emergency department with community-acquired pneumonia. *Annals of Emergency Medicine, 54*(5), 704–731.

Ranganathan, S., & Sonnappa, S. (2009). Pneumonia and other respiratory infections. *Pediatric Clinics of North America, 56*(1), 135–156.

UNIT

6

Pharmacotherapy for Gastrointestinal Tract Disorders

Nausea and Vomiting

Nausea and vomiting are common complaints in humans. The severity of the event can range from a slight discomfort or queasiness to uncontrollable, forceful vomiting. Despite this range, all are perceived to be uncomfortable and troublesome and should be treated in a proper and timely manner. Patients may refer to this experience by many different names: *upchuck, urp, queasy, throw-up, puke,* to name a few. There are many different causes of nausea and vomiting, such as motion sickness, pregnancy, and medications. Likewise, many treatment options can be used to manage this complication. People of all ages experience emesis, although the etiology may be related to age-specific factors. Drugs are most frequently used for the treatment of nausea and vomiting, but alterations of non-drug factors may decrease the severity of emesis. This chapter reviews the pathophysiology and pharmacotherapy of specific types of nausea and vomiting.

CAUSES

There are multiple causes for nausea and vomiting; however, some of the most common are from the ingestion or administration of substances or drugs, gastrointestinal (GI) disorders, neurologic processes, and metabolic disorders. The presence of noxious stimuli is frequently a cause of nausea and vomiting. Supratherapeutic digoxin (Lanoxin) and theophylline (Theo-Dur or Slo-Phyllin) are known to produce emesis. Nausea and vomiting occur more frequently with high-dose chemotherapy than with moderate doses of the same drugs. Erythromycin and some penicillin derivatives are acknowledged for inducing uncomfortable GI complications. Emesis can also result from excessive ethanol intake. It is well known that other sensory experiences, such as pungent odors or gruesome sights, can induce nausea and vomiting. **Box 28.1** presents specific etiologies for nausea and vomiting.

Patient-specific factors that increase susceptibility to nausea and vomiting include age, previous nausea and vomiting experiences, and sex. Most of the research identifying these characteristics was done in patients receiving chemotherapy. Poor control of nausea and vomiting with previous surgeries or chemotherapy predisposes a patient to subsequent episodes of emesis, also referred to as *anticipatory nausea and vomiting*. This form of emesis is often difficult to treat with standard antiemetics.

One study of patients with cancer reports a threefold increase in the incidence of emesis in patients previously treated with chemotherapy compared with chemotherapy-naive patients treated with identical chemotherapy regimens (Pisters & Kris, 1992).

Adult patients younger than age 30 have an increased incidence of emesis compared with their older counterparts. In addition, the younger patient population is more likely to experience extrapyramidal reactions from the drugs used to treat their nausea and vomiting. In patients who received the same chemotherapy and antiemetic premedications, women experienced more nausea and vomiting than men (Pisters & Kris, 1992).

Chronic ethanol intake exceeding 100 g/d (roughly five beers or mixed drinks per day) is associated with better emesis control and decreased incidence. A history of motion sickness may increase the risks of nausea and vomiting in another situation, such as with chemotherapy or surgery. Children in general experience nausea and vomiting more frequently than adults. Obesity and anxiety have also been associated with heightened emesis incidence.

The prevalence of nausea and vomiting may complicate 11% to 73% of surgical procedures. Prevalence is also increased by the use of certain inhalation agents (nitrous oxide, in particular) and by concomitant use of opiate medications; the use of propofol as an intravenous anesthetic agent lowers the risk of postoperative nausea and vomiting (PONV). PONV is more likely to occur after general than regional anesthesia, and its prevalence increases in parallel with the duration of surgery and anesthesia. PONV is especially common after gynecologic and middle ear surgery and also occurs more commonly with abdominal and orthopedic surgery than with laparoscopic or other extra-abdominal operations. PONV is also more likely in those with a history of PONV or motion sickness.

PATHOPHYSIOLOGY

The pathophysiology of nausea and vomiting is complex (**Figure 28-1**) and involves the modulation of medullary sites and neurotransmitters. Many sensory centers accept noxious stimuli from the body, including the chemoreceptor trigger zone (CTZ), visceral afferent nerves, cerebral cortex, limbic system, vestibular system, and midbrain intracranial pressure receptors.

BOX 28.1

Etiologies of Nausea and Vomiting

Therapy-induced causes
  Chemotherapy
  Radiation therapy
  Opiates
  Anticonvulsants
  Ipecac
  Antibiotics
  Digitalis or digoxin toxicity
  Theophylline
  Nonsteroidal anti-inflammatory drugs
  Hormonal therapies
Drug withdrawal
  Opiates
  Benzodiazepines
Metabolic disorders
  Addison disease
  Water intoxication
  Volume depletion
  Diabetic ketoacidosis
  Hypercalcemia
  Renal dysfunction–uremia
Gastrointestinal mechanisms
  Mechanical gastric outlet obstruction
    Peptic ulcer disease
    Gastric carcinoma
    Pancreatic disease
  Motility disorders
    Gastroparesis
    Drug-induced gastric stasis
    Irritable bowel syndrome
    Postgastric surgery
    Idiopathic gastric stasis
  Intra-abdominal emergencies
    Acute pancreatitis
    Acute pyelonephritis
    Acute cholecystitis

Acute cholangitis
Acute viral hepatitis
Intestinal obstruction
Acute gastroenteritis
  Viral gastroenteritis
  Salmonellosis
  Shigellosis
  Staphylococcal gastroenteritis (enterotoxins)
Cardiovascular disease
  Acute myocardial infarction
  Congestive heart failure
  Shock and circulatory collapse
Neurologic processes
  Cerebellar hemorrhage
  Increased intracranial pressure
    Hematoma
    Subdural effusion
    Tumor (benign or malignant)
    Hydrocephalus
    Reye syndrome
  Headache
    Migraine
    Severe hypertension
  Head trauma
  Vestibular disorders
Psychogenic causes
  Anorexia nervosa
  Anticipatory
Miscellaneous causes
  Pregnancy
  Noxious odors
  Ingestion of an irritant
  Operative procedures
  Septicemia
  Nicotine

Modulation of Nausea and Vomiting

These stimuli are transmitted to the vomiting center, also called the *emetic center*, which coordinates the sensory inputs and the act of vomiting. The vomiting center is the key component in the modulation of nausea and vomiting. Located in the lateral reticular formation of the medulla, it receives afferent impulses from the aforementioned sensory centers. On activation of the vomiting center, efferent impulses are sent to the nucleus tractus solitarius, an intertwined neural network that innervates the salivary, vasomotor, and respiratory centers and cranial nerves VIII and X. Efferent impulses are also sent

to the stomach, abdominal muscles, diaphragm, and associated sphincters to execute the involuntary act of vomiting. Much like the sensory centers that stimulate it, the vomiting center is rich in dopamine, histamine, serotonin, and acetylcholine receptors and can also be affected by binding to opiate and benzodiazepine receptors. An intact vomiting center is essential for coordination of the vomiting act.

Stimulatory Centers

The CTZ is one of the most important chemosensory organs responsible for the detection of noxious stimuli. It is uniquely

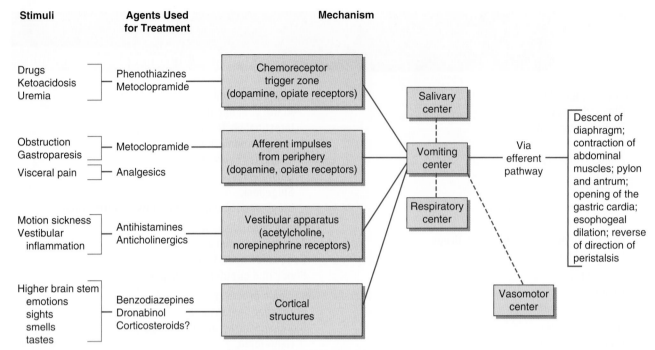

FIGURE 28–1 Pathophysiology of nausea and vomiting. (From Koda-Kimble, M. A., & Young, L. Y. [2004]. Nausea and vomiting. In M. A. Koda-Kimble, L. Y. Young, & B. J. Guglielmo [Eds.], *Applied therapeutics: The clinical use of drugs* [8th ed.]. Philadelphia: Lippincott Williams & Wilkins.)

located in the area postrema in the floor of the fourth ventricle of the (medulla) brain and is exposed to both blood and cerebrospinal fluid (CSF). Thus, toxins in both the blood and CSF can stimulate a response by the CTZ. These toxins may be drugs (chemotherapy, opiates, digoxin), poisons, or substances found naturally in the body (excess calcium, hormones). The CTZ is rich in neurotransmitter receptors for dopamine, serotonin, histamine, and acetylcholine. An antiemetic effect is elicited when these receptors are blocked.

Gastrointestinal Tract

The GI tract and pharynx are sites of origin for the stimulation of nausea and vomiting. Visceral afferent nerves, also referred to as *splanchnic nerves*, from the pharynx and GI tract transmit impulses from local neuroreceptors along the vagus nerve to the vomiting center. The GI tract is rich in local dopamine, histamine, and serotonin receptors. The visceral afferent nerves are also responsible for transmitting stimuli from other peripheral sites such as the heart, lungs, and testes; hence, the vomiting response may occur when a person has been punched in the abdomen or kicked in the groin. Abdominal surgery is another example in which visceral afferent nerves are involved in nausea and vomiting.

Central Nervous System

Motion sickness is primarily a central nervous system (CNS) response mediated by the vestibular system. Acetylcholine and histamine receptors have been found in the vestibular center. Blockade of these receptors provides some degree of protection from emesis. The cerebral cortex, the largest portion of

the brain, is responsible for the motor coordination of the body, sensory perception, learning, memory, and many other functions. Afferent impulses from specific sites of the cerebral cortex can result in emesis. The cerebellum is responsible for the regulation of balance, equilibrium, and coordination. Disruption of this portion of the brain can lead to temporary or chronic nausea and vomiting. These structures may also play a role in anticipatory emesis.

Limbic System

The limbic system and the midbrain intracranial pressure receptors can stimulate nausea and vomiting, although their mechanisms are not fully understood. In humans, the primary function of the limbic system is associated with the expression of mood, emotions, and feelings, as well as memory recall. Anxiety, fear, and other emotions may play a role at this site in the perception of nausea and vomiting. Head trauma, intracranial bleeding, and mass effect from a benign or malignant tumor can produce increased pressure in the brain. This increased intracranial pressure can cause nausea and vomiting. The optimal treatment in these situations is a reduction in intracranial pressure through surgery or corticosteroids.

DIAGNOSTIC CRITERIA

The three identified phases of emesis are nausea, retching, and vomiting. Nausea is the unpleasant physical sensation of impending retching or vomiting. Nausea often occurs without the other two steps of emesis, although they are all treated with the same pharmacologic agents. Common symptoms accompanying nausea are flushing, pallor, tachycardia, and hypersalivation. Gastric stasis, decreased pyloric tone, mucosal blood flow, and contractions of the duodenum with reflux into the stomach are physiologic responses to nausea. Retching, the second phase of emesis, is the involuntary synchronized labored movement of abdominal and thoracic muscles before vomiting. Vomiting is the coordinated contractions of the abdominal and thoracic muscles to expel the gastric contents. The lower esophageal sphincter contracts, allowing GI retroperistalsis. The actual expulsion of gastric contents differentiates vomiting from retching.

The acuteness of the symptomatology is based on history and physical examination. Several issues need to be addressed such as whether this is an acute emergency, such as mechanical obstruction, perforation, or peritonitis, clinical clues that the problem is likely to be self-limited, such as would be expected with viral gastroenteritis or a potentially offending medication. The goal is to determine whether empiric treatment with an antiemetic, a gastric acid-suppressing, or a prokinetic agent would be beneficial or whether the patient should be admitted to the hospital to correct fluid and electrolyte imbalance.

Acute nausea and vomiting differs considerably from that of chronic nausea and vomiting so symptom duration is important. Acute onset of nausea and vomiting suggests gastroenteritis, pancreatitis, cholecystitis, or a drug-related side effect. When nausea and vomiting are associated with diarrhea, headache, and myalgias, the cause is viral gastroenteritis; in this instance, symptoms should resolve spontaneously within 5 days. A more insidious onset of nausea without vomiting is suspicious of gastroparesis, a medication-related side effect, metabolic disorders, pregnancy, or even gastroesophageal reflux disease. Nausea and vomiting are considered chronic when their duration is longer than 1 month.

Timing and description of the vomiting are important. Vomiting that occurs in the morning before breakfast is typical of that related to pregnancy, uremia, alcohol ingestion, and increased intracranial pressure. Projectile vomiting suggests intracranial disorders, especially those that result in increased intracranial pressure. In this case, vomiting may not be preceded by nausea.

The onset of vomiting caused by gastroparesis or gastric outlet obstruction tends to be delayed, usually by more than 1 hour, after meal ingestion. Vomiting may be suggestive of psychiatric disorders.

Associated symptoms, such as abdominal pain, fever, diarrhea, vertigo, or a history of a similar contemporaneous illness among family, friends, or associates are important data to gather.

The physical examination looks at vital signs for signs of dehydration. Jaundice, lymphadenopathy, abdominal masses, and occult blood in the stool may reveal features suggestive of thyrotoxicosis or Addison disease. The abdominal examination should look for distention, visible peristalsis, and abdominal or inguinal hernias. Areas of tenderness are important: tenderness in the midepigastrium suggests an ulcer; in the right upper quadrant, cholecystitis or biliary tract disease. Auscultation may demonstrate increased bowel sounds in obstruction or absent bowel sounds in ileus.

INITIATING THERAPY

The treatment of nausea, retching, or vomiting in any patient begins with an evaluation and correction of possible causes. Most sources of nausea and vomiting may be reversed or palliated by surgery or medical interventions. Infectious causes should be promptly treated with antibiotics, and metabolic disorders require medical management. Some drug toxicities may be treated with antidotes, such as digoxin toxicity reversed with digoxin immune Fab (Digibind). The following section discusses medications used to treat nausea and vomiting. They should be used with definitive treatments when possible.

Alterations in a patient's daily activities may aid in managing nausea and vomiting and decrease the resources used to control the problem. Nonpharmacologic management of nausea and vomiting should be tailored to the presumed etiology.

Changes in a patient's diet may affect the frequency or severity of nausea and vomiting, such as avoidance of spicy foods and excessive grease or oil, and decreased caffeine intake. Professional counseling or group therapy may prove favorable for patients with psychogenic nausea and vomiting.

Hypnosis, behavior modification, and imagery are beneficial tools in controlling nausea and vomiting that has an anxiety component, such as chemotherapy-related anticipatory emesis. However, prevention of anticipatory nausea and vomiting is the optimal form of management.

Goals of Drug Therapy

The goals of drug therapy are simple: to alleviate the subjective feeling of nausea and the objective act of vomiting and their associated complications (**Box 28.2**). It is important to rely on the patient's subjective response when evaluating the efficacy of a specific therapy for nausea. Secondary goals are to minimize drug toxicity/adverse events and contain costs. The prevention of nausea and vomiting is the goal in the setting of chemotherapy and certain surgical procedures. Control or improvement in nausea and vomiting should occur within 5 to 60 minutes of a pharmacologic intervention. If this does not ensue, another method should be used promptly. **Table 28.1** reviews available antiemetic agents, dosages, comparable efficacy, and adverse effects. Pregnancy risk factors are included in the discussion of each drug class and in the pregnancy-related nausea and vomiting section.

Phenothiazines

Phenothiazines are a commonly used class of drugs to treat nausea and vomiting. Prochlorperazine (Compazine) and promethazine (Phenergan) are the most frequently used drugs in this class.

Mechanism of Action

Their mechanism of action presumably involves dopamine receptor blockade in the CTZ. Anticholinergic activity in the vomiting and vestibular centers of the brain may also contribute to the mechanism of action.

BOX 28.2

Complications of Nausea and Vomiting

Metabolic abnormalities
- Dehydration
- Alkalosis
- Hypokalemia
- Hypomagnesemia
- Hyponatremia
- Hypochloremia
- Malnutrition

Structural damage
- Wound dehiscence
- Esophagogastric tears/Mallory-Weiss tears
- Increased bleeding under skin flaps
- Tension on suture lines

Patient dissatisfaction
- Noncompliance
- Poor oral intake; anticipatory nausea and vomiting
- Delayed ambulation after surgery/procedures
- Fatigue
- Depression

Increased use of resources
- Prolongation of hospital stay
- Unexpected hospital admission
- Alteration or additional therapy

Aspiration pneumonia

Venous hypertension

The phenothiazines may be used as monotherapy for mild to moderate nausea and vomiting or in combination with other antiemetics for more severe nausea and vomiting. A dose–response quality has been noted for this drug class; however, the incidence of adverse effects such as extrapyramidal effects and sedation can also be associated with higher doses. Promethazine has activities of an antihistamine antiemetic and could also be classified with the antihistamine–anticholinergic class of drugs. The phenothiazines are a viable and practical option for long-term treatment of nausea and vomiting. Products are available in oral, rectal, and injectable formulations. To improve tailoring of the drug regimen to the patient, oral preparations are available as tablets, sustained-release capsules, and liquids. Rectal suppositories are useful in patients who cannot retain oral medications and when intravenous (IV) access is not an option. Suppositories should be avoided in patients who are thrombocytopenic because of the increased risk of bleeding or hemorrhage.

Contraindications

Caution should be used in patients taking concomitant drugs that cause CNS depression, such as sedatives, hypnotics, and opiates, because further sedation may result. Phenothiazines may exacerbate the symptoms of Parkinson disease. The safety of phenothiazines during pregnancy is controversial; most studies find phenothiazines to be safe for the mother and fetus if used occasionally in low doses. Most phenothiazines are in pregnancy risk category C. Phenothiazines may decrease the seizure threshold and should be used cautiously in patients with seizure disorders.

The phenothiazines are relatively inexpensive in relation to most of the other drug classes, with the exception of the sustained-release phenothiazine preparations, which tend to be costly.

Adverse Events

The most common adverse event of phenothiazine use is drowsiness or sedation. Phenothiazines also have the ability to evoke extrapyramidal symptoms (EPSs) by blocking the central dopaminergic receptors involved in motor function, particularly at higher doses. EPSs may present as dystonic reactions, feelings of motor restlessness, and parkinsonian signs and symptoms. Masklike face, drooling, tremor, cogwheel rigidity, pill-rolling motion, lack of ability to initiate voluntary movement, and gait abnormalities are all severe examples of parkinsonian presentations. Dystonic reactions may include spasm of the neck muscles or torticollis, extensor rigidity of back muscles, mandibular tics, difficulty swallowing or talking, and perioral spasms, often with protrusion of the tongue. Motor restlessness may consist of agitation, jitteriness, tapping of feet, and insomnia. Extrapyramidal reactions can be easily treated with the use of diphenhydramine (Benadryl) 25 mg orally or parenterally 3 to 4 times a day or benztropine (Cogentin) 1 to 4 mg orally or parenterally twice a day. Autonomic responses, such as hypotension and tachycardia, have been observed with IV phenothiazine use, particularly chlorpromazine. Hypotension and sedation are less likely to occur with prochlorperazine, thiethylperazine, and perphenazine, but these three agents are associated with a higher frequency of EPSs. Dry mouth, urinary retention, blurred vision, and other anticholinergic effects may occur with phenothiazine use. Reversible agranulocytosis is rarely associated (<1%) with phenothiazine therapy. This effect occurs more frequently in women and with chronic phenothiazine use. Cholestatic jaundice and photosensitivity are reactions that can occur rarely within the first few months of chronic phenothiazine use. These are more frequently observed in phenothiazine use for psychiatric conditions rather than emesis control.

Monitoring parameters include EPSs and parkinsonian symptoms. Doses may need to be decreased in severe hepatic dysfunction. Complete blood counts should be regularly monitored in chronic phenothiazine use. (See **Table 28.1.**)

Interactions

These drugs potentiate CNS depression with alcohol and other CNS depressants. They potentiate the action of α blockers and levels of the drug can be increased with propranolol. Anticonvulsant drug doses may have to be adjusted. They may antagonize oral anticoagulants.

TABLE 28.1 Overview of Selected Antiemetic Agents

Generic (Trade) Name and Dosage	Selected Adverse Events	Contraindications	Special Considerations
Phenothiazines			
chlorpromazine (Thorazine) 10–25 mg q4–6 h prn PO 25–50 mg q4–6h prn IV, IM 50–100 mg q6–8h prn rectal	Sedation or drowsiness EPSs: agitation, insomnia, motor restlessness, spasms of facial muscles, protrusion of tongue, and mandibular tics Anticholinergic effects: dry mouth, urinary retention, blurred vision	Hypersensitivity Cautious use with other CNS depressants, Parkinson syndrome, poorly controlled seizure disorder, severe hepatic dysfunction	Increased incidence of autonomic response with IV administration Higher incidence of EPSs
fluphenazine (Prolixin) 0.5–5 mg q6–8h prn PO, IM	Same as above	Same as above	
perphenazine (Trilafon) 2–6 mg q4–6h prn PO 5–10 mg q6h prn IM	Same as above	Same as above	Higher incidence of EPSs compared with other phenothiazines
prochlorperazine (Compazine) 5–10 mg q4–6h prn PO, rectal, IM, IV 10–30 mg bid PO sustained-release capsule	Same as above	Same as above	Sustained-release capsule more expensive Higher incidence of EPSs compared with other phenothiazines
promethazine (Phenergan) 12.5–25 mg q4–6h prn PO, rectal, IM, IV	Same as above	Same as above	
Antihistamines and Anticholinergics			
benzquinamide (Emete-con) 50 mg q3–4h prn IM 25 mg q3–4h prn IV	Sedation or drowsiness, confusion Anticholinergic effects: dry mouth, tachycardia, blurred vision, urinary retention, constipation	Hypersensitivity Caution in narrow-angle glaucoma, asthma, prostatic hypertrophy	IV preparation not recommended
dimenhydrinate (Dramamine) 50–100 mg q4–6h prn PO, IM, IV	Same as above	Same as above	Do not exceed 200 mg/d
diphenhydramine (Benadryl) 25–50 mg q6–8h prn PO 10–50 mg q2–4h prn IM, IV	Same as above	Same as above	Do not exceed 200 mg/d
hydroxyzine (Atarax, Vistaril) 25–100 mg q4–6h prn PO, IM	Same as above	Same as above	
meclizine (Antivert, Bonine) 25–50 mg q24h prn PO	Same as above	Same as above	
scopolamine (Transderm-Scop) 1.5 mg q3d transdermal patch	Same as above	Same as above	
trimethobenzamide (Tigan) 250 mg q6–8h prn PO 200 mg q6–8h prn IM, rectal	Same as above	Same as above	
Benzodiazepines			
lorazepam (Ativan) 0.5–2 mg q4–8h prn PO, IM, IV	Drowsiness or fatigue, confusion, constipation	Same as above	Dose should be low in frail, elderly, or critically ill patients
diazepam (Valium) 2–5 mg bid–qid prn PO, IM, IV	Same as above	Same as above	Same as above

(continued)

TABLE 28.1   **Overview of Selected Antiemetic Agents (*Continued*)**

Generic (Trade) Name and Dosage	Selected Adverse Events	Contraindications	Special Considerations
Serotonin Antagonists			
dolasetron (Anzemet) 100 mg PO 1 h before chemotherapy 100 mg IV 30 min before chemotherapy 12.5 mg IV 15 min before cessation of anesthesia 100 mg PO 2 h before surgery	Headache, diarrhea, ECG changes	Hypersensitivity Use with caution in patients with severe cardiac dysfunction	Very expensive (IV > PO) Use only when indicated
granisetron (Kytril) 10 μg/kg IV 30 min before chemotherapy 1 mg PO bid (q12h)—start before chemotherapy (Sancuso) patch—3.1 mg/24 h (1 patch)	Same as above	Same as above	Very expensive (IV > PO) Use only when indicated IV dose often rounded to 1- or 2-mg doses
ondansetron (Zofran) 0.15 mg/kg IV 30 min before chemotherapy and at 4 and 8 h	Same as above	Same as above	Very expensive (IV > PO) Use only when indicated
Other Antiemetics			
dexamethasone (Decadron) 8–20 mg IV/PO before chemotherapy; 4–8 mg IV bid (delayed nausea and vomiting)	Hyperactivity, GI irritation, mood swings, depression, hyperglycemia, anxiety	Hypersensitivity Use with caution in diabetic patients, history of ulcers, young male patients	Give IV over 5–15 min Administer orally with food Avoid chronic administration
methylprednisolone (Solu-Medrol) 125–500 mg IV q6h	Same as above	Same as above	Same as above
dronabinol (Marinol) 5–15 mg/m² PO 1–3 h before chemotherapy and q4h × 6 2.5–10 mg PO bid	Sedation, confusion, dysphoria, increased appetite	Use with caution if patient is receiving other CNS depressants	Controlled substance
antacids 15–30 mL q2–4h prn	Diarrhea, constipation	Renal dysfunction	May decrease absorption of other drugs
metoclopramide (Reglan)	EPSs		Side effects are dose dependent
20–30 mg PO qid prn, 1–2 mg/kg IV before chemotherapy and q2–4h (high-dose)	Diarrhea Drowsiness		EPS reversible with diphenhydramine

Antihistamines–Anticholinergics

A plethora of agents are available in the antihistamine–anticholinergic drug class. These agents are most useful for mild nausea, such as motion sickness. Hydroxyzine (Vistaril, Atarax), meclizine (Bonine, Antivert), dimenhydrinate (Dramamine), and scopolamine (Transderm Scop) are some of the more common agents of this class. Unlike most of the other classes of agents discussed in this chapter, some of the antihistamine–anticholinergic agents are available without a prescription.

Mechanism of Action

The mechanism of action appears to be interruption of visceral afferent pathways that are responsible for stimulating nausea and vomiting. These drugs are most frequently administered orally, but some can be given IV, intramuscularly, transdermally, or rectally.

The antihistamines are particularly useful for the treatment and prevention of motion sickness. For this indication, it is recommended that a dose be taken at least 30 to 60 minutes before the event (e.g., boating, air flight, car ride) and then repeated at regular intervals several times a day. The scopolamine patch is a highly useful agent for the prevention of motion sickness. A patch should be applied to clean, dry skin 1 to 2 hours before the potentially emetogenic event, and a new patch may be reapplied every 3 days.

Many of the antihistamines and anticholinergics have been used for the treatment of nausea in pregnancy.

Contraindications

Precautions are recommended with asthma, glaucoma, and GI or urinary obstruction. Antihistamines–anticholinergics are not recommended for nursing mothers.

Adverse Events

Adverse effects limit the use of anticholinergics–antihistamines. Patients frequently experience sedation, drowsiness, or confusion. The anticholinergic effects are troublesome, including blurred vision, dry mouth, urinary retention, and tachycardia. These anticholinergic effects are also dose related and occur more frequently as the dose increases or the drug is given more often. Caution is warranted in patients with narrow-angle glaucoma, prostatic hypertrophy, and asthma because these patients are more prone to the anticholinergic effects of these drugs.

Anticholinergic effects may be managed by nondrug therapies. Chewing gum or sucking on ice chips or hard candy may refresh a dry mouth. The intake of a high-fiber diet and adequate daily fluid consumption may curb constipation.

Monitoring for anticholinergic effects is of paramount importance. Severe effects may warrant discontinuation of the drug. Symptoms of overdose may include dilated pupils, tachycardia, hypertension, CNS depression, flushed skin, or, more seriously, respiratory failure and circulatory collapse. Adverse effects occur more commonly in patients with renal or hepatic dysfunction.

Interactions

These drugs can potentiate CNS depression with alcohol, tranquilizers, and sedative–hypnotics.

Benzodiazepines

Often used for other indications, benzodiazepines offer useful qualities to the antiemetic armamentarium. Not only do these agents treat and prevent emesis, they can cause anxiolysis and amnesia. These latter effects are particularly beneficial in anticipatory nausea and vomiting associated with chemotherapy.

Lorazepam (Ativan) is the most frequently used benzodiazepine for nausea and vomiting. Its mechanism of action is not fully elucidated; however, it probably acts centrally to inhibit the vomiting center. Lorazepam has only moderate antiemetic properties and is usually used in combination with other agents to control chemotherapy-associated anticipatory nausea and vomiting and delayed chemotherapy-associated nausea and vomiting.

Dosage

Both oral and parenteral forms of lorazepam are available. Patient-specific variables should be considered when identifying an appropriate dose. Usual oral or IV doses range from 0.5 to 2 mg at least 30 minutes before start of chemotherapy. As-needed (prn) antiemetic doses range from 0.5 to 3 mg IV or orally every 4 to 6 hours. To prevent oversedation, patients with poor performance status, the elderly, or frail individuals require low initial doses of lorazepam. Patients with compromised pulmonary or poor cardiac function should receive IV lorazepam with caution and have close monitoring of respiratory and cardiac status.

Contraindications

Lorazepam is not recommended for use in patients with hepatic or renal failure. Several studies have indicated that diazepam (Valium) may also cause fetal toxicity when administered to pregnant women, and thus should be avoided in this patient population. The benzodiazepines are in pregnancy risk category D.

Adverse Events

For benzodiazepines, CNS depression occurs most often, with drowsiness, fatigue, memory impairment, impaired coordination, and confusion occurring frequently. Lorazepam has an amnesic effect that for some patients is a benefit, whereas others may find it unacceptable. Paradoxical CNS stimulation resulting in restlessness, anxiety, nightmares, and increased muscle spasticity may occur. The drug should be discontinued if paradoxical stimulation occurs. Other adverse effects include constipation, headache, and increased or decreased appetite. Parenteral administration may cause hypotension, bradycardia, or apnea, particularly in the elderly and critically ill. (See **Table 28.1.**)

Monitoring parameters include cardiovascular and respiratory status for initial doses. Because the liver metabolizes the benzodiazepines, liver function tests should be assessed before dosing. The presence of adverse CNS effects should be evaluated with each clinic or hospital visit.

Interactions

These drugs potentiate CNS depression when used with other drugs that depress the CNS and alcohol.

Serotonin Antagonists

The serotonin antagonists are another class of antiemetics. Ondansetron (Zofran), granisetron (Kytril, Sancuso), palonosetron (Aloxi), and dolasetron (Anzemet) are available in the United States.

Mechanism of Action

These agents work by antagonizing the type 3 serotonin ($5HT_3$) receptors centrally in the CTZ and also peripherally at the vagal and splanchnic afferent fibers from the enterochromaffin cells in the upper GI tract. The serotonin antagonists were initially indicated for the treatment and prevention of chemotherapy-induced nausea and vomiting. They have changed the way nausea and vomiting are treated and have greatly improved the quality of life for patients receiving highly emetogenic chemotherapy regimens. Radiation-induced nausea and vomiting and PONV are two other areas where the serotonin antagonists have been studied. The unequivocal efficacy and lack of significant adverse effects make these agents ideal for select indications.

The serotonin antagonists are available orally as tablets and liquids and parenterally for IV use. Because these agents are used to prevent nausea and vomiting, oral administration in this situation is encouraged, even with highly emetogenic chemotherapy. There have been few data to support superior efficacy of one agent over another when used at recommended dosages. All of the serotonin antagonist preparations are costly and should be used conservatively and appropriately. Many institutions have created antiemetic guidelines to identify the approved indications of serotonin antagonists to optimize care and resources. The appropriateness of these agents in specific circumstances is discussed later.

Contraindications

There are inadequate human data for use in pregnancy; however, animal studies do not reveal evidence of harm to the fetus. Two case reports cite the efficacy of ondansetron in the treatment of hyperemesis gravidarum, without adverse sequelae to the fetus. The serotonin antagonists are in pregnancy risk category B. The serotonin antagonists should be used with caution in breast-feeding mothers; once again, human data are lacking, but ondansetron is distributed into the milk of lactating rats.

Adverse Events

Mild to moderate headache can occur in patients receiving oral or parenteral serotonin antagonists, followed in frequency by diarrhea. A few patients experience severe headaches requiring discontinuation of the drug. Other adverse effects that occur in less than 10% of patients are abdominal or epigastric pain, increased serum hepatic enzyme levels on liver function tests, hypertension, malaise or fatigue, constipation, pruritus, and fever. Rare cardiovascular effects have been reported, although a definite causal relationship has not been established. All three of the agents can cause electrocardiographic (ECG) alterations (prolonged PR interval and QT interval and widened QRS complex). This is best documented in the studies of dolasetron, but these ECG changes were deemed to be clinically nonsignificant by the authors (Audhuy, et al., 1996). Conservatively, in patients with severe cardiac dysfunctions such as arrhythmia and heart block, the serotonin antagonists should be used cautiously.

Important monitoring parameters for serotonin antagonists include baseline and follow-up liver function tests. Dosage reductions may be made for severe hepatic dysfunction. To avoid ECG-related complications, electrolyte assessment and correction of hypokalemia and hypomagnesemia are indicated. (See **Table 28.1.**)

Interactions

Caution is used when given with drugs that prolong cardiac conduction interval, diuretics, and cumulative high-dose anthracycline.

Metoclopramide and Other Antiemetics

Metoclopramide (Reglan) has been used to treat nausea and vomiting caused by several different stimuli. It is a highly useful agent in the treatment of diabetic gastric stasis, postsurgical gastric stasis, and gastroesophageal reflux, which may be associated with some degree of nausea.

Mechanism of Action

For these indications, metoclopramide enhances motility and gastric emptying by increasing the duration and extent of esophageal contractions, the resting tone of the lower esophageal sphincter, gastric contractions, and peristalsis of the duodenum and jejunum. Metoclopramide is also used in the prevention and treatment of chemotherapy-induced nausea and vomiting. Its mechanism of action is dopamine receptor inhibition in the CTZ. The central and peripheral actions of this agent make it efficacious in multiple clinical situations. Metoclopramide can be administered orally, IV, and intramuscularly. A sugar-free syrup exists for diabetic patients who cannot take the pills. Because metoclopramide is eliminated primarily by the kidneys, the dose of this drug should be decreased by 50% if the patient's creatinine clearance is less than 40 mL/min. Subsequent doses are based on the patient's clinical response. Periodic assessment of renal function is prudent. Patients should be informed of the sedative qualities of this agent and that use of other CNS depressants could potentiate this effect.

Adverse Events

The most clinically concerning adverse effects of metoclopramide are EPSs. Much like the effects seen with high doses of phenothiazines, facial spasms, rhythmic protrusions of the tongue, involuntary movements of limbs, motor restlessness, agitation, and other dystonic reactions can occur. These effects occur most commonly in children and young adults, in men more than women, and at high doses of metoclopramide. Twenty-five percent of adults ages 18 to 30 experience dystonic reactions after receiving high-dose metoclopramide for treatment of chemotherapy-induced emesis. EPSs occur within 24 to 48 hours of the initial dose and subside within 24 hours of drug discontinuation. High-dose metoclopramide is usually defined as 2 mg/kg per dose. EPSs can be prevented or treated with the addition of diphenhydramine 25 to 50 mg IV or orally. IV administration of diphenhydramine is preferred for serious presentations. Other reversal agents are benztropine and diazepam. Secondary to its actions in the intestinal tract, metoclopramide can cause diarrhea. Management of diarrhea includes discontinuation or dosage reduction of metoclopramide, increased fluid resuscitation, and electrolyte replacement. The use of metoclopramide may not be a prudent choice in a patient who already has diarrhea. Drowsiness and fatigue are noted in approximately 10% of patients. There are inadequate data for the use of metoclopramide in pregnancy; however, supratherapeutic doses in rats did not produce evidence of fetal harm. Metoclopramide is in pregnancy risk category B. Metoclopramide is known to be distributed into breast milk but does not appear to present a risk to the infant if the mother is taking 45 mg/d or less.

Interactions

A hypertensive crisis can occur when metoclopramide is used with monoamine oxidase inhibitors. Additive sedation can be seen when used with alcohol or other CNS depressants. These drugs are antagonized by anticholinergics and narcotics. They may diminish gastric and accelerate intestinal absorption of drugs and food.

Corticosteroids

Corticosteroids are usually reserved for chemotherapy-induced nausea and vomiting. Appreciation of the antiemetic properties of this class of agents occurred when clinicians observed decreased episodes of nausea and vomiting with Hodgkin disease protocols that included prednisone compared with protocols that did not include prednisone.

Mechanism of Action

The true mechanism of action in the relief of nausea and vomiting is unknown, but one postulated theory is the inhibition of prostaglandins. In nausea and vomiting secondary to increased intracranial pressure, corticosteroids provide relief by decreasing inflammation. Dexamethasone (Decadron) and methylprednisolone (Solu-Medrol) are the two most common corticosteroids used; however, the addition of prednisone (Deltasone) to lymphoma and leukemia chemotherapy regimens can provide heightened control of emesis. These corticosteroids are almost always used in combination with other agents in the control or prevention of emesis from highly emetogenic regimens.

Corticosteroids are available orally and parenterally. The oral form is beneficial for low doses or prolonged administration, but may cause significant GI toxicity. Patients should be encouraged to take oral corticosteroids with food to minimize GI irritation and complications. IV administration is ordinarily used in the prevention of nausea and vomiting, primarily to avoid GI complications. IV preparations should be infused over 5 to 15 minutes to prevent burning, flushing, and itching sensations associated with the phosphate salt dissociation. Of the corticosteroids studied, the utility of dexamethasone has been best defined. In clinical trials, single-agent dexamethasone was superior to prochlorperazine and comparable with high-dose metoclopramide when used for mildly to moderately emetogenic chemotherapy regimens. The combination of dexamethasone and high-dose metoclopramide was the standard of care for prevention of cisplatin-induced emesis until the introduction of the serotonin antagonists.

IV doses of dexamethasone as a premedication range from 8 to 20 mg.

Corticosteroids should be used with caution in uncontrolled diabetic patients. Sliding-scale insulin or careful alterations of oral hypoglycemic agent regimens may be used for unacceptably high blood glucose levels.

Adverse Events

Although very useful, the corticosteroids are associated with many toxicities and adverse effects. Mental disturbances range from mood swings, depression, anxiety, and aggression to frank psychosis and personality changes. Men are particularly susceptible to this aggressive behavior. Headache, restlessness, and insomnia are not infrequent, particularly with higher doses of corticosteroids. Patients and family members and loved ones will benefit from knowing that these effects may occur with therapy. Sleep aids may be necessary for secondary insomnia. Temazepam (Restoril) or diphenhydramine are viable options. Variable increases in blood glucose and decreased glucose tolerance result from glucocorticoid use. Regular evaluation of blood glucose in diabetic patients is warranted. Glucocorticoids, especially in large or chronic doses, can increase the susceptibility to and mask the symptoms of infection, such as fever. Many consequences of long-term corticosteroid use can be detrimental. Muscle wasting, adrenocortical insufficiency, fluid and electrolyte disturbances, cataract formation, and atrophy of the protein matrix of bone resulting in osteoporosis, vertebral compression fractures, aseptic necrosis of femoral or humeral heads, and pathologic fractures are some of the most serious complications of chronic corticosteroid use. Whenever possible, chronic corticosteroid use should be curtailed.

Interactions

Glucocorticoids may decrease effects of barbiturates, hydantoins, rifampin, and ephedrine. Potassium levels should be monitored when glucocorticoids are used with potassium-depleting diuretics.

Cannabinoids

Cannabinoids are indicated only for nausea and vomiting associated with chemotherapy. In the 1970s, it was observed that patients on chemotherapy who smoked marijuana experienced a lower incidence of nausea and vomiting. Investigators then determined that tetrahydrocannabinol (THC) has antiemetic properties.

Mechanism of Action

The true mechanism of action of THC is unknown, but it is most likely related to effects on the vomiting center and the opiate receptors in the CNS and cerebral cortex, but probably does not involve the CTZ. The agent available in the United States is dronabinol (Marinol).

The cannabinoids can be used to treat and prevent chemotherapy-induced nausea and vomiting. Because it is necessary to reach therapeutic blood levels of THC before chemotherapy administration to prevent emesis, administration of the cannabinoids should occur at least 6 to 12 hours before chemotherapy. Emesis can be controlled from mildly to moderately emetogenic chemotherapy regimens, and cannabinoids may provide some relief to patients where other agents have failed. When used with mildly to moderately emetogenic regimens, THC has been found to be superior to placebo, prochlorperazine, low-dose metoclopramide, and haloperidol. These agents are seldom front-line therapy because of their incidence and severity of adverse effects.

Patients should be cautioned about the deleterious CNS effects and told not to drive or operate machinery. Dosages can be reduced if the patient is experiencing CNS toxicities. Patients should avoid alcohol and other CNS depressants.

Adverse Events

Most of the adverse effects of the cannabinoids are CNS related and include sedation, ataxia, and dysphoria. Dysphoria may be expressed as confusion, hallucinations, anxiety, fear, memory loss, time distortion, and other undesired occurrences. Orthostatic hypotension, blurred vision, and tachycardia have been observed with the use of these drugs. With repeated doses, the patients usually become tolerant to most of the CNS adverse effects, but not to the antiemetic activity. There is a correlation between antiemetic response and a psychological "high." Younger patients and patients who have had previous experiences with recreational cannabinoids appreciate greater antiemetic efficacy from this drug class. The side effects of the cannabinoids occur more frequently than with many of the other agents and are particularly distressing to older adults. One potentially beneficial adverse effect is appetite stimulation, which may prove useful in hematology and oncology patients. The cannabinoids are in pregnancy risk category D and should be avoided in pregnancy or lactation.

Antacids

Over-the-counter (OTC) antacid preparations may provide relief to patients experiencing mild nausea and vomiting. The general mechanism by which these agents exhibit their effects is by coating the stomach and neutralizing gastric acid. Most preparations contain one or several of the following: calcium carbonate, magnesium hydroxide, aluminum hydroxide, or aluminum carbonate. Between 15 and 30 mL orally of an antacid preparation may provide relief. Patients should be encouraged to seek medical attention if they experience continued nausea and vomiting, and the patient may need medical workup for more serious GI diseases.

Toxicities from OTC antacids are infrequent, but they do exist. The agents containing magnesium may cause diarrhea; conversely, the agents containing aluminum or calcium may cause constipation. These adverse effects are dose dependent. Calcium-containing antacids can cause phosphate depletion. Caution should be used in patients with renal dysfunction because aluminum and magnesium may accumulate. Antacids, by coating the GI tract, can decrease the absorption of many oral medications such as digoxin, some antibiotics, corticosteroids, and allopurinol

(Zyloprim), which may lead to decreased efficacy of therapy. (For additional information on antacids, see Chapter 29.)

Selecting the Most Appropriate Agent

Nausea and Vomiting Not Chemotherapy-Induced

It is necessary for the practitioner to assess the etiology of the nausea and vomiting. If an organic cause can be determined, the cause should be corrected to alleviate the symptoms. For example, if the nausea and vomiting is a side effect of a medication, the medication is to be discontinued. If the cause is diabetic ketoacidosis, insulin is given. **Figure 28-2** shows the treatment algorithm.

First-Line Therapy

An antiemetic is selected based on patient-specific factors. Initially, a phenothiazine is used for mild to moderate nausea and vomiting. Promethazine and prochlorperazine are usually effective.

Second-Line Therapy

If the above treatment is not effective, an antihistamine or anticholinergic preparation can be used. These are usually not as effective as phenothiazines but may be useful in mild nausea.

Third-Line Therapy

If the first two therapies are not successful, the patient should be reevaluated for a physiological cause that has not been treated and therapy based on patient data.

Table 28.2 lists the recommended order of treatment for nausea and vomiting.

Chemotherapy-Induced Nausea and Vomiting

Nausea and vomiting are two of the toxicities of chemotherapy that patients fear most. Although not usually a life-threatening complication, uncontrolled nausea or vomiting can greatly affect a patient's quality of life and attitude. Fortunately, new agents and combinations of agents make it possible to control emesis.

The severity of chemotherapy-induced emesis depends on numerous factors. Most significant is the intrinsic ability of the chemotherapy regimen to cause nausea and vomiting. Before the U.S. Food and Drug Administration approves a drug for use, phase 1 and 2 studies must be performed to prove efficacy and safety and identify adverse effects. The incidence and severity of nausea and vomiting are initially reported at this time, when the drug is given as a single agent. Each chemotherapy agent can be identified as having highly, moderately high, moderate, moderately low, and low emetogenic potential. Based on this information, antiemetic regimens can be tailored to the chemotherapy regimen to prevent emesis. Mechanisms to identify the emetogenicity of combination chemotherapy regimens are presented in this section. Other factors that may increase the incidence of chemotherapy-induced nausea and vomiting are previous exposure to chemotherapy, psychosocial factors such as anxiety and depression, poor performance status, and younger age (<30 years). A history of alcohol abuse and male sex may

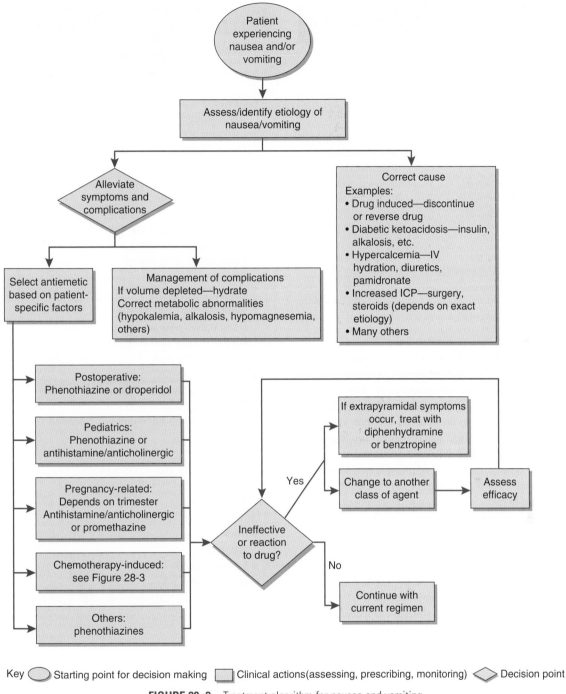

FIGURE 28–2 Treatment algorithm for nausea and vomiting.

correlate with a decreased incidence or severity of nausea and vomiting. The classifications of chemotherapy-induced nausea and vomiting include acute, delayed, and anticipatory.

Acute Emesis

Acute emesis is vomiting occurring within 24 hours of treatment. The onset of acute emesis is usually within 1 to 2 hours after the start of chemotherapy. It peaks within 4 to 10 hours and resolves within 24 hours, but these factors vary from agent to agent. This most common type of chemotherapy-induced nausea and vomiting is associated with a higher frequency and severity than the other two classifications. Acute emesis is strongly related to the agent or agents administered and the doses given (**Box 28.3** identifies the emetogenic potential of specific agents).

By definition, highly emetogenic chemotherapy agents induce emesis in greater than 90% of patients receiving that drug without antiemetic premedication. Chemotherapy agents

TABLE 28.2	Recommended Order of Treatment for Nausea and Vomiting*	
Order	Agents	Comments
First line	Phenothiazines	Most frequently used for mild to moderate nausea and vomiting Promethazine, prochlorperazine usually effective
Second line	Antihistamine Anticholinergic preparation	Usually not as efficacious as phenothiazines, but may be useful in mild nausea
Third line	Depends on response to other antiemetics	Tailor to patient-specific factors

*Consider patient-specific factors when choosing an antiemetic agent.

that have moderately high emetogenicity cause emesis in 60% to 90% of patients receiving chemotherapy. Chemotherapy that is moderately emetogenic has an incidence of 30% to 60%, moderately low has a 10% to 30% incidence of emesis, and low emetogenicity is defined as an incidence of less than 10%.

All patients receiving single agents that are moderately to highly emetogenic should be adequately pretreated to prevent the incidence of nausea and vomiting for at least 24 hours or the expected duration of nausea or vomiting. The current standard of care of antiemetic prophylaxis is the combination of a serotonin antagonist and a corticosteroid, such as granisetron or ondansetron with dexamethasone, at least 30 minutes before chemotherapy administration. Repeated doses may need to be given to prevent and treat emesis for 24 hours, depending on the pharmacokinetics of the agents used. Some practitioners use once-daily administration of serotonin antagonists, claiming that once the receptors are blocked, duration of receptor binding is the functional component rather than the plasma half-life. Because the purpose of these agents is to prevent nausea and vomiting, and the patient is not actively experiencing these effects, it is often acceptable to administer antiemetics orally. Combination regimens containing drugs that are moderately to highly emetogenic are given prophylactically in similar fashion. Although the aforementioned antiemetic combination is not universally effective, an estimated 70% to 90% of patients experience sufficient control. Examples of difficult clinical situations that may prohibit the use of a corticosteroid include poorly controlled diabetes and uncontrolled hypertension.

Contraindications to serotonin antagonists include hypersensitivity or severe cardiac dysfunction. Alternative prophylactic antiemetics must be chosen for patients who

BOX 28.3

Emetogenic Potential of Chemotherapy Agents

Highly emetogenic (>90%)
    Carmustine >250 mg/m^2
    Cisplatin >50 mg/m^2
    Cyclophosphamide >1,500 mg/m^2
    Dacarbazine
    Lomustine
    Mechlorethamine
    Streptozocin
Moderately high (60%–90%)
    Carboplatin
    Carmustine ≤250 mg/m^2
    Cisplatin ≤50 mg/m^2
    Cyclophosphamide ≤1,500 mg/m^2 or >750 mg/m^2
    Cytarabine >1,000 mg/m^2
    Doxorubicin >60 mg/m^2
    Methotrexate >1,000 mg/m^2
    Procarbazine oral
Moderate (30%–60%)
    Cyclophosphamide ≤750 mg/m^2
    Cyclophosphamide oral
    Doxorubicin 20–60 mg/m^2
    Idarubicin
    Ifosfamide
    Methotrexate 250–1,000 mg/m^2
    Mitoxantrone
    Topotecan
Moderately low (10%–30%)
    Docetaxel
    Etoposide
    5-Fluorouracil
    Gemcitabine
    Methotrexate >50 mg/m^2 or <250 mg/m^2
    Mitomycin
    Paclitaxel
Low (<10%)
    Bleomycin
    Busulfan
    Chlorambucil oral
    Cladribine
    Fludarabine
    Hydroxyurea
    Melphalan oral
    Thioguanine oral
    Vinblastine
    Vincristine
    Vinorelbine

have relative contraindications and are to receive emetogenic chemotherapy. High-dose metoclopramide with dexamethasone may be considered an option to a serotonin antagonist with dexamethasone because this was the gold standard for highly emetogenic regimens before the appearance of ondansetron. Once again, the antiemetic regimen should be tailored to the patient and the chemotherapy regimen.

Single-agent or combination chemotherapy regimens that are expected to be moderately low or low in emetogenic potential can be managed less aggressively. These drugs do not warrant the use of a serotonin antagonist. For some chemotherapy regimens and agents, such as the taxanes and fluorouracil, premedication frequently is not necessary; however, patients should be encouraged to use antiemetic medications as needed to control any nausea and vomiting after chemotherapy. Premedication with dexamethasone with or without a phenothiazine or metoclopramide may be used if a patient experiences nausea and vomiting from previous chemotherapy. All of these antiemetic drugs may be scheduled for a 24- to 36-hour period to prevent any nausea and vomiting. Patient-specific factors must be considered to identify an appropriate antiemetic regimen.

Regardless of the emetogenicity of a chemotherapy regimen or the use of premedications, antiemetics should be prescribed for prn or breakthrough use. Preferred prn antiemetics, such as prochlorperazine or metoclopramide, are effective, inexpensive, and easily administered. These agents provide reliable, safe control of mild nausea. These agents may be used before meals to alleviate anorexia secondary to nausea. Patients should be counseled about the common adverse effects of these agents, and each patient should be encouraged to report ineffective control of nausea and vomiting. When adhered to, the basic principles of chemotherapy antiemetic therapy (**Box 28.4**) are tremendously effective.

Delayed Emesis

Delayed nausea and vomiting is defined as emesis that begins or persists more than 24 hours after completion of chemotherapy. Some investigators suggest that because there is a "peak" in incidence at 18 hours after cisplatin-based chemotherapy, a revised definition of delayed emesis should include this timetable. The new-found, reliable control of acute emesis from highly to moderately emetogenic chemotherapy regimens has unveiled delayed nausea and vomiting as a more vexing problem. Many chemotherapy agents produce mild delayed nausea and vomiting, but cyclophosphamide, cisplatin, and the anthracyclines are particularly noted for their delayed emesis.

Delayed emesis usually is not as frequent or severe as acute emesis. The mechanism of delayed emesis is believed to be different from that of acute emesis. It is believed that delayed emesis is mediated by neurotransmitters, although serotonin does not play a major role. Combination antiemetic regimens have proven to be more effective than single-agent therapies. Single-agent serotonin antagonists were found to be equally as effective as metoclopramide or placebo and less effective

---

BOX 28.4

Basic Principles of Chemotherapy Antiemetic Therapy

- Consider emetogenic potential of chemotherapy regimen.
- Give appropriate antiemetics to prevent nausea and vomiting at least 30 min before emetogenic chemotherapy.
- Schedule antiemetics throughout anticipated period of nausea and vomiting risk.
- Always prescribe prn antiemetics for breakthrough nausea and vomiting between scheduled doses.
- Use antiemetic combinations with nonoverlapping mechanisms of action and adverse effects, when possible.
- Consider patient-specific variables when choosing a regimen (e.g., anxiety, performance status).
- Re-evaluate patients frequently during and between chemotherapy courses for efficacy and toxicity of antiemetic regimen.
- Consider nonpharmacologic interventions, especially in patients with anticipatory nausea and vomiting.

---

than dexamethasone, unlike their efficacy in preventing acute emesis. Regimens identified as most effective for delayed emesis include metoclopramide 0.5 mg/kg orally four times a day for 4 days with dexamethasone 8 mg orally twice a day for 2 days, followed by dexamethasone 4 mg orally twice a day for 2 days.

The use of scheduled phenothiazines (including long-acting phenothiazines) with dexamethasone is another effective option for the prevention of delayed nausea and vomiting. Addition of a benzodiazepine to the antiemetic regimen may prove useful for the control of emesis in anxious patients or patients with difficulty resting.

Anticipatory Emesis

Anticipatory nausea and vomiting occurs in up to 25% of patients receiving chemotherapy. It is usually associated with a history of uncontrolled nausea and vomiting with prior chemotherapy and is a conditioned response. Multiple factors can stimulate anticipatory nausea and vomiting, but most factors remind the patient of the previous unfavorable experience. For example, patients tell stories of becoming nauseated by the sight of their oncologist's office or by a smell that reminds them of receiving chemotherapy. Other triggers may be tastes, sounds, or thoughts of chemotherapy. Anticipatory nausea and vomiting most frequently occurs before the administration of chemotherapy, and it can lead to poorer control of nausea and vomiting with subsequent courses. The most effective treatment for delayed nausea and vomiting is prevention. It is crucial to premedicate adequately for highly to moderately emetogenic chemotherapy and to reassess control on a frequent and regular basis. This form of emesis is frequently refractory to standard antiemetic treatment; however, the benzodiazepines and butyrophenones may provide anxiolysis as well as antiemetogenicity. The addition of one of these agents is strongly encouraged for patients who have had previous unsatisfactory control of nausea and vomiting.

Many practice guidelines are available for the use of antiemetics in chemotherapy-induced nausea and vomiting. These guidelines are created by experts and are based on current literature (**Table 28.3** and **Figure 28-3**). To review treatment choices for other types of nausea and vomiting, see **Table 28.2** and **Figure 28-2**.

Special Population Considerations

Pediatric

The treatment of nausea and vomiting in children differs from that in adults. It is particularly important in the pediatric population to focus on treating the cause of the problem. The etiology of emesis can vary with age (**Box 28.5**). Because they are smaller, children are predisposed to dehydration and electrolyte abnormalities caused by emesis.

Pediatric patients experience more extrapyramidal or neuromuscular reactions to phenothiazines, particularly when the drugs are administered during an acute viral illness such as chickenpox, measles, or gastroenteritis. Because of its antihistamine quality, promethazine may be a viable phenothiazine option. Also, on a milligram-per-kilogram basis, children experience more extrapyramidal reactions from metoclopramide, even at IV doses as low as 0.5 mg/kg 4 times a day.

Most antiemetic agents are dosed according to milligram-per-kilogram of body weight or the age of the child, and many of the available agents are not recommended for use in patients younger than age 2 or 3. Some agents that are considered safe and effective in most situations are dimenhydrinate or oral or rectal trimethobenzamide (Tigan; IV not recommended). The phenothiazines are beneficial but should be used cautiously. For pediatric patients receiving chemotherapy, the prevention and treatment of emesis is similar to that in their adult counterparts, although specific pediatric dosing of the agents applies.

Women

Nausea and vomiting is experienced by more than 50% of pregnant women. A few women experience hyperemesis gravidarum, which can present as uncontrollable vomiting with inability to tolerate oral intake. These symptoms are most common in the first trimester of gestation but can occur at any time during pregnancy. Pregnancy-related emesis is believed to be modulated by CTZ stimulation.

Teratogenicity is the paramount concern when evaluating the safety of an agent in pregnant women. The first trimester of the pregnancy is when drugs or other exogenous substances can most affect embryonal development. Many of the studies performed to study the teratogenic effects of drugs encounter several difficulties. Most fetal malformations occur rarely, and frequently only a small sample size is obtained and reported. Mothers with underlying diseases, such as seizure disorder, hypertension, diabetes, and cancer, are known to have a higher incidence of infants with malformation. In these patient populations, the role of drugs versus the role of the disease in fetal abnormalities is unclear. Recall bias may play a factor

TABLE 28.3	Recommended Order of Treatment for Chemotherapy-Induced Nausea and Vomiting	
Order	**Agents**	**Comments**
Acute Prophylaxis for High, Moderately High, and Moderately Emetogenic Regimens		
First line	Serotonin antagonist + dexamethasone	May add other agents as needed
Second line	High-dose metoclopramide + dexamethasone	Prophylaxis for EPSs with metoclopramide
Third line	Depends on response to other antiemetics	Tailor to patient-specific factors
Acute Prophylaxis for Moderately Low and Low Emetogenic Regimens		
First line	No premedication or phenothiazine ± dexamethasone	Depends on chemotherapy regimen
Second line	Metoclopramide ± dexamethasone	Use low-dose metoclopramide
Third line	Depends on response to other antiemetics	Tailor to patient-specific factors
Delayed Nausea and Vomiting		
First line	Metoclopramide + dexamethasone	Continue 3–4 d after chemotherapy
Second line	Long-acting phenothiazine + dexamethasone	Monitor for EPSs
Third line	Depends on response to other antiemetics	Tailor to patient-specific factors

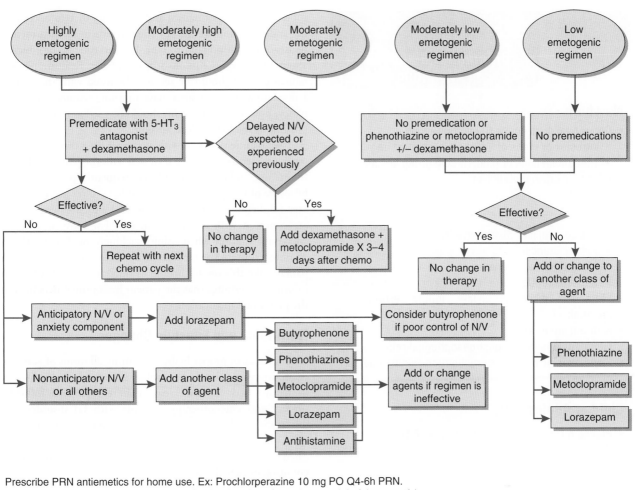

Prescribe PRN antiemetics for home use. Ex: Prochlorperazine 10 mg PO Q4-6h PRN.
Antiemetic regimen should be continued for the duration of emetic potential of the agent(s).

Key ⬭ Starting point for decision making   ▭ Clinical actions(assessing, prescribing, monitoring)   ◇ Decision point

FIGURE 28–3   Treatment algorithm for chemotherapy-induced nausea and vomiting.

in teratogenicity studies as well. Ultimately, current evidence-based information on the safety and risk of drugs during pregnancy should be used to make clinical decisions.

Agents that are used for mild to moderate nausea and vomiting in pregnancy include the phenothiazines, antihistamine–anticholinergic agents, and metoclopramide. Antihistamine drugs are generally believed to be safe for the pregnant women and her fetus, although there are incidental findings of malformations in fetuses exposed to antihistamines. Anticholinergic drugs have been proven to cause neonatal meconium ileus. Conversely, some anticholinergic agents such as scopolamine have not been associated with consistent teratogenesis.

Phenothiazines readily cross the placenta, but the bulk of evidence indicates their use is safe in this population. Antacids, such as calcium carbonate, may provide safe and reliable relief from mild nausea. Antihistamines, phenothiazines, metoclopramide, haloperidol, droperidol, and ondansetron

have all been used in hyperemesis gravidarum without adverse fetal sequelae. Drug classes that should be avoided in pregnant women are the benzodiazepines and cannabinoids. Increased rates of malformations and fetal complications have been associated with the use of these classes of agents; however, the use of other prescribed and illicit drugs by many of these mothers could cloud the picture. Corticosteroids are rarely used for the control of nausea and vomiting in pregnant women. The risks versus benefits of each drug and situation must be weighed carefully. Further studies to assess safety in this patient population are greatly needed.

MONITORING PATIENT RESPONSE

The best measure of nausea control is how the patient feels. To make evaluation of nausea more objective, nausea can be

Newborn

- Congenital obstructive GI malformations
  - Atresias or webs of esophagus or intestine
  - Meconium ileus or plug; Hirschsprung disease
- Inborn errors in metabolism

Infant

- Acquired or milder obstructive lesions
  - Pyloric stenosis
  - Malrotation and volvulus
  - Intussusception
- Metabolic diseases, milder inborn errors of metabolism
- Nutrient intolerances
- Functional disorders: gastroesophageal reflux
- Psychosocial disorders: rumination, injury due to child abuse

Child or Adolescent

- Please refer to adult etiologies (**Box 28.1**).

rated as none, mild, moderate, or severe. Another method is to ask the patient to rate the nausea on a scale from 0 to 10, with 0 equal to no nausea and 10 equal to severe nausea. These methods may help to compare nausea from day to day or week to week in the same patient. Vomiting is easily quantified by episodes per day and volume. If the volume of vomit exceeds 200 to 500 mL/d, the patient should be evaluated for electrolyte abnormalities.

PATIENT EDUCATION

It is pivotal to identify the cause of the nausea and vomiting and to educate the patient about actions that need to be taken. Many cases of mild nausea and vomiting can be alleviated without additional medications.

Drug Information

Some drugs may be taken with food to avoid GI discomfort, and dietary adjustments may prove to be helpful for some cases of nausea. This knowledge gives patients more control over their own well-being. Anxiety and mental illness are components of some occurrences of nausea and vomiting; therefore, counseling and education are the key components in the treatment of nausea and vomiting of this type. Patients can also be educated about the nonprescription drugs available. Realistic goals of nausea control should be set and discussed with the patient. For example, many women have morning sickness with pregnancy; however, medications should be used as infrequently as possible at the lowest dose possible.

With antiemetics, as with any other drug therapy, usual or serious toxicities should be reviewed with the patient. EPSs are frightening and uncomfortable; consequently, patients need to be aware of this potential effect and how to reverse it if necessary (diphenhydramine). Sedation and anticholinergic effects are common with many antiemetics. For most antiemetics, encourage caution when using machinery or driving. Proper administration of the medication should be reviewed. Will the patient take this on a schedule or only as needed? All of this information ensures that the patient has optimal benefit from the prescribed medication.

Nutritional and Lifestyle Changes

Maintenance of proper hydration during all forms of vomiting is important and should be emphasized to patients predisposed to nausea and vomiting (e.g., children, patients following surgery and chemotherapy, patients with GI disorders and infections). Rehydration with clear liquids is preferred over colas, milk, or caffeinated beverages. Patients should be educated on when to seek medical attention because of excessive vomiting or dehydration.

Complementary and Alternative Therapies

Patients suffering from nausea and vomiting of pregnancy (NVP) frequently do not receive therapy, in part because of fears of adverse effects of medications on the fetus. Several vitamin-based and herbal therapies have been shown to be effective and safe. Two randomized trials of vitamin B_6 have shown a benefit in reducing NVP. The recommended daily allowance is 1.3 to 2 mg/d. Women taking prenatal multivitamins are less likely to have severe NVP.

Ginger has been shown to reduce NVP. Ginger appears to work by inhibiting serotonin receptors in the GI tract and CNS. The dose of ginger for the powdered root form in motion sickness is 1 g up to 4 hours before an inciting event; in NVP, 250 mg four times a day; for chemotherapy-induced nausea and vomiting, 2 to 4 g daily; and for PONV, 1 g 1 hour before anesthesia induction.

Vitamin B_1 (thiamine) deficiency can lead to Wernicke encephalopathy in women with severe NVP. Replacement is needed for all women with vomiting of more than 3 weeks' duration. Prophylaxis with multivitamins and therapy with B_6, with or without doxylamine, are safe and effective therapies for NVP.

Case Study

S. B. is a 57-year-old African American man with newly diagnosed late-stage small-cell lung cancer. He has undergone radiation therapy to the brain for his metastases and is to start chemotherapy next week. His past medical history includes hypertension. He has no known drug allergies. A combination chemotherapy regimen has been chosen: cisplatin 100 mg/m^2 for one dose on the first day and etoposide 100 mg/m^2 IV every day for 3 days. He has experienced nausea and vomiting.

DIAGNOSIS: CHEMOTHERAPY-INDUCED NAUSEA AND VOMITING

1. List specific goals for treatment for S. B.
2. What drug therapy would you prescribe? Why?
3. What are the parameters for monitoring success of the therapy?
4. Discuss specific patient education based on the prescribed therapy.
5. List one or two adverse reactions for the selected agent that would cause you to change therapy.
6. What would be the choice for the second-line therapy?
7. What OTC and/or alternative medications would be appropriate for this patient?
8. What dietary and lifestyle changes should be recommended for this patient?
9. Describe one or two drug–drug or drug–food interactions for the selected agent.

BIBLIOGRAPHY

Starred references are cited in the text.

Antiemetic Subcommittee of the Multinational Association of Supportive Care in Cancer (MASCC). (1998). Prevention of chemotherapy and radiotherapy-induced emesis: Results of the Perugia Consensus Conference. *Annals of Oncology, 9*, 811–819.

*Audhuy, B., Cappelaure, P., Martin, M., et al. (1996). A double-blind, randomized comparison of the antiemetic efficacy of two intravenous doses of dolasetron mesylate and granisetron in patients receiving high-dose cisplatin chemotherapy. *European Journal of Cancer, 32A*, 807–813.

Gandara, D. R., Roila, F., Warr, D., et al. (1998). Consensus proposal for 5HT3 antagonists in the prevention of acute emesis related to highly emetogenic chemotherapy. *Supportive Care in Cancer, 6*, 237–243.

Gralla, R. J., Osoba, D., Kris, M. G., et al. (1999). Recommendations for the use of antiemetics: Evidence-based, clinical practice guidelines. *Journal of Clinical Oncology, 7*, 2971–2994.

Michelfelder, A., Lee, K., & Boding, E. (2010). Integrative medicine and gastrointestinal disease. *Primary Care: Clinics in Office Practice, 37(2)*, 255–267.

Navair, R. (2007). Overview of updated antiemetic guidelines for chemotherapy-induced nausea and vomiting. *Community Oncology, 4*(4, Suppl. 1), 3–11.

Nolte, M. J., Berkery, R., Pizzo, B., et al. (1998). Assuring the optimal use of serotonin antagonist antiemetics: The process of development and implementation of institutional antiemetic guidelines at Memorial Sloan-Kettering Cancer Center. *Journal of Clinical Oncology, 16*, 771–778.

*Pisters, K. M., & Kris, M. G. (1992). Management of nausea and vomiting caused by anticancer drugs: State of the art. *Oncology, 6*(2, Suppl.), 99–104.

Scorza, K., Williams, A., Phillips, J. D., & Shaw, J. (2007). Evaluation of nausea and vomiting. *American Family Physician, 76*(1), 76–84.

Gastroesophageal Reflux Disease and Peptic Ulcer Disease

Two related disorders of the gastrointestinal (GI) tract can cause abdominal discomfort: gastroesophageal reflux disease (GERD) and peptic ulcer disease (PUD). They are both common reasons for patients to present in primary care. The treatment for these diseases is with many of the same drugs.

GASTROESOPHAGEAL REFLUX DISEASE

GERD is a term used to describe signs or symptoms caused by reflux of stomach contents into the esophagus. It affects all segments of the population and is one of the most common conditions presenting in primary care. GERD refers to the abnormal exposure of the esophageal mucosa to retrograde gastric contents, resulting in symptoms or tissue damage. The concept of gastroesophageal reflux and its consequences was first described in a landmark article by Winkelstein (1935), who suggested that gastric secretions caused mucosal damage. In 1946, Allison used the term *reflux esophagitis* to identify the pathophysiologic process that results in inflammation of the esophagus through exposure to gastric refluxate. GERD is one of the most prevalent conditions in the GI tract, affecting approximately 360 out of 100,000 people (Shaheen & Provenzale, 2003). Over 60 million Americans have heartburn at least once a day. Of patients with GERD symptoms, 40% to 60% have reflux esophagitis and only 10% have erosive esophagitis. GERD accounts for 50% of noncardiac chest pain. Seventy-eight percent of patients with persistent hoarseness have GERD as do 82% of patients with asthma. Reflux is especially common during pregnancy. For most patients, GERD is a chronic disorder that significantly impairs quality of life and leads to high use of medical resources.

CAUSES

The cause of GERD is gastric contents entering and remaining in the lower esophagus because of transient relaxation of the lower esophageal sphincter (LES). Additional causes are an increase in intra-abdominal pressure, delayed gastric emptying, medication use, hiatal hernia, and poor esophageal acid clearance. The many risk factors for GERD are listed in **Box 29.1**.

PATHOPHYSIOLOGY

The fundamental abnormality of GERD is exposure of esophageal epithelium to gastric secretions, eliciting symptoms or resulting in histopathologic injury. Under normal circumstances, the LES, located at the gastroesophageal junction, provides an antireflux barrier. The mechanisms by which esophagogastric junction incompetence occur are:

- transient LES relaxation
- abdominal strain from increased gastric volume secondary to delayed gastric emptying
- aggressive refluxate passing through the patulous LES
- impaired esophageal epithelium defense mechanisms
- motility abnormalities causing impaired clearance of refluxed materials
- hiatal hernia.

Transient LES relaxation is part of a normal reflex that permits gas to escape from the stomach to facilitate belching. Stress

---

BOX **29.1**

Risk Factors for GERD

- Obesity
- Fatty foods
- Chocolate
- Peppermint
- Alcohol
- Nicotine
- Citrus juices
- Tomato products
- Caffeine
- Assuming recumbent position after eating
- Medications (anticholinergics, α-adrenergic agonists, β-adrenergic agonists, calcium channel blockers, dopaminergic agents, sedatives/tranquilizers, tricyclic antidepressants, theophylline, potassium chloride, ferrous sulfate, NSAIDs, alendronate)

reflux and free reflux become increasingly likely as LES pressure decreases as a result of exposure to fatty foods, gastric distention, alcohol consumption, and smoking. In addition, many medications used to treat other common medical conditions have been associated with altered LES tone. They include nitrates, theophyllines, oral contraceptives, calcium channel blockers, especially nifedipine (Procardia), and others, as listed in **Box 29.1**.

The composition and volume of gastroesophageal refluxate are important factors in GERD. It has been demonstrated that a high degree of esophagus exposure to acid facilitates esophageal mucosal injury and increases the severity of the disease.

One of the distinguishing characteristics between patients with GERD and others is the effectiveness of the esophageal defense mechanisms. There are four main defensive forces against development of reflux esophagitis:

- A competent gastroesophageal junction, as previously discussed
- Effective clearance of refluxed material
- Neutralization of acid by salivary bicarbonate and secretion of bicarbonate by submucosal esophageal glands
- An intact diffusion barrier of the esophageal mucosa

The defense mechanism most commonly altered in patients with GERD is prolonged acid clearance time. Normally, most fluid is cleared from the esophagus, leaving only a small amount that is eventually neutralized by swallowed saliva. In patients with GERD, the main contributors to impaired acid clearance are peristaltic dysfunction of the esophagus and re-reflux associated with hiatal hernia.

DIAGNOSTIC CRITERIA

For the most part, GERD is a clinical diagnosis that may be objectively confirmed by a very good history and some diagnostic tests. The symptoms of GERD are varied and range from the classic heartburn or regurgitation to atypical presentation of chest pain, hoarseness, asthma, or cough. Heartburn and regurgitation are very sensitive and specific for diagnosing GERD. However, up to 50% of patients with endoscopic evidence of esophagitis present with atypical symptoms. Symptoms that may predict more severe disease and complications include dysphagia and odynophagia. For a breakdown of the symptoms, see **Box 29.2**.

GERD can be classified as mild, moderate, or severe. Characteristics of each category are listed in **Box 29.3**.

Patients complaining of atypical symptoms, with or without the classic symptoms of GERD, present a diagnostic dilemma. Hoarseness may be the only manifestation of GERD. Asthma has been associated with GERD, especially when paroxysmal nocturnal exacerbations are reported.

The spectrum of endoscopic findings is varied as well. Approximately 50% of patients with GERD have a normal-appearing esophagus, whereas the other 50% have complications such as esophagitis, strictures, or Barrett esophagus.

The clinical diagnosis is made if symptoms are relieved with a therapeutic trial of antireflux therapy. Diagnostic testing includes barium x-rays, esophagoscopy, and pH monitoring.

BOX 29.2

Symptoms of GERD

Frequent Symptoms

- Heartburn
- Acid regurgitation
- Epigastric pain
- Belching
- Water brash

Atypical Symptoms

- Noncardiac chest pain
- Hoarseness
- Nausea
- Respiratory complications: asthma, nocturnal cough, wheezing, recurrent pneumonia, and lung abscesses

Alarm Symptoms

- Dysphagia
- Odynophagia
- Anemia
- Bleeding
- Weight loss

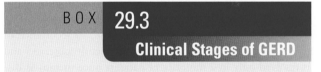

BOX 29.3

Clinical Stages of GERD

Mild

Heartburn fewer than 3 times weekly
No symptoms suggesting complicated disease

Moderate

Heartburn 3 or more times weekly
No symptoms suggesting complicated disease

Severe

Moderate GERD that fails appropriate therapy
Strictures, erosive esophagitis, or Barrett esophagus detected by endoscopy
Alarm symptoms suggesting complications (dysphagia, odynophagia, unexplained weight loss, iron-deficiency anemia, melena, hematemesis, hoarseness, asthma, unexplained lung disease)

INITIATING DRUG THERAPY

The cornerstones of therapy are lifestyle modifications that include elevating of the head of the bed, decreasing fat intake, stopping smoking, and avoiding recumbency for 3 hours after meals. These modifications may be sufficient for symptom control in patients with mild disease. However, the clinical efficacy of lifestyle changes alone is limited, and symptoms usually continue. Therefore, drug therapy is usually required in addition to lifestyle modifications.

Goals of Drug Therapy

The goals of drug therapy are to:

- relieve symptoms
- heal the esophageal mucosa
- prevent complications
- maintain remission.

An empirical trial of symptom-relieving medications may be the most expeditious way to diagnose GERD in those with classic symptoms. Those with classic symptoms are given 2 weeks of therapy with a histamine-2 receptor antagonist (H$_2$RA) or a proton pump inhibitor (PPI) 30 to 60 minutes before the first meal of the day. If the H$_2$RA twice a day does not relieve symptoms, the patient is switched to a PPI daily. If a PPI has been tried and the patient still has symptoms, the dose is increased or an additional dose is given 30 minutes before the evening meal. If there is response to therapy, the patient is continued on therapy for 8 to 12 weeks. The dosage is then tapered over 1 month to the lowest dose that gives the patient relief. If the symptoms recur, the patient is again given the initial effective medication and dose and further testing is recommended. If the initial therapy does not produce symptom relief, diagnostic testing is recommended.

GERD is a chronic, relapsing disease, so recurrence of reflux symptoms and esophagitis is frequently observed and is resolved only in a minority of patients once therapy is discontinued. Symptoms can recur quickly if therapy is stopped or the drug dose decreased. Long-term therapy is usually required. Drugs used to treat GERD act to decrease acid secretion and decrease or neutralize the acidity of gastric acid. They include:

- antacids, which raise the pH of refluxed gastric secretions and deactivate pepsin
- H$_2$RAs, which decrease gastric acid secretion by inhibiting stimulation of parietal cells by histamine
- PPIs, which suppress gastric acid.

PEPTIC ULCER DISEASE

It has been estimated that 1 in 10 Americans or approximately 10% of the population of the United States have had PUD at some time. It accounts for 1 million hospitalizations, 6,500 deaths a year, and a cost of about $6 billion annually. Thus, PUD is a significant cause of morbidity in the United States, and appropriate diagnosis and treatment can reduce medical expenditures associated with acute and chronic PUD and its complications.

CAUSES

Infection by the *Helicobacter pylori* bacterium and long-term use of nonsteroidal anti-inflammatory drugs (NSAIDs) are the major causes of PUD. Less common causes of PUD include cancer and other idiopathic or hypersecretory disorders such as Zollinger-Ellison syndrome.

Most cases of PUD can be linked to infection with *H. pylori*. The organism is present in approximately 10% to 20% of healthy adults younger than age 40 and approximately 50% to 80% of those older than age 60. Although *H. pylori* is a common infection, most people have asymptomatic and chronic antral gastritis but do not progress to the development of ulcers. Only about 15% of those infected eventually have an ulcer. Patients who have duodenal and gastric ulcers are infected with *H. pylori* in more than 90%, and 60% to 90% of cases, respectively. *H. pylori* infection is also associated with increased risk of gastric cancer and lymphoid lymphoma, and therefore the absence of infection in a patient with PUD suggests a more serious etiology and the need for an additional workup. The reasons for this are not clear.

The most significant risk factor for *H. pylori* infection is the socioeconomic status of the family during childhood. Evidence supports various routes of transmission (e.g., oral–oral, fecal–oral, iatrogenic), but no one route has been clearly identified as a more likely source. It appears alcohol consumption may be protective, coffee consumption may be associated with an increased prevalence, and smoking has no clear association with active *H. pylori* infection. One report also identified increasing age, lower income and education level, and musculoskeletal pain or headache as risk factors for recent active ulcers, whereas smoking more than one pack of cigarettes a day was a risk factor for chronic active ulcer disease.

NSAID-induced ulcerations are thought to occur in 10% to 30% of people taking the drugs. Serious complications of PUD, such as bleeding, occur in 2% to 4% of NSAID users. NSAIDs are one of the most commonly used prescription and nonprescription medications in the United States. NSAIDs are associated with the development of gastric ulcer twice as often as with duodenal ulcers.

Several factors increase the risk for development of GI complications from NSAIDs, including age (particularly patients older than age 75), history of PUD or ulcer bleeding, NSAID dosage and long duration of use, and concomitant drug therapy (e.g., anticoagulants, glucocorticoids). These serious complications are associated with increased hospitalization, mortality rates, and use of health care resources. It has been estimated that 15% to 35% of all complications of peptic ulcers are caused by the use of NSAIDs.

PATHOPHYSIOLOGY

Defensive mechanisms that protect the gastric mucosa from injury include mucus and bicarbonate secretion, mucosal blood flow, epithelial cell restitution and growth, and prostaglandins. Mucus protects underlying cells by acting as a barrier between the gastric mucosa and its contents and by preventing the back-diffusion of hydrogen ions from the gastric lumen into the mucosa. Gastric and duodenal epithelial cells secrete bicarbonate, which buffers the gastric mucosal surface. Mucosal blood flow in gastric and duodenal cells maintains the integrity of gastric mucosa by preventing ischemia. Rapid gastric epithelial cell turnover and epidermal growth factor aid in the restoration of damaged cells and wound healing, respectively. Prostaglandins play a key role in providing mucosal protection by stimulating and maintaining each of the aforementioned mucosal defense mechanisms.

When factors such as *H. pylori* and NSAIDs disrupt the normal mucosal physiology, peptic ulcers can form. It is likely that several factors, such as pathophysiologic abnormalities and environmental and genetic factors, act together to affect normal gastric and duodenal defense and healing mechanisms to result in ulcer formation.

H. pylori organisms are flagellated, spiral-shaped bacteria that burrow into the mucous layer of the gastric epithelium. The organism also produces urease, which neutralizes the hydrogen ions in gastric acid, making it uniquely protected against gastric acid and relatively inaccessible to antibiotics. Within 2 to 3 days after infection by *H. pylori*, an inflammatory response begins, acute gastritis ensues, and an antibody response is mounted. *H. pylori* induces ulcer formation as a result of increased gastrin secretion from the antral mucosa, increased acid secretion by the stomach, and increased acid load in the duodenum. The increased acid load, along with bacterial enzymes, toxins, and inflammatory mediators, is thought to weaken the protective mucous lining of the stomach or duodenum and result in ulcer formation. Immunoglobulin (Ig) A and IgG antibody titers can be used to detect infection by *H. pylori*, which is typically lifelong when left untreated. Humans are thought to be the principal carrier of *H. pylori* infection.

The NSAIDs induce gastroduodenal injury by two different mechanisms. NSAIDs cause a superficial irritation directly on the mucosa, as well as acting systemically by inhibiting the production of protective prostaglandins. NSAIDs inhibit cyclooxygenase (COX) in the arachidonic acid cascade, which in turn inhibits the production of mucosal prostaglandins. Recent data support the discovery of two subtypes of COX enzymes, COX-1 and COX-2. COX-1 plays an integral role in the maintenance of GI integrity and is found in the stomach, intestines, kidney, and platelets. COX-2 is inducible in areas of inflammation and is undetectable in most tissues. Until recently, all NSAIDs inhibited both COX enzymes. Newer NSAIDs selectively inhibit COX-2 to a great extent and have the potential for an improved GI side effect profile compared with older NSAIDs that inhibit both COX enzymes. Selective COX-2 inhibitors have comparable efficacy with older NSAIDs but may be associated with a lower risk for development of NSAID-induced ulcers. The basic understanding of topical versus systemic toxic effects of NSAIDs is still unclear. A considerable amount of debate continues in the literature regarding the relative roles each of these mechanisms play in the pathogenesis of NSAID-induced ulcers.

DIAGNOSTIC CRITERIA

Classically, PUD is characterized by symptoms of epigastric pain and dyspepsia. These are typical presenting symptoms that occur in approximately two thirds of patients with duodenal and one third of patients with gastric ulcer. The symptomatology of PUD is considered to be relatively nonspecific and does not assist in the differentiation of duodenal versus gastric ulcer. In addition, pain does not correlate well with ulcer presence or healing. NSAID-induced ulcers are less likely to cause symptoms compared with PUD associated with *H. pylori* infection.

Numerous methods, both invasive and noninvasive, are available for diagnosing infection by *H. pylori*. Urease tests, culture, and polymerase chain reaction, performed after endoscopy and biopsy, are considered to be invasive tests, whereas serology, stool antigen, and the urea breath test are considered noninvasive. Endoscopy is the gold standard test that, although invasive and expensive, is appropriate for initial evaluation of patients older than age 45 who present with significant dyspeptic symptoms (e.g., weight loss, poor appetite, vomiting) and no documented history of PUD. A follow-up endoscopy is neither cost effective nor practical for documenting eradication but may be useful to document refractory ulceration where recurrences are frequent. Culture is useful, particularly when it is suspected that antibiotic-resistant isolates are present or when retreatment is necessary after exposure to an antibiotic that fosters resistance, because sensitivity testing of *H. pylori* can be performed with selected antibiotics. Cultures, however, require an incubation period of up to 10 days. Enzyme-linked immunosorbent assay for IgA and IgG antibodies to *H. pylori* has been the most widely used noninvasive test for diagnosing *H. pylori* infection, but it is not reliable for documenting eradication because antibody titers fall slowly after antibiotic therapy. In addition, the results of serologic tests vary widely from one laboratory to the next. The more recently available noninvasive urea breath test is a reliable means of determining the presence of *H. pylori* as well as documenting eradication after treatment. This is a quick, simple test that is reported to have very high sensitivity and specificity, equal to those of endoscopy, for diagnosing *H. pylori* in adult patients. The stool antigen test has a sensitivity of about 94% and specificity of about 90%. This cannot be used to test for eradication until 6 to 8 weeks after therapy.

INITIATING DRUG THERAPY

Several pharmacologic options are available for treating PUD, depending on the etiology, symptoms, and diagnostic information (**Table 29.1**). A combination of antibiotics or

TABLE 29.1	Overview of Agents Used to Treat PUD and GERD

Generic (Trade) Name and Dosage	Selected Adverse Events	Contraindications	Special Considerations
Antibiotics			
amoxicillin (Amoxil) 500 mg qid	Diarrhea, nausea, hypersensitivity	Known allergy to penicillins, cephalosporins, or imipenem	Take without regard to meals.
clarithromycin (Biaxin) 500 mg bid–tid	Diarrhea, abnormal taste, nausea	Known allergy to macrolide antibiotics, concomitant use of astemizole, cisapride, or pimozide	Take without regard to meals. Consider avoiding use for retreatment if initial clarithromycin-containing regimen fails.
metronidazole (Flagyl) 250 mg qid	Peripheral neuropathy, metallic taste, nausea, disulfiram-like reaction if taken with alcohol	Known allergy to metronidazole	Avoid use of alcohol during therapy and for 1 d afterward. Available as Helidac (a patient-friendly kit containing bismuth subsalicylate, tetracycline) Take on an empty stomach with plenty of water and avoid ingestion of tetracycline simultaneously with dairy products, antacids, laxatives, or iron-containing products (these can be taken 2 h before or after tetracycline).
tetracycline (Sumycin) 500 mg qid	Diarrhea, esophageal ulcers, photosensitivity	Allergy Prescribe with caution in patients with renal or hepatic dysfunction.	May render oral contraceptives ineffective
H₂ Receptor Antagonists			
cimetidine (Tagamet) 300 mg qid, 400 mg bid, or 800 mg hs	Rarely, CNS side effects (e.g., headache, fatigue, dizziness, confusion), gynecomastia, impotence	Hypersensitivity to cimetidine or other H₂ antagonists	Take without regard to meals. Stagger doses if taking antacids. Patients should inform health care providers of any other drugs that are taken concomitantly because of the possibility of drug interactions.
famotidine (Pepcid) 20 mg bid or 40 mg hs	Rarely, CNS side effects (e.g., headache, fatigue, dizziness, confusion)	Hypersensitivity to famotidine or other H₂ antagonists	May be taken without regard to meals
nizatidine (Axid) 150 mg bid or 300 hs mg	Rarely, CNS side effects (e.g., headache, fatigue, dizziness, confusion)	Hypersensitivity to famotidine or other H₂ antagonists	May be taken without regard to meals
ranitidine (Zantac) 150 mg bid or 300 mg hs	Rarely, CNS side effects (e.g., headache, fatigue, dizziness, confusion)	Hypersensitivity to famotidine or other H₂ antagonists	May be taken without regard to meals, stagger doses if taking antacids
Proton Pump Inhibitors			
omeprazole (Prilosec, Zegerid) 40 mg qd or 20 mg bid	Diarrhea, headache	Hypersensitivity to omeprazole	Take 30–60 min before meals
lansoprazole (Prevacid) 30 mg bid–tid	Diarrhea, headache	Hypersensitivity to lansoprazole	Same as above
pantoprazole (Protonix) 40 mg qd	Diarrhea, headache, flatulence	Hypersensitivity to other proton pump inhibitors	Same as above
esomeprazole (Nexium) 20–40 mg qd	Diarrhea, headache	Same as above	Same as above
dexlansoprazole (Kapidex) 30-60 mg qd	Same as above	Same as above	Same as above
rabeprazole (AcipHex) 20 mg qd	Same as above	Same as above	Same as above

TABLE 29.1	Overview of Agents Used to Treat PUD and GERD (*Continued*)			
Generic (Trade) Name and Dosage	**Selected Adverse Events**	**Contraindications**	**Special Considerations**
Other Agents Used in PUD			
antacids Widely variable, depends on product contents and formulation	Rebound hyperacidity, diarrhea with magnesium-containing antacids, constipation with aluminum-containing antacids	None significant	Use magnesium–aluminum combination products to avoid diarrhea or constipation. Monitor for drug interactions between antacids and other drugs, such as fluoroquinolone antibiotics, tetracycline, ketoconazole, iron products.
sucralfate (Carafate) 1 g qid	Constipation	None significant	Take on an empty stomach (1 h before meals). Avoid antacids for 30 min before or after taking sucralfate.
misoprostol (Cytotec) 200 µg qid	Diarrhea, abdominal pain, nausea	Hypersensitivity to prostaglandins, pregnancy	Take with food. Reduce dose to 100 µg if diarrhea cannot be tolerated. Avoid use in pregnancy and in women trying to become pregnant.
bismuth subsalicylate (Pepto Bismol) 2 tabs qid for 7–14 d	Black stools, black tongue, constipation, tinnitus	Sensitivity to salicylates, coagulation disorder, influenza, varicella	Avoid in pregnancy and lactation.

antibiotic and antisecretory agents, antacids, H₂RAs, PPIs, misoprostol (Cytotec), and sucralfate (Carafate) can all be used appropriately for effective management of PUD. In the past, traditional antiulcer agents such as H₂RAs, PPIs, sucralfate, and antacids were used as empiric therapy for patients who presented with signs and symptoms of uncomplicated PUD. These agents are effective in healing ulcers if used appropriately, but relapses of PUD are common and can be prevented only by eradicating *H. pylori*.

The American Gastroenterological Association (AGA) cautions against empirical use of antisecretory agents for suspected PUD because such treatment may delay important diagnostic testing and appropriate long-term treatment. Nor does the AGA support treatment of *H. pylori*–induced ulcers without serologic or breath test results confirming *H. pylori*–induced infection.

When a treatment regimen is selected, it should be individualized based on a patient's age, comorbidities, concurrent medications, likelihood for adherence, and risk factors for complications from progressive ulcer disease and treatment.

Eradication of *H. pylori* facilitates ulcer healing, eliminates the need for maintenance therapy, and markedly reduces the risk of ulcer recurrence. Therefore, as suggested by a 1994 National Institutes of Health (NIH) consensus panel statement, antibiotic therapy is indicated for all patients with *H. pylori*–infected duodenal and gastric ulcers (NIH Consensus Development Panel, 1994). Available regimens are complex and expensive, have side effects, and require 7 to 14 days of at least three agents to achieve cure rates exceeding 80%. To complicate decision making, the study design and drug dosages

and schedules, and thus eradication rates, of trials evaluating regimens for treatment of *H. pylori* vary greatly.

Goals of Drug Therapy

The therapeutic goals of treatment for PUD associated with *H. pylori* are to relieve ulcer pain and dyspepsia, heal existing ulcers and erosions, and eradicate *H. pylori* to reduce recurrence and cure PUD.

Although the goals for treating NSAID-induced PUD are similar, an additional consideration is identifying an alternative to the NSAID for pain management, if possible, or prophylaxis to prevent further ulceration if treatment with an NSAID continues. Prophylaxis could include changing to an enteric-coated NSAID that can be taken with meals, adding misoprostol to the therapeutic regimen, or switching to an NSAID with COX-2 selectivity that may be associated with less GI toxicity.

DRUGS USED IN TREATMENT OF GERD AND PUD

Antibiotics

The antibiotics used to treat PUD work in various ways (**Table 29.2**).

Clarithromycin

Clarithromycin (Biaxin) is a macrolide antibiotic that, like azithromycin (Zithromax), is more acid-stable than

TABLE 29.2	Oral Drug Regimens Used to Eradicate *Helicobacter Pylori–* Induced Pud	
Therapy	**Duration**
Triple Therapy	
Clarithromycin 500 mg bid + amoxicillin 1 g bid + a PPI	7–14 d
Quadruple Therapy	
Bismuth subsalicylate 2 tablets (525 mg) or 30 mL qid + metronidazole 500 mg qid + tetracycline 500 mg qid +	14 d

erythromycin (Eryc) and inhibits bacterial protein synthesis. The half-life of clarithromycin is 3 to 4 hours, twice that of erythromycin but significantly shorter than that of azithromycin. Clarithromycin has significant activity against *H. pylori* when used as the sole antibiotic and especially when used in combination with at least one additional antibiotic and antisecretory agent. However, resistance to clarithromycin develops rapidly, so it should not be used in subsequent regimens once a treatment failure has occurred. Clarithromycin is commonly used at a dose of 500 mg twice daily. Clarithromycin can inhibit cytochrome P450 3A4 isoenzymes and should not be given concurrently with nonsedating antihistamines, such as loratadine (Claritin).

Metronidazole

Metronidazole (Flagyl) is active against various anaerobic bacteria and protozoa and is the mainstay of many commonly used *H. pylori* treatment regimens. Metronidazole is thought to enter the cells of microorganisms that contain nitroreductase, where the nitro group in metronidazole is reduced, attaches to deoxyribonucleic acid, inhibits synthesis, and causes cell death. The effectiveness of metronidazole is not dependent on pH. *H. pylori* is highly sensitive to metronidazole in areas where metronidazole use is low; however, where use is pervasive, up to 80% of *H. pylori* isolates can be resistant (Saledo & Al-Kawas, 1998). In a study evaluating resistant *H. pylori* organisms, 21% of patients had primary resistance to metronidazole (Adamek, et al., 1998). When used as a single agent, especially in areas where use is high, metronidazole results in very low eradication rates. Resistance is less likely to develop if metronidazole is used with bismuth or in combination with another antibiotic. It has been demonstrated that metronidazole-resistant *H. pylori* significantly affects the efficacy of quadruple therapy that includes metronidazole, colloidal bismuth subcitrate, tetracycline, and omeprazole (Prilosec). The half-life of metronidazole is 8 hours. Metronidazole is typically administered as 250 mg four times daily or 500 mg three times daily.

Amoxicillin

Amoxicillin (Amoxil) is an aminopenicillin that kills bacterial cells by interfering with cell wall synthesis. Although amoxicillin concentrations in gastric juices are high and *H. pylori* is highly sensitive to amoxicillin, monotherapy results in eradication rates of less than 20%. Amoxicillin is most active at a neutral pH, which may explain the low cure rate. When amoxicillin is used in combination with omeprazole, however, the concentration of amoxicillin in gastric juice increases substantially and results in a significantly higher eradication rate. Because amoxicillin has diminished activity at a low pH, the omeprazole-induced increase in gastric pH results in a substantial increase in bactericidal activity. Dual therapy with amoxicillin and omeprazole, however, has been associated with less-than-optimal eradication rates.

Amoxicillin is associated with higher eradication rates when it is used as one of three or four agents. In a nonrandomized study, one such regimen using omeprazole, amoxicillin, and metronidazole for 7 to 14 days was studied in over 300 British patients and resulted in a 90% eradication rate with few side effects (Bell, et al., 1995). *H. pylori* does not typically develop resistance to amoxicillin, so it can be used again in subsequent treatment regimens. Amoxicillin is typically administered at a dose of 500 mg four times daily.

Tetracycline

Tetracycline inhibits bacterial protein synthesis and is used for a wide variety of gram-positive and gram-negative bacterial infections. Tetracycline is stable at a low pH and acts topically against *H. pylori*. Although *H. pylori* is very sensitive to tetracycline and bacterial resistance has not been reported, it must be used with at least one other agent that has activity against *H. pylori* to achieve eradication. With significant variations in dosages and administration schedules, a bismuth compound, metronidazole, and either amoxicillin or tetracycline are drugs commonly used in a classic triple-drug regimen to eradicate *H. pylori*.

Tetracycline is usually given 2 hours before or 2 hours after food to increase systemic absorption. It has been recommended that tetracycline be administered along with bismuth subsalicylate (BSS) to facilitate binding, decreasing systemic absorption and increasing local exposure of tetracycline to the gastric mucosa. One study (Healy, et al., 1997), however, has determined that the tetracycline actually binds to a suspending agent called *veegum,* which is present only in the liquid form of BSS (Pepto-Bismol). The clinical significance of this interaction has yet to be determined in a clinical study. Because *H. pylori* resistance to tetracycline has not been reported, it may be used for retreatment, if necessary. The dose of tetracycline is usually 500 mg four times daily.

Histamine-2 Receptor Antagonists

All H$_2$RAs suppress gastric acid and pepsin secretion by competitively and reversibly occupying H$_2$ receptors. The H$_2$RAs differ in their relative potencies, with famotidine (Pepcid) being the most and cimetidine (Tagamet) being the least potent of the four. When administered in equipotent doses, the H$_2$RAs suppress gastric secretion equally. As a class, the H$_2$RAs are comparable in their volumes of distribution, serum half-lives, and clearance parameters. With the exception of nizatidine (Axid), the H$_2$RAs undergo extensive first-pass metabolism in the liver, and thus bioavailability is reduced to 30% to 80% of an administered dose. Although elimination occurs through both renal and hepatic routes, active renal tubular secretion is the primary mechanism of elimination for the H$_2$RAs; it therefore is recommended that doses be reduced in patients with severe renal impairment.

The H$_2$RAs achieve 70% to 95% healing rates in duodenal and gastric ulcers in 4 to 6 weeks when current dosing recommendations are followed. The published data are inconsistent in suggesting an advantage for any one H$_2$RA in producing initial healing. Multicenter, randomized, double-blinded, comparative studies of ranitidine (Zantac) with cimetidine, nizatidine, or famotidine have demonstrated equal efficacy and tolerability in treating and maintaining healed lesions in duodenal ulcers. Although the healing rates in gastric ulcers for the H$_2$RAs are relatively lower than in duodenal ulcers, the rates are very similar between the different agents used. As part of triple or quadruple therapy, the H$_2$RAs play an important role in treating PUD of an infectious origin. Symptom relief occurs more readily and efficacy rates may be higher when an antisecretory agent, such as an H$_2$RA, is added to a regimen.

The H$_2$RAs also may improve the activity of some antibiotics by increasing gastric pH. Ranitidine is the most widely studied H$_2$RA used in anti–*H. pylori* regimens and is available in combination with a bismuth compound as ranitidine bismuth citrate. The H$_2$RAs used in *H. pylori* regimens are usually dosed once or twice daily.

Adverse events associated with H$_2$RAs include thrombocytopenia, neutropenia, bradycardia, arrhythmias, confusion, depression, and gynecomastia. Cimetidine and ranitidine have been reported to cause dyskinesia, whereas famotidine and cimetidine can cause impotence, particularly at high doses.

Cimetidine is associated with more pharmacokinetic drug–drug interactions than the other H$_2$RAs, primarily because of its effect on drug-metabolizing enzymes. The interactions considered to be most important are those with cimetidine and warfarin (Coumadin), phenytoin (Dilantin), or theophylline (Slo-Phyllin). Other interactions, such as those with benzodiazepines and other drugs commonly used in elderly patients, can also be problematic. Large doses of ranitidine may inhibit one of the cytochrome P450 isoenzymes and interfere with metabolism of other drugs.

Proton Pump Inhibitors

The PPIs bind to the proton pump of the parietal call, inhibiting secretion of the hydrogen ion into the gastric lumen. The binding results in a profound inhibition of both basal and stimulated acid secretion. PPIs relieve pain and heal peptic ulcers more rapidly than the H$_2$RAs.

The PPIs are used once a day 30 to 60 minutes before the first meal of the day for treatment of GERD and are used once or twice a day for treatment of PUD. Notably, as with many other agents used in regimens for eradication of *H. pylori*, the overall effectiveness of the PPI regimen can be significantly affected by the dose of the drug. It has been suggested that because these drugs are thought to have direct activity against *H. pylori*, the use of higher doses may result in better eradication rates. The most commonly reported treatment-related adverse event during maintenance therapy is diarrhea. Drug interactions with the PPIs usually are not clinically significant.

Other Agents

Bismuth Subsalicylate

The mechanism of action of bismuth against *H. pylori* is complex and involves the inhibition of protein, cell wall, and adenosine triphosphate synthesis as well as a topical action to prevent adherence of *H. pylori* to gastric epithelial cells. With cure rates of approximately 10%, bismuth is not effective as a single agent for eradication. When used in combination with at least two additional antibiotics, however, significant eradication of *H. pylori* is achieved. In the United States, bismuth is formulated as BSS in chewable tablets and liquid and ranitidine bismuth citrate tablets (Tritec). Each BSS tablet and 15 mL of liquid contains 262 mg of bismuth, which is not absorbed, and 100 mg of salicylate, which is absorbed, similar to aspirin. Ranitidine bismuth citrate is available in 400-mg tablets and is approved by the U.S. Food and Drug Administration (FDA) for use with clarithromycin. In Europe, bismuth is available as colloidal bismuth subcitrate. Thus, many published studies conducted in countries other than the United States have involved administration of this compound to patients with PUD. The short half-life of bismuth results in the need for three to four times daily dosing of the product, although the ranitidine bismuth citrate dose is taken twice daily. Because *H. pylori* does not develop resistance to bismuth after repeated exposure, it may be used for retreatment when necessary.

Antacids

The numerous antacids available consist primarily of sodium bicarbonate, calcium carbonate, aluminum salts, and magnesium salts. The inorganic salts of antacids dissolve in gastric acid and release anions that partially neutralize the hydrochloric acid in the stomach. In usual doses, by increasing the gastric pH above 4, antacids inhibit the activity of pepsin. Antacids are minimally absorbed, and their neutralizing action on acid is local rather than systemic. When used to treat PUD, antacids must be administered many times daily in large doses. This frequent administration is not practical and can potentially decrease the absorption of many drugs. Antacids are not used to heal ulcers but may be helpful when used in combination with other antiulcer agents for intermediate, rapid relief of ulcer pain or dyspepsia.

The most frequent side effects associated with antacids are constipation or diarrhea. Sodium bicarbonate is limited to short-term use because of an increase in urinary sodium content as well as its potential to alter systemic pH. Calcium carbonate has been associated with hypercalcemia and acid production through the release of gastrin. Aluminum antacids may cause hyperaluminemia in patients with chronic renal failure. Similarly, hypermagnesemia, characterized by hypotension, nausea, vomiting, and electrocardiographic changes, may occur with continued administration of magnesium antacids in patients with renal impairment. Antacids may potentially cause drug interactions by altering the rate and the extent of absorption of concomitantly administered drugs.

Sucralfate

Sucralfate is a sulfated disaccharide compound with aluminum hydroxide that forms polyvalent bonds with damaged tissues as well as with normal GI mucosa. This complex adheres to an ulcer site, providing a barrier that prevents the penetration of acid, pepsin, and bile into gastric mucosa. Because sucralfate acts locally and is minimally absorbed from the GI tract, it is mostly excreted in the stool. Sucralfate, at 4 g/d, is as effective as ranitidine or cimetidine in promoting healing of duodenal and gastric ulcers and in rapidly relieving symptoms. Systemic adverse effects are rarely observed for sucralfate because of its minimal absorption. Of these side effects, constipation is most frequently reported. There has been concern over aluminum retention when sucralfate is administered to patients with impaired renal function. In addition, the aluminum released may chelate other drugs that are administered simultaneously. Although sucralfate is approved by the FDA for the treatment and maintenance of duodenal ulcers and is commonly used for stress ulcer prophylaxis, there is no role for sucralfate in the eradication of *H. pylori*.

Misoprostol

Misoprostol, a prostaglandin E$_1$ analog, inhibits the secretion of gastric acid, both basally and in response to food, histamine, pentagastrin, and coffee, by a direct action on parietal cells. Misoprostol has cytoprotective effects on the integrity of the gastric mucosa exposed to noxious stimuli. Misoprostol is an effective healing agent for patients with duodenal ulcers. However, it has FDA approval only for preventing NSAID-induced gastric ulcers.

Several placebo-controlled studies have demonstrated that misoprostol significantly reduces duodenal ulcer development in patients taking NSAIDs. When used to treat duodenal ulcers, misoprostol is not more effective than the H$_2$RAs, and it has a worse adverse effect profile. The MUCOSA trial demonstrated that misoprostol was significantly more effective than placebo, however, in preventing NSAID-induced ulcer complications in high-risk patients (Simon, et al., 1996).

Convincing data that misoprostol is effective in patients taking NSAIDs who have clinical ulcers are limited. These ulcers heal faster when the NSAID therapy is discontinued, but can be managed with an H$_2$RA or, ideally, with a PPI if the NSAID therapy continues.

Moreover, misoprostol does not relieve pain in patients with ulcers. Consensus panel recommendations suggest avoiding the use of NSAIDs in patients who develop ulcers while taking NSAIDs and misoprostol, although published data in this regard are limited. The dose of misoprostol does not need adjustment in patients with renal impairment.

The most frequently reported adverse event for misoprostol is diarrhea, which occurs in up to 40% of patients. The disorder can be severe enough to warrant the discontinuation of treatment. Studies indicate a dose–response relationship for diarrhea, ranging from 6% to 39% depending on the dosage regimen.

Misoprostol also may cause vaginal bleeding in postmenopausal women and should be avoided in women who are pregnant. Women taking misoprostol during childbearing years should be advised regarding appropriate use of contraception and should have a negative pregnancy test before beginning therapy.

Selecting the Most Appropriate Agent for GERD

Reflux esophagitis is a chronic disease that is likely to relapse, with 75% to 92% of patients reporting recurrence of symptoms 6 to 12 months after therapy is discontinued. Predictably, patients with more severe cases of GERD have higher relapse rates. Continued relapse puts the patient at risk for complications of esophagitis as well as deterioration of esophageal function; thus, maintenance acid-suppressive therapy is often necessary. Reducing the dosage of the medication or attempting maintenance with a less potent agent than used in healing also often results in recurrence.

Long-term suppression of acid secretion in patients infected with *H. pylori* appears to promote the proximal spread of the infection and the development of atrophic gastritis. This could in turn result in an increased risk of gastric cancer. Therefore, the European *Helicobacter pylori* Study Group (EHPSG, 1997) considered it *advisable* on the basis of *supportive evidence* that *H. pylori* should be eradicated when GERD requires long-term treatment with PPIs.

First-Line Therapy

In patients with mild GERD (symptoms fewer than three times a week), lifestyle changes are often effective, although drug therapy may be indicated. In moderate to severe GERD, drug therapy (**Table 29.3**) is needed along with lifestyle changes (**Figure 29-1**).

TABLE 29.3	Recommended Order of Treatment for GERD	
Order	**Agents**	**Comments**
First line	H₂ antagonists (cimetidine, ranitidine, famotidine, nizatidine)	For moderate GERD
	Proton pump inhibitors (omeprazole, lansoprazole, rabeprazole, esomeprazole, pantoprazole)	Rapid return of symptoms usually occurs if drug therapy stops.
		Works most effectively if given 2 times a day initially for 4–8 wk, then decreased to once a day
Second line	Referral for endoscopic examination	

Second-Line Therapy

H₂RAs are used as first-line therapy for mild GERD. The most effective treatment for initial therapy is twice-daily dosing, with the first dose in the morning and the second dose approximately 1 hour after the evening meal. If symptoms diminish by 90%, therapy is continued for 2 to 3 months. The dose is then tapered and the daily dose stopped. The drug may then be used on an as-needed basis. A PPI can be used in place of an H₂RA. These drugs provide more complete control of acid secretion than H₂RAs and are the most effective agents for treating GERD. Approximately 83% of patients report symptom relief. Treatment is recommended for 8 to 12 weeks.

Third-Line Therapy

If the first and second lines of therapy fail, the patient is referred to a gastroenterologist for endoscopy. In patients with esophagitis confirmed by endoscopy, PPI therapy begins immediately because of the superior healing rate associated with this drug class. If symptoms are eliminated, maintenance therapy is

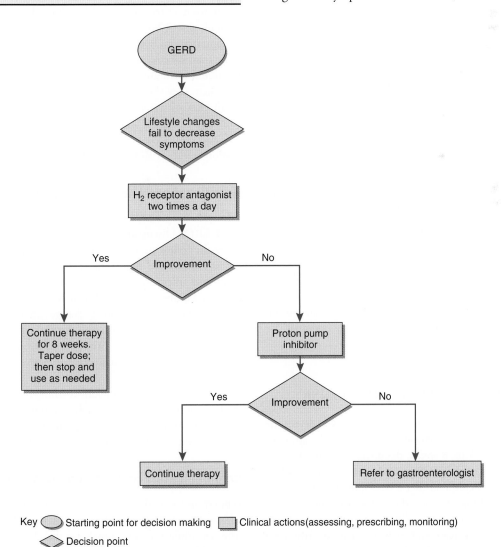

FIGURE 29–1 Treatment algorithm for GERD.

indicated at the lowest dosage necessary to prevent recurrence, continue healing, and eliminate the possibility of complications. In most cases, patients with erosive esophagitis cannot be weaned from acid suppression therapy because a rebound effect is common. (See **Table 29.3.**)

Special Population Considerations

Pediatric

Gastroesophageal reflux is common in healthy infants. These infants spit up or vomit after each feeding without discomfort. One half of infants outgrow this by age 6 months and the rest by age 18 months. Children with chronic gastroesophageal reflux exhibit poor growth, vomiting, hoarseness, coughing, and chronic sore throat. Treatment in infants is to thicken the formula or breast milk with 1 to 2 tablespoons of rice cereal per 2 ounces of liquid. The infant is burped after 1 to 2 ounces of formula or when changing the breast. The infant should be kept upright for 30 minutes after feeding. The head of the crib is raised 30 degrees.

Geriatric

Older patients often take drugs that decrease LES tone, causing symptoms of reflux. It is recommended that antacids containing sodium not be used in this population, nor are aluminum hydroxide–containing antacids recommended if the patient is constipated because their use can lead to hypophosphatemia, causing bone changes. Magnesium-containing antacids can be used if there is no renal disease present and may be helpful if the patient is also constipated.

Pantoprazole may have greater effect in elderly patients than in younger adults, and the dosage may have to be modified. In cases of liver disease, the dosage may also require adjustment because pantoprazole is metabolized and excreted by the hepatic system.

Women

Heartburn is a common occurrence in pregnancy. Antacids are generally safe when used in moderation; however, sodium bicarbonate is to be avoided because of the potential for alkalosis.

MONITORING PATIENT RESPONSE

Patients are seen 1 to 2 weeks after starting therapy to determine response. If the symptoms decrease, a full course of therapy continues for 8 weeks. After 8 weeks, the dosage is reduced to the lowest level that decreases symptoms and given once a day before meals. If symptoms continue after 8 weeks, the patient continues on therapy and may be referred to a gastroenterologist.

Because some patients may achieve remission after a single course of therapy, it is reasonable to attempt to identify these patients by a therapeutic trial and discontinuation of therapy. In most, symptoms recur, and endoscopy can be used to stratify

patients. Another approach would be to treat again, skipping endoscopy and following the patient's response. Patients who are started on empiric therapy without success as well as those with atypical symptoms who respond poorly to therapy should undergo endoscopy.

If symptom recurrence is frequent, the patient should be on a maintenance therapy regimen. Dosage should be titrated up to a level that eliminates symptoms, including increased or more frequent dosing of H$_2$RAs and twice-daily PPIs. It is rare for patients to continue to have symptoms despite high-dose acid suppression. Patients with continuing symptoms should be studied by 24-hour esophageal pH monitoring to confirm the GERD diagnosis. It may also be appropriate to suggest endoscopic surgery at this time.

PATIENT EDUCATION

Drug Information

Medication instruction should include the reason for taking antacids 1 to 2 hours after the H$_2$RA if these drugs are taken in combination. Reminders that antacids are not to be used for more than 2 weeks and that antacid tablets are not as potent as the liquid form are shared with the patient. If antacid tablets are taken, they should be thoroughly chewed and followed by a full glass of water. Effervescent tablets should be dissolved completely in water and drunk after the bubbles subside.

AstraZeneca has a Web site for patients with general information about GERD. It is www.gerd.com.

Nutritional and Lifestyle Changes

Lifestyle changes are as important as drug therapy in managing GERD. Discussion with the patient and family should cover the following important dietary changes: avoidance of excess alcohol and food intake; decreased amounts of chocolate and spicy, fried, or fatty foods eaten; and avoidance of the recumbent position for at least 3 hours after meals. Because these recommended changes involve many activities or foods that are pleasurable for the patient, they should occur gradually—one at a time. A nutritionist can be consulted to help the patient learn to choose and prepare less problematic foods.

Additional measures include teaching the patient to elevate the head of the bed approximately 4 to 6 inches (using blocks); to avoid tight, restrictive clothing; and to lose weight if necessary. Smoking cessation is another goal of patient education.

Complementary and Alternative Medicine

Peppermint is used by some for the treatment of GERD. It relaxes the sphincter of Oddi by reducing calcium influx and stimulates bile flow in animals by the chloretic action of its flavonoid components. The menthol has a direct spasmolytic effect on smooth muscle of the digestive tract.

Selecting the Most Appropriate Agent for PUD

For eradicating *H. pylori*, the ideal first-line regimen is one that is relatively cost-effective and easily adhered to by patients (**Figure 29-2**). The ideal second- and third-line regimens are those that are relatively cost-effective and easily followed by patients. Continuing antisecretory maintenance therapy for more than 2 weeks following antibiotic treatment is unnecessary after *H. pylori* eradication unless patients have concomitant GERD.

First-Line Therapy

There are several regimens used to treat *H. pylori*. Treatment is for 10 days. **Table 29.2** lists the regimens.

Second-Line Therapy

Longer duration therapy regimens (14 days) are second-line therapy. This improves the outcome by 10%.

Third-Line Therapy

Third-line therapy is endoscopy and biopsy to establish a definitive diagnosis.

Preventive Therapy in NSAID-Induced PUD

Clinical data do not support the use of misoprostol or a PPI to prevent ulcers in all patients taking NSAIDs. According to published guidelines from the American College of Gastroenterology, people at high risk for NSAID-induced ulcer, bleeding, and perforation should receive prophylaxis with misoprostol if they must continue receiving NSAID therapy.

The PPIs are acceptable alternatives for patients at risk for GI complications from NSAIDs. Factors that increase the risk for development of these complications include prior history of a GI event, age older than 60, use of a higher dose of an NSAID, and concurrent corticosteroid or anticoagulant use.

The H_2RAs are not recommended for prophylaxis because of their low efficacy in preventing gastric versus duodenal ulcers. For treating an NSAID-related ulcer, any drug that has the ability effectively to heal gastric or duodenal ulcer can be used.

Published guidelines recommend a PPI as the preferred therapy when an NSAID-induced ulcer needs to be healed, particularly when the NSAID cannot be discontinued.

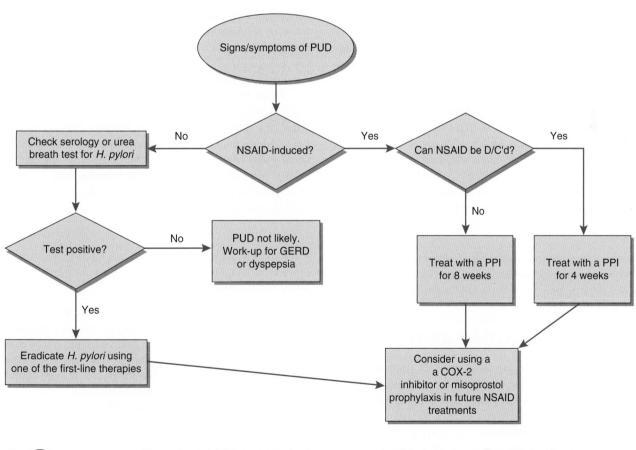

FIGURE 29–2   Treatment algorithm for PUD.

Special Population Considerations

It is important for the prescribing practitioner to be aware of unique considerations when dealing with the special populations of children, older adults, and women.

Pediatric

Epidemiologic data suggest that acquisition of *H. pylori* infection occurs in childhood, most likely before age 5. It is thought that the tissue damage and disease caused by *H. pylori* is progressive. Despite this suggestion, as well as the lack of evidence that preventing or treating infections acquired in youth produces long-term health benefits, children are not routinely screened for *H. pylori*. According to results of the limited number of small studies conducted in pediatric patients, eradication of *H. pylori* in children has been effective in curing PUD. However, there are no consensus guidelines for managing this infection in children. Recently published guidelines apply to adults only. Two regimens—MOC and clarithromycin, amoxicillin, and omeprazole—have both produced eradication rates greater than 80%. Because of the potential for significant adverse effects on teeth and bones, tetracycline should not be used in children younger than age 8.

Geriatric

The prevalence of *H. pylori* infection increases with age and eradication of *H. pylori* is necessary when gastric or duodenal ulcers are present in elderly patients. Age is a factor that significantly increases the risk for development of GI complications from NSAIDs. The presentation of PUD is often atypical in the elderly; hence, a high index of suspicion is necessary. Elderly patients are also at high risk for development of complications of PUD. Treatment of PUD in the elderly is similar to that in younger patients, although elderly patients are more likely to experience adverse effects and drug interactions from medications used to manage PUD. A heightened awareness and increased monitoring for these treatment-related complications are essential when treating the geriatric population.

Women

Women taking misoprostol during childbearing years should be advised regarding appropriate use of contraception and should have a negative pregnancy test before beginning therapy.

MONITORING PATIENT RESPONSE

Because the most common cause of PUD recurrence after treatment with antibiotics is failure to eradicate *H. pylori*, several issues should be considered in an attempt to prevent treatment failures. Noncompliance is a common cause for failure to eradicate *H. pylori*; thus, a primary treatment goal is ensuring patient adherence to an effective regimen for 7 to 14 days. Initial therapies to eradicate *H. pylori* are typically prescribed for 7 to 10 days, but in situations where retreatment is necessary because of recurrent disease, a minimum of 14 days

of therapy is often recommended. Adherence to a prescribed regimen is of paramount importance in achieving eradication rates quoted in the literature. Because many effective regimens are complex, some requiring up to 16 pills per day, it is important to individualize therapy as much as possible and to stress the importance of rigorous patient compliance and its link to successful eradication and thus treatment of PUD. Antibiotic resistance to metronidazole or clarithromycin can also lead to treatment failure. Finally, alterations in the dose or timing of administration of antibiotics can affect the success of an eradication regimen (e.g., tetracycline with regard to meals).

In addition to pretreatment screening to diagnose active infection by *H. pylori*, it is sometimes desirable to conduct a diagnostic test to determine the presence or absence of *H. pylori* after treatment. The urea breath test is particularly useful as a follow-up test in the early posttreatment period. Patients can be tested 4 to 6 weeks after the completion of antibiotic therapy using this noninvasive, simple test that is specific for active *H. pylori* infection. A urea breath test is widely available in the United States. Serology testing of IgG titers alone does not distinguish current infection from past infection until 6 months to 1 year after completion of treatment.

The practice of obtaining serial IgA titers has proven useful. In this study, drops in serum IgA titers at 3 months were adequately able to confirm eradication. This approach, however, is based on relative changes from pretreatment titers, and because results of the particular assay used in this study can vary greatly, a major disadvantage is the need to run both samples in parallel to minimize variation.

When the NSAID is discontinued in a patient with an NSAID-induced ulcer and appropriate ulcer treatment is initiated, the ulcer should heal after 8 weeks. Patients with an NSAID-induced ulcer should also be screened for the presence of *H. pylori* because it needs to be determined whether the ulcer is from the NSAID or due to infection with *H. pylori*. If *H. pylori* is present, treatment with a three- or four-drug anti–*H. pylori* regimen should be initiated.

PATIENT EDUCATION

Drug Information

Antacids can be used along with other antiulcer drugs for more immediate relief of symptoms of dyspepsia. Also, it is important for patients to understand that *H. pylori* infection can be cured with the appropriate antibiotic therapy. The adverse effects of the therapy can be unpleasant but the patient is to be encouraged to finish the therapy to ensure eradication.

Information for patients about PUD can be found at www.cdc.gov/ulcer/.

Nutritional and Lifestyle Changes

Patients diagnosed with PUD should be encouraged to eliminate cigarette smoking, NSAID use (if possible), and excessive caffeine and alcohol intake. Taking an NSAID with food, reducing the dose of the NSAID, or switching to a potentially less toxic agent such as acetaminophen or a COX-2 inhibitor are possible options in patients taking an NSAID. Stress management initiatives may also aid in PUD symptom relief.

Complementary and Alternative Medicine

Licorice has been used for PUD because of its anecdotal use for gastric irritation. However, licorice can be dangerous if consumed in large amounts. Consumption of 30 to 40 g/d for extended periods has resulted in electrolyte imbalances.

Case Study

J. G. is a 42-year-old white man presenting with a 2-month history of intermittent mid-epigastric pain. The pain sometimes wakes him up at night and seems to get better after he eats a meal. J.G. informs you that he was told by his doctor 6 months ago that he had an infection in his stomach. He never followed up and has been taking over-the-counter Zantac for 2 weeks without relief. He is concerned because the pain is continuing. He has no other significant history except he is a 20 pack-year smoker and he drinks 5 cups of coffee a day. He eats late at night and goes to bed about 30 minutes after dinner. He also takes Motrin twice a day for shoulder pain. He is allergic to penicillin.

DIAGNOSIS: PUD

1. List the specific goals for treatment for J. C.

2. What drug therapy would you prescribe for J. C.? Why?
3. What tests would you prescribe to determine the success of the therapy?
4. Discuss specific patient education based on the diagnosis and the prescribed therapy.
5. List one or two adverse reactions to the therapy that J. C. might have.
6. What would be the choice for second-line therapy?
7. What dietary and lifestyle changes should be recommended for this patient?
8. Describe one or two drug–drug or drug–food interactions for the selected therapy.

BIBLIOGRAPHY

*Starred references are cited in the text.

Ables, A., Simon, I., & Melton, E. (2007). Update on *Helicobacter* treatment. *American Family Physician, 75*(3), 351–358.

*Adamek, R. J., Suerbaum, S., Pfaffenbach, B., & Opfentuch, W. (1998). Primary and acquired *Helicobacter pylori* resistance to clarithromycin, metronidazole and amoxicillin. Influence on treatment outcome. *American Journal of Gastroenterology, 93,* 386–389.

*Allison, P. R. (1946). Peptic ulcer of the esophagus. *Journal of Thoracic Surgery, 15,* 308–317.

*Bell, J. D., Powell, K. U., Burridge, S. M., et al. (1995). Rapid eradication of *Helicobacter pylori* infection. *Alimentary Pharmacology and Therapeutics, 9,* 41–46.

*The European *Helicobacter pylori* Study Group (EHPSG). (1997). Current European concepts in the management of *H. pylori* infection: The Maastricht Consensus Report. *Gut, 41,* 8–13.

*Healy, D. P., Danserau, R. J., Dunn, A. B., et al. (1997). Reduced tetracycline bioavailability caused by magnesium aluminum salicylate in liquid formulations of bismuth subsalicylate. *Annals of Pharmacotherapy, 31,* 1460–1464.

*National Institutes of Health (NIH) Consensus Development Panel. (1994). *Helicobacter pylori* in peptic ulcer disease. *Journal of the American Medical Association, 272,* 65–69.

Oranu, A., & Vaezi, M. (2010). Noncardiac chest pain: Gastroesophageal reflux disease. *Medical Clinics of North America, 94*(2), 233–242.

Richter, J. (2007). The many manifestations of gastroesophageal reflux disease: Presentation, evaluation and treatment. *Gastrointestinal Clinics, 36*(3), 233–242.

Romakrishnan, K., & Salenos, R. (2007). Peptic ulcer disease. *American Family Physician, 75*(3), 1005–1012.

*Saledo, J. A., & Al-Kawas, F. (1998). Treatment of *Helicobacter pylori* infection. *Archives of Internal Medicine, 158,* 842–851.

*Shaheen, N., & Provenzale, D. (2003). The epidemiology of gastroesophageal reflux disease. *American Journal of Medicine Science, 326*(5), 264–273.

*Simon, L. S., Hatoum, H. T., Bittman, R. M., et al. (1996). Risk factors for serious nonsteroidal-induced gastrointestinal complications: Regression analysis of the MUCOSA trial. *Family Medicine, 28,* 204–210.

Wang, C., & Hunt, R. (2008). Medical management of gastroesophageal reflux disease. *Gastrointestinal Clinics, 37*(4), 879–899.

*Winkelstein, A. (1935). Peptic esophagitis: A new clinical entity. *Journal of the American Medical Association, 104,* 906–909.

CHAPTER 30

Veronica F. Wilbur

Constipation, Diarrhea, and Irritable Bowel Syndrome

Functional bowel disorders of the lower gastrointestinal (GI) tract can include symptoms of hypogastric cramping, abdominal pain, diarrhea, or constipation. Constipation and diarrhea can be self-limiting and are considered symptoms of possibly serious medical problems. Temporary dysfunctions of the bowel can include common GI upsets that can cause diarrhea or short-lived episodes of constipation. One of the most puzzling functional bowel disorders is irritable bowel syndrome (IBS). IBS typically presents with vague, crampy hypogastric pain and can be accompanied by alternating constipation and diarrhea. Similar pharmacologic agents are used to treat these symptoms, whether self-limited or chronic.

CONSTIPATION

Constipation is a common GI symptom that is defined as infrequent or difficult evacuation of stool. Every individual affected by constipation defines it differently, but normal defecation can vary from daily to three times a day or to every 3 days. Constipation can be a consequence of multiple factors, including diet, lifestyle, medications, and many disease states. In a systematic review of the epidemiology of constipation in North America by Higgins & Johanson (2004), the mean prevalence of constipation in the general population was found to be 12% to 19%. Constipation affects 2.2 females to 1 male and the incidence increases with age, especially in those over age 65. Shah, et al. (2008) reports an increase of 4 million ambulatory care visits for constipation between 2001 and 2004. Of these 4 million visits, the highest increase was in children younger than age 14. Dietary and lifestyle modifications are the preferred therapy for constipation, but many patients use over-the-counter (OTC) laxatives for relief. Americans spend over $1 billion for more than 150 types of OTC and prescription laxatives (Smith, et al., 2002; Stessman, 2003). Most of these laxatives are considered safe and effective, but overuse or abuse may have serious consequences.

CAUSES

Constipation may be initially diagnosed based on a thorough history and physical examination. If an identifiable cause is present, constipation is then classified as a secondary symptom. However, constipation may be a symptom of an underlying disease state (**Box 30.1**). The patient's lifestyle (e.g., diet, inactivity) or concomitant medications (**Box 30.2**) may also contribute to constipation. When no cause can be found for the symptoms of constipation, the disorder is categorized as idiopathic. Idiopathic constipation is usually caused by a reduction in the propulsive capacity of the colon (slow transit constipation) or a functional outlet. Although constipation is often a benign condition, it can be a symptom of a more serious problem. If left untreated in an elderly patient, constipation may lead to impaction, stercoral ulceration, anal fissures, megacolon, volvulus, and possibly carcinoma of the colon.

PATHOPHYSIOLOGY

The absorptive capacity and motility of the colon are major factors of bowel function. Approximately 9 L of fluid enters the small intestine daily from ingestion or intestinal secretions. The small intestine absorbs approximately 80% of this fluid load, which is approximately half of its capacity. The colon absorbs the remainder, with the exception of approximately 0.1 L of water that is passed in the stool. If absorption of the small intestine is reduced, the fluid load adds to the

---

BOX 30.1

Disorders Associated with Constipation

Bowel obstruction	Irritable bowel syndrome
Colonic tumors	Megacolon
Depression	Parkinsonism
Diabetes	Spinal injury
Diverticulitis	Stroke
Hypercalcemia	Uremia
Hypothyroidism	

BOX 30.2

Selected Medication Associated with Constipation

Activated charcoal
Antacids
  (aluminum- or
  magnesium-containing)
Anticholinergics
Antihistamines (sedating)
Antipsychotics
Bile acid sequestrants
Calcium supplements
Clonidine

Diuretics
Ferrous salts
HMG-CoA reductase
  inhibitors (i.e., statins)
Narcotic analgesics
Sodium polystyrene
  sulfonate
Sucralfate
Tricyclic antidepressants
Verapamil

BOX 30.3

History and Physical Examination for Chronic Constipation

Important history questions:
Onset and duration of symptoms
Patient's definition of constipation
Presence of abdominal cramping relieved by defeca-
  tion (*if yes, think irritable bowel syndrome*)
Presence of blood in the stool

Important aspects of the physical examination:
Evaluation of the perianal area for scars, fistulas,
  fissures, and external hemorrhoids
Observe the perineum at rest and while patient is
  bearing down.
Digital rectal examination—check for fecal impaction,
  stricture, or rectal masses.

burden of the colon, which is capable of absorbing 4 to 5 L of fluid per day. Fluid in excess of this amount results in diarrhea. Likewise, excessive reabsorption of water results in constipation.

The colon can be divided into three distinctive functional areas: (1) the cecum and proximal colon, (2) the transverse colon, and (3) the distal colon and rectum. Each area performs different roles in preparing the chyme for expulsion. The variation in the neurogenic tone of each area affects the capacity of the colon to retain or release the fecal material.

The motility of the bowel is affected by the flow of chyme from the coloileal reflex and its visceral hypersensitivity can contribute to the sense of urgency and tenesmus of proximal colonic transit. The neurogenic aspects of colon motility are poorly understood and need further study. Some of the stimuli thought to affect colonic activity are awakening from sleep or rest, ingestion of a high-calorie meal, and the sight or smell of food.

DIAGNOSTIC CRITERIA

The definition of constipation varies widely between health care providers and patients. Constipation can be idiopathic and is functionally defined as infrequent bowel movements accompanied by straining. Feces are hard, leading to straining and a feeling of incomplete evacuation of the rectum. An important distinction between chronic constipation and IBS is the absence of abdominal pain associated with the bowel pattern.

The diagnosis of constipation stems primarily from the history. A careful history (**Box 30.3**) can help the provider decide which diagnostic tests may be appropriate. Abrupt onset of constipation or onset in patients ages 45 to

50 suggests an organic cause and requires immediate attention (Dosh, 2002; Schiller, 2001; Stessman, 2003).

INITIATING DRUG THERAPY

Lifestyle modifications are preferred over pharmacologic therapy for treating constipation. Diet, exercise, and bowel habit training are usually targeted. However, research is inconclusive as to the value of increasing fluid intake and exercise (Muller-Lissner, et al., 2005). According to the National Center for Health Statistics, Americans eat 5 to 14 g of fiber daily, far short of the recommended 20 to 35 g recommended by the American Dietetic Association (American Dietetic Association, 2002; Dosh, 2002). Increased dietary fiber can be recommended for most patients without fear of colon obstruction. Fiber should be both soluble and insoluble in the form of fruits, vegetables, and whole grains, which cannot be digested by the body. Fiber should be slowly increased to 20 to 25 g per day over a 1- to 2-week period to improve compliance with therapy. Dietary fiber increases stool weight and shortens intestinal transit time. However, fiber therapy may not be effective for all patients. Fiber accelerates right colon transit, but there are few treatments for patients where the transit problem is the left colon.

One additional lifestyle modification includes establishing a regular pattern for bathroom visits. Patients should also be counseled not to ignore the urge to defecate, because this delay increases the time for absorption of fluid from the stool. Biofeedback, a method of retraining the pelvic floor muscles to relax during defecation, may be effective in selected patients.

Goals of Drug Therapy

An adequate trial of lifestyle modification should be attempted first. If this fails, pharmacologic management with laxatives may be appropriate. There is no evidence that laxatives cause dependency and should be withheld from long-term treatment (Medscape, 2005; Wald, 2006, 2007).

The goal of therapy for constipation is to increase the water content of the feces and increase motility of the intestines to promote comfortable defecation, using the lowest effective dose of a laxative for the least amount of time possible. Only if a patient fails therapy should the health care provider consider ordering colon transit studies to evaluate the transit time of stool in the intestine (Wald, 2006). Responses to laxatives vary and depend on the patient as well as the preparation. Several classes of laxatives are available for the symptomatic treatment of constipation: bulk-forming agents, saline laxatives, lubricant laxatives, surfactants (emollients), hyperosmotic laxatives, and stimulant laxatives. Proper selection of a laxative should be based on the individual clinical situation (**Table 30.1**).

Bulk-Forming Laxatives

Bulk forming laxatives work by binding to the fecal contents and pulling water into the stool. This ultimately softens and lubricates the stool, eases its passage, and reduces straining. Water is reabsorbed from fecal masses that stay in the colon for extended periods, and the result is dry stools. Bulk-forming agents hold water in the stool or swell and increase stool bulk. The bulk stimulates the movement of the intestines and facilitates the passage of intestinal contents. These types of laxatives are not useful when constipation results from the use of opioid medications.

Bulk-forming laxatives generally consist of psyllium seed husk, methylcellulose, polycarbophil, and wheat dextrin, which are made of polysaccharides, cellulose derivatives, or wheat starch such as methylcellulose (Citrucel) or psyllium (Metamucil). Polycarbophil (FiberCon) and wheat dextrin (Benefiber) have significant water-absorptive properties and also are used as antidiarrheals. All bulk-forming agents used for constipation should be taken with plenty of fluid (8 ounces) to increase efficacy. Malt soup extract (Maltsupex) made from barley malt reduces fecal pH. This may contribute to its laxative effect. Traditionally, these products have been marketed only as powders, which must be dissolved in water. Now many fiber products are available in powder, wafer, and caplet forms. Patients may need to try several before finding one that works for them. Brand names include Metamucil, FiberCon, and Citrucel. Metamucil is the preferred agent because it is the safest and most physiologic. Sugar-free methylcellulose and psyllium products are available for patients with diabetes. Patients with celiac disease or gluten intolerance should avoid using wheat dextrin products.

Contraindications to the use of bulking agents are symptoms of an acute surgical abdomen, intestinal obstruction or perforation, or inability to drink an adequate amount of fluid.

Action for all agents may begin in 12 to 24 hours, but a full effect is not usually seen for up to 3 days.

A half-cup to one bowl daily of wheat bran can provide adequate fiber supplementation, but synthetic forms of fiber are often better absorbed than food. Other foods can also add fiber to the diet and should be reviewed with the patient. The patient should be encouraged to drink adequate amounts of fluid throughout the day; if not contraindicated, up to 2,500 mL is preferred. These agents are more likely to be used as preventive measures. However given, they can take effect within 12 to 24 hours, and some acute relief of symptoms is possible.

Adverse Events

Overall, these agents are usually well tolerated, but compliance can be a problem because the most common side effect is increased flatulence, and some bloating can occur. With severe constipation, all agents can cause abdominal fullness and cramping. If these agents are used excessively, nausea and vomiting may occur.

Contraindications

Because bulk-forming laxatives have the most physiologic effect and are not systemically absorbed, they are the preferred agents for symptomatic treatment of constipation. However, these agents are not completely benign and should be avoided in patients with strictures of the esophagus, GI ulcerations, or stenosis secondary to the possibility of obstruction from increased bulk of intestinal contents. In addition, some bulk-forming agents may contain as much as 20 g of carbohydrates per dose. Sugar-free bulk-forming agents are available and are recommended for diabetic patients.

Interactions

The sugar-free preparations may contain aspartame, which is metabolized to phenylalanine and should be used cautiously with patients who must restrict their phenylalanine intake. Wheat gluten is a by-product of extracting the gluten from wheat; however, complete extraction cannot be guaranteed and should be avoided in patients with gluten intolerance. Concomitant administration of calcium-containing bulk laxatives may reduce the effectiveness of quinolone or tetracycline, so patients should separate the administration time of these agents.

Hyperosmotic Laxatives

Lactulose (Cephulac), sorbitol, polyethylene glycol/electrolyte solution (PEG-ES, Colyte), and polyethylene glycol (PEG, MiraLAX) are examples of hyperosmotic laxatives. These agents serve as or are metabolized to solutes in the intestinal tract. The increased concentration of solutes creates osmotic pressure by drawing fluid from a less concentrated gradient to the more concentrated gradient inside the GI tract. This increase in osmotic pressure stimulates intestinal motility and propulsion of fecal contents. The PEG products do not degrade colonic bacteria and therefore produce less bloating. Glycerin (Colace Suppository, Fleet Glycerin Suppository, Pedia-Lax Suppository) helps the stool

TABLE 30.1	Overview of Selected Laxatives		
Generic (Trade) Name and Dosage	**Selected Adverse Events**	**Contraindications**	**Special Considerations**
Bulk-Forming Laxatives			
methylcellulose (Citrucel) 2–6 g/d	Flatulence, stomach upset, fullness	GI obstruction	Take with plenty of water. Avoid in patients with GI ulceration.
psyllium (Metamucil) 3.4–10.2 g/d	Same as above	Same as above	Same as above Sugar-free formulation caution with phenylketonuria
polycarbophil (FiberCon) 1–6 g/d	Same as above	Same as above	Same as above Calcium content may interact with tetracycline or quinolone antibiotics.
malt soup extract (Maltsupex) 12–64 g/d	Same as above	Same as above	Same as above
wheat dextrin (Benefiber) Powder: 1 tbsp daily for age 6 and up Chewables: Age 12 – adult 3 tablets 3 times daily Ages 6 - 11 1 ½ tablets 3 times daily	Same as above	Same as above Not a good choice for those with possible celiac disease	Shelf life of 2 years Store in a cool environment. Less flatulence production than other bulking agents
Lubricants and Surfactants			
mineral oil 5–45 mL/d	Rectal seepage, irritation	Do not use with surfactants.	Impairs absorption of fat-soluble vitamins Caution in elderly and very young due to potential for development of lipid pneumonia
docusate sodium (Colace) 50–500 mg/d	Stomach upset	Do not use with mineral oil.	Most effective at preventing "straining" in high-risk patients (see text)
docusate calcium (Surfak) 50–240 mg	Same as above	Same as above	Same as above
docusate potassium (Dialose) 100–300 mg	Same as above	Same as above	Same as above
Saline Agents			
sodium phosphate enema (Fleet) 118 mL/d	Alterations in fluid/electrolyte balance, diarrhea	Caution in patients with congestive heart failure, hypertension, edema, and renal dysfunction	Care should be taken in the elderly and those with existing electrolyte disturbances.
sodium phosphate (Fleet Phospho-soda) 20–30 mL in water/d	Alterations in fluid electrolyte balance, dehydration, diarrhea	Same as above	Same as above Caution in renal dysfunction and the elderly
magnesium citrate 240 mL/d	GI upset, diarrhea	Caution in renal dysfunction	Stagger administration times of tetracycline and quinolone antibiotics.
magnesium hydroxide (Phillips Milk of Magnesia) 30–60 mL/d	GI upset, diarrhea	Same as above	Caution in renal dysfunction and the elderly Stagger administration times of tetracycline and quinolone antibiotics.
magnesium sulfate (Epsom salt) 1–2 tsp in ½ glass water	GI upset, diarrhea	Same as above	Caution in renal dysfunction and the elderly Stagger administration times of tetracycline and quinolone antibiotics.
Hyperosmotic Agents			
lactulose (Chronulac, Constilac, Duphalac) 15–60 mL	GI upset, diarrhea, flatulence	Caution in diabetic patients	Use lactulose with caution in patients with diabetes.
sorbitol 130–150 mL	GI upset, diarrhea, flatulence	Same as above	Caution in diabetic patients
Stimulants			
senna (Senokot) Tabs: 2–8/d Supp: 1 qhs Granules: 1–4 tsp/d	Griping, diarrhea, gas, discoloration of urine	GI obstruction	Caution: laxative abuse, cathartic colon
bisacodyl (Dulcolax) Tabs: 1–3/d Supp: 1 pr qd	Griping, diarrhea, gas	GI obstruction	Do not crush or chew tablets. Avoid concomitant administration of antacids and pH-lowering agents.
castor oil 15–60 mL/d	Stomach upset, diarrhea, colic	GI obstruction	Too potent for routine use

to evacuate by similar mechanisms, but also provides local rectal stimulation.

In addition to its osmotic effect, glycerin also has a local irritant effect in the suppository form. The irritant action adds to the osmotic action to stimulate bowel movement.

Lactulose is a disaccharide analog that is metabolized by bacteria to acids that increase osmotic pressure and acidify the contents of the colon. The result is increased intestinal motility and secretion.

In addition to its use for the symptomatic treatment of constipation, sorbitol is also used to prevent constipation in combination with activated charcoal for poisoning. Sodium polystyrene sulfonate (Kayexalate), a cation exchange resin used for treating hyperkalemia, is often combined with sorbitol to reduce the potential for constipation from the resin.

PEG-ES is a nonabsorbable solution that acts as an osmotic agent. It is usually used to evacuate the bowel before a GI examination such as a flexible sigmoidoscopy or colonoscopy. The solution is reconstituted with 1 gallon of tap water and should be chilled before consumption to increase palatability. The patient should begin drinking the solution at 4 PM the day before the procedure. One glass (8 oz) of the reconstituted solution should be consumed every 10 minutes over 3 hours until all 4 L are consumed. The patient should fast for 4 hours before ingesting the solution, and only clear liquids are allowed after ingestion.

Contraindications

Lactulose syrup should be used with caution in diabetic patients because it contains lactose and galactose. Lactose is also contraindicated in patients with appendicitis, acute surgical abdomen, fecal impaction, or intestinal obstruction. Caution must be used in diabetic patients because of sugar content.

Other osmotic agents such as magnesium hydroxide (Milk of Magnesia) or magnesium citrate (Citroma) can be used to promote defecation. Approximately 15% to 30% of the magnesium in these agents may be absorbed systemically; therefore, caution is needed in patients who have renal failure and decreased ability to excrete magnesium.

When taken appropriately, these agents are well tolerated. The most common adverse events are abdominal cramping and nausea. Evidence is lacking that extensive, long-term use of these agents can lead to laxative dependence (Brandt, et al., 2005). However, the use of these agents may be counterproductive in patients with changes in colonic transit time, IBS, or severe bloating and fullness (Wald, 2006).

In addition, sorbitol as a caloric sweetener has the potential to affect blood glucose levels and should be used with caution in diabetic patients. PEG-ES is not recommended in patients with gastric obstruction, bowel perforation, or colitis.

Adverse Reactions

Glycerin is among the safest laxative preparations available and is often used in infants and children. Rectal irritation is the most common side effect of glycerin suppositories. The most common side effects associated with lactulose and sorbitol include GI upset and diarrhea. PEG-ES rapidly cleanses the bowel and often causes nausea, abdominal fullness, cramps, and bloating.

Interactions

There are few documented interactions with the osmotic laxatives. However, because antacids may neutralize the acids produced from lactulose and interfere with its mechanism of action, concomitant administration of antacids should be avoided with lactulose. No other medications should be given within 1 hour of consumption of PEG-ES because the medication will likely be flushed from the GI tract.

Saline Laxatives

Like hyperosmotic laxatives, saline laxatives draw water into the intestine through osmosis. This creates an increase in intraluminal pressure and a resultant increase in intestinal motility. Magnesium citrate (Citrate of Magnesia), magnesium hydroxide (Phillips Milk of Magnesia), magnesium sulfate (Epsom salt), sodium phosphate, and sodium biphosphate (Fleet Phospho-soda) are examples of saline laxatives. Magnesium citrate and sodium phosphate and biphosphate are used as bowel evacuants for endoscopic examinations such as flexible sigmoidoscopy. A typical dose is one bottle of magnesium citrate at 4 PM the day before the test and two Fleet enemas 1 hour before leaving home the morning of the test.

Contraindications

Caution should be used when administering sodium phosphate salts to patients on sodium-restricted diets (e.g., hypertension, congestive heart failure, edema). In addition, phosphates can accumulate in patients with renal dysfunction, leading to serious complications such as hyperphosphatemia, hypokalemia, hypocalcemia, hypernatremia, metabolic acidosis, and coma.

Magnesium hydroxide and magnesium sulfate are commonly used for the symptomatic treatment of constipation. Because the kidneys eliminate magnesium, magnesium-containing laxatives should be used with caution in the elderly and in patients with decreased renal function. Excessive magnesium levels can result in central nervous system depression (drowsiness), muscle weakness, decreased blood pressure, and electrocardiographic changes.

Adverse Events

Dehydration is a concern with the use of saline laxatives, and these agents must be used with caution in patients who cannot tolerate excessive fluid loss and dehydration.

Interactions

Because Milk of Magnesia also has antacid properties and can increase the pH of the intestines, it should not be administered at the same time with agents that require an acidic environment to be absorbed. The most common example of this type of interaction is with the antifungals itraconazole (Sporanox) and ketoconazole (Nizoral). Therefore, administration of any antacid should be separated from administration of ketoconazole or itraconazole by at least 2 hours. In addition, the magnesium found in magnesium hydroxide and magnesium sulfate can bind with tetracycline and quinolone antibiotics to form a nonabsorbable complex that may reduce the effectiveness of the antibiotics. Administration of quinolones and tetracyclines should be separated from administration of magnesium-containing compounds.

Stimulant Laxatives

These laxatives vary in effects but act by increasing peristalsis through direct effects on the smooth muscle of the intestines and simultaneously promoting fluid accumulation in the colon and small intestine. Because of the irritating effect of the agents on the musculature, these agents should be avoided in long-term treatment. Stimulant laxatives include bisacodyl (Dulcolax) and senna concentrates (Senokot, Senokot S). Overall, stimulant laxatives have short-term usefulness and are not superior to bulking agents. There is little evidence that stimulant laxatives create permanent injury to the colonic mucosa (Brandt, 2005).

Contraindications

As with other laxatives, stimulants are contraindicated in patients with appendicitis, acute surgical abdomen, fecal impaction, or intestinal obstruction. Rectal fissures and hemorrhoids can be exacerbated by stimulation of defecation. Action begins 6 to 10 hours after oral administration and 15 minutes to 2 hours after rectal administration.

Adverse Events

These agents are not as well tolerated as the osmotic laxatives or bulking agents because of their side effects, which include nausea, vomiting, and abdominal cramping. These side effects can be more severe with cases of severe constipation. Long-term or excessive use can lead to laxative dependence.

Surfactant Laxatives

This class of laxatives reduces the surface tension of the liquid contents of the bowel. Ultimately, this promotes incorporation of additional liquid into the stool, forming a softer mass, and promotes easier defecation. However, stool softeners have insufficient data to support their efficacy, and fiber products may be superior to improve stool frequency (Brandt, 2005). Examples of this class include docusate sodium (Colace) and docusate calcium (Surfak). For patients who should not strain during defecation, this is the laxative of choice. Emollient laxatives only prevent constipation; they do not treat it. Combining these agents with fiber products helps promote defecation. Administration of emollient laxatives concomitantly with mineral oil is contraindicated because of increased absorption of the mineral oil. Action with these agents usually occurs between 1 and 3 days.

Contraindications

Docusate calcium or docusate potassium may be recommended for patients on sodium-restricted diets (e.g., hypertension, congestive heart failure). The sodium content of Colace (docusate sodium) is quite small (5.2 mg per capsule) and is likely insignificant.

Adverse Events

These agents are extremely well tolerated when used to prevent constipation. The most common side effect is stomach upset; other side effects, such as mild abdominal cramping, diarrhea, and throat irritation, are infrequent. Patients should take surfactants with plenty of water to improve effectiveness.

Interactions

Docusate, as a surfactant emollient laxative, may increase the absorption of mineral oil and potentially increase the risk for liver toxicity; therefore, this combination should be avoided.

Lubricant Laxatives

Mineral oil coats and softens the stool and prevents reabsorption of water from the stool by the colon. Lubricant laxatives are effective at preventing straining in high-risk patients (e.g., rectal surgery, labor and delivery, stroke, hemorrhoids, hernia, myocardial infarction).

Contraindications

Mineral oil may be aspirated and cause lipid pneumonia when administered to young, elderly, or bedridden patients. With the availability of safer laxative preparations, mineral oil should probably be avoided in these populations. If mineral oil is chosen, it should not be administered to patients before bedtime or when they are reclining to prevent aspiration.

Adverse Events

Mineral oil has an unpleasant taste, and because it is not absorbed, large single doses can seep through the anal sphincter and cause irritation. Dividing doses may prevent this.

Interactions

Mineral oil can impair the absorption of fat-soluble vitamins A, D, E, and K. Because warfarin (Coumadin) interferes with the synthesis of vitamin K–dependent clotting factors, a reduction in absorption of vitamin K may increase the effects of the anticoagulant. Although no direct interactions with oral anticoagulants have been reported, prothrombin levels may decrease. The docusates, as surfactant emollient laxatives, may increase the absorption of mineral oil and potentially increase the risk for liver toxicity; therefore, this combination should be avoided.

Chloride Channel Activators

Initially approved for chronic constipation in 2006, currently this class has only one drug, lubiprostone (Amitiza), and is derived from prostaglandin. While the entire mechanism is not understood, it appears to work by enhancing chloride-rich intestinal fluid without altering serum sodium and potassium concentrations. The activation of the chloride channel in the intestines pulls water into the lumen of the intestine. The drug is poorly absorbed systemically and appears to act locally on the intestines, improving stool consistency and motility. Lubiprostone is approved for treatment of adults with chronic constipation.

Contraindications

Lubiprostone is contraindicated in patients with potential mechanical obstruction, severe diarrhea, or hypersensitivity to components of the product. It is contraindicated in pregnant women and children.

Adverse Events

Nausea is the most common side effect of lubiprostone. The rate of nausea is dose dependent and was experienced by approximately 29% of patients. Other common GI side effects include diarrhea, abdominal pain, abdominal distention, and flatulence. The most commonly reported neurologic side effect is headache.

Interactions

No drug–drug interactions have been discovered with lubiprostone. In vitro studies showed the cytochrome P450 isoenzymes are not inhibited by the drug.

Selecting the Most Appropriate Agent

If lifestyle modification fails to reverse constipation, then selection of an appropriate laxative is necessary. The choice of laxative agent depends on several factors, including medical history, goal of therapy, concomitant medications, the potential for side effects, age, and personal preference.

Table 30.2 describes first-, second-, and third-line therapies (**Figure 30-1**).

First-Line Therapy

Provided no contraindications exist, a bulk-forming laxative is usually chosen as first-line therapy for constipation. Bulk-forming laxatives are not systemically absorbed. In addition, their pharmacologic effect is the most physiologic, meaning they have an effect similar to that of the natural effect of fiber from food on the GI tract. Their side effects are usually mild, and if necessary they can be administered safely for longer durations than other classes of laxatives such as the stimulants.

When hard or dry stools are the chief complaint or in situations where straining should be avoided (e.g., hernia, cardiovascular disease), a stool softener such as docusate is considered first-line therapy. Stool softeners also are not systemically absorbed and their side effects are usually minimal.

Glycerin suppositories have a local irritant effect on the rectum and are probably the safest of all preparations. This is preferred as first-line therapy in infants.

Second-Line Therapy

If a more rapid onset of action is desired, magnesium hydroxide may be chosen. Although it has a faster onset of action, dehydration from excessive use is a concern, particularly in patients unable to tolerate excessive fluid loss. In addition, magnesium-containing preparations should be avoided in patients with renal insufficiency or the elderly.

If the bulk-forming agents and magnesium hydroxide are ineffective or contraindicated, an osmotic laxative such as lactulose or sorbitol may be chosen. However, flatulence and the sweet taste limit compliance. In addition, lactulose and sorbitol should be used with caution in patients with diabetes.

TABLE 30.2	Recommended Order of Treatment for Constipation	

Order	Agents	Comments
First line	Bulk-forming agents (methylcellulose, psyllium, polycarbophil, malt soup extract, wheat dextrin)	Avoid in patients with GI obstruction or ulceration. Take with plenty of water.
	Docusate derivatives	Most effective at preventing straining at stool in high-risk patients (see text)
	Glycerin	Used most often in infants and small children
Second line	Milk of magnesia, magnesium sulfate	Caution in renal dysfunction and the elderly
	Lactulose, sorbitol	Use with caution in diabetic patients. Caution: laxative abuse, cathartic colon
Third line	Stimulant laxatives (senna, cascara sagrada, casanthranol, bisacodyl)	Impairs absorption of fat-soluble vitamins; used with caution in elderly and very young (lipid pneumonia)
	Mineral oil	Use with caution in congestive heart failure, hypertension, edema, and renal dysfunction.
	Sodium biphosphates	
	Magnesium citrate	Used as a bowel evacuant for endoscopic examinations
	Castor oil	Too potent to be used routinely for constipation

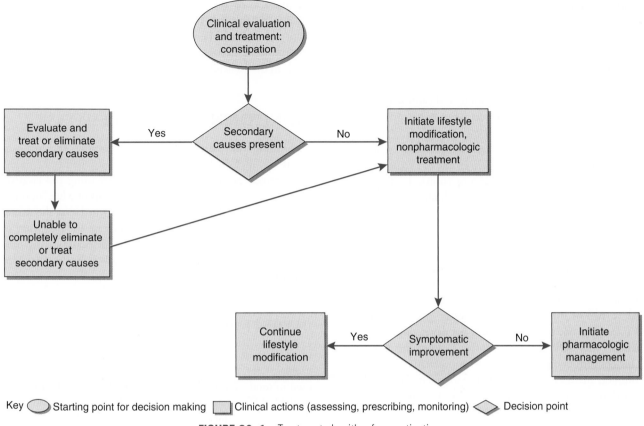

FIGURE 30–1 Treatment algorithm for constipation.

Third-Line Therapy

If bulk-forming or osmotic diuretics fail to work, a stimulant laxative may be chosen. Stimulant laxatives are very effective but have the highest potential for abuse. This high potential for abuse can cause serious complications. Therefore, stimulant laxatives should be reserved as third-line agents after other agents have failed or are contraindicated.

Mineral oil is effective as a lubricant laxative and may be an option in patients who should avoid straining. However, although mineral oil would seem safe, its ability to impair absorption of necessary vitamins and to cause aspiration pneumonitis limits its use. In addition, seepage is an inconvenient side effect that likely limits compliance. If an agent is necessary to soften the stool to prevent straining, docusate is a safer alternative.

Sodium biphosphate as an oral solution or enema is another option. These agents have the potential to cause fluid and electrolyte abnormalities and exacerbate concomitant disease states such as hypertension and congestive heart failure. Therefore, these agents should be used only after safer agents have failed. Because sodium biphosphate enemas and magnesium citrate solutions have a rapid onset of action, these agents are often preferred and are usually reserved for endoscopic procedures.

Castor oil is a potent cathartic that should not be used routinely for treating constipation.

Special Populations

Pediatric

Constipation can be distressing for children, particularly young children. Most children do not have an underlying pathophysiologic process. Stress over potty training or painful stools secondary to acute constipation can result in avoidance of defecation by the child. This in turn can result in larger, harder, and more painful stools, which eventually leads to soiling. Constipation and encopresis, a condition where soft stool is involuntarily lost, are often combined. Parents usually pay little attention to their child's bowel frequency unless incontinence occurs. The parents may become angry with the child, leading to further stress. To avoid constipation that may result in soiling, parents should be cognizant of their child's bowel habits.

Constipation may also result in urinary incontinence and urinary tract infections in children, particularly girls. Overflow incontinence may occur when the distended rectum presses on the bladder wall, causing bladder outflow obstruction. Fecal soiling in the external urethral opening predisposes constipated girls to infection. Treatment of constipation can reduce infection and incontinence.

Initially, manual evacuation of the rectum may be necessary; however, once this is done, it is necessary to use chronic laxative therapy (Borowitz, 2005). Treatment with pharmacologic agents in children is controversial, and few well-designed placebo-controlled trials have been conducted on the use of osmotic laxatives, fiber, formula-switching, sorbitol-containing juices, rectal stimulation by thermometer, or glycerin suppositories. The use of sodium phosphate enemas in children under 2 years of age has been associated with electrolyte disturbances, dehydration, and cardiac arrest.

For infants, malt soup extract or corn syrup (Karo) may be used at a dosage of 5 to 10 mL twice daily. For children older than 6 months, milk of magnesia, lactulose, or sorbitol at a dosage of 1 to 3 mL/kg/day given in one to two doses may be used. Senna syrup at a dosage of 5 to 10 mL/day for children ages 1 to 5 and 10 to 20 mL/day for children ages 5 to 15 is another option.

Geriatric

The choice of a laxative preparation may depend on the patient's attitude or beliefs about normal bowel habits. Normal bowel frequency can range from two or three bowel movements per day to two or three per week. However, many people think that less than one bowel movement per day is abnormal. These patients may seek an OTC laxative to keep them "regular." This concern about regular bowel movements is particularly common in the elderly. The self-reported incidence of constipation increases with advancing age, but the actual bowel movement frequency usually does not decline.

The overuse of laxatives in the elderly can be of particular concern because this population is more intolerant to the fluid and electrolyte abnormalities that accompany laxative abuse. In addition, many of the laxatives should be used with caution in elderly persons because they are more likely to have the disease states that some laxatives can exacerbate (e.g., heart failure, hypertension). Elderly patients are also more likely to take medications that may cause constipation, such as antipsychotics, tricyclic antidepressants, calcium supplements, and certain blood pressure medications.

Elderly patients should be carefully assessed to determine the cause of the constipation, and causative factors should be eliminated. Careful selection and judicious use of laxatives are necessary to avoid complications in this population.

Women

Girls and women with bulimia or anorexia nervosa may abuse laxatives as a means of reducing nutrient absorption to cause weight loss. Bulimia is 10 times more common in women than in men; it affects up to 3% of young women.

For the pregnant woman, the use of laxatives that are not absorbed into the systemic circulation, such as docusate and bulk-forming agents, should be considered as first-line therapy. Docusate sodium has not been found to be associated with fetal malformations and may be safe to use during pregnancy. Lactulose and sorbitol have not been found to be teratogenic in animals and may be safe to administer to pregnant women. Stimulant laxatives should be used only occasionally, if necessary. Cascara sagrada may cause loose stools in breast-fed

infants. Castor oil should be avoided in pregnant women because of the risk of stimulation of uterine contractions. Mineral oil should be avoided because its use can reduce the absorption of necessary vitamins by the mother, which may result in deficiencies for the neonate.

MONITORING PATIENT RESPONSE

Monitoring the patient's response to laxative therapy usually is accomplished by asking the patient whether he or she has regained normal bowel patterns after using the laxative. Different patients have different perceptions of what "normal" bowel habits are. Patients should be informed that the reason for treating with a laxative is not to increase the frequency of defecation but to promote comfortable defecation. Any misunderstanding by the patient on the goal of therapy may lead to chronic abuse of laxatives.

PATIENT EDUCATION

In most cases, the occasional use of laxatives poses no major problems for the patient. Laxatives are relatively safe when used in moderation. However, the fact that many laxatives are available OTC may give consumers the false impression that these agents are not dangerous and can be used routinely.

Health care providers should warn patients of the potential complications of laxatives. OTC laxatives carry a warning for the consumer not to use them for more than 7 days. For chronic constipation, use of a bulk-forming laxative may be a safer alternative, provided no contraindications exist. However, patients should be counseled that bulk-forming laxatives take time to work (up to 3 days). Because patients are usually looking for an immediate response, they may draw the conclusion that these agents are not effective if a bowel movement has not occurred within the first day. The next step taken by the patient is usually to look for a more potent agent such as a stimulant laxative, which may lead to chronic use and abuse.

Patient-Oriented Information Sources

Providing patients with information about constipation can help them understand constipation and their role in treatment. Patient education items are readily available on the Internet through the National Digestive Diseases Information Clearinghouse, which provides information to consumers on a wide variety of GI topics.

Nutrition/Lifestyle Changes

Patients should be educated on the lifestyle modifications discussed previously to reduce the need for a laxative. An increase in fluid intake improves the efficacy of most laxatives. Patients should also be educated on the potential for side effects of the laxative chosen as well as the appropriate method to administer the laxative.

Complementary and Alternative Medications

Little evidence exists that any specific herbal supplement or alternative treatment works to relieve constipation (Brandt, et al., 2005). However, senna is used as a laxative, acting similar to cascara, which was withdrawn from the market. It increases peristaltic activity in the lower bowel, has anti-absorptive properties, and stimulates secretions.

DIARRHEA

True diarrhea is an increase in frequency of loose, watery stools (three or more daily), usually over a period of 24 to 48 hours. It is a relatively common disorder of the GI tract that is experienced occasionally by most people. The organisms that cause diarrhea are easily transferred from person to person through food and water. Globalization and industrialization of the world has increased the ability of these organisms to spread. The Centers for Disease Control and Prevention (CDC) estimates that 211 million people experience acute diarrhea every year; an average of 16 million seek medical attention, resulting in 1.2 million hospitalizations and 600 deaths (Bushen & Guerrant, 2003). Children, the elderly, and those who are immunocompromised are most susceptible to the complications of diarrhea, and serious dehydration can result from the disorder. Proper hydration and symptomatic treatment as well as elimination of causative factors are necessary to prevent these complications. Ultimately, diarrhea can have a profound impact on public health, and proper diagnosis and treatment can prevent an epidemic.

CAUSES

Diarrhea may be caused by a host of different medications (**Box 30.4**), infective organisms (**Box 30.5**), or disease states or

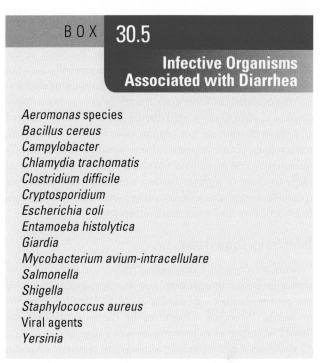

BOX 30.5

Infective Organisms Associated with Diarrhea

Aeromonas species
Bacillus cereus
Campylobacter
Chlamydia trachomatis
Clostridium difficile
Cryptosporidium
Escherichia coli
Entamoeba histolytica
Giardia
Mycobacterium avium-intracellulare
Salmonella
Shigella
Staphylococcus aureus
Viral agents
Yersinia

procedures (**Box 30.6**). Prompt attention to causative factors, as well as rehydration, prevents complications.

Medications

Antibiotics may cause diarrhea by direct irritation of the intestinal tract or disruption of the normal intestinal flora. The poor absorption of erythromycin (E-mycin) lends itself to irritation of the GI tract. Clarithromycin (Biaxin) and azithromycin (Zithromax) may cause less diarrhea than erythromycin. The clavulanic acid component of the combination of amoxicillin–clavulanic acid (Augmentin) is also a GI irritant, and diarrhea is

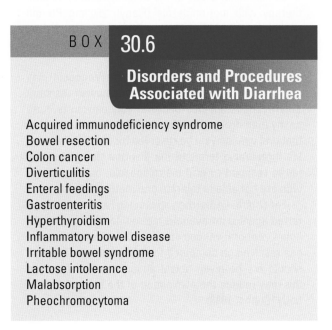

BOX 30.4

Medications Commonly Causing Diarrhea

Antacids (magnesium-containing)
Antibiotics
Antidepressants (selective serotonin reuptake inhibitors)
Cholinergic agents
Colchicine
Digoxin
Gastrointestinal stimulants (metoclopramide)
Laxatives
Metformin
Prostaglandins (dinoprostone)
Prostaglandin analog (misoprostol)
Quinidine

BOX 30.6

Disorders and Procedures Associated with Diarrhea

Acquired immunodeficiency syndrome
Bowel resection
Colon cancer
Diverticulitis
Enteral feedings
Gastroenteritis
Hyperthyroidism
Inflammatory bowel disease
Irritable bowel syndrome
Lactose intolerance
Malabsorption
Pheochromocytoma

a common side effect. Tetracycline and ceftriaxone (Rocephin) cause diarrhea by disrupting the normal balance of the gut flora.

Clostridium difficile, a normal part of the flora of the colon in up to 20% of hospitalized patients, normally does not cause disease unless chemotherapeutic medications or antibiotics trigger its toxins. Only certain antibiotics have been implicated in *C. difficile*–associated diarrhea. Less common causes of *C. difficile* diarrhea are vancomycin (Vancocin), erythromycin, tetracyclines, trimethoprim–sulfamethoxazole (TMP-SMZ), quinolones, and aztreonam (Azactam). The antibiotics most likely to cause *C. difficile* diarrhea are beta-lactam antibiotics (penicillins, cephalosporins, carbapenems) and clindamycin (Cleocin). **Box 30.7** gives more information.

Infectious Organisms

Patients traveling to a developing region may contract diarrhea from bacterial organisms. *Giardia* should be suspected if the patient travels to mountainous areas, recreational waters, or Russia. Pathogens transmitted by the fecal-to-oral route should be suspected in homosexual men (*Shigella, Salmonella, Campylobacter,* and intestinal protozoa) and in patients exposed to daycare centers (*Shigella, Giardia, Cryptosporidium*).

Traveler's diarrhea is usually a self-limiting, non–life-threatening illness; it affects 20% to 50% of people visiting developing countries. The cause is ingestion of fecally contaminated food products or water. High-risk areas include Latin America, Africa, Asia, and the Middle East. The typical duration is 2 to 3 days; symptoms include nausea and vomiting, cramps, and bloody stools. The most common pathogen is *Escherichia coli*; *Salmonella, Shigella,* and *Campylobacter* are the culprits less frequently.

Dietary restrictions are the main prevention for traveler's diarrhea. Travelers should avoid foods and beverages that are not steaming hot, raw vegetables, unpeeled fruit, tap water, and ice.

PATHOPHYSIOLOGY

Diarrhea may be classified by duration and category. Acute diarrhea lasts 1 to 14 days and is considered self-limiting. Persistent diarrhea lasts longer than 14 days but less than 30 days, and chronic diarrhea last more than 30 days. Diarrhea may also be categorized as osmotic, secretory, or exudative (inflammatory), or the diarrhea may be related to altered intestinal motility (transit). Some diarrheal illnesses involve more than one of these mechanisms. Diarrhea may also be a defense mechanism against toxins and invading organisms.

Osmotic Diarrhea

Osmotic diarrhea occurs when nonabsorbed solutes are retained in the lumen of the intestinal tract. The result is a hyperosmolar state that pulls water and ions into the intestinal lumen. Poorly absorbed salts (magnesium sulfate), lactose (in lactase deficiency), and large amounts of sugar substitutes (sorbitol) found in candy or chewing gum, diet foods, and soft drinks draw fluid into the intestinal tract, resulting in an overload of the colon.

Secretory Diarrhea

In secretory diarrhea, colonic absorption of fluid is secondary to active transport of Na^+ through Na^+-K^+-adenosine triphosphatase activity in the colonic epithelium. The colon absorbs chloride by exchanging it for HCO_3^2 and by uptake of sodium chloride. Any agent that increases concentrations of cyclic adenosine 3,5-monophosphate in the cells of the colon inhibits sodium chloride uptake and causes secretion of chloride. This results in secretion of fluid in the colon. Prostaglandins E2 and I2 and vasoactive intestinal peptide stimulate adenyl cyclase activity. Cholinergic agents and cholinesterase inhibitors cause secretion of sodium chloride and water. Secretory diarrhea can be classified as pure (e.g., cholera) or a part of a complex disease process (e.g., celiac disease, Crohn disease). Other stimuli that can cause secretory diarrhea include bacterial endotoxins, hormones from endocrine neoplasms, dihydroxy bile acids, hydroxylated fatty acids, and inflammatory mediators. Certain laxatives (senna, castor oil) and bile acids may also induce secretory diarrhea.

BOX 30.7

Treating *Clostridium Difficile* Diarrhea

C. difficile diarrhea may occur weeks after stopping antimicrobial therapy. The diarrhea may progress to colitis if left untreated. While awaiting the results of *C. difficile* toxin assay of the stool specimen, empiric therapy with metronidazole (Flagyl) 250 mg PO qid or vancomycin 125 to 250 mg PO qid for 5 to 7 days should be initiated. Clinical improvement should be seen within 3 days (Cunha, 1998).

Because routine use of vancomycin (Vancocin) may contribute to the emergence of vancomycin-resistant *Enterococcus* species and oral vancomycin is more costly than oral metronidazole, it has been suggested that oral vancomycin be reserved for the more severe, life-threatening forms of the disorder, for cases that fail to respond to oral metronidazole, or for patients who are not able to tolerate oral metronidazole.

For *C. difficile* diarrhea advancing to colitis, the preferred agent is intravenous metronidazole 1 g every 24 hours with oral vancomycin for 10 days or until colitis has resolved on computed tomography scan. Patients should not be given bowel antispasmodics because this may reduce the elimination of the toxins from the body (Cunha, 1998).

Exudative Diarrhea

Exudative (inflammatory) diarrhea may result from inflammatory diseases of the mucosa. Inflammation occurs due to the compromise of the tight junctions of the epithelial cells in the intestine. These diseases may cause an increase of blood, mucus, pus, and serum proteins that increase fluid and overload the colon, resulting in diarrhea. Enteritis, ulcerative colitis, and carcinoma are examples of inflammatory conditions that may result in exudative diarrhea.

Altered Intestinal Motility

Intestinal contents need to have sufficient time to be in contact with the lining of the intestinal tract for fluid, electrolytes, and nutrients to be absorbed adequately. Any factor that increases or decreases the motility of the intestinal tract may result in decreased absorption of fluid and electrolytes. Resection of the bowels, vagotomy, and certain agents (serotonin, laxatives, prostaglandins, prokinetic agents) can increase intestinal motility. Decreases in motility can result from autonomic injury or smooth muscle injury to the intestine and result in bacterial overgrowth, subsequently leading to diarrhea.

DIAGNOSTIC CRITERIA

A careful travel and social history is important to identify and treat specific causes, such as infection. Use of empiric antibiotic therapy is not recommended due to increasing resistance of many strains of bacteria. Selective testing of stool will be cost-effective while helping to guide the clinician in the use of specific therapy. According to the guidelines of the Infectious Disease Society of America (Guerrant, et al., 2001), diarrhea can be divided into three categories: community-acquired or traveler's diarrhea, nosocomial diarrhea, or persistent diarrhea. Each category can be specifically evaluated, leading to more precise therapy.

The fecal leukocyte, lactoferrin, or Hemoccult blood test is useful in patients with moderate to severe cases of acute infectious diarrhea because it supports the use of empiric antibiotic therapy in the febrile patient. However, measuring fecal leukocytes can be unreliable if specimens are transported, refrigerated, or frozen. Fecal lactoferrin, as a measure of polymorphonuclear neutrophils, has an advantage over fecal leukocytes as a highly sensitive and specific testing method for intestinal inflammation. Stool cultures have traditionally been used to identify the pathology of diarrhea, but the positive yields are very poor and incur high costs. Controversy exists regarding when to obtain stool cultures. The absence of vomiting with persistent diarrhea may also indicate the need for stool cultures. Hypotension, tachycardia, orthostasis, bloody stool, and abdominal pain and tenderness were not found to be good predictors of a positive stool culture.

Laboratory evaluation for ova and parasites should be performed in the following:

- A person not previously treated with empiric antiparasitic therapy
- A person with persistent diarrhea for more than 7 days
- A person who recently traveled to mountainous regions, Russia, or Nepal
- A person who was exposed to infants at daycare centers or who was exposed through a community water-borne outbreak
- A person with bloody diarrhea with few or no fecal leukocytes
- Homosexual men or patients with acquired immunodeficiency syndrome (AIDS)

For food- or water-borne pathogens, the incubation period and clinical features can give clues as to the source of infection.

Diarrhea and vomiting 6 hours after exposure to a food item suggests exposure to *Staphylococcus aureus* or *Bacillus cereus*. An incubation period of 8 to 14 hours suggests *Clostridium perfringens*. With an incubation period greater than 14 hours, with vomiting as the predominant feature, viral agents are suspected. In patients with fever greater than 101.3° F (38.5° C) plus leukocyte-, lactoferrin-, or Hemoccult-positive stools, or acute dysentery (grossly bloody stools), the most common pathogens identified by normal stool culture are *Shigella*, *Salmonella*, *Campylobacter*, *Aeromonas*, and *Yersinia*. Additionally, patients with grossly bloody stools should be tested for *E. coli* O157 or HUS.

INITIATING DRUG THERAPY

Most cases of diarrhea are self-limiting and can be self-treated. However, patients with profuse, watery diarrhea with dehydration, passage of blood and mucus, and fever exceeding 101.3°F should be evaluated for an inflammation-producing pathogen. These patients may benefit from antimicrobial therapy. In addition, a good history helps to determine the cause of illness. In diarrhea caused by infectious organisms, the pathogen should be identified so that therapy may be initiated to eradicate the organism and to prevent exposure to unnecessary antibiotics.

For traveler's diarrhea, prophylactic agents may be given to patients who should not, cannot, or will not comply with dietary restrictions. Chemoprophylaxis of traveler's diarrhea is controversial and usually is not recommended for patients unless the patient has an underlying illness (AIDS, prior gastric surgery), the purpose of the trip is particularly important (politicians, honeymoon), or the patient cannot or will not comply with dietary restrictions. In such cases, the use of bismuth subsalicylate (BSS; Pepto-Bismol), 2 tablets with meals and at bedtime, is recommended unless the reason for prophylaxis is a serious underlying illness. In these cases, a quinolone antibiotic should be used.

TABLE 30.3	**Indications for Empiric and Specific Antimicrobial Therapy in Infectious Diarrhea**
Indication for Antimicrobial Therapy	**Suggested Antimicrobial Therapy**
Fever (oral temperature >101.3° F [38.5° C]) together with one of the following: dysentery (grossly bloody stools) or those with leukocyte-, lactoferrin-, or Hemoccult-positive stools	Quinolone:*NF 400 mg, CF 500 mg, OF 300 mg bid for 3–5 d
Moderate to severe traveler's diarrhea	Quinolone:*NF 400 mg, CF 500 mg, OF 300 mg bid for 1–5 d
Persistent diarrhea (possible *Giardia* infection)	Metronidazole 250 mg qid for 7 d
Shigellosis	If acquired in the U.S., give TMP-SMZ 160/800 mg bid for 3 d; if acquired during international travel, treat as febrile dysentery (above); check to be certain of susceptibility to drug used.
Intestinal salmonellosis	If healthy host with mild or moderate symptoms, no therapy; for severe disease or that associated with fever and systemic toxicity or other important underlying condition, use TMP-SMZ 160 mg/800 mg or quinolone:*NF 400 mg, CF 500 mg, OF mg bid for 5–7 d depending on speed of response
Campylobacteriosis	Erythromycin stearate 500 mg bid for 5 d
Enteropathogenic *Escherichia coli* diarrhea (EPEC)	Treat as febrile dysentery
Enterotoxigenic *E. coli* diarrhea (ETEC)	Treat as moderate to severe traveler's diarrhea
Enteroinvasive *E. coli* diarrhea (EIEC)	Treat as shigellosis
Enterohemorrhagic *E. coli* diarrhea (EHEC)	Antimicrobials are usually withheld except in particularly severe cases, in which usefulness of these drugs is uncertain.
Aeromonas diarrhea	Treat as febrile dysentery
Noncholera *Vibrio* diarrhea	Treat as febrile dysentery
Yersiniosis	For most cases, treat as febrile dysentery; for severe cases, give ceftriaxone 1 g qd IV for 5 d.
Giardiasis	Metronidazole 250 mg qid for 7 d or (if available) tinidazole 2 g in a single dose or quinicine 100 mg tid for 7 d
Intestinal amebiasis	Metronidazole 750 mg tid for 5–10 d plus a drug to treat cysts to prevent relapses: diiodohydroxyquin 650 mg tid for 20 d or paromomycin 500 mg tid for 10 d or diloxanide furoate 500 mg tid for 10 d
Cryptosporidium diarrhea	None; for severe cases, consider paromomycin 500 mg tid for 7 d
Isospora diarrhea	TMP-SMZ 160 mg/800 mg bid for 7 d
Cyclospora diarrhea	TMP-SMZ 160 mg/800 mg bid for 7 d

TMP-SMZ, trimethoprim–sulfamethoxazole.
*Fluoroquinolones include norfloxacin (NF), ciprofloxacin (CF), and ofloxacin (OF).
From DuPont, H. L., and the Practice Parameters Committee of the American College of Gastroenterology. (1997). Guidelines on acute infectious diarrhea in adults. *American Journal of Gastroenterology, 92,* 1962–1975. Reprinted by permission from MacMillan Publishers LTD.

If prophylactic therapy is not prescribed, empiric therapy with a quinolone antibiotic at the first symptoms of diarrhea is recommended (**Table 30.3**). Patients should be properly hydrated, and BSS may be used to treat symptoms. Loperamide (Imodium) is a more effective option than BSS, but loperamide should be used with caution in the presence of fever or bloody stools because the antimotility effects of the drug may prolong disease by reducing the elimination of possible infectious pathogens. If an antidiarrheal medication is necessary, selection should be based on patient-specific variables, including potential side effects, convenience, efficacy, and the patient's symptoms. For patients with moderate or severe traveler's diarrhea, empiric antimicrobial therapy with a quinolone

antibiotic may be given. (See **Table 30.3.**) Patients with persistent diarrhea lasting 2 to 4 weeks without systemic symptoms or dysentery may be studied for the cause and treated, or given metronidazole (Flagyl) for empiric anti-*Giardia* therapy.

Goals of Drug Therapy

The goals of drug therapy are to reduce the symptoms of diarrhea and to make the patient as comfortable as possible. Causative factors should be identified and eradicated. Fluid and electrolyte replacement is particularly important to avoid serious complications from dehydration. Rehydration is discussed later in this chapter.

TABLE 30.4	Overview of Selected Antidiarrheals		
Generic (Trade) Name and Dosage	**Selected Adverse Events**	**Contraindications**	**Special Considerations**
Antimotility Agents			
diphenoxylate (Lomotil) 2.5–5 mg qid	Dry mouth, dry eyes, urinary retention, blurred vision, drowsiness, dizziness	Caution in patients with liver disease, fever, bloody stool, or fecal leukocytes	Drug Enforcement Administration Class V controlled substance
loperamide (Imodium) 4–16 mg/d in divided doses	Abdominal discomfort, constipation, drowsiness, dry mouth	Caution in patients with fever, bloody stools, or fecal leukocytes	May induce drowsiness; warn patients about driving or performing activities that require alertness.
Selected Antisecretory Agents			
bismuth subsalicylate (Pepto-Bismol) Start: 2 tablets or 30 mL Range: 2 tablets or 30 mL every 30 min to 1 h up to 8 doses	Black stools, darkening of tongue, tinnitus	Caution in patients who are aspirin sensitive or are taking medications that interact with warfarin Caution in children and teenagers with the flu or chickenpox	
polycarbophil (Fiber-Con) 1–6 g/d	Stomach upset, bloating, gas	Caution: Potential for drug interactions with tetracycline or quinolones	
kaolin, pectin, and bismuth salicylate (Kaopectate) Start: 30–120 mL of liquid or 2 tablets after each bowel movement Range: Up to 7 doses a day	Constipation, feeling of fullness, stomach bloating, gas	Do not use with children due to the salicylate component.	May adsorb nutrients and medications. Separate administration time of adsorbents and other medications.

Antidiarrheal Agents

Several types of drugs are used for the symptomatic relief of diarrhea; they include antimotility agents, adsorbents and absorbents, and the atypical antisecretory agent BSS. **Table 30.4** provides an overview of these drugs, and **Table 30.5** covers the recommended order of prescription.

Antimotility Agents

The antimotility agent loperamide is a congener of the narcotic analgesic meperidine (Demerol). It is not well absorbed and does not provide analgesic or euphoric effects. Loperamide slows GI motility by direct effects on circular and longitudinal muscles in the intestines. Another meperidine congener, diphenoxylate with atropine (Lomotil), is a controlled substance (Class V).

Contraindications

The antimotility effects may exacerbate infectious diarrhea by preventing the excretion of the infecting organism, allowing the organism more contact time in the intestines. Caution should be observed in using loperamide in patients with fever, bloody stools, or fecal leukocytes. In nondysenteric forms of diarrhea caused by invasive pathogens, loperamide can be used, provided antimicrobial therapy is administered.

Because loperamide undergoes extensive first-pass metabolism, caution should be used in patients with hepatic dysfunction because excessive side effects (central nervous system toxicity) may occur in these patients.

Because of the antimotility effects of diphenoxylate, it should be used with caution in patients with infectious

TABLE 30.5	Recommended Order of Treatment for Diarrhea	
Order	**Agents**	**Comments**
First line Second line	Loperamide Adsorbents or antisecretory agent	Easy to use, tablet or liquid Selection based on drug–drug interactions or allergies (e.g., aspirin sensitivity and bismuth subsalicylate)
Third line	Diphenoxylate	Side effect profile, especially with atropine added, lowers the utility of this agent.

diarrhea associated with fever or bloody stools. Diphenoxylate provides euphoric and analgesic effects at high doses but not at therapeutic doses. For this reason, diphenoxylate is combined with atropine to discourage abuse. Diphenoxylate should be used with caution in patients with liver impairment because the liver extensively metabolizes it.

Adverse Events

Adverse effects of loperamide include abdominal discomfort, constipation, and dry mouth. Although loperamide does not cross the blood–brain barrier, it may still induce drowsiness in some patients. Patients should be warned of the potential for drowsiness before driving or performing activities that require alertness. Although loperamide is usually well tolerated, it is not recommended in children younger than age 4 because shock, enterocolitis, fatal intestinal obstruction, and central nervous system toxicity have occurred.

Atropine has anticholinergic effects such as dry mouth, dry eyes, urinary retention, constipation, blurred vision, and tachycardia. Diphenoxylate may cause drowsiness or dizziness, and patients should be warned of these effects and should avoid activities that require alertness. The liquid formulation is recommended in children because the dose needs to be carefully tailored to the child based on age and weight. Diphenoxylate with atropine can cause respiratory depression in infants and young children and should be avoided in children younger than age 4.

Interactions

Diphenoxylate may potentiate the action of depressants such as alcohol, barbiturates, or benzodiazepines. In addition, atropine may potentiate the effects of other agents with anticholinergic properties such as tricyclic antidepressants, antipsychotics, and antihistamines. Diphenoxylate has a structure similar to that of meperidine, and when used concomitantly with monoamine oxidase inhibitors it can induce a hypertensive crisis.

Atypical Antidiarrheals

BSS has antisecretory, antimicrobial, and adsorbent properties, making it a reasonably useful agent for traveler's diarrhea.

Contraindications

BSS is broken down in the intestinal tract to salicylate; therefore, it should be used with caution in patients taking aspirin therapy or those hypersensitive to aspirin. In addition, caution should be used in children and adolescents with the flu or chickenpox because this population is at risk for aspirin-induced Reye syndrome.

Adverse Effects

Side effects of BSS include black stools, darkening of the tongue, and tinnitus, which can be a potential sign of salicylate toxicity.

Interactions

Because BSS has a salicylate component, it may interact with other medications that interact with aspirin (e.g., warfarin).

Adsorbents and Absorbents

Mechanism of Action

Kaolin, pectin, and attapulgite (Donnagel, Kaopectate) are all examples of adsorbents used alone or in combination in antidiarrheal preparations. These agents adsorb water and help to solidify loose stools. Adsorbents are usually given after each bowel movement until diarrhea is relieved or a maximum dose is reached. Dosages of different products and product combinations vary, but the dose of most adsorbents usually ranges from 30 to 120 mL or 2 tablets after each bowel movement up to six or seven doses per day for adults.

Polycarbophil (FiberCon, Fiberall), an absorbent, absorbs water in the GI tract and is used as an antidiarrheal. Its fiber content also makes it useful as a bulk-forming laxative when taken with plenty of water.

Adverse Events

The most common side effects of the adsorbents are constipation and a feeling of fullness. Absorbents may also produce upset stomach, bloating, and gas. Adsorbents and absorbents are generally considered safe because the medication works locally and is not absorbed systemically. However, adsorbents may not be as effective as antimotility agents at reducing the symptoms of diarrhea.

Interactions

Adsorbents are not selective and may adsorb nutrients and medications. This interaction must be taken into consideration because several doses may be necessary each day. Separating administration times of adsorbents and other medications is advised. Polycarbophil contains calcium and may interact with fluoroquinolone and tetracycline antibiotics.

Selecting the Most Appropriate Agent

The choice of antidiarrheal agent should be based on several factors, including the patient's history, potential side effects of the medication, potential for drug interactions, and efficacy of the available agents (**Table 30.5; Figure 30-2**).

First-Line Therapy

Although the adsorbents are not absorbed into the systemic circulation and are usually safe and well tolerated, they are not as effective at controlling diarrhea as loperamide. Therefore, loperamide may be considered as first-line therapy secondary to its efficacy. Loperamide is also reasonably well tolerated and has few drug interactions. However, patients should be warned about the potential for loperamide to cause drowsiness (particularly patients who must stay alert).

Because loperamide is an antimotility agent, it should be used with caution in patients with fever or bloody stools to

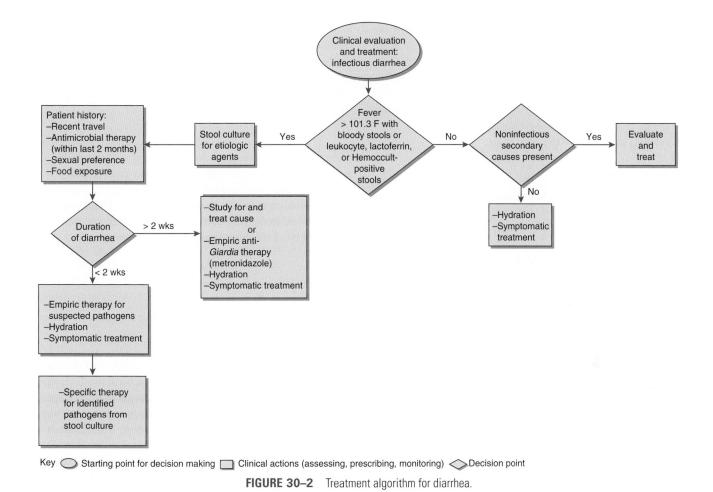

Key ⬭ Starting point for decision making ▢ Clinical actions (assessing, prescribing, monitoring) ◇ Decision point

FIGURE 30–2 Treatment algorithm for diarrhea.

avoid exacerbation of infectious diarrhea. In addition, caution should be used in patients with liver failure.

Second-Line Therapy

For patients who cannot tolerate loperamide or for those with contraindications, an adsorbent or antisecretory agent may be chosen.

Antisecretory agents such as BSS should be used with caution in patients taking warfarin and should be avoided in children or adolescents with the flu. Antisecretory agents should also be avoided in patients with a documented hypersensitivity to salicylates. Black stools, darkening of the tongue, and tinnitus are side effects that may be disturbing to the patient. BSS may be useful for prophylaxis against traveler's diarrhea and may be preferable over the adsorbents in a patient who also has indigestion or stomach upset that accompanies the diarrhea.

Although adsorbents may inhibit the absorption of nutrients from the diet and can cause some abdominal cramping, they are usually well tolerated.

Third-Line Therapy

Although diphenoxylate with atropine is an effective agent for treating diarrhea, the atropine component can cause significant anticholinergic effects that may exacerbate certain conditions and interact with other agents with anticholinergic activity. In addition, diphenoxylate is a Drug Enforcement Administration Schedule V drug, and its potential for abuse limits this agent to third-line therapy.

Special Populations

Pediatric

The American Academy of Pediatrics, Provisional Committee on Quality Improvement, Subcommittee on Acute Gastroenteritis(1996) published recommendations on the use of antidiarrheals in children. Their recommendations apply to children ages 1 month to 5 years who have no previously diagnosed disorders. They suggested that opiate and atropine combination drugs such as diphenoxylate with atropine be avoided in acute diarrhea in children because of the potential for side effects and the limited scientific evidence for efficacy. The committee also stated that loperamide and BSS are not recommended based on limited scientific evidence. Adsorbents are also not recommended based on limited evidence. The committee recognized that major toxic effects from adsorbents are in general not a concern, but the potential for poor absorption of nutrients and antibiotics is a potential disadvantage. The committee concluded that oral rehydration is most important and that routine use of antidiarrheal agents is not recommended based on lack of evidence or the potential for side effects.

If the health care provider still decides to choose diphenoxylate with atropine, the liquid formulation should be used because specific dosing is required based on the child's weight and age. In addition, diphenoxylate with atropine is contraindicated in children younger than age 2.

Geriatric

As with the pediatric population, rehydration is of paramount importance in the geriatric population. Elderly patients are likely to have multiple disease states that cause them to be intolerant of dehydration (e.g., congestive heart failure, diabetes, renal insufficiency). In addition, the antidiarrheal preparations may interact with agents that are commonly prescribed in the geriatric population. Diphenoxylate and loperamide may increase the sedative potential of benzodiazepines, antidepressants, anticholinergics, and antipsychotics. Adsorbents can reduce the absorption not only of important nutrients, but also of other medications. BSS should be used with caution in elderly patients taking aspirin and agents that interact with aspirin.

Women

As with constipation, antidiarrheals such as the adsorbents that are not absorbed systemically should be considered as first-line therapy for pregnant women with diarrhea. However, adsorbents can inhibit the absorption of important nutrients. Iron supplementation may be particularly important in pregnant women taking adsorbents for diarrhea. Loperamide has not been shown to be teratogenic in animals but has been inadequately studied in humans; therefore, the routine use of loperamide is not recommended. Diphenoxylate with atropine should be avoided because it has been shown to be teratogenic in animals. In addition, malformations in infants after first-trimester exposure have been reported. Both Lomotil and loperamide are excreted in breast milk. Salicylates have been shown to be teratogenic in animals. Therefore, use of BSS in the pregnant woman should be avoided.

MONITORING PATIENT RESPONSE

For most cases of diarrhea, the major concern is dehydration. Fluid and electrolyte depletion can lead to hypotension, tachycardia, and vascular collapse. Vascular collapse may occur quickly in the very old or the very young. Severe dehydration may result in decreased plasma volume and a decrease in perfusion, which may be of clinical significance, particularly in patients with congestive heart failure or chronic renal disease. Bicarbonate loss from excessive diarrhea may result in metabolic acidosis. This may be of particular concern in patients with type 1 diabetes mellitus who may be prone to ketoacidosis.

Patients should be monitored for signs of dehydration, such as orthostatic hypotension and poor skin turgor. The body weight of an infant is mostly water, and therefore infants may be weighed to determine significant fluid loss and dehydration from severe diarrhea. Monitoring serum electrolytes as well as intake of fluid and output of stools benefits patients who are hospitalized secondary to dehydration.

As stated earlier, the goal of therapy is not only to prevent dehydration but also to make the patient as comfortable as possible. Monitoring the effectiveness of an antidiarrheal preparation requires interviewing the patient to ensure a decrease in stool frequency and improved formation. Frequency and formation of stools vary from patient to patient, and determination of relief is subjective on the patient's part.

PATIENT EDUCATION

To avoid complications, patients should be educated about appropriate rehydration. In most cases, simple replacement of fluid and electrolytes with soda crackers, broths, and soups is all that is necessary in the nondehydrated adult with diarrhea. Oral rehydration solutions should also be considered because most sports drinks do not have enough sodium to replace losses from diarrhea (CDC, 2005). Additionally, food and drink high in sugar content should be avoided because it may increase the osmotic load and worsen the diarrhea. In the elderly or immunocompromised patient, solutions with sodium content in the range of 45 to 75 mEq/L are recommended. Boiled potatoes, noodles, rice, cereals, crackers, bananas, yogurt, soup, and boiled vegetables are recommended during the acute phase of diarrhea. The diet may return to normal as stools become formed.

Infants and children are particularly susceptible to dehydration with diarrhea. Oral replacement therapy is the preferred treatment to replace fluids and electrolytes in children with mild to moderate dehydration because it is less expensive than intravenous therapy and can be administered in many settings, including the home. Oral glucose–electrolyte solutions available in the United States (**Table 30.6**) are based on physiologic principles and should be recommended over commonly used nonphysiologic solutions such as colas, apple juice, chicken broth, and sports beverages.

Currently, oral replacement solutions (ORSs) are recommended for children with mild to moderate diarrhea (CDC, 2003). In addition, age-appropriate feeding should be continued and fluids encouraged. For children with mild to moderate dehydration (3% to 5% loss of total body weight), 50 to 100 mL/kg of ORS is recommended plus 10 mL/kg for each loose stool to replace continuing fluid losses. Severe dehydration (loss of 10% total body weight) can result in shock and is a medical emergency requiring intravenous therapy with normal saline or lactated Ringer's solution. In all situations, age-appropriate feeding should begin after dehydration is corrected.

TABLE 30.6	Commercially Available Oral Rehydration Solutions					
Product	**Carbohydrate (g/L)**	**Na$^+$ (mEq/L)**	**K$^+$ (mEq/L)**	**Cl$^-$ (mEq/L)**	**Base (mEq/L)**	**Calories (kcal)**
Infalyte* (Mead-Johnson)	30 (rice syrup solids)	50	25	45	34 (citrate)	126
Pedialyte[†] (Ross Laboratories)	25 (dextrose)	45	20	35	30 (citrate)	100
Rehydralyte (Ross Laboratories)	25 (dextrose)	75[‡]	20	65	30 (citrate)	100
WHO Solution[§] (Ianas Bros. Packaging Co.)	20 (glucose)	90[‡]	20	80	10 (citrate)	80

*Available in hospitals as 6-ounce nursing bottle.

[†]Available in hospitals as 8-ounce nursing bottle.

[‡]The American Academy of Pediatrics recommends these solutions with sodium contents of 75–90 mEq/L for replacement of deficit during initial rehydration (*Pediatrics*, 75, 358, 1985).

[§]Must be mixed with 1 L of boiled or treated water; packets available in stores or pharmacies in all developing countries.

Source: Manufacturer's product information.

From American Journal of Gastroenterology. (1997). Commercially available oral rehydration solutions. *American Journal of Gastroenterology, 92,* 1962–1975. Reproduced by permission from MacMillan Publishers Ltd.

Drug Information

Patients need to be aware of the potential side effects of antidiarrheal medications. Constipation can occur if these agents are taken for too long. Antidiarrheal agents taken in the setting of infectious diseases can prolong or worsen the disease. It is always best to contact a health care provider if diarrhea lasts more than 2 days.

Patient-Oriented Information Sources

Providing patients with information about acute diarrhea and what to expect can help them understand diarrhea and their role in the treatment. Patient education items are readily available on the Internet through the National Digestive Diseases Information Clearinghouse (NDDIC), which provides information to consumers on a wide variety of GI topics. The CDC also has a wide array of patient information about diarrhea.

Nutrition/Lifestyle Changes

It is not recommended to rest the gut. Oral intake and breast feeding should continue to replace lost calories during illness. Early feeding will stimulate enterocyte renewal, ultimately promoting a quicker recovery of the gut. Additionally, feeding decreases the potential risk of malnutrition.

Complementary and Alternative Medications

Probiotics have shown some efficacy in the treatment of diarrhea. The presumed mechanism of action is to alter the composition of the intestinal microflora and act against enteric pathogens (Guarino, 2009). Yogurt is a source of probiotics; however, not all brands have the active ingredients. Acidophilus capsules can be used to treat diarrhea resulting from antibiotic use. It restores the natural flora to the bowel. One to 10 billion viable organisms per day in three or four divided doses is appropriate.

IRRITABLE BOWEL SYNDROME

IBS is a functional bowel disorder that presents with abdominal discomfort and an alteration in bowel pattern. The disorder is an international health problem that can be one of the most perplexing chronic abdominal complaints reported to primary care providers and gastroenterologists. Epidemiologic studies in North America suggest a prevalence of 10% to 15%, with a 4:1 female predominance (Ringel, et al., 2001), while 7% to 10% have IBS worldwide (Brandt, et al., 2009). Newer data also suggest that veterans of the Gulf War have a high prevalence of IBS compared to the general population, which increases the prevalence of IBS in men (Brandt, et al., 2009).

Once thought to be associated primarily with psychological problems and stress, research is changing to an emphasis on motility of the gut, autonomic system imbalances, and increased visceral hypersensitivity (Akbar, 2009). A syndrome in childhood known as recurrent abdominal pain can be a hallmark of adult IBS. The majority of patients seeking care are ages 20 to 50, and symptoms can wax and wane over a lifetime.

CAUSES

For many years, the chief cause of IBS was thought to be primarily psychological. Now, however, research has identified physiologic but not pathologic causes that are accentuated by psychological stress. Symptoms generally are slow in onset, sometimes over weeks or months (Grundmann, 2010). Dysregulation occurs between the brain and the gut, leading to typical IBS symptoms. Commonly, the symptoms can be worse during times of physical and emotional stress, including sexual or physical abuse. In addition, some patients can identify foods that exacerbate the condition (e.g., lactose, caffeine, and fatty or spicy foods). Depending on the severity of the illness, pharmacotherapy may not be required and symptoms may respond solely to lifestyle changes. These lifestyle changes need to become incorporated into the patient's daily routines. Pharmacologic interventions may be required only intermittently to maintain symptom control.

PATHOPHYSIOLOGY

In general, the syndrome is believed to have the components of motility and sensory abnormalities. This leads to dysregulation of the bowel as modulated by the central nervous system (CNS). Many neuroimmune and neuroendocrine modulators, such as serotonin (5-HT), substance P, CCK, neurotensin, cytokines, and others, contribute to the increase in visceral sensitivity, central mechanisms controlling pain and dysregulation of the brain–gut axis. Local reflex mechanisms can also be responsible for mechanical distention of the gut in response to short chain fatty acids, affecting the emptying rate of the proximal colon. The prevailing theory is that the emptying rate of the proximal colon may be the key determination of overall colon function. The GI tract is innervated intrinsically and extrinsically by various neurohormonal agents from local or distant sources. Intrinsic factors include the neurons found in the enteric nervous system, which function similarly to the CNS. Bowel motor dysfunction can be associated with inflammation as well as changes in neurotransmitters, such as 5-hydroxytryptamine (5-HT3; serotonin). This neurotransmitter is found in the GI tract, and blocking it pharmacologically can decrease visceral pain, colonic transit, and GI secretions. External factors that can alter colonic activity are eating and drinking, stress, and endogenous hormones. Increased motility and abnormal contractions of the intestinal tract can result in either diarrhea or constipation-predominant IBS, due to either accelerated whole-gut transit times or delays in colonic transit. The IBS patient's sensory perception of colonic activity in response to balloon dilatation is more sensitive than that of patients with normal colonic activity. Sensory perception is also accentuated by external factors that lead to enhanced sensations that differ from those of healthy patients. However, evidence is increasing that IBS is not a psychological illness. This is supported by the fact that IBS exists in about 12% to 20% of the general adult population.

DIAGNOSTIC CRITERIA

The hallmark symptom of IBS is abdominal pain associated with a change in the consistency of stools that is relieved by defecation. Symptoms are usually first noticed in young adulthood and can be persistent or intermittent. Weight loss, rectal bleeding, fever, acute onset, and onset after age 50 are unusual in IBS and should raise suspicion of organic causes, not IBS. Diagnosis can be predominantly based on symptoms and appropriate treatment initiated, with reassessment in 3 to 6 weeks.

In 1978, the original Manning criteria proposed identifying IBS based on the presence of four symptoms: abdominal distention, pain relief with bowel action, more frequent stools with the onset of pain, and looser stools with the onset of pain. These criteria led to the establishment of an international group called the Multinational Working Teams for Diagnosis of Functional GI Disorders. This team identified key criteria for IBS, leading to the establishment of the Rome criteria (**Box 30.8**); the third revision focused on categorizing each type of IBS according to constipation, diarrhea, or mixed. However, the overall accuracy of the Rome criteria has led the American College of Gastroenterology (ACG) to simply define IBS as abdominal pain that occurs with altered bowel habits over a period of 3 months (Brandt, et al., 2009). Therefore, for IBS to be considered as a diagnosis the presenting clinical features may be sporadic, intermittent, or continuous but should be present for at least 3 months, as defined by the ACG. The Rome III criteria (**Box 30.8**) can be used to help verify the subtype, which can guide drug therapy.

The chief complaint most patients report is abdominal discomfort that can be relieved with defecation; however, symptom relief is often short-lived. Patients can also report abnormal bowel habits that alternate between diarrhea and constipation or are predominantly diarrhea or constipation; it is much more common to have bowel habits that are predominantly one type. Associated components can be abdominal distention, bloating, and gassiness. Extreme urgency after a meal can be common and can possibly result in an "explosive" bowel movement that relieves the overall discomfort.

BOX **30.8**

Rome III Criteria for Irritable Bowel Syndrome (2006)

Diagnostic criterion must be fulfilled for the last 3 months with symptom onset at least 6 months prior to diagnosis.

Recurrent abdominal pain or discomfort at least 3 days/month in the last 3 months associated with two of the following:

- Improvement with defecation
- Onset associated with change in frequency of stool
- Onset associated with a change in form (appearance) of stool

Organic symptoms of abdominal pain that do not suggest IBS are those that awaken the patient from sleep, initial onset in the elderly years, a change in abdominal pain that is not associated with bowel movements, significant weight loss, rectal bleeding, steatorrhea, and fever. In addition, steadily worsening symptoms should be considered atypical. These symptoms would suggest the need for additional studies. However, compared to the general population, IBS patients are not more likely to have organic causes for disease.

A key component of IBS treatment is a thorough history of symptoms, psychosocial stress, medications (because of GI symptoms from many drugs), and dietary habits (to identify nutritional patterns, gaps, and intolerances). Even in the general population, stress can result in GI symptoms. However, in the patient with IBS, these symptoms can become more pronounced. The relationship between psychological distress and GI symptoms has been well researched. Chronic and acute life stresses, including a history of verbal or sexual abuse, especially in childhood, may preclude early symptoms of IBS. These chronic stresses can contribute later in life to IBS symptoms.

Physical examination findings are often normal except for a slight diffuse abdominal tenderness with palpation, especially in the left lower quadrant near the sigmoid colon. Mild abdominal distention may also be present.

In 2009, the ACG Task Force, in an evidence-based position paper on the management of IBS in North America, reinforced the recommendation that minimal, if any, testing is necessary. Current treatments were evaluated and the conclusion was reached that care is often based on nonrandomized, non–placebo-controlled trials. The best available data show that only 1% of IBS patients have alarming symptoms signifying serious organic disease. Therefore, for patients without alarming features of IBS, routine diagnostic studies are not necessary. However, patients who are classified as IBS-D (diarrhea) or IBS-M (mixed) should be routinely tested for celiac sprue disease. Other studies such as abdominal ultrasound, flexible sigmoidoscopy, barium enema, or colonoscopy do not lead to any change in the proposed treatment and are therefore not recommended. Additional testing may be indicated for patients with the key symptoms previously identified or if the patient is older than age 50.

Types of IBS

According to the Rome III criteria (**Box 30.8**), patient subtypes can be identified according to presentation of diarrhea, constipation, mixed, or unspecified, although this is somewhat controversial. Therefore, along with the subtypes, patients can still be categorized according to *mild, intermittent, or continuous* IBS according to the predominant features of the patient's stool (Longstreth, 2006).

Mild IBS usually shows a sporadic pattern. Symptoms are worsened by stress and dietary factors. There is no alteration in the patient's daily activities because of the symptoms.

In *intermittent* IBS, the symptoms are worse and begin to affect the patient's daily life. It is more difficult to relate symptoms to specific precipitants, and a psychological component to the syndrome may be developing.

In *continuous* IBS, the symptoms affect every aspect of the patient's daily routines. An inability to pinpoint precipitants still exists, and there is a definite psychological component to the syndrome.

INITIATING DRUG THERAPY

Initial therapy is focused on establishing a therapeutic relationship and mapping out a long-term strategy. This provides the patient with knowledge regarding the disease process and lets the patient know that improvement may be a slow process, taking many months.

Patients with mild symptoms may be responsive to dietary and lifestyle changes (**Box 30.9**). Assessing the diet for potentially offending substances and removing those substances may improve symptoms. These substances may be lactose, caffeine, beans, cabbage, fatty foods, or alcohol (Simren, 2001). In a 1998 study, Versa and colleagues showed a positive correlation between IBS and lactose intolerance, female sex, and abdominal pain in childhood. A 2-week trial of a lactose-free diet is worth pursuing. Aspartame, an artificial sweetener found in many soft drinks and diet foods, may also provoke diarrhea. Trial elimination may also be worthwhile, especially in diarrhea-predominant IBS. However, with most IBS therapies the placebo effect is often just as successful as the therapy itself.

Maintaining a daily diary of food intake, bowel patterns, and emotional stressors can be helpful in the treatment of IBS. It serves to identify factors that can be addressed and evaluates the effectiveness of treatment. Lifestyle modification requires the patient to understand the stressors in his or her life and the effect these stressors have on physiologic functions. Identifying ways to reduce stress can be critical to improving IBS symptoms. Biofeedback can be used to decrease gut sensitivity, along with relaxation tapes to decrease stressors. Verne and Cerda (1997) and Daley, et al. (2008) showed some benefit of regular exercise in reducing stress and improving bowel transit. However, as previously discussed in the section on constipation, exercise has little benefit on bowel transit time.

BOX **30.9**

Dietary and Lifestyle Changes

Avoid foods that exacerbate the symptoms (e.g., lactose, caffeine, fatty or spicy foods).
Incorporate routine exercise into daily activities.
Explore the life stressors that aggravate the symptoms.
Learn ways to deal with stress, such as meditation, counseling, and biofeedback.

Goals of Drug Therapy

The pharmacologic agents used for IBS are the same as those discussed in the constipation and diarrhea sections of this chapter. The goal of pharmacotherapy for IBS is to alleviate or control the specific symptoms. Generally, clinical trials have been inadequate to establish a definite link between administration of specific drugs and relief of symptoms. In patients with IBS, between 50% and 75% still have symptoms after 5 years. Response rates to a placebo can be as high as 70% (Carlson, 1998; Mertz, 2003).

Bulk-Forming Laxatives

Previously, administration of dietary fiber in the form of a bulking agent was commonly the first agent prescribed in IBS (**Table 30.7**). However, administration of fiber to patients with IBS has become controversial. While the hypothesis exists that fiber increases colonic transit time and therefore lessens colon wall tension and ultimately abdominal pain, clinical trials on the use of fiber in IBS have had small sample sizes and have been short in duration. Also, fiber can exacerbate the diarrhea component of IBS. This led the ACG Task Force to conclude that fiber is no more effective than placebo and is not recommended for the treatment of IBS.

Hyperosmotic Laxatives

When the patient requires a laxative, it is preferable to administer one that is osmotic. (See **Table 30.7**.) These agents can work either as a disaccharide sugar, which produces an osmotic effect in the colon, resulting in colonic distention and promotion of peristalsis, or by an osmotic effect in the small intestine, drawing water into the lumen and softening the stool. Lactulose or sorbitol, disaccharide sugars, can be used for patients with predominant constipation. Polyethylene glycol 3350 (MiraLAX) is a glycolated laxative that can be safely used for a long period without adverse pharmacologic effects.

Contraindications

The same contraindications exist as when using these agents to treat chronic constipation. Lactulose is contraindicated in patients who must restrict their galactose intake and in patients with appendicitis, acute surgical abdomen, fecal impaction, or intestinal obstruction. Caution must be used with administration to diabetic patients because of sugar content.

Other osmotic agents such as magnesium hydroxide (Milk of Magnesia) or magnesium citrate (Citroma) can be used to promote defecation. Approximately 15% to 30% of the magnesium in these agents may be absorbed systemically; therefore, caution needs to be used in patients who have renal failure and a decreased ability to excrete magnesium.

Adverse Events

When taken appropriately, these agents are well tolerated. The most common adverse events are abdominal cramping or nausea. Extensive, long-term use of these agents can lead to laxative dependence.

Stimulant Laxatives

These laxatives vary in effects but act by increasing peristalsis through a direct effect on the smooth muscle of the intestines and by simultaneously promoting fluid accumulation in the colon and small intestine. Because of the irritating effect of the agents on the musculature, these agents should be avoided in long-term treatment. Stimulant laxatives include bisacodyl (Dulcolax) and senna concentrates (Senokot, Senokot S). As with other laxatives, stimulants are contraindicated in patients with appendicitis, acute surgical abdomen, fecal impaction, or intestinal obstruction. Rectal fissures and hemorrhoids can be exacerbated by stimulation of defecation. Action begins 6 to 10 hours after oral administration and 15 minutes to 2 hours after rectal administration. (See **Table 30.7**.)

These agents are not as well tolerated as osmotic laxatives or bulking agents because of their side effects, which include nausea, vomiting, and abdominal cramping. These side effects can be more severe with cases of severe constipation. Long-term or excessive use can lead to laxative dependence. Several OTC products use the brand name of Dulcolax. One has the main ingredient of bisacodyl and another is docusate sodium, which is a stool softener. This could be important, especially when the patient has been instructed to use the drug as bowel preparation for a GI study.

Surfactant Laxatives

This class of laxatives reduces the surface tension of the liquid contents of the bowel. Ultimately, this promotes incorporation of additional liquid into the stool, forming a softer mass, and promotes easier defecation. Examples of this class include docusate sodium (Colace, Dulcolax) and docusate calcium (Surfak). This is the laxative of choice for patients who should not strain during defecation. However, emollient laxatives only prevent constipation; they do not treat it. Administration of emollient laxatives concomitantly with mineral oil is contraindicated because of increased absorption of the mineral oil. Action with these agents usually occurs in 1 to 3 days. The practitioner should consider this class for prevention purposes, not for acute treatment. (See **Table 30.7**.) These agents are extremely well tolerated when used to prevent constipation. Side effects include mild abdominal cramping, diarrhea, and throat irritation, but these are infrequent.

Antidiarrheal Agents

Antidiarrheal agents for patients with IBS with predominant diarrhea can be used on an occasional basis. (See **Table 30.7**.) Loperamide HCl (Imodium) inhibits peristaltic activity, thereby prolonging transit time, and it can increase anal sphincter tone. Approximately 40% of the drug is absorbed from the GI tract and 75% is metabolized in the hepatic system; excretion is primarily in the feces. As previously discussed,

TABLE 30.7 Overview of Selected Agents Used to Treat Irritable Bowel Syndrome

Generic (Trade) Name and Dosage	Selected Adverse Events	Contraindications	Special Considerations
Selected Bulk-Forming Laxatives			
psyllium (Konsyl, Metamucil, Perdiem) Start: 1 tsp in 8 oz liquid bid–tid Range: 1–2 tsp in 8 oz liquid bid–tid	Abdominal fullness, increased flatus	Symptoms of acute surgical abdomen, intestinal obstruction, or perforation Inability to drink adequate amounts of water	Comes in granules, powder, or wafers Takes 12 h to 3 d to work
calcium polycarbophil (Equalactin, FiberCon, Mitrolan) Start: 500 mg tablets qd Range: 500–1000 mg qid	Abdominal fullness, increased flatus	Same as above	Takes 12 h to 3 d to work
methylcellulose (Citrucel) Start: 1 tsp in 8 oz liquid bid–tid Range: 1–2 tsp in 8 oz liquid bid or tid	Nausea, abdominal cramps	Same as above	Takes 12 h to 3 d to work
Hyperosmotic Laxatives			
lactulose (Duphalac) syrup Start: 15–30 mL PO daily Range: 15–60 mg/d	Flatulence, intestinal cramps, diarrhea, nausea, vomiting, electrolyte imbalances	Galactose-restricted diets, appendicitis, acute surgical abdomen, fecal impaction, or intestinal obstruction Use with caution in diabetic patients.	
magnesium citrate (Citroma) oral solution Start: 5 oz qhs Range: 5–10 oz qhs magnesium hydroxide	Abdominal cramping, nausea	End-stage renal disease	Can cause increased magnesium levels in patients with end-stage renal disease
(Milk of Magnesia/M.O.M.) Start: 15 mL qhs Range: 15–60 mL qhs	Abdominal cramping, nausea	End-stage renal disease	Same as above
Stimulant Laxatives			
bisacodyl (Dulcolax) Start: 10 mg PO in evening or before breakfast Range: 10–15 mg	Abdominal cramping, nausea, vomiting, burning sensation in rectum with suppositories		Oral: 6–8 h Rectal: 15–60 min
senna concentrates (Senokot) Start: 2 tabs or 1 level tsp at hs Range: 2–4 tabs or 1–2 tsp qhs	Abdominal cramping, nausea	Signs and symptoms of appendicitis, abdominal pain, nausea, vomiting	Elderly or debilitated, halve the dose
Surfactant Laxatives			
docusate calcium (Surfak) Start: 240 mg/d Range: 240 mg/d	None	None	May increase the systemic absorption of mineral oil
docusate sodium (Colace) Start: 50 mg/d Range: 50–200 mg/d	Bitter taste, throat irritation, nausea, rash	Signs and symptoms of appendicitis	Onset: 1–3 days Not to be used for acute relief of constipation
Antidiarrheal Agents			
diphenoxylate HCl with atropine sulfate (Lomotil) Start: 5 mg qid Range: 5–10 mg qid; maintenance may be 10 mg qd	Sedation, dizziness, dry mouth, paralytic ileus	Pseudomembranous enterocolitis, obstructive jaundice, diarrhea caused by organisms that penetrate intestinal mucosa Under 2 y of age Pregnancy category C	Onset 45–60 min
loperamide HCl (Imodium) Start: 4 mg after first loose stool then 2 mg after each following stool Range: 4–16 mg/d	Constipation	Acute dysentery	Peak levels 2.5 h after liquid and 5 h after capsule

(continued)

TABLE 30.7 **Overview of Selected Agents Used to Treat Irritable Bowel Syndrome (*Continued*)**

Generic (Trade) Name and Dosage	Selected Adverse Events	Contraindications	Special Considerations
Selected Antispasmodics (Anticholinergic Agents)			

belladonna alkaloids (Donnatal)
   Start: 1 tab or capsule tid or qid
   Range: 1–2 tabs/capsules tid or qid
	Drowsiness, anticholinergic effects, paradoxical excitement	Glaucoma, unstable coronary artery disease, GI or GU obstruction, paralytic ileus, severe ulcerative colitis	Antacids may inhibit absorption. Additive anticholinergic effects with other anticholinergics, antihistamines, narcotics, tricyclic antidepressants

dicyclomine HCl (Bentyl)
   Start: 20 mg qid
   Range: 20–40 mg qid if tolerated
	Same as above	Same as above	Same as above

clidinium (Librax)
   Start: 1 capsule qid—ac and qhs
 	
   Range: 1–2 capsules qid—ac and qhs
	Drowsiness, anticholinergic effects, paradoxical excitement, ataxia, confusion, jaundice	Glaucoma, GI or GU obstruction	Same as above

hyoscyamine sulfate (Levsin, Levbid, Levsin SL)
   Levsin
   Start: 1 tab q4h prn
   Range: 1–2 tabs q4h prn; max 12 tabs/d
   Levbid
   Start: 1 tab q12h
   Range: 1–2 tabs q12h; max 4 tabs/d
   Levsin SL
   Start: 1 tab swallowed or chewed q4h prn
   Range: max 12 tabs/d
	Same as above	Same as above	Same as above

Chloride Channel Activators			

lubiprostone (Amitiza) – 8 mg & 24 mg caplets
   Chronic constipation dose: 24 mg BID
   IBS-C: 8 mg BID
	Nausea, diarrhea, abdominal pain, dyspepsia		Pregnancy category C
			Not approved for children

the drug does not cross the blood–brain barrier into the CNS. Because of these properties, it is the preferred agent for treating diarrhea. Conversely, diphenoxylate hydrochloride with atropine (Lomotil) is an opiate similar to meperidine that increases smooth muscle tone in the GI tract, inhibits motility and propulsion, and diminishes gut secretions. It is absorbed orally and extensively metabolized by the liver. It can affect the CNS, and atropine has been added to discourage abuse.

Neither of these antidiarrheal agents should be used in a patient suspected of having diarrhea from pseudomembranous colitis or ulcerative colitis, or diarrhea resulting from poisoning or microbial infection. Diphenoxylate hydrochloride is contraindicated in patients who are hypersensitive to atropine or meperidine and patients with hepatic impairment. The atropine in Lomotil may aggravate glaucoma in patients with this disease. For additional discussion of contraindications and adverse events, see the diarrhea section.

Antispasmodic Agents

Treatment for patients with postprandial abdominal pain may require the use of antispasmodics. (See **Table 30.7.**) However, the efficacy of these medications remains unproven in controlled studies. The presumed desired action is by direct relaxation of the smooth muscle component of the GI tract. These agents competitively block the effects of acetylcholine at muscarinic cholinergic receptors that mediate the effects of parasympathetic postganglionic impulses. Examples of commonly used anticholinergics are dicyclomine hydrochloride (Bentyl) and hyoscyamine sulfate (Levbid, Levsin SL). Less commonly used are the belladonna alkaloids (Donnatal) and clidinium (Librax). Dosing of the anticholinergics is variable and general side effects are associated with the anticholinergic actions.

Contraindications

These agents are contraindicated in patients who have glaucoma, stenosing peptic ulcer, chronic obstructive pulmonary disease, cardiac arrhythmias, impaired liver or kidney function, and myasthenia gravis. Caution should be used in patients with hypertension, hyperthyroidism, and benign prostatic hyperplasia.

Adverse Events

Side effects include dry mouth, altered taste perception, nausea, vomiting, dysphagia, blurred vision, palpitations, and urinary hesitancy and retention. Anticholinergic side effects can be used as a measure of titration to achieve the desired pharmacologic end. It is important to monitor for signs of drug toxicity:

CNS signs resembling psychosis, accompanied by peripheral effects that include dilated, nonreactive pupils; blurred vision; hot, dry, flushed skin; dry mucous membranes; dysphagia; decreased or absent bowel sounds; urinary retention; hyperthermia; tachycardia; hypertension; and increased respiration.

Antidepressants

Antidepressants as a class have also been used in the treatment of IBS. It is not clear whether these agents work by improving a concomitant depression or by improving the anxiety and stress often associated with IBS. Initial work was done with use of the tricyclic agents such as imipramine (Tofranil), desipramine (Norpramin), and amitriptyline (Elavil) in patients with severe symptoms. Careful monitoring is important when tricyclic antidepressants are given to patients with IBS in which constipation predominates, because these agents can cause constipation. Newer agents in the selective serotonin reuptake inhibitor (SSRI) class may also prove beneficial. It has been suggested based on current investigations that antidepressants alter perceived pain thresholds, which are often abnormal in patients with IBS. See Chapter 40 for further discussion of these drugs.

Serotonin-3 Receptor Antagonists

A newer class of drugs has evolved to address the brain–gut–neurotransmitter (5-HT3 and 5-HT4) connection with regard to colonic transit time. Currently there is only one drug in this class.

The serotonin-3 receptor antagonist in animal models has been shown to decrease abdominal pain, slow colonic transit time, increase rectal compliance, and improve stool consistency. Alosetron (Lotronex) was initially marketed in 1999 but pulled from the market in November 2000 by the U.S. Food and Drug Administration (FDA) due to concerns regarding ischemic colitis and severe constipation. Alosetron is available only through providers who have officially signed with the pharmaceutical company (FDA, 2002) and is indicated for patients who have diarrhea and no constipation.

Chloride Channel Activators

Initially approved for chronic constipation in 2006, lubiprostone became approved for IBS in 2008 at a lower strength. It is only approved for women with IBS-C. This was the best replacement for Tegaserod, which was taken off the market in 2007.

Contraindications

Lubiprostone is contraindicated in patients with potential mechanical obstruction or hypersensitivity to components of the product.

Adverse Events

The side effect profile is similar to usage in chronic constipation; however, only GI effects are noted. Nausea is the most common side effect of lubiprostone. The rate of nausea is dose dependent and was experienced by approximately 8% of patients. Other common GI side effects include diarrhea, abdominal pain, and abdominal distention.

Interactions

No drug–drug interactions have been discovered with lubiprostone. In vitro studies showed the cytochrome P450 isoenzymes are not inhibited by the drug.

Selecting the Most Appropriate Agent

The emphasis in the care of patients with IBS should be multidimensional. IBS can present in many stages: mild, moderate, or severe. Selection of the most appropriate drug therapy should be based on the presenting symptoms. Each case needs to be evaluated, and treatment should be individualized (**Figure 30-3** and **Table 30.8**).

First-Line Therapy

First-line therapy is selected based on the presenting symptoms. Qualitatively, patients often feel the burden of this disease but believe this is not appreciated by primary care providers and specialists. Pharmacologic agents need to be considered only when an exacerbation of the disease occurs. Constipation-predominant IBS can be treated with an osmotic laxative on a long-term basis without adverse effects. Antidiarrheal agents are preferred in patients with diarrhea-predominant IBS. Loperamide is the preferred agent because it causes the least CNS activity and has the added benefit of improving anal sphincter tone. As with any chronic syndrome, use of low-level antidepressants may be helpful for symptom control.

With the additional problems of pain, gas, and abdominal bloating, a trial of an antispasmodic may relieve symptoms. Dicyclomine is the agent of first choice because of its shorter half-life, which may minimize the anticholinergic side effects of the class. Psychological symptoms associated with IBS may be treated by antidepressants. Selection of an antidepressant should be based on the specific symptoms of depression, stress, or anxiety. The SSRIs are the most commonly selected agents because of their safety profile and efficacy.

Second-Line Therapy

Unresolved complaints of predominant diarrhea can be treated with diphenoxylate hydrochloride, which has a longer duration of action but can be addictive because of its opioid properties and should be reserved for short-term use. For postprandial abdominal pain, gas, and abdominal bloating, longer-acting antispasmodics such as hyoscyamine sulfate can be considered. The second-line choice for psychological symptoms is the tricyclic antidepressants; these agents have more side effects than SSRIs.

Third-Line Therapy

The use of stimulant laxatives in cases of constipation-predominant IBS should be reserved for more resistant cases, but these agents should be used with caution. They should not be used for long periods, and they can aggravate abdominal cramping. The older anticholinergics such as the belladonna alkaloids and clidinium should be used very sparingly for postprandial abdominal pain, gas, and abdominal bloating because they produce more intense anticholinergic side effects.

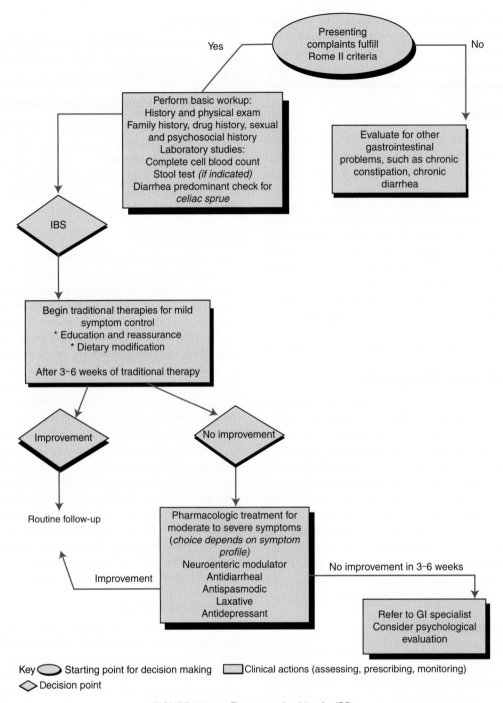

FIGURE 30–3 Treatment algorithm for IBS.

Special Considerations

Pediatric

Children with crampy abdominal pain, constipation, or diarrhea present a challenge to the practitioner. Although these symptoms sound like IBS, there are no established criteria for children. As previously discussed, some experts think that these children may acquire IBS later in life. Treatment for these symptoms can include some of the same approaches of increasing fiber and use of antidiarrheal agents and the newer antispasmodics. Close follow-up is an important aspect of care.

Geriatric

Initial presentation of IBS in people older than age 50 is rare. Abdominal pain in older patients should be considered a more ominous symptom unless they have been previously diagnosed with IBS or spastic colon, a version of colitis. Older patients may report a long-standing history of bowel trouble with any of these diagnoses.

Women

In Western society, women are more likely to have IBS and to seek care. A history of verbal or sexual abuse may also

TABLE 30.8	Recommended Order for Treatment for Irritable Bowel Syndrome	
Order	**Agents**	**Comments**
First Line		
Predominant constipation	Osmotic laxative—lactulose syrup, magnesium citrate, magnesium hydroxide	Milk of Magnesia is less expensive than citrate. Use magnesium products cautiously in patients with renal impairment. Use lactulose cautiously in diabetic patients.
Predominant diarrhea	Antidiarrheal—loperamide hydrochloride (Imodium)	May cause constipation Caution about drowsiness; may have a dry mouth
Abdominal bloating/gas	Antispasmodics—dicyclomine hydrochloride (Bentyl)	
Psychological symptoms	Antidepressants—selective serotonin reuptake inhibitors	Generally, as a class, these agents may be helpful with chronic syndromes. Cost may be an issue.
Second Line		Generalized central nervous system effects
Predominant constipation	Continue osmotic laxatives.	
Predominant diarrhea	Antidiarrheal—diphenoxylate hydrochloride (Lomotil)	Monitor for anticholinergic effects.
Abdominal bloating/gas	Antispasmodics—hyoscyamine sulfate (Levsin, Levbid, Levsin SL)	
Psychological symptoms	Antidepressants—tricyclic agents (imipramine, desipramine, amitriptyline (Tofranil, Norpramin, Elavil)	Onset of action and steady states vary with each drug.
Third Line		
Predominant constipation	Laxatives—bisacodyl (Dulcolax), senna concentrates (Senokot), emollient laxatives, docusate sodium (Colace), docusate calcium (Surfak), alosetron (Lotronex)	Caution with cardiac patients Can aggravate abdominal cramping Use only as additive to keep stools soft. Only approved providers can prescribe alosetron.
Abdominal bloating/gas	Antispasmodics—belladonna alkaloids (Donnatal), clidinium (Librax)	More severe generalized anticholinergic effects

contribute to IBS. Women have surgery more often when the origins of abdominal pains are unclear.

MONITORING PATIENT RESPONSE

Monitoring the patient's response to therapy should take place within 3 to 6 weeks of the initial evaluation. For patients with mild symptoms, the initial treatment includes working with the patient regarding dietary and lifestyle changes, education about the disease process, and reassurance about lack of organic causes. Patients with intermittent symptoms require the same initial approach, but addition of pharmacologic therapy can prove helpful, if only for the placebo effect of the drugs. Psychological counseling may also be helpful with these patients. Severe IBS requires all of these interventions and the addition of intensive psychotherapy. Patients with mild to intermittent symptoms can easily be managed in the primary care office with close monitoring initially, every 3 to 6 weeks, and then more routine care.

IBS is a disease of exacerbations and remissions, but up to 70% of patients respond to treatment within 12 to 18 months.

Those with a shorter duration of symptoms and fewer psychological symptoms have a better prognosis. Referral to a specialist should occur when there is no relief with any therapies, or when the patient has atypical symptomatology. Some patients do not respond. Continued symptoms rarely need a reappraisal of the diagnosis, but appropriate testing should be performed.

PATIENT EDUCATION

Patient education needs to cover dietary modifications, psychological stresses, and lifestyle changes. Begin by acknowledging the patient's fears and concerns and show that you take them seriously. According to current evidence-based research, patients can be reassured of the absence of organic disease based on the history and physical examination. The patient should be informed that this is a chronic disease and that IBS does not lead to cancer, colitis, or an altered life expectancy. Making the necessary dietary changes can be crucial for symptom relief, especially with mild symptoms. A multidisciplinary approach is often the best method of care, using the services of a dietitian and psychological counselor.

Drug Information

A variety of drugs are available to help control symptoms, and most have minimal side effects. However, the drugs need to be used in conjunction with stress relief techniques, identification of influencing factors, and education about the disease to help provide an improved quality of life.

Patient-Oriented Information Sources

Many resources exist for patients with IBS. One of the most comprehensive resources is the ACG, which covers many topics on GI health. The International Foundation of Functional Bowel Disorders also has a comprehensive website with resources for both patients and health care providers (**Box 30.10**).

BOX **30.10**

Patient Resources for Irritable Bowel Syndrome

http://www.gastro.org/generalPublic.html
http://www.aboutibs.org/
http://www.iffgd.org/index.html
http://digestive.niddk.nih.gov/ddiseases/pubs/ibs/

Nutrition/Lifestyle Changes

A major focus of caring for patients with IBS is helping them assess their diet, making adjustments as necessary. A trial of removing lactose foods from the diet poses no risks to the patient and may have a benefit if it relieves symptoms.

Case Study 1

C. J. is a 71-year-old woman who presents for follow-up. She complains of hard, dry stools over the past week. She remembers reading an educational brochure she picked up in her pharmacy that suggested increasing her fiber and fluid intake, but this has not alleviated her problem. C. J.'s past medical conditions include hypertension and chronic renal insufficiency. She had a stroke 1 year ago with little or no residual. Her medications include verapamil SR 240 mg daily, lisinopril 10 mg orally once daily, calcium carbonate 1,250 mg twice daily orally, and aspirin 325 mg orally once daily.

DIAGNOSIS: CONSTIPATION

1. List specific goals of treatment for this patient.
2. What drug therapy would you prescribe? Why?

3. What are the parameters for monitoring the success of the therapy?
4. Discuss specific patient education based on the prescribed therapy.
5. List one or two adverse reactions for the selected agent that would cause you to change therapy.
6. What would be the choice for second-line therapy?
7. What OTC or alternative medications would be appropriate for this patient?
8. What dietary and lifestyle changes should be recommended for this patient?
9. Describe one or two drug–drug or drug–food interactions for this patient.

Case Study 2

T. is a 34-year-old white man who presents with diarrhea of 2 days' duration. His other symptoms are nausea with vomiting and bloody stools for 1 day. The history reveals that the patient has just returned from a 3-day honeymoon in Mexico. He was careful to eat steaming hot foods and beverages but did have a frozen drink the last night of the trip.

DIAGNOSIS: TRAVELER'S DIARRHEA

1. List specific goals of treatment for this patient.
2. What drug therapy would you prescribe?

3. What are the parameters for monitoring the success of the therapy?
4. Discuss specific patient education based on the prescribed therapy.
5. List one or two adverse reactions for the selected agent that would cause you to change therapy.
6. What would be the choice for second-line therapy?
7. What OTC or alternative medications would be appropriate for this patient?
8. What dietary and lifestyle changes should be recommended for this patient?
9. Describe one or two drug–drug or drug–food interactions for this patient.

Case Study 3

S. C. is a 38-year-old woman who presents with intermittent diarrhea with cramping that is relieved by defecation. The diarrhea is not bloody or accompanied by nausea and vomiting. Review of past medical history includes some childhood "problems with my stomach," hypertension, and a recent cholecystectomy. She works as a housekeeper in a local inn and does not drink alcohol or smoke cigarettes.

DIAGNOSIS: IRRITABLE BOWEL SYNDROME

1. List specific goals of treatment for this patient.
2. What drug therapy would you prescribe?
3. What are the parameters for monitoring the success of the therapy?
4. Discuss specific patient education based on the prescribed therapy.
5. List one or two adverse reactions for the selected agent that would cause you to change therapy.
6. What would be the choice for second-line therapy?
7. What OTC or alternative medications would be appropriate for this patient?
8. What dietary and lifestyle changes should be recommended for this patient?
9. Describe one or two drug–drug or drug–food interactions for this patient.

BIBLIOGRAPHY

Starred references are cited in the text.

Abyad, A., & Mourad, F. (1996). Constipation: Common-sense care of the older patient. *Geriatrics, 51*(12), 28–36.

*Akbar, A. W. (2009). Visceral hpersensitivity in irritable bowel syndrome: Molecular mechanisms and therapeutic agents. *Alimentary Pharmacology and Therapeutics,* 423–435.

Alaimo, K., McDowell, M. A., Briefel, R. R., et al. (1994). *Dietary intake of vitamins, minerals and fiber of persons ages 2 months and over in the United States: Third National Health and Nutrition Examination Survey, Phase 1, 1988–91.* Hyattsville, MD: National Center for Health Statistics; Advance data from vital and health statistics: No 258.

*American Academy of Pediatrics, Provisional Committee on Quality Improvement, Subcommittee on Acute Gastroenteritis. (1996). Practice parameter: The management of acute gastroenteritis in young children. *Pediatrics, 97*(3), 424–435.

*American College of Gastroenterology Functional Gastrointestinal Disorders Task Force. (2002). Evidence-based position statement on the management of irritable bowel syndrome in North America. *American Journal of Gastroenterology, 97*(11), S1.

*American Dietetic Association. (2002). Position of the American Dietetic Association: Health implication of dietary fiber. *Journal of the American Dietetic Association,* 993–1000.

Annelis, M., & Koch, T. (2003). Constipation and the preached trio: Diet, fluid, intake, exercise. *International Journal of Nursing Studies, 40,* 843. Abstract obtained from Medline.

Baig, M., Zhao, R., Woodhouse, S., et al. (2002). Variability in serotonin and enterochromaffin cells in patients with colonic inertia and idiopathic diarrhea as compared to normal controls. *Colorectal Disease, 4,* 348.

Baker, S. S., Liptak, G. S., Colletti, R. B., et al. (1999). Constipation in infants and children: Evaluation and treatment. A medical position statement of the North American Society for Pediatric Gastroenterology and Nutrition. *Journal of Pediatric Gastroenterology and Nutrition, 29*(5), 612.

Barry, M. (2004). Review of the book *Travelers' Diarrhea. New England Journal of Medicine, 350,* 1801.

Bertram, S., Kurland, M., Lydick, E., et al. (2001). The patient's perspective of irritable bowel syndrome. *Journal of Family Practice, 50*(6), 521.

Besedovsky, A., & Bu, L. (2004). Across the developmental continuum of irritable bowel syndrome: Clinical and pathophysiologic considerations. *Current Gastroenterology Reports, 6*(3), 247. Abstract obtained from Medline.

Bonapace, E. S., & Fischer, R. S. (1998). Constipation and diarrhea in pregnancy. *Gastroenterology Clinics of North America, 27,* 197.

*Borowitz, S. (2005). Constipation. *eMedicine Specialties.* Retrieved from http://emedicine.medscape.com/article/928185-overview on September 10, 2010.

Bouhnik, Y., Neut, C., Raskine, L., et al. (2004). Prospective randomized, parallel-group trial to evaluate the effects of lactulose and polyethylene glycol-4000 on colonic flora in chronic idiopathic constipation. *Alimentary Pharmacology & Therapeutics, 19,* 889. Abstract obtained from http://ejournals.ebsoco.com. Retrieved on May 11, 2004.

Brandt, L. J., Bjorkman, D., Fennerty, M. B., et al. (2002). Systematic review on the management of irritable bowel syndrome in North America. *American Journal of Gastroenterology, 97*(11), S7.

*Brandt, L, Bjorkman, D., Fennerty, M. B., et al. (2005). American College of Gastroenterology functional disorders task force: An evidence based approach to the management of chronic constipation. *American Journal of Gastroenterology,* S1–S21.

*Brandt, L., Chey, W., Foxx–Orenstein, A., et al. (2009). American College of Gastroenterology Task Force on Irritable Bowel Syndrome. *American Journal of Gastroenterology,* S2.

*Brandt, L, Prather, C., Quigley, E., et al. (2005). Systematic review on the management of chronic constipation in North America. *American Journal of Gastroenterology,* S5–S22.

*Bushen, O., & Guerrant, R. (2003). Acute infectious diarrhea: Approach and management in the emergency department. *Topics in Emergency Medicine, 25,* 139.

Camilleri, M. (1999). Therapeutic approach to the patient with irritable bowel syndrome. *American Journal of Medicine, 107*(5A), 27S.

Camilleri, M., & Ford, M. (1998). Review article: Colonic sensorimotor physiology in health, and its alteration in constipation and diarrheal disorders. *Alimentary Pharmacology & Therapeutics, 12,* 287.

Camilleri, M., Mayer, E. A., Drossman, D. A., et al. (1999). Improvement in pain and bowel function in female irritable bowel patients with alosetron, a 5-HT$_3$ receptor agonist. *Alimentary Pharmacology & Therapeutics, 13,* 1149.

*Carlson, E. (1998). Irritable bowel syndrome. *Nurse Practitioner, 23*(1), 82–93.

Centers for Disease Control and Prevention. (1992). The management of acute diarrhea in children: Oral rehydration, maintenance, and nutritional therapy. *MMWR, 41*(No. RR-16).

*Centers for Disease Control and Prevention. (2003). *Managing acute gastroenteritis among children: Oral rehydration, maintenance and nutritional therapy.* Atlanta: MMWR.

*Centers for Disease Control and Prevention. (2005). *Guidelines for the management of acute diarrhea.* Washington, DC: Department of Health and Human Services.

Chaussade, S., & Minic, M. (2003). Comparison of efficacy and safety of two doses of two different polyethylene glycol-based laxatives in the treatment of constipation. *Alimentary Pharmacologic Therapeutics, 17,* 165.

Chen, B., Knowles, C., Scott, M., et al. (2002). Idiopathic slow transit constipation and megacolon are not associated with neurturin mutations. *Neurogastroenterology Motility, 14,* 513.

*Cunha, B. A. (1998). Nosocomial diarrhea. *Critical Care Clinics, 14,* 329–338.

*Daley, A., Grimett, C., Roberts, L., et al. (2008). The effects of exercise upon symptoms and quality of life in patients diagnosed with irritable bowel syndrome: A randomised control trial. *International Journal of Sports Medicine,* 778–782.

Dalton, C., & Drossman, D. (1997). Diagnosis and treatment of irritable bowel syndrome. *American Family Physician, 55*(3), 875.

DePontini, F., & Tonini, M. (2001). Irritable bowel syndrome: New agents targeting serotonin receptor subtypes. *Drugs, 61*(3), 317.

DeYoung, G. R. (2004). Tegaserod (Zelnorm) for irritable bowel syndrome. *American Family Physician, 69,* 363.

*Dosh, S. (2002). Evaluation and treatment of constipation. *Journal of Family Practice, 51.* Retrieved from http://www.jpoline.com/content/2002/06/jfp_0602_0555c.asp on June 30, 2004.

Drossman, D., & Thompson, W. G. (1992). The irritable bowel syndrome: Review and a graduated multicomponent treatment approach. *Annals of Internal Medicine, 116*(12), 1009.

*DuPont, H. L., and the Practice Parameters Committee of the American College of Gastroenterology. (1997). Guidelines on acute infectious diarrhea in adults. *American Journal of Gastroenterology, 92,* 1962–1975.

Ellis, M., & Meadows, S. (2002). What is the best therapy for constipation in infants? *Journal of Family Practice, 51,* 708. Retrieved from http://www.jpoline.com/content/2002/08/jfp_0802_0708c.asp on June 30, 2004.

El-Salhy, M., & Spangeus, A. (2002). Gastric emptying in animal models of human diabetes: Correlation to blood glucose level and gut neuroendocrine peptide content. *Upsala Journal of Medical Science, 107,* 89.

*FDA Talk Paper. (2002). FDA approves first treatment for women with constipation-predominant irritable bowel syndrome. Retrieved from http://www.fda.gov/bbs/topics/ANSWERS/2002/ANSO1160.html on May 23, 2004.

FDA Talk Paper. (2004). FDA updates Zelnorm labeling with new risk information. Retrieved from http://www.fda.gov/bbs/topics/ANSWERS/2004/ANSO1285.html on May 23, 2004.

Field, M. (2003). Intestinal ion transport and the pathophysiology of diarrhea. *Journal of Clinical Investigation, 111,* 931.

Fleming, K. A., Zimmerman, H., & Shubik, P. (1998). Granulomas in the livers of humans and Fischer rates associated with ingestion of mineral hydrocarbons: A comparison. *Regulatory Toxicology and Pharmacology, 27,* 75.

Gallagher, C. (2003). A guideline-based approach for managing acute gastroenteritis in children. *JSPN, 8*(3), 107.

Gattuso, J. M., & Kamm, M. A. (1994). Adverse effects of drugs used in the management of constipation and diarrhea. *Drug Safety, 10*(1), 47.

Greenberg, M., Amitrone, H., & Galiczynski, E. (2002). A contemporary review of irritable bowel syndrome. *Physician Assistant, 26*(8), 26.

*Grundmann, O. (2010). Irritable bowel syndrome: Epidemiology, diagnosis and treatment: An update for health-care practitioners. *Journal of Gastroenterology and Hepatology,* 691–699.

*Guarino, A. L. (2009). Probiotics as prevention and treatment for diarrhea. *Current Opinion in Gastroenterology,* 18–23.

*Guerrant, R., Van Gilden, T., Steines, T., et al. (2001). Practice guidelines for the management of infectious diarrhea. *Clinical Infectious Disease, 32,* 331.

Guthrie, E., & Thompson, D. (2002). ABC of psychological medicine: Abdominal pain and functional gastrointestinal disorders. *British Medical Journal, 325,* 701.

Hagemann, T. M. (1998). Gastrointestinal medications and breastfeeding. *Journal of Human Lactation, 14,* 259–262.

Hatari, D., Gurwitz, J. H., Avorn, J., et al. (1996). Bowel habit in relation to age and gender: Findings from the National Health Interview survey and clinical implications. *Archives of Internal Medicine, 156,* 315.

Hatari, D., Gurwitz, J. H., Avorn, J., et al. (1997). How do older persons define constipation? Implications for therapeutic management. *Journal of General Internal Medicine, 12,* 63–66.

*Higgins, P. D., & Johanson, J. F. (2004). Epidemiology of constipation in North America: A systematic review. *American Journal of Gastroenterology, 4,* 750–759. Abstract obtained from PubMed.

Holten, K. (2003). Irritable bowel syndrome: Minimize testing, let symptoms guide treatment. *Journal of Family Practice, 52*(12), 942.

Jancin, B. (2002). New evidenced-based guidelines target IBS: Diagnostic work-up simplified. *OB/GYN News, Dec. 1.* Retrieved from http://www.find-articles.com/cf_ds/mOCYD/2337/95514144/print.jhtml on February 6, 2004.

Kellow, J. E., Delvaux, M. M., Azpiroz, F., et al. (2000). Principles of applied neurogastroenterology: Motility/sensation. In D. A. Drossman, E. Corazziari, N. J. Talley, W. G. Thompson, & W. E. Whitehead (Eds.), *Rome II: The functional gastrointestinal disorders* (2nd ed., pp. 91–156). Lawrence, KS: Allen Press.

Larson, S. C. (1997). Traveler's diarrhea. *Emergency Medicine Clinics of North America, 15,* 179.

Lembo, A., & Camilleri, M. (2003). Current concepts: Chronic constipation. *New England Journal of Medicine, 345,* 1360.

Levron, J. C., Moing, L., & Chwetzoff, E. (1996). Example of active therapeutic follow-up: Itraconazole. *Therapie, 51,* 502–506.

Loening-Bauke, V. (1996). Encopresis and soiling. *Pediatric Clinics of North America, 43,* 279.

Loening-Bauke, V. (1997). Urinary incontinence and urinary tract infection and their resolution with treatment of chronic constipation of childhood. *Pediatrics, 100,* 228.

Loening-Bauke, V., Miele, E., & Staiano, A. (2004). Fiber (glucomannan) is beneficial in the treatment of childhood constipation. *Pediatrics, 113,* 259.

*Longstreth, G. E. (2006). Functional bowel disorders. *Gastroenterology,* 1480–1491.

McGilley, B. M., & Pryor, T. L. (1998). Assessment and treatment of bulimia nervosa. *American Family Physician, 57,* 2743.

*Medscape. (2005). Chronic constipation an expert interview with Dr. William Chey, MD. (D. W. Chey, Interviewer). Retrieved from http://www.medscape.com/viewarticle/563731 on September 10, 2010.

*Mertz, H. (2003). Irritable bowel syndrome. *New England Journal of Medicine, 349,* 2136.

Montgomery, L., & Scoville, C. (2002). What is the best way to evaluate diarrhea? *Journal of Family Practice, 51,* 575. Retrieved from http://www.jpoline.com/content/2002/06/jfp_0602_0575c.asp on June 30, 2004.

Moser, R. (1986). Irritable bowel syndrome: A misunderstood psychophysiological affliction. *Journal of Counseling and Development, 65,* 108.

*Muller-Lissner, S., Kamm, M., Scarpingato, C., & Wald, A. (2005). Myths and misconceptions about chronic constipation. *American Journal of Gastroenterology, 100*(1), 232–242.

National Digestive Diseases Information Clearinghouse. (2003). *What I need to know about constipation* [Brochure] (NIH publication No. 03-2754).

National Digestive Diseases Information Clearinghouse. (2004). *Constipation in children* [Brochure] (NIH publication No. 04-4633).

O'Sullivan, G. C. (2001). Probiotics. *British Journal of Surgery, 88,* 161.

*Ringel, Y., Sperber, A. D., & Drossman, D. A. (2001). Irritable bowel syndrome. *Annual Review of Medicine, 52,* 319.

*Schiller, L. (2001). Constipation. *Best Practice of Medicine, Oct. 22.* Retrieved from http://merck.praxis.md on February 6, 2004.

Schmulson, M., & Chang, L. (1999). Diagnostic approach to the patient with irritable bowel syndrome. *American Journal of Medicine, 107*(5A), 20S.

Shafik, A. (2003). Anorectal motility in patients with achalasia of the esophagus: Recognition of an esophagorectal syndrome. *BMC Gastroenterology, 3,* 28. Retrieved from http://www.biomedcentral.com/1471-230X/3/28.

Shafik, A., Shafik, A. A., & Ahmend, I. (2003). Effect of colonic distention on ileal motor activity with evidence of coloileal reflex. *Journal of Gastrointestinal Surgery, 7,* 701.

*Shah, N., Chitkara, D., Locke, G. R., et al. (2008). Ambulatory care for constipation in the United States 1993–2004. *American Journal of Gastroenterology, 103,* 1746–1753.

*Simren, M. E. (2001). Food related gastrointestinal symptoms in irritable bowel syndrome. *Digestion,* 108–115.

Sloots, C. E., & Felt-Bersma, R. J. (2003). Rectal sensorimotor characteristics in female patients with idiopathic constipation with or without paradoxical sphincter contraction. *Neurogastrology and Motility, 15,* 187.

*Smith, C., Hellebusch, S., & Mandel, K. (2002). Patient and physician evaluation of a new bulk fiber laxative tablet. *Gastroenterology Nursing, 26,* 31.

Steffen, R., DuPont, H., Heusser, R., et al. (1986). Prevention of diarrhea by the tablet form of bismuth subsalicylate. *Antimicrobial Agents and Chemotherapy, April,* 625.

*Stessman, M. (2003). Biofeedback: Its role in treatment of chronic constipation. *Gastroenterology Nursing, 26,* 251.

Talley, N. J., Jones, M., Nuyts, G., & Dubois, D. (2003). Risk factors for chronic constipation. *The American Journal of Gastroenterology, 98*(5), 1107. Abstract obtained from MedLine.

Thielman, N., & Guerrant, R. (2004). Acute infectious diarrhea. *New England Journal of Medicine, 350,* 38.

Toner, B., Emmott, S., Myran, D., & Drossman, D. (1999). *Cognitive-behavioral treatment of irritable bowel syndrome: The brain-gut connection.* New York: Guilford Press.

Tucker, M. (2000). First evidence-based guideline on constipation. *Family Practice News.* Retrieved from http://www.findarticles.com/cf_dis/mOBJI/2_30/59616045/print.jhtml on February 6, 2004.

U.S. Food and Drug Administration Center for Drug Evaluation and Research. (2002). *Medication guide for Lotronex tablets.* Retrieved from http://www.fda.gov/cder/drug/infopage/lotronex/medguide060502.htm.

*Verne, N., & Cerda, J. (1997). Irritable bowel syndrome: Streamlining the diagnosis. *Postgraduate Medicine, 102*(3), 197.

*Versa, T., Seppo, L., Marteau, P., et al. (1998). Relief of irritable bowel syndrome in subjective lactose intolerance. *American Journal of Clinical Nutrition, 67,* 710–715.

*Wald, A. (2006). Chronic constipation: Advances in management. *Neurogastroenterology and Motility,* 4–10.

*Wald, A. (2007). Appropriate use of laxatives in mangement of constipation. *Current Gastroentrology Reports,* 410–414.

CHAPTER 31

Liza Takiya

Inflammatory Bowel Disease

Inflammatory bowel disease (IBD) is a generic term used to describe two main chronic inflammatory conditions of the gastrointestinal (GI) tract: Crohn's disease (CD) and ulcerative colitis (UC). Although these conditions are similar in clinical presentation, CD is a chronic inflammatory disease characterized by transmural lesions located at any point on the GI tract, whereas UC is a chronic disease consisting of mucosal inflammation limited to the rectum and colon. IBD affects approximately 1 million Americans. In 2004, the prevalence of CD was estimated to be approximately 359,000, and for UC it is estimated to be 619,000 (National Institute of Diabetes and Digestive and Kidney Diseases, 2010). The incidence of UC has been relatively stable over the past 5 decades, whereas the incidence of CD is rising (Kornbluth & Sachar, 2010; Lichtenstein, et al., 2009). Both conditions are more common in whites than in any other race, and those of Jewish descent have a three- to six-fold greater incidence than the non-Jewish population. IBD shows no gender predilection and is usually first diagnosed in men or women between ages 15 and 25 (American Gastroenterological Association [AGA], 2001). Although the mortality rate is low for the disease, it significantly affects the patient's overall mental status, physical health, and quality of life. The most common emotional issues surrounding uncontrolled IBD appear to be anger, frustration, depression, and low self-esteem. These issues usually stem from the patient's inability to participate in routine activities, leading to a decreased quality of life. The disease has a negative impact on social interactions and daily functional status, leading to decreased productivity and attendance at work or school, decreased social engagements, and loss of independence. Health-related issues mirror those related to poor GI absorption, including nutritional deficiencies, electrolyte abnormalities, dehydration, cachexia, and iron deficiency anemia. Fatigue and lack of sleep are also common in patients with IBD. In addition, patients with long-standing CD may also be at risk for adenocarcinoma of the GI tract (Pederson, et al., 2010). All of these may result in frequent hospitalizations, altered lifestyle, and poor general health. Overall, in 2004, IBD had an estimated financial burden of $328 million in indirect health care costs and over $1.8 billion dollars in direct costs (Everhart, 2008).

CAUSES

The etiology of CD and UC is related to the dysregulation of immunologic mechanisms. The inflammatory nature of the condition has led researchers to believe that an autoimmune mechanism may predispose patients to IBD. The development of IBD may be attributed to a defect in the GI mucosal barrier that results in enhanced permeability and increased uptake of proinflammatory molecules and infectious agents. Tissue biopsies of the GI mucosal lining from patients with IBD reveal a high proportion of immunologic cytokines, including tumor necrosis factor (TNF), leukotrienes, and interleukin (IL)-1. A few bacterial and viral organisms have been associated with disease progression, including *Mycobacterium paratuberculosis*, measles virus, and *Listeria monocytogenes*; however, none has been definitively correlated with IBD.

Much of the recent evidence suggests that IBD is a complex genetic disorder. The high incidence of IBD in the Jewish population supports a genetic component of the etiology of CD and UC. A study comparing relatives of patients with IBD with the general population found a 10-fold increase in risk of development of IBD in those with familial occurrence. In addition, studies in twins support the notion that the disease course and occurrence of CD is genetically influenced (Halfverson, et al., 2007). Recently, the NOD2/CARD 15 gene has been associated with CD. Those who carry two copies of the risk alleles have been noted to be at higher risk for developing CD than others. The relationship between IBD and other genetic mutations and polymorphisms is currently being investigated. Until there is sufficient data to link a specific genetic mutation to IBD, the identification of genetic polymorphisms remains a research tool and not a clinical diagnostic tool.

Other factors, including psychological well-being and environmental triggers, may contribute to the exacerbation of IBD, although these factors do not have a predictable effect over a large population. Various studies have associated isolated mental instability or stressful events with IBD exacerbations, but a positive correlation between psychiatric illness and IBD is unsupported.

Environmental factors, including geographic location, dietary habits, drug-induced factors, and smoking status, are theorized to affect CD and UC exacerbations. IBD is more prevalent in the northern parts of the United States as well as in England and Scandinavian countries rather than the Mediterranean countries, suggesting that temperature or weather patterns may have an impact on CD or UC. Various dietary habits such as high sucrose consumption have been identified as exacerbating CD or UC, but no one particular food or group of foods seems to have a reliable effect in a large population. Oral contraceptive use and cigarette smoking have variable effects on CD versus UC; oral contraceptives and nicotine have been found to exacerbate CD, but not UC (Loftus, 2004). In addition, recently, the use of the anti-acne product isotretinoin (Accutane) has been associated with the development of IBD. The exact mechanism by which isotretinoin may cause IBD is unknown. However, isotretinoin does affect many immunologic mechanisms that may trigger IBD (Reddy, et al., 2006).

PATHOPHYSIOLOGY

Differentiating CD from UC is difficult because of their similar clinical presentations. Hallmark symptoms of IBD are bloody diarrhea, weight loss, and fever. Generally, CD can be distinguished from UC based only on endoscopic findings. The GI mucosal lining in CD is usually characterized by discontinuous, narrowed, thick, edematous, leathery patches with the presence of lesions, ulcerations, fissures, strictures, granulomas, and fibrosis. Fistulas and abscess formation occur most commonly in patients with deep transmural lesions. Granulomas and fistulas usually occur exclusively in patients with CD. UC usually affects the rectum and areas proximal, possibly extending throughout the entire large intestine with continuous, superficial uniform inflammation and ulceration. Other pathologic findings are rare in UC but may occur in patients with chronic, long-standing inflammation (**Table 31.1**).

Extraintestinal complications, including skin malformations, liver disease, joint deformities, and ocular manifestations, may also occur, although they are more common in CD than UC because of the more aggressive nature of CD, resulting in a higher probability of malabsorption of nutrients. (See **Table 31.1.**) Because the complications affect a variety of organ systems and result in nonspecific complaints, it is difficult to associate the complaints with CD or UC; however, it is important to be aware of the complications because their presence indicates poorly controlled disease.

DIAGNOSTIC CRITERIA

Because the clinical presentation of patients with CD or UC is nonspecific, definitive diagnosis relies on endoscopic or radiologic studies. Initial diagnosis of IBD must rule out other causes of bloody diarrhea such as infectious causes and other colitis conditions. Visualization techniques must be used to differentiate CD from UC because of their similar clinical pre-

TABLE 31.1 Common Signs and Symptoms of Crohn's Disease Versus Ulcerative Colitis

	Ulcerative Colitis	Crohn's Disease
Signs		
Abdominal mass	0	++
Fistulas	+/−	++
Strictures	+	++
Small bowel involvement	+/−	++
Rectal involvement	++	+/++
Extraintestinal disease		
Arthritis/arthralgia	++	++
Erythema nodosum	+/−	+/−
Abnormal liver function test values	++	++
Iritis/uveitis	+/−	+/−
Ankylosing spondylitis	+	+
Growth retardation	+	+
Toxic megacolon	+	+/−
Recurrence after colectomy	0	+
Malignancy	+	+/−
Symptoms		
Fever	+	++
Diarrhea	++	++
Weight loss	++	++
Rectal bleeding	++	+
Abdominal pain	+	++

Key: +, common; ++, very common; +/−, possible; 0, rare

sentations. Usually, endoscopic techniques are preferred over radiographs and radioactive isotopes because endoscopy permits direct visualization of the mucosal lining with increased specificity as to the extent of lesions, ulcerations, and inflammation, as well as providing the opportunity to obtain mucosal specimens for biopsy and further evaluation. The risk of mucosal perforation, however, may limit the use of endoscopic technology in patients with severely active disease.

Sigmoidoscopy or colonoscopy is preferred as a first-line diagnostic procedure; however, for CD, an endogastroduodenoscopy may also be required to visualize the upper GI tract. Radiologic studies with contrast, including either an upper GI series or barium enema, may be preferred in patients with severely active symptoms to decrease the risk of mucosal perforation.

Antibody tests are sometimes helpful in determining the diagnosis of CD or UC. The perinuclear antineutrophil cytoplasmic antibody (pANCA) and/or the anti-*Saccharomyces cerevisiae* antibody (ASCA) tests may be positive in patients with IBD, but there is a significant rate of false-negative results, since only 60% to 70% of patients with CD or UC are actually antibody positive (Kornbluth & Sachar, 2010). The combination of a positive pANCA and a negative ASCA may indicate the presence of UC, whereas the opposite may indicate CD.

However, the combined result still has a significant percentage of false negatives. Therefore, these tests are not used routinely to differentiate UC from CD.

INITIATING DRUG THERAPY

CD and UC share many clinical characteristics with pseudomembranous colitis, irritable bowel disease, peptic ulcer disease (PUD), traveler's diarrhea, colon cancer, and hemorrhoids. Evaluation of patients with suspected IBD must include a complete history focusing on recent use of antibiotics, recent international travel, diet history, use of laxatives or antidiarrheals, frequency and quality of daily bowel movements, history of PUD, and family history of IBD to rule out similar presenting conditions.

Physical examination should include assessment of vital signs and weight loss, a thorough abdominal examination, and special attention to extraintestinal complications. Guaiac testing and stool cultures may be helpful in ruling out PUD or infectious causes. Although there are no reliable surrogate laboratory markers that may indicate the presence of CD or UC, baseline laboratory studies, including electrolytes, liver panel, complete blood count (CBC), and hematology panel, are important in assessing the severity of the condition and patient well-being.

Initiation of proper drug therapy is based on the severity and extent of disease. CD may present as luminal or fistulizing disease. CD confined to the GI lumen can initially present as mild, moderate, or severe disease and is not predictable in its course. Fistulizing disease also has a varied clinical course, whereby certain patients may never experience a fistula and others may develop one early in the course of the disease. Treatment of fistulizing disease is typically more aggressive than luminal disease and may vary depending on the location of the fistula (bowel to bladder, bowel to skin, etc.). UC may be confined to the distal colon and rectum or may extend throughout the colon. Due to the location of the disease, treatment options for distal UC are greater than for extensive disease. The Working Definitions of Crohn's Disease Activity or the Criteria for Severity of Ulcerative Colitis may be used as a guide to determine severity (**Table 31.2** and **Table 31.3**). Both scales are frequently used in clinical trials; however, they are modified for use in clinical practice. There are many validated scales used to assess the severity of UC; however, there isn't one gold standard. Each scale highlights specific subjective and objective parameters that should be evaluated when assessing the progression of disease. Both scales highlight certain key features when predicting the severity of the condition, such as the frequency of stools per day and the presence of abdominal pain, fever, and anemia.

Treatment for IBD consists of aminosalicylates, corticosteroids, immunosuppressive agents, antibiotics, and biological agents. The decision to use one or a combination of these agents is based on the presence of CD versus UC, the severity of the disease, and whether treatment is targeted at active disease or maintenance of remission. In general, aminosalicylates are used

---

TABLE 31.2	Working Definitions of Crohn's Disease Activity

Mild to Moderate
- Ambulatory patients
- Able to tolerate oral alimentation
- No evidence of:
  - Dehydration
  - High fevers
  - Rigors
  - Prostration
  - Abdominal tenderness
  - Painful mass
  - Abdominal obstruction
- <10% weight loss

Moderate to Severe
- Failed treatment for mild to moderate disease OR
- Have
  - High fever
  - >10% weight loss
  - Abdominal pain/tenderness
  - Intermittent nausea or vomiting (without obstructive findings)
  - Significant anemia

Severe to Fulminant
- Persistent symptoms despite outpatient steroid therapy OR
- Have
  - High fever
  - Persistent vomiting
  - Intestinal obstruction
  - Rebound tenderness
  - Cachexia
  - Abscess

Remission
- Asymptomatic without inflammatory sequelae
- Not dependent on steroids

TABLE 31.3	Criteria for Severity of Ulcerative Colitis

Mild UC
- <4 stools daily (with or without blood)
- No presence of anemia, fever, or tachycardia
- Normal erythrocyte sedimentation rate (ESR)

Moderate UC
- >4 stools daily
- Minimal anemia, fever, or tachycardia

Severe UC
- >6 bloody stools daily
- Positive fever, tachycardia, anemia, or elevated ESR

Fulminant UC
- >10 stools daily
- Continuous bleeding
- Abdominal tenderness and distention
- Anemia requiring blood transfusion
- Colonic dilation

for treating mild to moderate exacerbations of UC and CD, as well as for maintaining remission in IBD. Corticosteroids are used to treat acute exacerbations and should not be used chronically to maintain remission. Immunosuppressive agents are used for the purposes of maintaining remission in IBD, whereas intravenous (IV) cyclosporine is used in a limited population to treat severely active, steroid-refractory UC. Antibiotics are reserved for treating and maintaining remission in patients with mild CD. Biologic agents are reserved for inducing and maintaining remission in patients with steroid-refractory CD. Infliximab is the only biological agent that has proven efficacy in managing patients with UC (**Table 31.4**).

Goals of Drug Therapy

Because no pharmacologic cure is available for CD or UC, the goals of treatment focus on symptom management and quality-of-life issues. With proper treatment, the patient should be able to:

- resume normal daily activities
- restore general physical and mental well-being
- attain appropriate nutritional status
- maintain remission of disease
- decrease the number and frequency of exacerbations
- decrease side effects related to medications
- increase life expectancy.

Ideally, patients should expect to recover from an acute exacerbation within 2 to 4 weeks, have minimal exacerbations throughout the year, and participate in any desired activity.

Aminosalicylates

Aminosalicylates remain the gold standard for the treatment of mild to moderate CD and UC. Although the exact mechanism of action is unknown, these drugs decrease inflammation in the GI tract by inhibiting prostaglandin synthesis, which results in a decrease in various immune mediators, including IL-1, cyclooxygenase, and thromboxane synthase. Therapy with these agents may improve symptoms within 1 week of initiating therapy or dosage adjustment. However, patients may need to take these agents long term to prevent exacerbations. Although they are safe for use in most patients, aminosalicylates are contraindicated in patients with aspirin allergy or glucose-6-phosphate dehydrogenase deficiency. Sulfasalazine is also contraindicated in patients who are hypersensitive to sulfa products. (See **Table 31.4.**) All of these agents must be used at maximum doses for maximum therapeutic benefit, although the incidence of side effects also increases with increased doses.

Sulfasalazine

Sulfasalazine (Azulfidine, Azulfidine EN) is efficacious and cost-effective for CD and UC therapy but has a limited role because of its unfavorable side effect profile. Sulfasalazine is a combination product that is cleaved in the proximal colon by bacterial azo-reductases to release sulfapyridine and mesalamine. The mesalamine compound is responsible for virtually all of the therapeutic effect, whereas sulfapyridine is responsible for many of the side effects associated with sulfasalazine. Sulfasalazine may be administered up to four times a day; the most effective and maximum daily dosage is 8 g daily.

Mesalamine

Mesalamine (Asacol, Rowasa, Pentasa, Lialda, Apriso, Canasa) is available in various formulations, including oral tablets, oral capsules, enemas, and rectal suppositories. Each formulation is released in various areas of the GI tract, allowing for targeted drug therapy; however, in clinical trials the capsules and tablets had similar efficacy at equivalent doses. Asacol, which is one of the oral tablet products, is formulated with an acrylic resin coating that disintegrates at a pH of 7, allowing the active ingredient to be released in the distal ileum and colon. Similarly, Lialda, another oral tablet formulation, has a coating that disintegrates at a pH of 6 to 7, and the core of the tablet forms a matrix that is released across a pH of 6.8 to 7.2. Pentasa, which is a sustained-released capsule, has ethylcellulose-coated granules that allow for the slow release of the drug beginning in the proximal small intestine and continuing throughout the colon. This formulation has slightly different pharmacokinetics than Apriso, which is also a delayed-release capsule. Apriso capsules are enteric-coated; they disintegrate at a pH above 6 and also contain granules that are formulated in a polymer matrix for extended release. Because each of the oral products has different pharmacokinetics, the dosing interval for the products ranges from once to four times a day. (See **Table 31.4**.) The rectal suppositories are used primarily for UC-associated proctitis, whereas the enema delivers mesalamine to the distal and sigmoid colon. The enema is typically given at bedtime to allow for direct contact of the drug with the mucosa for at least 8 hours. In patients with distal UC, a combination of oral and rectal mesalamine may be an appropriate therapeutic option. Studies have shown that combination mesalamine therapy is more effective than either single mesalamine formulation.

Olsalazine

Olsalazine (Dipentum), the third aminosalicylate preparation, consists of two mesalamine molecules joined by an azo-bond. As with sulfasalazine, the azo-bond is cleaved by bacterial azo-reductases in the GI tract, allowing the drug to be released in the proximal colon. It is administered twice daily, with patients taking up to 8 capsules per day for a total dosage of 2 g/d. Although each tablet of olsalazine has twice as much active ingredient as the mesalamine capsules, the efficacy is minimally enhanced.

Balsalazide

Balsalazide (Colazal) is a combination product consisting of 5-aminosalicylic acid (mesalamine), the therapeutically active portion of the molecule, and 4-aminobenzoyl-alanine, an inert moiety. The product is cleaved by bacterial azo-reductases in the colon to release the active compound. Each capsule

TABLE 31.4   **Overview of Agents Used to Treat Inflammatory Bowel Disease**

Generic (Trade) Name and Dosage	Selected Adverse Events	Contraindications	Special Considerations
Aminosalicylates			
sulfasalazine (Azulfidine, Azulfidine EN) Start: 500 mg twice daily Range: 1–8 g/d	Stevens-Johnson syndrome, rash, photosensitivity, nausea, vomiting, skin discoloration, agranulocytosis, crystalluria, hepatitis	Sulfa allergy, aspirin allergy, G6PD deficiency	Most efficacious at high doses Drug released in the proximal colon Available in enteric-coated tablets Dosage increases may occur as frequently as every other day.
oral mesalamine (Aprisol, Asacol, Lialda, Pentasa) Start: depends on product Range: 1– 4.8 g/d	Nausea, headache, malaise, abdominal pain, diarrhea	Aspirin allergy, G6PD deficiency	Products released differently in the GI tract May increase dose as frequently as every other day
rectal mesalamine (Rowasa Enema, Canasa suppository) Suppository Start: 1g at bedtime Range: 1 g/d Enema Start: 4 g at bedtime Range: 1–4 g/d	Malaise, abdominal pain	Aspirin allergy, G6PD deficiency	Only for distal ulcerative colitis, proctitis Suppository most effective in sigmoid colon, and enema may treat distal and sigmoid colon
olsalazine (Dipentum) Start: 500 mg twice daily Range: 1–2 g	Nausea, headache, malaise, abdominal pain, diarrhea	Aspirin allergy, G6PD deficiency	Drug released in proximal colon May increase dose as frequently as every other day Higher incidence of diarrhea
balsalazide (Colazide) Start: 1.5 g twice daily Range: 1.5–6.75 g	Headache, abdominal pain, diarrhea	Aspirin allergy, G6PD deficiency	Only approved for treatment of mild to moderate ulcerative colitis
Selected Corticosteroids			
prednisone (Orasone, Deltasone) Start: 40–60 mg daily Range: 10–100 mg	Hyperglycemia, increased appetite, insomnia, anxiety, tremors, hypertension, fluid retention, electrolyte imbalances	Active GI bleeding	Taper patient off steroids within 1–2 mo of initiation to decrease risk of long-term side effects.
oral methylprednisolone (Medrol) Start: 20–50 mg daily Range: 10–100 mg	Same as above	Same as above	Same as above
IV methylprednisolone (Solu-Medrol) Start: 5–10 mg q6h Range: 10–50 mg	Same as above	Same as above	IV treatment used for severe exacerbations Treatment duration should be a maximum of 7–14 d, then switch to oral therapy
rectal hydrocortisone suppositories (Anusol-HC) Start: 25 mg twice daily Range: 25–100 mg	Same as above		Used only for distal ulcerative colitis treatment
Hydrocortisone enema (Cortenema) Start: 100 mg bedtime Range: 100 mg/d			Enema is more effective than suppositories for distal colitis.
IV hydrocortisone (Solu-Cortef) Start: 50–100 twice daily Range: 25–150 twice daily	Same as above	Active GI bleeding	IV treatment used for severe exacerbations Treatment duration should be a maximum of 7–14 d, then switch to oral therapy
dexamethasone (Decadron) Start: 5–15 mg daily Range: 2–20 mg/d	Same as above	Same as above	Has longer onset of action than other agents
oral budesonide (Entocort EC) Start: 9 mg/day Maintenance: 6 mg/d for 3 mo	Minimal nausea	Same as above	Minimal systemic absorption Taper after 8 weeks of therapy. Effective for mild to moderately active luminal CD and maintenance

TABLE 31.4	Overview of Agents Used to Treat Inflammatory Bowel Disease (*Continued*)		
Generic (Trade) Name and Dosage	**Selected Adverse Events**	**Contraindications**	**Special Considerations**
Selected Immunosuppressives			

azathioprine (Imuran)
  Start: 50 mg/d
  Range: 2–2.5 mg/kg
	Pancreatitis, fever, arthralgias, nausea, rash, agranulocytosis, diarrhea, malaise, hepatotoxicity	Pregnancy, active liver disease, bone marrow suppression	Decrease dose for patients with severe renal dysfunction

6-mercaptopurine (Purinethol)
  Start: 50 mg/d
  Range: 1–2.5 mg/kg
	Same as above	Same as above	Same as above

oral methotrexate (Rheumatrex)
  Start: 5 mg 3 times a week
  Range: 5–7.5 mg 3 times a week
	Hepatic cirrhosis and fibrosis, neutropenia, pneumonitis, skin rash, nausea, diarrhea	Same as above	Same as above

IV cyclosporine Start: 4–8 mg/kg/d	Hypertension, nephrotoxicity, superinfection, hypomagnesemia	Renal failure, hepatic failure	Only used for severely acute UC refractory to steroids; total duration of therapy 7–10 d; has many drug interactions
Selected Antibiotics			

metronidazole (Flagyl)
  Start: 20 mg/kg/d
  Range: 10–20 mg/kg/d
	Nausea, diarrhea, disulfiram reaction, metallic taste, peripheral paresthesias, dizziness	Liver failure, renal failure, first trimester of pregnancy, uncontrolled seizure disorder	Should not be used with alcohol
			Most efficacious if used chronically >3 mo

ciprofloxacin (Cipro)
  Start: 500 mg twice daily
  Range: 500–2,000 mg/d
	Dizziness, nausea, diarrhea, photosensitivity	Children <12 y, pregnancy, uncontrolled seizure disorder	May cause arthropathies in patients <12 y
			Must be administered 2 h before or after divalent and trivalent cations

Tumor Necrosis Factor Inhibitors			

IV infliximab (Remicade)
  Start: 5 mg/kg
  Range: 5–10 mg/kg
	Infusion reactions (urticaria, dyspnea, hypotension), TB, invasive fungal infections, lymphoma, lupus-like syndrome	Class III/IV heart failure, active TB, hepatitis B or other infections	For severe, refractory UC and luminal and fistulizing CD; administered over 2 h as a single infusion
			Induction regimen dosed at weeks 0, 2, and 6; maintenance regimen dosed every 8 wk

adalilimumab (Humira)
  Start: 160 mg SQ
  Maintenance: 40 mg every week or every other week
	Opportunistic infections (TB, fungal, bacterial, viral), lymphoma and other cancers, injection-site reactions (erythema, pain, swelling)	Active TB, hepatitis B, or other infections	For luminal CD; induction regimen 160 mg initially and 80 mg at week 2

certolizumab pegol (Cimzia)
  Start: 400 mg at baseline, week 2, and week 4
  Maintenance: 400 mg every 4 wk
	Opportunistic infections (TB, fungal, bacterial, viral), lymphoma and other cancers, injection-site reactions (erythema, pain, swelling)	Active TB, hepatitis B, or other infections	For luminal CD

G6PD, glucose-6-phosphate dehydrogenase

contains granules of balsalazide that are insoluble in acid and designed to be delivered to the colon intact. It is administered three times a day, up to 9 capsules per day, for a total dosage of 6.75 g/d, equaling 2.4 g/d of pure mesalamine. Currently it has been studied only for use in mild to moderate ulcerative colitis in both adults and children. Side effects and contraindications are similar to those of mesalamine.

Adverse Events

Mesalamine, olsalazine, and balsalazide are poorly absorbed from the GI tract and thus are considered primarily topical agents, with limited systemic side effects and drug interactions. The major side effects of mesalamine include headache, malaise, abdominal pain, and diarrhea. Olsalazine has a similar side effect profile but has a higher incidence of diarrhea than mesalamine. Initially, diarrhea may not be easily distinguished from an IBD exacerbation, and therefore close monitoring of improvement of symptoms is essential. If the balsalazide capsules are opened and sprinkled in food, teeth staining may occur. In rare instances, mesalamine, olsalazine, and balsalazide have been associated with renal function impairment; therefore, renal function should be monitored during therapy. Sulfapyridine is absorbed systemically, accounting for many of the side effects and drug interactions incurred by sulfasalazine. Common adverse effects include nausea, vomiting, photosensitivity, oligospermia, and skin discoloration, which may be tolerable for most patients. Severe adverse reactions associated with sulfasalazine include Stevens-Johnson syndrome, agranulocytosis, crystalluria, pancreatitis, and hepatitis, which may necessitate discontinuation of therapy. Sulfasalazine is known to decrease folate levels; therefore, patients taking sulfasalazine should be supplemented with folic acid. Although drug interactions with sulfasalazine are limited, it may significantly decrease the effect of warfarin (Coumadin), and therefore close monitoring of the international normalized ratio is essential.

Corticosteroids

Corticosteroids are used intermittently to treat acute IBD exacerbations only. Corticosteroids allow for immunosuppression and prostaglandin inhibition when the disease fails to respond to aminosalicylate therapy. Corticosteroids may be used in conjunction with aminosalicylates, immunosuppressants, or biologic agents or as monotherapy to treat acute exacerbations. Corticosteroids with relatively quick onset of action and high glucocorticoid activity, such as prednisone (Orasone, Deltasone) and methylprednisolone (Medrol), are desirable in the treatment of CD or UC. Controlled-release oral budesonide (Entocort EC) is a unique corticosteroid due to its long-acting formulation and limited potential for absorption from the GI tract, thus theoretically leading to a localized effect in the GI lumen with minimal systemic side effects. Oral budesonide has been used as the treatment of choice in patients with mild to moderate exacerbations of CD in combination with aminosalicylates or as monotherapy.

Dosage

Doses equivalent to oral prednisone 40 to 60 mg/d are initiated in patients with mild or moderate exacerbations of CD or UC. A beneficial effect is usually seen with 7 to 10 days of therapy. Patients with mild to moderate exacerbations of distal UC can be treated with oral or rectal corticosteroids for approximately 4 to 8 weeks, after which drug dosages are tapered. Hydrocortisone is the only rectal corticosteroid enema formulation available for use in distal UC exacerbations. There are many tapering regimens that have been studied. The most common is a 5- to 10-mg weekly taper until a daily dose of 20 mg is reached, at which time the dose is tapered by 2.5 mg per week. In severe exacerbations, patients should receive 3 to 10 days of IV corticosteroid therapy and then switch to oral corticosteroid therapy for the remainder of the treatment period. (See **Table 31.4.**)

Adverse Events

Short-term corticosteroid use (<3 months) is associated with increased glucose levels, increased appetite, insomnia, anxiety, tremors, and increased fluid retention, leading to increases in blood pressure and electrolyte imbalances. Although discontinuation of therapy as a result of these side effects is not recommended with short-term corticosteroid treatment, routine monitoring is necessary.

Long-term corticosteroid use is associated with decreased bone density, leading to osteoporosis; fat redistribution, leading to the characteristic "buffalo hump"; decreased prostaglandin synthesis, resulting in gastric and duodenal ulcers; hypertriglyceridemia; hypokalemia; cataracts; and hirsutism. Therefore, long-term treatment with corticosteroids is not recommended. However, if patients are taking recurrent steroid therapy for recurrent exacerbations, monitoring for these side effects is imperative.

Interactions

Many corticosteroids are substrates of the cytochrome P450 isoenzyme 3A4, including prednisone, prednisolone, methylprednisolone, and budesonide. Therefore, agents that inhibit or induce this enzyme system, such as ketoconazole, clarithromycin, phenytoin, and pioglitazone, may alter the efficacy of the corticosteroid. Budesonide requires an acidic environment (pH <5.5) to be released, so agents that inhibit acid production or neutralize acid in the GI tract (i.e., histamine-2 antagonists, proton pump inhibitors, antacids) may limit the effectiveness of budesonide. Corticosteroids may also decrease the effectiveness of antidiabetic and antihypertensive agents due to their ability to increase blood glucose levels and blood pressure.

Immunosuppressive Agents

Immunosuppressive agents are used in IBD as adjunctive treatment with aminosalicylates to induce and maintain remission if exacerbations occur while the patient is being tapered off corticosteroid therapy or if frequent exacerbations occur with maximum dosages of aminosalicylates. IV cyclosporine is an exception: it is solely used to treat severe, acute exacerbations of UC when the patient is refractory to corticosteroids.

Azathioprine and 6-Mercaptopurine

Azathioprine (Imuran) and 6-mercaptopurine (Purinethol) are antimetabolites that act as purine antagonists to inhibit the synthesis of protein, ribonucleic acid (RNA), and deoxyribonucleic acid (DNA). By doing so, azathioprine and 6-mercaptopurine decrease the production of various inflammatory mediators. Because 6-mercaptopurine is the active metabolite of azathioprine, these agents are similar in efficacy, side effect profile, and dosing frequency. (See **Table 31.4.**) Although these agents have a short plasma half-life of approximately 1 to 2 hours, both have active metabolites with long half-lives of 3 to 13 days, resulting in optimal therapeutic effects within 10 to 15 weeks of initiation of therapy. 6-mercaptopurine is metabolized by the enzyme thiopurine methyltransferase (TPMT). The activity of this particular enzyme varies in patients based on a genetic polymorphism. Therefore, patients may be at a higher risk for certain side effects if they have low enzyme activity. TPMT testing is available to identify patients who may have low enzyme activity and, in turn, may experience more side effects.

These agents should be initiated during an acute exacerbation once the patient can tolerate oral medications to induce and maintain remission. Because of their slow onset of action, however, these agents are not effective for treating an acute exacerbation. The initial dosage of these agents is 50 mg/d in one dose; the dosage is increased every 2 weeks to a target dosage of 1 to 2 mg/kg/d for 6-mercaptopurine and 2 to 2.5 mg/kg/d for azathioprine. Because these agents are cleared by the renal system, dosages must be decreased in patients with creatinine clearance values under 50 mL/min. The dose for azathioprine and 6-mercaptopurine is usually decreased by 50% if the patient's creatinine clearance value falls below 50 mL/min to decrease the risk of accumulation and unwanted effects. Although these agents have the potential to cause significant adverse events, they are in general well tolerated. These agents should not be used in pregnancy or in patients with active liver disease.

Methotrexate

Methotrexate (Rheumatrex) has a therapeutic effect similar to that of azathioprine and 6-mercaptopurine; however, it inhibits intracellular dihydrofolate reductase, which results in inhibition of purine synthesis and suppression of IL-1 production. Both the intramuscular and oral preparations of methotrexate are efficacious in the induction and maintenance of CD remission, but similar efficacy has not been shown for UC. Doses of 25 mg/wk injected intramuscularly or 5 mg orally three times a week have been effective in inducing remission in patients with steroid-dependent CD after 12 to 16 weeks of therapy. At low doses, methotrexate is nearly completely absorbed when administered orally; therefore, there is no foreseen benefit in using the intramuscular preparation over the oral formulation during normal GI function.

Methotrexate dosages must be adjusted based on renal function. Patients with creatinine clearance values less than 50 mL/min should receive 50% of the normal dose. Methotrexate should not be prescribed to patients with active liver disease or pregnant women.

Cyclosporine

Cyclosporine (Sandimmune, Neoral) is reserved for the acute treatment of severe, steroid-refractory exacerbations of UC in hospitalized patients. Cyclosporine is a lipophilic, fungus-derived polypeptide that suppresses cell-mediated immunity by predominantly inhibiting IL-2 synthesis and release. Therapeutic effect is correlated with appropriate dosing. IV infusion of cyclosporine has been found effective at dosages of 4 to 8 mg/kg/d for UC. The use of cyclosporine in acute CD exacerbations is reported to have variable results. Because of poor systemic absorption, oral cyclosporine should not be used. Improvement of symptoms with IV therapy usually occurs within 2 to 3 days, and the duration of therapy is usually 7 to 10 days.

Adverse Events

Although azathioprine and 6-mercaptopurine are usually well tolerated, significant side effects may occur. These agents are associated with both allergic- and nonallergic-type side effects. Allergic-type side effects include pancreatitis, fever, rash, arthralgias, malaise, nausea, and diarrhea, which may occur regardless of dose. The main nonallergic-type side effects include bone marrow suppression and hepatotoxicity, which appear to be dose dependent. Pancreatitis may occur at any point in therapy and warrants discontinuation of therapy. The development of pancreatitis precludes the use of either 6-mercaptopurine or azathioprine in the future. Leukopenia and hepatotoxicity usually occurs during the initiation phase of therapy and may be managed by decreasing the dose. If a patient experiences side effects with either of these agents, it is not beneficial to switch the patient to the other agent.

Side effects of methotrexate include hepatic cirrhosis and fibrosis, bone marrow suppression, pneumonitis, folic acid deficiency, and rash. Nausea and diarrhea are also reported, but they occur more frequently with the oral formulation. Bone marrow suppression and liver dysfunction are dose dependent, and doses should be decreased in patients with these disorders. Folic acid should be administered concomitantly to limit folic acid deficiency.

Cyclosporine is most associated with nephrotoxicity, hypomagnesemia, and hypertension. Risk factors for nephrotoxicity are high-dose treatment, long-term treatment, and advanced age. Discontinuation of cyclosporine may restore renal function within 2 weeks. Other side effects of cyclosporine include nausea, vomiting, opportunistic infections, paresthesias, tremor, and seizures. Opportunistic infections occur because of the drug's immunosuppressive effects and may be managed by appropriate antibiotic therapy.

Interactions

Cyclosporine significantly interacts with various agents because of its metabolism through the cytochrome P450 3A4 isoenzyme system. Enzyme inhibitors, such as erythromycin (Eryc) and ketoconazole (Nizoral), increase blood levels of cyclosporine by inhibiting its metabolism, whereas enzyme inducers, such as phenytoin (Dilantin), carbamazepine (Tegretol), and rifampin (Rifadin), decrease cyclosporine blood levels. Grapefruit juice increases blood levels of cyclosporine, which may increase the incidence of side effects.

Antibiotics

The association between IBD and infectious causes has led to the use of antibiotics. Because the exact organism has not been isolated, it is difficult to determine which antibiotics are most appropriate for treatment. In general, an antibiotic that acts against gram-negative and *Mycobacterium* organisms with a low side effect profile and poor systemic absorption is desirable. Many agents have been studied, including broad-spectrum antibiotics, metronidazole (Flagyl), fluoroquinolones, antituberculars, and macrolides. However, based on the scarce published, controlled trials, mild to moderately active CD appears to respond only to metronidazole and ciprofloxacin (Cipro). (See **Table 31.4.**) Beneficial effects of antibiotic therapy have not been replicated in patients with UC.

Metronidazole showed efficacy in treating perianal CD. Since then, however, a few studies have found beneficial effects of metronidazole in the treatment of mild to moderately active luminal and fistulizing CD when used in combination with aminosalicylates or alone. The mechanism by which metronidazole alone exerts its beneficial effects in CD is unknown, although it is thought that the immune-modulating effects are more prominent than the antibacterial effects.

The normal dosage for treatment of mild to moderately active CD is 20 mg/kg/d. Once remission is attained, the dosage is titrated to 10 mg/kg/d for maintenance. The usual duration of therapy is up to 12 months, although remission is usually attained within 1 to 2 months. Although exacerbations of CD have been reported with the discontinuation of metronidazole, long-term use is associated with significant side effects.

Ciprofloxacin has also been studied for perianal and luminal CD with mixed results. Ciprofloxacin covers gram-negative organisms and *Mycobacterium* species as well as some gram-positive organisms and is usually well tolerated. Along with inhibiting DNA gyrase, which is its main antibacterial mechanism of action, ciprofloxacin also is reported to have immunosuppressive properties. A dosage of oral ciprofloxacin of 500 mg, twice daily, is as efficacious as 4 g of mesalamine daily in preliminary trials. Remission is attained after approximately 6 weeks of therapy. Ciprofloxacin is contraindicated in children and pregnant women.

Adverse Events

Short-term metronidazole therapy is associated with fairly benign side effects, including dry mouth, metallic taste, nausea, and vomiting. Abdominal distress, including cramping and diarrhea, may also occur, but these effects are difficult to distinguish from IBD symptoms. Long-term use of metronidazole is associated with neurotoxic effects such as peripheral paresthesias, dizziness, pruritus, and vertigo that may warrant discontinuation of therapy.

Ciprofloxacin is usually well tolerated. The most common side effects include nausea, diarrhea, dizziness, and rashes secondary to photosensitivity. However, long-term treatment may result in tendinitis and tendon rupture.

Interactions

Metronidazole is associated with severe nausea and vomiting (disulfiram effect) if taken concurrently with alcohol. Ciprofloxacin inhibits theophylline (Slo-Phyllin) metabolism, so theophylline serum levels may need to be monitored with chronic ciprofloxacin use. Any divalent or trivalent cation, such as calcium or iron, may interfere with the absorption of ciprofloxacin, therefore at least a 4-hour dosing interval should be maintained between these agents.

Biological Agents

Many biological agents are being investigated for the treatment of IBD, including TNF inhibitors, growth factors, lymphocyte inhibitors, and transcription inhibitors. Currently infliximab (Remicade), adalimumab (Humira), and certolizumab pegol (Cimzia), all of which are TNF inhibitors, are the only biological agents approved for the treatment of severe refractory luminal CD. Infliximab is also indicated for maintaining remission in CD as well as treating UC and fistulizing CD. The GI mucosal tissues of patients with active CD are found to overexpress numerous immunologic cytokines, including TNF. Biological TNF-α is a proinflammatory cytokine that stimulates the expression of various immunologic cytokines, such as IL-8 and interferon-γ. The TNF-α inhibitor agents produce their effect by neutralizing soluble forms of TNF-α and competitively inhibit its binding to the TNF receptor. In addition, TNF-α inhibitors may also induce apoptosis of activated monocytes.

Infliximab is a synthetically derived immunoglobulin (Ig) G monoclonal antibody consisting of 25% murine antibodies and 75% human antibodies. (See **Table 31.4.**) Infliximab is available only as an IV solution, and it is administered at a dosage of 5 mg/kg over a minimum of 2 hours. A single infusion dose at baseline, week 2, and week 6 is administered for the treatment of an acute exacerbation; infusions every 8 weeks are used to maintain remission. The infusions may be delivered in an inpatient or a monitored outpatient setting. Repeated doses of the product may increase the risk of immunogenicity and infusion-related reactions due to the murine component of the product. Infliximab has not been adequately studied in pregnant women, so caution should be used when prescribing it in pregnancy as well as in patients with heart failure.

Adalimumab is also a TNF-α inhibitor; however, it is a fully humanized IgG monoclonal antibody that binds specifically to human TNF. In general, fully humanized monoclonal antibodies are associated with less immunogenicity and infusion-related reactions. Adalimumab is administered as a subcutaneous injection every 2 weeks and may be increased to once weekly if necessary. (See **Table 31.4.**) In addition to patients with CD who are naïve to TNF-α inhibitors, adalimumab is effective in patients with CD who may not have responded to infliximab. It has not been well studied in UC or fistulizing CD or in children with UC or CD.

Certolizumab pegol is also a TNF-α inhibitor; however, it is not a full monoclonal antibody. Certolizumab pegol consists of only the FAB fragment of human-derived IgG, which is attached to polyethylene glycol. Since certolizumab pegol does not contain certain regions of a full antibody, it cannot cause antibody-dependent cell cytotoxicity or induce apoptosis as with infliximab or adalimumab. The polyethylene glycol portion of the product allows for a longer duration of action and thus a longer duration between injections. Certolizumab pegol is administered in two subcutaneous injections initially and weeks 2 and 4. For those who elicit a clinical response, certolizumab pegol may be used every 4 weeks to maintain remission. (See **Table 31.4.**) It has not been studied in the treatment of UC or fistulizing CD or in children.

Adverse Events

The primary side effects associated with TNF-α inhibitors are injection-site related reactions, which include erythema, itching, and swelling. Less common but significant side effects include the development of heart failure, tuberculosis (TB), hepatitis B reactivation, opportunistic infections, lymphoma and other malignancies, hepatotoxicity, vasculitis, and pancytopenia. Patients should be tested for latent TB and treated accordingly prior to treatment with TNF-α inhibitors. TNF-α inhibitors are contraindicated in patients with active TB and should be used cautiously in patients with heart failure.

Infliximab is also associated with infusion-related reactions, including transient hypersensitivity reactions, flushing, headache, dyspnea, rash, and fever, possibly secondary to the murine component of the product. These side effects may be managed by pretreating patients with antihistamines, acetaminophen, and/or corticosteroids. In addition, mild to moderate infusion reactions may be managed by decreasing the infusion rate.

Drug Interactions

Extensive drug interaction studies have not been performed to date, but due to their ability to alter the immunologic response, TNF-α inhibitors should not be administered along with live vaccines. Commonly, TNF-α inhibitors are administered to patients who are also taking immunosuppressive agents. The administration of other immunosuppressant agents (e.g., azathioprine, methotrexate) with these agents has been shown to be beneficial by decreasing the risk of immunogenicity (development of autoantibodies) and decreasing infusion-related reactions (Lichtenstein, et al., 2009). No significant drug interactions have been reported when TNF-α inhibitors are given with conventional IBD therapy.

Selecting the Most Appropriate Agent

For many diseases and disorders, there are drug treatment protocols that make clear distinctions between first-line, second-line, and third-line therapies. However, in IBD, the decision to use one therapeutic modality over another is based on the location of the inflammation, the severity and extent of disease, the patient's tolerance of the therapy, patient compliance, and cost (**Table 31.5**). The American College of Gastroenterology has developed guidelines for managing CD and UC (Lichtenstein, et al., 2009; Kornbluth & Sachar, 2010).

Crohn's Disease

Mild to moderately active luminal CD is typically treated with oral aminosalicylates alone or in combination with antibiotic therapy. However, monotherapy with budesonide has also been used with good results, especially in patients with ileal or right colonic disease. Oral agents are chosen over rectal agents because of the random presence of CD along the entire GI tract. Patients may be maintained on aminosalicylates or antibiotic therapy for months to years, but the goal is to

TABLE 31.5	Recommended Treatment Options for Crohn's Disease and Ulcerative Colitis			
Severity of Disease	**Distal UC**	**Extensive UC**	**Luminal CD**	**Perianal/Fistulizing CD**
Mild	Oral/rectal aminosalicylate OR Rectal corticosteroid	Oral aminosalicylate	Oral aminosalicylate WITH/WITHOUT Antibiotic therapy	Surgical drainage AND antibiotic therapy WITH/WITHOUT IV infliximab
Moderate	Oral aminosalicylate AND Rectal aminosalicylate Oral/rectal steroid	Oral aminosalicylate AND Oral steroid	Oral aminosalicylate AND Oral steroid (preferably budesonide)	
Severe	IV corticosteroid AND/OR IV cyclosporine	IV corticosteroid AND/OR IV cyclosporine	IV corticosteroid AND/OR TNF-α inhibitor	
Fulminant	IV corticosteroids AND/OR IV cyclosporine, IV infliximab	IV corticosteroid AND/OR IV cyclosporine, IV infliximab	IV corticosteroid AND/OR TNF-α inhibitor	
Remission	Oral/rectal aminosalicylate WITH/WITHOUT Oral immunosuppressive, IV infliximab	Oral aminosalicylate WITH/WITHOUT Oral immunosuppressive, IV infliximab	Oral aminosalicylate WITH/WITHOUT Oral immunosuppressive/TNF-α inhibitor	

taper the patient off the medication as soon as possible once remission is attained. Budesonide is indicated for 3 months to maintain remission in CD.

Treatment of moderate to severe CD usually consists of combination therapy with aminosalicylates and corticosteroids. Corticosteroid therapy is used acutely on a short-term basis for patients with moderate to severe disease to attain remission. Because of their high side effect profile, steroids are not used chronically to maintain remission. Oral agents may be used for patients with moderate to severe disease. The typical duration of therapy is 4 to 12 weeks at the full dose, and then doses are tapered by 5 to 10 mg weekly until discontinued. If patients have had multiple exacerbations and are steroid refractory or have fistulizing disease, TNF inhibitors may be indicated.

Severe to fulminant disease requires definitive drug therapy in addition to substantial supportive care measures due to poor oral absorption and rapid GI transit time. Oral therapy, including aminosalicylates, should not be administered until the patient can tolerate oral alimentation. IV corticosteroids are indicated to decrease inflammation and induce immunosuppression. For patients with moderate to severe or severe to fulminant disease whose disease is refractory to corticosteroids (either oral or IV), biological agents are an option. Supportive care measures, such as IV fluids, bowel rest, and parenteral nutrition, should also be considered.

Therapy to maintain remission should be considered in patients who have frequent exacerbations or who are "steroid-dependent." Immunosuppressive agents, including azathioprine, 6-mercaptopurine, methotrexate, and the TNF-alpha inhibitors, may be used with aminosalicylates to maintain remission in patients whose disease is refractory to aminosalicylate monotherapy. The immunosuppressant agents may take effect after 10 to 12 weeks. Therapeutic effect should be seen within 8 weeks of administration of the TNF-alpha inhibitors. Patients may be maintained on these agents for months to years, but the goal is to taper the patient off the medication as soon as possible due to the significant side effects. Antibiotics, specifically metronidazole and ciprofloxacin, have proved beneficial in maintaining remission of perianal and fistulizing CD with long-term use (**Figure 31-1**).

Ulcerative Colitis

For UC, guidelines specify various treatment approaches depending on the severity and location of disease. Distal colitis, identified as lesions below the splenic flexure, may be treated with oral, rectal, or IV agents depending on the severity of disease. Rectal agents should not be used in patients with extensive colitis due to the location of disease. The decision to use systemic or local preparations for distal colitis largely depends on patient preference; however, topical products allow for less systemic absorption, less frequent dosing, and a quicker onset of effect (**Figure 31-2**). Treatment of mild UC is best achieved with the use of aminosalicylates. The combination of oral and rectal aminosalicylates is more effective than either therapy alone. Corticosteroids may be used con-

currently with aminosalicylates for moderate UC exacerbations. Depending on the severity of the exacerbation and the location of the lesions, either rectal or oral preparations may be appropriate. Severe exacerbations may require hospitalization. Discontinuation of oral and topical therapy due to rapid GI transit time and the initiation of IV corticosteroid therapy are standard. If improvement in the condition is not seen in 7 to 10 days with IV corticosteroids, IV cyclosporine or IV infliximab may be considered. The use of IV cyclosporine is reserved for hospitalized patients who have not responded to IV steroids. Infliximab may be initiated in an outpatient or inpatient setting in patients with severe exacerbations after an adequate trial of steroids.

Surgery may be considered in patients whose disease fails to respond to drug therapy. The management of fulminant exacerbations is very similar to that of severe exacerbations, but the decision to perform a colectomy is considered at a much earlier stage for fulminant exacerbations. Along with definitive therapy, supportive measures including bowel rest, IV fluids, and adequate nutrition should be considered for those with severe and fulminant exacerbations. For those with frequent exacerbations or steroid dependence, immunosuppressive agents such as 6-mercaptopurine and azathioprine should be considered to induce and maintain remission. Typically, immunosuppressive agents are initiated after the patient can tolerate oral medications and are initiated along with aminosalicylate and corticosteroid therapy. The goal is to taper the corticosteroid and continue the aminosalicylate along with the immunosuppressive therapy for maintenance of remission.

Methotrexate has not been adequately studied in patients with UC and therefore is not recommended. Antibiotic therapy has not been shown to improve UC symptoms.

Drug Selection

Sulfasalazine was considered the first-line aminosalicylate because of its remarkable efficacy, low cost, and availability in oral liquid and tablet preparations; however, it must be taken four times a day and causes significant adverse drug reactions. For maximum therapeutic benefit, 4 to 8 g/d is necessary, so patients must take up to 16 tablets or 32 teaspoonfuls daily. In addition, immediate-release sulfasalazine has activity limited to the colon, making it less effective in conditions affecting the upper GI tract.

Mesalamine has emerged as the aminosalicylate of choice because of its availability in many formulations, dosing frequency, and its low side effect profile, but it is more expensive than sulfasalazine. Depending on the oral formulation and the severity of the disease, patients may need to take 6 to 16 pills daily to attain maximum therapeutic benefit. Normal dosages of oral mesalamine are 2 to 4.8 g/d. Olsalazine and balsalazide are not used as often because of their added cost without any significant clinical benefit.

The ideal corticosteroid for treating IBD would have high glucocorticoid activity, a low side effect profile, targeted

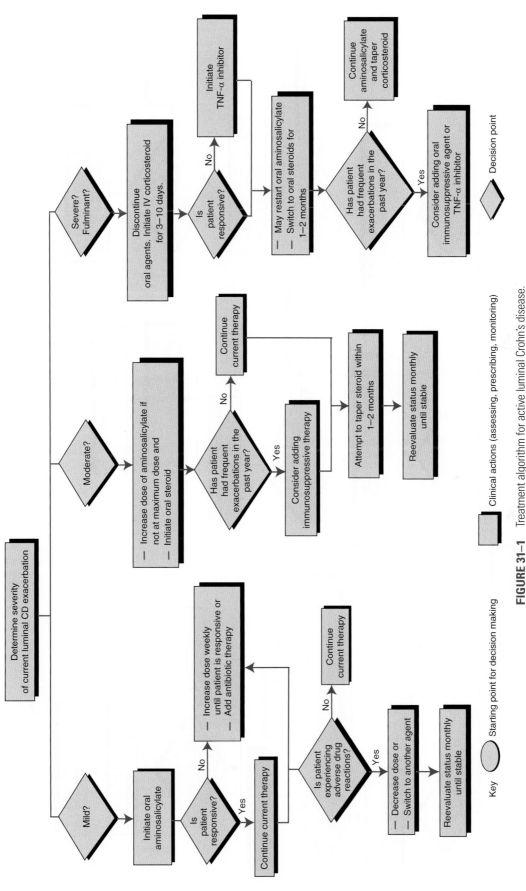

FIGURE 31–1 Treatment algorithm for active luminal Crohn's disease.

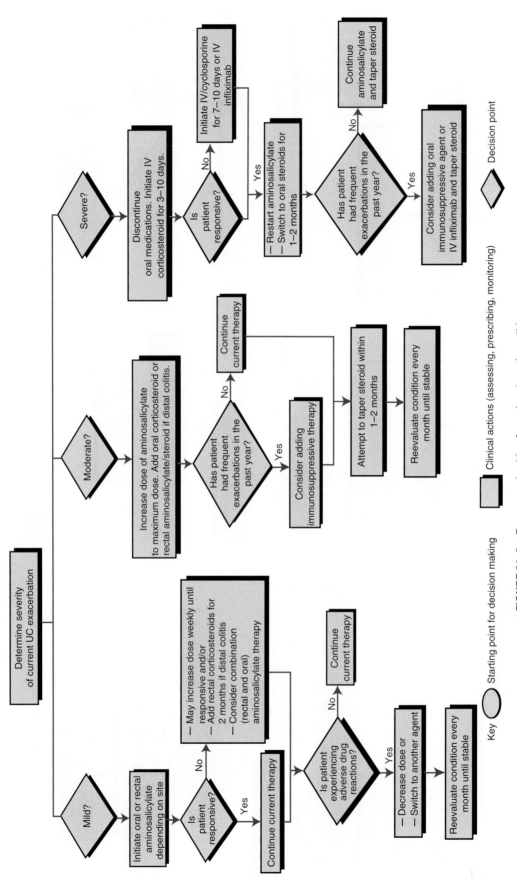

FIGURE 31–2 Treatment algorithm for active ulcerative colitis.

delivery to the diseased site and would be poorly absorbed from the GI tract, allowing for localized activity. Oral budesonide (Entocort) is approved specifically for the acute treatment of IBD due to its ideal characteristics, but due to its increased cost, other corticosteroids are used frequently to treat an acute exacerbation. The choice of steroid depends on the route of administration, onset of action, and glucocorticoid versus mineralocorticoid potency. In general, agents with more glucocorticoid activity are preferred over mineralocorticoid steroids because they have better anti-inflammatory action. Oral agents are used primarily in patients with localized or generalized disease with mild to moderate exacerbations, rectal formulations are reserved for patients with mild to moderate exacerbations of distal UC disease, and IV treatment may be initiated in patients with severe exacerbations of CD or UC.

The use of immunosuppressive agents varies based on the type of IBD and the severity of disease. Cyclosporine is reserved for the acute treatment of severe UC exacerbations because of the high cost of therapy, and high incidence of severe side effects. Because of a lack of comparative trials of methotrexate and azathioprine or 6-mercaptopurine, it is difficult to determine which agent would be considered first line; however, there are more data to support the use of azathioprine or 6-mercaptopurine than methotrexate for CD and UC. Azathioprine and 6-mercaptopurine are equally efficacious, with similar pharmacokinetic, adverse drug reaction, and cost profiles, so no great distinction can be made between the two.

The main distinction between methotrexate and the other two agents is its availability as an intramuscular injection and its dosing schedule. The infrequent dosing schedule of oral and intramuscular methotrexate may promote either compliance or noncompliance with the medication, depending on the patient. Combining these agents for the induction and maintenance of remission is not recommended because of overlapping side effect profiles and lack of improved efficacy data.

If antibiotic therapy is warranted, metronidazole or ciprofloxacin is an acceptable agent, depending on patient-specific factors.

There are a few differences among the TNF-α inhibitors that may make one agent more favorable in certain patients than others. Infliximab is the only product that is approved for the treatment of patients with severe, refractory UC or fistulizing CD. Therefore, it remains the best option in these patients at this time. For patients with luminal CD who are able to self-inject themselves, either adalimumab or certolizumab pegol may be an option. Adalimumab and certolizumab pegol are available as a prefilled syringe for convenience; however, adalimumab is administered subcutaneously as one injection every 2 weeks whereas certolizumab pegol is administered subcutaneously as two injections every 4 weeks. Infliximab may also be used for luminal CD; however, since it is an IV infusion, it must be administered by a health care practitioner in a monitored setting. Also, since adalimumab and certolizumab pegol are fully humanized monoclonal antibodies, the risk of infusion reactions, hypersensitivity, and development of autoantibodies are less likely than with infliximab. Adalimumab has also been found effective in patients who have previously not responded to infliximab (Sandborn, et al., 2007).

Special Population Considerations

Pediatrics

IBD is typically diagnosed early in life, usually during the second or third decade, leading to significant implications of IBD in the pediatric population. Treatment must be aggressive to limit the potential for nutritional deficiencies leading to stunted growth, malnutrition, and anemia. However, many of the medications lead to untoward effects or are not well studied in pediatrics. The use of long-term corticosteroids may lead to growth abnormalities, whereas ciprofloxacin use is contraindicated in children because it can cause arthropathy, resulting in poor bone formation. Infliximab is indicated for inducing or maintaining remission of CD in children older than age 6. The safety and efficacy of infliximab is not well studied in children with UC. Certolizumab pegol has not been studied in children. Adalimumab has been studied in children with CD but is not indicated in children at this time. Supplemental therapy including proper nutrition, iron therapy, and adequate hydration should also be considered to maintain growth and general health. Treating IBD in children involves aggressively managing the condition as well as the side effects with the limited options.

Pregnancy

The fertility rate in women with IBD is similar to the general population, but spontaneous abortions, stillbirths, and developmental defects are more common in pregnant women with active disease. Therefore, IBD should be treated aggressively in pregnant women to limit dehydration, anemia, and nutritional deficiencies that could adversely affect fetal outcomes. However, treatment options are limited for pregnant women due to the risk of teratogenicity or unwanted effects on the fetus. Methotrexate is absolutely contraindicated in pregnancy and lactation due to its potential for spontaneous abortions and teratogenicity. Data are controversial regarding the use of mercaptopurine and azathioprine during pregnancy. If either of these agents is necessary during pregnancy, an azathioprine dosage of 2 mg/kg/d or less is recommended to limit pancytopenia in the fetus. Azathioprine and mercaptopurine are contraindicated during nursing due to the potential of fetal immunosuppression. The use of cyclosporine should be reserved for severe refractory cases because it can cause growth retardation. The TNF inhibitors for IBD are all pregnancy category B; however, there are not adequate studies in humans to determine their safety in pregnancy. Therefore, they should only be reserved in patients with severe refractory disease whereby the benefits significantly outweigh the potential risks such as immunosuppression. Ciprofloxacin and metronidazole should also be avoided in pregnancy and lactation because they can cause fetal malformations. Corticosteroids may be used at the lowest doses possible to induce remission for the shortest period of time to limit adrenal suppression of the fetus. Women taking sulfasalazine should be given higher dosages of folate (2 mg/d) because sulfasalazine interferes with folate absorption. Preconception counseling is imperative to discuss the condition, lifestyle changes, nutritional issues, and treatment options with the patient. Special attention should be given to maintaining body weight before conception and preventing exacerbations during pregnancy.

MONITORING PATIENT RESPONSE

Various parameters must be monitored to detect efficacy and toxicity associated with therapy. Efficacy parameters include signs and symptoms of CD and UC, which are well defined in the Working Definition of Crohn's Disease Activity and Criteria for Severity of Ulcerative Colitis. Nutritional parameters such as weight, albumin, vitamin B_{12} levels, iron levels, and transferrin saturation should also be followed. Mental status and quality-of-life issues such as frequency of social interactions, attendance at work, and completion of activities of daily living all may indicate effectiveness of therapy. Although there are no definitive guidelines for the frequency of monitoring, it is important to monitor these endpoints when adjustments are made in drug therapy or when exacerbations occur.

Specific monitoring of drug toxicities is imperative for all pharmacologic agents. CBC and liver function tests should be performed periodically to detect asymptomatic undesired reactions in patients taking sulfasalazine. In addition, renal function (i.e., blood urea nitrogen, serum creatinine) should be monitored routinely with aminosalicylates to identify nephrotoxicity.

Corticosteroid treatment is associated with significant drug toxicities, but most occur with long-term use. In general, short-term corticosteroid treatment does not require intense monitoring. However, patients who have uncontrolled hypertension or who are glucose intolerant must have their blood pressure or fasting blood glucose level monitored periodically while taking corticosteroids. For patients taking corticosteroids on a long-term basis, baseline tests including a lipid panel, electrolytes, and fasting blood glucose studies should be performed every 6 to 12 months. A baseline bone density scan may be judicious and may be repeated yearly.

Azathioprine and 6-mercaptopurine are both associated with significant side effects, so it is important to acquire a baseline CBC with differential and serum creatinine, amylase, and liver function tests. The CBC should be monitored more frequently during the initiation of therapy (every 1 to 2 weeks for the first 3 months) and then less frequently (every 3 to 6 months) for the duration of therapy. Liver function tests should be monitored every 3 months for the first year or until a stable dosage has been achieved, then every 4 to 6 months for the duration of treatment. Creatinine clearance is an important parameter in guiding the dosing regimen of azathioprine or 6-mercaptopurine, so serum creatinine and creatinine clearance should be monitored annually if renal function is stable and more often if fluctuations in dosages or renal function occur. Amylase is not routinely ordered, but it may be checked upon patient complaints due to the risk of pancreatitis.

During the initial phase of methotrexate therapy, CBC and liver function tests should be performed every 2 to 4 weeks. If methotrexate therapy is continued beyond 16 weeks, CBC and liver function tests should be monitored every 4 to 8 weeks for the duration of therapy. Dosage adjustments must be made based on creatinine clearance, so serum creatinine must be monitored at baseline and at every dosage change. If renal function is stable, serum creatinine should be monitored annually at a minimum. Liver biopsies may be obtained once yearly if the patient is taking methotrexate, although formal recommendations have not been made.

IV cyclosporine therapy requires daily monitoring of cyclosporine blood levels (200 to 400 ng/mL), blood urea nitrogen, serum creatinine, and blood pressure. Although cyclosporine is extensively metabolized by the liver, it is eliminated by the kidneys and is highly associated with permanent renal dysfunction; therefore, renal function must be monitored closely. Dosages should be adjusted daily based on renal function and cyclosporine blood levels. Opportunistic infections may occur with high-dose cyclosporine use, so CBC, signs of infection, and temperature should also be monitored daily.

TNF-α inhibitors are associated with many side effects; however, most do not occur commonly. Due to the rare incidence of serious side effects, routine laboratory monitoring is not indicated; however, a heightened awareness of the clinical symptoms of adverse events is warranted. Patients and health care professionals should routinely monitor for symptoms of heart failure, vasculitis, TB, infection, hepatotoxicity, and lupus-like syndrome. Autoantibodies to the TNF-α inhibitors are known to develop and can be monitored via serum levels. Patients who develop autoantibodies may be more likely to develop lupus-like syndrome or have reduced efficacy with the agents (West, et al., 2008). Routine administration of TNF-α inhibitors and concomitant administration of immunosuppressants limit the development of autoantibodies.

Metronidazole and ciprofloxacin do not require significant drug monitoring, but long-term antibiotic treatment may lead to superinfection, so signs and symptoms of infection should be noted and treated. Patients receiving metronidazole therapy should also be monitored for peripheral paresthesias.

PATIENT EDUCATION
Drug Information

Patients and caregivers need to understand that uncontrolled IBD may affect quality of life, psychological well-being, and general physical health, so adherence to medication therapy is imperative. In addition, due to the increased GI transit time during an exacerbation, patients may not fully absorb oral medications for any of their conditions, which may lead to poor control of their other conditions during an IBD exacerbation.

Patients should swallow the enteric-coated sulfasalazine or mesalamine tablets and capsules whole so that the dosage form can penetrate the affected area. Sulfasalazine can discolor body fluids (e.g., urine and tears), which may stain clothing and contact lenses. When taking metronidazole, patients must abstain from alcohol to avoid severe nausea and vomiting.

Often patients request chronic corticosteroid therapy because of its beneficial results, but these patients need to be informed of the long-term complications of corticosteroids and should be advised regarding other medications that may be more appropriate for chronic therapy. Patients also need to be aware that immunosuppressants (azathioprine, 6-mercaptopurine, methotrexate) take 10 to 15 weeks to take effect; therefore, adherence to the medication regimen is imperative even though resolution of symptoms will not be apparent until weeks later.

Although the TNF-α inhibitors are quite efficacious for IBD, patients must be made aware of the significant risks associated with them. In addition, if patients are prescribed either adalimumab or certolizumab pegol, they must be instructed on the proper self-administration of a subcutaneous injection as well as sterile technique and safe needle disposal.

Patient-Oriented Information Sources

Along with their health care professionals, there are many other resources available for patients who are seeking information on IBD. A local support group may be a good resource for patients having trouble dealing with the illness. Many local hospitals as well as the Crohn's and Colitis Foundation of America organize support groups for patients with IBD. For general medical information regarding IBD, the following websites offer helpful patient-specific information:

- AGA: www.gastro.org
- American College of Gastroenterology: www.acg.gi.org
- Crohn's and Colitis Foundation of America: www.ccfa.org
- MedlinePlus: www.nlm.nih.gov/medlineplus/
- National Institute of Diabetes, Digestive, and Kidney Diseases: www.niddk.nih.gov

Preventive Care

Nutritional Status

Nutritional status is a significant issue for patients with active IBD and those with surgical resections. Patients with IBD are at risk for stunted growth, malnutrition, dehydration, weight loss, iron deficiency anemia, macrocytic anemia, osteopenia,

and other conditions. Nutrient deficiencies of iron, vitamin B_{12}, zinc, folate, calcium, and vitamin D may result from decreased oral intake, malabsorption, excessive losses, hypermetabolism due to infection, or drug-induced side effects. Concurrent administration of folate with methotrexate and sulfasalazine and administration of calcium and vitamin D with corticosteroids are recommended to limit the potential for nutritional deficiencies. Also, due to folate deficiencies, patients with IBD are at risk of hyperhomocystinemia, resulting in an elevated potential for thrombosis. Vitamin B_6 and vitamin B_{12} supplementation is recommended to decrease homocysteine levels. Folate supplementation is especially important in women of child-bearing age.

Many special dietary agents have been studied in patients with IBD with varying results. Diets high in short-chain fatty acids are associated with a small decrease in disease severity, potentially due to an anti-inflammatory effect. Fish oils, have been associated with a decreased frequency of exacerbations potentially due to their anti-inflammatory properties. An area of new research interest is the role of probiotics such as *Lactobacillus* and *Saccharomyces* in the treatment of IBD. By altering the GI flora, it is theorized that probiotic agents assist with controlling IBD exacerbations.

Enteral and parenteral routes of nutrition have been routinely used to improve the nutritional status of IBD patients. In general, enteral nutrition is preferred due to the complications of infection, thrombosis, and pancreatitis associated with parenteral nutrition. Along with correcting nutritional deficiencies, enteral nutrition has also been studied as a primary treatment measure in combination with aminosalicylates. Parenteral nutrition, however, is advocated in severe exacerbations when bowel rest is in order for proper healing of the IBD. In general, nutritional supplementation plays a large role in the management of IBD. Depending on the severity of weight loss and general health status of the patient, a combination of vitamin and mineral supplementation along with either enteral or parenteral nutrition should be advocated.

Vaccination

Vaccination status in patients with IBD is critical. Since IBD is an autoimmune disease and treatment is focused on immunosuppressant therapy, patients are at higher risk for developing infections. Vaccination records should be reviewed routinely and updated as necessary. Patients taking TNF inhibitors are at risk for hepatitis B reactivation; therefore, screening patients prior to therapy may be prudent. Patients taking an immunosuppressant cannot receive live vaccines; however, they are eligible for inactivated vaccines such as influenza, pneumococcal, meningococcal, tetanus, and hepatitis B (Kornbluth & Sachar, 2010).

Cancer Screening

Patients with IBD are at a higher risk for colorectal cancer (Eaden, et al., 2001). The extent of the risk depends on the extent, course, and duration of the disease in a particular individual. Due to the increased risk, patients with IBD for a minimum of 8 years should be screened for colorectal cancer with a colonoscopy and biopsy. Although the data are conflicting as to how often patients should be screened, the American College of Gastroenterology recommends either annually or biannually (Kornbluth & Sachar, 2010).

Complementary and Alternative Therapies

Alternative therapies are used by many patients with IBD: according to one study, 47% of patients with IBD had used alternative therapies for their condition. The most common alternative therapies used were Acidophilus and flaxseed, along with massage therapy, even though data are limited regarding the efficacy of these agents in IBD. Omega-3 fatty acids have also been studied for use in IBD. The National Institutes of Health reported variable results with the use of omega-3 fatty acids for IBD, so widespread use cannot be endorsed at this time (Agency for Healthcare Research and Quality, 2004).

Surgical options are considered in patients who are at risk for a further decline in physical health and quality of life resulting from frequent exacerbations that are unresponsive to conventional therapy. Surgical options include proctocolectomy for UC and a variety of ostomy procedures for patients

TABLE 31.6	Surgical Interventions
Procedure	**Area of Resection**
Sigmoid colostomy	Distal end of large intestine
Descending colostomy	Descending colon and rectum
Transverse colostomy	Small portion of transverse colon
Proctocolectomy/ileostomy	Entire rectum and large intestine

with CD, depending on the location of disease (**Table 31.6**). Proctocolectomy, the removal of the entire colon and rectum, is a curative intervention for UC. However, surgical procedures for CD are not curative because exacerbations may recur in existing areas of the GI tract, and surgery is used only to maintain remission.

For patients who have undergone surgery, the practitioner must pay close attention to general drug therapy issues. Because of the resection of the GI tract, these patients have issues similar to those of patients with short bowel syndrome. Rectally administered agents such as suppositories and enemas are ineffective in patients with any type of lower GI resection. Depending on the site of resection, sustained-released agents and medications targeted to specific areas of the GI tract also are ineffective in general.

Case Study

B. F., age 28, presents with diarrhea and abdominal pain. He says he feels weak and feverish. His symptoms have persisted for 5 days. He tells you he has 8 to 10 bowel movements each day, although the volume of stool is only about "half a cupful." Each stool is watery and contains bright-red blood. Before this episode, he had noticed a gradual increase in the frequency of his bowel movements, which he attributed to a new vitamin regimen. He has not traveled anywhere in the past 4 months and has taken no antibiotics recently. His medical history is significant for UC; his most recent exacerbation was 2 years ago. He is taking no medications except vitamins.

Examination findings include a tender, slightly distended abdomen. His BP is 122/84 sitting, 110/78 standing; HR 96 bpm; and temperature 100°F. Otherwise, physical findings are unremarkable. Laboratory study results reveal hemoglobin, 12 g/dL; hematocrit, 38%; white blood cell count, 12,000/mm³; platelet count, 242 k; sodium, 132; potassium, 3.6. All other study results are within normal limits. The most recent colonoscopy findings (4 years ago) revealed granular, edematous,

friable mucosa with continuous ulcerations extending throughout the descending colon.

DIAGNOSIS: EXACERBATION OF ULCERATIVE COLITIS

1. List specific goals of treatment for B. F.
2. What drug therapy would you prescribe? Why?
3. What are the parameters for monitoring success of the therapy?
4. Discuss specific patient education based on the prescribed therapy.
5. List one or two adverse reactions for the selected agent that would cause you to change therapy.
6. What would be the choice for the second-line therapy?
7. What over-the-counter and/or alternative therapies might be appropriate for B. F.?
8. What lifestyle changes would you recommend to B. F.?
9. Describe one or two drug–drug or drug–food interactions for the selected agent.

BIBLIOGRAPHY

*Starred references are cited in the text.

*Agency for Healthcare Research and Quality. (2004). *Effects of omega-3 fatty acids on lipids and glycemic control in type 2 diabetes and the metabolic syndrome, and on inflammatory bowel disease, rheumatoid arthritis, renal disease, systemic erythematous lupus, and osteoporosis.* Publication no. 04-E012-1. (URL: http://www.ahrq.gov/clinic/epcsums/o3lipidsum.htm.)

*American Gastroenterological Association. (2001). *The burden of gastrointestinal diseases.* Bethesda, MD: Author.

Cabre, E., & Gassull, M. A. (2003). Nutritional and metabolic issues in inflammatory bowel disease. *Current Opinions in Clinical Nutrition and Metabolic Care, 6,* 563–576.

Colombel, J. F., Lemann, M., Cassagnou, M., et al. (1999). A controlled trial comparing ciprofloxacin with mesalamine for the treatment of active Crohn's disease. *American Journal of Gastroenterology, 94,* 674–678.

Connell, W., & Miller, A. (1999). Treating inflammatory bowel disease during pregnancy: Risks and safety of drug therapy. *Drug Safety, 21*(4), 311–323.

*Eaden, J. A., Abrams, K. R., & Mayberry, J. F. (2001). The risk of colorectal cancer in ulcerative colitis: A meta-analysis. *Gut, 48,* 526–535.

*Everhart, J. E. (Ed.). (2008). *The burden of digestive diseases in the United States.* U.S. Department of Health and Human Services, Public Health Service, National Institutes of Health, National Institutes of Diabetes and Digestive and Kidney Diseases. Washington, DC: U.S. Government Printing Office; NIH Publication No. 09-6443.

Friedman, S., & Regueiro, M. D. (2002). Pregnancy and nursing in inflammatory bowel disease. *Gastroenterology Clinics of North America, 31,* 265–273.

Friend, D. R. (1998). Review article: Issues in oral administration of locally acting glucocorticosteroids for treatment of inflammatory bowel disease. *Alimentary Pharmacology and Therapeutics, 12,* 591–603.

Gassull, M. A. (2003). Nutrition and inflammatory bowel disease: Its relation to pathophysiology, outcome, and therapy. *Digestive Disorders, 211,* 220–227.

Graham, T. O., & Kandil, H. M. (2002). Nutritional factors in inflammatory bowel disease. *Gastroenterology Clinics of North America, 31,* 203–218.

*Halfverson, J., Jess, T., Bodine, L., et al. (2007). Longitudinal concordance for clinical characteristics in a Swedish-Danish twin population with inflammatory bowel disease. *Inflammatory Bowel Disease, 13,* 1536–1544.

Irvine, E. J. (1997). Quality of life issues in patients with inflammatory bowel disease. *American Journal of Gastroenterology, 92,* 18S–24S.

Klotz, U. (2000). The role of aminosalicylates at the beginning of the new millennium in the treatment of chronic inflammatory bowel disease. *European Journal of Clinical Pharmacology, 56,* 353–362.

*Kornbluth, A., & Sachar, D. B. (2010). Ulcerative colitis practice guidelines in adults: American College of Gastroenterology, Practice Parameters Committee. *American Journal of Gastroenterology, 105,* 501–523.

Lee, S. D., & Cohen, R. D. (2002). Endoscopy in inflammatory bowel disease. *Gastroenterology Clinics of North America, 31,* 119–132.

Lesko, S. M., Kaufman, D. W., Rosenberg, L., et al. (1985). Evidence for an increased risk of Crohn's disease in oral contraceptive users. *Gastroenterology, 89,* 1046–1049.

Lichtenstein, G. R., Abreu, M. T., Cohen, R., et al. (2006). American Gastroenterological Association institute technical review on corticosteroids, immunomodulators, and infliximab in inflammatory bowel disease. *Gastroenterology, 130,* 940–987.

*Lichtenstein, G. R., Diamond, R. H., Wagner, C. L., et al. (2009). Clinical trial: Benefits and risks of immunomodulators and maintenance infliximab for IBD-subgroup analyses across four randomized controlled trials. *Alimentary Pharmacology and Therapeutics, 30,* 210–226.

*Lichtenstein, G. R., Hanauer, S. B., & Sandborn, W. J. (2009). Management of Crohn's disease in adults. *American Journal of Gastroenterology.* e-pub ahead of print.

Liu, Y., van Kruiningen, H. J., West, A. B., et al. (1995). Immunocytochemical evidence of *Listeria, Escherichia coli,* and *Streptococcus* antigens in Crohn's disease. *Gastroenterology, 108,* 1396–1404.

*Loftus, E. V. (2004). Clinical epidemiology of inflammatory bowel disease: Incidence, prevalence, and environmental influences. *Gastroenterology, 126,* 1504–1517.

Murray, A., Oliaro, J., & Schlup, M. (1995). *Mycobacterium paratuberculosis* and inflammatory bowel disease: Frequency distribution in serial colonoscopic biopsies using the polymerase chain reaction. *Microbios, 83,* 217–228.

*National Institute of Diabetes and Digestive and Kidney Diseases. (2010). *Digestive disease statistics for the United States.* U.S. Department of Health and Human Services, Public Health Service, National Institutes of Health, National Digestive Disease Information Clearinghouse. NIH Publication No. 10-3873.

Orholm, M., Munkholm, P., Langholz, E., et al. (1991). Familiar occurrence of inflammatory bowel disease. *New England Journal of Medicine, 324,* 84–88.

*Pederson, N., Duricova, D., Elkjaer, M., et al. (2010). Risk of extra-intestinal cancer in inflammatory bowel disease: Meta-analysis of population-based cohort studies. *American Journal of Gastroenterology, 105,* 1480–1487.

Pullan, R. D., Rhodes, J., Ganesh, S., et al. (1994). Transdermal nicotine for active ulcerative colitis. *New England Journal of Medicine, 330,* 811–815.

*Reddy, D., Siegel, C. A., Sands, B. E., & Kane, S. (2006). Possible association of isotretinoin and inflammatory bowel disease. *American Journal of Gastroenterology, 101,* 1569–1573.

Rubin, D. T., & Hanauer, S. B. (2000). Smoking and inflammatory bowel disease. *European Journal of Gastroenterology and Hepatology, 12,* 855–862.

Safdi, M., DeMicco M., Sninsky, C., et al. (1997). A double-blind comparison of oral vs. rectal mesalamine vs. combination therapy in the treatment of distal ulcerative colitis. *American Journal of Gastroenterology, 92,* 1867–1871.

*Sandborn, W. J., Rutgeerts, P., Enns, R., et al. (2007). Adalimumab induction therapy for Crohn's disease previously treated with infliximab: A randomized trial. *Annals of Internal Medicine, 146,* 829–838.

Sandborn, W. J., & Targan, S. R. (2002). Biologic therapy of inflammatory bowel disease. *Gastroenterology, 122,* 1592–1608.

Sands, B. E. (2000). Therapy of inflammatory bowel disease. *Gastroenterology, 118,* S68–S82.

Sonnenberg, A., McCarty, D. J., & Jacobsen, S. J. (1991). Geographic variation of inflammatory bowel disease within the United States. *Gastroenterology, 100,* 143–149.

Stein, R. B., & Hanauer, S. B. (1999). Medical therapy for inflammatory bowel disease. *Gastroenterology Clinics of North America, 28*(2), 297–321.

Thompson, N. P., Montgomery, S. M., Pounder, R. E., et al. (1995). Is measles vaccination a risk factor for inflammatory bowel disease? *Lancet, 345,* 1071–1074.

Ursing, B., Alm, T., Barany, F., et al. (1982). A comparative study of metronidazole and sulfasalazine for active Crohn's disease: The Cooperative Crohn's Disease Study in Sweden. II: Results. *Gastroenterology, 83,* 550–562.

Walker, E. A., Roy-Byrne, P. P., Katon, W. J., et al. (1990). Psychiatric illness and irritable bowel syndrome: A comparison with inflammatory bowel disease. *American Journal of Psychiatry, 147,* 1656–1661.

*West, R. L., Zelinkova, Z., Wolbink, G. J., et al. (2008). Immunogenicity negatively influences the outcome of adalimumab treatment in Crohn's disease. *Alimentary Pharmacology and Therapeutics, 28*(9), 1122–1126.

Pharmacotherapy for Genitourinary Tract Disorders

Urinary Tract Infection

Urinary tract infection (UTI) is a broad term used to describe inflammation of the urethra, bladder, and kidney. Bacteria, yeast, or chemical irritants can cause inflammation in the urinary tract. UTIs are a common problem encountered in health care. UTIs occur across the life span. As many as 10% of women experience at least one episode of acute uncomplicated urinary infection in a year, and 60% have at least one episode during their lifetime. The peak incidence of infection occurs in young, sexually active women ages 18 to 24. Recurrent episodes are experienced by as many as 5% of women at some time during their life.

CAUSES

Women contract UTIs in a 30:1 ratio to men because of their short urethra and its proximity to the rectum. Sexual intercourse is a contributing factor. With intercourse, periurethral and urethral bacteria may ascend into the bladder. After age 65, the ratio of UTIs in women to men becomes closer to 1. Risk factors for UTIs in men include homosexuality, intercourse with an infected partner, and an uncircumcised penis.

Normal urine is sterile. Infection occurs when microorganisms, usually bacteria from the digestive tract, cling to the opening of the urethra and multiply. *Escherichia coli* is the causative pathogen in 85% to 90% of community-acquired UTIs. *Staphylococcus saprophyticus* accounts for approximately 5% to 20% of UTIs in young women.

Bacterial growth is decreased by dilute urine and a low urine pH. Glucose in urine is an enhanced medium for the growth of *E. coli*. The urine from pregnant women has a more suitable pH for growth of *E. coli*. Diaphragm and spermicide use (nonoxynol-9), estrogen deficiency, and constipation also are risk factors for UTIs. Inefficient bladder emptying causes UTIs because of stagnating urine. Underlying conditions that predispose to UTI are listed in **Box 32.1.**

PATHOPHYSIOLOGY

The development of a UTI depends on the virulence of the organism, the inoculum size, and the adequacy of the host's defense mechanisms. In general, the urinary tract is resistant to

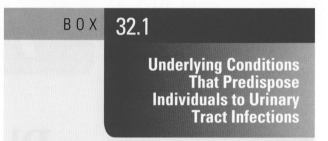

BOX 32.1

Underlying Conditions That Predispose Individuals to Urinary Tract Infections

- Female sex
- Pregnancy
- Diabetes
- Chronic degenerative neurologic conditions
- Paralysis
- Recurrent UTI
- Ineffective bladder emptying
- Estrogen deficiency
- Constipation
- Delayed postcoital micturition
- History of recurrent childhood UTI
- Sickle cell disease
- Polycystic kidney disease
- Structural defects of the urinary system
- Renal transplant

invading bacteria and rapidly eliminates organisms that reach the bladder. When bacteria enter the bladder, there is increased micturition and diuresis to empty the bladder.

Most pathogens enter the urinary tract and ascend the urethra to the bladder. Most of the microorganisms are from fecal flora, but the vagina is an important source of infecting organisms. Bacteria that cause UTIs originate in the fecal flora, colonize the vagina and periurethral introitus, and ascend to the urethra and bladder. In the bladder, the bacteria multiply and travel up the urethra to the renal pelvis and parenchyma, especially if there is vesicoureteral reflux. With cystitis, there is silent involvement of the kidneys in approximately 50% of cases.

The longer urethra in men increases the distance between the rectum and the urethral meatus, and the drier environment around the urethra and the antibacterial activity of prostatic fluid also decrease the risk of UTIs in men.

DIAGNOSTIC CRITERIA

In women of childbearing age, the most frequent presentation of cystitis is the classic triad of urinary urgency, frequency, and dysuria, with symptoms of abrupt onset. There may also be pressure or fullness in the suprapubic area and back pain. Pyelonephritis presents with flank pain, nausea and vomiting, and temperature greater than 100.4°F (38°C) with or without symptoms of cystitis.

Differentiation must be made between complicated and uncomplicated UTI before progressing with diagnostic evaluation. An uncomplicated UTI is defined as occurring in a premenopausal, sexually active, nonpregnant woman who has not recently had a UTI. A complicated UTI is one that occurs in a man, a postmenopausal or pregnant woman, or a patient with urinary structural defects, neurologic lesions, or a catheter. A UTI also is considered complicated if symptoms have persisted for more than 7 days. In sexually active men with symptoms of cystitis, urethritis must be ruled out. Pyelonephritis presents with recurrent fevers, chills, flank pain, and a positive urine culture.

The diagnosis of UTI is made after a careful history, physical examination, and limited laboratory studies. Because UTI is the most common infection for which adults receive antibiotics, its evaluation and management must be cost-effective. Cultures are not performed if the criteria for an uncomplicated UTI are met, because antimicrobial susceptibility profiles are predictable and culture results do not return until after the symptoms have resolved.

The leukocyte dipstick test is 75% to 95% sensitive in detecting pyuria. Examination of spun or unspun urine that does not show leukocytes should suggest a diagnosis other than UTI. Hematuria occurs in approximately half of all acute UTIs. Pretreatment and posttreatment cultures should be performed for male patients. Pretreatment cultures are ordered in suspected pyelonephritis; posttreatment cultures are performed only if symptoms recur within 2 weeks or if the symptoms do not resolve with treatment initially.

INITIATING DRUG THERAPY

A urine culture with 10^5/mL organisms or greater is a diagnostic indicator of UTI with or without symptoms. A patient who has symptoms and a culture with 10^2/mL organisms or greater is treated.

Although most UTIs resolve spontaneously if not treated, they are treated for symptom relief. The treatment for UTI is antibiotics. The choice of antibiotic and the length of treatment depend on whether the infection is uncomplicated or complicated and on the sex and age of the patient.

A short course of treatment increases compliance and decreases the cost and side effects. For women infected with susceptible *E. coli,* cure rates of 90% to 95% are achieved with 3 days of therapy. There is no benefit to treatment exceeding 3 days in uncomplicated UTIs in women unless nitrofurantoin is used; the length of treatment for this drug is 5 to 7 days.

Current resistance to ampicillin is near 50% in most regions of the United States. Therefore, it is not recommended for first-line therapy unless the organism is shown to be sensitive to it. Resistance to trimethoprim-sulfamethoxazole (TMP-SMZ) is up to 20% in some areas of the United States, but resistance to nitrofurantoin remains low.

Goals of Therapy

The goals of therapy for UTIs are to destroy the offending organism, relieve symptoms, and prevent complications.

Antibiotics are discussed in detail in Chapter 8. Those used to treat UTIs are listed in **Table 32.1.**

Urinary Analgesics

This class of drugs is used for the symptomatic relief of pain, urgency, burning, frequency, and discomfort associated with trauma to the lower urinary tract mucosa. They are used in infection, trauma, surgery, endoscopic procedures, and catheterization. They should not be used for more than 2 days and are not used for treatment of a UTI per se, but for symptom relief.

The azo dye in this class is excreted in the urine and exerts a rapid topical analgesic effect on the mucosa of the urinary tract. The urinary analgesics are used with caution in pregnancy and lactation and are contraindicated in renal insufficiency. For additional information, see **Table 32.1.**

Selecting the Most Appropriate Agent

A 3-day course of TMP-SMZ or trimethoprim alone continues to be recognized as first-line treatment. There are concerns, however, about rare but serious skin reactions to the sulfa component and about growing resistance (about 10% in Canada). This drug should be avoided in patients treated within 6 months because they are more likely to have resistant organisms.

Nitrofurantoin has a long history of good efficacy and continues as a first-line choice, even though a 7-day course is required. Despite heavy use, very little resistance to nitrofurantoin has developed. Fluoroquinolones have more recently been introduced to treat UTIs, and they are very effective in a 3-day course. Their cost and the potential for developing resistance, however, suggest that they should remain a second-line choice for treatment. Cephalosporins, ampicillin, and amoxicillin should not be used unless the cultured organism is sensitive to these agents.

Cystitis and pyelonephritis are treated with the same antibiotic, but the treatment course for pyelonephritis is longer. The most desirable antibiotic is one that is low in cost with an infrequent dosing schedule, lack of resistance in local pathogens, long duration in the urinary tract, and the potential to decrease the number of *E. coli* in the vaginal and fecal reservoirs. The antibiotic selected should spare the protective, natural bacterial flora of the vagina and gastrointestinal tract, and there should be a low side effect profile. Nonpregnant women with uncomplicated cystitis may be treated with a 3-day course of antibiotics (except with nitrofurantoin, which is 5 to 7 days). Postmenopausal women should be treated for

TABLE 32.1 **Overview of Selected Agents for Urinary Tract Infection**

Generic (Trade) Name and Dosage	Selected Adverse Events	Contraindications	Special Considerations
Antibiotics			
trimethoprim-sulfamethoxazole (Bactrim) Children: 5 mg/kg/d in divided doses for 10 d Adults: 1 DS ql2h for 10d	Nausea/vomiting, anorexia, megaloblastic anemia, hallucinations, depression, seizures	Megaloblastic anemia Pregnancy (category C) Breast-feeding mother Not recommended for children <2 mo G6PD deficiency	May consider newer macrolide antibiotics, such as clarithromycin and azithromycin
trimethoprim (Trimpex) 100 mg q12h for 3 d	Same as above	Megaloblastic anemia Pregnancy (category C) Breast-feeding mother Sulfa allergy	G6PD-deficient patients can have hemolysis. May cause falsely elevated creatinine Increase fluid intake.
nitrofurantoin (Macrobid, Macrodantin) Macrobid—100 mg q12h for 7 d Macrodantin—100 mg qid for 7 d	Nausea, pulmonary allergic reaction, dizziness, hemolytic anemia	Anuria Oliguria Pregnancy at term Nursing mother	Take with food to increase absorption.
ciprofloxacin (Cipro) 100–250 mg q12h for 3 d for uncomplicated cystitis and 7 d for complicated cystitis, and 500 mg for 10–14 d for uncomplicated pyelonephritis	Nausea, diarrhea, altered taste, dizziness, drowsiness, headache, insomnia, agitation, confusion Serious: pseudomembranous colitis, Stevens-Johnson syndrome	Allergy to fluoroquinolones Avoid in patients <18 y Pregnancy Use with caution in renal disease, central nervous system disease, breast-feeding (safety not established)	Raises serum level of theophylline Avoid taking with aluminum- or magnesium-containing antacids. Food slows absorption. Drug interacts with antacids, theophylline, warfarin, probenecid, digoxin, foscarnet, glucocorticoids.
ofloxacin (Floxin) 200 mg q12h for 3 d for uncomplicated cystitis and 7 d for complicated cystitis, and 200–300 mg for 10–14 d for uncomplicated pyelonephritis	Nausea, diarrhea, headache, insomnia, photosensitivity	Pregnancy (category C) Breast-feeding Not recommended in children	Take at least 30 min before or 2 h after meal. Avoid taking with aluminum- or magnesium-containing antacids or sucralfate, iron, and multivitamins with zinc because these can decrease absorption. Increase fluid intake significantly.
levofloxacin (Levaquin) 250 mg qd for 3 d for uncomplicated cystitis and 7 d for complicated cystitis, and 10–14 d for uncomplicated pyelonephritis	Nausea, diarrhea, photosensitivity	Same as above	Increase fluid intake significantly. Avoid taking with aluminum- or magnesium-containing antacids or sucralfate, iron, and multivitamins with zinc because these can decrease absorption.
norfloxacin (Noroxin) 400 mg q12h for 3 d for uncomplicated cystitis and 7 d for complicated cystitis and 10–14 d for uncomplicated pyelonephritis	Seizures, dizziness, nausea, headache, tendinitis/tendon rupture	Same as above	Same as above
cefixime (Suprax) 400 mg qd for 3 d for uncomplicated cystitis and 7 d for complicated cystitis, and 10–14 d for uncomplicated pyelonephritis	Diarrhea GI upset, rash, drug fever, pruritus, headache, dizziness, vaginitis	Known allergy to cephalosporins Use with caution in penicillin-allergic patients. Use with caution in patients with renal impairment, continuous ambulatory peritoneal dialysis, dialysis, GI disease.	Pregnancy category B

| TABLE 32.1 | Overview of Selected Agents for Urinary Tract Infection (*Continued*) | | | |

Generic (Trade) Name and Dosage	Selected Adverse Events	Contraindications	Special Considerations
Urinary Analgesics			
methenamine (Urised) 2 tabs qid	Rash, anticholinergic effects, xerostomia, flushing, difficulty in urinating, acute urinary retention with benign prostatic hyperplasia, tachycardia, dizziness, blurry vision, urine or fecal discoloration	Glaucoma Not recommended in patients <6 y Pregnancy (category C) Breast-feeding Bowel obstruction Urinary obstruction Cardiospasm	May cause blue-green discoloration of urine or feces Is not antibacterial
phenazopyridine (Pyridium) 200 mg tid	Headache, rash, GI upset, hemolytic anemia	Renal insufficiency	Discolors urine and clothes (red-orange) Is not antibacterial Take after meals.
flavoxate (Urispas) 100–200 mg tid–qid	Nausea and vomiting, anticholinergic side effects, vertigo, headache, drowsiness, urticaria, confusion, tachycardia	GI obstruction Obstructive uropathies Glaucoma	Reduce dose on improvement.

G6PD, glucose-6-phosphate dehydrogenase

7 days (**Figure 32-1, Table 32.2,** and **Table 32.3**). Men also require a 7-day treatment because of the increased chance of a complicated infection and prostatic infection.

First-Line Therapy

The first-line choice for cystitis is TMP-SMZ (Bactrim). This drug combination has little impact on normal vaginal flora but decreases the number of *E. coli* in vaginal and fecal reservoirs, decreasing the chance of reinfection. Trimethoprim appears to be similar in efficacy but with fewer side effects; it can also be used in patients with sulfa allergies. The sulfa ingredient may be more important for complicated cystitis and pyelonephritis.

Nitrofurantoin has a long history of good efficacy and continues as a first-line choice, even though a 7-day course is required. Despite heavy use, very little resistance to nitrofurantoin has developed.

Patients with cystitis can also be given urinary tract analgesics. This group includes methenamine (Urised), phenazopyridine (Pyridium, Uristat), or flavoxate (Urispas).

Uncomplicated pyelonephritis is usually treated in the outpatient setting because of the available oral antibiotics. The patient with pyelonephritis is admitted to the hospital only if he or she cannot take oral fluids or oral antibiotics, has a high fever or marked debility, or has a social situation incompatible with outpatient treatment. First-line therapy for pyelonephritis is an antibiotic, as mentioned previously, for 10 to 14 days. Fluoroquinolones are usually given first if culture results are not available because of their broad spectrum of activity. No follow-up is required if the symptoms resolve.

Second-Line Therapy

Fluoroquinolones and fosfomycin are options for empiric therapy of recurrent cystitis. If symptoms of cystitis do not resolve after 3 days of therapy, a 7-day course of antibiotics is recommended. Fluoroquinolones are not recommended as first-line agents for uncomplicated cystitis because of the increased cost and concerns over development of quinolone resistance. They should be reserved for treatment of UTIs in men and postmenopausal women and for patients with complicated UTIs and pyelonephritis.

In pyelonephritis, a culture is obtained after treatment. If the urine is not free of bacteria after initial therapy, 4 to 6 more weeks of therapy is prescribed.

Third-Line Therapy

The recurrence rate for UTIs is approximately 20%. At this point, a urine culture is done and treatment is based on the culture results. If the patient has fewer than two UTIs a year, treatment can be based on the previous culture results. Women who have three or more recurrences annually may be offered the option of self-treatment of recurrences. Postcoital use of antibiotic prophylaxis is effective for women who have recurrences related to intercourse. Continuous antibiotic prophylaxis in a single bedtime dose is also accepted practice for women who have frequent recurrences. Antibiotics that have been shown to reduce the number of recurrences to 0.3 or fewer per year are TMP-SMZ 40 mg/200 mg, TMP 100 mg, norfloxacin 200 mg, and nitrofurantoin macrocrystals 50 to 100 mg.

Special Population Considerations
Geriatric

In elderly patients, UTIs are commonly asymptomatic. Postmenopausal women are more prone to UTIs because there are uropathogen-dominant vaginal flora with the loss of estrogen. Lactobacilli diminish and pH increases. Elderly patients are at

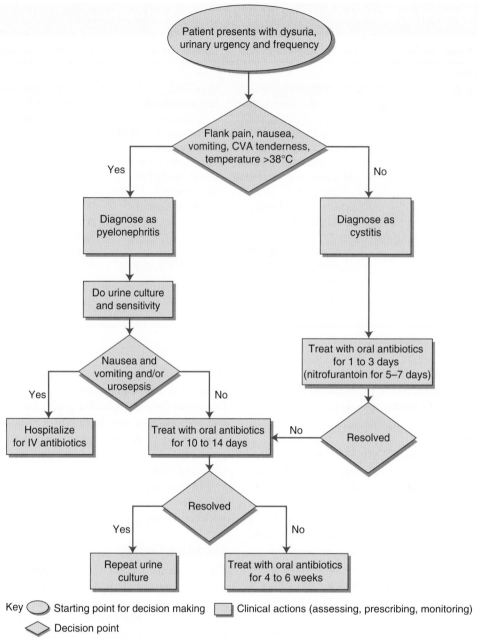

FIGURE 32–1 Treatment algorithm for UTI.

increased risk for UTIs. Approximately 10% to 20% of the population older than age 65 has bacteriuria related to factors such as fecal incontinence, incomplete bladder emptying, malnutrition, and increased urine pH. Any UTI in a man is considered complicated. *E. coli* and *Enterobacter* species are the usual organisms. In elderly men, *Proteus, Klebsiella, Serratia, Pseudomonas,* and *Enterococcus* species are also responsible for UTIs. UTIs in men are most often seen in conjunction with prostatic hyperplasia with partial obstruction or persistent prostatitis.

Nitrofurantoin is not recommended in the elderly because it requires a creatinine clearance of 40 mL/min. Treatment is for 7 to 10 days in women and 10 to 14 days in men with uncomplicated UTIs.

Women

Asymptomatic bacteriuria occurs in approximately 7% of pregnant women. Of these, pyelonephritis develops in 30% if the bacteriuria is not treated. Untreated UTIs can contribute to prematurity or stillbirth. Amoxicillin is effective in approximately two thirds of UTIs in pregnant women and is safe for the fetus. Also safe are cephalexin and nitrofurantoin (only during the first and second trimesters). Sulfonamides are safe except in the last trimester. In pregnancy, the urine is cultured 1 week after treatment and every 4 to 6 weeks during the pregnancy.

Physiologic changes in pregnancy increase the risk for pyelonephritis. The ureters become obstructed because of

TABLE 32.2	Recommended Order of Treatment for Uncomplicated Cystitis	
Order	**Agent**	**Comments**
First line	3-day oral therapy of • TMP-SMZ Or 7-d therapy of nitrofurantoin	Drink at least eight glasses of fluids. Initiate 7-d therapy in postmenopausal women and in men. May use urinary analgesics in combination with antibiotics Higher incidence of treatment failure with nitrofurantoin for 3 d, so 7-d use is recommended
Second line	7-day oral therapy of • TMP-SMZ May also use 7-d oral therapy of: • ciprofloxacin • levofloxacin • ofloxacin • norfloxacin	
Third line	Culture and sensitivity/ testing, then treat based on results	

TABLE 32.3	Recommended Order of Treatment for Uncomplicated Pyelonephritis	
Order	**Agents**	**Comments**
First line	Oral for 10–14 d: • ciprofloxacin • levofloxacin • enoxacin • norfloxacin • ofloxacin • sparfloxacin • TMP-SMZ • cefixime • cefpodoxime proxetil	Urine culture and sensitivity testing should be performed before treatment.
Second line	Oral therapy for 2–6 wk	
Third line	Hospitalization for IV therapy	For severe illness or possible urosepsis

blockage from the enlarged uterus. In addition, increased progesterone relaxes the smooth muscles of the ureter and bladder.

In 5% to 10% of women with UTI, there are no symptoms. Pregnant women should be screened for UTIs, and they must be treated regardless of whether they are symptomatic. Bacteriuria in pregnancy has been associated with a 20% to 30% incidence of pyelonephritis and premature delivery, intrauterine growth retardation, increased risk for death in the perinatal period, and congenital anomalies.

Children

UTIs in children may indicate a genitourinary anomaly. Accurate diagnosis usually requires invasive collection of urine, especially in very young children. It is important to start treatment quickly, especially in young children, because there is an increased risk of renal scarring in children under age 5 from UTIs. UTIs recur in 32% to 40% of children. Renal/bladder ultrasounds are recommended by the American Academy of Pediatrics in children under age 2 with a UTI. The American Academy of Pediatrics recommends 7 to 14 days of treatment for UTI in children.

MONITORING PATIENT RESPONSE

Cystitis that does not resolve or that recurs within a week after treatment requires culture and sensitivity testing and treatment with a fluoroquinolone for 7 days. UTIs recur within a year in approximately half of all women, although there is a very low incidence of pyelonephritis that develops as a result.

If pyelonephritis recurs within 2 weeks after treatment, a urine culture and sensitivity test and renal ultrasound or computed tomography scan should be performed to determine whether there is a urologic abnormality. If the organism is the same as the first, a 4- to 6-week course of antibiotics is recommended.

Patients who have three or more UTIs a year should be given prophylaxis, either continuous or postcoital. Continuous prophylaxis usually consists of TMP-SMZ 40 to 200 mg daily or three times a week. Postcoital therapy is indicated in women who identify intercourse as the cause of infection; the selected therapy is taken after intercourse. The use of estrogen replacement therapy in postmenopausal women decreases the number of recurrent UTIs. In cases of true relapse, the culture is repeated and therapy is prescribed for 2 to 4 weeks.

In pyelonephritis, a culture is repeated 1 to 2 weeks after completion of therapy. If there is a recurrence, therapy is recommended for 6 to 12 months.

PATIENT EDUCATION

Drug Information

Patients can get information about UTIs at http://kidney .niddk.nih.gov (National Institute of Diabetes and Digestive and Kidney Diseases); http://urinary-tract-infections.com; and http://www.urologychannel.com/uti.

Case Study

J . S., a 65-year-old woman with diabetes, seeks treatment for dysuria, frequent urination, flank pain, and costovertebral angle tenderness. She has a temperature of 102°F, and under the microscope her spun urine contains a large number of leukocytes.

DIAGNOSIS: CYSTITIS WITH POSSIBLE PYELONEPHRITIS

1. List specific goals for treatment for J. S.
2. What drug therapy would you prescribe? Why?
3. What are the parameters for monitoring success of the therapy?
4. Discuss specific patient education based on the prescribed therapy.
5. List one or two adverse reactions for the selected agent that would cause you to change therapy.
6. What would be the choice for second-line therapy?
7. What over-the-counter and/or alternative medications would be appropriate for J. S.?
8. What lifestyle changes would you recommend to J. S.?
9. Describe one or two drug–drug or drug–food interactions for the selected agent.

Lifestyle Changes

Various behavioral factors, such as voiding after intercourse, the direction of toilet paper use after bowel movements, type of menstrual protection used, and method of contraception, have been investigated to assess their impact on the frequency of UTIs. The use of spermicides changes the vaginal flora, increasing the colonization of *E. coli* and the frequency of UTIs. Women with recurrent UTIs should use a method of birth control that does not involve spermicides.

Other preventive measures include urinating before and after sexual intercourse and avoiding bubble baths and "feminine hygiene" products. Changing position while voiding helps to empty the bladder fully. Drinking six to eight glasses of water daily helps prevent UTIs. Urinating every 2 hours, taking the time to empty the bladder completely, also helps prevent UTIs. Foods that irritate the bladder should be avoided, including tea, coffee, alcohol, cola, chocolate, and spicy foods.

Complementary and Alternative Medicine

Cranberry juice concentrate or cranberry concentrate capsules have been recognized as alternatives to antibiotics or for the prevention of UTIs. Cranberry is believed to have anti-adherence properties in the urinary tract and acidifies urine. One 300- to 400-mg capsule is taken two times a day with a glass of water, or 8 to 16 ounces of preparations with at least 30% cranberry juice can be taken. Vitamin C, 500 mg every 4 hours for the duration of the UTI, has been suggested, with 1,000 to 1,500 mg/d for prevention of UTIs. Cranberry juice or tablets containing proanthocyanidin can reduce the rate of recurrences of UTI by one-half, exercising their effect by inhibiting adherence of *E. coli*.

Probiotics may decrease UTIs by restoring normal vaginal flora. Lactobacillus is thought to prevent colonization with *E. coli*.

BIBLIOGRAPHY

Clark, C., Kennedy, W., & Shortliffe, L. (2010). Urinary tract infections in children: When to worry. *Urology Clinics of North America, 37*(2), 229–241.

Drekonja, D., & Johnson, J. (2008). Urinary tract infections. *Primary Care: Clinics in Office Practice, 35*(2), 345–367.

Foster, R. (2008). Uncomplicated urinary tract infections in women. *Obstetric and Gynecologic Clinics, 35*(2), 235–248.

French, L., Phelps, K., Pothula, N., & Mushkbar, S. (2009). Urinary problems in women. *Primary Care: Clinics in Office Practice, 36*(1), 53–71.

Litza, J., & Brill, J. (2010). Urinary tract infections. *Primary Care: Clinics in Office Practice, 37*(3), 491–507.

Nicolle, L. (2008). Uncomplicated urinary tract infections in adults including uncomplicated pyelonephritis. *Urology Clinics of North America, 35*(1), 1–12.

Prostatic Disorders and Erectile Dysfunction

Disorders of the prostate appear as part of the normal aging process and also as abnormalities distinct from normal aging. Often it is not until age 40 that a man begins to show some form of noncancerous prostatic disorder, whereas prostate cancer usually is found after age 50. The incidence of prostatic disorders increases with age. It is estimated that 50% to 75% of men older than age 50 have benign prostatic hyperplasia (BPH), often with symptoms. Prostate cancer is the second most common type of cancer affecting men, with a lifetime prevalence of 17%. Black men have the highest incidence of prostate cancer. The age-adjusted death rate from prostate cancer is 64.4 per 100,000 for Black men compared to 26.6 per 100,000 for White men. Asian and Hispanic men are at lower risk than White men. In addition to race, other risk factors for prostate cancer are age and family history. The disease rarely occurs before age 45, but the incidence rises exponentially thereafter; nearly 70% of cases are diagnosed in men age 65 and older.

Prostate disorders are diagnosed through clinical manifestations and screening procedures to detect or rule out prostate cancer. Lack of knowledge about prostate cancer and lack of available screening procedures are the major deterrents to accurate and timely diagnosis of prostate cancer.

In a multinational epidemiologic study, 20% to 30% of men reported having a weak urine stream, hesitancy, urgency, incomplete emptying, or postvoid incontinence at least sometimes. Five percent to fifteen percent of men reported these same symptoms often (Coyne, et al., 2009).

Treatment of prostatic disorders itself may result in some untoward side effects, which must then also be managed. Often the man postpones seeking medical intervention and blames aging for many of the manifestations, thus delaying treatment. Some difficulties in seeking treatment can relate to the man's culture; sexuality—specifically, masculinity—can be perceived as synonymous with virility. For this reason, a man may choose not to discuss (even with a health care worker) clinical manifestations.

Prostatic disorders occur because of inflammation or infection (prostatitis), BPH, and prostate cancer; prostatitis can involve the bladder neck, thus becoming prostatocystitis. A bacterial infection is often the cause of prostatitis, although some nonbacterial forms of prostatitis do exist; inflammation can be chronic or acute.

Adenocarcinoma is the most common type of prostate cancer. Metastasis can follow slowly or quickly, and often the symptoms of metastasis are what lead the man to seek medical intervention.

Presenting manifestations of prostatic disorders are usually specific to the urinary tract and include difficulty in onset of urine flow with or without a low flow of urine, frequency or urgency in voiding, incontinence, distention of the bladder, and hematuria. Management of prostatic disorders is specific to the particular disorder (cancerous vs. noncancerous), with some overlap in treatment.

PROSTATITIS

CAUSES

Prostatitis is caused primarily by bacterial invasion, but some nonbacterial forms occur as well. This disorder can be acute or chronic. With acute bacterial prostatitis, the chief organisms involved are *Escherichia coli* and *Pseudomonas* species, although strains of staphylococci or streptococci also are seen. Chronic bacterial prostatitis is associated with *Pseudomonas, E. coli, Proteus mirabilis, Klebsiella pneumoniae,* and *Enterococcus* species, particularly *Enterococcus faecalis.* Nonbacterial prostatitis is essentially an inflammatory disorder.

PATHOPHYSIOLOGY

Often chronic, nonbacterial prostatitis is nonetheless problematic for the patient. Primary etiologies of this condition include two predominant patterns of inflammation. The first is that of an allergic condition and is associated with eosinophil infiltration. The second is a nonspecific form in which granulomatous inflammation by peculiar, large, pale macrophages is found.

In acute bacterial prostatitis, as with any type of bacterial invasion, the prostate becomes overwhelmed by the bacteria, leading to inflammatory response activation. Usually, acute bacterial prostatitis is seen as an infection ascending up the urinary tract, and younger men, ages 30 to 50, can be affected with this illness.

DIAGNOSTIC CRITERIA

Symptom manifestation revolves around urinary tract signs. There is pain in the lower abdomen, difficulty in bladder emptying with or without a small stream during urination, nocturia, and fever to 104°F (40°C). Along with the febrile state, as with other infections, general arthralgia and malaise can occur.

On examination and interview, the man often admits to painful ejaculation and pain in the rectal or perineal areas. All the symptoms are due to the edema associated with acute inflammation of the prostate. Because of the risk of generalized septicemia, pharmacotherapeutics are urgently warranted.

Culture isolation of prostatic urine is the most accurate method of diagnosis. Prostatic urine is defined as the third and fourth (urine) secretion specimens of four serial urine sample because prostatic fluid is at a significantly higher concentration in these last two of four serial voids. The four urine samples are obtained sequentially, beginning with the initial void, followed by a midstream urine specimen, prostatic massage secretion, and finally the urine voided after the prostatic massage. Standard laboratory culture techniques are applied to establish the causative organism.

Nonbacterial prostatitis is confirmed by negative prostatic urine cultures with a positive elevated white blood cell count and the presence of inflammatory cells in prostatic secretions. This condition and another nonbacterial type of prostatitis known as *prostatodynia* have the same symptoms as bacterial prostatitis. Treatment of the nonbacterial forms usually consists of symptom management without the use of antibiotics.

INITIATING DRUG THERAPY

Antibiotics are the required pharmacotherapy. (See Chapter 8.) Given that causative organisms are usually gram negative and, less commonly, gram positive, appropriate antibiotics are needed. The overall course of antibiotic therapy is of longer duration than that used to treat other systemic infections. Usually antibiotics are given for 4 to 6 weeks, but up to 12 weeks of therapy may be necessary. Because chronic bacterial prostatitis is a bacterial infection, an appropriate antibiotic with good tissue penetration in the prostate should be selected. Fluoroquinolones have demonstrated the best tissue concentration and are recommended as first-line agents. Although trimethoprim-sulfamethoxazole (TMP-SMZ) may be considered, the tissue penetration may not be as effective, and in many areas of the United States there is evidence of increasing uropathogenic resistance.

Second-line drugs include doxycycline, azithromycin, and clarithromycin. A 4- to 6-week course of therapy is usually recommended; however, a 6- to 12-week course is often needed

to eradicate the causative organism and to prevent recurrence, especially if symptoms persist after completion of the initial therapy. No guidelines exist for treating gram-positive organisms, but ciprofloxacin and levofloxacin have adequate gram-positive coverage as well as excellent gram-negative coverage, and both medications penetrate the prostate tissue well.

Adjunctive therapies that may be beneficial include the use of sitz baths, analgesics, stool softeners, and antipyretics, along with rest. Prostatic massage, voiding in a warm bath (to relax pelvic muscles), and discontinuation of alcohol and caffeinated beverages can also help to relieve symptoms. If possible, withdrawal from antidepressants, anticholinergics, or sedatives may also help bladder function.

Goals of Drug Therapy

The goal of pharmacotherapy for prostatitis is to eradicate the causative organism and restore the prostate to health. Prostatitis often becomes chronic, and therefore repeated trials with antibiotics or prolonged dosage schedules may be warranted.

Anti-Infectives

Table 33.1 depicts dosage information, adverse events, contraindications, and special considerations for the anti-infective management of bacterial prostatitis.

Trimethoprim–Sulfamethoxazole

This drug is a bacteriostatic combination product and is considered to be more powerful than its two components given separately. Also, when given as the combined form, resistance on the part of the causative organism arises less frequently. This agent ultimately adversely affects the production of proteins and nucleic acids of bacteria at the target (prostate) site. TMP-SMZ further inhibits growth of bacteria because of its antimetabolite property toward PABA (*para*-aminobenzoic acid). Drug–drug interactions can present when the patient is also taking phenytoin (Dilantin), oral hypoglycemics, or warfarin (Coumadin). Close monitoring of the seizure threshold, serum glucose level, or partial thromboplastin time is important in the patient on TMP-SMZ who is also taking these other agents.

Fluoroquinolones

Fluoroquinolones are also effective for bacterial prostatitis. Effective against gram-negative anaerobes and some gram-positive bacteria, these agents decrease the growth and replication of bacteria by inhibiting bacterial deoxyribonucleic acid (DNA) during synthesis. These agents may be the first choice for someone sensitive or allergic to TMP-SMZ.

The absorption of fluoroquinolones is reduced by milk, antacids (aluminum- or magnesium-based), iron or zinc salts, and sucralfate. For the patient who is also taking any of these medications, the dose should be taken either 2 hours after or 4 hours before the other medication.

Fluoroquinolones also affect the use of theophylline and warfarin. Elevated levels can occur, and thus a lower dosage of theophylline or warfarin may be necessary.

TABLE 33.1	Overview of Selected Antibiotics Used to Treat Acute Bacterial Prostatitis		
Generic (Trade) Name and Dosage	**Selected Adverse Events**	**Contraindications**	**Special Considerations**
trimethoprim-sulfamethoxazole (TMP-SMZ, Septra, Bactrim) 160 mg of TMP with 800 mg SMZ PO q12h	GI distress, rash	Allergy to sulfa and sulfa products	May prolong the INR for patients on oral anticoagulants
fluoroquinolones ciprofloxacin (Cipro) 500 mg BID norfloxacin (Noroxin) 400 mg bid levofloxacin (Levaquin) 250 mg daily	Headache, diarrhea, nausea, drowsiness, altered taste, insomnia, agitation, confusion Serious: pseudomembranous colitis, Stevens-Johnson syndrome	Allergy to macrolides Pregnancy and lactation Use with caution in patients with severe hepatic or renal disease.	May interfere with theophylline metabolism
doxycycline (Vibramycin) 200 mg PO as first dose, thereafter 100–200 mg PO q12h	GI distress, potential acute hepatotoxicity, potential for nephrotoxicity	Hypersensitivity to any of the tetracyclines Pregnancy and lactation	Decreased effectiveness with food and dairy products, so do not take with food unless side effects are significant. Can lead to diabetes insipidus because of antagonistic effect with antidiuretic hormone

Doxycycline

A long-acting tetracycline, doxycycline (Vibramycin) acts by inhibiting protein synthesis: binding of peptidyl transfer ribonucleic acid (tRNA) is blocked at ribosomal mRNA.

Many of the metal ions—aluminum, calcium, iron, magnesium, and zinc—can interfere by creating chelates with doxycycline. Thus, if these metals are given (and they often are as components of antacids), at least 2 hours should separate their use from the ingestion of doxycycline.

Azithromycin and Clarithromycin

These are macrolide antibiotics. Macrolides inhibits RNA-dependent protein synthesis by reversibly binding to the 50 S ribosomal subunits of susceptible microorganisms. They induce dissociation of tRNA from the ribosome during the elongation phase. Thus, RNA-dependent protein synthesis is suppressed, and bacterial growth is inhibited. Macrolides are mainly bacteriostatic but can be bacteriocidal depending on bacterial sensitivity and antibiotic concentration.

Selecting the Most Appropriate Agent

Oral antibiotics are the treatment agents of choice.

First-Line Therapy

The primary choice for first-line antibiotic therapy is a fluoroquinolone (**Table 33.2**). Therapy lasts for 4 to 6 weeks. See **Figure 33-1** for more information. TMP-SMZ may also be considered if treatment is in an area where there is not a high incidence of resistance.

Second-Line Therapy

Doxycycline, azithromycin, and clarithromycin are second-line agents. If the infection is not resolved with 4 to 6 weeks of drug treatment, therapy can be continued for up to 12 weeks.

Special Population Considerations

In older men who are taking fluoroquinolones, creatinine clearance must be monitored.

MONITORING PATIENT RESPONSE

As a group, anti-infective agents should begin to elicit results after the first week of therapy. Subjective response from the patient indicating alleviation of symptoms is helpful in monitoring the effectiveness of these medications. Some patients may not notice symptom resolution until after 2 weeks; they should be told this and encouraged to continue taking the

TABLE 33.2	Recommended Order of Treatment for Prostatitis	
Order	**Agents**	**Comments**
First line	Fluoroquinolones or TMP-SMZ	Ineffective against enterococci Treat for 4–6 wk
Second line	Doxycycline or azithromycin or clarithromycin	

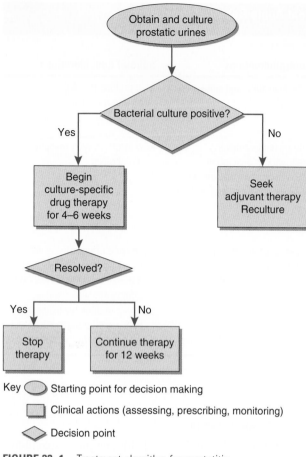

FIGURE 33–1 Treatment algorithm for prostatitis.

medication. Ultimately, 12 weeks of therapy may be required. Follow-up cultures may be obtained at the practitioner's discretion. Further diagnostic criteria may also be recommended for ongoing symptom manifestation.

PATIENT EDUCATION

The patient should understand potential side effects, interactions, and appropriate use of the medications. Literature can provide patients with a guide for such potential concerns as well as dosing information. With a prepared and knowledgeable patient, these medications are effective against prostatitis. Cost also can be a factor of concern to the patient. The practitioner should be aware of any financial constraints the patient may have, because compliance with medication is important for effective treatment of bacterial prostatitis.

BENIGN PROSTATIC HYPERPLASIA

BPH is the most common prostate problem in men older than age 50; the disease rarely causes symptoms before age 40. As life expectancy rises, so does the occurrence of BPH—an estimated

6.3 million men have BPH. In the United States alone, the disease accounts for 6.4 million doctor visits and more than 400,000 hospitalizations annually. Approximately 90% of men age 80 and older have histologic evidence of BPH, and more than 80% have BPH-related symptoms. Approximately 25% of men older than age 55 and 50% of men older than age 75 experience decreased urinary flow.

CAUSES

The cause of BPH is not well understood. It has been observed that BPH does not develop in men whose testes were removed before puberty. For this reason, some researchers believe that factors related to aging and the testes may spur the development of BPH. Men produce both testosterone and small amounts of estrogen. As men age, the amount of active testosterone in the blood decreases, leaving a higher proportion of estrogen. Studies performed on animals have suggested that BPH may occur because the higher amount of estrogen within the gland increases the activity of substances that promote cell growth. Another theory focuses on dihydrotestosterone (DHT), a substance derived from testosterone in the prostate, which may help control its growth. Some research has indicated that even with a drop in the blood's testosterone level, older men continue to produce and accumulate high levels of DHT in the prostate. This accumulation of DHT may encourage the growth of cells. Researchers have also noted that men who do not produce DHT do not develop BPH.

PATHOPHYSIOLOGY

The underlying pathophysiologic process of BPH is the formation of large, nonmalignant lesions at the periurethral region of the prostate gland. Prostatic hyperplasia is an overgrowth of normal cells in the stromal and epithelial tissues of the prostate gland. The hyperplasia originates in the transition zone of the prostate, which surrounds the prostatic urethra between the bladder and the anus. The etiology of the hyperplastic process is unknown, but it has been speculated that it is hormone-related because it occurs only in older men. The male aging process involves a decrease in testosterone production with a concomitant increase in estrogen; estrogen may be a sensitizer for the escalating hyperplasia.

Bladder control involves reflex activity of the peripheral autonomic nervous system (ANS). The reflex for normal micturition is housed in the brain stem and supported by descending and ascending pathways from the spinal cord. Both the external sphincter and the detrusor muscle are needed for bladder control. Reflex micturition is innervated at the S2 to S4 and T1 to L1 levels in the spinal cord. The cortical center of the brain appears to be important for inhibition or control of the micturition center to modulate contractile, filling, and expulsion activity.

Parasympathetic and sympathetic innervation is crucial to the role of the ANS in voiding. Parasympathetic interplay allows for the detrusor muscle to maintain tone and to contract, whereas sympathetic interplay allows for the bladder to expand and maintain a large filling capacity. It is for this reason that pharmacologic intervention is so effective in managing BPH—the ANS can be effectively manipulated by pharmacotherapy.

Disease manifests as urinary tract symptoms. Obstructed urine outflow, the predominant pattern, includes diminished force of the urine stream, an urgent need for nocturnal voiding, residual urine with or without overflow incontinence, and even a feeling of pressure in the abdomen. These manifestations result from either partial or complete compression of the urethra by the hyperplastic prostate. Bladder wall hypertrophy occurs, and herniation into the bladder can occur. Ultimately, if treatment is not initiated, a postrenal cause of renal failure can develop because of back-pressure on the renal system (i.e., the ureters) and the onset of hydronephrosis.

DIAGNOSTIC CRITERIA

Diagnosis of BPH usually begins with the patient seeking medical intervention because of the annoying symptoms. Along with a complete social history and physical examination, a digital rectal examination (DRE) is performed to palpate the prostate. The degree of prostate enlargement has not been found to correlate with the severity of symptoms; rather, the location of the enlargement is what leads to symptom manifestation.

The American Urological Association (AUA) has created a Symptom Index Scale (**Table 33.3**) to correlate symptom severity with prostate size. In this numeric scale symptoms are scored as mild (0 to 7 points), moderate (8 to 19 points), or severe (20 to 35 points). The AUA recommends that this scale be used on initial assessment and then for following the course of illness by periodic ongoing assessment of the patient. Such follow-up management enables the practitioner to initiate more acute or intensive therapy when the score increases. Patients with severe BPH symptoms should not be managed by this scale.

Postvoid catheterization is performed to ascertain the degree of urine retention; any amount of residual urine beyond 100 mL is considered significant. Uroflowmetry provides information about the force of the urine stream. Urodynamics can also be assessed using noninvasive pneumatic technology. Other diagnostic tools include x-ray films, digital ultrasound, computed tomography (CT) scans, magnetic resonance imaging (MRI), and radionuclide scans. Biopsies can be added to

TABLE 33.3	**AUA Symptom Index Scale**					
	AUA Symptom Score (Circle 1 Number on Each Line)					
Questions to Be Answered	**Not at All**	**Less Than 1 Time in 5**	**Less Than Half the Time**	**About Half the Time**	**More Than Half the Time**	**Almost Always**
1. Over the past month, how often have you had a sensation of not emptying your bladder completely after you finished urinating?	0	1	2	3	4	5
2. Over the past month, how often have you had to urinate again <2 h after you finished urinating?	0	1	2	3	4	5
3. Over the past month, how often have you found you stopped and started again several times when you urinated?	0	1	2	3	4	5
4. Over the past month, how often have you found it difficult to postpone urination?	0	1	2	3	4	5
5. Over the past month, how often have you had a weak urinary stream?	0	1	2	3	4	5
6. Over the past month, how often have you had to push or strain to begin urination?	0	1	2	3	4	5
7. Over the past month, how many times did you most typically get up to urinate from the time you went to bed at night until the time you got up in the morning?	0 (None)	1 (1 time)	2 (2 times)	3 (3 times)	4 (4 times)	5 (5 times or more)

the diagnostic workup for further clinical assessment of any hardened prostatic areas found by DRE. Laboratory monitoring of creatinine and blood urea nitrogen should be incorporated to determine whether renal involvement exists and, if so, to what degree. Prostate-specific antigen (PSA) levels can be elevated in patients with BPH.

Many symptoms of BPH stem from obstruction of the urethra and gradual loss of bladder function, which results in incomplete emptying of the bladder. The symptoms of BPH vary, but the most common ones involve changes or problems with urination, including a hesitant, interrupted, or weak stream; urgency, dribbling, or urinary retention; more frequent urination, especially at night; painful urination; and incontinence.

It is extremely important to evaluate men at risk for these symptoms. In 8 out of 10 cases, these symptoms suggest BPH, but they also can signal more serious conditions, such as prostate cancer.

INITIATING DRUG THERAPY

The two major classes of drugs used to treat BPH are α-adrenergic antagonists or α-blockers (doxazosin, terazosin, tamsulosin, and alfuzosin) and 5-α-reductase inhibitors (finasteride and dutasteride). Alpha-blockers relax the smooth muscle fibers of the bladder neck and prostate, thereby reducing the dynamic components of prostatic obstruction. Five-α-reductase inhibitors decrease levels of intracellular DHT (the major growth-stimulatory hormone in prostate cells) without reducing testosterone levels. This leads to prostatic size reduction of 20% to 30%. Symptom relief occurs within 2 weeks of initiating α-blockers, compared with several months with finasteride.

Management of BPH can include medical, surgical, and a combination of medical and surgical intervention. Pharmacotherapy is prescribed with both medical and surgical approaches to care. The progression of BPH is unique to the individual; the man often will "watch and wait" before proceeding further into active therapy because the process of hyperplasia can be slow. This is acceptable as long as the AUA score is 19 or less.

The Medical Therapy of Prostatic Symptoms (MTOPS) trial tested whether finasteride (Proscar), doxazosin (Cardura), or a combination of the drugs could prevent progression of BPH and the need for surgery or other invasive treatments. Physicians at 17 MTOPS medical centers treated 3,047 men with BPH for an average of 4.5 years. Participants were randomly assigned to receive doxazosin, finasteride, combination therapy, or a placebo. Vital signs, urinary symptoms, urinary flow, adverse effects, and medication use were assessed every 3 months. DRE, serum PSA level, and urinalysis were performed yearly. Prostate size was measured by ultrasound at the beginning and end of the study. Progression of disease was defined by one of the following: a 4-point rise in the AUA score, urinary retention, recurrent urinary tract infection, or urinary incontinence.

Finasteride, a 5-α-reductase inhibitor, and doxazosin, an α-1 receptor blocker, together reduced the overall risk of BPH progression by 66% compared with a placebo. The combined drugs also provided the greatest symptom relief and improvement in urinary flow rate. Doxazosin alone reduced the overall risk of progression by 39% and finasteride alone by 34% relative to a placebo. The risk of urinary retention was reduced 81% with combination therapy and 68% with finasteride alone. Doxazosin alone did not reduce the risk of urinary retention. The risk of incontinence was reduced 65% with combination therapy. Only five men developed urinary tract or blood infections. No patients developed impaired kidney function related to BPH.

Twenty-seven percent of men taking doxazosin, 24% of men taking finasteride, and 18% of men taking combination therapy stopped treatment early, primarily because of adverse effects. The most common adverse effects included sexual dysfunction in men treated with finasteride, and dizziness and fatigue in men treated with doxazosin.

Goals of Therapy

The goals of therapy include reduced bladder outlet obstruction, improved quality of life, fewer symptoms, and decreased residual urine volume.

The mainstay of medical management is pharmacotherapy. Pharmacotherapy is used for both controlling hyperplasia and managing annoying side effects, either as primary therapy or as an adjunct to surgical intervention. Management of hyperplasia is based on the premise that there are hormonal changes related to aging and that alpha-adrenergic receptors are present in prostate tissue, specifically smooth muscle. Pharmacotherapeutic interventions consist of hormonal manipulation and blocking effects achieved by alpha-adrenergic blockers. For dosage, adverse events, contraindications, and special considerations of drugs used for BPH, see **Table 33.4**.

5-Alpha-Reductase Inhibitors

Finasteride (Proscar) and dutasteride (Avodart), androgen hormone inhibitors, are used for managing the symptoms of BPH. They aid in the inhibition of androgen transformation from their steroid precursors.

Mechanism of Action

Five-α-reductase inhibitors act by specifically blocking 5-α-reductase, the enzyme that activates testosterone in the prostate. It impairs prostate growth by inhibiting the conversion of testosterone to DHT and causes changes in the epithelial cells of the transition zone. By preventing testosterone activation, 5-α-reductase inhibitors lessen or prevent urinary system symptoms. They also decrease prostatic volume and prevent the progression of the disease in men with a significantly enlarged prostate. There is a slow reduction of 80% to 90% in the serum DHT level. As a result, prostatic volume decreases by about 20% over 3 to 6 months of treatment. Dutasteride blocks both types 1 and 2 5-α-reductase.

TABLE 33.4	Overview of Selected Agents Used to Treat Benign Prostatic Hyperplasia			
Generic (Trade) Name and Dosage	Selected Adverse Events	Contraindications	Special Considerations	
α-Adrenergic Blockers terazosin (Hytrin) 　1–20 mg PO qd	Orthostatic hypotension, somnolence, dizziness	Hypersensitivity to terbutaline Tachyarrhythmias, hypertension, pregnancy, lactation Use with caution in patients with cardiac insufficiency.	Take at bedtime to avoid hypotension.	
doxazosin (Cardura) 　4–8 mg PO qd	Dizziness, headache, fatigue, malaise	Lactation Use with caution in patients with CHF, renal failure, hepatic impairment.	May have secondary benefit to client with cardiac disease Avoid combination with alcohol, nitrates, or other antihypertensive drugs.	
tamsulosin HCl (Flomax) 　0.4 mg/d PO qd; increase to 　0.8 mg/d PO qd	Orthostasis, headache, problems with ejaculation	Allergy to tamsulosin Prostatic cancer, pregnancy, lactation	Ejaculatory problems more common in higher dosage (0.8 mg/d) Interaction with cimetidine decreases clearance of tamsulosin.	
5-α-Reductase Inhibitor finasteride (Proscar) 5 mg daily dutasteride (Avodart) 0.5 mg daily	Impotence, decreased libido, smaller ejaculate volume	Not to be handled by pregnant women	Inform patient that effective outcome of therapy may take up to 6 mo.	

Studies have been done to determine the efficacy of finasteride and placebo. The larger Proscar Safety Plus Efficacy Canadian Two-Year Study (PROSPECT) found that treatment with finasteride led to significant improvements in urinary symptoms and flow rates (Nickel, et al., 1996). However, in the PROSPECT study, the improvements with finasteride were significantly less than those with any α blocker or surgery.

5-α-reductase inhibitors decrease PSA levels by 40% to 50%. In a patient taking finasteride who has PSA screening, PSA levels should be doubled and then compared in the usual fashion to age-related norms.

Dosage

The dosage for finasteride is 5 mg/day; that for dutasteride is 0.5 mg/day. These dosages are recommended for use as long-term therapy; studies have shown benefit beyond the usual 2-year period, with beneficial effects in the third year.

Adverse Events

Adverse events include decreased libido, impotence, ejaculatory failure, and gynecomastia. Finasteride can also falsify the PSA level after 6 months of therapy.

Alpha-Adrenergic Blockers

Alpha-adrenergic blockers include terazosin (Hytrin), doxazosin (Cardura), prazosin (Minipress), and tamsulosin (Flomax).

Mechanism of Action

As a pharmacologic classification, α-adrenergic blockers are functional antihypertensives with potential effects on glomerular filtration rate, renal perfusion, and heart rate. They are strongly linked with fluid retention. They relax the smooth muscle of the prostate and bladder neck without interfering with bladder contractility, thereby decreasing bladder resistance to urinary outflow. In general, weeks to months may pass before benefits from these medications are noted. However, benefits may last for up to 2 years, in some cases longer.

Adverse Events

Side effects can be a major concern, especially considering the potential for hypotension, specifically orthostatic hypotension, and fluid retention. However, cardiac output can actually improve, thus preventing heart failure. Of the four agents, prazosin has more potential for causing orthostatic hypotension than the others.

Side effects such as dizziness, postural hypotension, fatigue, and asthenia affect 7% to 9% of patients treated with nonselective alpha blockers. Side effects can be minimized by bedtime administration and slow titration of the dosage.

Tamsulosin (Flomax) is a highly selective α_{1A}-adrenergic antagonist that was developed to avoid the side effects of nonselective agents. Some patients who do not respond to nonselective α blockers may respond to tamsulosin and, because of the selectivity, may have fewer side effects.

TABLE 33.5	Recommended Order of Treatment for Benign Prostatic Hyperplasia	
Order	**Agents**	**Comments**
First line	If AUA score is 7 or less, watchful waiting	
Second line	α-adrenergic blocker or 5-α-reductase inhibitor	α-adrenergic blocker can be prescribed for patients with hypertension; 5-α-reductase inhibitor is recommended if prostate enlargement exceeds 40 g.
Third line	Combination of α blocker and 5-α-reductase inhibitor	

Selecting the Most Appropriate Agent

The most appropriate agent is the one that achieves symptom control and produces the fewest adverse effects (**Table 33.5** and **Figure 33-2**).

First-Line Therapy

If symptoms are mild (AUA score <7), no medical treatment is recommended. The man should limit his fluid intake after dinner, avoid decongestants, massage the prostate after intercourse, and void frequently.

Second-Line Therapy

Pharmacotherapy is initiated when the AUA score is more than 7. An α-adrenergic blocker or a 5-α-reductase inhibitor can be prescribed. To limit the number of daily drugs, it may be prudent to use an α-adrenergic blocker in the patient who is also hypertensive. A 5-α-reductase inhibitor may be prescribed if the prostate is enlarged to 40 g or more.

Analyzed together, the results of multiple studies suggest that 5-α-reductase inhibitors may work best in men with a large gland, whereas α blockers are effective across the range of prostate sizes.

Third-Line Therapy

Combination therapy with a 5-α-reductase inhibitor and alpha blocker may show greater improvement.

Fourth-Line Therapy

Referral to a urologist for possible surgery is recommended if other therapy fails.

The prevailing surgical intervention is prostatic resection or prostatectomy. Transurethral resection of the prostate (TURP) is the most common surgical intervention. Regardless of the surgical technique used (i.e., retrograde, perineal, or suprapubic approach), removal of the prostate is not without potential complications. The primary side effect, which can be permanent, is impotence from nerve damage. Incontinence is rare and usually only temporary; retrograde ejaculation can occur. Prostatectomy using laser technique is also an option, as is balloon dilatation or urethral stent implantation. Laser

surgery requires only an overnight stay; stent insertion is recommended for the man with cardiac or pulmonary morbidities, although it does not address the underlying problem of BPH itself.

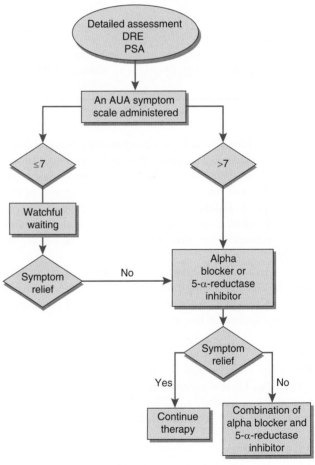

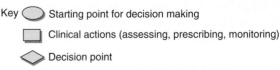

FIGURE 33–2 Treatment algorithm for benign prostatic hyperplasia (BPH).

Transurethral microwave thermotherapy is performed on an outpatient basis. Although anesthesia is not required, use of a local or general antianxiety agent may be helpful because the procedure is performed by catheter insertion into the prostate, through the urethra. This procedure uses heat derived from microwave energy (approximately 45°C) to remove or destroy excess cells of the prostate while cool water is circulated to preserve surrounding tissue.

TABLE 33.6	Alternative Therapies for Benign Prostatic Hyperplasia	
Agent	**Dosage**
Saw palmetto	Doses vary based on manufacturer
Pygeum	50–100 mg PO bid
Zinc	150 mg PO qd for 2 mo, 50–100 mg qd thereafter

MONITORING PATIENT RESPONSE

As noted previously, the AUA symptom score can be used to monitor men with mild or even moderate BPH. Abatement of symptoms is used to evaluate the success of pharmacotherapy. If side effects become evident with a chosen agent, a different agent can be tried. The patient's blood pressure should be monitored frequently during the first 2 weeks of treatment to observe for an untoward hypotensive response. In addition, the practitioner should not pass off subjective complaints related to sexual health, because it could lead to medication noncompliance.

PATIENT EDUCATION

Drug Information

With terazosin use, an improvement in urine flow may begin within 1 to 2 weeks; thus, the patient must be informed that urine flow improvement will not occur overnight. The man should rise slowly from a sitting or standing position and quickly sit down or recline if abrupt vertigo occurs.

Lifestyle Changes

Patients with BPH can obtain symptomatic relief with regular, relaxed, and frequent voiding; decreasing fluid intake several hours before bedtime; and avoiding diuretics and alcohol. Other medications to avoid include anticholinergics, antihistamines, and antidepressants.

Alternative Therapies for BPH

Many men are using herbal and nutritional therapies to support prostate health. Men are encouraged to lose weight if overweight, to eat a low-fat, high-fiber diet, and to drink a minimum of 2 quarts of water daily. Supplements to maintain prostate health include saw palmetto, pygeum, and zinc (**Table 33.6**). Because these are not found in standard pharmacologic compendiums, dosages for saw palmetto and pygeum should follow the manufacturer's recommendations.

Saw palmetto, an herb derived from the dark berries of a palm tree native to the southern United States, is reported to have been in use since the 1700s. Purportedly, it is useful for the management of prostate inflammation by a threefold mechanism. First, it inhibits testosterone conversion to DHT, resulting in the prevention of prostate enlargement. Second,

it stops DHT binding to receptor sites; third, it has a general inhibitory effect on both estrogen and androgen receptors. There is no evidence of deleterious effects on PSA levels with the use of saw palmetto. Saw palmetto is available in capsule, liquid, or softgel form and as a tea; the tea is not believed to be effective for BPH. Saw palmetto often is used in combination with pygeum (http://www.sawpalmetto.com).

Pygeum is the ground and powdered bark of the pygeum tree, an evergreen of southern Africa. It is prepared as a tea for easing complaints related to the genitourinary system. Widely used in Europe for symptom relief in BPH and thus postponement of surgery or the use of stronger medications, the efficacy of pygeum is being researched at the University of Southern California. Dosage recommendations are 50 to 100 mg twice daily; gastrointestinal irritation is a rare side effect (http://www.mothernature.com).

Zinc also plays a role in BPH, improving general prostate health by preventing or even decreasing prostate enlargement. Research has supported that doses of zinc sulfate lead to the inhibition of 5-α-reductase, the enzyme for conversion of testosterone to DHT. The recommended dosage for zinc sulfate is 150 mg/day for 2 months followed by a maintenance dose of 50 to 100 mg/day.

PROSTATE CANCER

In the decade from 1980 to 1990, the incidence of prostate cancer increased by 50%, although this is actually perceived as a positive development, indicating enhanced screenings rather than a truly increased incidence of disease. This disease is more common in African-American men than in white men and, in general, in men from North, Central, and South America, Africa, and the Near East. Ironically, in African-American men, prostate cancer develops at a significantly higher rate than in their native African counterparts. Men of Asian heritage have a low incidence of prostate cancer and low death rates from the disease. Once again, Asian-American men have a slightly higher incidence of prostate cancer than their native Asian counterparts.

Incidence reports estimate that 1 of every 11 men will have cancer of the prostate; as the man ages, the risk of developing prostate cancer also increases. Greater than 80% of the diagnosed prostate cancers have been in men age 65 or older (Bullock & Henze, 2000).

CAUSES

The disease seems to be closely aligned with the aging process; the exact cause is not well understood, although a genetic predisposition has been found. Thus, sons of men who have had prostate cancer are at higher risk for developing prostate cancer themselves. No link between prostate cancer and BPH has been uncovered. From an environmental and occupational perspective, association with cadmium in the workplace is correlated with the later onset of prostate cancer.

Essentially 95% of prostate cancers are adenocarcinomas, with most occurring at the prostate's periphery. How aggressive the neoplasm becomes seems to be more highly correlated with the degree of anaplasia, or lack of differentiation, of the cancer cells as opposed to tumor size. Progression of the cancer begins with local extension, but metastasis to distant sites occurs through blood and lymphatic vessels. Given the anatomic location of the prostate, it is easily understood how progression to the pelvis and rectum, lumbar and thoracic spine and ribs, and femur can ensue.

PATHOPHYSIOLOGY

In many cases, symptoms present only with advanced disease. As with BPH, bladder-associated problems occur first—slow urine stream, inadequate emptying of bladder, painful urination, frequency, and nocturia. However, with prostate cancer, unlike BPH, there is no remission from these symptoms. Difficulty in defecation, and even obstruction of the large bowel, can also occur depending on how the tumor is spreading, but again this is usually seen with advanced disease.

DIAGNOSTIC CRITERIA

Early detection of prostate cancer is crucial. Enhanced screening has alerted many men to seek medical intervention for prostate cancer well before symptom manifestation. African-American men are still diagnosed at a more advanced stage, and their rate of survival is poorer than among Whites. Thus, public education targeting African-American men is of paramount importance.

Three screening methods are commonly used. The first is the DRE; the second is the serum level of PSA. When either result is abnormal, an ultrasound study is performed transrectally. The man should be cautioned to avoid ejaculation for 48 hours before obtaining a PSA because false-positive results may be obtained. The diagnostic yield rises dramatically when ultrasound is incorporated with DRE and PSA. It is recommended that all men older than age 40 undergo an annual DRE, and all men older than age 50 also have their PSA level tested annually in addition to the DRE. Normal PSA values should be less than 2.7 in men younger than age 40 and 4.0 or less in men older than age 40.

However, for confirmation of cancer, and with suspect findings, further diagnostic investigation is warranted. This includes a biopsy to confirm the diagnosis and identify the cancer's histologic type, after which MRI and CT scans are necessary to determine the extent of metastasis.

Treatment options include surgery, chemotherapy, and radiation, either alone or in combination. Regardless of the treatment modality, loss of physiologic function can occur. This loss of function varies from temporary loss of urinary control to permanent incontinence. In addition to loss of urinary control, fecal incontinence can also result. Sexual dysfunction frequently occurs and involves the ability to attain an erection or have emission or ejaculation. Return to normal physiologic function often occurs over time, but some permanent dysfunction can result.

INITIATING DRUG THERAPY

Pharmacologic intervention can also help the patient return to normal physiologic function after other treatments, such as partial or radical prostatectomy, which are options based on the cancer's histologic type and the extent of metastasis. Often, surgery is performed after a period of radiation or chemotherapy. A main postoperative concern is that bladder dysfunction will persist; this manifests as incomplete emptying, incontinence, decreased force of stream, and urinary scarring.

Bilateral orchiectomy has also been used for advanced disease to decrease the risk of complications and spread of prostate cancer, but it is not considered curative in the setting of metastasis or advanced disease. Bilateral orchiectomy is radical surgery used to extend the man's life; it provides relief from symptoms. There is minimal morbidity and mortality associated with the surgery, but it may have a negative impact on the man's self-esteem and sense of identity. Postsurgical pharmacologic management is crucial to promoting the man's self-esteem and correcting, as much as possible, the altered physiologic function.

ERECTILE DYSFUNCTION

Erectile dysfunction (ED) is the most common sexual problem in men. It is defined as the repeated inability to achieve or maintain an erection that is firm enough for sexual intercourse. ED can be a total inability to achieve erection, an inconsistent ability to do so, or a tendency to sustain only brief erections. The incidence of ED increases with age: about 5% of men age 40 experience ED, compared with 15% to 25% of men age 65. However, ED is not an inevitable part of aging.

It is estimated that at least 10 to 20 million American men suffer from ED. Laumann and colleagues (1999) showed that the prevalence of male sexual dysfunction approached 31% in a population survey of approximately 1,400 men ages 18 to 59.

CAUSES

An erection requires a precise sequence of events, and ED can occur when any of the events are disrupted. The sequence includes nerve impulses in the brain, the spinal column, and the area around the penis and response in muscles, fibrous tissues, veins, and arteries in and near the corpora cavernosa. Damage to nerves, arteries, smooth muscles, and fibrous tissues (often as a result of disease) is the most common cause of ED. Chronic diseases such as diabetes, kidney disease, chronic alcoholism, multiple sclerosis, atherosclerosis, vascular disease, and neurologic disease account for about 70% of ED cases. Between 35% and 50% of men with diabetes experience ED. Psychological issues can also lead to ED, and it is often a combination of physical and psychological issues. **See Box 33.1** for a list of risk factors for ED.

Surgery (especially radical prostate surgery for cancer) can injure nerves and arteries near the penis, thus causing ED. Injury to the penis, spinal cord, prostate, bladder, and pelvis can lead to ED by harming nerves, smooth muscles, arteries, and fibrous tissues of the corpora cavernosa.

Many common drugs such as antihypertensives, antihistamines, antidepressants, tranquilizers, appetite suppressants, and cimetidine can have ED as an adverse event. Psychological factors such as stress, anxiety, guilt, depression, low self-esteem, and fear of sexual failure cause 10% to 20% of ED cases. Other possible causes of ED include smoking, which affects blood flow in veins and arteries, and hormonal abnormalities, such as low testosterone levels.

PATHOPHYSIOLOGY

The penis is innervated by both autonomic and somatic nerves. Sympathetic and parasympathetic fibers in the cavernous nerves regulate blood flow into the corpus cavernosum during erection and detumescence. Erection, at the level of the penis, begins with transmission of impulses from parasympathetic nerves and nonadrenergic, noncholinergic nerves. This neural stimulus leads to the release of nitric oxide from the nonadrenergic, noncholinergic nerves and possibly the endothelial cells. Nitric oxide increases intracellular levels of cyclic guanosine monophosphate (cGMP) in the cavernosal smooth muscle, which acts to relax cavernosal tissue, perhaps by activating protein kinase G and stimulating phosphorylation of the proteins that regulate corporal smooth muscle tone. The actions of the parasympathetic nervous system, nitric oxide, and cGMP permit rapid blood flow into the penis and the development of an erection. As pressure within the corporal body increases, small emissary veins traversing the tunica albuginea are occluded, trapping blood in the corpus cavernosum. The erection is maintained until ejaculation, which usually leads to detumescence.

Phosphodiesterases (PDEs) are hydrolytic enzymes that play a critical role in regulating physiologic processes by terminating signal transduction through their hydrolytic action on cyclic nucleotides. They play a key role in the physiology of erection.

Significant changes in penile structure occur with aging. Collagen and elastic fibers in the tunica albuginea are key structures that permit increases in the girth and length of the penis during tumescence, and ultra-structural analysis of penile biopsies has shown that the concentration of elastic fibers decreases with age. This decrease results in a reduction in elasticity, which could contribute to ED in elderly men. Additionally, there is a decrease of up to 35% in the smooth muscle content of the penis in men older than age 60. Decreases in the ratio between corpus cavernosum smooth muscle and connective tissue has been associated with increased likelihood of diffuse venous leak that may contribute to ED. It has also been noted that the concentration of type III collagen decreases and that of type I collagen increases in the aging penis. It has been suggested that this change makes the corpus cavernosum less compliant, reduces filling of vascular spaces, and also contributes to veno-occlusive dysfunction. It has also been hypothesized that changes in the collagen content of the penis may result in chronic ischemia that leads to loss of smooth muscle cells. Any condition, disease, medication, or injury or surgery that affects the ability to initiate erections or to fill the lacunar space or store blood may cause ED.

BOX 33.1

Risk Factors for Erectile Dysfunction

Advancing age
Cardiovascular disease
Cigarette smoking
Diabetes mellitus
History of pelvic irradiation or surgery, including radical prostatectomy
Hormonal disorders (e.g., hypogonadism, hypothyroidism, hyperprolactinemia)
Hypercholesterolemia
Hypertension
Illicit drug use (e.g., cocaine, methamphetamine)
Medications (e.g., antihistamines, benzodiazepines, selective serotonin reuptake inhibitors)
Neurologic conditions (e.g., Alzheimer's disease, multiple sclerosis, Parkinson disease, paraplegia, quadriplegia, stroke)
Obesity
Peyronie disease
Psychological conditions (e.g., anxiety, depression, guilt, history of sexual abuse, marital or relationship problems, stress)
Sedentary lifestyle
Venous leakage

ED involves multiple organic and psychogenic factors, which often coexist. Psychogenic factors are the most common causes of intermittent ED in younger men, but these are usually secondary to or may coexist with organic factors in older men. Other factors contributing to ED include vasculogenic, neurogenic, endocrinologic, structural (traumatic), and pharmacologic causes and lifestyle factors, such as obesity, a sedentary lifestyle, and alcohol and tobacco use. Many of the conditions that contribute to ED are chronic and systemic, involving multiple avenues of damage. These conditions include cardiovascular disease, hypertension, diabetes mellitus, and depression. Many of the diseases linked to ED involve endothelial dysfunction.

There are many drugs that can affect erectile function. These include:

- alcohol
- analgesics
- anticholinergics
- anticonvulsants
- antidepressants
- antihistamines
- antihypertensives
- anti-parkinson agents
- corticosteroids
- diuretics
- nicotine
- tranquilizers

DIAGNOSTIC CRITERIA

A thorough history is paramount to diagnosing ED. Every male patient should be asked about medical conditions, medications, and sexual function. Initial diagnostic workup should usually be limited to a fasting serum glucose level and lipid panel, thyroid-stimulating hormone test, and morning total testosterone level.

INITIATING DRUG THERAPY

ED can be very traumatic to men. There are now drugs that can assist with achieving and maintaining an erection that is firm enough for sexual intercourse. Testosterone levels should be determined and a complete cardiac history and evaluation should be done to determine whether there are contraindications to these medications. Approximately one third of men with ED do not respond to therapy with phosphodiesterase-5 (PDE5) inhibitors.

Goals of Drug Therapy

The goals of drug therapy for ED are to enable the patient to achieve sexual satisfaction and to achieve and maintain an erection.

Phosphodiesterase-5 Inhibitors

PDE5 inhibitors promote penile erection by inhibiting the breakdown of one of the messengers involved in the erectile response. PDE5 is the main cGMP-catalyzing enzyme in human trabecular smooth muscle. It is also expressed in vascular smooth muscle, lung, platelets, and a wide variety of other tissues but is not present in cardiac muscle cells. Human corpus cavernosum also contains PDE types 2, 3, and 4 enzymes. PDE5 inhibitors are contingent on the presence of cGMP in the smooth muscle cell. In the presence of sexual stimulation, PDE5 inhibitors reinforce the normal cellular signals that increase cyclic nucleotide concentrations by blocking cyclic nucleotide hydrolysis, thereby facilitating the initiation and maintenance of an erection.

Dosage

The recommended dosage of sildenafil is 50 mg 30 to 60 minutes before intercourse, but doses range from 25 to 100 mg. The maximum is one dose a day. Food can delay absorption.

The recommended dose of tadalafil is 10 mg, but doses range from 5 to 20 mg. Tadalafil can be taken without restriction on food or alcohol intake.

The recommended dose of vardenafil is 10 mg, but doses range from 2.5 to 20 mg. It is taken 60 minutes before intercourse. Food can delay absorption.

Time Frame for Response

Sildenafil and vardenafil are rapidly absorbed, reaching maximum plasma concentrations within 30 to 120 minutes (median 60 minutes) of oral dosing in the fasted state; a high-fat meal has been found to reduce the rate of absorption. The elimination half-life is approximately 4 hours, and no more than one dose should be taken per 24-hour period.

Tadalafil has an onset of action of 30 minutes and allows intercourse for at least 30 hours. This is significant because it may eliminate the need for planning sexual activity.

Contraindications

PDE5 inhibitors can potentiate the vasodilatory properties of nitrates, so their administration in patients who use nitrates in any form is contraindicated. In an emergency situation, nitrates can be used 24 hours after administration of sildenafil and vardenafil and 48 hours after tadalafil.

PDE5 inhibitors are contraindicated in patients with unstable angina, hypotension with a systolic blood pressure below 90 mm Hg, uncontrolled hypertension of more than 170/110 mm Hg, history of recent stroke, life-threatening arrhythmia, myocardial infarction (MI) within 6 months, and severe cardiac failure. They are also contraindicated in patients with severe hepatic impairment or end-stage renal disease requiring dialysis.

Sildenafil has a relative contraindication with the concomitant use of α blockers and should not be taken within 4 hours of an α blocker and at a dose no greater than 25 mg. Tadalafil should not be taken with an α blocker other than

TABLE 33.7 **Overview of Selected Agents Used to Treat Erectile Dysfunction**

Generic (Trade) Name and Dosage	Selected Adverse Events	Contraindications	Special Considerations
tadalafil (Cialis) 5–20 mg/d	Headache, flushing, GI disturbance, nasal congestion, rash, priapism	Nitrates and α blockers except tamsulosin 0.4 mg once a day	Food and alcohol make no difference in absorption. May remain in system for 36 h.
vardenafil (Levitra) 5–20 mg/d	As above	Nitrates and α blockers	High-fat meal delays absorption.
sildenafil (Viagra) 25–100 mg/d	As above and color disturbances	Nitrates and within 4 h of an α blocker and at a dose no >25 mg	As above

tamsulosin, 0.4 mg once a day. Vardenafil is contraindicated with any α blocker.

Adverse Events

Most adverse events are vasodilatory, including headache, flushing, and nasal congestion. Dyspepsia has also been reported. With sildenafil, abnormal color vision has been reported.

Interactions

Potent CYP3A4 inhibitors can cause increased levels of PDE5 inhibitors. They may also be affected by amlodipine, beta blockers, cimetidine, diuretics, and erythromycin.

Selecting the Most Appropriate Agent

It is important to include the significant other in counseling about ED. A complete cardiac history must be taken. If there is any question as to the stability of the cardiac status, further testing must be done. Testosterone, serum glucose (or alternatively glycosylated hemoglobin), and serum lipid levels must be determined in all cases of ED. Depending on patient history and physical examination findings, more extensive laboratory tests may be necessary. If testosterone levels are abnormal, testosterone replacement is needed. See **Table 33.7** for selected agents.

The patient with the following factors is considered at low risk for a cardiac event with the use of PDE5 inhibitors: fewer than three risk factors for coronary artery disease, controlled hypertension, mild, stable angina, uncomplicated MI more than 8 weeks previously, mild valvular disease, and New York Heart Association class 1 heart failure. See **Box 33.2** and **Figure 33-3**.

First-Line Therapy

First-line therapy for ED is aimed at lifestyle changes and modifying pharmacotherapy that may contribute to ED. A PDE5 inhibitor is also prescribed (**Table 33.8**).

Second-Line Therapy

If PDE5 inhibitors are not successful in treating ED, the patient should be referred to a urologist. Alternative therapies include penile intracavernosal injection therapy, a medical intraurethral system for erections, a vacuum erection device, and penile prostheses.

MONITORING PATIENT RESPONSE

The patient should be followed in 6 months to determine the effectiveness of therapy and to reevaluate his cardiac status. If the patient does not meet the criteria for low risk, the PDE5 inhibitors are discontinued.

PATIENT EDUCATION

Drug Information

With sildenafil and vardenafil, a high-fat meal has been found to reduce the rate of absorption. Food and alcohol have no effect on the absorption of tadalafil.

Sildenafil has a relative contraindication with the concomitant use of α blockers and should not be taken within 4 hours of an α blocker and at a dose no greater than 25 mg. Tadalafil should not be taken with an α blocker other than tamsulosin 0.4 mg once a day. Vardenafil is contraindicated with any α blocker.

BOX 33.2

Low-Risk Factors for Cardiac Events from PDE5 Inhibitors

Fewer than three risk factors for coronary artery disease
Controlled hypertension
Stable angina
Uncomplicated MI more than 8 weeks previously
Mild valvular disease
New York Heart Association class 1 heart failure (see Chapter 22)

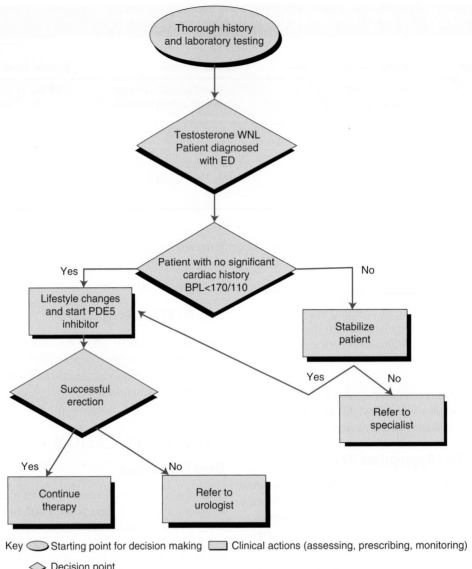

FIGURE 33–3 Treatment algorithm for erectile dysfunction.

TABLE 33.8	Recommended Order of Treatment for Erectile Dysfunction	
Order	**Agent**	**Comment**
First line	PDE5 inhibitors	Contraindicated if on nitrates, unstable hypertension, unstable cardiac condition
Second line	Referral to urologist	Procedures available include penile intracavernosal injection therapy, medical intraurethral system for erections, vacuum erection device, penile prostheses

Complementary and Alternative Medicine

Yohimbine, an agent derived from the bark of the African yohimbe tree, has been found to be beneficial in some cases of ED. It is reported to act by both peripheral and central mechanisms, acting peripherally as a presynaptic stimulant at parasympathetic NANC nerves and presynaptically as an adrenergic depressant at sympathetic alpha$_1$-adrenoceptors, both mechanisms augmenting penile blood flow. It also appears to have central nervous system activity, with blockade of the erection-suppressing α_2-adrenoceptors; several studies have reported a more favorable response with yohimbine compared with placebo in ED of psychogenic origin.

Case Study

M. P., age 45, works as an accountant in a busy firm. He is of African-American descent. He and his wife have been married for 25 years and have two children, ages 21 and 18. His father is alive and well at age 68 but was diagnosed with BPH 5 years ago. M. P. considers himself to be in good health and has no allergies; he is approximately 15% overweight. His wife insisted that he seek medical intervention because of urinary symptomatology: he has difficulty starting his stream of urine, burning on urination, nocturia, and lower back and pelvic discomfort. The result of a PSA test, his first in over 2 years, is 3.1.

DIAGNOSIS: BPH

1. List specific goals for treatment for M. P.
2. What drug therapy would you prescribe? Why?
3. What are the parameters for monitoring the success of the therapy?
4. Discuss specific patient education based on the prescribed therapy.
5. List one or two adverse reactions for the selected agent that would cause you to change therapy.
6. What would be the choice for second-line therapy?
7. What over-the-counter and/or alternative medications would be appropriate for this patient?
8. What dietary and lifestyle changes should be recommended for this patient?
9. Describe one or two drug–drug or drug–food interactions for the selected agent.

BIBLIOGRAPHY

*Starred references are cited in the text.

*Bullock, B. A., & Henze, R. L. (2000). *Focus on pathophysiology*. Philadelphia: Lippincott Williams & Wilkins.

*Coyne, K. S., Sexton, C. C., Thompson, C. L., et al. (2009). The prevalence of lower urinary tract symptoms (LUTS) in the USA, the UK and Sweden: Results from the Epidemiology of LUTS (EpiLUTS) study. *British Journal of Urology International, 104*(3), 352–360.

Fagelman, E. (2002). Herbal medicines to treat benign prostatic hyperplasia. *Urology Clinics of North America, 29*(1), 23–29.

Gammoch, J. (2010). Lower urinary tract symptoms. *Clinics in Geriatric Medicine, 26*(2), 249–260.

Heidelbaugh, J. (2010). Management of erectile dysfunction. *American Family Physician, 81*(3), 305–312.

Hua, V. N. (2004). Acute and chronic prostatitis. *Medical Clinics of North America, 88*(2), 483–494.

Jewett, M., & Klotz, L. (2007). Advances in medical management of benign prostatic hypertrophy. *Canadian Medical Association Journal, 176*(13), 1850–1851.

*Laumann, E., Paik, A., & Rosen, R. C. (1999). Sexual dysfunction in the United States: Prevalence and predictor. *Journal of the American Medical Association, 281*(6), 537–544.

*Nickel, J. C., Fradet, Y., Boake, R., et al. (1996). Efficacy and safety of finasteride therapy for benign prostatic hyperplasia: Results of a 2-year randomized controlled trial (the PROSPECT study). *Canadian Medical Journal, 155*(9), 1251–1259.

Selvin, E., Burnett, A., & Platz, E. (2007). Prevalence and risk factors for erectile dysfunction in the U.S. *American Journal of Medicine, 120*(2), 151–157.

Sharp, V., Takas, E., & Powell, C. (2010). Prostatitis: Diagnosis and treatment. *American Family Physician, 82*(4), 397–406.

Stefel, A. D. (2004). Erectile dysfunction: Etiology, evaluation and treatment options. *Medical Clinics of North America, 88*(2), 387–416.

Thorne, M. B., & Geraci, S. (2009). Acute urinary retention in elderly men. *American Journal of Medicine, 122*(9), 815–819.

Overactive Bladder

Overactive bladder (OAB) is a highly prevalent yet underreported condition that transcends the boundaries of race, gender, and socioeconomic class. OAB is loosely defined by the International Continence Society (ICS) as a constellation of symptoms that include primarily urinary urgency usually accompanied by frequency (voiding eight or more times per 24 hours) and nocturia (awakening two or more times at night to void), with or without urge urinary incontinence. The most recent data suggest that OAB affects between 16% and 17% of adults in the United States, or about 34 million people. However, given the substantial underreporting and the inherent challenges in identifying sufferers of OAB, the actual prevalence is likely markedly higher. Women and men tend to be affected by OAB proportionately; however, women are more likely than men to present with the symptom of incontinence as part of their clinical picture. The incidence of OAB increases linearly with age and is predicated on a number of factors that are impacted by aging. However, OAB with or without incontinence is not considered a normal part of aging; OAB symptomatology and any instance of urgency is always considered pathologic.

OAB syndrome has extensive ramifications with respect to morbidity, mortality, and economic impact. A preponderance of literature supports the assertion that OAB is associated with increased rates of depression, decreased self-esteem, social isolation, general fragility, and falls and fracture. Upon development of OAB symptoms, patients tend to engage in avoidance behaviors in order to escape the social stigma and embarrassment associated with urinary incontinence or urinary urgency. Eventually this translates into substantial lifestyle changes and the potential for social isolation. Total costs attributable to OAB as of 2007 are estimated to be $65.9 billion ($49.1 billion direct medical, $2.3 billion direct nonmedical, and $14.6 billion indirect) (Ganz, et al., 2010). A leading cause of morbidity in the elderly population and the most commonly cited reason for assisted living and long-term care facility admission, OAB needs to be assessed in the primary care setting preemptively.

The terms OAB, detrusor overactivity (DO), and urinary incontinence (UI) are frequently used interchangeably erroneously. UI is a possible symptom in the symptomatology construct that comprises OAB; it does not necessarily need to be present in patients diagnosed with OAB. While urgency is the cardinal symptom of OAB and must be present in order to yield a diagnosis of OAB, only about 25% to 35% of patients experience *incontinence* as well. DO implies an involuntary and inappropriate contraction of the bladder; however, it is considered a surrogate marker of OAB that may or may not correlate with urgency. There is considerable overlap between nonpharmacologic and pharmacologic treatments for OAB, UI, and DO; therefore, urinary incontinence subtypes will be discussed. The accepted nomenclature for UI differentiates between the underlying pathophysiology and the nature of the urine loss. Urge urinary incontinence (UUI) implies a strong and sudden urge to urinate that cannot be deferred and results in involuntary loss of urine. Stress urinary incontinence (SUI) occurs when an internal or external force impacts the bladder or the musculature that supports it. Common examples of such pressures include coughing, sneezing, heavy lifting, or prolapsed pelvic organs. Mixed urinary incontinence is a combination of both SUI and UUI. The historical term *overflow incontinence,* which suggested some level of obstruction or voiding difficulty, has been replaced with bladder outlet obstruction (BOO) and is no longer part of the classification schema.

CAUSES

The exact cause of the OAB symptom constellation is multifactorial and not completely elucidated. There are numerous underlying anatomic, physiologic, and comorbidity-related factors that precipitate or exacerbate OAB. The majority of cases are considered idiopathic, with the remainder being attributed to myogenic or neurogenic causation.

PATHOPHYSIOLOGY

The bladder and the corresponding micturition cycle is controlled by a complex, coordinated interplay among the central nervous system (CNS), peripheral nervous system, and the anatomic components of the lower urinary tract (LUT). The LUT is composed of the bladder, urethra, bladder outlet, internal and external urethral sphincters, and the musculature of the pelvic floor (**Figure 34-1**). The discord between the continuous production of urine (1 to 2 L/day) and the episodic nature of voiding necessitates the storage of urine. The bladder (detrusor muscle) is a highly compliant, viscoelastic hollow

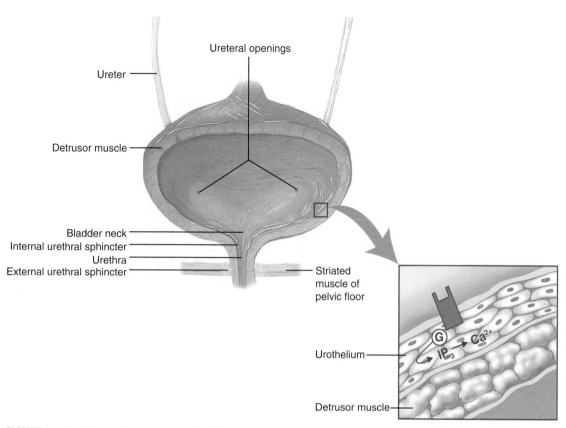

FIGURE 34–1 M_3 receptors are coupled to G proteins, which activate phospholipase, generating inositol triphosphate (IP_3). IP_3 causes the release of stored Ca2+, which stimulates bladder contraction.

organ that expands to accommodate the storage of urine while maintaining a constant pressure throughout this filling phase. As the bladder fills, it maintains a pressure that is lower than that of the urethra, therefore facilitating the development of a pressure gradient that prevents urine from being expelled. The normal urge to void is under voluntary control and therefore only when the bladder reaches a critical volume, or about 75% of total capacity, will an individual feel the desire to void. This urge, which is different from pathologic urgency and is under different neural control, can be deferred until an appropriate time. Upon conscious and deliberate urination, the urethral resistance decreases and phasic contractions in the bladder result in increased bladder pressure and the subsequent voiding of urine.

The LUT is innervated by efferent and afferent neuronal complexes involving sympathetic, parasympathetic, and

Nerve	Anatomic Location	Nervous System	Spinal Cord Origin	Physiologic Function
TABLE 34.1	**Bladder and Urethral Innervation**			
Pudendal	External sphincter	Somatic	S2, S3, S4	Maintains tone in pelvic floor
				Excitatory innervation to external urethral sphincter
Pelvic	Urethra	Parasympathetic	S2, S3, S4	Relaxes sphincter
Hypogastric	Urethra	Sympathetic	T1–L2	Stimulates sphincter closure
Pelvic	Bladder neck	Parasympathetic	S2, S3, S4	Relaxes sphincter
Hypogastric	Bladder neck	Sympathetic	T1–L2	Stimulates sphincter closure
Pelvic	Bladder	Parasympathetic	S2, S3, S4	Contraction of detrusor during micturition
Hypogastric	Bladder	Sympathetic	T1–L2	Relaxes detrusor during filling phase

somatic nerves. The *sympathetic* nervous system primarily stimulates urethral sphincter closure and detrusor relaxation during filling, while the *parasympathetic* system influences contraction of the detrusor and relaxation of the urethral sphincters during the emptying phase. Somatic innervation maintains the tone of the striated pelvic floor muscles and the external urethral sphincter (**Table 34.1**). The bladder is continuously bombarding the CNS with afferent signals during the filling phase via Aδ fibers and C fibers. These normal impulses indicate when the bladder is filling and also when it is nearing capacity. The impulses are transmitted to higher brain centers such as the cortex, pons, and brainstem, which also exert some level of control over micturition. The sensations generated by this neurotransmission will result in variable degrees of the normal urge to urinate. The Aδ fibers generally respond to the mechanical stretch of the bladder during the filling phase. However, during pathologic conditions, it is thought that the unmyelinated C sensory fibers may precipitate abnormal OAB sensations. The C sensory fibers are dappled with vanilloid receptors (which can be stimulated by capsaicin), purinergic receptors or P2X$_2$ and P2X$_3$ (which can be stimulated by adenosine triphosphate),

and neurokinin receptors (which can be stimulated by neurokinin A and substance P). See **Figure 34-2**.

Acetylcholine-mediated activation of muscarinic receptors is the predominant physiologic mediator of detrusor contraction. Muscarinic receptor subtypes M$_1$, M$_2$, and M$_3$ are found in the urinary bladder; however, it is the M$_3$ subtype that is primarily responsible for bladder contraction. These receptors, particularly the M$_3$ subtype, have become drug targets for purposes of treating OAB.

Any aberration of any individual component or combination of components involved in the micturition reflex can result in OAB or UI, as can separate comorbid conditions or physiologic states. Transient and reversible conditions or behaviors may contribute to symptoms consistent with OAB; namely increases in fluid intake or increases in caffeine or alcohol consumption. Benign prostatic hyperplasia (BPH) or obstruction can manifest in incontinence. Sacral nerve damage can lead to urinary retention. Irrespective of the etiology of OAB, the common themes include increased bladder pressure at low volumes during filling, altered response to stimuli, amplified myogenic activity and contraction, and changes in the smooth muscle anatomy.

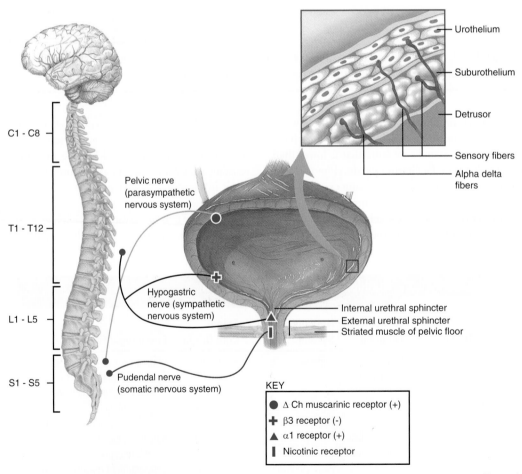

FIGURE 34–2 The bladder is innervated by the sympathetic, parasympathetic, and somatic nervous systems. The pudendal nerve maintains external sphincter and pelvic muscle tone. The pelvic nerve stimulates bladder contraction. The hypogastric nerve stimulates internal sphincter closure and detrusor relaxation.

Owing to the poor electrical coupling between smooth muscle bundles in the bladder, the highly innervated bladder is able to ignore some of the errant impulses that would otherwise cause unwanted contraction. Patchy denervation and morphologic changes in the electrical coupling may result in bladder hypertrophy and incomplete emptying. Abnormal micturition can be stimulated by damage to the afferent neurons in the dorsal root ganglia as well, which can then confer an abbreviated delay in the micturition reflex. Ischemic conditions such as diabetic neuropathy, peripheral vascular disease, and urethral stricture may also result in compromised blood flow and ultimately neuronal death with subsequent detrusor hyperactivity. Inevitable physiologic changes that occur during the aging process may also contribute to impaired cortical inhibition of bladder contraction. Stroke, Alzheimer's disease, and multiple sclerosis have been implicated in contributing to the disease process as well. Non-neurogenic conditions may also yield OAB symptoms; polyuria may be produced by uncontrolled diabetes, and nocturia may be precipitated by sleep apnea (**Box 34.1**).

Once OAB symptoms have emerged, a self-propelling cycle of factors can further exacerbate the condition. Urgency, a central feature of OAB, increases the frequency of micturition and therefore reduces the volume of each micturition provided that fluid intake remains constant. This sometimes leads to incomplete bladder emptying and subsequent residual volume that promotes the urgency and increased frequency of urination. Similarly, DO can result from neurogenic or myogenic causes. The contractions tend to be weak, which results in incomplete bladder emptying, a reduced bladder capacity, and therefore increased urinary frequency.

DIAGNOSTIC CRITERIA AND EVALUATION

OAB is a markedly underreported condition, owing mostly to the embarrassment and stigma with which it is associated. It tends to elude the typical clinical assessments and patient interviews that comprise the primary care visit and is generally diagnosed only when it is reported by the patient. The only diagnostic criteria that have been firmly established are the presence of urgency with or without nocturia and frequency. These criteria are inherently subjective; however, there have been attempts to impose objective measurements and ratings in order to determine whether a symptom is pathologic.

Current recommendations suggest that pointed questioning should be integrated into the patient interview during routine primary care visits in order to capture urinary symptoms that may otherwise be overlooked. If patient complaints or interview-generated information is suggestive of OAB, the practitioner should perform a genitourinary exam and urinalysis as well as a more in-depth medical history that is germane to urinary health. One of the major goals of this interview would be the establishment of potential causative factors acutely or

---

BOX 34.1

Factors That May Precipitate or Worsen Overactive Bladder

Neurologic Conditions
Stroke
Spinal cord injury
Diabetic neuropathy
Alzheimer's disease
Multiple sclerosis

Systemic or Metabolic Conditions
Sleep disorders (apnea)
Venous insufficiency/heart failure
Diabetes mellitus

Behavioral Considerations
Excessive fluid or caffeine consumption
Constipation
Impaired mobility

Psychological Conditions
Depression

Medications
Diuretics
Narcotic pain relievers
Calcium channel blockers
Alpha-adrenergic antagonists
Anticholinergics
Alpha-adrenergic agonists

Miscellaneous
Prostate enlargement
Estrogen deficiency

Urinary Tract Pathology
Urinary tract infection
Urinary obstruction

---

chronically (acute infection, changes in fluid intake, menstrual history, obstetric history, prostate pathology). The urinalysis is intended to assist in ruling out hematuria or an infection.

Since abnormalities or pathology in the LUT can precipitate OAB symptoms, it is imperative to evaluate the bladder, urethra, and pelvic floor muscles as well. In patients at risk for urinary retention (diabetics, spinal cord injury patients, patients with BPH), more invasive testing may be required. A residual urine volume of more than 100 ml suggests urinary retention, and these patients may need to be evaluated by cystoscopy to rule out malignancy. OAB is a constellation of symptoms, all of which could be reasonably attributed to other conditions. Therefore, OAB is often diagnosed after the exclusion of other pathology. Primarily infections, cancers (bladder, prostate), structural abnormalities (urethral, prostate), and urinary retention should be ruled out during the evaluation process.

BOX **34.2**

Diagnostic Differential

Bladder cancer, bladder calculus, interstitial cystitis
Endometriosis
Prostate cancer
Urethral calculus
Bacterial cystitis, prostatitis, urethritis
Urinary retention, polyuria, psychogenic urinary frequency

A neurologic exam, with emphasis on the sacral neuronal pathways, is recommended because OAB may be caused by neurogenic LUT dysfunction. In addition to assessments of gait, abduction/dorsiflexion of toes, and sensory innervation to the LUT, a rectal exam will provide some information relevant to voluntary sphincter control. In males specifically, a measurement of prostate specific antigen (PSA) and administration of the American Urological Association's subjective symptoms assessment (AUA-7) should occur (**Box 34.2**).

One of the tools with the highest level of clinical evidence is the "bladder diary" or "voiding diary," a patient-generated daily log that includes fluid intake and urinary output with corresponding times. Typically, entries are made by the patient over either a 3- or 7-day period. It yields information regarding urinary habits, estimation of bladder capacity, volume voided with each micturition, diurnal and nocturnal frequency, urgency, and incontinence. A number of clinical trials have used this tool to assess outcomes and have found that bladder diaries are an accurate measure of OAB symptoms, including urgency. Another parameter that is thus far not validated is "warning time," the length of time between an initial perception of the urge to void and the time at which it can no longer be deferred.

The use of urodynamic testing (UDT), the comprehensive evaluation of bladder and urethral performance during micturition, has been met with some controversy. UDT consists of a collection of urodynamic assessments that range from simple direct observations to complex, sophisticated, invasive evaluations. In order to best assess a LUT dysfunction or OAB, the symptoms need to be reproducible in a clinical setting. **Table 34.2** provides a list of the possible components of UDT. UDT is not required for a diagnosis of OAB; however, it may be indicated if there is suspicion of a bladder outlet obstruction, neurogenic voiding dysfunction, or an uncertain diagnosis.

INITIATING DRUG THERAPY

Once a diagnosis of OAB has been established, the subsequent steps include an assessment of the degree of impairment or annoyance resulting from OAB, initiation of empiric or disease-specific therapy if required, treatment of comorbid conditions, and referral to a specialist if warranted. If it is determined that the patient is significantly bothered by OAB and/or has begun

TABLE 34.2	**Urodynamic Testing**	
Component	**Description**	**Clinical Utility**
Uroflowmetry	Measurement of the volume over urine voided, speed at which voiding occurs, and duration of void	Obstruction is likely if speed is <10 mL/s.
Post-void residual (PVR)	After voiding, determination of PVR made via ultrasound or through catheterization	<25 mL is considered normal and >100 mL is abnormal.
Multichannel filling cystometry	Evaluation of bladder capacity, bladder compliance, and at what volume the urge to void occurs; accomplished by filling the bladder with normal saline and measuring detrusor pressure	Bladder pressure during filling should be <10 cm H_2O; dysfunction is diagnosed if the pressure rises at an unacceptable rate.
Leak point pressure	Evaluation of the first urine leakage and the abdominal pressure at which it occurs; the patient is instructed to perform Valsalva maneuver (e.g., coughing); patient is observed for urine leakage	Low readings (<40 cm H_2O) are associated with sphincter weakness.
Pressure flow study	Assesses the interaction among the bladder, bladder outlet, pelvic floor, and urethra during voiding; patient is instructed to void with all catheters in place (catheters include urethral catheterization and possibly vaginal or rectal catheterization)	Useful for diagnosing bladder outlet obstructions
Electromyography	Assessment of the coordination between the perineal muscles and the bladder	Useful in diagnosing neurogenic etiology of OAB

to engage in avoidance behaviors that are compromising quality of life, drug therapy should be initiated (**Table 34.3**).

The *anticholinergic* or anti-muscarinic drugs (oxybutynin, tolterodine, trospium, darifenacin, solifenacin, fesoterodine) have the greatest level of evidence with respect to their safety and efficacy in treating OAB. Their clinical use is sometimes limited, however, by their inherent anticholinergic adverse effects, most commonly dry mouth, blurred vision, constipation, cognitive dysfunction, and urinary retention. This is particularly challenging because the population with the highest prevalence of OAB is the elderly, an age cohort that is also more predisposed to cognitive dysfunction, urinary retention, and visual disturbances.

TABLE 34.3 **OAB Medication Overview**

Medication	Usual Dose	Uroselectivity	Clinical Considerations	Level of Evidence
Anticholinergics/Antimuscarinics				
oxybutynin (Ditropan)	5–15 mg orally three times daily	No	Dry mouth occurs in up to 66% of patients. Indicated for neurogenic and non-neurogenic detrusor overactivity	1A
oxybutynin ER (Ditropan XL)	5–15 mg orally once daily	No	Dry mouth occurs in up to 66% of patients. Indicated for neurogenic and non-neurogenic detrusor overactivity	1A
oxybutynin (Oxytrol transdermal patch)	3.9 mg/patch twice weekly (every 3–4 d)	No	Dry mouth occurs half as frequently as compared to the oral formulation.	1A
tolterodine (Detrol)	2 mg orally twice daily	Yes	Incidence of dry mouth is 20% to 25%.	1A
tolterodine ER (Detrol LA)	4 mg orally once daily	Yes	Dry mouth occurs in <20% of patients.	1A
trospium (Sanctura)	20 mg orally twice daily	Yes	Take before meals or on an empty stomach. No CYP P450 metabolism	1A
trospium extended release (Trospium XR)	60 mg orally once daily	Yes	Take before meals or on an empty stomach. No CYP P450 metabolism	1A
solifenacin (Vesicare)	5–10 mg orally once daily	Yes		1A
darifenacin hydrobromide (Enablex)	7.5–15 mg once daily (may titrate up to 15 mg after 2 wk if tolerated)	Yes	Possibly less impact on cognitive function than other antimuscarinics	1A
fesoterodine (Toviaz)	4–8 mg orally daily	No	Less CYP2D6 interaction potential	1A
Tricyclic Antidepressants				
imipramine (Tofranil)	10–25 mg orally three times daily	No	High interaction potential	3C
Serotonin-Norepinephrine Reuptake Inhibitors				
duloxetine (Cymbalta)	40–80 mg orally once daily	No	Avoid concomitant administration with other serotonergic drugs.	1A
Alpha-Adrenergic Antagonists				
alfuzosin (Uroxatral)	2.5 mg orally three times daily	No		4D
doxazosin (Cardura)	1–16 mg orally once daily	No	Dizziness occurs in up to 20% of patients.	4D
prazosin (Minipress)	1–10 mg orally twice daily	No		4D
tamsulosin (Flomax)	0.4–0.8 mg orally once daily	No		4D
terazosin (Hytrin)	1–10 mg orally at bedtime	No		4D
silodosin (Rapaflo)	8 mg orally once daily	No	Retrograde ejaculation occurs in up to 28% of patients.	4D
Miscellaneous				
1 tablet vaginally (estradiol) daily for 2 wk, then 1 tablet twice weekly 0.5 g cream applied nightly for 2 wk, then twice weekly				
estrogen	Vaginal ring: 2 mg intravaginally; following insertion, ring should remain in place for 90 dNo	No	Risk of worsening estrogen-responsive malignancies Potential for CHD risk	4D
desmopressin	20–40 µg spray intranasally at bedtime 0.1–0.4 mg orally 2 h prior to bedtime	No	Risk of worsening estrogen-responsive malignancies Potential for CHD risk	1B

If tolerability issues preclude the use of anticholinergic drugs, tricyclic antidepressants (TCAs; imipramine), desmopressin, topical estrogens for females, and alpha-adrenergic antagonists for males are appropriate alternatives. There is emerging evidence about the role of selective serotonin reuptake inhibitors (SSRIs) and serotonin-norepinephrine reuptake inhibitors (SNRIs) in treating OAB syndrome. Vanilloids and afferent nerve inhibitors such as capsaicin or resiniferatoxin are in the investigation phases to assess their utility in managing OAB.

The combination of pharmacologic and nonpharmacologic treatment tends to yield superior outcomes and clinical success. "Bladder training" encompasses pelvic floor exercises, scheduled voiding, urge suppression skills, and extensive patient education. Over 70% of patients who are considered cognitively competent experience a meaningful reduction in incontinence episodes over a 2- to 3-month period as a result of employing bladder training and pelvic floor exercises (Ouslander, 2004). Benefit may still be derived from prompted scheduled voiding in patients who are cognitively impaired. In refractory cases of OAB, biofeedback devices that deliver electrical stimulation via vaginal or rectal probes augment the pelvic floor exercises. In severe or refractory patients, surgical interventions, such as neural ablation, slings, and neuromodulating device implantation, may be attempted. This will be further discussed.

Compensatory behaviors such as limiting fluid intake or reducing the frequency of diuretics are not recommended, although patients frequently engage in these behaviors. Self-imposed fluid restriction may precipitate dehydration and subsequent increased fall risks, cognitive impairment, worsened renal function, and changes in drug metabolism. Altering diuretic administration could negatively impact the treatment of other conditions or result in fluid overload. The use of absorbent pads or undergarments may help to mitigate the social stigma aspect of OAB, especially in patients who experience incontinence. Rushing to find a restroom when urgency occurs also predisposes patients to falls and fractures (**Box 34.3**).

Goals of Drug Therapy

The intended outcome of pharmacologic therapy is primarily resolution of symptoms (urgency, frequency, nocturia), cessation of incontinence episodes (if present), and a full return to previous level of social functioning. In the event of a comorbid mood disorder (depression, anxiety) that emerged as a consequence of OAB, goals of therapy would include resolution of this disorder as well. Patients suffering from OAB are at an increased risk for urinary tract infections, and those with associated incontinence are at risk for perineal skin infections. These corresponding issues may resolve spontaneously upon treatment of the OAB and/or incontinence; however, additional drug therapy may be required (**Table 34.4**).

Anticholinergic/Antimuscarinic Drugs

As a class, antimuscarinic drugs are the mainstay of pharmacologic therapy for OAB and UI. Anticholinergic drugs are considered first-line therapy and typically will be used even after clinical failure or intolerance to an initial anticholinergic medication. The class is divided into tertiary and quaternary amines, differing with respect to lipophilicity, molecular size, and charge. High lipophilicity, small molecular size, and low charge confer upon the tertiary amines (oxybutynin, tolterodine, solifenacin, darifenacin, fesoterodine) easy transfer into the CNS via the blood-brain barrier. The quaternary amine trospium tends to not be as well absorbed and has limited ability to cross the blood-brain barrier (**Table 34.5**).

Mechanism of Action

The mechanism of action of each of the medications is relatively similar, with the exception of oxybutynin. Generally, anticholinergics mediate a pharmacologic action by antagonizing the parasympathetic muscarinic receptors in the bladder with relative selectivity for the M_3 and M_1 subtypes. Antagonism of the M_3 muscarinic receptors manifests as a reduction in spontaneous myocyte activity, a decrease in frequency, and a reduction in contraction intensity. They effectively increase bladder capacity, decrease the intensity and frequency of bladder contractions, and delay the initial urge to void. Oxybutynin is both an antimuscarinic and an antispasmodic (secondary to direct muscle relaxation) as well as a local anesthetic.

Oxybutynin boasts a lengthy and robust history of efficacy with respect to OAB and UI. A tertiary amine, oxybutynin is highly lipophilic and easily crosses the blood-brain barrier, thereby conferring higher rates of CNS and anticholinergic adverse effects. The potential for cytochrome P450 enzyme interactions is relatively high as well. Secondary to these adverse effects and interaction potential, oxybutynin may not be well tolerated in all patient populations. Oxybutynin undergoes extensive first-pass metabolism to its active metabolite, N-desmethyl oxybutynin, which is purported to produce most of the pharmacologic activity and adverse effects. Up to 80% of patients will report at least one significant muscarinic-mediated adverse effect during therapy, up to 20% of whom will subsequently discontinue therapy. Xerostomia, experienced by up to 70% of patients, is dose-related but is also the most common reason cited for discontinuing oxybutynin therapy. Despite these inherent limitations, the use of oxybutynin remains prevalent among all available formulations. The extended-release (ER; Ditropan XL) formulation of oxybu-

BOX 34.3

Behavioral Modifications

Reduce fluid consumption.
Reduce alcohol consumption.
Reduce caffeine consumption.
Start bladder training.
Perform pelvic floor exercises.

TABLE 34.4	Medication Pharmacokinetics and Clinical Considerations

Drug	Metabolism	Interactions	Contraindications	Clinical Considerations
Antimuscarinics				
oxybutynin	Minor substrate of CYP3A4	CYP3A4 inhibitors or inducers Pramlintide may enhance the anticholinergic effects of anticholinergics.	Narrow-angle glaucoma, urinary retention	Xerostomia (29%–71%; dose related) Constipation (7%–15%)
tolterodine	Major substrate of CYP2D6 and 3A4 Minor substrate of CYP2C9 and 2C19	Strong CYP2D6 or 3A4 inhibitors or inducers Systemic azole antifungals may decrease metabolism of tolterodine. Tolterodine may enhance the anticoagulant effect of warfarin.	Urinary retention, narrow-angle glaucoma	Prolonged QTc interval at supratherapeutic doses CYP2D6 poor metabolizers more likely to exhibit QTc prolongation Dosage adjustment for renal impairment Dry mouth (35%; ER capsules, 23%)
trospium	Not fully elucidated; thought to be metabolized by esterase hydrolysis and conjugation	Pramlintide may enhance the anticholinergic effect of anticholinergics.	Bladder flow obstruction, narrow-angle glaucoma	Dosage adjustment of IR trospium in renal impairment Avoid use of ER trospium in patients with renal impairment.
solifenacin	Major CYP3A4 substrate	Major inhibitors or inducers of CYP3A4 Grapefruit juice may increase the serum level effects of solifenacin.	Bladder flow obstruction, narrow-angle glaucoma	Dosage adjustment for severe renal impairment (CrCl <30 mL/min)
darifenacin	Major substrate of CYP3A4 and minor substrate of 2D6 Moderate inhibitor of 2D6 and minor inhibitor of 3A4	CYP3A4 or 2D6 inhibitors or inducers	Uncontrolled narrow-angle glaucoma; urinary retention, paralytic ileus, GI or GU obstruction Concomitant administration of thioridazine	Xerostomia (19%–35%), constipation (15%–21%)
fesoterodine	Parent compound metabolized to active metabolite (5-HMT) by nonspecific esterases 5-HMT metabolized by CYP2D6 and CYP3A4	CYP3A4 or 2D6 inhibitors or inducers	Bladder-flow obstruction, narrow-angle glaucoma	Dose adjustment in patients with severe renal impairment (CrCl <30 mL/min)
Tricyclic Antidepressants				
imipramine	Major substrate of CYP2D6 (minor substrate of 1A2, 2B6, 2C19)	CYP2D6 inhibitors or inducers Metoclopramide (may enhance TCA toxicity) QTc-prolonging drugs (ex: tetrabenazine, ziprasidone, thioridazine)	Concurrent use of MAO inhibitors (within 14 d) Concurrent use of dronedarone	Orthostatic hypotension, confusion, drowsiness, ECG changes, urinary retention
Serotonin-Norepinephrine Reuptake Inhibitors				
duloxetine	Major substrate of CYP1A2 and 2D6 Moderate inhibitor of 2D6	CYP1A2 or 2D6 inhibitors or inducers MAO inhibitors Thioridazine	Concomitant use or within 2 wk of MAO inhibitors; uncontrolled narrow-angle glaucoma	Ulcerogenic potential increased with NSAIDs (increased risk of bleeding) Serotonin syndrome or neuroleptic malignant syndrome risk Not recommended when CrCl <30 mL/min
Alpha-Adrenergic Antagonists				
alfuzosin	Major substrate of CYP 3A4	Strong CYP3A4 inhibitors	Strong CYP3A4 inhibitors (itraconazole, ketoconazole, ritonavir)	Avoid concomitant use with other alpha-1-antagonists Potential to cause dizziness

(continued)

TABLE 34.4	Medication Pharmacokinetics and Clinical Considerations (*Continued*)			
Drug	**Metabolism**	**Interactions**	**Contraindications**	**Clinical Considerations**
doxazosin	Major substrate of CYP3A4	Strong CYP3A4 inhibitors	Strong CYP3A4 inhibitors (itraconazole)	Dizziness may occur in up to 28% of patients.
prazosin	Major substrate of CYP3A4	Strong CYP3A4 inhibitors	Strong CYP3A4 inhibitors (itraconazole)	Dizziness
tamsulosin	Major substrate of CYP3A4	Strong CYP3A4 inhibitors	Strong CYP3A4 inhibitors (itraconazole)	Dizziness
terazosin	Major substrate of CYP3A4	Strong CYP3A4 inhibitors	Strong CYP3A4 inhibitors (itraconazole)	Dizziness
silodosin	Major substrate of CYP3A4	Strong CYP3A4 inhibitors	Strong CYP3A4 inhibitors (itraconazole)	Retrograde ejaculation

tynin has been clinically shown to be equally efficacious but is associated with less adverse effects than the conventional formulation. The transdermal oxybutynin patch (Oxytrol) causes roughly 75% less dry mouth as compared to ER tolterodine.

Tolterodine (Detrol) is a competitive antagonist of muscarinic receptors that causes increased residual urine volume and decreased detrusor pressure. It is associated with clinically meaningful reductions in micturition frequency as well as incontinence episodes. In comparison to oxybutynin, tolterodine use yields less dosage changes, adverse effects, and treatment-related therapy discontinuations. Tolterodine ER (Detrol LA) is 18% more effective in reducing the incidence of incontinence as compared to the regular formulation and is responsible for 23% less xerostomia (Robinson & Cardozo, 2010). ER oxybutynin, however, is significantly more efficacious than ER tolterodine in reducing micturition frequency.

Trospium (Sanctura) is a nonselective muscarinic receptor antagonist that improves urinary frequency, episodes of incontinence, urgency, and volume voided. A quaternary ammonium compound, trospium crosses the blood-brain barrier only to a limited extent, which confers a reduced likelihood of cognitive sequelae.

Solifenacin (Vesicare) is a bladder-selective M_3 receptor antagonist that has been shown to be statistically significantly more efficacious than ER tolterodine with respect to urge incontinence, overall incontinence, and urgency. In another pivotal study, solifenacin was shown to reduce episodes of urgency and increase warning time. It is postulated that solifenacin may provide a greater level of efficacy as compared to other drugs within the class. However, despite its bladder selectivity, solifenacin causes dry mouth in over 20% of patients and xerostomia-related treatment discontinuation in almost 5% (Robinson & Cardozo, 2010).

Darifenacin (Enablex), a tertiary amine, is a highly selective M_3 receptor antagonist that is effective in reducing frequency of micturition, increasing bladder capacity, reducing frequency and severity of urgency, and reducing the number of episodes of incontinence.

Fesoterodine (Toviaz), a prodrug, is converted to its active metabolite 5-hydroxymethyl tolterodine (5-HMT), which exerts a pharmacologic effect as a competitive antagonist at the muscarinic receptors. Tolterodine (Detrol) is metabolized to 5-HMT via a cytochrome P450 (CYP) 2D6-mediated oxidation, and both tolterodine and 5-HMT are responsible for the pharmacologic effect of Detrol. Fesoterodine, however, does not require CYP2D6 activation and therefore may have less potential for pharmacokinetic variability and CYP2D6-specific drug interactions.

TABLE 34.5	Molecular Properties of Antimuscarinic Drugs		
Drug	**Molecular Classification**	**Corresponding Molecular Characteristics**	**Clinical Characteristics**
oxybutynin tolterodine solifenacin darifenacin fesoterodine	Tertiary amine	High lipophilicity Small molecular size Low charge	Extensive transfer into CNS Increased risk of cognitive adverse effects
trospium	Quaternary amine	Low lipophilicity Large molecular size High charge	Limited transfer into CNS Reduced risk of cognitive adverse effects

Time Frame for Response

Expected therapeutic response is variable among members of this class. Generally, a meaningful response would be realized within about 2 weeks. However, evidence suggests that patients taking tolterodine ER experienced reduced micturition, urgency episodes, and incontinence by day 5 of therapy. Trospium may exert a clinical effect as early as day 1 with regard to incontinence, day 3 for urgency, and day 5 for micturition frequency.

Contraindications

Anticholinergic medications are capable of precipitating or worsening urinary retention as well as worsening narrow-angle glaucoma. Both of these conditions, if present in the patient prior to therapy, represent contraindications to the use of antimuscarinics. Antagonism of muscarinic receptors and subsequent down-regulation of acetylcholine activity can result in paralysis of smooth muscle in the bladder or gastrointestinal tract. Additionally, mydriasis can occur with increased intraocular pressure; therefore, anticholinergics should be avoided in patients with narrow-angle glaucoma. Tolterodine, trospium, solifenacin, and fesoterodine require a dosage reduction in the case of severe renal impairment (creatinine clearance [CrCl] < 30 mL/minute). However, the ER formulation of trospium should be avoided in patients with severe renal impairment (**Table 34.6**).

Adverse Events

The expected adverse event profile includes traditional anticholinergic effects such as xerostomia, constipation, and urinary retention. Antimuscarinic drugs exert an action mainly during the storage phase of the micturition cycle when there is an absence of parasympathetic activity in the detrusor. During the emptying phase of micturition, there is a massive release of acetylcholine, which effectively blunts the drug's action. If this did not occur, the presence of the active drug would undoubtedly decrease the ability of the bladder to contract to promote urinary retention. Prescribing these drugs within the confines of acceptable dosing typically does not precipitate urinary retention; however, overdose or pharmacokinetic interactions may do so.

TABLE 34.6	Antimuscarinic Medication Dosing Considerations					
	Oxybutynin	**Tolterodine**	**Trospium**	**Solifenacin**	**Darifenacin**	**Fesoterodine**
Usual Dose	IR: 5–15 mg orally three times daily ER: 5–15 mg orally once daily Patch: 3.9 mg/patch twice weekly (every 3–4 d)	IR: 2 mg orally twice daily ER: 4 mg orally once daily	IR: 20 mg orally twice daily ER: 60 mg once daily ≥75: 20 mg orally once daily	5–10 mg orally once daily Dosage adjustment with concomitant CYP3A4 inhibitors: Maximum dose 5 mg/d	7.5–15 mg once daily Dosage adjustment with concomitant potent CYP3A4 inhibitors (ex: azole antifungals, erythromycin, protease inhibitors): 7.5 mg/d	4–8 mg orally daily
Renal Insufficiency		**Use with caution **CrCl 10–30 mL/min: IR: 1 mg twice daily ER: 2 mg daily	CrCl ≤30 mL/min: IR: 20 mg once daily at bedtime ER: Use not recommended	CrCl <30 mL/min: Maximum dose: 5 mg/d		Severe renal impairment (CrCl <30 mL/min): 4 mg
Hepatic Insufficiency		IR: 1 mg twice daily ER: 2 mg daily		Moderate (Child-Pugh class B): Maximum dose: 5 mg/d Severe (Child-Pugh class C): Use not recommended	Moderate impairment (Child-Pugh class B): Daily dosage should not exceed 7.5 mg/d Severe impairment (Child-Pugh class C): use not recommended	Severe hepatic impairment (Child-Pugh class C): Use not recommended
CYP Interactions	CYP3A4 inhibitors or inducers	Strong CYP2D6 or 3A4 inhibitors or inducers Azole antifungals		Major inhibitors or inducers of CYP3A4	CYP 2D6 and 3A4 inhibitors	Strong CYP 3A4 inhibitors

Interactions

Most antimuscarinic drugs are metabolized by one or more CYP P450 isoenzymes, the most common of which are CYP3A4 and CYP2D6. Heterozygous or CYP2D6 homozygous patients are considered "extensive metabolizers," which implies an innate ability to appropriately metabolize drugs via this isoenzyme. However, patients who are poor metabolizers with respect to CYP2D6 may be at an increased risk for drug-related toxicity secondary to their inability to fully metabolize CYP2D6-metabolized drugs. Trospium is metabolized exclusively by nonspecific esterases independent of the hepatic CYP P450 system. Notable drug interactions within the anticholinergic class tend to involve pharmacokinetic interactions at the enzyme level and typically manifest as increases or decreases in drug metabolism. Solifenacin and tolterodine are capable of causing prolonged QTc, particularly in supratherapeutic dosing. Concomitant administration of other QTc-prolonging medications can potentiate a pharmacodynamic interaction that may result in arrhythmia.

Tricyclic Antidepressants

Despite its traditional indication, imipramine (Tofranil) also has anticholinergic activity and has been used in the treatment of OAB. Imipramine has established utility in treating nocturnal enuresis in children with success rates as high as 70%. Regardless of the apparent clinical success in mitigation of enuresis, there are no randomized, controlled trials that support the use of imipramine in OAB.

Mechanism of Action

Imipramine, a TCA, blocks the reuptake of serotonin and norepinephrine by the presynaptic neuronal membrane.

Adverse Events, Contraindications, and Interactions

The use of monoamine oxidase (MAO) inhibitors within 14 days of initiation of imipramine is contraindicated because this increases the risk of serotonin syndrome. Imipramine may cause orthostatic hypotension and numerous cardiotoxic effects, which include a prolonged QTc interval and proarrhythmic potential. Concomitant administration of drugs that are capable of prolonging the QT interval represents an interaction risk level X and therefore would be contraindications as well (dronedarone). Strong CYP2D6 and CYP2C19 inhibitors should be avoided as well.

Serotonin-Norepinephrine Reuptake Inhibitors

Venlafaxine (Effexor) and duloxetine (Cymbalta), SNRIs, have been evaluated as nontraditional therapies for OAB.

Mechanism of Action

Serotonin facilitates urine storage, augmenting parasympathetic innervation and inhibiting sympathetic innervation to the bladder. During the filling phase, glutamate is released and acts upon Onuf's nucleus. Onuf's nucleus is a discrete confluence of neurons in the anterior horn of the sacral region of the spinal cord, which is involved in the micturition reflex, continence, and muscular contraction during orgasm. The action of glutamate in Onuf's nucleus activates the pudendal nerve and subsequent release of acetylcholine, which elicits contraction of the external urethral sphincter. The dense population of the nucleus with serotonin and norepinephrine receptors implies a facilitator role for these monoamines with regard to the micturition reflex and urine storage. Duloxetine enhances urethral sphincter activity and is associated with dose-dependent decreases in episodes of incontinence and improvements in quality of life. It is believed that duloxetine exerts this effect by increasing the availability of serotonin and norepinephrine in the synaptic clefts of Onuf's nucleus. Nausea occurs in about 25% of patients but tends to subside by day 7 of treatment. Numerous studies support the use of SNRIs alone or in combination with pelvic-floor muscle exercises.

Contraindications, Adverse Events, and Interactions

Duloxetine may not be used concurrently with MAO inhibitors or within 2 weeks of discontinuing an MAO inhibitor. Duloxetine is metabolized in the liver by CYP3A4 and CYP2D6 and therefore is subject to pharmacokinetic interactions with strong inhibitors of these isoenzymes. It is not to be coadministered with thioridazine because there is a significant CYP2D6-mediated interaction that may result in increased concentrations and toxicity in both drugs. Concomitant administration of duloxetine with other medications that have serotonergic or noradrenergic actions may increase the risk of serotonin syndrome or neuroleptic malignant syndrome.

Alpha-Adrenergic Antagonists

The α-adrenergic antagonists have proven efficacy and tolerability with respect to treating BPH in males. However, some studies suggest that tamsulosin may reduce bladder pressure, increase the flow rate, and provide symptomatic improvement in patients with OAB and a confirmed obstruction. The extent to which OAB symptoms are relieved is appreciably less than the resolution of symptoms of obstruction. Use in women is controversial because α-adrenergic antagonists may precipitate stress incontinence in female patients.

Mechanism of Action

Alpha-adrenergic antagonists, or alpha blockers, competitively inhibit postsynaptic alpha$_1$-adrenergic receptors in prostate and bladder tissue. The antagonism reduces the sympathetic–mediated urethral stricture that is associated with BPH or bladder outlet obstruction symptoms.

Adverse Events

Postural hypotension is one of the most clinically relevant adverse effects that may occur. All of the drugs in this class have the potential to induce this effect; however, doxazosin precipitates postural hypotension in upwards of 30% of patients. It is of special concern since the majority of patients who would likely be taking an alpha-1-antagonist are elderly and are predisposed to postural hypotension and subsequent falls.

Interactions

The alpha-1-antagonists are metabolized by CYP3A4, and concomitant administration with strong CYP3A4 inhibitors should be avoided. Also, secondary to the potential to cause hypotension, more than one alpha blocker should not be used concurrently.

Estrogens

Despite the dearth of anecdotal evidence supporting the use of estrogens for symptomatic improvement of OAB and incontinence in females, randomized, controlled trials have yielded contradictory results at best. Unopposed systemic estrogen therapy or combination estrogen/progesterone therapy is associated with an increase in SUI and UUI episodes, as was evidenced by several large multinational studies. Topical estrogen therapy in the form of vaginal estradiol tablets (Vagifem) or the estrogen-releasing vaginal ring (Estring) has, however, demonstrated some symptomatic improvement. The vaginal tablet improved urgency, frequency, urge incontinence, and stress incontinence. The vaginal ring improved urge incontinence, stress incontinence, and nocturia. The therapeutic effect is attributed to increasing the maximum urethral pressure, although some clinicians hypothesize that it is due to reversal of urogenital atrophy and not direct bladder or urethral activity.

Mechanism of Action

Topical estradiol exerts a local action that improves tone and elasticity of female urogenital anatomy by increasing secretion of the cervical mucosa, thickening vaginal mucosa, and proliferation of the endometrium. Both the vaginal tablet and the vaginal ring are indicated for urinary urgency and dysuria.

Contraindications

Patients with undiagnosed vaginal bleeding, a history of breast carcinoma or estrogen-dependent tumors, thromboembolic disorders (deep vein thrombosis, pulmonary embolism, stroke, myocardial infarction), or patients who are pregnant should not use estrogens.

Adverse Events

Administration of topical estrogens for OAB and incontinence symptoms is not without risk. Well-designed, large-scale, randomized, controlled trials have clearly demonstrated the cardiovascular sequelae that can result from utilizing hormone replacement therapy (HRT) for primary prevention of cardiovascular disease. Since the advent of the Women's Health Initiative study, the use of HRT has dramatically declined. However, in selected individuals, HRT is still used for the treatment of menopause-related symptoms, which include urogenital complaints (vaginal atrophy, dysuria, incontinence).

Risks of administration include the potential for thromboembolic complications, aggravation of existing estrogen-responsive malignancies or development of estrogen-responsive cancers, changes in libido, mood dysregulation, irritability, or syncope.

Antidiuretic Drugs

Mechanism of Action

Desmopressin (1-desamino-8-D-arginine vasopressin; DDAVP), a synthetic vasopressin analogue, had been indicated for nocturnal enuresis in adults and children. It possesses profound antidiuretic properties without any appreciable pressor activity; DDAVP can diurese without impacting blood pressure in a clinically significant way. Exploiting the hypothesis that a relative absence of nocturnal vasopressin and subsequently increased nocturnal urine production underlies the predisposition to suffer from enuresis, DDAVP reduces urine volume and osmolality. In addition to the established indication for enuresis in children, DDAVP has been shown to be efficacious in treating adult patients with nocturia of polyuric origin.

Contraindications and Adverse Events

Patients with hyponatremia or a history of hyponatremia or moderate to severe renal impairment (CrCl <50 mL/min) should avoid DDAVP. Adverse effects are mild and rare. However, there is a risk of water retention with or without hyponatremia. Sodium monitoring is recommended in elderly patients prior to treatment and several days into therapy.

Interactions

There are no significant drug interactions associated with DDAVP. Several medications (lithium, TCAs, SSRIs, nonsteroidal anti-inflammatory drugs, carbamazepine) may enhance the toxic effects of DDAVP, but none of the risks are particularly likely.

New and Emerging Therapies

Vanilloid receptors on afferent neurons that innervate the bladder and urethra may be acted upon by capsaicin or resiniferatoxin. Capsaicin-mediated activation of the afferent neurons results in an initial excitation phase immediately followed by a protracted blockade that effectively desensitizes the neurons to normal stimuli. A capsaicin analogue, resiniferatoxin, can also impact the afferent neurons and the Aδ fibers. This transient physiologic "damage" to sensory nerves results in more prolonged retention of urine and improvement in OAB and DO of neurogenic and idiopathic origin.

Botulinum toxin A blocks the release of acetylcholine from the presynaptic neuron, which, in turn, decreases muscle contractility and increases muscle atrophy locally.

Selecting the Most Appropriate Agent

First-Line Therapy

As previously stated, there is an absence of published clinical guidelines for OAB in the United States. Therefore, the choice of an initial drug therapy is generally based on clinical experience, clinical trials, and recommendations from the ICS. In the absence of contraindications, anticholinergic medications are considered first-line therapy for OAB and symptoms of incontinence. Nonpharmacologic interventions, such as bladder training, typically are recommended prior to initiating drug therapy. Oftentimes if the behavioral modifications do not suitably resolve the symptoms of OAB, a medication will be added to the nondrug intervention.

Antimuscarinics as a class have an established reputation with regard to efficacy and safety. They effectively reduce bladder pressure, increase bladder capacity and compliance, increase the volume threshold for desire to urinate, and reduce inappropriate bladder contractions. Tolerability issues involving anticholinergic adverse effects (dry mouth, constipation) may limit clinical utility in some patient populations, but largely does not significantly impact therapy. There is no unequivocal evidence that recommends the use of one member of this class over another; however, there have been smaller studies that suggest some differential benefits. In terms of efficacy, the larger body of literature supports relative equivalence among antimuscarinics. ER formulations have demonstrated improved efficacy compared to their immediate-release (IR) counterparts. Some recent meta-analyses have insinuated that solifenacin may offer superior clinical efficacy compared to oxybutynin ER and tolterodine ER (Robinson & Cardozo, 2010). When considering the anticholinergic side-effect potential, oxybutynin is undeniably responsible for the most xerostomia and constipation. Trospium and darifenacin promote fewer cognitive sequelae than oxybutynin, tolterodine, or solifenacin. Trospium is not metabolized by the CYP P450 system and therefore is associated with far fewer drug interactions than the rest of this class, which is metabolized primarily by CYP. New evidence suggests that fesoterodine may be more effective than tolterodine in terms of efficacy and improvement in quality of life. Tolterodine is currently the market leader in the majority of countries.

Second- and Third-Line Therapy

Failure or intolerance to the initial anticholinergic medication generally warrants the trial of a second anticholinergic medication. Since there are some appreciable differences among anticholinergics in terms of side-effect profiles and tolerability, a switch to another anticholinergic typically precedes a switch to a different class.

Duloxetine has demonstrated some success in OAB, but to a greater extent with stress incontinence. Incontinence (generally urge incontinence) is part of the OAB symptom constellation and is alleviated by duloxetine treatment. A similar scenario exists for the use of estrogens for OAB. Estrogens are primarily used for SUI and other urogenital symptoms but have demonstrated utility in OAB.

Imipramine's clinical success is comparable to that of oxybutynin; however, the potential for more serious adverse effects (cardiotoxicity, life-threatening drug interactions, and mortality risk in overdose) relegates this option to a last resort. Additionally, imipramine is indicated for urinary incontinence in children; there is no officially labeled indication for OAB symptoms in adults currently.

Botulinum A toxin is indicated for neurogenic and non-neurogenic DO as well as neurogenic spasm of the urethra due to spinal cord injury or secondary to DO. Injection of 100 to 300 U directly into the detrusor muscle promotes an effect for 3 to 9 months. The need for repeat injections, the potential for adverse effects, and product and administration costs have resulted in reduced usage for OAB.

Surgical intervention is arguably the last option in terms of management of OAB; it is generally attempted after failure of all reasonable pharmacologic options. This is mostly due to the inherent risks in abdominal or pelvic operation, namely impacts on renal function, sexual function, and on any abdominal or pelvic pathology. In addition, surgical intervention is generally most effective in cases of isolated stress incontinence where there is underlying bladder or urethral pathology. In females, surgery usually involves repositioning the urethra so that it is more amenable to pressure changes or providing artificial support or resistance to the urethra by way of a sling. In males, surgery involves implantation of a manually controlled artificial silicone urethral sphincter.

Refractory OAB

Depending upon the underlying etiology of OAB, some patients may not be successfully treated with first- or even second-line options. If multiple antimuscarinic drugs fail, as well as appropriate second- and third-line options, more invasive interventions might become necessary. Implantable neurostimulator devices or sacral neuromodulator placement are moderately successful but costly alternatives. Electrical stimulation of the peripheral nervous system has been shown to positively impact urinary urgency and urge incontinence. Both anal and vaginal transcutaneous stimulation play a role in the treatment of OAB. Direct electrical stimulation of the third and sometimes fourth sacral nerves via a surgically implanted modulator delivers continuous stimulation directly to a nerve with which it is in close contact. Augmentation cystoplasty surgery involves the anastomosis of a segment of bowel to the bisected bladder. This procedure increases bladder capacity and decreases bladder pressure. Serious risks include kidney or bladder infections, new recurrent urinary tract infections, or metabolic abnormalities. Surgical augmentation cystoplasty, neobladder construction, and urinary diversion techniques involve more risk and tend to be reserved for severe, refractory cases.

Another therapeutic consideration is the somewhat controversial dual antimuscarinic drug therapy. This has been studied in both adults and children and has been found to be safe and effective. Dual therapy does not appear to contribute to increased incidence of adverse effects; however, in some patients, the addition of a second anticholinergic drug precipitated post-void residual volume increases but not urinary retention (Bolduc, et al., 2009).

In male patients with OAB in the setting of bladder outlet obstruction secondary to BPH, the combination of α-adrenergic blockers and 5-α-reductase inhibitors (finasteride, dutasteride) may offer some clinical utility.

Special Considerations

Pediatric

Isolated incontinence tends to manifest in young children as nocturia or enuresis. This is generally due to underlying deficits in learned neural control, delayed development of the nervous system, or potentially a more complex issue involving multiple systems. OAB symptoms of urgency or frequency in children commonly occur as a result of fecal impaction or underlying structural abnormalities. Children can present with voiding dysfunction, urgency, frequency, or incontinence. Oxybutynin IR and ER formulations are the only pharmacologic options approved by the U.S. Food and Drug Administration for OAB in children, although tolterodine IR and ER and trospium have been evaluated in clinical trials. All of the medications yielded successful outcomes in terms of reductions in diurnal incontinence, urgency episodes, micturition, and increases in bladder capacity. The adverse effects are similar to those experienced by adults and consisted mainly of dry mouth. Cognitive effects are not significant with respect to memory, cognition, speed of processing, or attention. DDAVP nasal spray has been the cornerstone of therapy for children with enuresis and has demonstrated clinical efficacy, safety, and tolerability.

Geriatric

As was previously mentioned, there is an inherent challenge with regard to OAB in the elderly patient. Numerous nonurinary factors such as anatomic, physiologic, age-related, or iatrogenic elements predispose elderly patients to the development of OAB or the worsening of existing OAB. The incidence of OAB is highest in the elderly population, and yet the preferred pharmacologic modality for treating this syndrome tends to impact cognition to an extent that may limit utility in this population. Despite these clinical considerations, antimuscarinic therapy is still considered first line. If the adverse effects are intolerable or if the antimuscarinic agent aggravates an existing condition, an alternate medication should be given. If pharmacologic options are exhausted or are not feasible, surgical interventions can be considered in surgical candidates or the syndrome can be managed less aggressively. Less aggressive options include scheduled voiding, bladder training, and the use of absorbent pads or undergarments.

Women

True OAB syndrome affects men and women relatively equally; however, the symptom of incontinence tends to present more frequently in women. Furthermore, within postmenopausal symptomatology, vaginal atrophy and other urogenital changes may underlie urgency, frequency, and urge or stress incontinence that frequently accompanies menopause. SUI affects 78% of women with incontinence episodes (Basu & Duckett, 2009). SUI may be predicated on intrinsic urethral sphincter deficiency or urethral hypermobility secondary to the loss of vaginal support structures. Antimuscarinic medications are first line; however, in appropriately selected patients, topical estrogens may offer some therapeutic benefit. Duloxetine has been extensively studied in women with stress incontinence secondary to urethral dysfunction or vaginal atrophy. There is an established correlation between SUI and female sexual dysfunction.

MONITORING PATIENT RESPONSE

Despite the seemingly impressive efficacy of anticholinergic drug therapy, there is roughly a 50% placebo response rate, which complicates the assessment of patient response. As the majority of OAB symptomatology is subjective in nature, patient-generated feedback is the most valuable assessment tool with which to measure success. The domains related to the pathology itself that should be assessed include symptoms, symptom severity, and quality of life. If drug therapy has been initiated, drug-specific parameters such as treatment-emergent side effects or drug interactions need to be assessed as well.

There are numerous validated symptom inventories and quality of life assessment tools that have been employed in clinical trials as well as in practice to monitor patient response to treatment. The ICS highly recommends that symptom assessment and quality of life inventories be used throughout the treatment process in order to assess and guide therapy. The OAB-q assesses both the symptoms and quality of life impact in men and women. The reduced version of this scale includes 8 bladder symptom items and 25 health-related quality of life (HRQOL) items, which include symptom bother, coping skills, concerns and worries, sleep, social interaction, and HRQOL total. In females, the Urogenital Distress Inventory (UDI-6), the Incontinence Severity Index (ISI), and the BFLUTS questionnaire are used to assess the symptom of urinary incontinence specifically. In males, the ICS_{male} and DAN-PSS will assess the symptom of urinary incontinence. The UDI-6 assesses 19 LUT symptoms as well as the degree of anxiety or bother that is experienced as a result of the incontinence episodes. This scale may have predictive value with respect to urodynamic studies, especially in stress incontinence, bBOO, and DO. The ISI is a simple index that generates a numerical product based on frequency and volume of urine loss. The product is associated with the level of severity of the incontinence. BFLUTS evaluates incontinence symptoms and LUT symptoms as well as the degree of bother associated with each. Both the ICS_{male} and DAN-PSS assess LUT symptoms and the extent to which the patient is bothered. Unfortunately, there is no consensus regarding at which point or how frequently these assessment tools should be administered to yield optimal information about treatment response.

Ongoing assessment of potential treatment-related adverse effects is highly recommended. This can be accomplished by clinician-led patient interviews or patient-generated complaints. The drugs most frequently used to treat OAB have the potential to cause bothersome or sometimes serious adverse effects. Since the patient population most often affected by OAB is usually also affected by polypharmacy, multiple medical conditions, predisposition to falls, and predisposition to anticholinergic adverse effects, diligent monitoring of iatrogenic effects is paramount.

PATIENT EDUCATION AND PATIENT-ORIENTED INFORMATION SOURCES

Although OAB tends to affect the elderly more frequently than younger patients and may be partially caused or worsened by seemingly normal processes associated with aging, OAB is *not* considered a normal part of aging. Patients need to be made aware of this and their symptoms need to be validated. One of the challenges in diagnosing OAB is the reluctance of patients to complain of the symptoms or the patient's misconception about the symptoms being a normal part of aging. Once a patient is diagnosed with OAB, it is exceptionally important to emphasize that the symptoms need not be tolerated and that ongoing assessment of symptoms and symptom bother is essential to successful treatment.

Once a treatment modality has been mutually agreed upon by the patient and the care provider, the risks and benefits need to be clearly explained to the patient. More often than not, the treatment will consist of a medication and lifestyle changes or bladder training. The medications used to treat OAB (usually anticholinergics) will likely cause at least some minor anticholinergic adverse effects such as dry mouth or constipation. Severe xerostomia can be treated with adequate hydration as well as saliva substitutes. Constipation can be avoided by maintaining adequate hydration or remedied by using a stool softener (docusate) or a stimulant laxative (senna, bisacodyl). Patients should be warned about potentially severe anticholinergic effects such as urinary retention and advised to seek medical attention if symptoms consistent with urinary retention present. Antimuscarinic drugs may potentially augment anticholinergic effects of other anticholinergic medications. Therefore, in the case of multiple physicians, patients should be advised to make their care providers aware of any and all medications prescribed by all members of the healthcare team.

Aside from the OAB and medication information that may be provided by the patient's care provider, there are numerous reputable sources for patient-oriented information. The American Urogynecology Society maintains a patient-friendly website that explains pelvic-floor disorders, incontinence, and OAB. It also provides a list of frequently asked questions, tools for patients, bladder diary support, medications and other treatment options, and a search engine for locating a care provider. The National Association for Continence is another reputable website that offers useful information regarding underlying causes of OAB, treatment options, frequently asked questions, and a public bathroom finder. The bathroom finder tool is a Google Maps™–powered application that allows the user to input a city or zip code and will then generate a graphical representation of the location of public restrooms.

Nutrition/Lifestyle Changes

Generally before the initiation of drug therapy, patients will be encouraged to adopt some clinician-guided lifestyle changes to minimize the impact of diet or behavior on OAB. It is *not* recommended that patients attempt to remedy OAB on their own by modifying behavior as was previously discussed. Uninformed and unmonitored changes (such as cessation of diuretic use) may detrimentally impact other aspects of the patient's care or may instigate a nascent problem. All of the nutritional or lifestyle changes should be recommended by the care provider and should be monitored; none of these changes should be initiated by the patient.

Compounds that irritate the bladder may exacerbate or precipitate OAB. Tomatoes, artificial sweeteners, grapes, carbonated beverages, strawberries, apple juice, vinegar, weight loss supplements, and spicy foods all may contribute to OAB pathology. Alcohol and caffeine not only act as bladder irritants but they also inhibit antidiuretic hormone (ADH) release, which in turn, will increase the production of urine and contribute to urgency and frequency. Moderation of the consumption of these foods, beverages, or products will likely reduce some of the added pressures that may be contributing to OAB symptoms.

Maintenance of a healthy body weight will also aid in the mitigation of OAB symptoms as excess weight puts increased pressure on the bladder. Pelvic-floor exercises and bladder training are also shown to be effective in treating OAB as monotherapy or in combination with medications.

Complementary and Alternative Medications

Numerous natural compounds and botanicals have been evaluated for purposes of treating OAB; however, there is a paucity of evidence to support their use. OAB or urinary dysfunction that is associated with BPH may be further remedied by adjunctive treatment with saw palmetto extract. Saw palmetto or American dwarf plant (*Serenoa repens*) is thought to inhibit 5-α-reductase as its primary pharmacologic action. 5-α-reductase is responsible for the conversion of testosterone to dihydrotestosterone (DHT). DHT is among the androgens that contribute to prostate growth and, in BPH, contributes to pathologic prostate growth. Inhibition of 5-α-reductase opposes the pathologic enlargement of the prostate and subsequently eases the pressure on the urethra at the bladder neck. This effectively reduces or removes the bladder outlet obstruction and improves LUT symptoms in males. Saw palmetto extract would not be an appropriate therapeutic option in patients who do not have an underlying BPH-mediated bladder outlet obstruction.

To date, three active comparator trials have evaluated the efficacy and safety of saw palmetto extract as compared to 5-α-reductase inhibitors or α1-receptor antagonists. Saw

Case Study

C. J. is a 55-year-old postmenopausal woman presenting with a 2-year history of incontinence. She reports that she often cannot get to the bathroom in time when she feels the urge to urinate. She also wets herself when she laughs or sneezes. She is very embarrassed about this problem and has decreased her excursions from the house because of it. She drinks six cups of coffee a day and takes hydrochlorothiazide for hypertension.

DIAGNOSIS: STRESS INCONTINENCE

1. List specific goals for treatment for C. J.
2. What drug therapy would you prescribe? Why?
3. What are the parameters for monitoring the success of the therapy?
4. Discuss specific patient education based on the prescribed therapy.
5. List one or two adverse reactions for the selected agent that would cause you to change therapy.
6. What would be the choice for second-line therapy?
7. What OTC and/or alternative medications would be appropriate for this patient?
8. What dietary and lifestyle changes should be recommended for this patient?
9. Describe one or two drug–drug or drug–food interactions for the selected agent.

---

palmetto and finasteride both improved the score on the International Prostate Symptom Score (IPSS), improved quality of life, and increased peak urinary flow rate. Unlike finasteride, saw palmetto did not impact prostate volume or PSA. The trial comparing saw palmetto to tamsulosin did not find a difference between the two groups in terms of IPSS reduction, maximal flow rate, and irritative or obstructive symptoms (Suzuki, et al., 2009).

BIBLIOGRAPHY

Starred references are cited in the text.

Bartoli, S., Aguzzi, G., & Tarricone, R. (2010). Impact on quality of life of urinary incontinence and overactive bladder: A systematic literature review. *Urology, 75*(3), 491–500.

*Basu, M., & Duckett, J. R. (2009). Update on duloxetine for the management of stress urinary incontinence. *Clinical Interventions in Aging, 4,* 25–30.

*Bolduc, S., Moore, K., Lebel, S., et al. (2009). Double anticholinergic therapy for refractory overactive bladder. *Journal of Urology, 182*(4 Suppl.), 2033–2038.

Campbell, J. D., Gries, K. S., Watanabe, J. H., et al. (2009). Treatment success for overactive bladder with urinary urge incontinence refractory to oral antimuscarinics: A review of published evidence. *BMC Urology, 9,* 18.

Chapple, C. R., Artibani, W., Cardozo, L. D., et al. (2005). The role of urinary urgency and its measurement in the overactive bladder symptom syndrome: Current concepts and future prospects. *British Journal of Urology International, 95*(3), 335–340.

Chu, F. M., & Dmochowski, R. (2006). Pathophysiology of overactive bladder. *American Journal of Medicine, 119*(3 Suppl. 1), 3–8.

Fry, C. H., Meng, E., & Young, J. S. (2010). The physiological function of lower urinary tract smooth muscle. *Autonomic Neuroscience, 19;154*(1–2), 3–13.

*Ganz, M. L., Smalarz, A. M., Krupski, T. L., et al. (2010). Economic costs of overactive bladder in the United States. *Urology, 75*(3), 526–32, 532.e1–e18.

Gillespie, J. I., van Koeveringe, G. A., de Wachter, S. G., et al. (2009). On the origins of the sensory output from the bladder: The concept of afferent noise. *British Journal of Urology International, 103*(10), 1324–1333.

International Continence Society. (2005). *3rd International Consultation on Incontinence.* Plymouth, UK: Health Publications Ltd.

Irwin, D. E., Abrams, P., Milsom, I., et al., and EPIC Study Group. (2008). Understanding the elements of overactive bladder: Questions raised by the EPIC study. *British Journal of Urology International, 101*(11), 1381–1387.

Michel, M. C., & Chapple, C. R. (2009). Basic mechanisms of urgency: Preclinical and clinical evidence. *European Urology, 56*(2), 298–307.

Miller, J., & Hoffman, E. (2006). The causes and consequences of overactive bladder. *Journal of Women's Health, 15*(3), 251–260.

*Ouslander, J. G. (2004). Management of overactive bladder. *New England Journal of Medicine, 350*(8), 786–799.

*Robinson, D., & Cardozo, L. (2010). New drug treatments for urinary incontinence. *Maturitas, 65*(4), 340–347.

*Suzuki, M., Ito, Y., Fujino, T., et al. (2009). Pharmacological effects of saw palmetto extract in the lower urinary tract. *Acta Pharmacologica Sinica, 30*(3), 227–281.

Tsakiris, P., Oelke, M., & Michel, M. C. (2008). Drug-induced urinary incontinence. *Drugs & Aging, 25*(7), 541–549.

Tyagi, S., Thomas, C. A., Hayashi, Y., et al. (2006). The overactive bladder: Epidemiology and morbidity. *Urology Clinics of North America, 33*(4), 433–438, vii.

Ward-Smith, P. (2009). The cost of urinary incontinence. *Urologic Nursing, 29*(3),188–190, 194.

Yamaguchi, O., Nishizawa, O., Takeda, M., et al. (2009). Clinical guidelines for overactive bladder. *International Journal of Urology, 16I*(2), 126–142.

Sexually Transmitted Infections

Sexually transmitted infections (STIs) are among the most common illnesses in the world. They have far-reaching health, social, and economic consequences. Our knowledge about the global prevalence and incidence of these infections is limited by the quality and quantity of data available from throughout the world. STIs remain a major public health concern in the United States. An estimated 19 million infections occur each year. The economic burden is impressive: direct medical costs are estimated as high as $15.5 billion annually. Women and infants are disproportionately affected (Hollier & Workowski, 2008).

People at high risk for contracting STIs are those aged 18 to 28. The highest rate of gonorrhea and chlamydia infections is among females aged 15 to 19. It is also important to bear in mind that STIs rank among the top five risks of international travelers, along with diarrhea, hepatitis, and motor vehicle accidents (Frenkl & Potts, 2008).

In 2006, the Centers for Disease Control and Prevention (CDC) updated the guidelines for treating STIs (**Table 35.1**). Available from the CDC, these guidelines are one of the most widely used documents published by that organization. The guidelines emphasize the development of management strategies that are adaptable to the managed care environment. Because the guidelines are considered the gold standard for treating STIs, most of the information in this chapter is based on them. The goals of therapy for all STIs are to eradicate the causative organism and prevent complications.

The accurate and timely reporting of STIs is integrally important for assessing morbidity trends, targeting limited resources, and assisting local health authorities in partner notification and treatment. STIs, human immunodeficiency virus (HIV), and acquired immunodeficiency syndrome (AIDS) cases should be reported in accordance with state and local statutory requirements. Syphilis, gonorrhea, chlamydia, chancroid, HIV infection, and AIDS are reportable diseases in every state. The requirements for reporting other STIs differ by state, and clinicians should be familiar with state and local reporting requirements. Reporting can be provider or laboratory based.

Intrauterine or perinatally transmitted STIs can have severely debilitating effects on pregnant women, their partners, and their fetuses. All pregnant women and their sex partners should be asked about STIs, counseled about the possibility of perinatal infections, and ensured access to treatment, if needed.

All pregnant women in the United States should be tested for HIV infection as early in pregnancy as possible. Testing should be conducted after the woman is notified that she will be tested for HIV as part of the routine panel of prenatal tests, unless she declines the test.

CHLAMYDIAL INFECTION

Chlamydial infection is the most prevalent STI in the United States, with 3 to 4 million cases reported annually. The detection and treatment of this disease is important because the complications can be serious.

CAUSES

Chlamydial infection is caused by *Chlamydia trachomatis*, which shares properties of both bacteria and viruses. The organism is transmitted sexually or perinatally. Repeated infections are common.

In infants, perinatal exposure to the mother's cervix causes the infection. The prevalence is greater than 5% regardless of race, ethnicity, or socioeconomic status. In preadolescent children, sexual abuse must be considered as a causative factor for chlamydial infection; infection of the nasopharynx, urogenital tract, and rectum may persist for greater than 1 year. Because criminal investigation is always a possibility, cultures should be confirmed by microscopic fluoroscopy, which can detect conjugated monoclonal antibodies specific for *C. trachomatis*.

Chlamydial infections occur most frequently in women younger than age 25. All adolescents and young women should be screened for chlamydia yearly, as should any woman who has new or multiple sex partners.

PATHOPHYSIOLOGY

Chlamydial organisms are like viruses in that they are obligate intracellular parasites. They resemble bacteria by containing both deoxyribonucleic acid (DNA) and ribonucleic acid, by dividing by binary fission, and by having cell walls that resemble those of gram-negative bacteria. Species of chlamydial

TABLE 35.1	Pharmacotherapy for Sexually Transmitted Infections	
Infection	**Treatment**	**Comments**

Chlamydial infection	azithromycin 1 g PO once *or*
	doxycycline 100 mg PO bid for 7 d
	Alternative
	    erythromycin base 500 mg PO qid for 7 d *or*
	    erythromycin ethylsuccinate 800 mg PO qid for 7 d *or*
	    ofloxacin 300 mg bid for 7 d *or*
	    levofloxacin 500 mg PO for 7 days
		Use amoxicillin, erythromycin, *or* azithromycin in pregnancy.

Genital herpes	*Initial episode treatment* for 7–10 d
	    acyclovir 400 mg PO tid *or*
	    acyclovir 200 mg PO 5 times a day *or*
	    famciclovir 250 mg PO tid *or*
	    valacyclovir 1 g PO bid
	Recurrent treatment for 5 d
	    acyclovir 400 mg PO *or*
	    acyclovir 200 mg PO 5 times a day *or*
	    acyclovir 800 mg bid *or*
	    famciclovir 125 mg PO bid *or*
	    valacyclovir 500 mg PO bid *or*
	    valacyclovir 1 g once a day
	Suppressive treatment
	    acyclovir 400 mg bid *or*
	    famciclovir 250 mg bid *or*
	    valacyclovir 500 mg or 1,000 mg qd
		Treatment can be extended if healing is not complete after 10 d.

Gonorrhea	cefixime 400 mg PO once *or* ceftriaxone 125 mg IM once *or* ciprofloxacin 500 mg PO once *or* levofloxacin 250 mg PO once *or* ofloxacin 400 mg PO once plus azithromycin 1 g PO once *or* doxycycline 100 mg PO bid for 7 d *Alternative* spectinomycin 2 g IM once	

Human papilloma virus	*Patient applied*
	    podofilox 0.5% solution or gel for 3 d, then 4 d of no therapy
	    imiquimod 5% cream 3 times a week up to 16 wk
	Provider applied
	    podophyllin resin 10%–25% in compound of tincture of benzoin weekly as needed
	    trichloroacetic acid or bichloracetic acid 80%–90% weekly as needed
		Solution applied with cotton swab and gel with finger to visible warts. This is done for 3 d, then 4 d with no therapy, and may be repeated four times.
		Area should be washed with mild soap and water 6–10 h after application.
		Allow to air dry. Wash off 1–4 h after application.
		Apply only to warts and let dry; white "frosting" appears; powder with talc or sodium bicarbonate to remove unreacted acid.

Pelvic inflammatory disease	ofloxacin 400 mg PO bid *or* levofloxacin 500 mg daily *and* metronidazole 500 mg PO bid for 14 d *or* ceftriaxone 250 mg IM once *or* cefoxitin 2 g IM *and* probenecid 1 g PO once *and* doxycycline 100 mg PO bid for 14 d	

Syphilis	*Early primary, secondary, or latent syphilis <1 y*
	    Adult: benzathine penicillin G 2.4 million U, IM single dose
	    Child: 50,000 U/kg, IM, single dose up to 2.4 mil unit
	Latent disease >1 y or unknown duration
	    Adult: benzathine penicillin G 2.4 million U, IM, for 3 doses at 1-wk intervals
	    Child: 500,000 U/kg, IM, for 3 doses at 1-wk intervals
	Allergic to penicillin and not pregnant doxycycline 100 mg PO bid for 14 d *or* tetracycline 500 mg PO bid for 14 d
	Allergic to penicillin and pregnant Desensitization followed by treatment with penicillin	

Centers for Disease Control and Prevention. (2006). Sexually transmitted treatment guidelines, 2006. *Morbidity and Mortality Weekly Reports, 55*(RR-11), 1-93.

organisms include *Chlamydia psittaci* and *C. trachomatis*, the latter of which has a number of serotypes. These species cause numerous diseases, including lymphogranuloma venereum, blinding trachoma, conjunctivitis, nongonococcal urethritis, cervicitis, salpingitis, proctitis, epididymitis, and newborn pneumonia.

DIAGNOSTIC CRITERIA

The infection may be silent: more than half of infected patients have no clinical signs or symptoms. In symptomatic women, the clinical presentation includes vaginal discharge, mucopurulent cervicitis with edema and friability, urethral syndrome or urethritis, pelvic inflammatory disease (PID), ectopic pregnancy, infertility, and endometritis. Men may report a thin, clear discharge and dysuria. Chlamydial organisms are the major causes of nongonococcal urethritis and epididymitis in young men.

In infants ages 1 to 3 months, chlamydial infection presents in the mucous membranes of the eye, oropharynx, urogenital tract, and rectum and as subacute, afebrile pneumonia; in neonates, it presents as an asymptomatic infection of the oropharynx, genital tract, and rectum. However, chlamydial infection most commonly presents as conjunctivitis 5 to 12 days after birth and is the most frequent identifiable infectious cause of ophthalmia neonatorum. Therefore, for all infants with conjunctivitis who are no older than 30 days, a chlamydial etiology should be considered.

Diagnostic tests for chlamydial ophthalmia neonatorum include tissue cultures and nonculture tests. Ocular exudate should also be tested for *Neisseria gonorrhoeae*.

Chlamydial infection is diagnosed by examination, culture, and antigen detection methods, including direct fluorescent monoclonal antibody staining, enzyme-linked immunosorbent assay, DNA probe assay, and polymerase chain reaction.

INITIATING DRUG THERAPY

Treatment for all STIs consists of antimicrobial therapy followed by preventive education.

Goals of Drug Therapy

Patients are treated to eradicate the organism and prevent transmission to sex partners or to a newborn during birth. Because chlamydial infections often are accompanied by gonococcal infections, patients may be treated for both infections.

Antibiotic Therapy

Antibiotic treatments are prescribed to cure infection and usually relieve symptoms (CDC, 2006). Azithromycin (Zithromax) and erythromycin (E-mycin), macrolide antibiotics; doxycycline (Vibramycin), a tetracycline antibiotic; and ofloxacin (Floxin), a fluoroquinolone, are drugs of choice for chlamydial infections.

If therapeutic compliance is in question, azithromycin should be used for treatment because it is prepared as a single-dose drug. Doxycycline, however, has been used more extensively and is less expensive. Erythromycin is less efficacious and has gastrointestinal (GI) side effects. Ofloxacin is as efficacious as doxycycline and azithromycin but is more expensive and has no advantage with regard to dosing regimen. Other fluoroquinolones are not effective or have not been adequately tested (**Table 35.2**).

In infants, erythromycin base treatment has an efficacy of 80%. A second course of therapy may be required, and follow-up of the infant is recommended.

Mechanism of Action

Azithromycin and erythromycin bind to bacterial ribosomes to block protein synthesis. The drugs are also bactericidal, depending on their concentration. (For more information on antibiotic actions, see Chapter 8.) Doxycycline is thought to act in a similar way, whereas ofloxacin kills bacteria by blocking DNA gyrase and inhibiting DNA synthesis.

Dosages

A single 1-g dose of azithromycin or 100 mg of doxycycline twice a day for 7 days is the usual initial therapy.

Contraindications

Sensitivity to erythromycin or other macrolides is the main contraindication to therapy.

The safety and efficacy of azithromycin in pregnant and lactating women are not known. Doxycycline and ofloxacin are contraindicated in pregnant women.

Adverse Events

In some patients, GI side effects (nausea, vomiting, diarrhea, abdominal discomfort) cause them to discontinue therapy.

Selecting the Most Appropriate Agent

The most appropriate therapy is the one that best matches the needs of the patient in different situations or stages of life. **Figure 35-1, Table 35.1,** and **Table 35.2** summarize treatment options.

Special Population Considerations

Pediatric

To prevent chlamydial infection among neonates, prenatal screening is recommended. In general, patients appropriate for screening include pregnant women younger than age 25 with new or multiple sex partners.

C. trachomatis infection of neonates results from perinatal exposure to the mother's infected cervix. The prevalence of *C. trachomatis* infection among pregnant women does not vary by race/ethnicity or socioeconomic status. Neonatal ocular prophylaxis with silver nitrate solution or antibiotic ointments does not prevent perinatal transmission of *C. trachomatis* from

| TABLE 35.2 | Overview of Drugs Used to Treat Chlamydial Infections* | | | |

Generic (Trade) Name and Dosage	Selected Adverse Events	Contraindications	Special Considerations

azithromycin (Zithromax)
  Adult: 1 g PO single dose
  Pregnancy: 1 g PO in a single dose
  Child (≥45 kg, <8 y): 1 g PO in a single dose
  Child (≥8 y): 1 g PO in a single dose (or doxycycline as below)
	GI upset, abdominal pain, pseudomembranous colitis, angioedema, cholestatic jaundice	Hypersensitivity to azithromycin, erythromycin, or any macrolide antibiotic
		Use with caution with impaired hepatic or renal function.
			Do not take with aluminum- or magnesium-containing antacids.

doxycycline (Vibramycin)
  Adult: 100 mg bid for 7 d
  Child (≥8 y): 100 mg PO bid for 7 d
	Superinfection, photosensitivity, GI upset, enterocolitis, rash, blood dyscrasias, hepatotoxicity	Pregnancy, lactation, hypersensitivity to any of the tetracyclines	Monitor blood, renal, and hepatic function in long-term use.
			Use of drug during tooth development may discolor teeth.
			Advise patient to avoid excessive sunlight or ultraviolet light.
			Caution patient that drug absorption is reduced when taken with food or bismuth subsalicylate.

amoxicillin (Augmentin) Pregnancy: 500 mg tid for 7 d	Hypersensitivity reactions, pseudomembranous colitis, GI upset, rash, urticaria, vaginitis	History of Augmentin-associated cholestatic jaundice, hepatic dysfunction, or allergic reactions to any penicillin	Monitor blood, renal, and hepatic function in long-term use.
ofloxacin (Floxin) 300 mg bid for 7 d	Rash, hives, rapid heartbeat, difficulty swallowing or breathing, photosensitivity, angioedema, dizziness, lightheadedness	Pregnancy, hypersensitivity to ofloxacin or quinolones Use with caution with hepatic or renal insufficiency.	Do not take with food. Drink fluids liberally.
levofloxacin (Levaquin) 500 mg daily for 7 d	Same as above	Same as above	Same as above

erythromycin base (E-mycin)
  Adult: 500 mg qid for 7 d
  Pregnancy: 500 mg qid for 7 d or 250 mg qid for 14 d
  Children: 50 mg/kg/d PO divided into 4 doses daily for 10–14 d
	GI upset, pseudomembranous colitis, hepatic dysfunction, cardiac dysrhythmias, CNS disturbances, urticaria, skin eruptions, hearing loss, superinfection and local irritation	Known hypersensitivity to erythromycin
		Prescribe with caution for patients with impaired hepatic function and children who weigh <45 kg.
			Effectiveness of treatment is approximately 80%; a second course of therapy may be required.
			Use for prophylaxis of ophthalmia neonatorum and infant pneumonia.

erythromycin ethylsuccinate (E.E.S.)
  Adult: 800 mg qid for 7 d
  Pregnancy: 800 mg qid for 7 d or 400 mg qid for 14 d
	Same as above	Same as above	Same as above

*In adults, pregnant women, children, ophthalmia neonatorum, and infant pneumonia

mother to infant. However, ocular prophylaxis with those agents does prevent gonococcal ophthalmia and therefore should be continued.

Initial *C. trachomatis* perinatal infection involves mucous membranes of the eye, oropharynx, urogenital tract, and rectum. *C. trachomatis* infection in neonates is most often recognized by conjunctivitis that develops 5 to 12 days after birth. Chlamydia is the most frequent identifiable infectious cause of ophthalmia neonatorum. *C. trachomatis* also is a common cause of subacute, afebrile pneumonia

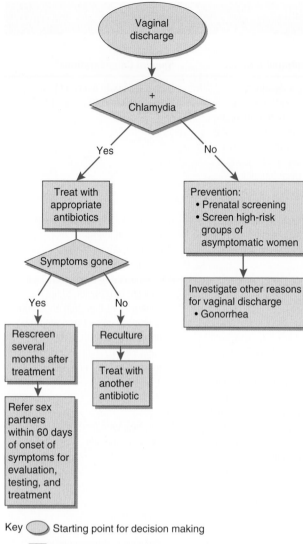

Key ⬭ Starting point for decision making

▭ Clinical actions (assessing, prescribing, monitoring)

◇ Decision point

FIGURE 35–1   Treatment algorithm for chlamydial infection.

MONITORING PATIENT RESPONSE

Because therapy with azithromycin or doxycycline is highly efficacious, patients do not need to be retested after treatment is completed. However, 3 weeks after completion of treatment with erythromycin (or amoxicillin–clavulanate), a test of cure may be considered because the drugs are not highly efficacious and the frequent side effects may discourage patient adherence. (Women retested after several months of treatment showed high rates of infection, presumed to be a result of reinfection. Therefore, rescreening women several months after treatment may help to detect further morbidity.)

Screening for *C. trachomatis* should be performed in high-risk groups when the practitioner performs a pelvic examination. High-risk groups include sexually active adolescents and women ages 20 to 24, particularly those who have new or multiple sex partners, those attending family planning clinics, prenatal clinics, or abortion facilities, or those in juvenile detention centers. Screening for high-risk men should be considered when they seek health care.

PATIENT EDUCATION

The patient's sex partner must be treated. Patients should abstain from sexual intercourse for 7 days after single-dose therapy or until the 7-day regimen is completed. Abstinence should also continue until the patient's sex partner has been treated, to prevent reinfection. Sex partners should be treated if they have had sexual contact with the patient during the 60 days preceding onset of symptoms in the patient or the diagnosis of chlamydial infection. The most recent sex partner should be treated even if the time of the last sexual contact was greater than 60 days before onset or diagnosis.

GONORRHEA

Approximately 1 million new infections with *N. gonorrhoeae* occur each year in the United States. They are the major causes of PID, tubal scarring, infertility, ectopic pregnancy, and chronic pelvic pain in the United States. Most men seek treatment before serious complications develop, but not soon enough to prevent transmission to others. In women, symptoms may not develop until complications such as PID occur. Screening of men and women at high risk for STIs is an important component of gonorrhea control (CDC, 2006). Patients infected with *N. gonorrhoeae* frequently are coinfected with *C. trachomatis*; this finding has led to the recommendation that patients treated for gonococcal infection also be treated routinely with a regimen that is effective against uncomplicated genital *C. trachomatis* infection. Because the majority of gonococci in the United States are susceptible to doxycycline and azithromycin, routine cotreatment might

with onset from ages 1 to 3 months. Asymptomatic infections also can occur in the oropharynx, genital tract, and rectum of neonates.

A chlamydial etiology should be considered for all infants aged 30 days or less who have conjunctivitis.

Pregnancy

The recommended regimen for pregnancy is erythromycin base 500 mg orally four times a day for 7 days or amoxicillin 500 mg orally three times daily for 7 days.

Alternative regimens are erythromycin base 250 mg orally four times a day for 14 days; erythromycin ethylsuccinate 800 mg orally four times a day for 7 days or 400 mg orally four times a day for 14 days; or azithromycin 1 g orally, single dose. Erythromycin estolate is contraindicated during pregnancy because of drug-related hepatotoxicity.

also hinder the development of antimicrobial-resistant *N. gonorrhoeae*.

CAUSES

Gonorrhea is caused by *N. gonorrhoeae,* a gram-negative diplococcal bacterium. It is transmitted by sexual contact, and the rate of male-to-female transmission is higher than female-to-male or male-to-male. Women with gonorrhea have a high prevalence of other STIs, including chlamydial infection, trichomoniasis, bacterial vaginosis, and herpes genitalis.

Uncomplicated anogenital gonorrhea in women can involve the endocervix, urethra, Skene's glands, Bartholin's glands, and anus. The endocervix is the most common site of infection. Pharyngeal infection can also occur and is usually asymptomatic.

PATHOPHYSIOLOGY

Several strains of gonorrhea have been identified. Gonococcal sensitivity and resistance to antibiotics are clinically significant. Certain strains of the organism are resistant to sulfonamides. Penicillinase-producing *N. gonorrhoeae* and chromosomal-resistant *N. gonorrhoeae* are resistant to penicillin, and tetracycline-resistant *N. gonorrhoeae* is resistant to tetracycline.

DIAGNOSTIC CRITERIA

In the United States, an estimated 600,000 new *N. gonorrhoeae* infections occur each year. Most infections among men produce symptoms that cause them to seek curative treatment soon enough to prevent serious sequelae, but this may not be soon enough to prevent transmission to others. Among women, many infections do not produce recognizable symptoms until complications such as PID have occurred. Up to 30% of women with gonorrheal infection have symptoms. Signs and symptoms include purulent or mucopurulent cervical discharge, dysuria, anal bleeding, menorrhagia, and pelvic discomfort. Men may have discharge and regional lymphadenopathy.

Gonorrhea is diagnosed by examination and culture for *N. gonorrhoeae*. Diagnosis is confirmed by identification of the organism on culture, positive oxidase reaction, and gram-negative diplococcal morphology on Gram's stain.

INITIATING DRUG THERAPY

Preventive education is always offered. Sex partners should be referred for evaluation and treatment of *N. gonorrhoeae* and *C. trachomatis* infection if their last contact with the patient was within 60 days before onset of symptoms or diagnosis

of infection. The patient's most recent sex partner should be treated even if the patient's last sexual intercourse was more than 60 days before onset of the symptoms or diagnosis. All patients diagnosed with gonorrhea should be tested for syphilis.

Patients treated for gonococcal infection are also treated for chlamydial infection because patients with gonorrhea are commonly coinfected with *C. trachomatis*. The occurrence of fluoroquinolone-resistant *N. gonorrhoeae* in the United States is rare. Patients with treatment failure should undergo culture and susceptibility testing, and the local health department should be notified (CDC, 2006).

Goals of Drug Therapy

The goal of drug therapy is to eradicate disease and prevent complications and spread of infection to others.

Antibiotics

The CDC describes recommended regimens for uncomplicated gonococcal infections of the cervix, urethra, and rectum (**Table 35.3**).

Cefixime

Cefixime (Suprax) covers an antimicrobial spectrum similar to that of ceftriaxone (Rocephin), but cefixime 125 mg intramuscularly (IM) provides a higher and more sustained bacterial level than the 400-mg oral dose of cefixime. The advantage of cefixime is that it can be administered orally, and clinical trials have shown a 97.1% cure rate for uncomplicated urogenital and anorectal gonococcal infections.

Ceftriaxone

A single injection of 125 mg of ceftriaxone provides sustained, high antibacterial levels in the blood. Extensive clinical experience shows that the drug is safe and effective for treating uncomplicated gonorrhea at all sites, with a cure rate of 99.1% in clinical trials for uncomplicated urogenital and anorectal infections.

Fluoroquinolones

Ciprofloxacin (Cipro) is safe and relatively inexpensive, can be administered orally, and is effective against most strains of *N. gonorrhoeae*. A 500-mg single dose provides sustained antibacterial levels in the blood. It has a cure rate of 99.8% in clinical trials of uncomplicated urogenital and anorectal infections.

Ofloxacin is also effective against most strains of *N. gonorrhoeae*. Clinical trials show the 400-mg dose to be effective for treating uncomplicated urogenital and anorectal infections, with a cure rate of 98.4%. Levofloxacin 250 mg in a single dose is also effective.

Quinolones should not be used to treat men having sex with men or heterosexuals who have recently traveled. The recommended treatment is ceftriaxone 125 mg IM in a single dose or cefixime 400 mg orally in a single dose.

TABLE 35.3   Overview of Selected Drugs Used to Treat Uncomplicated Gonococcal Infections in Adults and Children*

Generic (Trade) Name and Dosage	Selected Adverse Events	Contraindications	Special Considerations
ceftriaxone (Rocephin) Adult: 125 mg IM in a single dose Child: ophthalmia neonatorum: 25–50 mg/kg IV or IM in a single dose, not to exceed 125 mg Child: 125 mg IM in a single dose or 50 mg/kg (maximum dose 1 g) IM or IV in a single dose daily for 7 d or 50 mg/kg (maximum dose 2 g) IM or IV in a single dose daily for 10–14 d Child (<45 kg with bacteremia or arthritis): 50 mg/kg: max 1 g IM or IV in a single daily dose for 7 d Child (>45 kg with bacteremia or arthritis): 50 mg/kg, max 2 g, IM or IV in a single daily dose for 10–14 d	Pseudomembranous colitis, rash, GI upset, hematologic abnormalities	Known allergy to cephalosporins Prescribe with caution to penicillin-sensitive patients. Prescribe with caution to hyperbilirubinemic infants, especially premature infants.	Use for uncomplicated gonococcal infection of the pharynx. Prescribe prophylactically in infants whose mothers have gonococcal infection.
cefixime (Suprax) 400 mg PO in a single dose	Pseudomembranous colitis, GI upset, skin rash, headache, dizziness	Known allergy to cephalosporins Prescribe with caution to penicillin-sensitive patients and patients with renal impairment or GI disease. Prescribe with caution in patients on hemodialysis or continuous ambulatory peritoneal dialysis.	
ciprofloxacin (Cipro) 500 mg PO in a single dose	Pseudomembranous colitis, photosensitivity, dizziness, lightheadedness, restlessness, GI upset	Hypersensitivity to ciprofloxacin or fluoroquinolones	Advise patient to take 2 h after meals, drink fluids liberally, and avoid taking antacids, which interfere with absorption. Prescribe for uncomplicated gonococcal infection of the pharynx.
ofloxacin (Floxin) 400 mg PO in a single dose	Rash, hives, rapid heartbeat, difficulty swallowing and breathing, photosensitivity, angioedema, dizziness, lightheadedness	Pregnancy Hypersensitivity to ofloxacin or fluoroquinolones Prescribe with caution in patients with hepatic or renal insufficiency.	Advise patient to take drug on empty stomach and drink fluids liberally. Prescribe for uncomplicated gonococcal infection of the pharynx.
levofloxacin (Levaquin) 250 mg in a single dose	Same as above	Same as above	Same as above
spectinomycin (Trobicin) Adult: 2 g IM in a single dose Child: 40 mg/kg (max dose 2 g) IM in a single dose	Pain at injection site, urticaria, transient rash, pruritus, dizziness, headache, GI upset, chills, fever, nervousness, insomnia, rare anaphylaxis, low Hg, high BUN and ALT levels	Hypersensitivity to spectinomycin Administer with caution in patients with hypersensitivity or allergies.	Prescribe for patients who cannot tolerate cephalosporins or fluoroquinolones. Unreliable against pharyngeal infections Unreliable for treating pharyngeal infections in children Perform follow-up culture after treatment.

Drug	Adverse reactions	Contraindications and cautions	Nursing considerations
ceftizoxime (Cefizox) 500 mg IM	Eosinophilia, thrombocytosis; high AST, ALT, alkaline phosphatase, and BUN levels; GI upset, pseudomembranous colitis, headache, dizziness, tinnitus	Known allergy to ceftizoxime; Prescribe with caution for patient with hypersensitivity to penicillin or allergies or GI disease.	Monitor renal function.
cefotaxime (Claforan) 500 mg IM	Pseudomembranous colitis, rash, pruritus, fever, GI upset	Hypersensitivity to cefotaxime or cephalosporins; Prescribe with caution to penicillin-sensitive patients and those with GI disease and renal impairment.	
cefotetan (Cefotan) 1 g IM	Pseudomembranous colitis, GI upset, hypersensitivity reactions	Known allergy to cephalosporins; Prescribe with caution to penicillin-sensitive patients and those with GI disease.	Avoid drinking alcohol during therapy.
cefoxitin (Mefoxin) with probenecid (Benemid) 2 g IM: 1 g PO	*cefoxitin:* Pseudomembranous colitis, thrombophlebitis, rash, pruritus, eosinophilia, fever, dyspnea, hypotension, GI upset; *probenecid:* Headache, dizziness, GI upset, hypersensitivity, acute gouty arthritis, nephrotic syndrome, uric acid stones	*cefoxitin:* Hypersensitivity to cefoxitin or cephalosporins; Prescribe with caution to penicillin-sensitive patients and those with GI disease. *probenecid:* Hypersensitivity to probenecid; Children <2 y, blood dyscrasias, uric acid kidney stones; Prescribe with caution to patients with peptic ulcer.	
enoxacin (Penetrex) 400 mg PO in a single dose	Pseudomembranous colitis, GI upset, headache, dizziness	Hypersensitivity to enoxacin, tendinitis or tendon rupture associated with use of enoxacin or fluoroquinolones	Do not take antacids, bismuth subsalicylate, iron, or multivitamins with zinc for 8 h before or 2 h after taking drug. Avoid caffeine. Drink fluids liberally.
lomefloxacin (Maxaquin) 400 mg PO in a single dose	Severe photosensitivity, pseudomembranous colitis, dizziness, lightheadedness, hypersensitivity	Hypersensitivity to lomefloxacin or fluoroquinolones	Advise patient to drink fluids liberally, avoid mineral supplements or vitamins with iron 2 h before or after taking drug. Avoid sucralfate or antacids 4 h before or 2 h after taking drug.
norfloxacin (Noroxin) 800 mg PO in a single dose	Pseudomembranous colitis, dizziness, lightheadedness, photosensitivity, hypersensitivity, headache, GI upset	Hypersensitivity to norfloxacin, tendinitis or tendon rupture associated with the use of the drug or fluoroquinolones	Take 1 h before or 2 h after a meal or milk ingestion; drink fluids liberally; avoid multivitamins, antacids, iron, or zinc 2 h before or after taking the drug.
azithromycin (Zithromax) 2 g PO; Uncomplicated gonococcal infection of the pharynx: 1 g PO in a single dose	GI upset, abdominal pain, pseudomembranous colitis, angioedema, cholestatic jaundice	Hypersensitivity to azithromycin, erythromycin, or any macrolide antibiotic; Prescribe with caution in patients with impaired hepatic or renal function.	Take 1 h before or 2 h after meals for greatest absorption. Avoid taking with aluminum- or magnesium-containing antacids. Comes in powder form
doxycycline (Vibramycin) 100 mg PO bid for 7 d	Superinfection, photosensitivity, GI upset, enterocolitis, rash, blood dyscrasias, hepatotoxicity	Pregnancy, lactation, hypersensitivity to any of the tetracyclines	Monitor blood, renal, and hepatic function in long-term use. Because of photosensitivity, patient should avoid sunlight or UV light. Use of drug during tooth development may discolor teeth. Absorption is reduced when drug is taken with food or bismuth subsalicylate (Pepto-Bismol). Prescribe for uncomplicated gonococcal infection of the pharynx.

*Infections of the cervix, urethra, and rectum; uncomplicated gonococcal infection of the pharynx; ophthalmia neonatorum; and gonococcal infection in children

Other

The CDC also recommends several alternative treatments. Spectinomycin (Trobicin) has been effective for uncomplicated urogenital and anorectal gonococcal infections, curing 98.2% in clinical trials. However, the drug is expensive and must be injected IM in a 2-g single dose. It is used for patients who cannot tolerate cephalosporins and quinolones.

The CDC also recognizes other antimicrobials for use against *N. gonorrhoeae*. A single dose of azithromycin (Zithromax) 2 g orally is effective for uncomplicated gonococcal infection, but it is expensive and causes GI distress. Doxycycline 100 mg twice daily for 7 days is also effective.

The regimen recommended by the CDC for uncomplicated gonococcal infections of the pharynx is summarized in **Table 35.1** and **Figure 35-2.** These infections are more difficult to treat than urogenital and anorectal infections. Few drugs can reliably cure these infections more than 90% of the time. Treatment for gonorrhea and chlamydial infection is suggested, even though chlamydial coinfection of the pharynx is unusual.

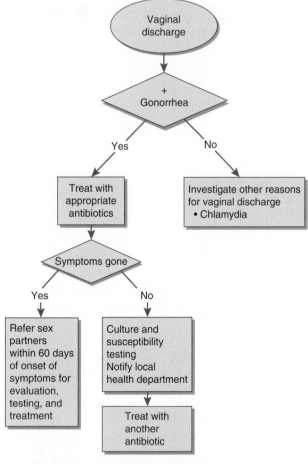

Key — Starting point for decision making

— Clinical actions (assessing, prescribing, monitoring)

— Decision point

FIGURE 35–2 Treatment algorithm for gonorrheal infection.

Selecting the Most Appropriate Agent

Therapy for uncomplicated gonococcal infections includes a cephalosporin or fluoroquinolone, as follows:

- Single-dose cefixime 400 mg orally, or
- Single-dose ceftriaxone 125 mg IM, or
- Single-dose ciprofloxacin, 500 mg, or
- Single-dose ofloxacin 400 mg, or
- Single-dose levofloxacin 250 mg

PLUS

- Single-dose azithromycin 1 g, or
- Doxycycline 100 mg orally twice daily for 7 days

The choice is based on the practitioner's assessment of the patient's reliability, allergies, and preferences. If there is a question regarding the patient's reliability, ceftriaxone IM may be the treatment of choice because it is administered in the office.

Special Population Considerations

Pediatric

Gonococcal infection may be transmitted to infants exposed to infected cervical exudate at birth. The infection presents as an acute illness 2 to 5 days after birth. The prevalence in infants depends on the prevalence of infection in pregnant women, whether pregnant women are screened for gonorrhea, and whether newborns receive prophylactic treatment. Manifestations of the infection in newborns include ophthalmia neonatorum, which may result in perforation of the ocular globe and blindness, sepsis with arthritis, and meningitis, rhinitis, vaginitis, urethritis, and inflammation at fetal monitoring sites. Cultures should be taken when typical gram-negative diplococci are identified in conjunctival exudate, and testing for chlamydial organisms should be done in all cases of neonatal conjunctivitis. Presumptive treatment can be given for newborns who are at increased risk for gonococcal ophthalmia or who have conjunctivitis but no gonococci in a Gram-stained smear of conjunctival exudate. Infants with gonococcal ophthalmia should be hospitalized and monitored for signs of disseminated infection. Many physicians prefer to continue therapy until cultures are negative for gonococcal organisms at 48 to 72 hours.

To prevent ophthalmia neonatorum, prophylactic agents, including silver nitrate, erythromycin, and tetracycline, are recommended for instillation in the eyes; this is required by law in most states, regardless of whether delivery was vaginal or cesarean (**Table 35.4**).

In preadolescent children, sexual abuse is the most frequent cause of gonococcal infection. Vaginitis is the most common manifestation, followed by anorectal and pharyngeal infections, which are commonly asymptomatic. Standard culture procedures should be used to diagnose the infection, and nonculture gonococcal tests should not be used alone.

Follow-up cultures are not needed if ceftriaxone is used. Only parenteral cephalosporins are recommended for use in children. Quinolones are not approved for use in

| TABLE 35.4 | Prophylaxis for Ophthalmia Neonatorum |

Topical Agent	Adverse Events	Contraindications	Special Considerations
silver nitrate 1% aqueous solution in a single application	Mild chemical conjunctivitis With repeated applications, cauterization of the cornea and blindness may occur.	Hypersensitivity to silver nitrate	Instill one of these preparations into both eyes of the neonate as soon as possible after birth. Use single-use tubes of the agent. Preparation is caustic and irritating to skin and mucous membranes.
erythromycin (Ilotycin) 0.5% ophthalmic ointment in a single application	Sensitivity reactions	Hypersensitivity to erythromycin	Same as above
tetracycline (Achromycin) 1% ophthalmic ointment in a single application	Dermatitis, increased lacrimation, transient stinging or burning, foreign body sensation	Hypersensitivity to tetracycline	Same as above

children because of concerns regarding toxicity. A follow-up culture is needed to ensure that treatment was effective if spectinomycin is used. All children with gonococcal infections should be evaluated for syphilis and chlamydial coinfection.

Women

Women who are pregnant should not be treated with fluoroquinolones or tetracycline. An alternate cephalosporin can be used, and if the patient cannot tolerate a cephalosporin, a single 2-g dose of spectinomycin IM can be substituted. For presumptive or diagnosed *C. trachomatis* infection, azithromycin or amoxicillin is recommended.

MONITORING PATIENT RESPONSE

Patients who have had uncomplicated gonorrhea and who were treated with any of the recommended regimens do not need to return for test of cure. If symptoms persist after treatment, the patient is evaluated by culture for *N. gonorrhoeae*, and isolated gonococci should be tested for antimicrobial susceptibility. If infection is identified, its source is usually reinfection rather than treatment failure. In patients treated with spectinomycin for pharyngeal infection, culture should be performed 3 to 5 days after treatment because spectinomycin is not highly effective against these infections.

PATIENT EDUCATION

Patient education concentrates on prevention. All patients should be encouraged to adopt meticulous hygiene and practice safe sex, to insist that partners seek treatment, and to schedule and keep follow-up health care appointments.

SYPHILIS

In the 1990s, syphilis reemerged in endemic forms in the United States, with a significant increase in the incidence of primary, secondary, and congenital syphilis. The increase has been attributed to greater use of illicit drugs, most notably crack cocaine, and high-risk sexual behavior related to drug use. Approximately 120,000 cases of primary and secondary syphilis occur annually in the United States (CDC, 2006).

CAUSES

Syphilis is a chronic, infectious disease caused by the spirochete *Treponema pallidum*. Infection may be active, and characterized by symptoms, or inactive (latent). The latent stage has no clinical symptoms. During the latent stage, infections can be detected by serologic testing. Early latent syphilis is defined as latent syphilis acquired within the preceding year. Any other cases of latent syphilis are either late latent syphilis or syphilis of unknown duration (CDC, 2006).

PATHOPHYSIOLOGY

T. pallidum is considered a bacterium because of its cell wall and response to antibiotic therapy. *T. pallidum* is not readily grown in vitro and cannot be seen by light microscopy.

DIAGNOSTIC CRITERIA

Patients who contract syphilis may seek treatment for signs or symptoms of primary infection, which include an ulcer or chancre at the infection site. The chancre erupts approximately 3 weeks after exposure. Signs and symptoms of secondary syphilis are low-grade fever, malaise, sore throat, hoarseness, headache, anorexia, rash, mucocutaneous lesions, alopecia, and adenopathy. Signs and symptoms of tertiary infection include cardiac, neurologic, ophthalmic, auditory, or gummatous lesions. Definitive methods for diagnosing early syphilis include dark-field examination and direct fluorescent antibody study of the chancre's exudate or tissue. The serologic tests used to confirm the syphilis diagnosis are nontreponemal and treponemal. The nontreponemal tests are the Venereal Disease Research Laboratory (VDRL) test and the rapid plasma reagin test. The treponemal tests include the fluorescent treponemal antibody absorption test and the microhemagglutination assay for antibody to *T. pallidum*. The two serologic tests are necessary because false-positive nontreponemal test results occur on occasion secondary to certain medical conditions. Treponemal test antibody titers do not correlate accurately with disease activity and should not be used to assess treatment response.

A single test cannot be used to diagnose all cases of neurosyphilis. The diagnosis is made using a combination of tests, including combinations of reactive serologic test results; abnormalities of cerebrospinal fluid (CSF) cell count or protein; or reactive VDRL-CSF with or without clinical manifestations (CDC, 2006).

INITIATING DRUG THERAPY

Although sexual transmission occurs only when mucocutaneous syphilitic lesions, including the rash, are present, people exposed in any stage should be evaluated clinically and serologically. Treatment should be given to those who were exposed within 90 days preceding the diagnosis of primary, secondary, or early latent syphilis in a sex partner, because the partner might be infected even if he or she is seronegative. Treatment should also be given to those who were exposed more than 90 days before the diagnosis of primary, secondary, or early latent syphilis in a sex partner if serologic test results are unavailable and follow-up tests and treatments are uncertain. Patients who have syphilis of unknown duration and who have high nontreponemal serologic test titers are considered to have early syphilis. Sex partners should be notified and treated. Long-term partners of patients with late syphilis should have a clinical and serologic evaluation and should be treated based on the findings.

For all stages of syphilis, penicillin is the preferred treatment. The stage and clinical manifestations of the disease determine the preparation used as well as the dosage and duration of treatment. However, no adequate trials have been performed to determine the optimal penicillin regimen. The only therapy with documented efficacy for syphilis during pregnancy or neurosyphilis is parenteral penicillin G benzathine. Penicillin G has been used for the past five decades to achieve a local cure and to prevent late sequelae.

Goals of Drug Therapy

The goal of treatment for primary and secondary syphilis is cure. The goal of treatment for latent syphilis is to prevent occurrence or progression of late complications. There is limited evidence supporting specific regimens for penicillin, even though clinical experience has shown the effectiveness of penicillin in achieving these goals.

Antibiotics

Penicillin

Adults with primary or secondary syphilis should be treated with penicillin G benzathine (Bicillin). Other choices for unusual situations include doxycycline, tetracycline (Achromycin), ceftriaxone, and erythromycin (**Table 35.5**).

Mechanism of Action

Penicillins are bactericidal. They disrupt synthesis of the bacterial cell wall and bind to enzyme proteins, interfering with the biosynthesis of mucopeptides and preventing the structural components of the cell wall from leaking out. As such, the bacteria cannot lay protein cross-links in the cell wall. In addition, autolytic enzymes, which promote lysis of bacteria, are activated.

Contraindications

Penicillin is contraindicated in patients with allergies to penicillin, cephalosporin, or imipenem (Primaxin).

Adverse Events

Hypersensitivity, urticaria, laryngeal edema, fever, eosinophilia, anaphylaxis, hemolytic anemia, leukopenia, thrombocytopenia, neuropathy, and nephropathy are some of the adverse effects of the penicillins.

Interactions

Penicillin decreases the effect of oral contraceptives. Hyperkalemia can result from concurrent use of potassium-sparing diuretics, angiotensin-converting enzyme inhibitors, and potassium supplements with parenteral penicillin G.

Doxycycline, Tetracycline, and Others

Nonpregnant patients with latent syphilis who are allergic to penicillin should be treated with doxycycline or tetracycline. Both drugs should be given for 2 weeks if the infection is of less than 1 year's duration; otherwise they should be given for 4 weeks. Patients who are not pregnant but who are allergic to penicillin and who have primary or secondary syphilis should be treated with doxycycline or tetracycline. For patients who cannot tolerate these, ceftriaxone is recommended. Although erythromycin is less effective than other regimens, it can be used for nonpregnant, compliant patients. Patients whose compliance is questionable or pregnant patients who are allergic to penicillin should be desensitized and treated with penicillin. For more information (see Chapter 8).

TABLE 35.5	Overview of Selected Drugs Used to Treat Syphilis			
Generic (Trade) Name and Dosage	**Selected Adverse Events**	**Contraindications**	**Special Considerations**
Nonallergic Adults			
penicillin G benzathine (Bicillin) *Primary, secondary, and early latent infection:* 2.4 million U IM single dose *Late latent infection, infection of unknown duration, or tertiary infection:* 7.2 million U; total 3 doses of 2.4 million U IM each at 1-wk intervals	Hypersensitivity, urticaria, laryngeal edema, fever, eosinophilia, serum sickness–like reactions, anaphylaxis, hemolytic anemia, leukopenia, thrombocytopenia, neuropathy, nephropathy	Hypersensitivity to any penicillin or procaine	Use with caution with patients with allergies or asthma. Do not inject into or near an artery or nerve.
Nonallergic Children			
Primary, secondary, and early latent infection: 50,000 U/kg IM up to adult dose of 2.4 million U in a single dose *Late latent infection, infection of unknown duration:* 50,000 U/kg IM up to adult dose of 2.4 million U administered as 3 doses at 1-wk intervals (total 150,000 U/kg up to adult dose of 7.2 million U)	Same as above	Same as above	Same as above
Nonpregnant, Penicillin-Allergic Patients			
doxycycline (Vibramycin) 100 mg PO bid for 2 wk *Latent syphilis:* 100 mg PO bid for 4 wk (if infection is <1 y, give for 2 wk)	Superinfection, photosensitivity, GI upset, enterocolitis, rash, blood dyscrasias, hepatotoxicity	Pregnancy, lactation Hypersensitivity to any of the tetracyclines	Monitor blood, renal, and hepatic function in long-term use. Avoid sunlight or UV light. Use of drug during tooth development may cause dental discoloration. Absorption is reduced when taken with food or bismuth subsalicylate.
tetracycline (Achromycin) 500 mg PO qid for 2 wk *Latent syphilis:* 500 mg PO qid for 4 wk (if infection is <1 y, give for 2 wk)	Photosensitivity, GI upset, glossitis, dysphasia, enterocolitis, pancreatitis, anogenital lesions, elevated hepatic enzymes, hepatic toxicity, rash, hypersensitivity, dizziness, tinnitus, visual disturbances	Hypersensitivity to any tetracyclines	Use of drug during tooth development may cause dental discoloration. Use of tetracycline may render oral contraceptives less effective.
ceftriaxone (Rocephin) 1 g PO qd for 8–10 d	Pseudomembranous colitis, rash, GI upset, hepatologic abnormalities	Known allergy to cephalosporins	Prescribe with caution to penicillin-sensitive patients.
erythromycin (Ilosone) 500 mg PO qid for 2 wk	GI upset, abdominal pain, anorexia, hepatic dysfunction, rash, superinfection, pseudomembranous colitis	Hypersensitivity to erythromycin Hepatic disease	Prescribe with caution in patients with hepatic disease or myasthenia gravis, or patients who are breast-feeding.

Selecting the Most Appropriate Agent

Penicillin G therapy is the first and usually only choice for patients who have syphilis and who are not allergic to penicillin. For patients who are allergic to penicillin and who are not pregnant, first-line therapy relies on doxycycline or tetracycline. There are no proven alternative drugs for pregnant women who have syphilis and who are allergic to penicillin. These women should be desensitized and then treated with penicillin (**Figure 35-3**).

Special Population Considerations

Pediatric

Children with syphilis should have a CSF examination for asymptomatic neurosyphilis. To assess for congenital or acquired syphilis, birth and maternal records should be reviewed. Children who have primary or secondary syphilis should have an evaluation, consultation with child protection services, and treatment with a pediatric regimen.

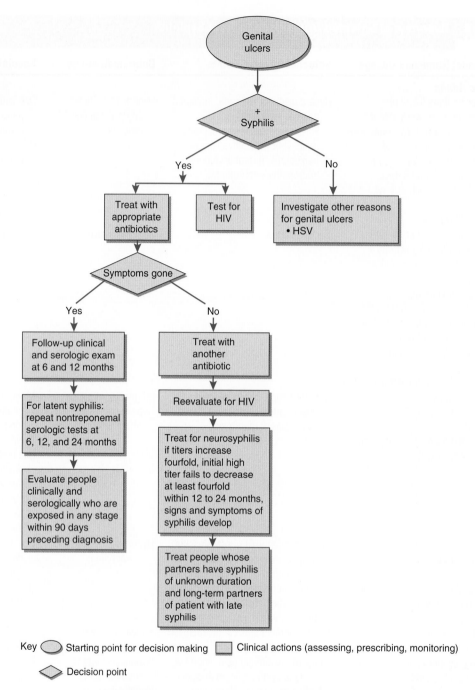

FIGURE 35–3 Treatment algorithm for syphilis.

Women

Pregnant women should be screened and treated for syphilis to protect the fetus and the newborn from exposure to syphilis. Screening is performed at the time pregnancy is confirmed. If the patient is in a high-risk group, testing should also occur at 28 weeks and at delivery. Pregnant patients who are allergic to penicillin should be desensitized and treated with penicillin.

At-Risk Populations

All patients with syphilis should be tested for HIV infection. In areas where the prevalence of HIV is high, patients with primary syphilis should be retested for HIV after 3 months if the first HIV result was negative.

MONITORING PATIENT RESPONSE

Patients should have a clinical and serologic examination at 6 and 12 months, or more frequently if follow-up results are uncertain. Those who fail to respond to treatment or who were reinfected, those who have signs that persist or recur, or those who have a sustained fourfold increase in nontreponemal test titer values within 6 months after treatment for primary or

TABLE 35.6 Overview of Drugs Used to Treat Neurosyphilis			
Generic (Trade) Name and Dosage	**Selected Adverse Events**	**Contraindications**	**Special Considerations**
aqueous crystalline penicillin G 18–24 million U/d, give as 3–4 million U IV q4h for 10–14 d	Similar to penicillins	Hypersensitivity to penicillin	This penicillin preparation is the drug of first choice in treating neurosyphilis; second-line therapy is procaine penicillin.
procaine penicillin (Bicillin with probenecid, Benemid) 2.4 million U IM/d, plus probenecid 500 mg PO qid, both for 10–14 d	Similar to other penicillins *Probenecid:* Headache, dizziness, GI upset, hypersensitivity reactions, acute gouty arthritis, nephrotic syndrome, uric acid stones	Hypersensitivity to penicillin or probenecid Children <2 y: blood dyscrasias, uric acid kidney stones	If compliance can be ensured, avoid IV, intravascular, or intra-arterial administration. *Probenecid:* Use caution in prescribing for patients with peptic ulcer.

secondary syphilis should be retreated after evaluation for HIV infection. Treatment with three weekly injections of penicillin G benzathine is recommended if additional follow-up results are uncertain, unless CSF examination identifies neurosyphilis.

Patients with latent syphilis should be evaluated for tertiary disease. All patients with latent syphilis should have quantitative nontreponemal serologic tests repeated at 6, 12, and 24 months.

Patients should be evaluated for neurosyphilis and treated if titer values increase fourfold, an initially high titer fails to decrease at least fourfold within 12 to 24 months, or signs and symptoms related to syphilis develop. Patients with symptoms of neurologic or ophthalmic disease should be evaluated for neurosyphilis and syphilitic eye disease and treated appropriately according to the results (**Table 35.6**).

PATIENT EDUCATION

Teaching patients about preventive strategies is important in deterring the transmission of disease. All patients with a diagnosis of syphilis should be advised to undergo HIV testing as well.

GENITAL HERPES SIMPLEX VIRUS INFECTION

In the United States, genital herpes is the most prevalent genital ulcer disease. It is associated with a higher risk of HIV infection. This infection has been diagnosed by serologic tests in at least 45 million people in the United States. More than 500,000 new cases occur each year. Most infected people remain undiagnosed. They have mild or unrecognized infections that shed the virus in the genital tract intermittently. Although some first episodes of genital herpes may be characterized by severe disease requiring hospitalization, many people are unaware they have the infection or are asymptomatic when transmission occurs. The disease can be controlled, not cured. It recurs periodically. Viral infections, for which curative therapy is not

available, have been stable or increasing in prevalence. With 500,000 new cases each year, herpes simplex virus (HSV) is one of the most common viral STIs.

CAUSES

Genital herpes simplex is caused by HSV, which has two serotypes: HSV-1 and HSV-2. The infection is transmitted by contact with an infected person by kissing or sexual intercourse, or during vaginal birth. Recurrent outbreaks may be triggered by injury to the infected area, an illness that alters immune status, emotional stress, or menses.

PATHOPHYSIOLOGY

Recurrent genital herpes is usually caused by HSV-2. After the virus enters the body through a susceptible mucosal surface, it resides and remains dormant in the cells of the nervous system until activated later. Exacerbations of varying frequency may or may not occur. In general, recurrent outbreaks are less severe than the initial episode.

DIAGNOSTIC CRITERIA

A diagnostic evaluation for herpes includes a health history and physical examination. In addition to serologic testing for HSV, patients should have a serologic test for syphilis. HIV testing should be considered as well. Specific tests for genital herpes include culture or antigen test for HSV. In addition, a POCkit-HSV-2 test can be performed.

The patient seeking treatment may report any one of three genital HSV syndromes. The first is primary infection, which is the first infection with genital HSV characterized by no preexisting antibodies to either HSV-1 or HSV-2. Symptoms include genital pain, vesicles, fever, malaise, regional adenopathy, and, in women, lesions on the cervix. The second syndrome is nonprimary first episode infection, which is the first clinically evident infection in women who have had a previous infection with the heterologous strains. The symptoms include fewer lesions, few constitutional symptoms, and a shorter, milder course. The third syndrome is recurrent infection, which usually has no constitutional symptoms, a shorter duration of viral shedding, and a shorter healing time.

INITIATING DRUG THERAPY

The only effective therapy for genital herpes is drug therapy. Patient education is an important measure for preventing spread of the disease.

Goals of Drug Therapy

Treatment goals for first clinical episodes, recurrent episodes, and daily suppressive therapy aim to control the symptoms of the herpes episodes. The drugs do not eradicate the latent virus, and once discontinued they do not affect the risk, frequency, or severity of recurrences. Treatment trials show acyclovir (Zovirax), valacyclovir (Valtrex), and famciclovir (Famvir) to be beneficial for treating genital herpes. The use of topical acyclovir is discouraged because it is substantially less effective than the systemic drug. The recommended acyclovir-dosing regimens have been approved by the U.S. Food and Drug Administration and reflect substantial clinical experience and expert opinion for initial and recurrent episodes (**Table 35.7**).

Antivirals: Acyclovir, Famciclovir, and Valacyclovir

The three first-line systemic agents used to control genital herpes infections are acyclovir, famciclovir, and valacyclovir. These drugs inhibit viral DNA replication and are highly effective.

Acyclovir, which has low bioavailability, works only in the cells infected by HSV. Famciclovir, a prodrug of penciclovir, is well absorbed. It is converted to penciclovir by first-pass metabolism. Valacyclovir, a prodrug of acyclovir, is converted rapidly by first-pass metabolism to acyclovir. It has a 50% bioavailability; it also deactivates viral DNA polymerase.

Because antiviral medications are excreted by the renal system, caution should be used in patients with renal disease. They should also be prescribed cautiously for pregnant patients and are contraindicated in breast-feeding patients. These antivirals interact with probenecid, which increases the effect of the antiviral agent, and with zidovudine (Retrovir), which may cause drowsiness. For a detailed discussion of the roles that acyclovir, famciclovir, and valacyclovir play in controlling HSV-1 and HSV-2, see Chapter 13.

TABLE 35.7	Overview of Selected Drugs to Treat Genital Herpes		
Generic (Trade) Name and Dosage	**Selected Adverse Events**	**Contraindications**	**Special Considerations**
acyclovir (Zovirax) *First clinical episode:* 400 mg tid for 7–10 d or 200 g 5 times a day for 7–10 d *Recurrence:* 400 mg tid for 5 d or 200 mg 5 times a day for 5 d or 800 mg bid for 5 d *Daily suppressive therapy:* 400 mg bid *Severe disease:* 5–10 mg/kg IV q8h for 5–7 d or until clinical resolution occurs	GI upset (nausea, vomiting), headache, CNS disturbances, rash, malaise, vertigo, arthralgia, fatigue, viral resistance	Hypersensitivity to acyclovir Use with caution with renal impairment, pregnancy, breast-feeding mothers.	Do not exceed maximum dose.
famciclovir (Famvir) *First clinical episode:* 250 mg tid for 7–10 d *Recurrence:* 125 mg bid for 5 d *Daily suppressive therapy:* 250 mg bid	Headache, fatigue, GI upset With chronic use: pruritus, rash, laboratory test abnormalities, paresthesias	Hypersensitivity to famciclovir Pregnancy, lactation Use with caution in patients with renal dysfunction.	Easy to administer for prolonged treatment May be affected by drugs metabolized by aldehyde oxidase
valacyclovir (Valtrex) *First clinical episode:* 1 g PO bid for 7–10 d *Recurrent episodic infection:* 500 mg PO bid for 5 d *Daily suppressive therapy:* 500 mg PO qd (<9 episodes a year) or 1,000 mg PO qd	GI upset, headache, dizziness, abdominal pain	Hypersensitivity to valacyclovir Do not use in children Use with caution with renal impairment, pregnancy, lactation.	Valacyclovir 500 mg qd is less effective than other valacyclovir regimens in patients with ≥10 episodes yearly. Be alert for renal or CNS toxicity in patients taking other nephrotoxic drugs.

Selecting the Most Appropriate Agent

Therapy progresses from selecting treatment for the first clinical episode of infection to prescribing an antiviral agent for suppressive therapy (**Figure 35-4**).

First-Line Therapy

Treatment for the first clinical episode of genital herpes includes antiviral therapy and counseling about the natural history of the virus, sexual and perinatal transmission, and methods to reduce transmission. Antiviral therapy for the initial outbreak includes the following:

- Acyclovir 400 mg three times daily for 7 to 10 days, or
- Acyclovir 200 mg five times a day for 7 to 10 days, or
- Famciclovir 250 mg three times a day for 7 to 10 days, or
- Valacyclovir 1.0 g two times a day for 7 to 10 days

The choice is based on the cost of medication, patient preference, or scheduling issues.

Second-Line Therapy (Recurrent Episodes)

Most patients with genital herpes infection have recurrent episodes of genital lesions. Episodic or suppressive antiviral therapy may shorten the duration of lesions or prevent recurrences. Episodic therapy is beneficial for recurrent disease if the treatment is started during the prodromal phase or within 1 day after onset of the lesions. When given episodic treatment, the patient should also be given additional antiviral therapy so the treatment can be initiated at the first sign of prodrome or genital lesions. Recurrent episodes are treated with:

- Acyclovir 400 mg three times a day for 5 days, or
- Acyclovir 800 mg two times a day for 5 days, or
- Acyclovir 800 mg three times a day for 2 days, or
- Famciclovir 125 mg two times a day for 5 days, or
- Famciclovir 1,000 mg twice a day for 1 day, or
- Valacyclovir 500 mg two times a day for 3 days, or
- Valacyclovir 1.0 g once a day for 5 days

Third-Line Therapy (Suppressive Therapy)

Third-line therapy is also known as suppressive therapy for HSV. The frequency of recurrent symptoms, or outbreaks, can be reduced by 75% or more with daily suppressive therapy, although suppressive therapy does not eliminate subclinical viral shedding. This therapy is used for patients with more than six episodes a year. Acyclovir has documented safety and efficacy for use for as long as 6 years, valacyclovir and famciclovir for 1 year. Discontinuation of therapy should be discussed with the patient after 1 year of continuous suppressive therapy to determine the rate of recurrence and the patient's psychological adjustment. In many patients, the frequency of recurrence decreases over time.

Asymptomatic viral shedding is reduced but not eliminated with suppressive treatment with acyclovir. Therapy is not discontinued in patients who are HIV positive.

Suppressive therapy is:

- Acyclovir 400 mg two times a day, or
- Famciclovir 250 mg two times a day, or
- Valacyclovir 500 or 1,000 mg once a day

Valacyclovir 500 mg once a day may be less effective than other regimens for prolonged suppression.

Severe or Complicated Disease

For patients with severe disease or complications requiring hospitalization, intravenous (IV) therapy is indicated. The recommended regimen is acyclovir 5 to 10 mg/kg body weight IV every 8 hours for 5 to 7 days or until clinical resolution is attained.

Special Population Considerations

Pediatric

The risk of HSV infection in the neonate is not completely eliminated with cesarean delivery. Infants exposed to HSV during birth should be followed carefully. Before clinical signs develop, the CDC recommends that the infant have surveillance cultures of mucosal surfaces to detect HSV infection. Infants born to women who acquired genital herpes near term should receive acyclovir therapy. Infants with neonatal herpes should be treated with acyclovir 30 to 60 mg/kg/d for 10 to 21 days.

Women

During pregnancy, the first clinical episode of genital herpes may be treated with oral acyclovir. IV administration of acyclovir is indicated for life-threatening maternal HSV infection. Acyclovir is not recommended for routine administration in pregnant women who have a history of recurrent genital herpes. The safety of systemic acyclovir and valacyclovir in pregnant women is unknown.

Women who acquire genital herpes close to the time of delivery (30% to 50%) are at high risk for transmitting the disease to the neonate. Those who have recurrent herpes at term or those who acquire genital HSV during the first half of pregnancy (3%) are at low risk for transmitting the disease to the neonate.

Sex partners who are symptomatic should have an evaluation and treatment similar to patients who have genital lesions. Most people who have genital HSV infection have no history of genital lesions. Therefore, asymptomatic sex partners of patients with newly diagnosed genital herpes should be interviewed regarding histories of typical and atypical genital lesions and encouraged to perform examinations and seek medical attention immediately if lesions appear.

MONITORING PATIENT RESPONSE

Response to therapy is monitored by symptom relief and resolution of lesions.

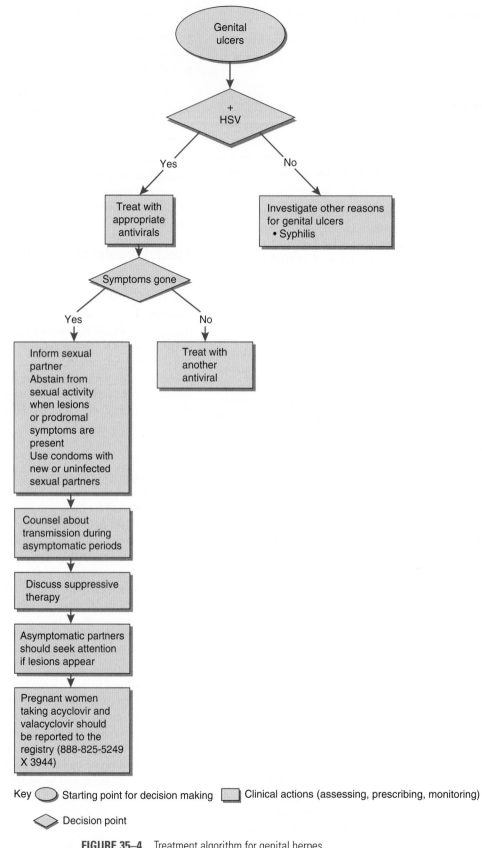

FIGURE 35–4   Treatment algorithm for genital herpes.

PATIENT EDUCATION

Patients should inform their sex partners that they have genital herpes and should abstain from sexual activity when lesions or prodromal symptoms are present. The practitioner can also discuss use of condoms with sex partners. Patients should also be counseled about transmission of HSV during asymptomatic periods.

The risk of neonatal infection should be discussed with both sexes, and women who are pregnant should advise their health care providers about the infection. Patients should also be advised that episodic antiviral therapy may shorten the duration of lesions during recurrent episodes and that recurrent outbreaks can be ameliorated or prevented with suppressive antiviral therapy. Prevention of neonatal herpes should be emphasized during late pregnancy and counseling provided regarding unprotected genital and oral sexual contact at this time.

Patients who have genital herpes should be educated about the natural history of the disease, with emphasis on the potential for recurrent episodes, asymptomatic viral shedding, and the attendant risks of sexual transmission. All persons with genital HSV infection should be encouraged to inform their current sex partners that they have genital herpes and to inform future partners before initiating a sexual relationship. Persons with genital herpes should be informed that sexual transmission of HSV can occur during asymptomatic periods. Asymptomatic viral shedding is more frequent in genital HSV-2 infection than genital HSV-1 infection and is most frequent in the first 12 months of acquiring HSV-2.

PELVIC INFLAMMATORY DISEASE

It is estimated that PID affects 1 million women each year. Approximately 250,000 of these women are hospitalized and more than 150,000 major surgical procedures are performed. The disease is associated with significant long-term consequences, including tubal-factor infertility, ectopic pregnancy, and chronic pelvic pain. Risk factors for PID include previous episodes of PID, presence of *N. gonorrhoeae, C. trachomatis*, or bacterial vaginosis in the lower genital tract, multiple sex partners, use of an intrauterine contraceptive device, adolescence, sexual intercourse during the last menstrual period, douching, and cigarette smoking. Oral contraceptives are thought to afford some protection against PID.

CAUSES

The most common etiologic agents for PID are *N. gonorrhoeae* and *C. trachomatis*. Other microorganisms that are part of the vaginal flora can also cause PID, as well as *Mycobacterium hominis* and *Ureaplasma urealyticum*.

PATHOPHYSIOLOGY

PID consists of several inflammatory disorders of the upper female genital tract that include any combination of endometritis, salpingitis, tubo-ovarian abscess, and pelvic peritonitis. It is an ascending infection that spreads from the lower genital tract to the endometrium, to the fallopian tubes, and to the peritoneal cavity.

DIAGNOSTIC CRITERIA

In all settings, no single historical, physical, or laboratory finding is sensitive and specific enough to make the diagnosis of acute PID. Many cases of PID are not recognized because they are asymptomatic or because the patient or health care provider fails to recognize mild or nonspecific symptoms.

The following diagnostic criteria are from the CDC (2006) guidelines. Empiric treatment of PID should be given to sexually active young women and others who are at risk for STIs if all of the following minimum criteria are present with no other causes for the illness: lower abdominal tenderness, adnexal tenderness, and cervical motion tenderness. Additional criteria may be used to enhance the specificity of the minimum criteria, including oral temperature exceeding 101°F (38.3°C), abnormal cervical or vaginal discharge, elevated erythrocyte sedimentation rate, elevated C-reactive protein, and laboratory documentation of cervical infection with *N. gonorrhoeae* or *C. trachomatis*. In selected cases, the following definitive criteria for diagnosing PID are warranted: histopathologic evidence of endometritis on endometrial biopsy; transvaginal sonography or other imaging techniques showing thickening, fluid-filled tubes with or without free pelvic fluid or tubo-ovarian complex; and laparoscopic abnormalities consistent with PID.

INITIATING DRUG THERAPY

Treatment for PID is prescribed when the patient's signs and symptoms meet the diagnostic criteria. Treatment includes empiric, broad-spectrum coverage of likely pathogens, including *N. gonorrhoeae, C. trachomatis*, anaerobes, gram-negative facultative bacteria, and streptococci. The CDC (2006) recommends patients be hospitalized when surgical emergencies cannot be excluded and when the patient is pregnant; does not respond clinically to oral antimicrobials; cannot tolerate an outpatient oral regimen; has severe illness, nausea and vomiting, or high fever; has a tubo-ovarian abscess; or is immunodeficient. There are no efficacy data that compare parenteral with oral regimens, and clinical experience should guide the decision to switch from parenteral to oral therapy, which may occur within 24 hours of clinical improvement.

Goals of Drug Therapy

In addition to ameliorating infection or preventing the progression of disease, the goal of drug therapy is to preserve the patient's reproductive health or at least minimize the effects of infection. Treatment should begin as promptly as possible because prevention of long-term sequelae has a direct correlation with immediate antibiotic coverage. Factors to consider in selecting treatment include drug availability and cost, patient acceptance, and antimicrobial susceptibility.

Antimicrobials and Appropriate Treatment Choices

For the most part, antimicrobial regimens for PID are those used for patients with chlamydial and gonorrheal infections.

Refer to the sections on chlamydial infection and gonorrhea in this chapter, and also see **Table 35.8** for an overview of drug therapy in PID and **Figure 35-5** for a synopsis of the treatment. For women with PID of mild or moderate severity, parenteral therapy and oral therapy appear to have similar clinical efficacy.

Special Population Considerations

So that the mother and fetus can be closely monitored, pregnant women with suspected PID should be hospitalized and treated with parenteral antibiotics.

TABLE 35.8	Overview of Selected Drugs to Treat Pelvic Inflammatory Disease		
Generic (Trade) Name and Dosage	**Selected Adverse Events**	**Contraindications**	**Special Considerations**
cefoxitin (Mefoxin) Mefoxin plus probenecid (Benemid) 2 g IV q6h Mefoxin plus doxycycline (Vibramycin) 100 mg PO for 14 d	*cefoxitin:* Pseudomembranous colitis, thrombophlebitis, rash, pruritus, eosinophilia, fever, dyspnea, hypotension, GI upset *doxycycline:* Superinfection, photosensitivity, GI upset, enterocolitis, rash, blood dyscrasias, hepatotoxicity	Hypersensitivity to cefoxitin or cephalosporins Pregnancy, lactation, hypersensitivity to any of the tetracyclines	Prescribe with caution to penicillin-sensitive patients and those with GI disease. Monitor, blood, renal, and hepatic function in long-term use. Avoid sunlight or UV light. Use of drug during tooth development may cause dental discoloration. Absorption is reduced when taken with food or bismuth subsalicylate.
doxycycline (Vibramycin) 100 mg PO bid for 14 d or clindamycin (Cleocin) 450 mg PO qid for 14 d	Same as above	Same as above	Parenteral therapy may be discontinued 24 h after patient improves clinically. Clindamycin is used with tubo-ovarian abscess rather than doxycycline.
ofloxacin (Floxin) 400 mg PO bid for 14 d	Rash, hives, rapid heartbeat, difficulty swallowing or breathing, photosensitivity, angioedema, dizziness, lightheadedness	Pregnancy Hypersensitivity to ofloxacin or fluoroquinolones	Use with caution with hepatic or renal insufficiency. Do not take with food.
metronidazole (Flagyl) 500 mg PO bid for 14 d	CNS stimulation, phototoxicity, GI upset, insomnia, headache, dizziness, tendinitis or tendon rupture, local reactions	Hypersensitivity to metronidazole Pregnancy, lactation	Take on empty stomach with full glass of water and maintain adequate hydration throughout therapy. Avoid excessive sunlight or UV light. Monitor blood, renal, and hepatic function in long-term use. Use with caution with CNS disorders that increase seizure risk, and in renal or hepatic impairment.
ceftriaxone (Rocephin) 250 mg IM once	Pseudomembranous colitis, rash, GI upset, hematologic abnormalities	Known allergy to cephalosporins	Prescribe with caution to penicillin-sensitive patients.

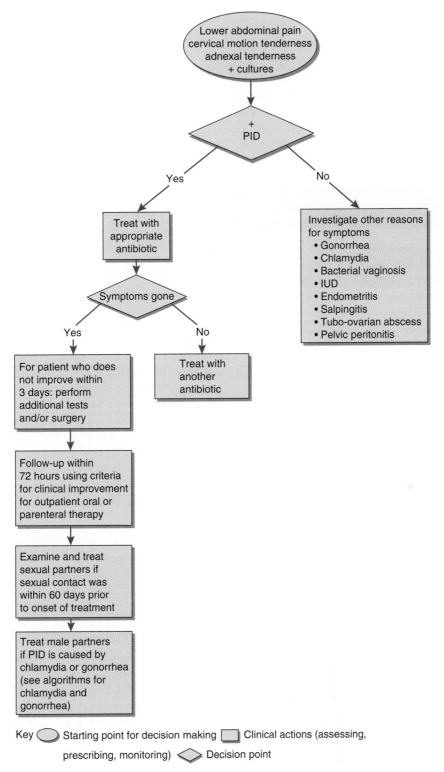

FIGURE 35–5   Treatment algorithm for pelvic inflammatory disease (PID).

MONITORING PATIENT RESPONSE

Patients treated with oral or parenteral therapy should demonstrate substantial clinical improvement within 3 days after therapy has been initiated. Those who do not improve in this period usually require additional diagnostic tests or surgical intervention. The patient should be seen after 1 week of antibiotic therapy to check for residual pelvic abnormalities. Outpatient oral or parenteral therapy also requires a follow-up examination performed within 72 hours, using the criteria for clinical improvement.

PATIENT EDUCATION

If *N. gonorrhoeae* or *C. trachomatis* is present, the practitioner needs to explain to patients with PID that their sex partners should be examined and treated if they have had sexual contact with the patient during the 60 days before the onset of the patient's symptoms. Male partners of women with PID caused by *C. trachomatis* or *N. gonorrhoeae* are often asymptomatic and should be treated empirically with regimens that are effective against both infections.

HUMAN PAPILLOMA VIRUS INFECTION

The detection of human papilloma virus (HPV) infection has increased in frequency in the genital tracts of men and women. Genital warts, known as *condylomata acuminata,* have been detected with widely increasing frequency as well. One million new cases of HPV are diagnosed each year, and the prevalence of this disease is between 24 and 40 million cases.

CAUSES

More than 30 HPVs are associated with infection of the genital tract. The sexual transmission of HPV is well documented, with the highest prevalence in young, sexually active adolescents and adults. Risk factors include the presence of other STIs, an increased number of sex partners, and use of oral contraceptives without other protection.

PATHOPHYSIOLOGY

Most HPVs cause no symptoms, are subclinical, or remain unrecognized. Warts that are visible in the genital tract are usually caused by HPV types 6 or 11, which also cause warts (that cannot be seen externally) on the uterine cervix and in the vagina, urethra, and anus. These viruses, which can produce symptoms, have also been associated with conjunctival, nasal, oral, and laryngeal warts. They are rarely associated with invasive squamous cell carcinoma of the external genitalia. Genital warts can be painful, friable, or pruritic, depending on their size and anatomic location.

Cervical dysplasia has been strongly associated with other HPV types in the anogenital region, including types 16, 18, 31, 33, and 35. These are found occasionally in visible genital warts and have been associated with external genital squamous intraepithelial neoplasia and vaginal, anal, and cervical intraepithelial dysplasia and squamous cell carcinoma. Visible genital warts can be infected simultaneously with multiple HPV types.

DIAGNOSTIC CRITERIA

Genital warts are diagnosed definitively by biopsy, which is needed only if the diagnosis is uncertain, if the lesions do not respond to standard therapy, if the disease worsens during therapy, if the patient is immunocompromised, or if the warts are pigmented, indurated, fixed, and ulcerated. The literature does not support HPV nucleic acid tests for use in the routine diagnosis or management of visible genital warts. For women who have exophytic cervical warts, high-grade squamous intraepithelial lesions must be ruled out before initiating treatment for genital warts (CDC, 2006).

INITIATING DRUG THERAPY

There is no evidence that current treatments eradicate or affect the natural history of HPV infection or the development of cervical cancer. Removal of warts may or may not decrease infectivity. Warts that are not treated may resolve on their own, remain unchanged, or increase in number and size. Treatment is guided by patient preference, cost of treatment and available resources, experience of the health care practitioner, wart size and number, anatomic location of wart, wart morphology, convenience, and adverse effects. No single treatment is ideal for all patients, nor is one superior to another.

Visible genital warts may be self-treated by the patient if they are accessible or by the health care practitioner. Nonpharmacologic therapies include surgery or laser therapy. Carbon dioxide laser is used for extensive warts or intraurethral warts and for patients who do not respond to other treatments. Pharmacotherapy may include podophyllin resin (Podofin), imiquimod (Aldara), trichloroacetic acid (TCA), bichloracetic acid (BCA), or intralesional interferon (Intron A).

Goals of Drug Therapy

The primary goal in treating visible genital warts is the removal of symptomatic warts and prevention of HPV transmission. Removal can induce wart-free periods in most patients. Often, genital warts are asymptomatic. Pharmacologic therapy may include podofilox (Condylox), imiquimod, TCA, and BCA (**Table 35.9**).

Podofilox and Podophyllin Resin

Visible genital warts can be self-treated by the patient with podofilox. The patient must be able to identify and reach the warts to be treated. Podofilox in 0.5% solution or gel is safe, inexpensive, easy to use, and efficacious on mucosal surfaces.

A stronger preparation for application only by the health care provider is podophyllin resin, which may be administered at a 10% to 25% concentration in a compound with tincture of benzoin. The CDC does not recommend use of podophyllin by the patient because of rare but potential toxicity involving systemic absorption, bone marrow suppression, or serious GI upset. The preparation is applied weekly as needed. Again, to guard against potential toxicities, the CDC recommends washing the preparation from the application site 1 to 4 hours after application. The most common adverse effect, which indicates the preparation is working, is local irritation. The preparation has not been established as safe for use during pregnancy.

TABLE 35.9	Overview of Selected Drugs and Procedures Used to Treat Genital Warts		
Generic (Trade) Name and Dosage	**Selected Adverse Events**	**Contraindications**	**Special Considerations**
Patient Applied			
podofilox solution or gel (Condylox) 0.5% bid for 3 d followed by 4 d of no therapy; repeat cycle as needed for a total of 4 cycles	Mild or moderate pain or local irritation	The safety of podofilox during pregnancy has not been established.	Apply solution with cotton swab or apply gel with finger. Total wart area should not exceed 10 cm^2, and total volume of podofilox should not exceed 0.5 mL/d.
imiquimod cream (Aldara) 5% cream applied three times a week for up to 16 wk	Mild to moderate local inflammatory reactions	The safety of imiquimod during pregnancy has not been established.	Apply with finger at bedtime. Wash area with mild soap and water 6 to 10 h after application of cream. May clear area of warts in 8 to 10 wk or sooner
Practitioner Applied			
cryotherapy	Pain, necrosis, blistering	Use of cryoprobe in the vagina is not recommended because of risk of vaginal perforation and fistula formation.	Repeat applications every 1–2 wk. Use local anesthetic. Indicated for urethral meatus warts, anal warts, oral warts
podophyllin or resin in compound tincture of benzoin 10% to 25% (Podofin)	Local irritation	The safety of podophyllin during pregnancy has not been established. Use with caution vaginally because of potential systemic absorption.	Apply small amount to each wart and allow site to air dry. Limit to ≤0.5 mL of podophyllin or ≤10 cm^2 of warts per therapy session. Wash off preparation 4 h after application to reduce local irritation. Repeat application weekly if necessary. With vaginal warts, allow to dry before removing speculum and treat with ≤2 cm^2 per session. For warts on the urethral meatus, treatment area must be dry before preparation comes in contact with normal mucosa.
trichloroacetic acid or bichloracetic acid 80%–90%	Can spread rapidly and damage adjacent tissue; pain		Apply small amount only to warts and allow site to dry. White "frosting" will develop. Use talc with baking soda to remove unreacted acid if an excess amount is applied. Repeat treatment weekly as needed. Indicated for vaginal warts

Imiquimod

Like podofilox, imiquimod may be self-administered by the patient. This antimitotic preparation enhances the immune response to HPV. Imiquimod can be topically applied three times weekly for 3 to 4 months. As with podophyllin, the imiquimod site should be washed with mild soap and water 6 to 10 hours after application. Warts should disappear in 8 to 10 weeks. During imiquimod therapy, sexual contact should be avoided to prevent viral transmission. Adverse effects include a local inflammatory reaction. The safety of use during pregnancy has not been established.

TCA and BCA

TCA and BCA are applied by the health care provider. These are strong, 80% to 90% acids that flow onto the wart site quickly, and the fluid can spread equally quickly. Application requires particular care and skill. The acid is applied only to the warts and left to air-dry. A white "frosting" appears at the site. The practitioner can use talc or sodium bicarbonate powders to neutralize acid that falls on healthy tissue. TCA and BCA can be used effectively on keratinized areas and are safe for use during pregnancy. They are associated with low systemic toxicity.

Intralesional Interferon

Interferon is ineffective when used systemically. However, the use of intralesional interferon appears to be effective, and recurrence rates after therapy are comparable to those with other treatment modalities. Intralesional therapy appears to be effective because of interferon's antiviral or immunostimulating effects.

Selecting the Most Appropriate Agent

Treatment of genital warts should be guided by the preference of the patient, the available resources, and the experience of the health care provider. No definitive evidence suggests that any one of the available treatments is superior to the others, and no single treatment is ideal for all patients or all warts. Most patients have 10 or fewer genital warts. These warts respond to most treatment modalities. Factors that may influence selection of treatment include wart size, wart number, anatomic site of wart, wart morphology, patient preference, cost of treatment, convenience, adverse effects, and provider experience. Many patients require a course of therapy rather than a single treatment. In general, warts located on moist surfaces or in intertriginous areas respond better to topical treatment than do warts on drier surfaces. **Figure 35-6** outlines the most appropriate patient- or practitioner-applied drug therapies in the most appropriate order.

Special Population Considerations

Pediatric

Laryngeal papillomatoses in infants and children are caused by HPV 6 and 11. The prevention value of cesarean section is unknown, and the route of transmission is not completely understood.

Women

Many experts recommend removing warts during pregnancy because they can proliferate and become friable.

MONITORING PATIENT RESPONSE

If the warts are not completely clear after six treatments or the patient has not improved significantly after three practitioner-administered treatments, the treatment plan should be changed. Evaluation of the risk/benefit ratio of treatment

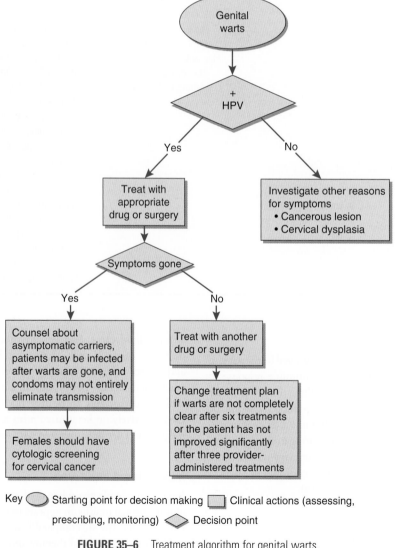

FIGURE 35–6 Treatment algorithm for genital warts.

should occur throughout the course of therapy to avoid over-treatment. Women with genital warts should have cytologic screening for cervical cancer.

Once warts are eradicated, follow-up evaluations are not mandatory. Patients should monitor for recurrences, especially in the first 3 months. Patients who have concerns regarding recurrences can have a follow-up evaluation 3 months after treatment. Earlier follow-up visits may help to verify a wart-free state and monitor or treat complications, and can be used for patient education and counseling.

PATIENT EDUCATION

The practitioner needs to provide precise instruction and guidance for applying topical antimitotic preparations, such as by showing how to apply podofilox solution with a cotton swab and the gel with a finger to visible warts. Patients should also be informed that HPV organisms persist despite resolution of lesions. Sex partners do not need to be examined because reinfection is most likely minimal and treatment to reduce transmission is not realistic in the absence of curative therapy. However, partners should be counseled about having a partner with genital warts and should be informed that the patient may remain infectious even when the warts are gone. The use of condoms may not eliminate the risk of transmission.

Patients should be warned that ablative therapies may cause scarring in the form of persistent hypopigmentation or hyperpigmentation. Depressed or hypertrophic scars rarely occur. Disabling chronic pain syndromes can also occur but are rare.

Case Study

J. R. is a 36-year-old white, middle-class woman who has been sexually active with one partner for the past 2 years. She and her partner have no history of STIs, but her partner has a history of fever blisters. She reports genital pain, genital vesicles and ulcers, and fever and malaise for the last 3 days. Examination reveals adenopathy and vaginal and cervical lesions.

DIAGNOSIS: GENITAL HERPES

1. List specific goals for treatment for J. R.
2. What drug therapy would you prescribe? Why?
3. What are the parameters for monitoring the success of the therapy?
4. Discuss specific education for J. R. based on the diagnosis and prescribed therapy.
5. List one or two adverse reactions for the selected agent that would cause you to change therapy.
6. What, if any, would be the choice for second-line therapy?
7. What OTC or alternative medicines would you recommend?
8. What dietary and lifestyle changes should be recommended for this patient?
9. Describe one or two drug–drug or drug–food interactions for the selected agent.

BIBLIOGRAPHY

Starred references are cited in the text.
Biggs, W., & Williams, R. (2009). Common gynecological infections. *Primary Care: Clinics in Office Practice, 36*(1), 33–51.
Brill, J. (2010). Sexually transmitted infections in men. *Primary Care: Clinics in Office Practice, 37*(3), 509–525.
*Centers for Disease Control and Prevention. (2006). Sexually transmitted treatment guidelines, 2006. *Morbidity and Mortality Weekly Reports, 55*(RR-11), 1–93.
*Frenkl, T., & Potts, J. (2008). Sexually transmitted infections. *Urologic Clinics of North America, 35*(1), 33–46.
*Hollier, L. M., & Workowski, K. (2008). Treatment for sexually transmitted diseases in women. *Infectious Disease Clinics of North America, 22*(4), 665–691.
Rosen, T., Vandergriff, T., & Hurting, M. (2009). Antibiotic use in sexually transmitted diseases. *Dermatology Clinics, 27*(1), 49–61.
Shafii, T., & Burnstein, G. (2009). The adolescent sexual health visit. *Obstetrics and Gynecology Clinics, 36*(1), 99–117.
Trigg, B., Kerndt, P., & Aynalem, G. (2008). Sexually transmitted infection and pelvic inflammatory disease in women. *Medical Clinics of North America, 92*(5), 1083–1113.
VanVranken, M. (2007). Prevention and treatment of sexually transmitted diseases: An update. *American Family Physician, 76*(12), 1827–1832.

Pharmacotherapy for Musculoskeletal Disorders

CHAPTER 36

Lauren K. McCluggage
Carol Gullo Mest

Osteoarthritis and Rheumatoid Arthritis

The term *arthritis* means inflammation of a joint and is a generic catch-all term used to describe more than 100 conditions that affect the bones, joints, and muscles, with osteoarthritis being the most common. Unfortunately, many times a patient's specific arthritic condition is not differentiated, which can then lead to pain and disability. According to the Centers for Disease Control and Prevention, arthritis is the leading cause of disability in adults in the United States, and the prevalence of arthritis is projected to increase to 67 million patients by 2030.

Although arthritis once was accepted as an expected part of the aging process, research has discovered treatments that can be prescribed to patients of all ages. However, most forms of arthritis can only be treated and not cured. In order to receive the best treatment, the specific type of arthritis must be determined since treatment for one type may be ineffective for another. Two of the major arthritis conditions, osteoarthritis (OA) and rheumatoid arthritis (RA), are discussed in this chapter.

OSTEOARTHRITIS

OA, formerly known as *degenerative joint disease,* is the most common joint problem in the United States. Based on U.S. data from 2005, OA affects approximately 14% of adults older than age 25 and one-third of adults older than age 65. Although prevalent, OA is often undiagnosed because clinical signs and symptoms are typically attributed to the normal aging process. In population-based studies in which asymptomatic patients were screened, the incidence of radiographic-defined OA was consistently higher than the incidence of symptomatic OA in the hands, knees, and hips.

OA is a progressive disease that can result in chronic pain, restricted range of motion, and muscle weakness, especially if a weight-bearing joint is affected. The joints commonly affected by OA include the knees, hips, cervical and lumbar spine, distal interphalangeal (DIP) joints, and the carpometacarpal joint at the base of the thumb.

CAUSES

There are two forms of OA. *Primary,* or idiopathic, OA arises from physiologic changes that occur with normal aging. *Secondary* OA usually results from traumatic injuries or inherited conditions and may present as hemochromatosis, chondrodystrophy, or inflammatory OA.

There are several modifiable and nonmodifiable risk factors that contribute to the development of OA. Of all the risk factors, obesity is the greatest in the development of OA of the knees and hips, especially in women. This is due to mechanical stress on weight-bearing joints. There may also be a metabolic effect of excess fat on articular cartilage that may account for some of the significance of obesity as a systemic risk factor. Other modifiable risk factors include prior joint injury and occupations that require excessive mechanical stress or heavy lifting. For patients with a past knee injury, the lifetime risk of knee OA is 57% compared to 45% in patients with no previous injury.

The nonmodifiable risk factors include gender, age, race, and genetics. Women have a higher overall risk for developing OA, but men tend to have disease onset at an earlier age. Increasing age is a risk factor until age 75, at which point the risk levels off. OA of the DIP and carpometacarpal joints is more common in white women; OA of the knees occurs more frequently in African-American women. Genetics may determine approximately one-fourth of knee OA cases and one-half of hip and hand OA cases.

PATHOPHYSIOLOGY

OA must be differentiated from other forms of arthritis because the physiologic changes specific to the condition dictate disease management. Although most forms of arthritis, including OA, result in degeneration of articular cartilage, the subsequent formation of new bone is a change specific to OA.

The physiologic changes associated with OA begin with deterioration of the articular cartilage, which reduces joint friction during movement by diffusing mechanical stress to the underlying bone. Normal articular cartilage is smooth and is supported by subchondral bone. The subchondral bone serves as a flexible base to absorb mechanical force.

Articular cartilage consists of chondrocytes, connective tissue cells that are embedded in an extracellular matrix. The matrix is made up of collagen, water, and proteoglycans (macromolecules). The proteoglycans provide elasticity and flexibility to the matrix, which allows the articular cartilage to resist direct pressure. In OA, there is a reduction in proteoglycans in the extracellular matrix, leading to a decrease in resiliency to mechanical stress. In time, the articular cartilage becomes friable. The underlying subchondral bone responds to this change through a process termed *remodeling*. Remodeling involves the production of new bone that is thicker than the original bone. If remodeling occurs at the joint margins, an osteophyte (bone spur) may develop. The adjacent cortical bone becomes fortified with new bone, resulting in an irregular narrowing of the joint space. Sclerosing and cyst formation may ensue.

In addition to cartilaginous changes, concomitant changes in the synovial fluid must be considered. Synovial fluid, the main lubricant of joints, is produced and excreted from the cartilage. Destruction of the proteoglycans in OA renders the mechanism of synovial release ineffective, thereby further impairing the smooth mechanical operation of the joint. **Figure 36-1** demonstrates the mechanism of cartilage destruction.

DIAGNOSTIC CRITERIA

The American College of Rheumatology (ACR) published criteria for the diagnosis of OA of the knee (1986), hip (1991), and hand (1990) (**Box 36.1**). Often, a thorough history and physical examination provide enough data to diagnose OA. The most common symptom is joint pain; the patient in an early stage of OA usually describes the pain as insidious, intermittent, and mild. As the disease progresses, the patient may describe the pain as more constant and more disabling. Most patients report remittance of pain with rest and exacerbation of pain with joint movement.

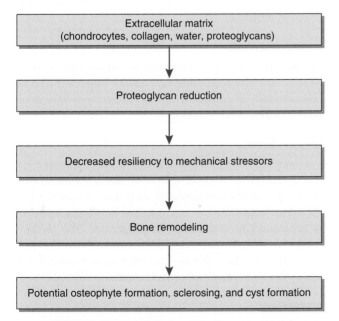

FIGURE 36–1 Destruction of cartilage in osteoarthritis.

BOX 36.1

Diagnostic Criteria for Osteoarthritis

- Hand: Pain, aching, or stiffness and 3 of the following
  - Hard tissue enlargement of >2 joints
  - Hard tissue enlargement of >2 DIP joints
  - <3 swollen MCP joints
  - Deformity of >1 selected joint
- Hip: Pain and 2 of the following
  - ESR <20 mm/h
  - Radiographic femoral or acetabular osteophytes
  - Radiographic joint space narrowing
- Knee
  - Clinical diagnosis: Knee pain and 3 of the following
    - >50 y old
    - Stiffness <30 min
    - Crepitus
    - Bony tenderness
    - Bony enlargement
    - No palpable warmth
  - Clinical and radiographic diagnosis: Knee pain + osteophytes and 1 of the following
    - >50 y old
    - Stiffness < 30 min
    - Crepitus
  - Clinical and laboratory diagnosis: Knee pain and 5 of the following
    - Age >50 y old
    - Stiffness <30 min
    - Crepitus
    - Bony tenderness
    - Bony enlargement
    - No palpable warmth
    - ESR <40 mm/h
    - RF <1:40
    - Synovial fluid signs of OA (clear, viscous, or WBC count <2,000/mm^3)

Although the symptoms of OA are localized, associated pain may be referred. For example, it is common for OA of the hip to be referred to the medial knee. Another symptom associated with OA is crepitus, a painless "crackling" in the joint. Crepitus most commonly affects the knee, but it may be heard in other joints affected by OA as well. As OA progresses to later stages of articular damage, deformity of the joint may be observed. The deformity usually appears as an enlargement of the joint, which may result from either increased bone production or synovitis. Other deformities resulting from OA of the knee include varus (bow-legged knees) and valgus (knock-kneed legs).

OA of the cervical spine may present with pain that radiates to the supraclavicular or upper trapezius areas. Depending on the level of nerve involvement, symptoms may progress to include pain in the distal upper extremities. OA of the lumbar spine may produce symptoms of neurogenic claudication.

On physical examination, decreased range of motion is the most common finding. This finding may be absent in the early stages of the disease but gradually progresses as the condition worsens. In later stages of the disease, joint contractures may occur, resulting in varus and valgus deformities. Patients with severe OA of the hip may present with gait disturbances.

Because OA is a progressive disease, complications such as joint effusion and enlargement may occur. Occasionally, radicular problems may occur secondary to changes in the cervical vertebrae.

Joint enlargement due to the formation of osteophytes may be observed. Osteophyte formation in the DIP joint is called *Heberden's nodes*; in the proximal interphalangeal joint, it is referred to as *Bouchard's nodes*.

Radiologic findings in OA may be used to confirm the suspected diagnosis. Narrow joint spaces with osteophyte formation are common findings.

Typical laboratory data are unaffected by OA, which is not a systemic disease, though there is promising information regarding a new biochemical marker, the collagen fragment CTX-II. This marker may be a valuable tool for diagnosing and monitoring the progression of OA. CTX-II is a type II collagen peptide fragment associated with cartilage destruction. In a controlled study, researchers found that patients with elevated CTX-II levels were more likely to be diagnosed with OA. These findings were independent of age, sex, and body mass index. Changes that occur in CTX-II with treatment have not yet been studied.

INITIATING DRUG THERAPY

Before initiating drug therapy, the practitioner should recommend appropriate physical activity or physical therapy. The goals of physical therapy are to reduce pain, improve motion, and maintain functional ability (**Box 36.2**).

BOX 36.2

Physical Therapies for Osteoarthritis

- Moist heat to help diminish muscle spasm and relieve stiffness
- Weight loss if the patient is overweight
- Exercises to strengthen the muscles surrounding the involved joint(s) and a fitness program to maintain flexibility of the involved joint through swimming, walking, cycling, and isometric exercises
- Use of assistive devices to help with ambulation and activities of daily living

---

The goals of pharmacotherapy for OA are to maintain function, prevent further joint damage, and diminish associated pain. The degree of joint involvement and the severity of the symptoms usually dictate proper interventions for individual patients.

Acetaminophen

First-line pharmacotherapy for OA is geared toward analgesia, specifically with acetaminophen (Tylenol). Due to acetaminophen's cost-effectiveness and safety, it is currently the first-line treatment recommended in guidelines by the ACR, the European League against Rheumatism (EULAR), and others.

Mechanism of Action

Acetaminophen exerts its action within the central nervous system (CNS). It is thought to inhibit central cyclooxygenase (COX), which results in decreased prostaglandin synthesis. Through this prostaglandin inhibition, acetaminophen exerts analgesic and antipyretic effects but does not have anti-inflammatory effects.

Dosage

The recommended dose is 650 mg every 4 to 6 hours or 1,000 mg every 6 to 8 hours around the clock. The key to acetaminophen dosing for OA is to schedule the dose regardless of the patient's pain. To be most effective it must be taken regularly.

The recommended dose of up to 4 g/d is safe for patients with normal liver function. Higher doses have been associated with hepatotoxicity. Patients with a history of liver disease or who are chronic alcohol drinkers should not take more than 1,800 to 2,000 mg/d.

Time Frame for Response

If taken as scheduled, patients can experience pain relief within 1 week of initiation.

Contraindications

The only absolute contraindication to acetaminophen use is hypersensitivity to acetaminophen. Acetaminophen should be used cautiously in patients with hepatic disease or who drink more than 3 alcoholic drinks daily.

Adverse Events

Acetaminophen is typically well tolerated with the most common adverse events being dizziness and rash. For patients who take more than the recommended daily dose, acetaminophen can induce hepatic failure as a result of the accumulation of the hepatotoxic metabolite acetylimidoquinone. Also, patients need to be educated about the risk of accidental overdose with combination products that also contain acetaminophen. Renal toxicity has also been observed with chronic overdosages.

Interactions

With chronic doses of greater than 1.3 g daily, acetaminophen can increase the international normalized ratio (INR) of a patient on warfarin. If a patient is on chronic acetaminophen and warfarin, the INR should be monitored more frequently upon initiation and discontinuation of acetaminophen. Isoniazid may increase the risk of hepatotoxicity of acetaminophen.

Nonsteroidal Anti-inflammatory Drugs

Second-line therapy for OA includes nonsteroidal anti-inflammatory drugs (NSAIDs), the most commonly used class of drugs in the world. NSAIDs are further classified according to their chemical structure (**Table 36.1**). Although these classes have subtle differences, they all basically act by inhibiting COX. These drugs may be prescribed if patients do not respond well to acetaminophen or if an inflammatory process has begun.

Mechanism of Action

There are two mechanisms by which NSAIDs exert their anti-inflammatory action (**Figure 36-2**). One is by inhibiting the conversion of arachidonic acid to prostaglandin, prostacyclin, and thromboxanes—all of which are mediators of pain and inflammation. The other is by interfering with protein kinase activation (especially when taken at higher doses).

COX is the enzyme that converts arachidonic acid to prostaglandin G_2. The COX enzyme is present in two forms, COX-1 and COX-2. Most NSAIDs unselectively inhibit both COX-1 and COX-2, except for celecoxib, which is more selective for COX-2. COX-1 enzymes are found in the gastrointestinal (GI) tract and kidney and produce protective prostaglandins, which is why most research focuses on preserving the activity of COX-1. COX-2 is produced at nonspecific sites of inflammation as well as in the kidneys. Inhibition of COX-2 produces anti-inflammatory and analgesic effects without affecting the GI tract. COX-2 produces protective prostaglandins in the kidney that are responsible for maintaining adequate blood perfusion via vasodilation of the afferent arteriole. Therefore, inhibition of either COX-1 or COX-2 can result in decreased renal perfusion and impaired kidney function.

Dosage

Dosing of NSAIDs is variable. The drugs are classified into short-, intermediate-, and long-acting categories. NSAIDs require five half-lives to reach peak therapeutic levels and five half-lives to be fully excreted. Categories with a longer half-life require longer periods to reach therapeutic levels.

Some common agents used to treat OA are diclofenac, ibuprofen, or the COX-2 inhibitor celecoxib. Diclofenac is given at 50 mg twice daily, and ibuprofen is usually given at 400 mg four times daily. The typical dose of celecoxib is 100 mg twice daily or 200 mg once daily. Patients should be encouraged to use the prescribed NSAID consistently for 2 to 3 weeks to determine its effectiveness. **Table 36.1** gives information about other agents and dosing considerations.

Time Frame for Response

Patients' responses to NSAIDs are quite variable. Patients who do not respond to one NSAID may respond to another, even one in the same class. This response variability is also seen in the side effect profile of NSAIDs. The practitioner should be familiar with several of the NSAIDs from each class and should try to individualize therapy based on symptom management and side effects.

Contraindications

NSAIDs are contraindicated in patients allergic to aspirin, in patients with alcohol dependence, or in pregnant patients. Further, since celecoxib contains a sulfa moiety, it is contraindicated in patients with a sulfa allergy. Caution should be used when prescribing NSAIDs to patients with renal or hepatic impairment or the elderly. Due to the increase in cardiovascular adverse events, all NSAIDs carry a black box warning emphasizing that they are contraindicated for perioperative pain treatment in patients undergoing coronary artery bypass graft surgery.

Adverse Events

NSAIDs have gained a reputation as innocuous agents because of their over-the-counter (OTC) availability and widespread use. However, this class of drugs is far from benign, and patient education materials should highlight potential adverse events. The side effect profile of NSAIDs is quite extensive.

Visual changes, weight gain, headache, dizziness, nervousness, photosensitivity, weakness, tinnitus, easy bruising or bleeding, and fluid retention are adverse events that have been associated with use of NSAIDs. Again, cautious use and frequent monitoring, particularly of elderly patients, is of paramount importance for safe NSAID use. The most common adverse events of NSAIDs occur in the GI and renal systems.

Adverse GI events may run the gamut from minor GI irritation to ulcers, GI bleeding, perforation, and gastric outlet obstruction. These GI effects are why NSAIDs remain a second-line approach to OA treatment. Concomitant use of misoprostol (Cytotec) has been shown to decrease the incidence of ulcer disease and GI complications. Misoprostol, a prostaglandin analog, is given at 200 mg four times daily. Its use should be limited to patients at high risk for GI complications (age >65, comorbid medical conditions, history of peptic ulcer disease or upper GI bleeding, oral glucocorticosteroids, or anticoagulants).

Studies of the treatment of GI effects as a result of NSAIDs have compared the efficacy of proton pump inhibitors and histamine-2 (H_2) receptor antagonists. Yeomans, et al. (1998) determined that omeprazole (Prilosec), a proton pump inhibitor, healed existing ulcers and prevented further ulcer development more effectively than ranitidine (Zantac), an H_2 receptor antagonist. Similarly, Hawkey, et al. (1998) found omeprazole and misoprostol equally successful at treating ulcers and other GI symptoms associated with NSAID use. However, omeprazole was better tolerated and was associated with an improved relapse rate.

Another option for patients experiencing GI adverse events with nonselective NSAIDs is celecoxib. In a study conducted by Chan, et al. (2010), patients randomized to celecoxib had a lower incidence of upper or lower GI events compared to patients treated with diclofenac plus omeprazole.

TABLE 36.1   Overview of Selected Nonsteroidal Anti-Inflammatory Agents Used to Treat Osteoarthritis and Rheumatoid Arthritis

Generic (Trade) Name	Dosage	Contraindications	Special Considerations
Short-Acting NSAIDs*			
ibuprofen (Motrin)	1,200–3,200 mg/d PO in 3-4 divided doses	Allergy to the drug, salicylates, or other NSAIDs; pregnancy, lactation; use cautiously with impaired hepatic or renal function	Therapeutic response may occur over several weeks.
fenoprofen (Nalfon)	800–3,200 mg/d PO in 3-4 divided doses	Same as above	Patient should have ophthalmic examination periodically during long-term therapy.
indomethacin (Indocin)	50–200 mg/d PO in 2-3 divided doses	Same as above, and also GI bleeding with history of proctitis or rectal bleeding	Increased toxic effects if taken concomitantly with lithium; decreased diuretic effect with loop diuretics; potential decreased antihypertensive effect with beta blockers
tolmetin (Tolectin)	600–2,000 mg/d PO in 3-4 divided doses	Pregnancy, lactation; use cautiously with allergies, renal, hepatic, CV, and GI conditions	May affect results (false positive) of proteinuria tests using acid precipitation tests; patient should have ophthalmic examination periodically during long-term therapy.
meclofenamate (Meclomen)†	200–400 mg/d PO in 3-4 divided doses	Same as above	Patient should have ophthalmic examination periodically during long-term therapy.
diclofenac sodium (Voltaren) diclofenac potassium (Cataflam)	OA: 100–150 mg/d PO in 2–3 divided doses RA: 100–200 mg/d PO in 2-4 divided doses	Significant renal impairment, pregnancy, lactation; use cautiously with impaired hearing; allergies; hepatic, CV and GI conditions	Increases serum levels of lithium and risk of lithium toxicity
Intermediate-Acting NSAIDs*			
aspirin (Bayer, others)	2.4-3.6 g/d PO in 4-6 divided doses; maximum daily dose is 5.4 g	Allergy to salicylates, other NSAIDs, tartrazine, hemophilia and other bleeding disorders, pregnancy (possibly teratogenic), and more; do not use in children after illness because of association with Reye's syndrome	Increased risk of bleeding when taken concomitantly with anticoagulants and other NSAIDs Consult package insert for extensive list of interacting drugs and effects.
naproxen (Naprosyn)	500–1,500 mg/d PO in 2 divided doses	Allergy to naproxen, salicylates, other NSAIDs Pregnancy, lactation Use cautiously in patients with asthma, chronic urticaria, CV dysfunction, hypertension, GI bleeding, peptic ulcer, impaired hepatic or renal function.	May take with meals if GI upset occurs. Patient should have ophthalmic examination periodically during long-term therapy. Increased serum levels of lithium and risk of lithium toxicity
sulindac (Clinoril) oxaprozin (Daypro)	300 mg/d PO in 2 divided doses 600–1,200 mg/d PO	Same as above Significant renal impairment; pregnancy; lactation; use cautiously with impaired hearing, allergies, hepatic, CV and GI conditions	Same as above
Long-Acting NSAIDs*			
nabumetone (Relafen)	750–2,000 mg/d PO in 1-2 divided doses	Same as above	May be taken in divided dose
piroxicam (Feldene)	10–20 mg/d PO	Pregnancy and lactation; use cautiously with allergies, renal, hepatic, CV and GI conditions	May be taken with or without food
diflunisal (Dolobid)	500–1,500 mg/d PO in 2-3 divided doses	Same as above	Because therapeutic response progresses over several weeks, evaluate therapeutic response after 2 wk.
etodolac (Lodine)	IR: 600 –1,000 mg/d PO in 2 or 3 divided doses ER: 400–1,000 mg/d PO	Same as above	
COX-2 Selective NSAIDs			
celecoxib (Celebrex)	200–400 mg/d PO in 2 divided doses	Allergy to the drug or to sulfonamides, NSAIDs, or aspirin Significant renal impairment Pregnancy, lactation	Elimination of the drug occurs primarily through hepatic metabolism; therefore, patients with symptoms suggesting liver dysfunction should be carefully monitored.

*Drugs in the short-acting group have serum half-lives of approximately 1–4 h; in the intermediate-acting group, approximately 10–20 h (dose dependent); and in the long-acting group: approximately 45 h for piroxicam and 72 h for phenylbutazone.
† Brand name only available in Canada.

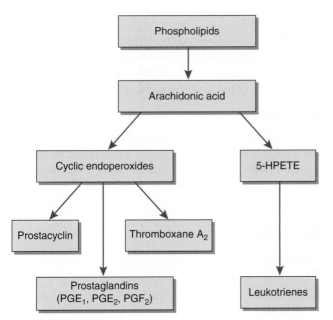

FIGURE 36–2 Mechanism of nonsteroidal anti-inflammatory drug action.

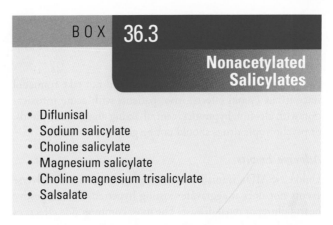

Patients with renal disease, congestive heart failure, cirrhosis, and volume depletion may experience renal aberrations, particularly related to renal blood flow. These adverse events underscore the need for frequent monitoring of patients on long-term NSAID therapy.

Controversy surrounds the issue of increased risk of cardiovascular events, including thrombotic events, myocardial infarction, and stroke due to NSAID use. This increased risk led to the market removal of two COX-2 selective agents, rofecoxib and valdecoxib. All NSAIDs have a black box warning regarding this increased risk and warn that patients with cardiovascular disease risk factors may be at an increased risk. In multiple analyses, naproxen seems to have little to no increased cardiovascular risk, whereas diclofenac consistently demonstrates an increased risk.

Interactions

NSAIDs have the potential to increase bleeding so they need to be used cautiously with other anticoagulants, specifically warfarin. Also, due to the risk of hypertension, NSAIDs may counteract the effect of antihypertensives. If possible, patients with hypertension should not be on NSAIDs. The combination of NSAIDs and angiotensin-converting enzyme inhibitors or angiotensin receptor blockers may result in decreased renal function and should be avoided. For patients who take aspirin daily, NSAIDs must be taken 30 minutes to 2 hours after or 8 hours before the aspirin in order for the aspirin to be cardioprotective.

Nonacetylated Salicylates

Nonacetylated salicylates (**Box 36.3**) are especially beneficial in patients who are sensitive to the GI irritation caused by long-term aspirin use. Diflunisal (Dolobid), the most commonly used nonacetylated salicylate, is an effective COX-1

inhibitor with anti-inflammatory and analgesic properties, but its antipyretic activities are weak. In terms of symptom relief, the nonacetylated salicylates are probably as effective as aspirin in treating inflammatory disorders.

Analgesics

When the pain associated with OA progresses and is no longer responsive to acetaminophen or NSAIDs, analgesics are the next option. Analgesics can also be used in patients who cannot tolerate acetaminophen or NSAIDs or in whom they are contraindicated. Analgesics only decrease pain and have no effect on inflammation. These drugs should be prescribed for a limited time because of potential dependence and withdrawal symptoms. Analgesics used for OA other than tramadol and tapentadol, detailed below, include codeine in combination with acetaminophen.

Tramadol

Mechanism of Action

Tramadol exerts multiple effects to induce pain relief. It is a mu opioid receptor agonist similar to other opioids such as morphine. By binding to the mu opioid receptor, ascending pain pathways are inhibited, resulting in decreased pain sensation. In addition, tramadol also inhibits the reuptake of serotonin and norepinephrine. These neurotransmitters are also involved in the ascending pain pathway.

Dosage

Tramadol is available as an immediate-release tablet (Ultram), extended-release tablet (Ultram ER), and in combination with acetaminophen (Ultracet). For the immediate-release tablet, patients can take 50 to 100 mg every 4 to 6 hours as needed for pain with a maximum daily dose of 400 mg. For patients taking the extended-release tablet, the starting dose is 100 mg daily with an increase every 5 days to the maximum of 300 mg per day. All forms of tramadol need to be dose adjusted for renal and hepatic dysfunction.

Time Frame for Response

Patients may feel a decrease in pain as soon as 1 hour after taking an immediate-release tramadol dose with a maximum effect at 2 hours. The extended-release tablet takes about 12 hours for the maximum effect to be seen.

Contraindications

Patients with an opioid dependency should not take tramadol since it has opioid effects. Also, patients with acute intoxication with alcohol, hypnotics, central-acting analgesics, opioids, or psychotropic drugs should not be given tramadol.

Adverse Events

Unlike NSAIDs, tramadol does not produce serious GI adverse events nor does it aggravate existing hypertension, congestive heart failure, or renal disease. The most common side effects of tramadol include nausea, dizziness, drowsiness, and sweating. Due to the opioid receptor agonism, tramadol has the potential to exert similar adverse events as other opioids, such as constipation, dependency, euphoria, and respiratory depression.

Interactions

Tramadol is metabolized by CYP2D6, and any medication that inhibits or induces this enzyme will interact with tramadol. Also, because it inhibits serotonin reuptake, tramadol has the potential to induce serotonin syndrome when used in combination with other serotonergic agents, such as selective serotonin reuptake inhibitors, tricyclic antidepressants, monoamine oxidase (MAO) inhibitors, or linezolid.

Tapentadol

Mechanism of Action

Similar to opioids, tapentadol is an agonist for the mu opiate receptor. In addition, tapentadol also inhibits the reuptake of norepinephrine.

Dosage

For patients starting tapentadol (Nucynta), the recommended dose for the first day of therapy is 50 to 100 mg every 4 to 6 hours as needed with the option of giving the second dose as soon as 1 hour after the first dose, if needed. After the first day of therapy, the recommended dose is 50 to 100 mg every 4 to 6 hours as needed with a maximum daily dose of 600 mg. The dosing interval should be increased to every 8 hours or longer in patients with moderate hepatic impairment. Tapentadol is not recommended in patients with severe hepatic or renal impairment.

Time Frame for Response

Patients are likely to experience pain relief within 1 to 2 hours of taking the dose.

Contraindications

Due to the opioid receptor agonism, tapentadol is contraindicated in patients with impaired pulmonary function who are not in a monitored setting. Also, patients with paralytic ileus should avoid use due to the risk of opioid-induced constipation. Last, since tapentadol inhibits norepinephrine reuptake, it cannot be used within 14 days of a MAO inhibitor.

Adverse Events

The adverse event profile of tapentadol is similar to that of other opioids and tramadol. The most common adverse events are dizziness, somnolence, constipation, nausea, and vomiting. There is a risk of respiratory depression and CNS depression.

Interactions

Tapentadol needs to be used cautiously with other CNS depressants due to additive effects. As mentioned above, tapentadol and MAO inhibitors cannot be used within 14 days of each other. Using tapentadol with serotonergic agents increases the risk of serotonin syndrome.

Topical Agents

Capsaicin

Mechanism of Action

For the relief of arthritic pain, capsaicin exerts its effect through the depletion of substance P. Initially, capsaicin releases substance P from the peripheral sensory neurons. However, with repeated use, substance P becomes depleted, and capsaicin prevents reaccumulation of substance P. Substance P is a chemomediator responsible for pain transmission from the periphery to the CNS. Therefore, by depleting peripheral neurons of substance P, the pain impulse will not be transmitted centrally.

Dosage

Capsaicin is available as an OTC product in a patch, cream, gel, liquid, or lotion. The directions for the patch are to apply it to the affected area three to four times a day for 7 days. The patch can remain on the area for up to 8 hours. The cream, gel, liquid, and lotion forms should be applied at least three times a day for maximal efficacy.

Time Frame for Response

The maximal effect is seen after 2 to 4 weeks of continual use.

Contraindications

There are no absolute contraindications for topical capsaicin. Patients should be advised to not apply capsaicin to broken or irritated skin.

Adverse Events

The most common adverse event is burning and irritation at the application site. The burning typically subsides within days of continual use. Due to the initial release of substance P, patients may experience some pain with initial use and should be advised to expect this.

Topical NSAIDS

Diclofenac is currently the only commercially available topical NSAID. It is available as a 1.5% solution (Pennsaid) for the relief of OA pain of the knee and as a 1% topical gel (Voltaren) for the relief of OA pain in joints amenable to topical therapy.

Mechanism of Action

The mechanism of action for topical diclofenac is the same as for oral NSAIDs. The benefit is that minimal diclofenac is absorbed when applied topically, which then decreases the risk of adverse events. Data has shown that only 6% to 10% of the topical gel and 2% to 3% of the solution is absorbed.

Dosage

The dosage of topical diclofenac is dependent on the formulation and location. For the gel, if used on the lower extremities, 4 g should be applied four times a day; if used on the upper extremities, 2 g should be applied four times a day. The entire total daily dose should not exceed 32 g/d. For the topical solution, 40 drops should be applied to the affected knee(s) four times a day. The solution should be applied in 10-drop increments to limit spillage. It can be first applied to the hand and then rubbed on the knee. Regardless of formulation, it is imperative that the entire affected area be covered to achieve maximal effect.

Contraindications

Topical diclofenac carries the same warnings and contraindications as oral NSAIDs, although the risk is less. Also, topical diclofenac is contraindicated on nonintact or damaged skin.

Adverse Events

The most common adverse events are application site reactions and include pruritus, rash, dry skin, pain, and exfoliation.

Interactions

Topical diclofenac should be used cautiously with medications that interact with oral NSAIDs since some of the topical medication is absorbed.

Corticosteroids

If symptoms of OA are restricted to one or two joints that have not responded to first- or second-line treatment, intra-articular corticosteroids may be helpful. Aseptic technique and a local anesthetic are required. The amount of drug injected depends on the size of the joint. Careful technique that avoids the surrounding soft tissues is imperative to avoid tissue atrophy. The side effect of localized pain may be treated with an NSAID or another appropriate analgesic. Injection of corticosteroids usually produces symptom relief within a few days, and the relief may last up to several months. Because of the potential for cartilage destruction and osteonecrosis with repeated injections, this therapy should be used judiciously.

SELECTING THE MOST APPROPRIATE AGENT

In selecting therapies for OA, the prescriber should consider patient variables such as age, childbearing status, progression of arthritis, and underlying illnesses. The recommended treatment order appears in **Table 36.2** and **Figure 36-3**.

First-Line Therapy

Acetaminophen, 1 g every 6 hours, has been shown to be effective in reducing the pain of OA within 4 weeks and lasting for up to 2 years. There is conflicting data regarding the analgesic effect of acetaminophen compared to NSAIDs for OA pain. Some trials indicate that NSAIDs are superior, especially in patients with more severe disease, whereas other trials indicated equivalence. Regardless of the analgesic effect, NSAIDs result in more adverse effects. Therefore, acetaminophen is

TABLE 36.2	**Recommended Order of Treatment for Osteoarthritis**	
Order	**Agents**	**Comments**
First line	Acetaminophen	Useful as long as symptoms remain mild, intermittent, and do not affect the range of motion of affected joint(s)
	Topical capsaicin or diclofenac	Useful for localized mild pain
Second line	Low-dose NSAIDs, such as celecoxib, ibuprofen, diclofenac, or the combination drug diclofenac and misoprostol	Begin NSAID therapy if inflammatory response has occurred as manifested by more constant and disabling pain or if acetaminophen therapy has failed.
Third line	Intra-articular corticosteroids	Therapeutic option that depends on size of joint involved and degree of inflammation. A single joint should not receive an injection more than once every 6 mo.
	Analgesics such as tramadol, tapentadol, or codeine	Centrally acting analgesics useful for moderate to moderately severe pain
		Used for a limited time because of potential for dependence and withdrawal

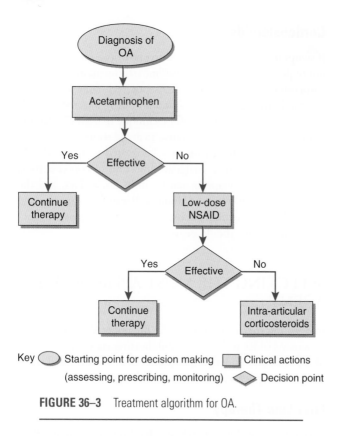

Key ⬭ Starting point for decision making ▭ Clinical actions
(assessing, prescribing, monitoring) ◇ Decision point

FIGURE 36–3 Treatment algorithm for OA.

considered first-line treatment for patients with OA due to its efficacy and safety.

If pain is mild and localized, topical capsaicin or diclofenac can be initiated to prevent systemic adverse events associated with other systemic therapies.

Second-Line Therapy

For patients without risk factors for GI disturbance, if acetaminophen therapy fails to provide relief, ibuprofen or a similar nonselective NSAID should be considered for second-line therapy. Since there is no evidence that one NSAID is more effective than another, the choice of the specific NSAID should be based on the cost and convenience of therapy. For patients at increased risk for GI disorders, such as peptic ulcer disease, a COX-2 inhibitor may be a better second-line choice. Alternatively, the use of a traditional NSAID coupled with a proton pump inhibitor may be sufficient to provide analgesia along with gastric protection.

Third-Line Therapy

For patients who have failed to obtain pain control with acetaminophen or NSAIDs or those in which these therapies are contraindicated, opioid or nonopioid analgesia can be tried. The addition of codeine to acetaminophen may further reduce pain, but often patients discontinue this combination due to the side effects associated with codeine (constipation, drowsiness). Tramadol or tapentadol may be tried, realizing that patients may experience similar adverse effects as they do to opioids.

Intra-articular steroids may be useful when an effusion is present and there are clear signs of local inflammation.

Special Populations

Geriatric

For elderly patients, the practitioner usually prescribes an NSAID with a shorter half-life in a smaller dosage than for a younger adult. Patients over age 65 should be considered at risk for GI hemorrhage and treated with either a COX-2 inhibitor or a combination of a COX-1 NSAID and a gastric protective agent, such as misoprostol, or a proton pump inhibitor.

Women

Many of the NSAIDs are pregnancy category C agents during the first 30 weeks of gestation. After gestational week 30, most NSAIDs are categorized as class D agents, indicating that there is evidence of harm to the fetus and should only be used in life-threatening illnesses.

MONITORING PATIENT RESPONSE

In addition to routine questions about the efficacy of the drug (e.g., pain relief), baseline and ongoing monitoring for specific drug therapy should be done. If a patient is taking acetaminophen, baseline liver function tests should be checked and monitored periodically. Monitoring for NSAID therapy includes a complete blood count (CBC), urinalysis, and serum creatinine. These studies should be repeated at 1 to 3 months and then every 3 to 6 months thereafter for the duration of therapy. In patients at risk for GI hemorrhage, the clinician should consider evaluating the patient for stool occult blood, anemia, and other signs of bleeding.

PATIENT EDUCATION

Drug Information

For patients taking acetaminophen, they need to be educated that it is most effective if taken around the clock regardless of pain. Also, patients need to be cognizant of other products that may contain acetaminophen and ensure they are not exceeding the daily limit. Last, for patients taking scheduled acetaminophen, alcohol intake should be minimized or avoided.

Patients taking NSAIDs need to be aware of their potentially harsh effects on the GI system, ranging from mild GI discomfort to gastric bleeding. The practitioner may emphasize strategies for dealing with some of these adverse events, including taking NSAIDs with food or milk or at meals. Patients should be reminded that a specific NSAID should be used regularly for 2 to 3 weeks before switching to another NSAID. This period is needed to assess whether the medication is effective.

Patients receiving a corticosteroid injection for joint pain need to be informed that a single joint should not be injected more frequently than every 6 months. Patients should be cautioned to limit activity of the injected joint for several days after the injection. Otherwise, the reduced pain perception of the joint may allow the patient to cause further joint damage, enhancing the progression of OA.

Patient-Oriented Information Sources

The National Institute of Arthritis and Musculoskeletal and Skin Diseases (NIAMS) is a government-sponsored group that provides information on OA and its treatment (http://www .niams.nih.gov/hi/topics/arthritis/oahandout.htm). This information is also available in Spanish. The Arthritis Foundation (http://www.arthritis.org/conditions/DiseaseCenter/oa.asp) provides information on the web and in print.

Nutrition/Lifestyle Changes

The practitioner should provide the patient with information about the continued use of physical therapy, exercise, and weight loss.

Complementary and Alternative Medications

Glucosamine, a form of an amino acid, is a naturally occurring substance in the body. It is believed to be involved in the development and repair of cartilage. Exogenous replacement of this substance is thought to help build on existing cartilage. Evidence-based reviews of this agent suggest that moderate improvements in pain relief and function can be achieved when administered at 1,500 mg/d. This effect is thought to be similar in magnitude to that of low-dose NSAIDs or acetaminophen.

Chondroitin, a large protein-like molecule that can impart elasticity to collagen, has shown similar, but slightly less, efficacy compared to glucosamine. The dosage of chondroitin used in most of the studies was 800 to 1,200 mg/day.

The most common adverse effects associated with these products are GI discomfort, including diarrhea, heartburn, nausea, and vomiting. A concern exists that glucosamine may negatively affect blood glucose; however, this has not been proven in trials. Also, because of its uncertainty, glucosamine is not recommended in patients with poorly controlled diabetes. Since they are considered food supplements, there is little U.S. Food and Drug Administration regulation, and the preparations may vary in potency and effectiveness.

RHEUMATOID ARTHRITIS

RA is a chronic autoimmune inflammatory disease characterized by symmetric polyarthritis and joint changes, including erythema, effusion, and tenderness. The course of RA is characterized by remissions and exacerbations. RA can affect several organs, but it usually involves synovial tissue changes in the freely movable joints (diarthroses). RA most commonly affects small joints, including the wrists, second through fifth metatarsophalangeal joints, proximal interphalangeal joints, and metacarpophalangeal joints. RA may also affect large joints, including the elbows, shoulders, neck, hips, knees, and ankles.

In 2008, approximately 0.6% of the adult population in the United States had RA, with the prevalence in women about twice of that in men (Helmick, et al., 2008). New onset of RA is seen throughout the life span, including infancy, but most cases occur in the fifth or sixth decade. Recent data have shown that diagnosis is occurring later in life, and the overall prevalence is decreasing. Previous data have shown that patients with RA have a higher rate of disability and mortality compared to patients of similar age without RA. However, with the increased use of disease-modifying antirheumatic drugs (DMARDs), especially early in the disease process, these risks appear to have normalized (Kroot, et al., 2000).

CAUSES

The cause of RA continues to be the subject of research. Theories of causation include genetic factors, infectious agents, environmental factors, and an antigen–antibody response. It is unlikely that a single factor is responsible for all cases of RA.

PATHOPHYSIOLOGY

The major physiologic changes associated with RA include synovial membrane proliferation followed by erosion of the subarticular cartilage and subchondral bone. Although the precise etiology of RA is unknown, mounting evidence points to a series of immunologic events. It is unclear whether an infectious, viral, or genetic agent prompts these events.

Specific major histocompatibility complex class II alleles and human leukocyte antigen are seen more frequently in patients with RA. These molecules are responsible for processing and presenting antigenic material to CD4+ T cells. The exact antigen that initiates the following cascade is unknown, but could be an exogenous or endogenous protein. T-cell activation stimulates monocytes, macrophages, and synovial fibroblasts to produce proinflammatory cytokines, including tumor necrosis factor (TNF) alpha, interleukin (IL)-1, and IL-6. During this process, matrix metalloproteinases are also released, causing major destruction in the joint cartilage. The activated T cells stimulate B cells, which then produce immunoglobulins, including rheumatoid factor (RF). The activation of the macrophages, monocytes, and synovial fibroblasts along with the release of cytokines stimulate angiogenesis in the synovial membrane. TNF-alpha is a key inflammatory mediator because it induces further production of pro-inflammatory cytokines and stimulates expression of adhesion molecules on endothelial cells. The expression of adhesion molecules promotes recruitment of leukocytes and more inflammatory cells. The result is a self-perpetuating inflammatory cycle.

Early Phase

In the early phase of RA, the synovium becomes more vascularized, and proliferation and hypertrophy begin. This results in the synovial tissue becoming edematous and exhibiting frond-like villi. As leukocytes proliferate, the synovial fluid becomes less viscous.

Progression

As RA progresses to the chronic form, continued hyperplasia and hypertrophy of the synovial lining occur. The thickness of the synovial lining increases up to fivefold from the normal one or two cell layers. The proliferation of the synovium persists, with lymphocytic tissue and plasma cells forming around blood vessels. This proliferative tissue extends into the joint space, joint capsule, ligaments, and tendons (Firestein, 1998; Moncur & Williams, 1995).

Severe, Chronic Rheumatoid Arthritis

In severe RA, pannus forms as a result of the release of lysosomal enzymes. Pannus is granulation tissue composed of lymphocytes, plasma cells, fibroblasts, and macrophages. Growing much like a tumor, pannus can invade the cartilage, activate chondrocytes, and release enzymes that can degrade cartilage and bone. This destructive process begins at the synovium and extends to the unprotected area at the junction of the cartilage and subchondral bone. These inflammatory cells can erode surrounding tissue, tendons, and cartilage. When pannus invades the joint margins, decreased range of motion and ankylosis may ensue. Pannus is a specific feature of RA, differentiating it from other forms of arthritis.

DIAGNOSTIC CRITERIA

In 2010, the ACR and EULAR collaborated on defining classification criteria for RA (**Table 36.3**). The goal of the criteria is to identify patients early who have a high probability of persistent RA and in whom early treatment would be beneficial. The emphasis of the classification criteria is on new patients with synovitis not explained by other conditions. Components of these criteria include joint involvement, serologic testing, acute phase reactants, and duration of symptoms.

The serology test can be either RF or anti-citrullinated protein antibody (ACPA, also know as *anti-cyclic citrullinated peptide* or *anti-CCP*), and the acute phase reactant test can be either erythrocyte sedimentation rate (ESR) or C-reactive protein (CRP). For serology tests, results are divided into three categories: negative, low-positive (above normal but less than 3 times the upper limit of normal [ULN]), or high-positive (greater than 3 times the ULN). The acute phase reactants are either normal or abnormal. None of these tests alone are sufficient to diagnose RA, but each is a component of diagnosis.

Other classic symptoms experienced by patients with RA include morning stiffness in involved joints persisting for at least 1 hour and subsiding with activity, symmetric joint involvement, and painful, swollen joints. Although RA characteristically affects joint structures, it is a systemic disease with potential extra-articular manifestations. Throughout the disease, the patient also may have generalized symptoms such as weakness, fatigue, mild fever, anorexia, and weight loss. End-organ involvement may occur in patients with high RF titers.

TABLE 36.3	Classification Criteria for Rheumatoid Arthritis

A score of ≥6/10 = definite RA
Patients must meet the following 2 criteria prior to scoring criteria A–D

1.	Have at least one joint with clinical synovitis	
2.	Synovitis cannot be explained by another condition	
A.	Joint involvement	
	1 large joint	0
	2–10 large joints	1
	1–3 small joints	2
	4–10 small joints	3
	>10 joints with at least 1 small joint	5
B.	Serology	
	Negative RF and negative ACPA	0
	Low-positive RF or low-positive ACPA	2
	High-positive RF or high-positive ACPA	3
C.	Acute phase reactants	
	Normal CRP and ESR	0
	Abnormal CRP or abnormal ESR	1
D.	Duration of symptoms	
	<6 wk	0
	≥6wk	1

RF, rheumatoid factor; ACPA, anti-citrullinated protein antibody; CRP, C-reactive protein; ESR, erythrocyte sedimentation rate

The most common extra-articular manifestation of RA is joint nodules. These occur in 15% to 20% of patients with RA and are most commonly seen in patients with erosive disease. These subcutaneous nodules may develop in any area of the body exposed to pressure. Some of these areas are the olecranon bursa, knuckles, ischial spines, Achilles tendon, extensor surfaces of the forearm, and the bridge of the nose (in patients who wear glasses). These nodules may also form internally on the heart, lungs, and intestinal tract. The nodules are firm and rubbery, occur in clusters, and may be either freely mobile or attached to underlying connective tissue. The treatment of the nodules is confined to the treatment of the underlying disease. These nodules may occur in other connective tissue diseases (e.g., systemic lupus erythematosus), so alone they are not criteria for diagnosing RA.

An ocular manifestation of RA is sicca syndrome; patients have a sensation of grittiness in the eyes, accumulation of dried mucus, and decreased tear production. Scleritis and episcleritis are occasional sequelae of sicca syndrome. Additional extra-articular manifestations of RA include vasculitis, pulmonary fibrosis, and pericarditis.

INITIATING DRUG THERAPY

Physical and occupational therapies are considered mainstays of nonpharmacologic therapy in patients with RA. These therapies help protect the joints and maintain strength, function, and mobility. Reduction of joint stress is an additional goal of therapy. Patients should engage in activity to their fullest possible extent, with adequate rest after activity, but they should avoid vigorous exercise and heavy labor during acute exacerbations of the disease. Hydrotherapy and hot and cold packs may be used to relax muscle spasms and facilitate joint movement. Warm showers and paraffin treatments may help relieve morning stiffness.

In 2008, the ACR published guidelines for the initiation of nonbiologic and biologic DMARDs and indicated that all patients with RA should be started on a DMARD (Saag, et al., 2008). Evidence has shown that the earlier in the disease process that DMARDs are started, the greater the chance of reducing disability and disease progression. The use of NSAIDs and corticosteroids can still be considered for symptom control, but do not have disease-modifying characteristics.

Goals of Drug Therapy

The goals of drug therapy for RA include reducing pain, stiffness, and swelling; preserving mobility and joint function; and preventing further joint damage.

Nonsteroidal Anti-Inflammatory Drugs

NSAIDs are typically used to help relieve pain and improve symptoms during the diagnostic process. These agents are continued through the initiation of a DMARD to maintain reduced symptoms. This approach allows NSAIDs to exert their anti-inflammatory action while the DMARD takes effect. See the discussion of NSAIDs in the Osteoarthritis section of this chapter; also see **Table 36.1.**

Corticosteroids

Low-dose corticosteroids (prednisone 10 mg or equivalent) are beneficial in patients who are beginning DMARD therapy. Because the therapeutic effect of DMARDs may not be seen until several weeks to months after initiating therapy, corticosteroids may be used to provide almost immediate symptom relief. Corticosteroids are also indicated in elderly patients with recent onset of RA. Last, higher doses of corticosteroids are beneficial in acute flares to regain control of inflammation and pain.

The difficulty in therapy with corticosteroids lies in the fine dosing line that divides therapeutic effects from long-term side effects. Low doses, such as prednisone 5 to 7.5 mg every morning, may be beneficial. The lowest dose possible should be given by gradually decreasing the dose in 1-mg decrements.

Injectable corticosteroids can be used if symptoms are restricted to one or two joints that have not responded to first-line treatment. They may also be of limited benefit for acute flare-ups of RA.

The most common adverse events of corticosteroid therapy include cataracts, glaucoma, mild glucose intolerance, and cutaneous atrophy. Less common adverse events include myopathy, hypothalamic–pituitary–adrenal axis dysfunction, and osteoporosis. Osteoporosis may be avoided by taking a calcium supplement (1,500 mg/d) along with vitamin D (800 mg/d).

Disease-Modifying Antirheumatic Drugs

As stated previously, the early use of DMARDs is advocated because of the high degree of inflammation that is present early in the disease (**Table 36.4**). Radiographic evidence of joint damage usually is present in the first year of the disease, and functional deterioration due to this damage may be irreversible. Therefore, early initiation of DMARD therapy may be the best course of action to take in meeting the long-range goals of treatment. DMARD therapy should be initiated within 3 months after onset of symptoms. There are several DMARDs to select from; the ones described here are the DMARDs currently recommended by the ACR. Due to lack of data or high adverse events profile, cyclophosphamide, D-penicillamine, cyclosporine, azathioprine, and gold compounds are not currently recommended for patients with RA. They can be used in patients who have failed the traditional treatments discussed below.

Methotrexate

The most commonly prescribed DMARD is methotrexate (Rheumatrex). The patient best suited for treatment with methotrexate is one who has morning stiffness and synovitis.

Mechanism of Action

Methotrexate, a folic acid antagonist, is thought to affect leukocyte suppression, decreasing the inflammation that results from immunologic by-products. When treatment stops, exacerbation of symptoms may occur as early as 2 weeks after cessation.

Dosage

Methotrexate is available for oral, subcutaneous, intramuscular, or intravenous (IV; reserved for chemotherapy) use. For most patients, a starting dose of 7.5 mg orally once per week is recommended. If a significant decrease in symptoms is not noted by week 6 of therapy, the dosage is increased by 2.5 mg/wk every 2 to 4 weeks until symptom control is attained. Most patients respond to 12.5 to 15 mg/wk. The maximum weekly oral dose is 25 mg. Injectable methotrexate may be used if there is an inadequate response to oral therapy or if the weekly dose needs to exceed 25 mg.

Time Frame for Response

Approximately 70% to 75% of patients respond favorably to methotrexate therapy, but it may take 3 to 8 weeks before improvement is noted. More than 50% of patients stay on the treatment for more than 5 years. However, if patients have difficulty tolerating side effects, methotrexate should be discontinued or the dosage should be lowered.

Contraindications

Methotrexate is contraindicated in pregnant and breast-feeding patients and those with leukopenia (white blood cell [WBC] count of less than 3,000 cells/mm^3), acquired immunodeficiency syndrome, renal impairment (creatinine clearance <30 mL/min), or liver disease (liver enzymes > two times the ULN). Methotrexate also has many black box warnings, including the risk of hepatotoxicity, renal impairment, pneumonitis,

TABLE 36.4 Overview of Selected Disease-Modifying Antirheumatic Drugs

Generic (Trade) Name and Dosage	Selected Adverse Events	Contraindications	Special Considerations
Preferred DMARDs			
methotrexate (Rheumatrex) 7.5 mg/wk in single dose, up to 25 mg/wk	GI effects, leukopenia, oral ulcers, thrombocytopenia, pulmonary toxicity, hepatotoxicity	Pregnancy and 1 mo before conception; caution in alcohol drinkers and liver disease	May take 3–8 wk to achieve clinical benefit; can induce spontaneous abortion and birth defects; monitoring includes CBC, serum creatinine, and liver function tests at 4- to 8-wk intervals
sulfasalazine (Azulfidine) 500–1,000 mg/d in divided doses; may increase up to maximum 3 g/d	GI effects, heartburn, dizziness, head-ache, rash, neutropenia, thrombocy-topenia, orange-yellow color of skin	Contraindicated in intestinal or urinary obstruction Safety in pregnancy not established in RA treatment, although drug has proved safe in patients with inflammatory bowel disease in pregnancy	May take 1–4 mo to achieve clinical effect; causes reversible sterility in men; recommend that men cease therapy 90 d before starting a family; monitoring includes liver enzyme evaluation; CBC is necessary early in therapy but required less with prolonged use
hydroxychloroquine (Plaquenil) 400–600 mg/d in divided doses	GI effects, rash, CNS effects, ocular effects	Use caution in pregnancy and with lactation.	Six months may be needed for clinical effect. Can trigger exacerbation of psoriasis; prolonged therapy may cause retinal damage Monitoring should include periodic CBC and eye examination every 3–6 mo to monitor for retinal damage.
leflunomide (Arava) 100 mg PO daily for 3 days; 20 mg daily thereafter	Diarrhea, hair loss, weight loss, rash, infection	Pregnancy	If 20 mg daily is not tolerated, then 10 mg daily may be used. Long half-life; cholestyramine will enhance elimi-nation if agent is to be discontinued.
Nonpreferred DMARDs			
D-penicillamine (Depen, Cuprimine) 125 mg/d as single dose; may increase at monthly intervals to maximum daily dose of 1.5 g	GI effects, rash, itching, renal effects, autoimmune reactions, cytopenia	Not recommended in pregnancy or lactation—causes damage to fetal connective tissue	From 4 to 6 mo may be needed to establish clinical effect of therapy Monitoring should include CBC with differential and platelets and urinalysis every 2–6 wk.
azathioprine (Imuran) 50–100 mg in single daily dose; can increase after 6–8 wk; 3.5 mg/kg is maximum daily dose	GI effects, bone marrow suppression, infection, hepatotoxicity, alopecia	Renal disease; avoid during pregnancy and lactation	From 6 to 8 and up to 12 wk may be needed to establish clinical effect. Monitoring should include CBC with differential and platelets weekly for the first month, then biweekly for the second and third months, then monthly.
cyclophosphamide (Cytoxan, Neosar) 1 mg/kg/d increased to 2 mg/kg/d after 6 wk	Alopecia, hemorrhagic cystitis, sterility, GI effects, increased susceptibility to infection, thrombocytopenia	Contraindicated for RA during pregnancy and lactation	In renal impairment, decrease dose. Four months may be needed to establish clinical effect. Monitoring includes CBC with differential, plate-lets, urinalysis for blood repeatedly, erythrocyte sedimentation rate, BUN, serum creatinine.

Drug/Dosage	Adverse Effects	Contraindications	Special Considerations
cyclosporine A (Sandimmune, Neoral) 5 mg/kg/d divided into 2 doses	Hypertension, tremor, nephrotoxicity, hepatotoxicity, increased susceptibility to infection, hyperkalemia	Contraindicated for RA during pregnancy and lactation	Approximately 8 wk may be needed to establish clinical effect. Decrease dose by 50% if hypertension or nephrotoxicity results. Monitoring includes CBC with differential, BUN, serum creatinine, serum bilirubin, liver enzymes repeatedly.
gold compounds *Injectable:* aurothioglucose (Solganal); gold sodium thiomalate (Myochrysine) 10 mg/wk IM, up to a total dose of 1 g: maintenance dose ~50 mg/mo *Oral:* auranofin (Ridaura) 3 mg bid	GI effects, rash, itching, stomatitis, vasomotor reactions, bone marrow suppression, nephritis, pneumonitis, exfoliative dermatitis, proteinuria	Uncontrolled diabetes; liver and renal disease, systemic lupus erythematosus, blood dyscrasias; lack of long-term studies in pregnant women, so not recommended during pregnancy or lactation	May take 6–8 wk for injectable form and 3–6 mo for oral form of drug to establish effectiveness. Monitoring includes routine CBC with differential, platelet count; urinalysis to measure protein; renal and liver function tests.

Biologic DMARDs

Drug/Dosage	Adverse Effects	Contraindications	Special Considerations
etanercept (Enbrel) 25 mg SQ twice weekly or 50 mg SQ weekly	Upper respiratory tract infections, pain at the injection site, headache	Concurrent infections or hypersensitivity to medication	Use caution in patients predisposed to infection. Concomitant immunosuppressants can increase risk of serious infection.
infliximab (Remicade) 3 mg/kg IV infusion at baseline, 2 wk, 6 wk, then every 8 wk thereafter	Urticaria, infusion reactions, dyspnea, hypotension	Same as above	Same as above
adalimumab (Humira) 40 mg SQ every other week; 40 mg weekly as monotherapy	Redness, swelling, bruising, or pain at the site of injection, headache, upset stomach, diarrhea, infection, rash	Same as above	Same as above
golimumab (Simponi) 50 mg SQ monthly in combination with methotrexate	Injection site reactions, infection, dizziness, antibody formation	Same as above	Same as above
certolizumab pegol (Cimzia) 400 mg SQ at weeks 0, 2, and 4 then 200 mg every other week	Injection site reactions, headache, nausea, infection	Same as above	Same as above
anakinra (Kineret) 100 mg SQ daily	Redness, swelling, bruising, or pain at the site of injection, headache, upset stomach, diarrhea, infection, rash	Sensitivity to *Escherichia coli*–derived proteins; preexisting infection	Routine monitoring of white blood cells is recommended; concomitant immunosuppressants can increase risk of serious infection
abatacept (Orencia) 500–1,000 mg (based on weight) IV at weeks 0, 2, and 4, and then every 4 wk	COPD exacerbations, headache, hypertension, infusion reactions, infections, anaphylaxis	Hypersensitivity to abatacept; use caution in patients with history of infections or COPD	Concomitant immunosuppressants increases risk of infection. Reserved for patients unresponsive to other therapy
tocilizumab (Actemra) 4-8 mg/kg IV every 4 wk	Increased LDL and transaminase, decreased WBC, infusion-related reactions	Untreated latent TB or hepatitis	Indicated for patients who did not respond to TNF-alpha inhibitor

bone marrow suppression, diarrhea, ulcerative stomatitis, dermatologic reactions, and opportunistic infections. The ACR also lists acute serious bacterial infections, latent tuberculosis (TB), active fungal infections, active herpes-zoster viral infection, platelets less than 50,000 cells/mm³, treated lymphoproliferative disease within 5 years, and acute or chronic hepatitis B or C as contraindications to methotrexate therapy.

Adverse Events

The most commonly reported adverse events of methotrexate are nausea and abdominal pain. These effects may be minimized by switching to parenteral therapy. Oral ulcers, leukopenia, anemia, and thrombocytopenia are also common. However, these adverse reactions may be minimized by administering 1 mg of folic acid daily. Although methotrexate may inhibit folic acid metabolism, it does not seem to affect the efficacy of the therapy.

The most serious adverse event of therapy is liver toxicity, which occurs more frequently in patients with diabetes, obesity, alcohol use, and existing liver disease. Pneumonitis is another potentially serious side effect of therapy. A baseline chest x-ray may be obtained, and patients should be instructed to report the new onset of a dry cough, dyspnea, or fever. Methotrexate should be immediately discontinued if the patient has pulmonary problems because immutable pulmonary damage may occur.

Baseline laboratory values should be obtained before initiation of therapy and should include a CBC, liver function tests, blood urea nitrogen (BUN), and serum creatinine. During therapy, the CBC should be monitored every 4 weeks, and creatinine, BUN, and liver function tests should be monitored every 3 months. A transient yet marked increase in liver enzymes may be seen, with stabilization occurring with continued treatment or dose reduction. If liver enzymes persist at concentrations of two to three times the ULN, then methotrexate should be discontinued and a liver biopsy obtained.

Methotrexate is classified as pregnancy category X due to the risk of fetal death or severe abnormalities and has implications for both males and females. Therefore, women who wish to conceive should stop taking methotrexate at least one ovulatory cycle before attempting to become pregnant. Men must discontinue methotrexate at least 3 months before trying to conceive. Men and women of childbearing age who are not sterilized should use a reliable form of contraception.

Interactions

Concurrent use with NSAIDs may increase the risk of bone marrow suppression and GI toxicity. The combination should be avoided when taking moderate to high doses of methotrexate. Medications such as penicillins, tetracyclines, probenecid, and sulfonamides that compete with methotrexate for renal tubular secretion will enhance the effects of methotrexate and should be used cautiously. Methotrexate may increase the concentrations of mercaptopurine and theophylline. Concomitant use of cholestyramine decreases the absorption of methotrexate.

Sulfasalazine

Like methotrexate, sulfasalazine (Azulfidine) is an effective DMARD that relieves symptoms relatively quickly. The best candidates for treatment are patients with significant synovitis but no poor prognostic factors.

Mechanism of Action

Sulfasalazine's mechanism of action is not clearly understood but is thought to be due to its conversion to sulfapyridine and 5-acetylsalicylic acid in the gut. Research has shown the anti-inflammatory features of this conversion, as well as its ability to decrease inflammatory cytokine and immunoglobulin M RF production.

Dosage

Sulfasalazine is available in oral form in 500-mg tablets. Dosing is started at 1,000 mg/d in two divided doses. The daily divided dose is gradually increased to 2,000 mg over 2 weeks. After 12 weeks of 2,000 mg daily, if the response is still not adequate, then the dose can be increased to 3,000 mg daily. Enteric-coated tablets are recommended for the treatment of RA to reduce the risk of GI-related adverse events.

Time Frame for Response

Patients may start to notice an effect as early as 1 month, but the full effect may take up to 4 months.

Contraindications

Due to its sulfa component, sulfasalazine is contraindicated in patients with a sulfa allergy. Also, once a pregnant woman is at full term, sulfasalazine is classified as a pregnancy category D and should be avoided. Patients with a GI or genitourinary tract obstruction or those with porphyria should not use this medication. Platelet count of less than 50,000 cells/mm³, liver enzymes greater than two times the ULN, or hepatitis B or C infection resulting in Child-Pugh class B or C hepatic function are contraindications, according to the ACR guidelines.

Adverse Events

The most common adverse events to sulfasalazine are dose dependent and include nausea and diarrhea. Other reported adverse events include dizziness, intestinal or urinary obstruction, oral ulcers, thrombocytopenia, orange-yellow pigmentation of the skin, headache, and depression. Any of these common adverse events may become intolerable and cause discontinuation of the drug. Reversible sterility has been reported in men; therapy should be discontinued 3 months before attempting to father a child.

Agranulocytosis, the gravest adverse event to sulfasalazine, has been reported in fewer than 2% of patients, but it dictates immediate discontinuation. Before initiating sulfasalazine therapy, the practitioner should obtain baseline laboratory test values, including a CBC and liver enzymes. These values should be monitored every 2 weeks for 1 month after initiation of therapy and then monthly for 5 months. If laboratory values remain stable for the first 6 months of therapy, a CBC should be checked every 3 months.

Interactions

The risk of bone marrow suppression will be enhanced if used with other suppressive agents such as azathioprine, methotrexate, or mercaptopurine. Sulfasalazine may increase the effects of oral hypoglycemics and oral anticoagulants; therefore, patients should be monitored closely if on concurrent therapy. Sulfasalazine may decrease the concentration of cyclosporine.

Antimalarials

The antimalarial agents hydroxychloroquine (Plaquenil) and chloroquine are attractive because of their low adverse event profile, with the drugs being discontinued in fewer than 9% of patients. However, because these drugs cannot limit the progression of RA, they are currently used as an adjunct to methotrexate therapy or as single-agent therapy in early, mild RA without bone erosion.

Mechanism of Action

Antimalarials inhibit antigen processing by elevating cellular pH, which changes antigen degeneration. Thus, the presentation of the antigen to T cells is impaired.

Dosage

Hydroxychloroquine and chloroquine are available in oral form and are rapidly and completely absorbed. Dosing is calculated by patient weight, but the typical dosage for hydroxychloroquine is 200 mg twice daily or 400 mg daily.

Time Frame for Response

Therapeutic effects are usually noted within 2 to 6 months of treatment.

Contraindications

Patients with preexisting retinal field changes should not use antimalarials due to the ocular effects of long-term therapy.

Adverse Events

The most common adverse events of antimalarials are nausea, diarrhea, and abdominal discomfort. Less common adverse events include photosensitivity and skin pigmentation changes. A maculopapular, pruritic rash encompassing the entire body may occur and cause extreme discomfort. Although neuromyopathy has been reported rarely, deep tendon reflexes should be monitored regularly for diminished activity.

After absorption, these drugs concentrate in the retina, kidneys, bone marrow, and liver. The concentration of antimalarials in specific organs dictates baseline and ongoing monitoring during therapy. Specifically, eye examinations should be performed every 6 to 12 months because of potential retinal accumulation of the drug. A CBC should be performed periodically.

Interactions

Antimalarial agents can decrease the metabolism of beta blockers with some exceptions, including atenolol and nadolol. For patients on beta blockers, consider switching to atenolol prior to initiating antimalarial therapy. Also, cyclosporine and digoxin concentrations may be increased, requiring more frequent monitoring. Antimalarial doses should be separated from magnesium-containing products by 2 to 4 hours due to decreased absorption of the antimalarials.

Leflunomide

Leflunomide (Arava) exerts anti-inflammatory and antiproliferative actions, retarding erosions and joint space narrowing.

Mechanism of Action

Leflunomide is a prodrug that undergoes rapid conversion to its active metabolite. The drug is a competitive inhibitor of dihydrofolate reductase. This inhibition decreases the production of pyrimidines (amino acid building blocks), decreasing T-cell and B-cell proliferation. This action is similar to methotrexate, making this agent a reasonable alternative for patients who cannot tolerate or who have an inadequate response to methotrexate. Since leflunomide inhibits pyrimidine synthesis and methotrexate inhibits purine synthesis, these agents may be used in combination.

Dosage

Since the half-life of the active metabolite is 15 to 18 days, therapy with leflunomide is usually initiated with a 100-mg loading dose for 3 days, and then the agent is continued at 20 mg/d if tolerated. If the patient cannot tolerate 20 mg per day, the dose can be lowered to 10 mg/d. The loading dose can be omitted in patients at increased risk for hepatic or hematologic toxicity.

Time Frame for Response

Benefit from leflunomide can be seen as early as 4 weeks but may take up to 3 months.

Contraindications

Like other DMARDs, leflunomide is contraindicated in pregnancy. Since the half-life is so long, a typical washout period for women who wish to conceive is about 2 years. However, agents interrupting the enterohepatic recirculation (e.g., activated charcoal or cholestyramine) can be used to reduce the half-life of the metabolite to about 1 day. The dosing of cholestyramine, as recommended by the manufacturer, is 8 g three times a day for 11 days. To ensure appropriate clearance, plasma concentrations should be <0.02 mg/L measured twice at least 14 days apart.

Due to hepatotoxicity, patients with a history of alcoholism or with preexisting liver disease should not take leflunomide.

Adverse Events

About 5% of patients receiving leflunomide monotherapy have elevated liver enzymes. While this number appears low, there are reports of more than 10 patients dying while on leflunomide therapy; the deaths are thought to be related to the hepatotoxicity of the agent.

More common adverse events include GI symptoms, weight loss, alopecia, and hypertension. Leflunomide also has been associated with bone marrow suppression, including anemia, thrombocytopenia, and agranulocytosis.

A CBC and liver function tests should be taken as a baseline and then monthly for the first 6 months of therapy. If test results remain stable, monitoring can be every 6 to 8 weeks thereafter.

Interactions

Leflunomide is a weak inhibitor of the CYP2C9 enzyme and therefore may increase the levels of agents metabolized through this pathway, including warfarin. Rifampin may increase the concentration of leflunomide's active metabolite. The use of bile acid sequestrants decreases the enterohepatic recycling of leflunomide, decreasing its effectiveness.

Biologic Disease-Modifying Antirheumatic Drugs

Biologic agents are developed from living sources, such as humans, animals, or microorganisms. The introduction of various biologics effective against RA has changed the management of RA. These agents target multiple components involved in the pathogenesis of RA, such as TNF-alpha, T-cell activation, IL-1, and IL-6.

Tumor Necrosis Factor Inhibitors

Etanercept (Enbrel), infliximab (Remicade), adalimumab (Humira), golimumab (Simponi), and certolizumab pegol (Cimzia) are TNF-alpha inhibitors used in RA treatment.

Mechanism of Action

These agents act by binding the circulating TNF-alpha and render it inactive. This then reduces the chemotactic effect of TNF-alpha by reducing IL-6 and CRP, resulting in reduced infiltration of inflammatory cells into joints. Also, when these agents bind to surface TNF-alpha, cell lysis occurs.

Dosage

All five of these agents are injectables. Etanercept is self-administered subcutaneously at 25 mg twice weekly or 50 mg weekly as combination therapy or monotherapy. Infliximab is an IV infusion with a recommended dose of 3 mg/kg at 0, 2, and 6 weeks and then every 8 weeks thereafter. Doses of infliximab have ranged from 3 to 10 mg/kg every 4 to 8 weeks. Infliximab is indicated in conjunction with methotrexate because infliximab antibodies develop when administered as monotherapy. Adalimumab is given at 40 mg every other week as a subcutaneous injection. Adalimumab may be administered concomitantly with methotrexate, glucocorticoids, or NSAIDs. It may also be used as monotherapy; however, the dose may need to be increased to 40 mg weekly. Certolizumab pegol is administered as a subcutaneous injection at a dose of 400 mg at 0, 2, and 4 weeks and then 200 mg every other week thereafter.

An alternative maintenance dosing regimen is 400 mg every 4 weeks. Golimumab is only indicated for use in combination with methotrexate, and the recommended dose is 50 mg subcutaneously one time a month.

Time Frame for Response

All of the TNF-alpha inhibitors produce a rapid response, within days to weeks.

Contraindications

Patients should be assessed at baseline for infections or risk factors for infections. There have been reports of TB developing in patients taking infliximab; the theory is that the immunomodulation allows latent TB to flare. This usually occurs within the first 2 to 5 months of therapy. Therefore, all patients must be evaluated for latent TB with a tuberculin skin test prior to beginning therapy. Other serious infections, including fungal and opportunistic infections, have also occurred with these agents, and careful consideration of the patient's history is important when prescribing them.

Adverse Events

Adverse events include injection-site reactions (certolizumab pegol, golimumab, etanercept, adalimumab) or infusion reactions (infliximab). Caution must be used when administering these agents to patients predisposed to infection. Sepsis and fatal infections have occurred in patients receiving TNF-alpha inhibitors. If a patient develops an infection while taking a TNF-alpha inhibitor, the agent should be discontinued until the infection resolves.

Interactions

TNF-alpha inhibitors should not be used in combination with abatacept or anakinra due to the increased risk of infection. As a result of immunosuppressive effects, patients should not receive live vaccinations while being treated with a TNF-alpha inhibitor. Also, the response to other vaccines may be diminished while on therapy.

Anakinra

Anakinra (Kineret) is a recombinant form of human IL-1 receptor antagonist, but differs by the addition of methionine at one of the N-terminals.

Mechanism of Action

The levels of naturally occurring IL-1 receptor antagonists are not adequate to compete with the elevated amount of IL-1 present in the synovium of RA patients. With limited competition, IL-1 can promote inflammation and degrade cartilage. By exogenously providing this antagonist to RA patients, the joint inflammation process is interrupted.

Dosage

Anakinra is given 100 mg subcutaneously daily. In patients with severe renal dysfunction (creatinine clearance below 30 mL/min), it should be administered every other day.

Time Frame for Response

In patients who responded to anakinra, the effect was seen within 12 weeks.

Contraindications

The primary contraindication to anakinra is sensitivity to *Escherichia coli*–derived proteins. Similar to the other immunomodulators, preexisting infection or risk of infection may be a contraindication since there is an increased risk of infection in patients taking anakinra. Anakinra should not be administered in combination with TNF-alpha inhibitors due to the increased risk of infection.

Adverse Events

The most common adverse event of anakinra is skin irritation, including erythema, inflammation, and pain at the injection site. This occurs in more than half of patients and usually resolves within a few weeks. Although rare, there is a possibility of hypersensitivity reactions, including anaphylaxis and angioedema. Also, patients are at an increased risk for infection.

Patients also may experience a decrease in WBCs. Routine monitoring is recommended at baseline and then monthly for the first 3 months, and then quarterly for the first year.

Interactions

No known pharmacokinetic drug interactions exist. Pharmacodynamically, agents that suppress the immune system should be used with caution, if at all, due to the increased risk of serious infections. Anakinra should not be used in combination with TNF-alpha inhibitors.

Abatacept

Abatacept (Orencia) is indicated for the treatment of moderate to severe RA unresponsive to other DMARD therapy as monotherapy or combination therapy.

Mechanism of Action

Abatacept is a costimulation modulator that binds to CD80 and CD86 on antigen-presenting cells. This binding blocks the CD28 interaction between the antigen-presenting cell and T cells necessary for T-cell activation. Therefore, abatacept decreases the activation of T cells.

Dosage

Abatacept is give as an IV infusion over 30 minutes and is dosed based on weight (<60 kg: 500 mg; 60 to 100 kg: 750 mg; >100 kg: 1,000 mg). It is dosed at weeks 0, 2, and 4 and then every 4 weeks thereafter.

Time Frame for Response

The onset of action for abatacept ranges from 1 to 3 months.

Contraindications

The only absolute contraindication associated with abatacept is hypersensitivity to it or any component of the formulation.

Abatacept should be used cautiously in patients with a history of infection or chronic obstructive pulmonary disease (COPD). Patients need to be screened for hepatitis and latent TB prior to initiation due to the risk of reactivation.

Adverse Events

Patients with COPD experienced a higher rate of exacerbations, cough, pneumonia, and dyspnea. Common adverse events include headache, hypertension, and infusion-related reactions. Similarly to other immunomodulators, abatacept is associated with a higher risk of infections. Although rare, abatacept can cause anaphylaxis.

Interactions

Patients should not receive a live vaccine while on abatacept or for up to 3 months after discontinuing the drug. Abatacept should not be used in combination with TNF-alpha inhibitors or anakinra due to the increased risk of immunosuppression.

Tocilizumab

Tocilizumab (Actemra) is the first IL-6 receptor inhibitor on the market and is indicated for adult patients with moderate to severe RA after not responding to at least one TNF-alpha inhibitor.

Mechanism of Action

Tocilizumab is a humanized anti-IL-6 receptor monoclonal antibody. By inhibiting IL-6 activity, B-cell and T-cell activation is decreased as well as acute phase reactant production and osteoclast activation.

Dosage

Tocilizumab is administered as an IV infusion at a dose of 4 to 8 mg/kg every 4 weeks.

Time Frame for Response

It may take up to 3 months for patients to feel the effect of tocilizumab.

Contraindications

There are no absolute contraindications associated with tocilizumab. Similar to the other biologic agents, patients should be screened for TB and hepatitis prior to initiation.

Adverse Events

Overall, tocilizumab is well tolerated. There have been laboratory abnormalities associated with tocilizumab that include increased low-density lipoprotein cholesterol, elevated transaminase, and decreased WBCs. Approximately 8% of patients experienced an infusion-related reaction.

Based on laboratory abnormalities, a CBC and liver function tests need to be monitored at baseline and then every 4 to 8 weeks while on therapy. A lipid panel should be checked at baseline, 4 to 8 weeks into therapy, and then every 6 months while being treated with tocilizumab.

Interactions

Avoid using tocilizumab with leflunomide due to concern for increased hematologic toxicity. Patients should not receive live vaccines while on therapy and for at least 3 months after discontinuing treatment. Also, patients may not be able to respond appropriately to inactivated vaccines administered while on therapy. Due to the risk of infection, tocilizumab should not be used with any TNF-alpha inhibitors, anakinra, abatacept, or other immunosuppressants.

Selecting the Most Appropriate Agent

In 2008, the ACR published recommendations regarding the use of nonbiologic and biologic DMARDs for the treatment of RA. It is important to note that tocilizumab, golimumab, and certolizumab pegol were not available when these recommendations were created and that anakinra was not included due to lack of data at that time.

Decisions regarding appropriate therapy are based on disease duration, poor prognostic factors, and disease activity. Disease duration is divided into less than 6 months (early), 6 to 24 months (intermediate), and greater than 24 months (late). Poor prognostic factors include functional limitation, extra-articular disease, RF positivity, positive ACPA, or bony erosions on radiography. Last, disease activity is divided into low, moderate, or high based on several questionnaire instruments.

In selecting a DMARD or combining DMARDs, the clinician needs to consider the toxicities of the medications, including the interactions with other prescribed drugs. Some patients may have difficulty adhering to monitoring requirements for some of the more toxic drugs. Other patients may not be able to adhere to a strict dosing schedule. In addition, the time required to achieve benefit can be protracted with certain DMARDs, which may be unacceptable to the patient. Finally, the cost of the various therapies varies widely.

Symptomatic Treatment

NSAIDs and/or corticosteroids are recommended for acute symptoms associated with RA. These agents are particularly helpful while a patient is undergoing diagnostic assessment. These agents do not have disease-modifying abilities; therefore, once a definite diagnosis is made, DMARD therapy should be started. NSAIDs and steroids can be continued until the DMARD takes effect.

First-Line Therapy

Methotrexate or leflunomide are options as monotherapy for patients of all disease durations and disease activity regardless of poor prognostic factors. Sulfasalazine monotherapy is an option for patients who do not have poor prognostic factors. Hydroxychloroquine is reserved for patients with early to intermediate disease of low activity without poor prognostic factors. For early disease, TNF-alpha inhibitors plus methotrexate can be used for patients with high disease activity for 3 to 6 months regardless of prognostic factors or for patients with high disease activity for less than 3 months with poor prognostic factors. Dual or triple DMARD therapy can be considered in patients with intermediate disease with moderate to high activity, intermediate disease with low activity with poor prognostic factors, or long disease duration. **Table 36.5** outlines the indications for initiating DMARD therapy.

Second-Line Therapy

For patients who fail one DMARD, an alternate can be tried. This second DMARD can either be added or switched for the first DMARD, especially if tolerability is a concern. Monotherapy with a TNF-alpha inhibitor is recommended for patients with disease duration of longer than 6 months who fail methotrexate monotherapy with high disease activity or who have moderate activity with poor prognostic factors.

Third-Line Therapy

For patients who failed methotrexate combination therapy or sequential DMARD therapy and have low disease activity, further nonbiologic DMARDs should be tried. If they have moderate or high disease activity without poor prognostic factors, either another nonbiologic DMARD or a TNF-alpha inhibitor can be started. For those patients with moderate to high disease

TABLE 36.5	Initial DMARD Options for Patients with RA
MTX or LEF	All durations, low, moderate, or high activity, ± poor prognostic factors
SSZ	All durations, low, moderate, or high activity, − poor prognostic factors
HCQ	Duration <24 mo, low activity, − poor prognostic factors
MTX + HCQ	All durations, moderate to high activity, ± poor prognostic factors
	Long duration, low activity, ± poor prognostic factors
MTX + LEF	>6 mo duration, high activity, ± poor prognostic factors
	Long duration, low activity, + poor prognostic factors
MTX + SSZ	All durations, high activity, + poor prognostic factors
HCQ + SSZ	Intermediate duration, high activity, − poor prognostic factors
Triple DMARD	All durations, moderate to high activity, + poor prognostic factors
	>6 mo duration, high activity, ± poor prognostic factors
TNF-alpha inhibitor + MTX	Early disease, high activity for <3 mo, + poor prognostic factors
	Early disease, high activity for 3 to 6 mo, ± poor prognostic factors

MTX, methotrexate; LEF, leflunomide; SSZ, sulfasalazine; HCQ, hydroxychloroquine; DMARD, disease-modifying antirheumatic drug; TNF, tumor necrosis factor

activity with poor prognostic factors, therapy with abatacept, a TNF-alpha inhibitor, or rituximab should be initiated.

Tocilizumab is indicated for patients who have failed at least one TNF-alpha inhibitor. Golimumab was proven to be effective in patients who had failed a previous TNF-alpha inhibitor also.

Special Populations

Geriatric

Caution should be used when starting elderly patients on NSAIDs due to the increased risk of GI hemorrhage. Further, many elderly patients have decreased renal function, and NSAIDs may contribute to a decline in this function. Several DMARDs and some immunomodulators are renally excreted, and doses should be adjusted in the elderly due to decreased renal function.

Pediatric

In children, aspirin therapy is stopped if the child is exposed to varicella or influenza because of the risk of Reye's syndrome. Also, children receiving vaccinations may have a diminished response if they are taking immunomodulators such as anakinra.

Women

Women with RA who plan on having children need to discuss treatment options with their physician and understand the risks of conception. Certain medications, including methotrexate, leflunomide, abatacept, and rituximab, cannot be used during pregnancy because of known teratogenicity. DMARDs with the most data to support their use during pregnancy are antimalarials, sulfasalazine, azathioprine, and cyclosporine. These medications can be used as monotherapy or in combination with corticosteroids or NSAIDs. If corticosteroids are used during pregnancy, the dose should not exceed 15 mg/d because higher doses increase the risk of intrauterine infection and premature delivery. NSAIDs should be avoided after 30 weeks of gestation because of the increased risk of premature closure of the ductus arteriosus in the fetus. TNF-alpha inhibitors are all classified as pregnancy category B, indicating there were not teratogenic effects in animals and limited or no data in humans. There have been case reports of congenital malformations in children exposed to TNF-alpha inhibitors as a fetus. Therefore, TNF-alpha inhibitors need to be used cautiously in pregnant women.

MONITORING PATIENT RESPONSE

Because the drugs used for treating arthritis have many adverse events and because most are used for long-term treatment, monitoring should include baseline studies against which later results can be compared. CBC with differential, urinalysis, creatinine, serum bilirubin, liver enzymes, ESR, BUN, platelet studies, and eye examinations are among the tests performed periodically during therapy.

PATIENT EDUCATION

Patient education depends on the type of agent selected. The patient should know that routine blood work is important to detect adverse events before they become serious and life-threatening. Patients taking DMARDs and immunomodulators should report illness immediately, as the risk of serious infections is increased in these patients. Patients need to understand that there is a delay between initiating therapy and experiencing the full clinical effects and that therapy must be continued in order to be effective.

Patient-Oriented Information Sources

Support groups, education of family members, and assistive devices can help with activities of daily living. The American Rheumatism Association (800-282-7023) can provide information and assistance. The National Institutes of Health, in conjunction with the American Society of Health-System Pharmacists and the United States Pharmacopeia, has a drug information website with information about thousands of medications (http://www.nlm.nih.gov/medlineplus/druginformation.html).

Nutrition/Lifestyle Changes

Weight loss programs and healthy habits such as adequate rest are key to the success of a treatment program. Patients should consider occupational therapy as needed to help with household chores. The patient should avoid repetitive joint motion and vibrations from electrical appliances or tools to reduce exacerbations. Splinting the affected joint helps relieve pain and prevent deformity. Patients should remove the splint at least once daily and for any exercise activities. Patients should be instructed on strategies to avoid physical and emotional stress, which may precipitate an exacerbation.

Complementary and Alternative Medications

Folk remedies have been used for RA for many years. Although most of these remedies cause no harm, there is little scientific evidence supporting their efficacy. Some of the more commonly used approaches include shark cartilage, chondroitin, herbs, vitamins, acupuncture, magnet therapy, climate therapy, and several diets. Clinicians should be aware of the therapies being considered or used by the patient; joint treatment goals should be established and monitored. Just as in traditional medicine, patients using complementary approaches either alone or as adjunctive therapy require ongoing monitoring for safety and efficacy of the selected approach.

Chiropractic treatment has helped many patients with RA, and more insurance carriers are reimbursing for chiropractic services. Chiropractic treatment as an adjunct to traditional measures should be viewed as mainstream therapy.

A recent review of the literature suggests that gamma-linolenic acid (GLA) may have a moderate effect on reducing pain and joint tenderness. This agent is found in borage seed oil (9% GLA), black currant oil (6% GLA), or evening primrose oil (2% GLA). The dose should be about 540 mg/d of GLA.

Case Study 1

J. W., a 46-year-old African-American woman, presents to your office with the chief complaint of bilateral stiffness of the shoulders, hands, and wrists in the morning. She reports she is otherwise healthy, takes no medications, and is employed as a systems analyst for a large bank. She recalls having some minor flu-like symptoms approximately 3 weeks before her visit. The stiffness makes it difficult for her to work for any extended period. She has also started wearing a wig because she cannot raise her arms in the morning to fix her hair. She has lost 10 pounds over the past 8 months but has not consciously dieted. She finds it increasingly difficult to drive, particularly when making turns and driving in reverse.

DIAGNOSIS: RHEUMATOID ARTHRITIS OF THE SHOULDERS, HANDS, AND WRISTS

1. List specific goals of treatment for J. W.
2. Which NSAID and which DMARD (assuming RA is confirmed) would you prescribe, and why?
3. How would you monitor J. W. in terms of efficacy and adverse effects? Specifically, what laboratory tests would you order?
4. List one or two adverse reactions for the selected agent that would cause you to change therapy.
5. If the above occurred, what would be the choice for second-line therapy, and why?
6. Discuss specific patient education based on your first-line therapy choices.
7. Describe one or two drug–drug or drug–food interactions for both the NSAID and the DMARD.
8. What dietary and lifestyle changes should be recommended for J. W.?
9. What over-the-counter and/or alternative medications would be appropriate for J. W.?

Case Study 2

G. P., a 66-year-old, right-handed white man, seeks treatment for swelling and decreased range of motion in the third finger of his right hand. He tells you he retired at age 65 after 40 years of assembly-line work. He reports that his physical activity has decreased and his weight has increased 20 pounds since retiring. His hobbies include woodworking and playing cards.

Although he describes several years of joint pain that gradually worsened, his activities were not limited until approximately 6 months ago, when he noted an insidious onset of swelling in the right third DIP joint. Over the years, he has sporadically taken acetaminophen, aspirin, and ibuprofen to control the pain. He reports that none of the drugs provided better relief than the others. He is concerned that he will continue to lose movement in the finger that is already affected, as well as in the fingers of his left hand. His medical history is remarkable for hypertension and three episodes of gout.

DIAGNOSIS: OSTEOARTHRITIS

1. List specific goals of treatment for G. P.
2. What drug therapy would you prescribe, and why?
3. How would you monitor in terms of efficacy and adverse effects? Specifically, what laboratory tests would you order for G. P.?
4. List one or two adverse reactions for the selected agent that would cause you to change therapy.
5. If the above occurred, what would be the choice for the second-line therapy, and why?
6. Discuss specific patient education based on your first-line therapy choice.
7. Describe one or two drug–drug or drug–food interactions for your chosen drug therapy.
8. What dietary and lifestyle changes should be recommended for this patient?
9. What over-the-counter and/or alternative medications would be appropriate for G. P.?

BIBLIOGRAPHY

*Starred entries are cited in text.

Aletaha, D., Neogi, T., Silman, A. J., et al. (2010). 2010 rheumatoid arthritis classification criteria. *Arthritis and Rheumatism, 62*(9), 2569–2581.

Altman, R., Alarcon, G., Appelrouth, D., et al. (1990). The American College of Rheumatology criteria for the classification and reporting of osteoarthritis of the hand. *Arthritis and Rheumatism, 33*(11), 1601–1610.

Altman, R., Alarcon, G., Appelrouth, D., et al. (1991). The American College of Rheumatology criteria for the classification and reporting of osteoarthritis of the hip. *Arthritis and Rheumatism, 34,* 505–514.

Altman, R., Asch, E., Bloch, D., et al. (1986). The American College of Rheumatology criteria for the classification and reporting of osteoarthritis of the knee. *Arthritis and Rheumatism, 29,* 1039–1049.

American College of Rheumatology. (2000). Recommendations for the medical management of osteoarthritis of the hip and knee. *Arthritis and Rheumatism, 43*(9), 1905–1915.

American College of Rheumatology (2002). Guidelines for the management of rheumatoid arthritis. *Arthritis and Rheumatism, 46*(2), 328–346.

American College of Rheumatology Ad Hoc Committee on Clinical Guidelines. (1996). Guidelines for monitoring drug therapy in rheumatoid arthritis. *Arthritis and Rheumatism, 39,* 723–731.

Blackburn, W. D. (1996). Management of osteoarthritis and rheumatoid arthritis: Prospects and possibilities. *American Journal of Medicine, 100*(Suppl.), 24S–30S.

*Chan, F. K., Lanas, A., Scheiman, J., et al. (2010). Celecoxib versus omeprazole and diclofenac in patients with osteoarthritis and rheumatoid arthritis (CONDOR): A randomized trial. *Lancet, 376,* 173–179.

Easton, B. T. (2001). Evaluation and treatment of the patient with osteoarthritis. *Journal of Family Practice, 50*(9), 791–797.

*Firestein, G. S. (1998). Rheumatoid arthritis. *Scientific American, 21,* 1–14.

Gardner, G. C., & Gilliland, B. C. (1998). Rheumatoid disorders. In E. B. Larsen & P. G. Ramsey (Eds.), *Medical therapeutics* (3rd ed., pp. 790–794). Philadelphia: Lippincott-Raven.

*Hawkey, C. J., Karrasch, J. A., Szczepanski, L., et al. (1998). Omeprazole compared with misoprostol for ulcers associated with nonsteroidal anti-inflammatory drugs. *New England Journal of Medicine, 338,* 727–734.

*Helmick, C. G., Felson, D. T., Lawrence, R. C., et al. (2008). Estimates of the prevalence of arthritis and other rheumatic conditions in the United States: Part 1. *Arthritis and Rheumatism, 58*(1), 15–25.

Kellick, K. A., Martins-Richards, J., & Chow, C. (1998). Management of arthritis. *Primary Care Practice, 2*(1), 66–80.

*Kroot, E. J., van Leeuwen, M. A., van Rijswijk, M. H., et al. (2000). No increased mortality in patients with rheumatoid arthritis: Up to 10 years of follow up from disease onset. *Annals of Rheumatic Disease, 59,* 954–958.

Lawrence, R. C., Felson, D. T., Helmick, C. G., et al. (2008). Estimates of the prevalence of arthritis and other rheumatic conditions in the United States: Part II. *Arthritis and Rheumatism, 58*(1), 26–35.

Marlowe, S. M. (1998). Evaluating rheumatic complaints. *Primary Care Practice, 2*(1), 3–19.

Moen, M.D. (2009). Topical diclofenac solution. *Drugs, 69*(18), 2621–2632.

*Moncur, C., & Williams, H. J. (1995). Rheumatoid arthritis: Status of drug therapies. *Physical Therapy, 75,* 511–525.

National Center for Chronic Disease Prevention and Health Promotion. (2010). Arthritis: Meeting the challenge. www.cdc.gov/arthritis.

Oddis, C. V. (1996). New perspectives on osteoarthritis. *American Journal of Medicine, 100,* 10S–15S.

O'Dell, J. R. (1996). Rheumatoid arthritis: When more than one DMARD is needed. *Journal of Musculoskeletal Medicine, 13*(12), 21–28.

O'Dell, J. R. (2004). Drug therapy: Therapeutic strategies for rheumatoid arthritis. *New England Journal of Medicine, 350*(25), 2591–2602.

Olsen, N. J., & Stein, C. M. (2004). Drug therapy: New drugs for rheumatoid arthritis. *New England Journal of Medicine, 350*(21), 2167–2179.

Ostensen, M. (2009). Management of early aggressive rheumatoid arthritis during pregnancy and lactation. *Expert Opinion in Pharmacotherapy, 10*(9), 1469–1479.

Ross, C. (1997). A comparison of osteoarthritis and rheumatoid arthritis. *Nurse Practitioner, 22,* 20–39.

*Saag, K. G., Teng, G. G., Patkar, N. M., et al. (2008). American College of Rheumatology 2008 recommendations for the use of nonbiologic and biologic disease-modifying antirheumatic drugs in rheumatoid arthritis. *Arthritis and Rheumatism, 59*(6), 762–784.

Soeken, K. K., Miller, S. A., & Ernst, E. (2003). Herbal medicines for the treatment of rheumatoid arthritis. *Rheumatology, 42*(5), 652–659.

*Yeomans, N. D., Tulassay, Z., Laszlo, J., et al. (1998). A comparison of omeprazole with ranitidine for ulcers associated with nonsteroidal anti-inflammatory drugs. *New England Journal of Medicine, 338,* 719–726.

CHAPTER 37

Susan M. Schrand
Betty E. Naimoli

Fibromyalgia

Fibromyalgia (FM) is a chronic condition of widespread musculoskeletal pain characterized by diffuse aches and stiffness, soft tissue tender points, fatigue, and nonrestorative sleep. It has been estimated that nearly 7 to 10 million Americans have FM, with women being 20 times more likely than men to acquire this condition. Most patients experience an onset of symptoms around the second or third decade of life, but FM has been identified as affecting people of all ages (Colorado Health Net, 1996).

Reiffenberger & Amundson (1996) reported that 5% to 6% of patients receiving care in family practice and general medicine offices are diagnosed with FM, and suggested that this condition may be present in up to 5% of the general population. Patients with FM are often seen by rheumatologists, and the number of office visits is only slightly less than for patients with rheumatoid arthritis. For family health care providers, Maurizio & Rogers (1997) stated that FM may be one of the most common conditions encountered. With a continued rise in prevalence of FM, Jones & Burckhardt (1997) estimated an annual financial toll of $15.9 billion in both direct and indirect health care costs, causing a significant public health concern.

CAUSES

There is no known cause or cure for FM, and its etiology has been long debated. Because of this lack of understanding and direction in disease management, people with FM may be among the more challenging patients for primary care providers. Patients often have a difficult time distinguishing specific events that precede their symptoms. Common factors precipitating FM include a flu-like viral illness, physical or emotional trauma, and withdrawal of corticosteroids. Symptoms that coincide with FM include migraine or tension-type headaches, irritable bowel, waking with stiffness and achiness, feeling under-rested or unrefreshed after a full night of sleep, hypersensitivity to cold or heat, environmental sensitivities, abdominal pain, sensations of numbness and tingling in hands and feet, and anxiety and depression (Maurizio & Rogers, 1997).

PATHOPHYSIOLOGY

Three possible explanations for this syndrome that are being explored are deficiencies in pain mechanisms, changes in the central nervous system (CNS), and muscular abnormalities. Allodynia, or a reduction in pain threshold, is commonly associated with FM, but as Jones & Burckhardt (1997) noted, researchers are still trying to explain the origins of chronic pain symptoms. It has been discovered, for example, that peripheral pain nerves (nociceptors) in muscle tissue that has experienced repeated stretching or pressure can release neurotransmitters in the spinal cord. As these neurotransmitters enter the CNS, the result is allodynia, with its symptoms of increased response to and duration of pain after noxious stimuli. Research on this theory continues.

Because patients with FM commonly experience sleep disturbances and chronic pain, researchers are also focusing on neurohormones as a factor in the disease etiology. Neurohormones, including serotonin, endorphins, or substance P, can have effects on sleep patterns, mood, and pain response. With substance P being influenced by serotonin, any deficiency could lead to an exaggerated sensory perception of stimuli. Goldenberg (1998) cited one study that showed patients with FM having a threefold increase in substance P. The sleep disturbance may also disrupt the production of growth hormone, a substance essential for tissue repair, which is produced during non–rapid eye movement (REM) or stage 4 sleep.

More recently, Wassem & Stillion-Allen (2003) suggested that recent studies may classify FM into a disease of the immune and CNS activation. Some research has documented inconsistencies in the growth hormones somatomedin C and IGF-1, the sympathoadrenal systems, and the neuroendocrine axis.

Muscular changes have been identified through biopsy, but the results reveal only nonspecific changes. On microscopic examination, a "moth-eaten" appearance of muscle noted in patients with FM has been associated with nonpathologic conditions and disuse (Jones & Burckhardt, 1997). No evidence of an inflammatory process was found in either tendon or muscle tissue.

Psychological factors, especially depression, play a role in FM, but no universal pattern or striking psychological abnormalities have been documented (Rosenblum, et al., 1996).

Because the etiology is unknown and the objective findings are nonspecific, FM is frequently considered a psychosomatic disorder. Anxiety about illness stemming from chronic pain, along with the uncertainty of the diagnosis, is more likely to be a precipitating factor for psychological distress in patients with FM than a specific individual trait (Jones & Burckhardt, 1997).

DIAGNOSTIC CRITERIA

The term *fibromyalgia* has evolved from earlier terms, such as fibrositis, fibromyositis, muscular rheumatism, psychogenic rheumatism, and primary FM. To simplify matters, FM is now the only term used to describe this syndrome.

In 1990, the American College of Rheumatology (ACR) developed classification criteria to help clinicians better distinguish FM from other rheumatologic disorders, such as rheumatoid arthritis or neck or back pain syndromes, and to provide a better exclusion system for conducting research. To be diagnosed with FM, a patient usually meets the criteria listed in **Box 37.1.** Jones & Burckhardt (1997) warned that clinicians should use clinical judgment to best explain their patients' signs and symptoms rather than rule out FM if the patient does not meet the exact ACR criteria.

INITIATING DRUG THERAPY

The chronic nature and lack of visible outward signs of FM make it reasonable and helpful to involve family and friends of the patient in education about the disease. Understanding that FM is a disease process is a crucial factor in promoting health and improvement for patients with FM. In most cases, FM interferes with the patient's quality of life, either in personal relationships or the ability to work and be a productive member of society. The fact that others recognize the patient's physical and psychological suffering can be most beneficial (Carette, 1996). Patients and their families should be encouraged to understand that FM is not crippling. With supportive environments, both at home and in the health care system, the patient can learn to take an active, self-help approach to controlling the disorder. Practitioners need to emphasize wellness rather than illness (Simms, 1996).

Most current research about FM suggests that patient education should be a primary focus in managing patients with FM. Many patients express a sense of relief when their symptoms finally have a name (Jones & Burckhardt, 1997). Keeping patients up to date on information regarding new research findings and treatment modalities while encouraging them to participate in support groups can give them the tools needed to gain self-efficacy.

Several alternatives to traditional drug therapy have been tried at various times by various patients. Low-impact exercise is one of the few therapies studied that proves significantly beneficial in managing symptoms. Hence, encouraging a system-

---

BOX 37.1

American College of Rheumatology Diagnostic Criteria for Fibromyalgia

History of widespread pain (defined as pain in the left side of the body, in the right side of the body, above the waist and below the waist)

In addition to widespread pain, axial skeletal pain (cervical spine, anterior chest, or thoracic spine or low back). Shoulder and buttock pain is categorized with the side pains. Low back pain is categorized as lower segment pain.

Pain on digital palpation in at least 11 of 18 "tender points" (9 bilaterally). Tender points include:

- Occiput: bilateral, at the suboccipital muscle insertions
- Low cervical: bilateral, at the anterior aspects of the intertransverse spaces at C5–C7
- Trapezius: bilateral, at the midpoint of the upper border
- Supraspinatus: bilateral, at origins, above the scapular spine near the medial border
- Second rib: bilateral, at the second costochondral junctions, just lateral to the junctions on upper surfaces
- Lateral epicondyle: bilateral, 2 cm distal to the epicondyles
- Gluteal: bilateral, in upper outer quadrants of buttocks in anterior fold of muscle
- Greater trochanter: bilateral, posterior to the trochanteric prominence
- Knee: bilateral, at the medial fat pad proximal to the joint line

---

Adapted with permission from Wolfe, F., et al. (1990). The American College of Rheumatology 1990 criteria for the classification of fibromyalgia: Report of the Multicenter Criteria Committee. *Arthritis and Rheumatism, 33,* 160–172.

---

atic, supervised exercise regimen is one of the most beneficial therapies that can be offered. However, patients with FM need to avoid any "impact-loading" exercises that involve jumping up and down, such as running sports. Walking, swimming, and bicycling are activities that can improve physical conditioning and minimize symptoms. Having the patient receiving adequate pharmacologic and psychological support prior to starting an exercise regimen will most likely promote adherence and increased tolerance to the recommended regimen (Wassem & Stillion-Allen, 2003). Even for the healthy person, commitment to a routine exercise program can be challenging, so encouraging and implementing an exercise regimen for people who live with chronic pain and an impaired quality of life may prove to be even more difficult for the practitioner.

Pacing is an important concept to relay to patients with FM. Learning to take life's activities more slowly—alternating days of rest and exercise and avoiding stressful situations—usually improves their sense of well-being (Bennett & McCain, 1995).

There is no generally applicable algorithm for the pharmacologic management of FM, so the goal is relief from or control of symptoms. Most of the reviewed literature suggests beginning with low-dose tricyclic antidepressants (TCAs). TCAs are not approved for FM by the U.S. Food and Drug Administration (FDA) but have been widely used to manage symptoms. TCAs block the reuptake of serotonin and/or norepinephrine and have demonstrated moderate overall efficacy for many FM symptoms, including pain, stiffness, tenderness, fatigue, and sleep quality (Arnold, et al., 2004). These agents most consistently improve sleep, and their efficacy may be due in large part to their sedative effects. However, their effects wane over time, and many patients have problems with tolerating side effects, including dry mouth, sedation, weight gain, and cardiac arrhythmias (Huynh, et al., 2008). Patients who benefit from low-dose TCAs may avoid these side effects, but additional treatment options are needed for patients who do not receive adequate relief at a low dosing level.

There are some data suggesting that patients with a mixed FM and depression will do moderately well with TCA treatment. There appears to be a functional reduction in serotonergic activity in patients with FM, and antidepressants might enhance the activity of serotonin and norepinephrine neurotransmitters in the descending inhibitory pain pathways, leading to a reduction in pain.

Antidepressants

Tricyclic Antidepressants

Amitriptyline hydrochloride (Elavil) increases non-REM stage 4 sleep by inhibiting reuptake of serotonin rather than acting in an antidepressant manner (Maurizio & Rogers, 1997). Low doses of amitriptyline appear to cause REM suppression and prolong stages 3 and 4 of non-REM sleep.

Because the goal of FM therapy differs from that of depression therapy, drug dosages and onset of action differ significantly. Prescribing 10 mg of amitriptyline 2 to 3 hours before bedtime helps the patient gain more restful sleep and minimizes any "hangover" feeling the next day. Dosing may start as low as 5 mg/d for patients sensitive to anticholinergic side effects. (See Chapter 40 for details of anticholinergic side effects.) If the patient does not respond to the 10-mg daily dose after 1 week, the dosage is increased to 20 mg/d, and increments of 10 mg on a weekly basis are added. Doses that exceed 50 mg/d provide little additional benefit. Patients experiencing significant improvements should continue the dosage effective for them for approximately 3 months. After

this time, a tapering regimen of 10 mg/month should begin until the minimum effective dosage is achieved. Patients may maintain their dosage regimen for years without complications, but abrupt discontinuation of a TCA may lead to rebound insomnia. Tapering of this medication is recommended (Simms, 1996).

Nortriptyline hydrochloride (Pamelor) is another drug in the TCA class that has provided symptomatic relief for patients with FM (**Table 37.1**). Similarly, doxepin may be used. The doses of these agents, like amitriptyline, are lower than those used for depression. These agents could be considered alternatives to amitriptyline, though there are no data suggesting that one is more effective than another for the treatment of FM.

Dual Neurotransmitter Reuptake Inhibitors

Serotonin and norepinephrine mediate the transmission of painful stimuli in the CNS pathways and may modulate the neuroendocrine system's sensitivity to and processing of painful stimuli. Thus, serotonin/norepinephrine reuptake inhibitors (SNRIs) and norepinephrine/serotonin reuptake inhibitors (NSRIs) may be useful in the management of FM and are currently the first- and second-line pharmacologic choices for patients with FM (Huynh, et al., 2008). These agents are more specific than TCAs and therefore lack the high side effect profile and potential drug interactions of TCAs. Duloxetine (Cymbalta; an SNRI) was FDA-approved for the treatment of FM in 2008. In 2009, milnacipran (Savalla; an NSRI) was the first drug approved specifically for FM treatment.

Selective Serotonin Reuptake Inhibitors

Fluoxetine (Prozac), a selective serotonin reuptake inhibitor (SSRI), has been studied as a potential antidepressant agent for FM therapy, but it was found to contribute to sleep disturbances because of its stimulating characteristics (Simms, 1996). The full dosage of an SSRI would be recommended as therapy for patients with FM who have concomitant depression, but the decline in sleep quality may cause problems. Some clinicians manage this by prescribing an SSRI in the morning and a TCA at bedtime (Bennett & McCain, 1995). In a 12-week, flexible-dose, placebo-controlled trial, Arnold et al. (2002) found fluoxetine to be effective on most outcomes (i.e., Fibromyalgia Impact Questionnaire total score and the McGill Pain Questionnaire), and it was well tolerated.

New-Generation Anticonvulsants

The anticonvulsants gabapentin (Neurontin) and pregabalin (Lyrica) often are used to manage FM symptoms. Pregabalin was the first agent to receive FDA approval for the treatment of the disorder. These agents exert their influence by binding to the alpha 2-delta subunit of voltage-gated calcium channels of neurons, reducing calcium influx at nerve terminals and therefore inhibiting the release of neurotransmitters (Stahl, 2004).

TABLE 37.1   Pharmacologic Therapy for Fibromyalgia

Generic (Trade) Name	Starting Dose and Range	Side Effects	Contraindications	Special Considerations
amitriptyline (Elavil)	Start at 5 mg/d. Increase by increments of 10 mg/wk if no relief after 1 wk of therapy. Continue effective dose for 3 mo, then begin taper of 10 mg/mo until minimum effective dose is achieved. Safe to maintain above dose for years	See Chapter 40, Table 40.4, for complete listing of side effects.	Hypersensitivity to any tricyclic drug Concomitant therapy with MAO inhibitors Recent MI Pregnancy Lactation	Abrupt discontinuation of drug may lead to rebound insomnia. Due to different dosing methods, there is no suggested plasma concentration to follow. Avoid alcohol. SSRI combination use may increase levels of TCAs. FDA approved for fibromyalgia
cyclobenzaprine (Flexeril)	10–40 mg/d in divided doses	CNS: drowsiness, dizziness, fatigue GI: dry mouth, nausea, constipation	Recovering MI Use caution in patients with urinary retention.	Avoid alcohol. Report any dizziness, blurred vision, or other CNS symptoms.
doxepin (Sinequan)	10–50 mg once daily	See Chapter 40, Table 40.4, for complete listing of side effects.	Hypersensitivity to any tricyclic drug Concomitant therapy with MAO inhibitors Recent MI Pregnancy Lactation	Abrupt discontinuation of drug may lead to rebound insomnia. Due to different dosing methods, there is no suggested plasma concentration to follow. Avoid alcohol.
fluoxetine (Prozac)	Start at 20 mg in a.m. May increase by weekly increments.	See Chapter 40, Table 40.4, for complete listing of side effects.	Hypersensitivity to any SSRI drug	
gabapentin (Neurontin)	300 mg daily to 1,200 mg tid	Weight gain, dizziness, sedation	Contraindicated if patient has hypersensitivity to drug	Pregnancy category C; increased incidence of seizures when discontinued abruptly
nortriptyline hydrochloride (Pamelor)	10–50 mg once daily	See Chapter 40, Table 40.4, for complete listing of side effects.	Same as for amitriptyline	Same as for amitriptyline
tramadol (Ultram)	25–300 mg/d	Dizziness, constipation, nausea, headaches, sleepiness	Do not use in patients for whom opioid use is contraindicated.	Pregnancy category C; do not use in patients with seizure risk or respiratory depression.
pregabalin (Lyrica)	150–225 mg bid; start at 75 mg bid (may increase to 150 mg bid within 1 wk); max dose 225 mg bid	Dizziness, somnolence, dry mouth, edema, blurred vision, weight gain, difficulty with concentration/attention	Contraindicated if patient has hypersensitivity to drug	Pregnancy category C Increased risk of suicidal thoughts
duloxetine (Cymbalta)	60 mg/d; start 30 mg/d for 1 wk, increase to 60 mg/d (Doses >60 mg/d did not show benefit and had increased incidence of side effects.)	See Chapter 40, Table 40.4, for complete listing of side effects.	Hypersensitivity to any SSRI drug	
milnacipran (Savella)	50 mg bid; start 12.5 mg/d (increase on day 2 to 12.5 mg bid, on day 4 to 25 mg bid, after day 7 to 50 mg bid); max dose 100 mg bid	Nausea, headache, constipation, dizziness, insomnia, hot flush, hyperhidrosis, vomiting, palpitations, heart rate increase, dry mouth, hypertension	Contraindicated in patients taking an MAO inhibitor or in patients with narrow-angle glaucoma	Pregnancy category C Increased risk of suicidal thoughts

The results of a 14-week randomized, double–blind, placebo-controlled trial demonstrated that pregabalin is effective across a wide range of FM symptoms (Arnold, et al., 2008). Compared with placebo-treated patients, pregabalin-treated (300 mg/d or 450 mg/d) patients had significantly greater mean changes in pain scores, and more pregabalin-treated patients reported improvements in the Patients' Global Impression of Change scale (a measure of the clinical significance of treatment effect). Pregabalin-treatment patients also had significant improvements in sleep and total Fibromyalgia Impact Questionnaire scores compared with the placebo-treated patients. The most commonly reported adverse events were dizziness and somnolence, which tended to be dose-related (Arnold, et al., 2008).

Skeletal Muscle Relaxants

Cyclobenzaprine hydrochloride (Flexeril, Cycloflex), a TCA structurally similar to amitriptyline, shows some short-term efficacy in FM. This drug, which has properties that reduce brain stem noradrenergic function and motor neuron efferent activity, is usually marketed as a muscle relaxant (Simms, 1996). Because of the lack of substantial drug trials, dosing recommendations vary in the literature. One study cited by Simms (1996) reported some benefits with dosing beginning at 10 mg/d for 1 week, 25 mg/d for weeks 2 through 12, and 50 mg/d for weeks 13 through 24. Dosing described by Goldenberg (1998) started at 10 to 40 mg/d in divided doses. Patients taking cyclobenzaprine in this regimen showed improvement in pain, fatigue, sleep, and tender point count. Bedtime dosing is highly recommended with this agent because of its potential to cause impairment and drowsiness.

Cyclobenzaprine, having similar properties to the TCAs, can cause anticholinergic side effects such as drowsiness, dizziness, lightheadedness, dry mouth, and muscle weakness and should usually be avoided when a patient is already taking TCAs.

Anti-Inflammatory Agents

Nonsteroidal anti-inflammatory drugs (NSAIDs) are commonly used for analgesia, but because there does not seem to be any inflammatory process associated with FM, minimal relief is obtained with their use (Wassem & Stillion-Allen, 2003). In light of the associated symptoms of irritable bowel, NSAIDs are not the analgesics of first choice. Acetaminophen may be better tolerated for analgesia, especially in patients who have irritable bowel syndrome. Studies are underway to assess the combination of TCAs and NSAIDs for symptom relief, but at this time the combination cannot be suggested for therapy. See Chapter 36 for more information on NSAIDs.

Narcotic Analgesics

Because of the chronic nature of FM, narcotic analgesic drugs should be avoided for pain control because of their addiction potential. There may be some clinical situations that require management with narcotics, especially during disease flare-ups or during initiation of new therapies. Yunus & Arslan (2004)

reserved use for patients who have failed to respond to other therapy attempts. Narcotics must be reserved for short-term use and with close collaboration with the prescriber. Yunus and Arslan reported that they had success using oxycodone, 10 to 30 mg/d in divided doses every 12 hours, with codeine, 30 mg, two to four times daily. They suggested avoiding this class of medication altogether in patients with known addiction potential. See Chapter 7 for more information regarding narcotic analgesics.

Selecting the Most Appropriate Agent

Figure 37-1 provides an algorithm for treating FM. Drug treatment is individualized to meet the patient's needs. First- and second-line therapies are summarized in **Table 37.2**.

First-Line Therapy

TCAs are generally considered first-line therapy; however, if they are ineffective or intolerable due to side effects, there are more options now than ever before.

Amitriptyline is the first line of medication suggested for short-term treatment of FM, although nortriptyline or cyclobenzaprine may be tried as well. Once a minimum effective dosage is achieved, therapy may continue for years. Discontinuation of therapy should be gradual (tapered) to avoid untoward effects.

Second-Line Therapy

The development of new drugs for FM has significantly improved the management of this difficult pain syndrome. There are currently three medications approved by the FDA for the management of FM: the alpha-2-delta ligand, pregabalin, and the serotonin and norepinephrine reuptake inhibitors duloxetine and milnacipran (Arnold, 2010).

Third-Line Therapy

When first- or second-line therapy is unsuccessful, the practitioner may add an analgesic. Analgesics are effective for some patients. Tramadol, with or without acetaminophen, has been effective in patients with FM (Nickerson, 2009). Tramadol is a centrally acting opioid analgesic that exerts its effect through the binding of parent drug M1 metabolites to the mu opioid receptors and through the weak inhibition of norepinephrine and serotonin reuptake. Tramadol should be used with caution due to the possibility of typical opiate withdrawal symptoms with discontinuation and the risk of abuse and dependence (Nickerson, 2009). NSAIDs may be useful as adjunctive therapy; however, there is no evidence that they are effective when used alone. This is probably because FM pain is not caused by an inflammatory process (Nickerson, 2009).

Special Population Considerations
Geriatric

Care must be taken when prescribing TCAs to patients older than age 65. The anticholinergic effect can worsen existing glaucoma and benign prostatic hyperplasia in men.

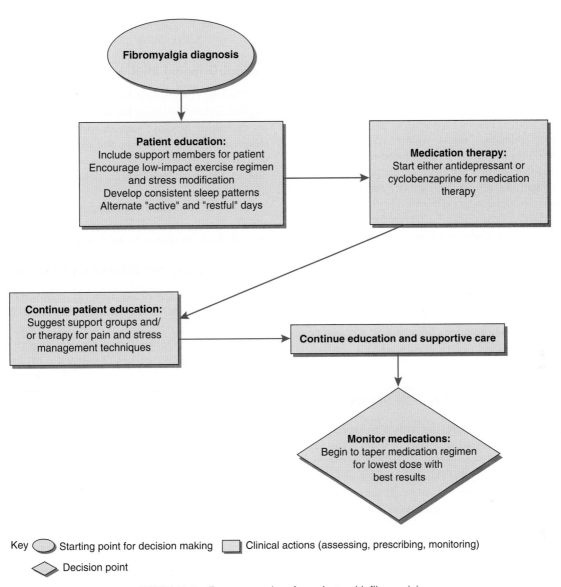

FIGURE 37-1   Treatment options for patients with fibromyalgia.

TABLE 37.2	Recommended Order of Treatment for Fibromyalgia	
Order	**Agents**	**Comments**
First line	Tricyclic antidepressants (TCAs) initially for short term. Suggested agents include amitriptyline, nortriptyline, and cyclobenzaprine.	Dosage schedules of these medications are adjusted to meet patient needs and are not in accord with recommended dosage for depression therapy. Patient should be monitored for side effects associated with TCAs and educated to recognize and report adverse events.
Second line	Additional therapy with a selective serotonin reuptake inhibitor such as fluoxetine (Prozac)	Dosage schedules of these medications are adjusted to meet patient needs and are not in accord with recommended dosage for depression therapy. Patients should be educated to recognize and manage possible side effects.

The sedative effects can affect a patient's ability to perform activities of daily living. Dosages above those recommended can cause confusion. Similarly, narcotic analgesia should be used with caution in the elderly due to the side effect profile.

Women

This disease primarily affects women. A recent review (Yunus, 2001) showed that the ratio of women to men is 9:1. He reported that women had more tender points than men, but in men with the disease, pain severity and physical functioning were not significantly different. He did not offer convincing evidence of the reason for the gender differences but postulated that there might be a complex interaction between physiology, psychology, and environmental factors.

The clinician must consider the dangers of prescribing teratogenic medications to women of childbearing age. Amitriptyline is a category D medication, and caution should be taken when prescribing it to this age group (Lacy, et al., 1996–1997). Cyclobenzaprine (Flexeril) is a category B medication.

MONITORING PATIENT RESPONSE

Keeping in close contact with the patient to monitor pain relief, sleep quality, and general feelings of sickness and teaching the patient to recognize signs of anticholinergic effects are keys to careful monitoring. No radiologic studies are indicated for monitoring patients with FM, although annual liver function tests and baseline electrocardiograms are suggested for monitoring the use of TCAs.

PATIENT EDUCATION

FM is a disease commonly seen by the primary care provider. Helping patients understand its chronic nature and encouraging them to focus on their wellness is vital in managing the condition. Low-impact exercise, stress reduction, established sleep patterns, and strong support systems are essential factors for improving quality of life for people with this disease. The practitioner needs to be aware of pharmacologic and nonpharmacologic alternatives to assist patients with health promotion. As more research is done on FM, practitioners hope to gain a better understanding of how to manage care of patients with this disorder without becoming frustrated by its chronicity.

Drug Information

Since there is no specific treatment for FM, the practitioner should seek traditional sources of drug information such as the FDA, the *Physicians' Desk Reference, Drug Facts and Comparisons*, and the manufacturer of a specific agent. The practitioner can access information about ongoing clinical trials for FM at ClinicalTrials.gov (http://clinicaltrials.gov/ct/gui/action/FindCondition?ui=D005356&recruiting=true).

Patient-Oriented Information Sources

The National Fibromyalgia Association's website (http://fmaware.org/fminfo/brochure.htm) has information related to improving the quality of life of patients with FM. This site provides information about the disease and clinical trials involving FM treatment, along with products to support patients with the disease. The association has an online newsletter and offers support groups.

The National Library of Medicine (http://www.nlm.nih.gov/medlineplus/tutorials/fibromyalgia.html) has an online tutorial about the diagnosis and treatment of FM.

Complementary and Alternative Medications

Nearly 33% of Americans turn to complementary and alternative medicine to help manage their health (Eisenberg, et al., 1993). Patients with complicated disease processes who feel that conventional medicine is failing to treat their symptoms effectively turn to alternative therapy to seek additional relief. Twenty FM patients involved in a pilot study reported improvement in pain, function, and mood with the use of a mind-body intervention combining patient education, meditation techniques, and movement therapy (Singh, et al., 1998).

Various methods of alternative medicine such as acupuncture, transcutaneous electrical nerve stimulation, massage, biofeedback, and hypnotherapy produced some pain relief and have shown some efficacy in randomized controlled clinical trials (Ebell & Beck, 2001). Acupuncture has been examined in a meta-analysis and proved to be a useful adjunctive treatment for many patients with this disease. Millea & Holloway (2000) reported that although acupuncture is not curative, it can help to improve quality of life. A recent report from the Agency for Healthcare Quality and Research (2003) concluded that there was insufficient evidence to support the use of acupuncture in the treatment of FM.

One herbal remedy is being looked at as a topical anesthetic. Capsaicin (Zostrix) is a cream that comes in 0.025% or 0.075% strengths. The active ingredient comes from dried, ripe fruits of Capsicum and functions as a counter-irritant that depletes substance P from sensory nerve fibers. This cream is being investigated in various painful conditions, including diabetic neuropathy, postherpetic neuralgia, stump pain, and postmastectomy pain, to name a few. Markovits and Gilhar (1997) found capsaicin to be successful with pain relief and suggested that it might help to reduce the use of NSAIDs. They reported that the use of capsaicin 0.025% four times a day for 5 weeks led to relief of neck and shoulder pain in patients with FM, although no exact statistics were reported specific to FM pain relief. They mentioned that 74% of patients reported mild burning associated with capsaicin use. Evidence at this time remains inconclusive regarding its use in FM therapy, and it cannot be recommended.

Case Study

S. S., a 28-year-old white female, comes to you as a new patient with her chief complaint being chronic pain and poor sleep patterns. During your interview, you discover that she has been fighting global, diffuse body pain and feeling depressed for the past 2 years. She just recently received health insurance and would like to figure out why she is feeling so poorly. After a complete history and physical and a full panel of labs, you find all of her results to be within normal limits, with the exception of global tenderness.

Using the diagnostic criteria from the ACR, you note that she has 15 of the 18 tender points, widespread pain, and morning stiffness and fatigue. After diagnosing her with FM, you begin to form a plan of care.

1. List at least two specific goals for the treatment of this patient.
2. Which agent would you prescribe, and what were some considerations that led you to this choice?
3. How would you monitor the success of your treatment, and when would you do so?
4. List one or two adverse reactions for the selected agent that would cause you to change therapy.
5. Describe one or two drug–drug or drug–food interactions for the selected agent.
6. What would be the choice for second-line therapy should the adverse reactions you considered occurred?
7. Are there any over-the-counter or alternative medications you would recommend she consider adding to your regimen?
8. How would you respond if this patient asked about the use of acupuncture to treat her disease?

BIBLIOGRAPHY

Starred references are cited in the text.

*Agency for Healthcare Quality and Research. (2003). Technology assessment Report: Acupuncture for fibromyalgia. http://www.cms.hhs.gov/coverage/download/id83.pdf. Accessed July 7, 2004.

Arnold, L. M. (2010). Fibromyalgia: Expert insights on improving treatment adherence. *Medscape Education Rheumatology*, CME/CE Released: 07/09/2010, http://www.medscape.org/viewarticle/724281.

*Arnold, L. M., Hess, E. V., Hudson, J. I., et al. (2002). A randomized, placebo-controlled, double-blind, flexible-dose study of fluoxetine in the treatment of women with fibromyalgia. *American Journal of Medicine, 112,* 191–197.

Arnold, L. M., Keck, P. E. Jr., & Welge, J. A. (2000). Antidepressant treatment of fibromyalgia: A meta-analysis and review. *Psychosomatics, 41,* 104–113.

*Arnold, L. M., Lu, Y., Crofford, L. J., et al. (2004). A double-blind, multi-center trial comparing duloxetine with placebo in the treatment of fibromyalgia patients with or without major depressive disorder. *Arthritis & Rheumatology, 50,* 2974–2984.

*Arnold, L. M., Russell, I. J., Diri, E. W., et al. (2008). A 14 week, randomized, double blinded, placebo-controlled monotherapy trial of pregabalin in patients with fibromyalgia. *Journal of Pain, 9,* 792–805.

*Bennett, R. M., & McCain, G. A. (1995). Coping successfully with fibromyalgia. *Patient Care, 15,* 29–45.

*Carette, S. (1996). Chronic pain syndromes. *Annals of Rheumatic Disease, 55,* 497–501.

*Colorado Health Net. (1996). Fibromyalgia definitions, facts and statistics. [On-line]. Available: http://www.coloradohealthnet.org/site/idx_fibro.html.

Cymbalta (duloxetine) package insert. (2009). Indianapolis, IN: Eli Lilly and Co.

*Ebell, M., & Beck, E. (2001). How effective are complementary/alternative medicine (CAM) therapies for fibromyalgia? *Journal of Family Practice, 50,* 401.

*Eisenberg, D. M., Kessler, R. C., Foster, C., et al. (1993). Unconventional medicine in the United States: Prevalence, costs and patterns of use. *New England Journal of Medicine, 328,* 246–252.

*Goldenberg, D. L. (1998). Fibromyalgia and related syndromes. In J. H. Klippel & P. A. Dieppe (Eds.), *Rheumatology* (2nd ed., pp. 1–12). Philadelphia: C. V. Mosby.

*Huynh, C. N., Yanni, L. M., & Morgan, L. A. (2008). Fibromyalgia: Diagnosis and management for the primary health provider. *Journal of Women's Health, 17,* 1379–1387.

*Jones, K. D., & Burckhardt, C. S. (1997). A multidisciplinary approach to treating fibromyalgia syndrome. *Pain Management, 12,* 7–14.

*Lacy, C., Armstrong, L. L., Ingrim, N., & Lance, L. L. (1996–1997). *Drug information handbook: Pocket* (pp. 10, 59–61, 265–266). Cleveland: Lexi-Comp.

Lyrica (pregabalin) package insert. (2009). New York: Pfizer Inc.

*Markovits, E., & Gilhar, A. (1997). Capsaicin: An effective topical treatment in pain. *International Journal of Dermatology, 36,* 401–404.

*Maurizio, S. J., & Rogers, J. L. (1997). Recognizing and treating fibromyalgia. *Nurse Practitioner, 22,* 18–31.

*Millea, P. J., & Holloway, R. L. (2000). Treating fibromyalgia. *American Family Physician, 62,* 1575–1580.

Nickerson, B. (2009). Recent advances in the treatment of pain associated with fibromyalgia. *US Pharmacist 34*(9), 49–55.

Practicing Clinicians Exchange. (2009). Emerging issues in primary care. *Fibromyalgia: Assessment and Treatment,* (Volume 2), 49–60. Available: http://www.practicing clinicians.com.

*Reiffenberger, D., & Amundson, L. (1996). Fibromyalgia syndrome: A review. *American Family Physician, 53,* 1698–1704.

*Rosenblum, R., Campbell, S., & Rosenbaum, J. (1996). *Clinical Neurology of Rheumatic Diseases* (pp. 12–13). Boston: Butterworth-Heinemann.

Savella (milnacipran) package insert. (2009). St. Louis, MO: Forest Pharmaceuticals, Inc.

*Simms, R. W. (1996). Fibromyalgia syndrome: Current concepts in pathophysiology, clinical features, and management. *Arthritis Care and Research, 9,* 315–328.

*Singh, B. B., Berman, B. M., Hadhazy, V. A., & Creamer, P. (1998). A pilot study of cognitive behavioral therapy in fibromyalgia. *Alternative Therapies in Health and Medicine, 4*(2), 67–70.

*Stahl, S. M. (2004). Mechanism of action of alpha2delta ligands: Voltage sensitive calcium channel (VSCC) modulators. *Journal of Clinical Psychiatry, 65,* 1033–1034.

*Wassem, R. A., & Stillion-Allen, K. A. (2003). Evidence-based management of the fibromyalgia patient. In search of optimal functioning. *Advance for Nurse Practitioners,* 34–41.

*Yunus, M. B. (2001). The role of gender in fibromyalgia syndrome. *Current Rheumatology Reports, 3*(2), 128–134.

*Yunus, M. B., & Arslan, S. (2004). Fibromyalgia syndrome: Can it be treated? *Consultant,* 289–302.

UNIT

9

Pharmacology for Neurological/ Psychological Disorders

CHAPTER 38

Kelleen N. Flaherty
Elyse L. Dishler

Headaches

Headache is one of the most common complaints presenting in primary care. The pain of a headache can range from mild to severe, be acute or chronic, and may be hours to days in duration. While there are three categories of headaches according to the most recent International Classification of Headache Disorders (Headache Classification Subcommittee of the International Headache Society, 2004), the most commonly encountered headaches seen in primary care are the primary and secondary headaches (**Box 38.1**). A primary headache is one with no identifiable underlying organic disease process; a secondary headache is one for which a specific etiology has been identified. The practitioner must first rule out a secondary headache and then accurately diagnose the type of primary headache. In some instances, a primary and secondary headache can occur simultaneously. This chapter will focus on diagnosing and treating tension-type headache (TTH) and migraines, the most common forms of primary headache presenting in clinical practice.

Tension headaches have a dull quality, with pain that radiates bilaterally from the forehead to the occiput in a band-like fashion. The pain often radiates down the neck and sometimes even into the trapezius muscle. The pain is mild to moderate and can last from 30 minutes to several days in severe cases. Tension headaches are not typically present upon awakening, but begin later in the day and progress with time. The pain of these headaches is rarely debilitating, but it can affect a person's ability to function, especially if prolonged or chronic. There are no associated symptoms of nausea, vomiting, photophobia, or phonophobia. Migraine is a neurologic syndrome causing not only throbbing head pain but also nausea, appetite change, photophobia, and phonophobia. The pain generally ranges from moderate to severe and can be debilitating. About 14% of women and 6% of men in the world are estimated to have migraine (Stovner, et al., 2007), although some 50% are also estimated to be undiagnosed (Solomon & Lipton, 1999). The age of onset is from 15 to 35, but peak prevalence is from ages 35 to 45. Family histories of migraines, usually along the female line, are common in migraine patients. It is estimated that some 25% of individuals suffering from migraines are absent from school or work approximately six times a year (migraine ranks 19th in disabling conditions in the world based on World Health Organization criteria), resulting in an estimated annual medical cost of $1,600 for each individual and a combined direct and indirect cost to society of approximately $5 to $17 billion (1992 dollars) per year (Osterhaus, et al., 1992; Clouse & Osterhaus, 1994; Leonardi, et al., 2005).

Cluster headaches may be chronic or acute and episodic and are far less common than migraine or tension headaches, occurring in less than 1% of the population. It is approximately four times more common in males than in females, and the acute/episodic variety approximately six times more common than chronic cluster headache (Fischera, et al., 2008). While the pathophysiology of cluster headache is incompletely understood, hypothalamic dysfunction is believed to be involved; consequently, circadian rhythms are disrupted. Cluster headaches often occur at specific times during sleep-wake cycles, another indication of hypothalamic involvement (Francis, et al., 2010). The pain is disabling, burning, or boring and centered around one eye and is described by patients as being more severe than childbirth or passing a kidney stone. Attacks are unilateral, generally lasting from 15 to 180 minutes, and may occur one to eight times per day. Associated ipsilateral symptoms may include lacrimation, nasal congestion, rhinorrhea, miosis, ptosis, eyelid edema, or conjunctival injection. Restlessness and agitation may also accompany an attack (Headache Classification Subcommittee, 2004). A patient with symptoms suggestive of cluster headache should be referred to a neurologist or headache specialist.

CAUSES OF TENSION HEADACHES

There are multiple causes of these common headaches, many likely still undiscovered. It has been suggested that tension headaches result from underlying psychological issues, but data do not exist to support this. In fact, anxiety and depression may be a result rather than a cause of recurring headache pain (Breslau, et al., 2000). Inadequate sleep is a common precipitating factor, causing tension headache in 39% of healthy volunteers after sleep deprivation (Blau, 1990). Cigarette smoking has also been correlated with an increased number of days of headache per week (Payne, et al., 1991). Underlying muscle tension in the cervical or pericranial muscles occurs more frequently in tension headache sufferers than in headache-free controls (Hatch, 1992).

Although more common in migraine patients, one cause of recurrent tension headaches is the overuse of over-the-counter (OTC) and prescription analgesic medications, leading to medication overuse headache (MOH) (Headache Classification Subcommittee, 2004). The headache recurs as

Primary Headaches

Migraine

Tension-type headache (TTH)

Cluster headache (CH) and other trigeminal autonomic cephalalgias (TACs)

Other primary headaches (primary stabbing headache, primary cough headache, primary exertional headache, primary headache associated with sexual activity, hypnic headache, primary thunderclap headache, hemicrania continua, and new daily-persistent headache [NDPH])

Secondary Headaches

Headache attributed to head and/or neck trauma

Headache attributed to cranial or cervical vascular disorder

Headache attributed to nonvascular intracranial disorder

Headache attributed to a substance or its withdrawal

Headache attributed to infection

Headache attributed to disorder of homeostasis

Headache or facial pain attributed to disorder of cranium, neck, eyes, ears, nose, sinuses, teeth, mouth, or other facial or cranial structures

Headache attributed to psychiatric disorder

Cranial Neuralgias, Central and Primary Facial Pain, and Other Headaches

Cranial neuralgias and central causes of facial pain

Other headache, cranial neuralgia, central or primary facial pain

Modified from: International Classification of Headache Disorders, 2nd Edition (2004). *Cephalgia, 24* (Suppl. 1), 1–160.

each dose of medication wears off, causing the patient to take another analgesic and thus continue the cycle of pain. Treating more than two headaches, either migraine or tension, per week can lead to development of chronic daily headache.

PATHOPHYSIOLOGY OF TENSION HEADACHES

The physiology of tension headaches is poorly understood and an active area of research. The most common hypothesis is that the pain of these headaches is muscular and related to increased resting pericranial muscle tone. The flaw in this hypothesis is that electromyographic studies do not consistently detect elevated resting muscle tone in patients with chronic tension headaches. Recent evidence has shown that central pain processing is an important part of TTH pathophysiology (Cathcart, et al., 2010).

One study showed increased muscle hardness in patients with chronic TTH that was present with or without the headache being present (Ashina, et al., 1999a). What is unknown is whether this muscle hardness is the cause or the result of the pain. Further research implicates nitric oxide (a vasodilator) as a local mediator of TTH. Blocking nitric oxide production led to decreased pericranial muscle hardness and headache pain in patients with chronic TTH (Ashina, et al., 1999b). Sustained peripheral pain signals coming from the pericranial myofascial tissue eventually lead to increased central nervous system (CNS) sensitization, lowering pain thresholds. The increased tenderness, centralized pain, and lowered pain threshold together contribute to the development of chronic TTH (Bezov, et al., 2011).

DIAGNOSTIC CRITERIA

The first step in determining the type of headache a patient has is to take a detailed headache history. The history should include the patient's age; the time of day when the attack occurs; the duration and frequency of attacks; precipitating or relieving factors; the quality, location, and intensity of the pain; and associated symptoms. The social history and family history are also important. The results of physical and neurologic examinations should be unremarkable in a patient with primary headache, other than revealing possible tenderness of pericranial muscles. Diagnosis is mostly of exclusion: all possible secondary headaches or migraine headache are ruled out. Tension headaches may be diagnosed as primary, secondary, or both (Headache Classification Subcommittee, 2004). Diagnostic alarms in the evaluation of a headache patient that require further testing include headache onset after age 50, sudden-onset headache, accelerating headache pattern, headache with fever and stiff neck, and abnormal results on the neurologic examination. ICHD-2 diagnostic criteria for frequent episodic tension headache can be seen in **Box 38.2**.

INITIATING DRUG THERAPY FOR TENSION HEADACHES

Before initiating drug therapy, it is critical to determine the type and frequency of OTC medication use. Patients with tension headaches and headaches in general frequently self-medicate and may present when experiencing MOH. Treating more than two headaches per week for more than a few consecutive weeks can lead to development of a chronic daily headache pattern. Caffeine and butalbital products are notorious contributors to MOH. The initial treatment of MOH consists of withholding all analgesics for 1 to 2 weeks.

BOX 38.2

Diagnostic Criteria for Frequent Episodic Tension Headache

A. At least 10 episodes occurring on ≥1 but <15 days per month for at least 3 months (≥12 and <180 days per year) and fulfilling criteria B through D
B. Headaches lasting from 30 minutes to 7 days
C. Headache has at least two of the following characteristics:
 1. Bilateral location
 2. Pressing/tightening (nonpulsating) quality
 3. Mild or moderate intensity
 4. Not aggravated by routine physical activity such as walking or climbing stairs
D. Both of the following:
 1. No nausea or vomiting (anorexia may occur)
 2. No more than one of photophobia or phonophobia
 3. Not attributed to another disorder

Headache Classification Subcommittee of the International Headache Society. (2004). The international classification of headache disorders, 2nd ed. *Cephalalgia, 24* (Suppl. 1), 1–160.

It is also important to help identify headache triggers and to encourage a healthy lifestyle. Often simple changes, such as eating and sleeping in a consistent pattern, decreasing alcohol and tobacco use, and using good posture, can decrease headache severity and frequency.

Adjuncts to pharmacologic therapy include relaxation therapy, biofeedback, self-hypnosis, and cognitive therapy. Data from a large meta-analysis show positive results with the use of biofeedback, particularly when combined with relaxation (Nestoriuc, et al., 2008). Some techniques of relaxation are progressive muscle relaxation and the use of autogenic phrases. With progressive muscle relaxation, patients learn to contract and then relax all of the major muscles from head to toe. Using autogenic phrases involves repeating statements about calmness, warmth, and heaviness, allowing the patient to relax deeply. Patients may also benefit from acupuncture or cervical physical therapy in the case of chronic tension headaches.

Goals of Drug Therapy for Tension Headaches

The primary goals of drug therapy should be to reduce the severity and frequency of headaches, thus improving the patient's quality of life and ability to function. The goals for patients with episodic tension headaches are to select appropriate analgesic agents that will have the fewest side effects. Prophylactic therapy should be considered in addition to abortive analgesic agents for patients with more than two significant headaches per week. In a patient with MOH, it is appropriate to start a prophylactic agent and abruptly stop abortive analgesic medications (other than barbiturate drugs, which must be tapered) simultaneously. It is important to educate patients about MOH and to limit the use of analgesics to 2 days per week. Regular and frequent treatment with analgesics may cause development of chronic headache. It is important that patients do not overuse analgesics, as this is likely to interfere with the efficacy of preventive treatment (Headache Classification Subcommittee, 2004).

Acetaminophen and Aspirin

Acetaminophen at a dose of 1,000 mg can be very effective in treating mild to moderate tension headaches, although given the hepatotoxic qualities of the drug, a U.S. Food and Drug Administration (FDA) advisory committee in 2009 voted to lower the recommended single dose to 650 mg (making 1,000-mg tablets available by prescription only) and to lower the maximum daily limit from its presently recommended 4,000 mg (Schilling, et al., 2010). The advantage of this drug is that it is well tolerated and has few drug–drug interactions and side effects. Acetaminophen should be avoided in patients with heavy alcohol consumption or chronic liver disease, as the drug is metabolized through the liver. Chronic use of acetaminophen or use of acetaminophen at high doses can cause liver damage, particularly in the elderly; the leading cause of acute liver failure in the United States is acetaminophen overdose (and the leading drug overdose seen in emergency departments is with acetaminophen). Prolonged use of acetaminophen and aspirin or nonsteroidal anti-inflammatory drugs (NSAIDs) should be avoided. The amount of acetaminophen should be limited to 2 g/day for patients taking warfarin (Coumadin) because the combination could increase the International Normalized Ratio (INR) and the risk of bleeding. Acetaminophen overdose is often accidental; patients need to be cautioned not to exceed 4,000 mg/day (preferably less) and to take care not to take other acetaminophen-containing medications in the same day (Schilling, et al., 2010).

Aspirin can also alleviate mild to moderate tension headaches. It inhibits prostaglandin synthesis, reducing the inflammatory response and platelet aggregation. Contraindications to aspirin use include a history of bleeding disorders, asthma, and hypersensitivity to salicylates or NSAIDs. Patients should avoid combining aspirin with other NSAIDs because decreased serum concentrations of NSAIDs result when both drugs are used together. The most common adverse effects associated with aspirin are gastrointestinal in nature, such as nausea, vomiting, or heartburn.

Nonsteroidal Anti-Inflammatory Drugs

NSAIDs work well for moderate tension headaches. They work by inhibiting the enzyme cyclooxygenase-2 (COX-2), responsible for prostaglandin synthesis, thereby reducing inflammation. These drugs take effect in 30 to 60 minutes, similar to aspirin and acetaminophen. Commonly used NSAIDs are ibuprofen, naproxen, ketoprofen, and indomethacin.

Common side effects of NSAIDs are abdominal cramps, nausea, indigestion, and even headache. Occasionally these drugs cause peptic ulcers and GI hemorrhage. Many NSAIDs contain boxed warnings about cardiovascular effects, GI effects, and/or use in patients with renal impairment. COX-2 inhibitors are not indicated specifically for headache but are indicated for acute pain and have shown efficacy in stabbing headache (Ferrante, et al., 2010) and migraine (Wentz, et al., 2008). COX-2 inhibitors also carry black box warnings, particularly for cardiovascular events.

Any given NSAID should be tried in a patient twice before deciding whether it is successful or not. It is not uncommon for a patient to respond poorly to one NSAID and extremely well to another.

Antiemetic Agents

Although patients with tension headaches rarely suffer from nausea, antiemetic agents can augment the pain-relieving properties of analgesics. Commonly used antiemetics are promethazine and prochlorperazine. These medications can be sedating and have numerous other potential side effects, including rare but serious neurologic and bone marrow effects. Patients should be educated about these possible effects before starting on these medications and should be encouraged to use them sparingly.

Other Abortive Agents

For patients whose headaches do not respond to the above agents, certain combination agents can be considered. Some patients have a good response to OTC agents containing acetaminophen, aspirin, and caffeine (such as Excedrin Extra Strength®). However, these agents have a high rate of analgesic MOH when used regularly and probably should not be used more than 1 to 2 days per week.

Prescription combinations that can be used include butalbital/acetaminophen/caffeine (Fioricet® and others) and butalbital/aspirin/caffeine (Fiorinal® and others). Butalbital is a barbiturate, which is sedating and potentially habit-forming; these medications should not be used in patients with a history of substance abuse. Fiorinal and Fioricet very commonly cause MOH and should not be used for more than 3 days per month. If a patient is taking many butalbital-containing pills per day, they must be slowly tapered to avoid withdrawal symptoms. Patients taking these medications should be closely monitored. **Table 38.1** gives an overview of selected drugs used to abort TTH.

Combination acetaminophen/narcotic products such as Vicodin® and Percocet® are not recommended; the FDA has recommended their removal from the market or an inclusion of a black box warning if the drugs remain on the market (FDA, 2009).

Prophylaxis of Tension Headaches

If a patient has more than two tension headaches per week, prophylaxis should be considered. Antidepressant medications are commonly used for headache prophylaxis. Abundant evidence exists for the efficacy of amitriptyline. There are data from a few trials supporting the use of venlafaxine, but data supporting the use of other antidepressants for headache prophylaxis (including migraine) are lacking. Smaller uncontrolled trials or case studies have shown efficacy with other tricyclic antidepressants (TCAs), such as imipramine, doxepin, and protriptyline. While there have been trials conducted on the efficacy of fluoxetine as headache prophylaxis, neither it nor the other selective serotonin reuptake inhibitors (SSRIs) have been shown to be effective as headache prophylaxis despite having a more favorable side effect profile as compared to TCAs. There are data showing efficacy of the selective norepinephrine reuptake inhibitor (SNRI) venlafaxine, which may represent an optimal choice over amitriptyline given the fewer side effects associated with its use (Zissis, et al., 2007). Other antidepressants, such as monoamine oxidase (MAO) inhibitors and serotonin antagonists, have been studied, but safety issues and side effect profiles make them an inappropriate choice for headache prophylaxis. Antidepressants for which little support exists as a headache medicine should only be considered if the headache being treated is comorbid with depression. Alleviation or palliation of one comorbidity, however, will not necessarily resolve the other (Smitherman, et al., 2010). Prophylactic medications should be started at low dosages and increased slowly. It can take 4 to 8 weeks before the full effect of these prophylactic agents is seen. Finding the appropriate prophylactic agent for a patient is a process of trial and error, as medications work differently in different patients.

Amitriptyline, a TCA, is the medication most commonly used to prevent tension headaches. It can be used in doses much lower than those used for treating depression, ranging from 10 to 75 mg. Common side effects include sedation, constipation, blurred vision, and dry mouth. Amitriptyline should be used with caution in patients with a history of coronary artery disease, urinary retention, glaucoma, and seizures. Usually only low doses of amitriptyline are needed, making discontinuation because of side effects uncommon. Higher doses of amitriptyline are typically used in headache patients with concomitant depression (Smitherman, et al., 2010). Given its anticholinergic properties, amitriptyline is an inappropriate choice for use in elderly patients.

Fluoxetine (Prozac®) and venlafaxine (Effexor®) are used with some success in patients with chronic tension headaches. For headache prophylaxis, fluoxetine is commonly used in doses of 20 to 40 mg/d, and venlafaxine is recommended at 150 mg/d (Bendtsen, et al., 2010). Venlafaxine has performed significantly better vs. placebo for TTH in one trial at a dose of 150 mg/d (Zissis, et al., 2007).

These drugs may also concurrently treat depression and anxiety. Common side effects are nausea, somnolence, and insomnia, which often diminish after a few weeks. Patients may also experience sexual dysfunction, increased sweating, or nervousness; these side effects may or may not diminish with time. Fluoxetine and venlafaxine can interact with many medications. These medications must be tapered down slowly and not abruptly stopped, as withdrawal symptoms may occur.

TABLE 38.1	Overview of Selected Drugs to Abort Tension-Type Headaches		
Generic (Brand) Name and Dosage	**Selected Adverse Events**	**Contraindications**	**Special Considerations**
acetaminophen 325–650 mg q4h–6h limit dose to 3,250 mg/d	Severe hepatotoxicity on acute overdose, potential liver damage w/ chronic daily dosing, nephrotoxicity, agranulocytosis, rash	Chronic alcohol use, alcoholic liver disease, impaired liver or renal function, G6PD deficiency	Avoid using w/alcohol.
aspirin 325–650 mg q4h–6h, not to exceed 4,000 mg/d	GI upset (stomach pain, nausea, heartburn, vomiting); GI bleeding and angioedema (uncommon)	Platelet or bleeding disorders, renal dysfunction, erosive gastritis, peptic ulcer disease, asthma, rhinitis, nasal polyps, severe hepatic or renal failure, or sensitivity to salicylates	Avoid using w/NSAIDs, alcohol, during pregnancy, and in children <16 y with viral infections. Discontinue 1–2 wk prior to surgery.
NSAIDs ibuprofen 200–400 mg q4h–6h, not to exceed 1,200 mg/d; under clinical supervision not to exceed ≤2,400 mg/d *Note*: Use lower doses in patients w/renal or hepatic disease.	3%–9%: Dizziness, rash, epigastric pain, heartburn, nausea, tinnitus	**WARNING: NSAIDs are associated with an increased risk of adverse cardiovascular thrombotic events, including MI, stroke, and new onset or worsening of preexisting hypertension. Use is contraindicated for treatment of perioperative pain in the setting of CABG surgery.** Recent GI bleed, 3rd trimester of pregnancy, renal disease	Use w/caution if history of CHF, HTN, GI bleeding. Monitor for anemia w/ long-term use. Elderly are at increased risk for AEs even at low doses. Withhold for at least 4–6 half-lives prior to dental or surgical procedures. May increase risk of GI irritation, inflammation, ulceration, bleeding, and perforation
naproxen initial: 500 mg, then 250 mg q6h–8h not to exceed 1,250 mg/d *Note*: enteric-coated formulations not recommended for tx of acute migraine (Matchar, et al., 2000)	3%–9%: Edema, dizziness, drowsiness, headache, pruritus, skin eruption, ecchymosis, fluid retention, abdominal pain, constipation, nausea, heartburn, hemolysis, tinnitus, dyspnea	Same as above, including **BOXED WARNING**	Same as above
ketoprofen 25–50 mg q6h–8h	>10%: Dyspepsia, abnormal LFTs; 3%–9%: Headache, abdominal pain, constipation, diarrhea, flatulence, nausea, renal dysfunction	Same as above, including **BOXED WARNING**	Same as above
Barbiturates Fioricet: butalbital 50 mg, caffeine 40 mg, acetaminophen 325 mg 1–2 tabs q4h, not to exceed 6 tabs/d *Note:* Do not use butalbital for management of acute migraine.	Drowsiness, lightheadedness, dizziness, sedation, shortness of breath, nausea, vomiting, abdominal pain, intoxicated feeling	Hepatic or renal dysfunction, peptic ulcer disease, history of substance abuse, porphyria, pregnancy, concomitant use w/alcohol or other CNS depressants	Contains acetaminophen. Use w/caution when taking other acetaminophen-containing drugs; do not exceed a total daily dose of 3,250 mg acetaminophen. May be habit-forming or subject to abuse; avoid prolonged use or using w/other sedating medications. Not recommended for use in the elderly.

| TABLE 38.1 | Overview of Selected Drugs to Abort Tension-Type Headaches (*Continued*) |

Generic (Brand) Name and Dosage	Selected Adverse Events	Contraindications	Special Considerations
butalbital 50 mg/ caffeine 40 mg/ aspirin 325 mg (Fiorinal®) 1–2 tabs q4h, not to exceed 6 tabs/d *Note*: Do not use butalbital for management of acute migraine.	Drowsiness, lightheadedness, dizziness, sedation, shortness of breath, nausea, vomiting, abdominal pain, and intoxicated feeling	Hemorrhagic diathesis (e.g., hemophilia, hypoprothrombinemia, von Willebrand's disease, thrombocytopenias, thrombasthenia and other ill-defined hereditary platelet dysfunctions, severe vitamin K deficiency, and severe liver damage) Nasal polyps, angioedema and bronchospastic reactivity to aspirin or other NSAIDs Peptic ulcer or other serious GI lesions Porphyria	Use w/caution in the debilitated; severe impairment of renal or hepatic function, coagulation disorders, head injuries, elevated intracranial pressure, acute abdominal conditions, hypothyroidism, urethral stricture, Addison's disease, or prostatic hypertrophy. Not recommended for use in the elderly.

An additional caution when considering the use of any antidepressant is that of suicidal ideation, particularly in adolescents. In 2007, the FDA required black box warnings in all antidepressant-prescribing information "…about increased risks of suicidal thinking and behavior, known as suicidality, in young adults ages 18 to 24 during initial treatment (generally the first 1 to 2 months)" (FDA, 2007). **Table 38.2** lists prophylactic agents for TTH.

First-Line Therapy for Tension Headaches

Aspirin and acetaminophen are appropriate first-line agents. They should be used no more than 2 days per week, as with any other analgesic agents, to avoid MOH. Acetaminophen should be used at a maximum single dose of 650 mg and a maximum daily dose of 3,250 mg. If used judiciously, these agents have few adverse effects and are very well tolerated. They work best for mild to moderate headaches.

Second-Line Therapy for Tension Headaches

NSAIDs are the next option for treatment of TTH. If one agent fails for two consecutive headaches, another agent in this class should be tried. NSAIDs seem to work well for more stubborn TTH. If they provide incomplete relief, an antiemetic agent may be added to augment their effect.

Another second-line agent to try is an OTC caffeine-containing analgesic. These medications should be used infrequently and may be alternated with NSAIDs for different headaches.

Third-Line Therapy for Tension Headaches

If the above agents fail, then butalbital-containing compounds (Fioricet or Fiorinal) may be used in patients without specific risk factors for these medications. These agents may also be reserved as backup if the above-mentioned agents fail to relieve a more severe TTH. Again, butalbital-containing agents should never be used more than 3 days per month, as they easily trigger MOH.

As mentioned earlier, any patient requiring treatment for two or more headaches per week or who has particularly severe TTH should be considered for a prophylactic agent (**Table 38.3** and **Figure 38-1**).

CAUSES OF MIGRAINE HEADACHE

Why some patients experience migraines while others do not is unknown, but it is clear that there is a genetic component to migraines and that migraines tend to cluster in families (Kallela, et al., 2001). There are many possible migraine triggers, and each patient's triggers are unique. Triggers range from certain foods to too much or too little sleep to medications to hormonal factors and others. In some patients, no obvious triggers are found. Estrogen is thought to play a role in the development of migraines, which explains the predominance of migraines in females. About 25% of migraine attacks occur within 4 days of menses, when estrogen has fallen to a low level (Fox & Davis, 1998). The best way to pinpoint triggers is to have the patient keep a diary of what he or she ate and did in the 12 hours before getting the headache to see if any patterns emerge. **Box 38.3** lists migraine triggers.

PATHOPHYSIOLOGY OF MIGRAINE HEADACHES

While previously believed to be vasculogenic in nature, neurogenic mechanisms are now recognized as the underlying cause of migraine pathophysiology. According to this concept, migraine pain is thought to originate from the trigeminovascular system of the cerebrum. This system is a network of fibers that surrounds cranial blood vessels in close proximity, allowing for regulation of the environment of the vessel wall. The trigeminovascular system is an initiator and promoter of tissue inflammation, and, when activated, releases neuropeptides that cause vasodilation and inflammation. Noradrenergic and, more significantly, serotonergic

| TABLE 38.2 | Overview of Selected Drugs Used to Prevent Tension-Type Headaches |

Generic (Brand) Name and Dosage	Selected Adverse Events	Contraindications	Special Consideration
amitriptyline initial: 10–25 mg qhs, usual dose 150 mg qhs; reported dosing ranges 10–400 mg/d (higher doses in patients w/ concomitant depression)	Degree of anticholinergic effects (urinary retention, dry mouth, constipation) are higher in amitriptyline than in other TCAs; drowsiness/sedation (sometimes significant), orthostasis, conduction abnormalities	**WARNING:** **Antidepressants increase the risk of suicidal thinking and behavior in children, adolescents, and young adults (ages 18 to 24) with major depressive disorder and other psychiatric disorders.** Not FDA-approved for children <age 12	Most widely used. Use w/caution in patients w/ history of CVD (stroke, MI, tachycardia, or conduction abnormalities). Use w/caution in patients w/BPH, glaucoma, urinary retention, xerostomia, visual problems, constipation, or history of bowel obstruction. Use w/caution in patients with diabetes, seizures, hyperthyroidism (or thyroid supplementation), or hepatic or renal dysfunction. Effects may be intensified by use of other CNS drugs or alcohol. Use w/caution in the elderly.
fluoxetine 20–40 mg daily w/ tapered discontinuation	Insomnia, nausea, dry mouth, sexual symptoms	**See BOXED WARNING above** Pregnancy, concomitant use of MAO inhibitors, pimozide, or thioridazine MAO inhibitor use must be stopped 14 d before initiation of fluoxetine. Fluoxetine must be discontinued 5 wk prior to start of MAO inhibitors, mesoridazine, and thioridazine.	Monitor for suicidality and serotonin syndrome or neuroleptic malignant syndrome-like reactions. Monitor for rash, anaphylaxis, and pulmonary syndromes. Asses for mania/hypomania prior to use. Monitor for seizures, altered appetite and weight, bleeding, hyponatremia, anxiety, and insomnia.

neurons regulate this activity. Modulation of pain control is disrupted, contributing to allodynia (Smitherman, et al., 2010). The trigeminovascular system may be activated by the "migraine generator" in the brain stem. The "migraine generator" includes the neuromodulatory locus coeruleus (noradrenergic), dorsal raphe nucleus (serotonergic), and periaqueductal gray region (pain modulation). Once triggered, impulses travel out through cranial nerve VII and ultimately result in dilated meningeal blood vessels and release of neuroinflammatory compounds, which subsequently results in more vasodilation (Smitherman, et al., 2010). The "migraine generator" may receive its trigger(s) from the cerebral cortex, thalamus, or hypothalamus in response to emotion or stress, circadian rhythm disruption, or environmental factors, including lights, strong odors, and loud noises (Lance, 1993).

DIAGNOSTIC CRITERIA FOR MIGRAINE HEADACHE

The first step in making a precise diagnosis of migraine is to obtain a thorough headache history. Evaluation of the history should include age at onset; time of day when attacks occur; duration of attack; precipitating or relieving factors; nature, intensity, and location of headache pain; and any associated symptoms. The patient should also be questioned about any aura symptoms, such as visual symptoms (flashing lights, loss of peripheral vision, diplopia) or other sensory symptoms (vertigo, tinnitus, paresthesias, or hemiparesis). Because a family history is evident in many patients, asking if anyone in the family experiences migraines aids in the diagnosis. Specific diagnostic criteria for migraine with aura (classic migraine) and without aura (common migraine) are given in **Box 38.4**.

TABLE 38.3	Recommended Order for Treatment of Tension-Type Headaches	
Order	**Agents**	**Comments**
First line	Aspirin or acetaminophen	Not to be used more than 2 days a week
Second line	NSAIDs and/or caffeine-containing analgesics	Antiemetic may be added if needed
Third line	Butalbital-containing compounds	Not to be used more than 3 days a month

Patients most frequently experience migraines in the early morning, but a migraine attack can come at any time of the day. Migraines are more often unilateral than bilateral, with the pain occurring around the eye or the temple. Migraine pain generally peaks 2 to 12 hours into the attack. Common symptoms accompanying migraine include nausea, anxiety, depression, irritability, fatigue, light and noise sensitivity, diarrhea or constipation, and hunger or anorexia. Patients may describe the pain of migraine as pounding, pulsating, or throbbing. A migraine sufferer often seeks refuge in a dark, quiet place.

INITIATING DRUG THERAPY FOR MIGRAINE HEADACHES

Practitioners must consider many factors when designing a treatment regimen for patients with migraine, such as the severity of the pain, duration of attack, concomitant disease states, current medication use, and any triggers. Migraine treatment needs to be highly individualized. **Table 38.4** gives an overview of selected drugs used for abortive treatment of migraine headaches; **Figure 38-2** provides a treatment algorithm for acute management of migraine.

The most effective treatment for migraines involves both nonpharmacologic and pharmacologic approaches. Nonpharmacologic approaches include various psychological techniques that aid in managing the migraine attack. Relaxation, stress management, and biofeedback are some techniques used to reduce migraine severity and frequency. Progressive muscle relaxation and the use of autogenic phrases are examples of relaxation techniques. (See section on tension headaches.) It helps for patients to keep a diary detailing their headaches and the circumstances surrounding them to uncover any triggers or patterns.

Goals of Drug Therapy

The main goal of pharmacologic therapy is to relieve the migraine attack with minimal or no side effects. Short-term goals include decreasing the severity and duration of the headache and relieving nausea, if present. Long-term goals established by the U.S. Headache Consortium include reducing attack frequency and severity, reducing disability, improving quality of life, preventing headache, avoiding headache medication escalation, and educating and enabling patients to manage their disease (Matchar, et al., 2000). Efficacy endpoints in the management of migraine (i.e., in clinical trials) are generally recognized as being pain-free (no pain) or headache relief (improvement) response at 2 hours post-dose, reduction in 24-hour recurrence rate, and favorable adverse event profile (Johnston & Rapoport, 2010).

Nonsteroidal Anti-Inflammatory Drugs

First-line agents for mild to moderate migraines are NSAIDs and aspirin. These medications, like all migraine medication, work best when taken early in the attack. The most common side effects are gastrointestinal. The same doses as used for tension headaches are appropriate for migraines. Aspirin may be used in initial dosages of up to 900 mg. Aspirin alone is effective in up to 40% of migraine patients (Silberstein, 2002). As with tension headaches, a given NSAID should be used on more than one occasion before deciding whether it is efficacious.

Caffeine-Containing Compounds

Over-the-counter caffeine-containing compounds (such as Excedrin Extra Strength® or Excedrin Migraine®) are also effective for milder migraines, but they can easily cause MOH and should be used no more than 3 days per month or for more than 48 hours at a time. These preparations also contain acetaminophen (250 mg per tablet), so caution is required if acetaminophen or many of the other OTC or prescription acetaminophen-containing preparations are being used (Schilling, et al., 2010).

5-HT$_1$ Receptor Agonists (Triptans)

Triptans are migraine-specific drugs that work as 5-HT$_1$ serotonin receptor agonists. These receptors are located on intracranial blood vessels, presynaptically on CNS sensory neurons, and trigeminal terminals. Triptans cause cerebral vasoconstriction and can treat both the pain and nausea of migraine.

Triptans are indicated for acute treatment of migraine with or without aura, and they are used for moderate to severe migraines or for milder migraines that do not respond to NSAIDs, aspirin, or the above combination drugs. Triptans vary in their time to peak concentration, half-lives, adverse event profiles, formulation, and route of administration, which helps guide the selection of a triptan for a particular patient. Given the highly individualized nature of migraine, different medications may be more effective than others in any given patient. If a triptan fails on two separate occasions, another triptan should be tried. Triptans work best when given early in the course of a migraine, but unlike many other agents, they may be effective even when given late in the course of a migraine.

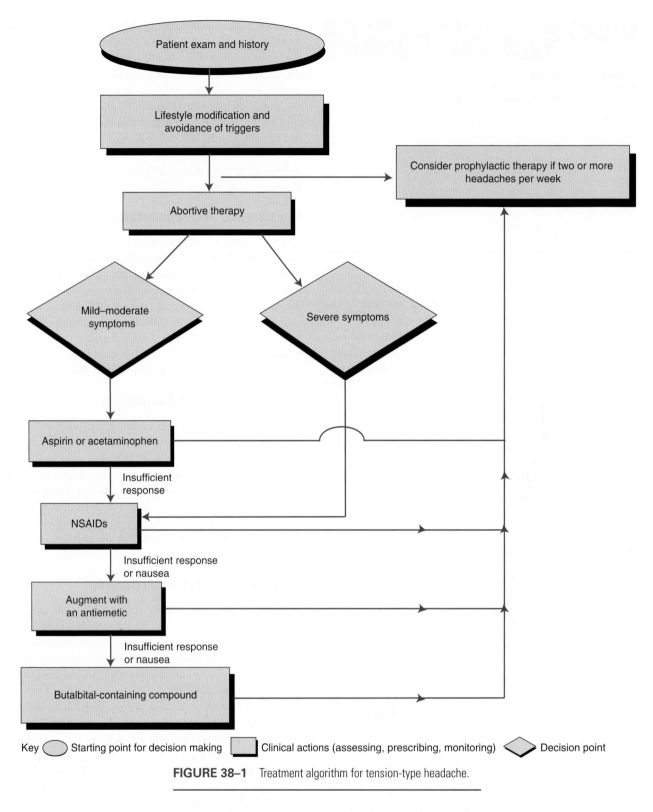

FIGURE 38–1 Treatment algorithm for tension-type headache.

Triptans should not be used more than 9 days per month and should not be used within 24 hours of any other vasoconstricting drug, such as ergotamine. Use of these medications is considered to be a better choice than use of the ergot derivatives as potency is similar, but adverse events are significantly fewer in number (Khoury & Couch, 2010). Triptans should

be avoided in patients with basilar, hemiplegic, or retinal migraines; they must also be avoided in patients with coronary artery disease, cerebrovascular disease, or severe peripheral vascular disease.

The seven triptan drugs are sumatriptan, zolmitriptan, naratriptan, rizatriptan, almotriptan, eletriptan, and

BOX 38.3

Factors That May Trigger Migraine Headaches

PSYCHOLOGICAL FACTORS

Anxiety
Depression
Stress

MEDICATIONS

Cimetidine
Cocaine
Hormones (contraceptives, hormone replacement therapy)
Indomethacin
Mestranol
Nicotine
Nifedipine
Nitroglycerin
Reserpine

DIETARY FACTORS

Alcohol
Aspartame
Caffeine
Chocolate
Monosodium glutamate
Tyramine-containing foods (e.g., red wine)

ENVIRONMENTAL FACTORS

Bright, flashing lights or glare
High altitude
Loud noises
Strong odors
Tobacco smoke
Weather changes

LIFESTYLE FACTORS

Dieting/skipping meals
Strenuous exercise
Too much or too little sleep

HORMONAL FACTORS

Menopause
Menses
Pregnancy

BOX 38.4

Diagnostic Criteria for Migraine (ICHD –2)

MIGRAINE WITHOUT AURA

A. At least five attacks fulfilling criteria B–D
B. Headache attacks lasting 4–72 hours (untreated or unsuccessfully treated)
C. Headache has at least two of the following characteristics:
   1. unilateral location
   2. pulsating quality
   3. moderate or severe pain intensity
   4. aggravation by or causing avoidance of routine physical activity (e.g., walking or climbing stairs)
D. During headache, at least one of the following:
   1. Nausea and/or vomiting
   2. Photophobia and phonophobia
E. Not attributed to another disorder

MIGRAINE WITH AURA

A. At least two attacks fulfilling criteria B–D
B. Aura consisting of at least one of the following, but no motor weakness:
   1. fully reversible visual symptoms, including positive features (e.g., flickering lights, spots or lines) and/or negative features (i.e., loss of vision)
   2. fully reversible sensory symptoms including positive features (i.e., pins and needles) and/or negative features (i.e., numbness)
   3. fully reversible dysphasic speech disturbance
C. At least two of the following:
   1. homonymous visual symptoms and/or unilateral sensory symptoms
   2. at least one aura symptom develops gradually over ≥5 minutes and/or different aura symptoms occur in succession over ≥5 minutes
   3. each symptom lasts ≥5 and ≤60 minutes
D. Headache fulfilling criteria B–D for *Migraine without Aura* begins during the aura or follows aura within 60 minutes
E. Not attributed to another disorder

Data from Headache Classification Subcommittee of the International Headache Society. (2004). The international classification of headache disorders, 2nd ed. *Cephalalgia*, *24*(Suppl. 1), 1–160.

TABLE 38.4 Overview of Selected Drugs for Acute Migraine Treatment

Generic (Trade) Name and Dosage	Selected Adverse Events	Contraindications	Special Considerations
aspirin 325–650 mg q4h-6h, not to exceed 4,000 mg/d	GI upset (stomach pain, nausea, heartburn, vomiting); GI bleeding and angioedema (uncommon)	Platelet or bleeding disorders, renal dysfunction, erosive gastritis, peptic ulcer disease, asthma, rhinitis, nasal polyps, severe hepatic or renal failure, or sensitivity to salicylates	Avoid using w/ NSAIDs, alcohol, during pregnancy, and in children <16 y with viral infections. Discontinue 1–2 wk prior to surgery.
NSAIDs See Table 38.1.	See Table 38.1.	See Table 38.1 (including **BOXED WARNING**).	See Table 38.1.
OTC caffeine-containing compounds (Excedrin® Extra-Strength or Excedrin® Migraine; acetaminophen 250 mg/aspirin 250 mg/caffeine 65 mg) 1–2 tabs q24h; do not use for longer than 48 h	Insomnia, agitation	Uncontrolled HTN	Avoid use with other vasoconstriction agents.
Triptans sumatriptan (Imitrex®) 25, 50, 100 mg PO at headache onset, may repeat dose up to 100 mg in 2 h 6 mg subcutaneous, may repeat dose in 2 h 5 or 20 mg intranasal; may repeat dose in 2 h	PO: 3% – >10%: Malaise/fatigue, jaw pain/lightness/pressure, paresthesia, pressure/lightness/heaviness, warm/cold sensation SC: >10%: Dizziness, warm/hot sensation, pain at injection site, paresthesia; 3%–10%: chest pain/lightness/heaviness/pressure, burning, feeling of heaviness, flushing, pressure sensation, feeling of tightness, drowsiness, neck, throat, and jaw pain/lightness/pressure, mouth/tongue discomfort, weakness, numbness, throat discomfort IN: >10%: Bad taste, nausea, vomiting; 5-10%: nasal discomfort/disorder	Pregnancy, uncontrolled HTN, ischemic heart disease, stroke, TIA, PVD, severe hepatic impairment, basilar or hemiplegic migraine Use within 24 hr of use of ergot derivatives, or within 2 wk of (or concomitant) use of MAO inhibitors. Do not use as prophylactic treatment for migraine. Not for IV use.	Use w/caution in history of CAD, HTN, seizure disorder (or low seizure threshold), or hepatic impairment. Use caution with concomitant use of other serotonergic drugs (SSRIs, SNRIs, other triptans) or proserotonergic drugs (tryptophan). Use at lowest possible doses.
zolmitriptan (Zomig®) tablet: 2.5 mg at onset orally disintegrating tablet: 2.5 mg at onset nasal spray: 1 spray (5 mg) at onset	PO: 3%–10%: Chest pain, dizziness, somnolence, pain, nausea, xerostomia, dyspepsia, paresthesia, weakness, warm/cold sensation, neck/throat/jaw pain, diaphoresis	Pregnancy, ischemic heart disease or vasospastic CAD, uncontrolled HTN, symptomatic Wolff-Parkinson-White syndrome or other arrhythmias associated w/ accessory cardiac conduction pathway disorders Use within 24 hr of (or concomitant) use of another 5HT₁ agonist, or use within 2 wk of (or concomitant) use of MAO inhibitors Concomitant use w/ergot derivatives or sibutramine Management of basilar or hemiplegic migraine Additional contraindications for IN use: stroke, TIA, PVD	High risk factors for heart disease (HTN, high cholesterol, obesity, diabetes, smoking, strong family history of heart disease, postmenopausal women, and males >40 years old)

Drug/Dosing	Adverse Effects	Contraindications	Precautions/Comments
naratriptan (Amerge®) 2.5 mg q4h to max of 5 mg/d	1%–10%: Dizziness, drowsiness, malaise/fatigue, nausea, vomiting, paresthesia, pain/pressure in throat or neck	Pregnancy, uncontrolled HTN, ischemic heart disease, PVD, severe hepatic or renal impairment Use within 24 hr of (or concomitant) use of ergot derivatives or sibutramine Treatment of basilar or hemiplegic migraine	Use w/caution in patients w/risk factors for CAD, smoking (decreases serum concentrations), cerebral/subarachnoid hemorrhage, stroke, peripheral vascular ischemia, and history of HTN. Not recommended for use in elderly Use lowest possible dose.
rizatriptan (Maxalt®) oral tablet and Maxalt-MLT®, orally disintegrating tablet) tablet: 5–10 mg q2h to max of 30 mg/d (patients taking concomitant propranolol: max of 15 mg/d) orally disintegrating tablet: 5–10 mg q2h to max of 30 mg/d (patients taking concomitant propranolol: max of 15 mg/d) *Note:* Patients w/cardiac risks should be administered first dose in the physician's office under observation.	>10%: Dizziness, drowsiness, fatigue (dose-dependent) 1%–10%: Increase in BP, chest pain, palpitations, flushing, mild increases in GH, hot flashes, abdominal pain, xerostomia, nausea, dyspnea	Documented ischemic heart disease or Prinzmetal's angina or uncontrolled HTN Use within 24 hr of (or concomitant) use of another 5HT₁ agonist, or use within 2 wk of (or concomitant) use of MAO inhibitors, or concomitant use w/ergot derivatives Treatment of basilar or hemiplegic migraine	Reconsider migraine diagnosis if patient does not respond to first dose, patients w/ symptoms of angina post-dose should be evaluated for CAD or Prinzmetal's angina before receiving a second dose. Do not administer to patients w/risk factors for CAD (e.g., HTN, hypercholesterolemia, smoking, obesity, diabetes, strong family history of CAD, menopause, males >age 40) w/o adequate cardiac workup. Evaluate cardiovascular status periodically. Use w/caution in the elderly or in patients w/hepatic or renal impairment (including dialysis). Avoid concomitant use of other serotonergic drugs (SSRIs/SNRIs, other triptans) and serotonin precursors (tryptophan).
almotriptan (Axert®) 6.25–12.5 mg q2h to max of 25 mg/d *Note:* Patients taking potent CYP3A4 inhibitors should only take 6.25 mg as a starting dose to a max of 12.5 mg/d.	3%–10%: Somnolence, dizziness, nausea	Pregnancy, known or suspected ischemic heart disease, stroke TIA, PVD, uncontrolled HTN Use within 24 hr of (or concomitant) use of another 5HT₁ agonist or concomitant use w/ergot derivatives, MAO inhibitors, or sibutramine Treatment of basilar or hemiplegic migraine	Do not use for migraine prophylaxis or cluster headache; if patient doesn't respond to first dose, reconsider migraine diagnosis. Use w/caution in patients w/sulfonamide allergy (blindness may occur). Do not administer to patients w/risk factors for CAD (e.g., HTN, hypercholesterolemia, smoking, obesity, diabetes, strong family history of CAD, menopause, males >age 40) w/o adequate cardiac workup. Evaluate cardiovascular status periodically. Use w/ caution in patients w/ hepatic or renal impairment, avoid concomitant use of other serotonergic drugs (SSRIs/SNRIs, other triptans).
eletriptan (Relpax®) 20–40 mg q2h to max of 80 mg/d	3%–10%: Chest pain/tightness, dizziness, somnolence, headache, nausea, xerostomia, weakness, paresthesia	Pregnancy, ischemic heart disease or signs or symptoms of ischemic heart disease, stroke, TIA, PVD, or uncontrolled HTN Severe hepatic impairment Concomitant use within 24 hr of an ergot derivative or another 5HT₁ agonist, or within 72 hours of potent CYP3A4 inhibitors or sibutramine Treatment of basilar or hemiplegic migraine. Migraine prophylaxis	If patient doesn't respond to first dose, reconsider migraine diagnosis. Do not administer to patients w/risk factors for CAD w/o adequate cardiac workup. Evaluate cardiovascular status periodically. Use w/caution in patients w/mild to moderate hepatic impairment. Avoid concomitant use of other serotonergic drugs (SSRIs/SNRIs, other triptans) or serotonin precursors (tryptophan).

(continued)

TABLE 38.4 **Overview of Selected Drugs for Acute Migraine Treatment** *(Continued)*

Generic (Trade) Name and Dosage	Selected Adverse Events	Contraindications	Special Considerations
frovatriptan (Frova®) 2.5 mg q2h to max of 7.5 mg/d	3%–10%: Flushing, dizziness, fatigue, headache, hot or cold sensation, xerostomia, paresthesia, skeletal pain	Ischemic heart disease or signs and symptoms of ischemic heart disease, stroke, TIA, PVD, or uncontrolled HTN Concomitant use within 24 h of an ergot derivative or another 5HT₁ agonist Concomitant use w/ sibutramine Treatment of hemiplegic or basilar migraine	Not intended for migraine prophylaxis or cluster headache; rule out underlying neurologic disease in patients w/ atypical headache or migraine (w/ no prior history of migraine), or inadequate clinical response to first dose. Do not administer to patients w/risk factors for CAD w/o adequate cardiac workup. Evaluate cardiovascular status periodically. Slow onset, longest half-life of the triptans.
Ergot Derivatives			
ergotamine tartrate (Ergomar®) 2 mg SL at start of migraine, then 1 tab q30min if needed, to 3 tab/d and 5 tab/wk	Serious vasoconstrictive distress (ischemia, cyanosis, absence of pulse, cold extremities, gangrene, precordial distress and pain, ECG changes and muscle pains), transient tachycardia or bradycardia and hypertension, nausea, vomiting, paresthesias, numbness, weakness, vertigo, localized edema, itching, rare fibrosis (retroperitoneal, pleuropulmonary, and heart valve)	**WARNING: Serious and/or life-threatening peripheral ischemia has been associated with the coadministration of ergotamine tartrate with potent CYP3A4 inhibitors, including protease inhibitors and macrolide antibiotics. Because CYP3A4 inhibition elevates the serum levels of ergotamine tartrate, the risk for vasospasm leading to cerebral ischemia and/or ischemia of the extremities is increased. Hence, concomitant use of these medications is contraindicated.** Pregnancy category X PVD, coronary heart disease, or HTN Impaired hepatic or renal function Sepsis	Withdrawal and MOH may occur with prolonged use.
dihydroergotamine (Migranal®) IM/SC: 1 mg first sign of headache, repeat hourly to a max dose of 3 mg total, to a max dose of 6 mg/wk IV: 1 mg first sign of headache, repeat hourly to a max dose of 2 mg total, to a max of 6 mg/wk Intranasal: 1 spray (0.5 mg) each nostril, repeat q15min if necessary, to a max of 4 sprays to a max of 6 sprays/d and a max of 8 sprays/wk	Nasal spray >10%: Rhinitis; 3%–10%: Dizziness, somnolence, nausea, taste disturbance, vomiting, application site reaction, pharyngitis	**See BOXED WARNING above** Pregnancy category X Ischemic heart disease (angina pectoris, history of MI, or documented silent ischemia) Patients w/clinical symptoms or findings consistent w/ coronary artery vasospasm, including Prinzmetal's variant angina Uncontrolled HTN Use of 5HT₁ agonists, ergotamine-containing or ergot-type medications or methysergide within 24h Treatment of hemiplegic or basilar migraine PAD Sepsis Following vascular surgery Severely impaired hepatic or renal function	Use only when a clear diagnosis of migraine headache has been established. Not for prolonged use. Use with caution in the elderly.

Drug/Dose	Side Effects	Contraindications	Comments
caffeine/ergotamine (Cafergot®) PO: 1 mg ergotamine/100 mg caffeine; 1–2 tabs at onset; may repeat after 1h to max of 6 tabs/d rectal: 2 mg ergotamine/100 mg caffeine: 1 supp PR; may repeat after 1 h to max 2 supp/d	Nausea, vomiting, irritability, palpitations, paresthesias, MOH, dizziness tingling of the extremities, rare MI	**WARNING Serious and/or life-threatening peripheral ischemia has been associated with coadministration of Cafergot with potent CYP3A4 inhibitors (e.g., protease inhibitors, macrolide antibiotics). Because CYP3A4 inhibition elevates serum levels of Cafergot, the risk of vasospasm leading to cerebral ischemia and/or ischemia of the extremities is increased. Concomitant use of these medications is contraindicated.** HTN, PVD, and CAD Pregnancy Impaired hepatic or renal function Sepsis	Use w/caution with concomitant use of less potent CYP3A4 inhibitors. Avoid excessive or prolonged use. Not indicated for migraine prophylaxis. Monitor use in mild to moderate hepatic impairment. MOH may be associated w/ prolonged and uninterrupted use.
Barbiturates—See Table 38.1			
Opioids butorphanol nasal spray (1 mg) 1 spray in 1 nostril, may repeat in 1 hr; can repeat initial dosing sequence q3–4h PRN adjust for renal and hepatic impairment: 1 mg at onset, 1 mg 60–90 min later, then at intervals of no less than 6 hr	>10%: Somnolence, dizziness, nausea and/or vomiting, nasal congestion, insomnia	History of substance abuse	Use w/caution in impaired renal, hepatic, or pulmonary function. Use w/caution in the elderly.
acetaminophen w/codeine (Tylenol® w/codeine) 1–2 tabs q4h to a max of 12 tabs/d Tylenol w/codeine 3: 30 mg codeine, 300 mg acetaminophen Tylenol w/codeine 4: 60 mg codeine, 300 mg acetaminophen	Severe hepatotoxicity on acute overdose, potential liver damage w/ chronic daily dosing, nephrotoxicity, agranulocytosis, rash, drowsiness, constipation	Chronic alcohol use, alcoholic liver disease, or impaired liver or renal function G6PD deficiency History of substance abuse Pregnancy (prolonged use or high doses at term)	May be used sparingly in pregnancy Do not exceed 3,250 mg acetaminophen/d (including concomitant use of other acetaminophen-containing drugs). Decrease dose in patients w/renal impairment. Use w/caution in patients w/respiratory disorders, CNS depression/coma, head trauma, morbid obesity, prostatic hyperplasia, urinary stricture, thyroid dysfunction, or severe renal or liver insufficiency. May cause CNS depression or hypotension Use w/ caution in patients w/ hypovolemia or cardiovascular disease. Abrupt discontinuation after prolonged use may result in withdrawal.
Steroids dexamethasone single dose of 4 mg or 4 mg bid ×2 d then 4 mg daily ×3 d w/tapered discontinuation	Nausea, GI upset, insomnia, mood swings, rare and serious steroid psychosis, peptic ulcer disease, CHF	Pregnancy Systemic fungal infections Do not use w/acute head injury. Avoid concomitant use w/aldesleukin, BCG, dronedarone, everolimus, natalizumab, nilotinib, nisoldipine, pazopanib, ranolazine, romidepsin, tolvaptan, and live vaccines	Use as rescue medication only. Use w/caution in thyroid disease, hepatic and renal impairment, CVD, DM, glaucoma, cataracts, myasthenia gravis, GI diseases, and in patients at risk for osteoporosis or seizures. Use w/caution in the elderly at the lowest possible dose for a short duration.

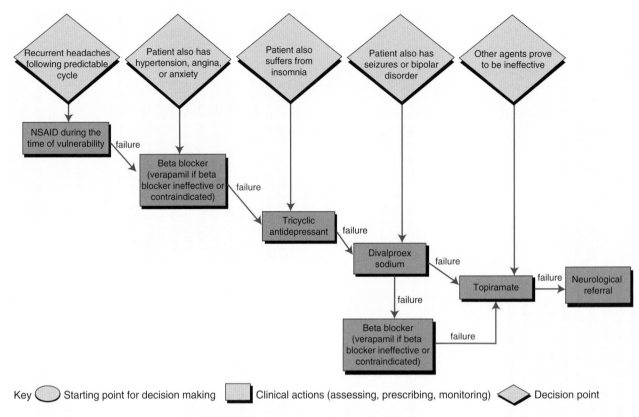

Key ◯ Starting point for decision making ▢ Clinical actions (assessing, prescribing, monitoring) ◇ Decision point

FIGURE 38–2 Treatment algorithm for migraine prophylaxis.

frovatriptan. Sumatriptan and zolmitriptan are available as a nasal spray, and sumatriptan has a subcutaneous form. These are useful for patients with severe nausea who cannot tolerate an oral medication. Rizatriptan is also available as an orally disintegrating tablet. The injectable form of sumatriptan has the fastest onset of action of any of the triptans, but has a short half-life, often giving limited headache relief. Sumatriptan is also associated with more adverse events than the other trip-tans. Frovatriptan has the longest half-life of the triptans, at 26 hours, making it useful for patients with long-lasting migraines. Use of the triptans in the early, mild stages of migraine (but not during aura) results in greater relief (up to 70% pain–free in clinical trials) than use of the drugs during moderate or severe migraine (up to 30% pain–free in clinical trials), but the patient needs to be able to recognize onset of migraine and distinguish it from TTH. Use of a triptan for more than 9 days per month may result in MOH, during which time preven-tive therapy will be ineffective (Tfelt-Hansen, 2007; Khoury & Couch, 2010).

Sumatriptan

Sumatriptan (Imitrex®) was the first triptan on the market (FDA-approved in 1992 and now available as a generic) and still offers the fastest relief of all the triptans presently available. In its subcutane-ous form, it offers the highest therapeutic gain of all the triptans in clinical trials. It is safe and well tolerated (available OTC in the UK) (Tfelt-Hansen, 2007; Johnston & Rapoport, 2010; Antonaci,

et al., 2010). Sumatriptan is available in tablets (25, 50, and 100 mg), a nasal spray (20 mg), and a subcutaneous injection (6 mg). (See **Table 38.4**.)

Injectable sumatriptan offers the quickest onset of action (10 minutes), whereas the effects of the tablet take longer (30 to 90 minutes). Injectable sumatriptan is associated with more adverse events than oral sumatriptan (Johnston & Rapoport, 2010). If the headache recurs, the patient can take a second dose of medication, but only after a certain time and without exceeding the maximum dose of 200 mg/d. Patients with migraine with aura cannot take sumatriptan until the headache actually begins because the drug has no effect on relieving aura symptoms. In one trial, 2 hours after oral admin-istration of 100 mg sumatriptan, 58% of patients improved and 35% were pain–free; after injection of 6 mg sumatriptan, 71% of patients improved within 1 hour, 79% improved within 2 hours, and 43% were pain–free after 1 hour and 60% after 2 hours (Ferrari, 1998). Patients with nausea and vomiting tend to find the nasal formulation easier to take. Pain relief may be dose-dependent, but with increased doses come increased adverse events (Johnston & Rapoport, 2010).

Zolmitriptan

Zolmitriptan (Zomig®; FDA-approved in 1997 and now avail-able as a generic) is available in tablet form, nasal spray, and oral disintegrating form. The recommended initial dose of zolmitrip-tan is 2.5 mg. (See **Table 38.4**.) The onset of effect is attained within 45 minutes, resulting in a rapid therapeutic response. Its half-life is 3 hours, longer than that of sumatriptan, and it is extremely potent at serotonin receptors. Zolmitriptan has been shown in clinical trials to be similar in efficacy to sumatriptan (5 mg vs. 100 mg, respectively), and at a dose of 2.5 mg, it is similar in efficacy to sumatriptan 50 mg, almotriptan 12.5 mg, eletriptan 40 mg, and rizatriptan 10 mg. Therapeutic gain is slightly higher in nasal and orally disintegrating formulations. Efficacy may be dose-dependent, with a concomitant increase in adverse events. Contraindications and adverse effects are similar to the other triptans. (See **Table 38.4**.)

Naratriptan

Naratriptan (Amerge®; FDA-approved in 1998 and now available as a generic) is marketed as an alternative agent for patients who are taking repeated doses of other migraine therapies, specifically those who have recurrent headache or chest tightness when using oral sumatriptan. Naratriptan is available only in 1 mg and 2.5 mg tablet formulation (see **Table 38.4**) and reaches peak serum concentrations in 2 to 3 hours. While onset is slow, duration of action is longest of all the triptans; because of its long half-life of 6 hours, headache recurrences are not common. Therapeutic gain at 4 hours (as compared with 2) tends to be higher in this triptan. In the original clinical trial, headache relief was experienced by 68% of patients 4 hours post-dose, and was maintained for 8 to 24 hours. Given its availability only in low dosages, its side effect profile in clinical trials was comparable to placebo, making this triptan a good option for patients experiencing intolerable side effects with other triptans (Johnston & Rapoport, 2010; Mathew, et al., 1997).

Rizatriptan

Rizatriptan (Maxalt®; FDA-approved in 1998) is available in a tablet (5 and 10 mg) and oral disintegrating tablet (Maxalt-MLT; 5 and 10 mg), offering an alternative way to treat a migraine. Onset of action is rapid, particularly with the orally disintegrating tablet. Rizatriptan 10 mg produces faster relief than sumatriptan 50 mg and naratriptan 2.5 mg, and is similar in efficacy to almotriptan 12.5 mg, eletriptan 40 mg, and zolmitriptan 2.5 mg. Effects of rizatriptan can be observed within 30 minutes and last from 14 to 16 hours. In the original clinical trial, 62% of patients taking the 5-mg dose and 71% of patients taking the 10-mg dose experienced pain relief 2 hours post-dose. Complete relief was achieved in 33% of patients taking a 5-mg dose and 42% of patients taking the 10-mg dose. The drug is well tolerated, even at 10 tablets per month. Recurrence rates in the literature have been mixed (Johnston & Rapoport, 2010; Teall, et al., 1998). Contraindications to the use of rizatriptan can be found in **Table 38.4**.

Almotriptan

Almotriptan (Axert®; FDA-approved in 2001) is a rapidly absorbed triptan with a moderately long half-life (3 to 4 hours). Its efficacy is similar to the other triptans, but its potential for drug–drug interactions is reduced, given that it is metabolized by three separate metabolic pathways. It is a well-tolerated drug with few adverse events and is a good choice for triptan-naïve patients or as an alternate drug for patients who need to be switched over from other triptans due to intolerable side effects (Johnston & Rapoport, 2010). Contraindications to the use of almotriptan can be found in **Table 38.4**.

Eletriptan

Eletriptan (Relpax®; FDA-approved in 2002) is available in 20- and 40-mg tablets. The recommended initial dose is 40 mg at the onset of migraine. If relief is not obtained in 2 hours, the dose may be repeated, to a maximum of 80 mg/d. Onset of action is rapid, and elimination half-life is moderately long (4 hours)—shorter only than naratriptan and frovatriptan. While essentially comparable in efficacy to the other triptans, eletriptan at a dose of 40 mg is the only triptan shown to have greater efficacy than sumatriptan at 100 mg. Both efficacy and adverse events are dose-dependent, although trials have reported adverse events to be transient and mild to moderate in nature. Contraindications and adverse effects are similar to the other triptans. (See **Table 38.4**.)

Frovatriptan

Frovatriptan (Frova®; FDA-approved in 2001) has a half-life of 26 hours, by far the longest of all the triptans. Hence, its therapeutic gain is better assessed at 4 hours rather than 2; the 40-hour headache response rate for frovatriptan is 66%. Like naratriptan, its onset is somewhat slower (although this is not the case in all patients taking the medication in early migraine), but its effects are more sustained. Frovatriptan is also metabolized both by the kidney and hepatic CYP1A2, reducing the likelihood for drug–drug interactions. It has also been shown to be particularly effective in menstrually related migraine, not only as acute relief, but as a 2-day "miniprophylaxis." It is available as a 2.5-mg tablet, which is the recommended dose. If a first dose provides some relief but the headache recurs, another dose may be taken no sooner than 2 hours after the preceding dose, to a maximum of 7.5 mg/day. Contraindications and adverse effects are similar to the other triptans (Johnston & Rapoport, 2010). (See **Table 38.4**.)

Sumatriptan and Naproxen

Sumatriptan and naproxen (Treximet®; FDA-approved in 2008) is an oral tablet combination medication containing 85 mg sumatriptan and 500 mg naproxen. It is more efficacious than monotherapy with sumatriptan or naproxen alone (as is combined use of individual sumatriptan and naproxen tablets). In clinical trials, 57% to 65% reported headache relief at 2 hours, as well as absence of photophobia (32% to 58%), phonophobia (56% to 61%), and nausea (71% in one study but not significantly different from placebo in another study). Sustained pain relief at 24 hours was also significantly better than monotherapy with either sumatriptan or naproxen. It follows the sumatriptan dosing recommendations (one tablet at migraine onset; if relief is not obtained, a second dose may be taken at least

2 hours later, with a maximum of two tablets in 24 hours), and its adverse events, contraindications, and warnings are the same as those for each of its individual components (including the boxed warning for the naproxen component) (Brandes, et al., 2004; Khoury & Couch, 2010). (See **Table 38.4**.)

Ergot Derivatives

The first migraine-specific drugs to be developed were the ergot derivatives (ergotamine tartrate and dihydroergotamine, with a variety of trade names). They are generally recognized as safe and effective, but have fallen out of favor because of unpredictable patient responses and greater adverse events as compared with the safer triptans. Ergot derivatives have partial agonist, antagonist, or both types of activity for serotonergic, dopaminergic, and alpha-adrenergic receptors, resulting in constriction of peripheral and cranial vessels. Ergot derivatives are typically used to treat infrequent, longstanding migraines in patients that have had multiple relapses when using triptans, but care should be taken to prescribe the medication infrequently, at recommended doses, and in careful consideration of contraindications (e.g., they are pregnancy category X drugs and are absolutely contraindicated in patients with cardiovascular or cerebrovascular disease, and in patients taking concomitant medications metabolized by the CYP3A4 pathway, such as protease inhibitors, azole antifungals, and certain macrolide antibiotics). While generally found to be less efficacious than oral sumatriptan in clinical trials, rectal ergotamine was found to have superior efficacy than rectal sumatriptan (73% vs. 63%, respectively). Ergotamine/caffeine combinations are also available in oral, sublingual, and rectal formulations, although evidence of efficacy for these preparations is inconsistent or conflicting (Wilson, 2007; Bigal & Tepper, 2003).

Ergotamine tartrate (Ergostat®, Ergomar®) is available in 2-mg sublingual tablets. Ergotamine is not an optimal choice, given its side effect profile (nausea may be sufficient enough for discontinuation). It is associated with more side effects than dihydroergotamine, and use of the medication more than 10 times per month may cause MOH. Dihydroergotamine (Migranal®) is available intramuscularly (1 mg), intravenously (1 mg), subcutaneously (1 mg), and as a nasal spray (0.5 mg). There are no oral formulations. This drug is mainly used to treat severe, refractory migraines, recurring migraines, MOH, or status migrainosus (debilitating migraine attacks lasting longer than 72 hours) and is usually managed by specialists. Cafergot®, a combination of caffeine and ergotamine, is available in oral (1 mg ergotamine, 100 mg caffeine) and suppository (2 mg/100 mg) forms. Cafergot can also increase the incidence of migraines and should be used infrequently (Monteith & Goadsby, 2011; Wilson, 2007; Tfelt-Hansen, 2007; Morren & Galvez-Jimenez, 2010). See **Table 38.4** for side effects and contraindications.

Barbiturates

Butalbital-containing compounds such as Fiorinal® (butalbital 50 mg/aspirin 325 mg/caffeine 40 mg) and Fioricet®

(butalbital 50 mg/acetaminophen 325 mg/caffeine 40 mg) should be used sparingly and only if the migraine-specific agents have repeatedly failed. There are no data to support the efficacy of these medications, and if overused (as infrequently as 5 times per month), these agents can lead to addiction, MOH, development of chronic daily headache, and withdrawal symptoms. These drugs have been removed from the market in the European Union, Asia, and Latin America due to their lack of efficacy and associated risks. Fioricet should particularly be used with caution given its acetaminophen content if it is used concomitantly with other acetaminophen-containing drugs (Tepper & Spears, 2009). See **Table 38.4** for side effects and contraindications.

Opioids

Opioids are useful when used as rescue medications for severe migraines that do not respond to the above medications. They are also useful in patients who have infrequent migraines and have contraindications to other agents. They may be used sparingly for moderate to severe migraines during pregnancy. They are in general not recommended for the treatment of migraine, and if used as rescue medications should be used only a few times per year. Overuse can lead to MOH, status migrainosus, or development of chronic daily headache. These are C-IV medications, and the potential for dependence or abuse should also be taken into account when considering them for use. Examples of these medications include butorphanol (generic nasal spray, 1 mg/spray) and acetaminophen plus codeine (Tylenol® plus codeine; acetaminophen 300 mg/codeine 30 mg or 40 mg) for mild to moderate pain. The acetaminophen content per dose is 300 mg, which needs to be considered when used concomitantly with other acetaminophen-containing drugs so that a maximum daily dose of 3,250 mg is not exceeded (Tepper & Spears, 2009; Wilson, 2007). See **Table 38.4** for side effects and contraindications.

Steroids

If a patient has a severe, persistent migraine or status migrainosus that seems refractory to any abortive medications, a brief course of steroids (typically dexamethasone 6 mg for 5 days) may be used as a rescue medication until the patient is headache–free for 24 hours. There are few good data supporting the efficacy of steroid use, but they have been used with good results (Tepper & Spears, 2009; Wilson, 2007). See **Table 38.4** for side effects and contraindications.

Antiemetic Agents

The antiemetic agents prochlorperazine and metoclopramide are effective adjunctive therapies for patients experiencing an acute migraine with or without nausea and vomiting. Prochlorperazine comes in a suppository form, which is useful for patients unable to tolerate oral medications. These medications augment the effects of the above-mentioned abortive agents and may be taken before or together with these agents.

PROPHYLACTIC DRUG THERAPY FOR MIGRAINES

Prophylactic medications are used to reduce the frequency and severity of migraine attacks. A therapeutic trial of a given agent should last for 2 to 3 months before the efficacy of the agent is assessed. The main classes of agents are beta blockers, calcium channel blockers, TCAs, anticonvulsants, serotonin antagonists, and NSAIDs. The choice of prophylactic agent should be based on the patient's comorbidities, and the efficacy and side effect profile of the medication. See **Figure 38-3** for a migraine prophylaxis algorithm. **Table 38.5** gives an overview of selected drugs used to prevent migraines.

The current recommendations for starting prophylactic therapy are recurring migraines that affect the patient's functioning and quality of life despite acute symptomatic treatments, intolerance or failure of multiple acute treatments, overuse of acute medications, MOH, special circumstances such as hemiplegic migraines, and more than two headaches per week (Silberstein, 2002; Pringsheim, et al., 2010).

Medications should be started at low doses and titrated slowly until the desired effects occur. Dosages may need to be lowered if side effects occur. A full therapeutic trial takes at least 2 months. It may take months until an effective agent is found.

Beta Blockers

Beta blockers are often considered first-line agents for prophylactic treatment of migraines. Propranolol (Inderal®), metoprolol (Lopressor®), atenolol (Tenormin®), nadolol (Corgard®), and timolol have been used for migraine, all with similar efficacy. Only propranolol and timolol have been approved by the FDA for migraine prophylaxis. Beta blockers are contraindicated in patients with uncompensated congestive heart failure, bradycardia, second- or third-degree atrioventricular block, and asthma. Side effects include fatigue, vivid dreams, depression, impotence, bradycardia, and hypotension. Many pathways of the cytochrome P450 enzyme system metabolize beta blockers. Beta blockers have numerous drug interactions, and practitioners should consult a reference before prescribing them to avoid such interactions.

Tricyclic Antidepressants

TCAs can also be used as first-line agents for migraine prophylaxis. The agents most commonly used include imipramine (Tofranil®), nortriptyline (Pamelor®), and amitriptyline (Elavil®). Patients usually need only low doses for prophylaxis, lower than those generally used to treat depression. Patients should avoid use if they are currently taking an MAO inhibitor, have glaucoma, or are pregnant. Anticholinergic side effects commonly occur and include sedation, constipation, blurred vision, hypotension, and slowed conduction in the atrioventricular node. Tricyclic antidepressants also have many potential drug interactions; prescribers should consult a reference before administering them.

Anticonvulsants

Valproic acid (Depakene®) and divalproex sodium (Depakote®) can reduce the frequency, severity, and duration of migraines (Mathew, et al., 1995). Use of these drugs is contraindicated in patients with liver disease. Side effects such as tremor, weight gain, nausea, and hair loss limit their use as agents for prophylaxis. Numerous drug interactions can result when valproic acid or divalproex sodium is administered with other anticonvulsants. Increased effects or toxicity of valproic acid are seen with the administration of CNS depressants and aspirin. Valproic acid is contraindicated in pregnancy because it is toxic to the fetus.

Before starting valproic acid, a baseline complete blood count and liver function tests should be obtained. The dose should be increased very gradually, and follow-up liver function tests and valproate levels should be monitored. If tremor appears, the dose should be lowered.

Topiramate (Topamax®) has been shown to be effective in migraine prophylaxis and is particularly effective for patients who have chronic daily headache or who have failed to respond to many other prophylactic treatments. Topiramate has many potential side effects that limit its use, such as concentration and memory impairment, significant somnolence, mood disturbance, and tremor. It should be used with caution in patients with renal or hepatic impairment.

Calcium Channel Blockers

Verapamil (Calan®) is the calcium channel blocker most commonly used in migraine prophylaxis; however, it provides only a slight benefit in reducing the frequency of attacks. It is often considered a second- or third-line agent, for use when other agents are ineffective or contraindicated. The mechanism of action is believed to be the inhibition of serotonin release, which is not achieved until after up to 8 weeks of therapy. Its use is contraindicated in patients with bradycardia, heart block, ventricular tachycardia, or atrial fibrillation. Side effects include constipation, fluid retention, bradycardia, and hypotension. Numerous drug interactions are associated with calcium channel blockers; prescribers must consult a reference before administering.

Nonsteroidal Anti-Inflammatory Drugs

NSAIDs may be used for prophylaxis. Naproxen sodium is the most common agent used. NSAIDs can be used to prevent headaches that occur with a regular pattern (e.g., menstrual migraine). Therapeutic effects are believed to result from inhibition of prostaglandin synthesis and inflammation originating in the trigeminovascular system. These agents may cause GI and renal toxicity if used for a prolonged period and carry a boxed warning about the increased risk of adverse cardiovascular thrombotic events, including myocardial infarction (MI), stroke, and new onset or worsening of preexisting hypertension, as well as use for perioperative pain in coronary artery bypass graft surgery. If the patient requires an NSAID on a chronic basis, renal function should be monitored.

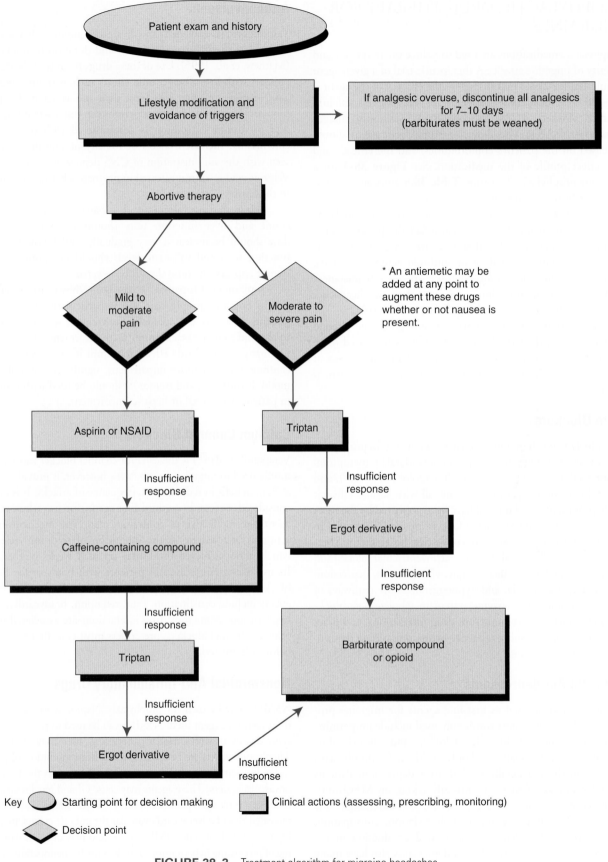

FIGURE 38–3 Treatment algorithm for migraine headaches.

TABLE 38.5 Overview of Selected Drugs Used for Migraine Headache Prophylaxis

Generic (Brand) Name and Dosage	Selected Adverse Events	Contraindications	Special Considerations
Beta Blockers			
propranolol (long-acting) start 80 mg daily; goal 160–240 mg daily; increase dose gradually and taper discontinuation, discontinue after 6 wk if no satisfactory response Note: Adjust dose in hepatic impairment	Common: Drowsiness or fatigue, cold hands and feet, weakness or dizziness, dry mouth, eyes, and skin	**WARNING: Beta blocker therapy should not be withdrawn abruptly (particularly in patients with CAD), but gradually tapered to avoid acute tachycardia, hypertension, and/or ischemia.** Pregnancy Uncompensated CHF, cardiogenic shock, severe sinus bradycardia or 2nd- or 3rd-degree heart block Severe asthma or COPD	Useful if there is history of coexisting HTN or CAD. Use w/caution in patients w/PVD or w/concomitant beta blocker use. Use w/caution in patients w/DM, myasthenia gravis, psychiatric disease, and renal or hepatic dysfunction.
timolol initial: 10 mg bid to a max of 30 mg/d	Anaphylaxis (serious); >3%: fatigue/tiredness, bradycardia; AEs in CAD population more numerous Asthenia or fatigue, heart rate <40 beats/min, cardiac failure-nonfatal, hypotension, claudication, cold hands and feet, nausea or digestive disorders, dizziness	**See BOXED WARNING above** Bronchial asthma or history of bronchial asthma, or severe COPD Sinus bradycardia, 2nd- and 3rd-degree AV block, overt cardiac failure, or cardiogenic shock	Use w/caution in impaired hepatic or renal function, marked renal failure, muscle weakness, or cerebrovascular insufficiency. Use w/caution w/concomitant use of catecholamine-depleting drugs, NSAIDs, calcium antagonists, digoxin and either diltiazem or verapamil, quinidine, and clonidine.
Tricyclic Antidepressants amitriptyline—See Table 38.1			
Anticonvulsants valproic acid (Depakene®, Stavzor®) Depakene 250 mg softgel capsule Stavzor delayed release 125, 250, and 500 mg softgel capsules initial: 250 mg bid to a max of 1,000 mg/d	≥5%: Headache, asthenia, fever, nausea, vomiting, abdominal pain, diarrhea, anorexia, dyspepsia, constipation, somnolence, tremor, dizziness, diplopia, amblyopia/blurred vision, ataxia, nystagmus, emotional lability, thinking abnormal, amnesia, flu syndrome, infection, bronchitis, rhinitis	**WARNING: May cause teratogenic effects such as neural tube defects (e.g., spina bifida). Hepatic failure resulting in fatalities has occurred in patients; children <age 2 are at considerable risk. Cases of life-threatening pancreatitis, occurring at the start of therapy or following years of use, have been reported in adults and children.** Hepatic disease or significant hepatic dysfunction Known urea cycle disorders	Monitor for hypothermia and thrombocytopenia. Monitor psychiatric patients for suicidal ideation. Use w/caution w/ concomitant use of carbapenem, topiramate, aspirin, or lamotrigine. Drug interactions are also known for felbamate, rifampin, amitriptyline/nortriptyline, carbamazepine, clonazepam, diazepam, ethosuximide, phenobarbital, phenytoin, tolbutamide, warfarin, and zidovudine. Use w/caution in the elderly.
divalproex (Depakote®) initial: 250 mg bid, up to 1,000 mg/d	>10%: Nausea, somnolence, dizziness, vomiting; >5%–10% Asthenia, abdominal pain, dyspepsia, rash	See **BOXED WARNING, above**	See above

(continued)

TABLE 38.5   Overview of Selected Drugs Used for Migraine Headache Prophylaxis (*Continued*)

Generic (Brand) Name and Dosage	Selected Adverse Events	Contraindications	Special Considerations
topiramate (Topamax®) initial: 25 mg qhs for first wk, increased weekly by increments of 25 mg; recommended therapeutic dose 100 mg/d in 2 divided doses *Note:* Taper gradually	>5%: paresthesia, anorexia, weight decrease, fatigue, dizziness, somnolence, nervousness, psychomotor slowing, difficulty w/ memory, difficulty w/concentration/attention, confusion; renal calculi, rare acute-angle glaucoma >5% in migraine trials: paresthesia, taste perversion	None	Decreases effectiveness of oral contraceptives. Monitor for acute myopia, oligohidrosis and hyperthermia, suicidal behavior and ideation, metabolic acidosis, cognitive/neuropsychiatric dysfunction, and hyperammonemia. Use caution w/ concomitant administration of valproic acid, oral contraceptives, metformin, lithium, and other carbonic anhydrase inhibitors.
Calcium Channel Blockers verapamil 40–80 mg tid	>1%: Headache, URI, fatigue, nausea, constipation, dizziness, edema	Severe left ventricular dysfunction, hypotension or cardiogenic shock, sick sinus syndrome, 2nd- or 3rd-degree AV block, atrial flutter or atrial fibrillation and an accessory bypass tract (e.g., Wolff-Parkinson-White, Lown-Ganong-Levine syndromes)	Useful if there is coexisting HTN Monitor LFTs periodically, use w/caution in patients w/ impaired renal or hepatic function, and in patients w/ decreased neuromuscular transmission. Use caution w/ concomitant administration of erythromycin, ritonavir, alcohol, aspirin, grapefruit juice, beta blockers, digitalis, other antihypertensive agents, disopyramide, flecainide, quinidine, lithium, carbamazepine, and rifampin, phenobarbital, cyclosporine, theophylline, inhalation anesthetics, neuromuscular-blocking agents, telithromycin, clonidine

Other Prophylactic Agents

Monoamine oxidase inhibitors can also be used for migraine prophylaxis, but because they have multiple serious side effects, their use should be managed by a neurologist.

Gabapentin (Neurontin®) has recently been established to be effective in the treatment of chronic daily headache at dosages of 1,800 to 2,400 mg/d. Angiotensin-converting enzyme inhibitors and angiotensin receptor blockers are also being studied as potential prophylactic agents.

SSRIs, such as venlafaxine and fluoxetine, have been used with some success; they are particularly useful in patients also suffering from anxiety or depression.

Selecting the Most Appropriate Agent

It is important to initiate therapy at the first sign of a migraine. The following section discusses the recommended therapy for migraines (**Table 38.6**).

First-Line Therapy

Nonsteroidal anti-inflammatory drugs and aspirin are appropriate first-line therapy for mild to moderate migraine. They are inexpensive and generally well tolerated. Triptans are first-line therapy for moderate to severe migraine with or without an antiemetic. NSAIDs may be tried for more severe migraines, but they are often unsuccessful.

Second-Line Therapy

Over-the-counter caffeine-containing compounds are appropriate treatment options for mild to moderate migraines that have not responded to the above agents. They can also be used as rescue medications if NSAIDs or aspirin fail to relieve a given attack. For more severe migraines, an ergot derivative along with an antiemetic can be used as second-line therapy if multiple triptans have failed in past treatment efforts.

TABLE 38.6	Recommended Order for Treatment of Migraine Headaches	
Order	Agents	Comments
First line	NSAIDs or aspirin	With moderate to severe migraines, can use antiemetic as needed
Second line	Triptans	*First tier* • sumatriptan 50–100 mg • almotriptan 12.5 mg • rizatriptan 10 mg • eletriptan 40 mg • zolmitriptan 2.5 mg *Slower effect/better tolerability* • naratriptan 2.5 mg • frovatriptan 2.5 mg
Third line	Triptans plus an NSAID	Can use antiemetic as needed
	Infrequent headache: • ergotamine 1–2 mg • dihydroergotamine 2 mg nasal spray	*For headache recurrence:* • ergotamine 2 mg, most effective rectally/usually w/caffeine • naratriptan 2.5 mg • almotriptan 12.5 mg • eletriptan 40 mg

Data from Goadsby, P. J., & Sprenger, T. (2010). Current practice and future directions in the prevention and acute management of migraine. *Lancet Neurology, 9*(3), 285–298.

Third-Line Therapy

If the above agents are ineffective in treating mild to moderate migraines, triptans should be tried. For severe migraines that have not responded to triptans or ergot derivatives and antiemetics, butalbital-containing compounds or opioids may be considered.

CLUSTER HEADACHES

Patients suspected of having cluster headaches should be promptly referred to a neurologist. There is clinical evidence for the efficacy of several medications for the acute and prophylactic treatment of cluster headache. Subcutaneous sumatriptan 6 mg, zolmitriptan nasal spray 5 and 10 mg, and 100% oxygen 6 to 12 L/min are recommended for the management of acute attacks. Data also exist supporting the use of sumatriptan nasal spray 20 mg and oral zolmitriptan 5 and 10 mg. Data (although the strength of the evidence is somewhat lower) suggest there is efficacy for the use of suboccipital steroid injections, verapamil 360 mg, lithium 900 mg, and melatonin 10 mg. Octreotide (Sandostatin®), a somatostatin receptor agonist, has also been shown to be efficacious at 100 mcg subcutaneously in an outpatient trial (Goadsby, 2005; Francis, et al., 2010).

SPECIAL POPULATION CONSIDERATIONS

Pediatric

The most common headache type seen in children is migraine. Migraines may present differently in children than in adults. Prevalence is higher in boys prior to puberty, but higher in girls thereafter. Epidemiologic studies have shown that prevalence increases with age, hitting a peak in adolescence. Average age of onset is 7 in boys and 11 in girls, and the incidence of migraine with aura peaks before migraine without aura. The pain is throbbing and pulsating but tends to be bifrontal or bitemporal. Children may have severe nausea and vomiting along with the pain. The headache usually persists for 1 to 3 hours but may last for longer than a day. A particular challenge with pediatric patients is distinguishing migraine from a host of other possible disorders (e.g., epilepsy, or vascular or metabolic disorders), further complicated by interpreting the complaint from the child or his or her parents. Cheese, chocolate, and citrus fruits are common triggers of migraine in children. Nonpharmacologic approaches to migraine management, such as developing good sleeping habits and routines, are important. Pediatric migraines are usually best managed by simple analgesics such as acetaminophen and ibuprofen, with an antiemetic added if necessary. Patients and their caregivers, however, need to be cautioned not to use the medication too frequently; use of OTC analgesics more than five times per week can lead to MOH or development of chronic daily headache. Triptans are not indicated for use in children, although safety and efficacy of the nasal formulations of sumatriptan and zolmitriptan and oral formulations of rizatriptan and almotriptan have been demonstrated in clinical trials in patients ages 12 to 17. Amitriptyline is a popular drug of choice for prophylaxis of pediatric migraine, and topiramate is gaining in popularity; its efficacy is well supported by clinical trials. Divalproex sodium and propranolol are also used as prophylactic agents (Lewis, 2009).

Tension headaches do occur in children. Recurrent tension headaches should prompt a search for underlying stressors at home or at school. A vision examination should also be performed. Tension headaches are usually best managed by simple analgesics, taking care not to overuse the medication.

Geriatric

New-onset migraines do not often occur in the geriatric population. Changes in renal and hepatic function often occur with advancing age, so if a geriatric patient is experiencing migraines, adjustment of drug dosages is recommended.

A new headache pattern in an elderly patient should make the practitioner suspicious of organic disease or a medication side effect. Many of the medications used to treat migraine are contraindicated for use in older populations (naratriptan is not recommended for use in the elderly, and rizatriptan should be used with caution) or need to be used at a lower dose. Comorbidities and polypharmacy need to be considered carefully prior to choosing pharmacologic management.

Women

As noted earlier, migraines occur more often in women than in men; likely an estrogen-related phenomenon. Pregnancy is a primary concern if drug therapy is to be initiated, even though migraines can diminish during the second and third trimesters. Practitioners should consider drug therapy for pregnant women using the risk-versus-benefit approach. The agents selected should be those that are safe to use during pregnancy. Triptans and ergot derivatives are *strongly contraindicated* in pregnancy. Acetaminophen is the safest analgesic to use during pregnancy, but it is usually minimally effective. For more severe migraines, ibuprofen may be used in the first and second trimester only. Tylenol with codeine may be used sparingly throughout the pregnancy.

Menstrual migraines are a common problem that may be particularly responsive to triptans. Frovatriptan, in particular, has been used with success as "miniprophylaxis" for menstrually related migraine (Johnston & Rapoport, 2010). Women may also be particularly vulnerable to migraine during perimenopause and menopause, when estrogen levels dramatically decline. In one cross-sectional analysis, women using hormone replacement therapy were found to be 40% more likely to have migraines than those who were not taking hormone replacement (Misakian, 2003). If a woman wishes to stay on hormone replacement therapy despite migraines, she can be given a reduced dose and can be switched to pure estradiol or synthetic ethinyl estradiol. Using continuous dosing instead of interrupted dosing may also reduce migraine frequency.

MONITORING PATIENT RESPONSE

Careful monitoring of therapy is important. The practitioner should document the frequency, intensity, and duration of migraines before starting any new therapy and should evaluate the patient periodically after implementing any drug or lifestyle change to assess its effectiveness. Prescribers should monitor how frequently patients are taking abortive therapies to ensure they are not using them excessively. Patients should return to the office after a few attempts with a therapy to assess its effectiveness, and practitioners should switch to another agent if the therapy is unsuccessful. Practitioners also need to evaluate prophylactic therapies for patient compliance and effectiveness. They should note in the chart side effects to therapy and treatment failures to avoid repeating ineffective therapies.

PATIENT EDUCATION

Drug Information

Practitioners need to educate patients about their headaches and what they should realistically expect from treatment. The prescriber should attempt to identify headache triggers (i.e., diet,

medication, or environmental factors) by encouraging patients to keep diaries and pay close attention to when migraines start, and should encourage the patient to avoid or minimize these triggers.

Practitioners also must educate patients about their drug therapy. They should tell patients how frequently they can take an abortive therapy, what the maximum daily dose is, and what side effects to expect from the medication. If the patient will be using a nasal spray or injectable medication, the prescriber should demonstrate proper administration technique. Also, prescribers need to encourage patients to take their prophylactic therapies as scheduled, emphasizing that taking prophylactic therapies on an as-needed basis will not improve the condition. If switching to a new therapy, the prescriber should remind the patient to stop using the old therapy and not to use the two therapies simultaneously (unless this is intended). Patients must be strongly cautioned about drug–drug interactions, the dangers of concomitant use with some medications, and the use of any medications or food additives they may not report. Acetaminophen overdose is common; patients must ensure that they are not taking a combined dose of acetaminophen from two or more medications that exceeds a maximum daily dose of 3,250 mg.

Nutrition

Foods that can trigger headaches include aspartame, caffeine, chocolate, monosodium glutamate, and red wine and other alcohol. The patient should be aware of any foods that trigger his or her headaches and should avoid them. Some medications should be taken with food, and taking some (oral) medications on a full stomach may slow absorption of the drug.

Complementary and Alternative Medicine

Some patients use feverfew to prevent migraines. The active ingredients in feverfew are the sesquiterpene lactones, which have an anti-inflammatory effect that blocks the transcription of inflammatory proteins and inhibits the release of serotonin. A minimum of 0.2% is the recommended dosage. Side effects include nausea, flatulence, diarrhea, and indigestion. Withdrawal symptoms when stopping long-term use can include muscle stiffness, anxiety, and rebound migraines. It also has anticoagulant properties, so prothrombin time and INR levels should be checked periodically, and it should be stopped 2 weeks before surgical procedures.

Another nutritional supplement used for migraine prophylaxis is butterbur. This contains petasin and isopetasin, which have vasodilation properties and inhibit leukotriene synthesis, reducing inflammation. A dosage of 50 mg twice daily has been shown to reduce migraines (Grossman & Schmidramsl, 2001). There should be at least 7.5 mg petasin in the preparation. Side effects include abdominal pain, distended abdomen, and reduced urinary output.

Magnesium, high-dose riboflavin (vitamin B_2), and coenzyme Q10 have also been shown to reduce migraines (Goadsby & Sprenger, 2010).

Case Study

J. J., age 24, presents to your practice for the first time. She reports constant headaches. She smokes a pack of cigarettes a day but is in good health otherwise. She states that the headaches usually occur in the morning and last a few hours. The pain, localized to an area near her right temple, has a throbbing quality. The headache often results in nausea and vomiting and sensitivity to bright lights. She has tried to treat the headaches with acetaminophen, ibuprofen, and naproxen unsuccessfully. The headaches are causing her to miss work and she is afraid she will lose her job.

DIAGNOSIS: MIGRAINE HEADACHES WITHOUT AURA

1. List specific goals of therapy for J. J.
2. What drug therapy would you prescribe? Why?

3. What are the parameters for monitoring success of the therapy?
4. Discuss specific patient education based on the prescribed therapy.
5. List one or two adverse reactions for the selected agent that would cause you to change therapy.
6. What would be the choice for the second-line therapy?
7. What OTC and/or alternative medicines might be appropriate for this patient?
8. What dietary and lifestyle changes might you recommend?
9 Describe 1 or 2 drug–drug or drug–food interactions for the selected agent.

BIBLIOGRAPHY

Starred references are cited in the text.

*Antonaci, F., Dumitrache, C., De Cillis, I., et al. (2010). A review of current European treatment guidelines for migraine. *Journal of Headache Pain, 11*(1), 13–19.

*Ashina, M., Bendtsen, L., Jensen, R., et al. (1999a). Muscle hardness in patients with chronic tension-type headaches: Relation to actual headache state. *Pain, 75*(2–3), 201–205.

*Ashina, M., Lassen, LH., Bendtsen, L., et al. (1999b). Effect of inhibition of nitric oxide synthetase on chronic tension-type headaches: A randomized crossover trial. *Lancet, 353*(9149), 287–289.

*Bendtsen, L., Evers, S., Linde, M., et al. (2010). EFNS guideline on the treatment of tension-type headache—Report of an EFNS task force. *European Journal of Neurology, 17*(11), 1318–1325.

*Bezov, D., Ashina, S., Jensen, R., & Bendtsen, L. (2011). Pain perception studies in tension-type headache. *Headache, 51*(2), 262–271.

*Bigal, M. E., & Tepper, S. J. (2003). Ergotamine and dihydroergotamine: A review. *Current Pain and Headache Reports, 7*(1), 55–62.

*Blau, J. N. (1990). Sleep deprivation headache. *Cephalgia, 10*(4), 157–160.

*Brandes, J. L., Saper, J. R., Diamond, M., et al. (2004). Topiramate for migraine prevention. *JAMA, 291*(8), 964–973.

*Breslau, N., Schultz, L. R., Stewart, W. F., et al. (2000). Headaches and major depression: Is the association specific to migraine? *Neurology, 54*(2), 308–313.

*Cathcart, S., Winefield, A. H., Lushington, K., & Rolan, P. (2010). Stress and tension-type headache mechanisms. *Cephalalgia, 30*(10), 1250–1267.

*Clouse, J. C., & Osterhaus, J. T. (1994). Healthcare resource use and costs associated with migraine in a managed healthcare setting. *Annals of Pharmacotherapy, 28*(5), 659–664.

*Ferrante, E., Rossi P., Tassorelli, C., et al. (2010). Focus on therapy of primary stabbing headache. *Journal of Headache Pain, 11*(2), 157–160.

*Ferrari, M. D. (1998). Migraine. *Lancet, 351*(9108), 1043–1051.

*Fischera, M., Marziniak, M., Gralow, I., et al. (2008). The incidence and prevalence of cluster headache: A meta-analysis of population-based studies. *Cephalalgia, 28*(6), 614–618.

*Food and Drug Administration. (2007). Antidepressant use in children, adolescents, and adults. http://www.fda.gov/drugs/drugsafety/informationbydrugclass/ucm096273.htm. Updated 8-12-2010, accessed December 21, 2010.

*Food and Drug Administration. (2009). Summary Minutes of the Joint Meeting of the Drug Safety and Risk Management Advisory Committee, Nonprescription Drugs Advisory Committee, and the Anesthetic and Life Support Drugs Advisory Committee June 29 and 30, 2009. http://www.fda.gov/downloads/AdvisoryCommittees/CommitteesMeetingMaterials/Drugs/DrugSafetyandRiskManagementAdvisoryCommittee/UCM179888.pdf. Accessed December 21, 2010.

*Fox, A. W., & Davis, R. L. (1998). Migraine chronobiology. *Headache, 38*(6), 436–441.

*Francis, G. J., Becker, W. J., & Pringsheim, T. M. (2010). Acute and preventive pharmacologic treatment of cluster headache. *Neurology, 75*(5), 463–473.

*Goadsby, P. J. (2005). New targets in the acute treatment of headache. *Current Opinions in Neurology, 18*(3), 283–288.

*Goadsby, P. J., & Sprenger, T. (2010). Current practice and future directions in the prevention and acute management of migraine. *Lancet Neurology, 9*(3), 285–298.

*Grossman, W., & Schmidramsl, H. (2001). An extract of Petasites hybridus is effective in the prophylaxis of migraine. *Alternative Medicine Review, 6*(3), 303–310.

*Hatch, J. P. (1992). The use of EMG and muscle palpation in the diagnosis of tension-type headache with and without pericranial muscle involvement. *Pain, 49*(2), 175–178.

*Headache Classification Subcommittee of the International Headache Society. (2004). The international classification of headache disorders, 2nd ed. *Cephalalgia, 24*(Suppl. 1), 1–160.

*Johnston, M. M., & Rapoport, A. M. (2010). Triptans for the management of migraine. *Drugs, 70*(12), 1505–1518.

*Kallela, M., Wessman, M., Havanka, H., et al. (2001). Familial migraine with and without aura: Clinical characteristics and co-occurrence. *European Journal of Neurology, 8*(5), 441–449.

*Khoury, C. K., & Couch, J. R. (2010). Sumatriptan–naproxen fixed combination for acute treatment of migraine: A critical appraisal. *Journal of Drug Design, Development and Therapy, 18*(4), 9–17.

Lacy, C. F., Armstrong, L. L., Goldman, M. P., et al. (2010). *Drug information handbook* (19th ed.). Hudson, OH: Lexi–Comp.

*Lance, J. W. (1993). Current concepts of migraine pathogenesis. *Neurology, 44*(Suppl. 3), 11–15.

*Leonardi, M., Steiner, T. J., Scher, A. T., et al. (2005). The global burden of migraine: Measuring disability in headache disorders with WHO's Classification of Functioning, Disability and Health (ICF). *Journal of Headache Pain, 6*(6), 429–440.

*Lewis, D. W. (2009). Pediatric migraine. *Neurology Clinics, 27*(2), 481–501.

*Matchar, D. B., Young, W. B., Rosenberg, J. H., et al. (2000). Evidence–based guidelines for migraine headache in the primary care setting: Pharmacological management of acute attacks. U.S. Headache Consortium (©2000 AAN). http://www.aan.com/professionals/practice/pdfs/gl0087.pdf. Accessed on January 7, 2011.

*Mathew, N. T., Saper, J. R., & Silberstein, S. D. (1995). Migraine prophylaxis with divalproex. *Archives of Neurology, 52*(3), 281–286.

*Mathew, N. T., Asgharnejad, M., Peykamian, M., et al. (1997). Naratriptan is effective and well tolerated in the acute treatment of migraine. Results of a double-blind, placebo-controlled, crossover study. The Naratriptan S2WA3003 Study Group. *Neurology, 49*(6), 1485–1490.

*Misakian, A. L. (2003). Postmenopausal hormone therapy and migraine headache. *Journal of Women's Health, 12*(10), 1027–1036.

*Monteith, T. S., & Goadsby, P. J. (2011). Acute migraine therapy: New drugs and new approaches. *Current Treatment Options in Neurology, 13*(1), 1–14.

*Morren, J. A., & Galvez–Jimenez, N. (2010). Where is dihydroergotamine mesylate in the changing landscape of migraine therapy? *Expert Opinion on Pharmacotherapy, 11*(18), 3085–3093.

*Nestoriuc, Y., Rief, W., & Martin, A. (2008). Meta-analysis of biofeedback for tension-type headache: Efficacy, specificity, and treatment moderators. *Journal of Consulting and Clinical Psychology, 76*(3), 379–396.

*Osterhaus, J. T., Gutterman, D. L., & Plachetka, J. R. (1992). Healthcare resource and lost labour costs of migraine headache in the US. *Pharmacoeconomics, 2*(1), 67–76.

*Payne, T. J., Stetson, B., Stevens, V. M., et al. (1991). The impact of cigarette smoking on headache activity in headache patients. *Headache, 31*(5), 329–332.

*Pringsheim, T., Davenport, W. J., & Becker, W. J. (2010). Prophylaxis of migraine headache. *Canadian Medical Association Journal, 182*(7), E269–E276.

*Schilling, A., Corey, R., Leonard, M., et al. (2010). Acetaminophen: Old drug, new warnings. *Cleveland Clinic Journal of Medicine, 77*(1), 19–27.

*Silberstein, S. D. (2002). *Clinician's manual on migraine* (2nd ed.). Philadelphia: Current Medicine, Inc.

*Silberstein, S. D. (2009). Preventive migraine treatment. *Neurologic Clinics, 27*(2), 429–443.

*Smitherman, T. A., Walters, A. B., Maizels, M., et al. (2010). The use of antidepressants for headache prophylaxis. *CNS Neuroscience and Therapeutics,* [Epub ahead of print] doi: 10.1111/j.1755–5949.2010.00170.

*Solomon, S., & Lipton, R. B. (1999). Headaches and face pain as a manifestation of Munchausen Syndrome. *Headache, 39*(1), 45–50.

*Stovner, L. J., Hagen, K., Jensen, R., et al. (2007). The global burden of headache: A documentation of headache prevalence and disability worldwide. *Cephalalgia, 27*(3), 193–210.

*Teall, J., Tuchman, M., Cutler, N., et al. (1998). Rizatriptan (MAXALT) for the acute treatment of migraine and migraine recurrence. A placebo-controlled, outpatient study. Rizatriptan 022 Study Group. *Headache, 38*(4), 281–287.

*Tepper, S. J., & Spears, R. C. (2009). Acute treatment of migraine. *Neurologic Clinics, 27*(2), 417–427.

*Tfelt–Hansen, P. (2007). Acute pharmacotherapy of migraine, tension-type headache, and cluster headache. *Journal of Headache Pain, 8*(2), 127–134.

*Wentz, A. L., Jimenez, T. B., Dixon, R. M., et al. and CXA20008 Study Investigators. (2008). A double-blind, randomized, placebo-controlled, single-dose study of the cyclooxygenase-2 inhibitor, GW406381, as a treatment for acute migraine. *European Journal of Neurology, 15*(4), 420–427.

*Wilson, J. F. (2007). In the clinic. Migraine. *Annals of Internal Medicine, 147*(9), ITC11–1–ITC11–16.

*Zissis, N. P., Harmoussi, S., Vlaikidis, N., et al. (2007). A randomized, double-blind, placebo-controlled study of venlafaxine XR in out-patients with tension-type headache. *Cephalalgia, 27*(4), 315–324.

Seizure Disorders

Epilepsy is a common neurologic condition affecting approximately 1% of the population worldwide, with 5% to 7% of adults experiencing one seizure in their lifetime and an estimated annual cost in the United States of $12.5 billion. Epilepsy is best defined as recurrent seizure activity. A single seizure does not constitute epilepsy unless a brain abnormality is identified, which may result in future seizure episodes. It is a multifaceted disease with various physical manifestations, prognoses, outcomes, and responses to treatment. Frequent seizures can lead to neuronal damage, which may lead to changes in memory and other cognitive functions. Therefore, it is important for the practitioner to be aware of the various etiologies and to screen patients appropriately with accurate and reliable diagnostic testing. With appropriate diagnosis and treatment, more than 90% of people with epilepsy lead normal, healthy, and productive lives.

CAUSES

Seizures can occur at any age, with etiology varying by age. The most common cause of epilepsy is idiopathic, accounting for about 65% of all cases. Other causes of epilepsy include vascular abnormalities (11%), congenital malformations (8%), and trauma (5%). Seizures from degeneration, infection, and neoplasm are considerably less prevalent. In newborns and infants, perinatal injuries, metabolic defects, congenital malformations, and infection are more likely causes of epilepsy, but still less frequent than the idiopathic diagnoses.

Some cases of epilepsy are hereditary or congenital (present at birth), and some are acquired (e.g., serious head injury, a central nervous system [CNS] infection, stroke, or dementia). However, not all people with these disorders develop epilepsy. This suggests that there is a certain threshold that plays a role in the development of epilepsy and may be based on individual biochemistry. Why a person may have a seizure at one time rather than another relates to cause. This further suggests that there may be immediate triggers that can provoke an attack in a predisposed person (e.g., sudden seizure activity in people who are playing video games, working with a calculator, or listening to a particular piece of music). These sensory triggers are uncommon and are often referred to as *reflex epilepsy*.

Predisposing factors that may cause epilepsy more often are sleep deprivation, hyperventilation, fever from underlying illness, hormonal changes occurring during menses, and drug or alcohol ingestion. All of these may lower the seizure threshold and provoke seizures in people who are predisposed.

Several acute metabolic, infectious, medication-related, and other disorders (e.g., alcohol or drug withdrawal, viral meningitis, or hypoglycemia from an overdose of insulin) are associated with seizures. However, upon recovery from these disorders, a person is not necessarily predisposed to future seizures. These are known as *secondary* or *acute* seizures rather than epilepsy.

Pathophysiology

To understand the pathophysiologic process of an epileptic seizure, it is necessary to understand normal neuronal conduction. Normal cellular transmission between nerve cells is dependent on a normal distribution of positively or negatively charged ions between the inside and the outside of the cell. In normal human physiology, there is a resting membrane potential (270 microvolts) that leaves the inside of the cell negatively charged with respect to the outside of the cell. A stimulus is needed to produce a cellular discharge, and once stimulated, an action potential is generated. After the generation of the action potential, there is a brief period during which the nerve cell membrane is hyperpolarized, which makes it more difficult for a second action potential to be generated until the normal resting membrane ionic gradient is restored.

Communication between neurons occurs through highly specialized structures called *synapses*. There are hundreds of synapses on each neuron. In these synapses, neurotransmitters are released from vesicles in the neurons where they are stored and then diffuse across the synaptic region to contact specific receptors. Once stimulated, the receptors can open or close a specific ion channel. There are two types of ion channels—excitatory and inhibitory. The channels consist of a number of different protein substances. The main inhibitory neurotransmitter in the CNS is gamma-aminobutyric acid (GABA). There are several excitatory neurotransmitters as well, including glutamate and aspartate. These chemicals can activate several different receptors that, depending on their action, can excite or inhibit a group of nerve cells.

To produce an actual seizure, a large group of nerve cells (neurons) must fire abnormally and together. It is thought that this firing occurs within certain highly organized areas of the brain that tend to support seizure activity. This is known as an *epileptic focus*. When epileptic discharges (focus) occur, normal inhibitory circuits (GABA-ergic) begin to fire, which tends to limit the size of the focus. The implication is that a seizure may result from impairment of the inhibitory brain nerve cells or conditions in which there is abnormal excitation. The epileptic focus that is produced may lead to a focal seizure only in the involved area of the brain, or the discharge may travel through other pathways to become more generalized and involve the entire brain. Clinical manifestations of a seizure can be classified by type of seizure, but the manifestations depend on the balance between abnormal, excitatory, and inhibitory neuronal firing, the location of the epileptic focus, and the patterns and degree of spread of the epileptic focus.

Classification of Seizures

The International Classification of Epileptic Seizures (ICES) categorizes seizures in two major groups: partial seizures and generalized seizures. The terminology used by the ICES, however, is not always the same as that used by many clinicians. For instance, many practitioners call the ICES "absence" seizure a *petit mal,* and the designation "tonic-clonic" is often referred to as a *grand mal* seizure. A complex partial seizure is often referred to as a *psychomotor* or *temporal lobe* seizure, and a simple partial seizure has been called *focal* or *Jacksonian*.

Furthermore, classifying epileptic seizures by seizure type is difficult because seizures often appear within a cluster of other signs and symptoms. To help classify seizure type, physicians may look for precipitating factors, age of onset, severity, chronicity, diurnal or circadian cycling, anatomic location of seizure focus, and physical manifestations to help define the patient's treatment and prognosis.

Partial (Focal, Local) Seizures

Partial seizures begin in a localized area of the brain, although there may be generalization to involve both hemispheres. Simple partial (focal) seizures typically result in no alteration of consciousness, and the first clinical and electroencephalogram (EEG) change indicates an initial activation of nerve cells in a limited part of one cerebral hemisphere.

The patient's symptoms are determined by the anatomic location of the seizure focus. There may be motor, sensory, autonomic, or psychic symptoms. These may evolve into complex partial or secondary generalized tonic-clonic seizures. An EEG recorded during this time may show some low-voltage fast activity, rhythmic spikes, and slow-wave activity.

Complex partial seizures (psychomotor) are associated with impaired consciousness and with some form of automatic behavior (automatisms). This type of seizure can evolve from a simple partial seizure and can generate into a secondarily generalized tonic-clonic seizure. The EEG may show a unilateral or bilateral, low-voltage, fast activity with rhythmic spikes and slow waves. Complex partial seizures may be preceded by an aura.

Generalized (Convulsive or Nonconvulsive) Seizures

Generalized seizures involve both hemispheres of the brain from the onset, and they result in early loss of consciousness. Generalized seizures may involve only loss of consciousness (similar to absence seizures), or they may result in generalized tonic-clonic, clonic, or myoclonic seizures.

Absence seizures (petit mal) usually have a sudden onset, are brief (often lasting less than 10 seconds), and interrupt ongoing activities. The patient exhibits a blank stare and is usually unresponsive when spoken to, although at times the patient may be able to relate what was said to him or her during the initial phase of the seizure. There may be some mild clonic or tonic jerking, but it is not prolonged. There is abrupt onset and discontinuation. There is no postictal confusion, which may be characteristic of other seizure types, and there are no other associated symptoms. The EEG shows a very rhythmic, 3 cycles/second spike-wave discharge during the event. There is often confusion as to the diagnosis of absence seizures versus complex partial seizures. Absence seizures are usually restricted to childhood and are provoked by hyperventilation.

A subtype of absence seizure is the *atypical absence seizure,* in which the alteration of consciousness may not be complete. A child experiencing this type of seizure may continue with some activities. There may be an associated loss of muscle tone of the face and neck muscles and there may be mild clonic twitching of the eyelids and mouth. The onset and discontinuation of this type of seizure is gradual.

Tonic-clonic seizures (grand mal) are associated with abrupt loss of consciousness. There may be some vague, ill-defined warning signs but no true aura. The patient experiences a sudden, sharp, bilaterally symmetric contraction of muscles and may cry, fall, or do both. The patient's head may be extended and appear cyanotic. There may be associated tongue biting and incontinence. Depressed consciousness that can be prolonged (several hours) characterizes the postictal period, during which the patient exhibits bilaterally symmetric clonic jerking of the extremities, increased salivation and frothing at the mouth, and deep respiration and relaxation of muscles. After the postictal period, the patient usually reports waking with muscle stiffness and headache. The EEG typically shows generalized high-voltage, spike-wave activity.

Clonic seizures consist of rapidly repetitive bilateral jerking of the extremities and facial muscles with loss of consciousness. The postictal phase is usually short.

Atonic seizures (drop attacks or astatic seizures) are characterized by a sudden loss of muscle tone, which may be only fragmentary. This type of seizure may be brief and not associated with loss of consciousness. It can occur in a repetitive, rhythmic, and successive manner and may be seen in patients with more diffuse neurologic insult and psychomotor retardation. Atonic seizures are frequently associated with Lennox-Gastaut syndrome.

Myoclonic seizures are sudden, brief, shock-like muscular contractions. They may be generalized or they may be confined to the face and trunk muscles, to one or more of the extremities, or to individual muscle groups. Myoclonic seizures can occur regularly in a repetitive manner, or they can be sporadic. These seizures may accompany other neurologic conditions, such as metabolic or toxic states, as well as epilepsy.

Tonic seizures consist of brief, generalized tonic contractions with associated head extension, possible stiffening of the back, and stiffening of all four extremities. These seizures can be associated with autonomic symptoms, a rapid heart rate, and cessation of breathing followed by cyanosis. This type of seizure is also seen in Lennox-Gastaut syndrome and may be precipitated during slow-wave sleep.

Status Epilepticus

Status epilepticus is a life-threatening emergency that requires immediate identification and treatment. The standard definition is seizure activity persisting for more than 30 minutes or two or more sequential seizures without recovery between them. In clinical practice, any seizure activity persisting for more than 5 minutes is typically considered status epilepticus and treated as such. Status epilepticus can be classified as either partial or primary generalized. Precipitating factors include drug noncompliance and sudden withdrawal from antiepileptic drugs (AEDs), fever, withdrawal from alcohol or sedative drugs, metabolic disorder, sleep deprivation, and possibly a new cerebral pathologic process.

Diagnostic Criteria

The accurate diagnosis of a seizure helps the health care provider decide whether to initiate or withhold drug treatment and which medications to prescribe. A well-conducted history and physical and neurologic examinations may allow a diagnosis of epilepsy to be made without further diagnostic or laboratory testing. The initial assessment should include associated factors (e.g., age, medical history, precipitating events), symptoms during the seizure (e.g., aura, behavior, motor symptoms, loss of consciousness), and symptoms following a seizure (e.g., postictal state). Unfortunately, many of the manifestations of epilepsy are subtle, making diagnosis and classification difficult. In fact, no single test, clinical finding, or symptom is reliable by itself to discriminate between epilepsy and nonepileptic events.

One of the most useful and standard tests for assisting in the diagnosis of epilepsy is the EEG. The EEG is a brainwave tracing showing voltage fluctuations versus time that is recorded from scalp electrodes placed in specific locations on the head (i.e., montages). An EEG is recommended as part of the neurodiagnostic evaluation of children and adults presenting with an apparent unprovoked first seizure.

Neurologic imaging studies also help in the diagnosis of epilepsy. Computed tomography (CT) scanning of the brain is used to detect masses or lesions, bleeding, or stroke-like conditions. Magnetic resonance imaging (MRI), although helpful in diagnosing lesions, bleeding, and stroke-like states, also helps find more subtle brain abnormalities, including medial temporal sclerosis. Current guidelines recommend the use of CT or MRI as part of the initial neurodiagnostic evaluation

of adults presenting with an apparent unprovoked first seizure. MRI is the preferred imaging study for use in children. Other less frequently used tests include cerebral arteriography and positron emission tomography (PET). Cerebral arteriography may detect vascular malformation, aneurysms, and significant vascular disease. PET helps particularly in diagnosing partial epilepsy. PET scans measure regional cerebral blood flow and metabolism both during and between seizures. However, PET scanning is expensive, and some insurance carriers do not approve the test for reimbursement.

INITIATING DRUG THERAPY

The selection of the ideal AED depends on several factors, including seizure type and the age and sex of the patient. Treatment with AEDs starts after the diagnosis is confirmed and the patient has experienced two or more seizures. If a patient has one or more risk factors for recurrent seizures (EEG abnormalities, structural lesions, partial seizures, or a family history), then pharmacotherapy can be initiated.

Many epilepsy specialists advocate monotherapy as the first principle of management. If monotherapy fails, replacement by a second AED is recommended. Monotherapy has several advantages, including increased compliance. The most frequent cause of failure to control seizure activity is the patient's lack of adherence to drug therapy. Management of toxicity is easier with monotherapy because adverse events often can be correlated with serum drug levels. Some epilepsy specialists report that up to 75% of their patients have had complete seizure control on monotherapy.

Usually, when monotherapy with several drugs has failed, polytherapy may be tried. In contrast to monotherapy, polytherapy may increase the risk of chronic toxicity in the patient. Whenever two or more drugs are used simultaneously, decisions regarding therapy become more complex, and there is an increased risk of adverse events and drug interactions.

The particular drug selected depends on the seizure type and toxicity. **Table 39.1** and **Figure 39-1** outline the recommended treatment order and algorithm of treatment.

Surgical Treatment of Epilepsy

The surgical treatment of epilepsy has become an important therapeutic modality. Candidates for surgery are patients whose seizures are uncontrolled with medical therapy or who experience intolerable drug side effects. In general, patients with complicated epilepsy should be referred to a neurologist or epilepsy specialist for a decision regarding the need for surgical treatment.

Various surgical procedures can be performed, including anterior temporal lobectomy, amygdala-hippocampectomy, extratemporal focus removal, lesionectomy, corpus callosotomy, and hemispherectomy. Outcomes are generally good with approximately 70% of patients seizure-free after a temporal lobectomy.

TABLE 39.1	**Recommended Order of Treatment for Epileptic Seizures**			
	Partial (Both Simple and Complex) Seizures	**Generalized Tonic-Clonic Seizures**	**Absence Seizures**	**Atypical Absence, Myoclonic, and Atonic Seizures**
First-line therapy	carbamazepine, phenytoin, fosphenytoin, valproic acid, lamotrigine, topiramate, oxcarbazepine	carbamazepine, phenytoin, valproic acid, fosphenytoin	ethosuximide, valproic acid, lamotrigine	valproic acid
Second-line therapy (alternative therapy)	felbamate, gabapentin, lacosamide, levitiracetam, phenobarbital, pregabalin, primidone, tiagabine, vigabatrin	felbamate, gabapentin, lamotrigine, levitiracetam, phenobarbital, primidone, ethotoin, mephobarbital, mephenytoin, vigabatrin	clonazepam, paramethadione, trimethadione, methsuximide, phensuximide	clonazepam

Goals of Drug Therapy

The drug treatment of patients with epilepsy is designed to reduce the number of seizures. A realistic goal for most patients is to completely control seizures, ideally achieved with monotherapy. In addition to controlling seizures, another goal should be improving the patient's quality of life by allowing a return to normal activities of daily living without restriction (except driving; see Patient Education).

Hydantoins

Indications/Uses

One of the oldest and most effective AEDs is phenytoin (Dilantin). It is effective in treating a wide range of seizure types, including generalized tonic-clonic as well as simple or partial seizure activity. In either case, it can be used as a first-line drug for monotherapy. Phenytoin is one of the most commonly used anticonvulsants for generalized tonic-clonic (grand mal) seizure activity and for simple and complex partial seizures. It can also be used for preventing seizures after head trauma, neurosurgery, and hemorrhagic stroke.

Mechanism of Action

Phenytoin blocks post-tetanic potentiation by stabilizing neuronal membranes. It decreases seizure activity by increasing the efflux or decreasing the influx of sodium ions across cell membranes in the motor cortex during generation of nerve impulses. It also regulates neuronal excitability by inhibiting calcium conduction through altering calcium uptake in presynaptic terminals and preventing cyclic nucleotide accumulation and cerebellar stimulation.

Dosage

Phenytoin is available in multiple dosage forms, including chewable tablets, extended-release capsules, liquid, and intravenous (IV). Regardless of dosage form, a loading dose of phenytoin is typically given to achieve a therapeutic level as quickly as possible. The loading dose is 15 to 20 mg/kg/d in both adults and children. If given IV, the maximum infusion rate is 50 mg/min to avoid cardiovascular collapse or 25 mg/min in patients with pre-existing cardiac disease. If given orally, it is divided into 3 doses given every 2 to 4 hours to increase

tolerability. Following a loading dose, the normal maintenance dose is 5 to 6 mg/kg/d in adults and 5 to 12 mg/kg/d in children based on age. The therapeutic serum concentration of phenytoin is 10 to 20 mcg/mL in a person with a normal albumin level, while the therapeutic level of free, unbound phenytoin is 1 to 2 mcg/mL.

Phenytoin is unique because it is metabolized in a nonlinear manner, exhibiting Michaelis-Menten enzyme kinetics. The enzymes that metabolize phenytoin are saturable, meaning that as the amount of drug approaches this saturation point, small incremental increases in a dose can result in disproportionately high serum levels. Further, as the concentrations reach closer to the saturation point, the half-life of phenytoin increases. This must be considered when adjusting phenytoin doses.

Contraindications

There are no absolute contraindications for phenytoin other than allergy (**Table 39.2**).

Adverse Events

Phenytoin exhibits adverse effects specific to dosage form and serum concentration in addition to other adverse effects. Patients receiving IV phenytoin are subject to adverse events such as hypotension, bradycardia, cardiac arrhythmias, cardiovascular collapse (especially with rapid IV use), venous irritation, thrombophlebitis, and possibly death. Therefore, the maximum infusion rate is 50 mg/minute in most patients and 25 mg/minute in patients with underlying cardiac disease. Concentration-specific adverse effects of phenytoin are listed in **Table 39.3.**

Other adverse events include gingival hyperplasia, hirsutism, coarsening of facial features, rash, hepatitis, megaloblastic anemia, thrombocytopenia, mild sensory polyneuropathy, Stevens-Johnson syndrome, systemic lupus erythematosus (SLE), and folic acid deficiency.

Interactions

Phenytoin is a cytochrome P450 (CYP) 2C9 and CYP2C19 enzyme substrate and a CYP1A2, CYP2C9, CYP2D6, and CYP3A3/4 enzyme inducer. In addition to enzyme interactions, because of the high protein binding exhibited by phenytoin, it may be displaced by other highly protein-bound drugs, such as valproic acid and salicylic acid. Drug interactions occur

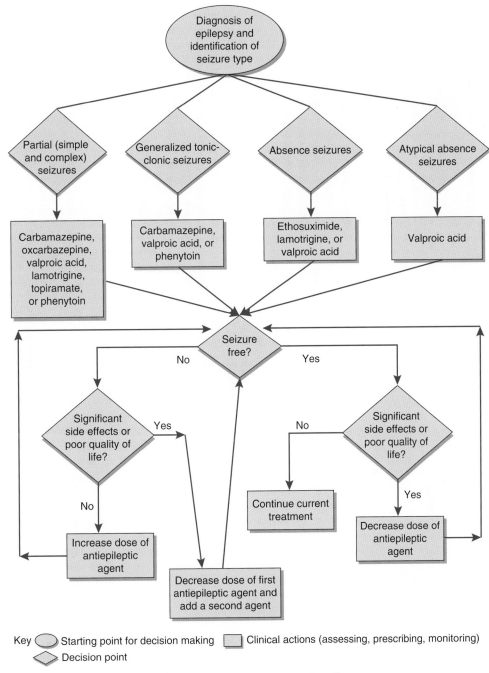

FIGURE 39-1 Treatment algorithm for epilepsy.

frequently with phenytoin and can have a significant impact on therapeutic outcomes. **Box 39.1** contains a list of non-AEDs that interact with phenytoin, and **Table 39.4** lists interactions between AEDs.

Fosphenytoin

Indications/Uses

Fosphenytoin (Cerebyx), the prodrug of phenytoin, is a parenteral drug indicated for controlling generalized convulsive status epilepticus and preventing and treating seizures occurring during neurosurgery. It is indicated only for short-term

(<5 days) administration when phenytoin is unavailable or inappropriate or deemed less advantageous.

Mechanism of Action

Fosphenytoin is converted to phenytoin by plasma esterases. Phenytoin is the active moiety of fosphenytoin and therefore the mechanism of action is the same.

Dosage

The dose, concentration in solutions, and infusion rates for fosphenytoin are expressed as phenytoin sodium equivalents.

TABLE 39.2 Overview of Drugs Used to Treat Seizures

Generic (Trade) Name and Dosage	Dose Adjustments	Selected Adverse Events	Contraindications	Special Considerations
phenytoin (Dilantin) Loading dose: 15–20 mg/kg in three divided doses q2–4h to decrease GI adverse events Maintenance dose: 300 mg/d or 5–6 mg/kg/d in three divided doses, or qd-bid using an extended-release form of the drug		Nystagmus, ataxia, cognitive impairment, lethargy, gingival hyperplasia, increase in body hair, coarsening of facial features, acne, folate deficiency, skin rash	Hypersensitivity to phenytoin, other hydantoins, or to any of its components; heart block; sinus bradycardia Pregnancy category D	Avoid IM and SQ administration due to pain, erratic absorption, and risk of local tissue damage. Maximum IV administration is 50 mg/min; 25 mg/min in the elderly and in patients with preexisting cardiovascular conditions An in-line 0.22–5 µg filter is recommended for IVPB solutions. Therapeutic ranges: Neonates: 8–15 µg/mL total phenytoin, 1–2 µg/mL free phenytoin Children and adults: 10–20 µg/mL total phenytoin, 1–2.3 µg/mL free phenytoin
fosphenytoin (Cerebyx) Loading dose 15–20 mg phenytoin equivalents/kg Initial daily maintenance dose: IV or, IM, 4–6 mg PE/kg/d		Nystagmus, dizziness, pruritus, ataxia, headache	Hypersensitivity to phenytoin or fosphenytoin or to any of its components; occurrence of any rash while on treatment (the drug should not be resumed if rash is bullous, purpuric, or exfoliative); not recommended for use in children <4 y Pregnancy category D	Maximum infusion rate: 150 mg/min IV filtration is not required. Therapeutic range: see phenytoin
carbamazepine (Tegretol) 6–12 y: 20–30 mg/kg/d in 2–4 divided doses per day; usual dose is 400–800 mg/d, maximum 1 g/d 12 y–adult: usual dose 800–1,200 mg/d in 3–4 divided doses		Hematologic abnormalities, drowsiness, fatigue, ataxia, SIADH, rash (Stevens-Johnson syndrome), GI upset, confusion, nystagmus, and seizures	Hypersensitivity to carbamazepine or tricyclic antidepressants, bone marrow suppression, recent use of an MAO inhibitor (≤14 d) Pregnancy category D	Oral suspension should not be administered simultaneously with other liquid medicinal agents or diluents. To avoid GI upset, take with food or water and divide doses. The appearance of a rash does not automatically rule out using carbamazepine. Therapeutic ranges: 6–12 µg/mL; 4–8 µg/mL if used in combination with other AEDs; toxic > 15 µg/mL
valproic acid (Depakote, Depakene) Children and adults: 30–60 mg/kg/d in 2–3 divided doses	Reduce dose in hepatic impairment and avoid in severe impairment.	Lethargy, GI upset, weight gain, alopecia, hepatitis	Hypersensitivity to valproic acid, its derivatives or any component; hepatic dysfunction; hepatic failure resulting in death has occurred, and children <2 y are at considerable risk Pregnancy category D	Therapeutic range: 50–100 mg/mL; toxic >200 µg/mL Seizure control may improve at levels >100 µg/mL. Toxicity may occur at levels of 100–150 µg/mL. Take with food or milk; do not administer with carbonated drinks.
ethosuximide (Zarontin) Children 3–6 y: 15–40 mg/kg/d in 2 divided doses Children > 6 y and adults: 20–40 mg/kg/d in 2 divided doses		Nausea, GI upset, hiccups, headache	Hypersensitivity to ethosuximide or its components Pregnancy category C	Seldom-used drug for absence seizures in children Therapeutic range: 40–100 mg/L

phenobarbital (Barbita, Solfoton) Infants: 5–8 mg/kg/d in 1–2 divided doses Children 1–5 y: 6–8 mg/kg/d in 1–2 divided doses Children 5–12 y: 4–6 mg/kg/d in 1–2 divided doses Children >12 y–adults: 1–3 mg/kg/d in 2–3 divided doses or 50–100 mg bid-tid		Sedation, ataxia, cognitive impairment, hyperactivity, rash, problems with sleep, megaloblastic anemia (responds to folic acid)	Hypersensitivity to phenobarbital or any of its components Preexisting CNS depression, severe uncontrolled pain, porphyria, severe respiratory disease with dyspnea or obstruction Use caution in patients with hypovolemic shock, congestive heart failure, hepatic impairment, respiratory dysfunction or depression, previous addiction to the sedative/hypnotic group, chronic or acute pain, renal dysfunction, and the elderly. (Because of its long half-life and addiction potential, phenobarbital is not recommended as a sedative in the elderly.) Pregnancy category D	Avoid rapid IV administration (>50 mg/min). Do not add IV form to acidic solutions. Avoid intra-arterial injection. CrCl <10 mL/min—administer q12–16 h. Tolerance, or psychological and physical dependence, may occur with prolonged use. Abrupt withdrawal in patients with epilepsy may precipitate status epilepticus. Therapeutic ranges: Infants and children: 15–30 µg/mL Adults: 20–40 µg/mL Toxic range: >40 µg/mL
primidone (Mysoline) Children <8 y: 10–25 mg/kg/d tid-qid Children a>8 y–adults: Start at 100–125 mg qhs for 3 d; then increase to 100–125 mg bid for 3 d; then increase to up to 250 mg tid		Same as above	Hypersensitivity to primidone, phenobarbital, or to any of its components; porphyria Use caution in renal or hepatic impairment or pulmonary insufficiency. Pregnancy category D	Abrupt withdrawal may precipitate status epilepticus. This drug is 20%–50% dialyzable; administer dose after dialysis or administer supplemental 30% dose. Folic acid as a supplement to avoid folic acid deficiency and megaloblastic anemia: Adults: 5–12 µg/mL Children <5 y: 7–10 µg/mL Toxic level: >15 µg/mL Be consistent with protein intake during primidone therapy. (Low-protein diets increase the duration of action.) Avoid foods high in vitamin C because of displacement of drug from binding sites.
gabapentin (Neurontin) 900–1,800 mg/d in 3 divided doses Children >12 y: 300 mg on day 1 at bedtime; 300 mg bid on day 2; 300 mg tid on day 3	Dose adjust for renal failure.	Ataxia, fatigue, dizziness, somnolence, weight gain, GI upset	Hypersensitivity to gabapentin or its components Pregnancy category C	Dosage adjustments for patients with renal impairment: CrCl >60 mL/min: 1,200 mg/d CrCl 30–60 mL/min: 600 mg/d CrCl 15–30 mL/min: 300 mg/d CrCl <15 mL/min: 150 mg/d

(continued)

TABLE 39.2 Overview of Drugs Used to Treat Seizures (*Continued*)

Generic (Trade) Name and Dosage	Dose Adjustments	Selected Adverse Events	Contraindications	Special Considerations
lamotrigine (Lamictal) Children 2–12 y with concomitant AEDs without valproic acid therapy: 5–15 mg/kg/d; max. 400 mg/d in 2 divided doses Adults: 100–400 mg/d in 1–2 doses/d	Children 2–12 y with concomitant valproic acid therapy: 1–5 mg/kg/d; max. 200 mg/d in 2 divided doses Adults with concomitant valproic acid therapy: 50–200 mg/d in 2 divided doses	Dizziness, headache, rash, ataxia, tremor, GI upset, diplopia, Stevens-Johnson's syndrome (rare)	Hypersensitivity to lamotrigine or any of its components Use with caution with lactation, hepatic or cardiac dysfunction, and in children. Pregnancy category C	Take without regard to meals; drug may cause GI upset. Immediately report development of a rash. Gradually decrease dosage (taper) over 2 wk when discontinuing drug therapy.
topiramate (Topamax) Adults: initial: 50 mg/d; titrate by 50 mg/d at 1-wk intervals to a target dose of 200 mg bid	CrCl <70 mL/min: administer 50% of dose and titrate more slowly.	Cognitive difficulties, tremor, dizziness, ataxia, headache, fatigue, GI upset, renal calculi	Hypersensitivity to topiramate or any of its components Pregnancy category C	Maintain adequate fluid intake.
tiagabine (Gabitril) Children 12–18 y: 4 mg qd for 1 wk; may increase to 8 mg daily in 2 divided doses for 1 wk; then may increase by 4–8 mg weekly to response or up to 32 mg in 2–4 divided doses/d Adults: 4 mg qd for 1 wk; may increase by 4–8 mg/wk to response or up to 56 mg in 2–4 divided doses/d		Dizziness, somnolence, asthenia, confusion, GI upset, anorexia, fatigue, impaired concentration, speech or language problems, confusion	Hypersensitivity to tiagabine or any of its components Pregnancy category C	Should be taken with food Use caution when taking with other CNS depressants.
oxcarbazepine (Trileptal) Initial dose: 300 mg bid; increased by 600 mg/d at weekly intervals Children 4–16 y: 8–10 mg/kg in 2 divided doses/d, not to exceed 600 mg/d		Dizziness, diplopia, ataxia, headache, weakness, rash, hyponatremia	Hypersensitivity to oxcarbazepine or any of its components	Very recent drug
levetiracetam (Keppra) 500 mg twice daily; max 1,500 mg daily		Somnolence, asthenia, fatigue, dizziness, ataxia, anorexia	Hypersensitivity to the agent; not indicated for children Hypersensitivity to sulfonamides; not indicated for children	No drug interactions, rapid titration; only as adjunct therapy Long half-life leads to long titration period of 100 mg every 2 wk.

TABLE 39.3	Relationship Between Total Serum Concentration of Phenytoin and Adverse Events
Serum Concentration	**Adverse Events**
>20 mcg/mL	Far lateral nystagmus
>30 mcg/mL	45 degrees lateral gaze nystagmus and ataxia
>40 mcg/mL	Decreased mentation and lethargy
>100 mcg/mL	Lethal

Fosphenytoin should always be prescribed in phenytoin sodium equivalents: 75 mg of fosphenytoin sodium = 50 mg of phenytoin sodium. (See **Table 39.2.**) Fosphenytoin is given as a loading dose of 15 to 20 phenytoin equivalents/kg followed by a maintenance dose of 4 to 6 phenytoin equivalents/kg/d. Advantages over phenytoin include the ability to give it as an intramuscular injection in those without IV access and at a maximum infusion rate of 150 phenytoin equivalents/minute.

Contraindications/Precautions

Contraindications to fosphenytoin include hypersensitivity to phenytoin or fosphenytoin or a rash that occurs during treatment (treatment should not be resumed if the rash is exfoliative, purpuric, or bullous). Caution must be used in patients with severe cardiovascular disease, hepatic disease, renal disease, diabetes mellitus, porphyria, fever, or hypothyroidism. It is not recommended for use in children younger than age 4.

BOX 39.1	Non-Antiepileptic Drugs That Interact with Phenytoin

Non-AEDs Affecting Phenytoin Levels
Decreases Phenytoin Levels
   Alcohol (long-term use)
   Antacids, folic acid, rifampin, tube feedings
Increases Free-Phenytoin Levels
   Aspirin, diazoxide, tolbutamide
Increases Total Phenytoin Levels
   Alcohol (shortly after intake), amiodarone, chloramphenicol, chlordiazepoxide, chlorpheniramine, cimetidine, disulfiram, fluconazole, fluoxetine, imipramine, isoniazid, metronidazole, omeprazole, propoxyphene, sulfonamides, ticlopidine, trazodone

Adverse Events

The adverse event profile of fosphenytoin consists of nystagmus, somnolence, dizziness, ataxia, local intolerance to injection, paresthesia, nephrotic syndrome, and hypotension. The dose-related effects are the same as those with phenytoin, as are drug interactions. Adverse events of overdosage include unsteady gait, tremors, hyperglycemia, chorea, gingival hyperplasia, gynecomastia, slurred speech, mydriasis, confusion, agranulocytosis, granulocytopenia, hyperreflexia, coma, SLE, hypotension, and encephalopathy. In the case of fosphenytoin, an IV filter is not required during administration, whereas a filter is needed for IV phenytoin administration.

Interactions

See the section regarding phenytoin.

Carbamazepine

Indications/Uses

Carbamazepine is indicated for the treatment of partial and generalized tonic-clonic seizures. It is a first-line drug choice for monotherapy in simple or complex partial seizures with secondary generalization.

Mechanism of Action

Carbamazepine's mechanism of action is not completely understood. It is believed to alter synaptic transmission by limiting the influx of sodium ions across cell membrane channels. Other potential mechanisms of action include depressing activity in the nucleus ventralis of the thalamus or decreasing summation of temporal stimulation.

Dosage

Carbamazepine is available as an immediate-release tablet, extended-release tablet, and oral suspension. The usual starting dosage of carbamazepine is 200 mg twice daily as tablets or 100 mg four times daily as a suspension. Doses should be increased weekly by increments of no more than 200 mg. The usual maintenance dose is 800 to 1,200 mg divided into 2 to 4 doses, depending on the dosage form chosen. The therapeutic plasma concentration is 4 to 12 mg/L. Carbamazepine undergoes autoinduction after 3 to 5 weeks of therapy, resulting in decreased serum concentrations without a change in dose. Frequent monitoring may be required following initiation or changes in dosing.

Contraindications

Contraindications to carbamazepine include hypersensitivity to carbamazepine or tricyclic antidepressants, bone marrow suppression, and recent use of a monoamine oxidase (MAO) inhibitor (≤14 days).

Adverse Events

Adverse events associated with carbamazepine include hematologic abnormalities, drowsiness, fatigue, ataxia, syndrome

TABLE 39.4 Summary of Interactions Between Select Antiepileptic Drugs

Added Drug	Effects of Added Drug on Other AED Levels								
	CBZ	GBP	LTG	PB	PHT	VPA	ESM	PRM	FBM
CBZ	Autoinduction	0	↓	↓, ↑	↓, ↑	↓	↓	↓ PRM ↑ PB	↓
GBP	0	—	0	0	0	0	?	?	?
LTG	0	0	—	0	0	↓	?	?	?
PB	↓ CBZ ↑ EPOX	0	↓	—	↓, ↑	↓	↓	X	↓
PHT	↓ CBZ ↑ EPOX	0	↓	↓, ↑	—	↓ Total, ↑ Free	↑	↓ PRM ↑ PB	↓
VPA	↑ EPOX	0	↑	↑	↓ Total, ↑ Free	—	Slightly ↑	↑ PB	↑
ESM	0	?	?	↑	Slightly ↑	0	—	0	?
PRM	↓ CBZ ↑ EPOX	?	?	X	↓, ↑	?	↓	—	?
FBM	↓ CBZ ↑ EPOX	?	?	?	↑	↑	?	?	—

AED, antiepileptic drug; CBZ, carbamazepine; EPOX, CBZ epoxide metabolite; ESM, ethosuximide; FBM, felbamate; GBP, gabapentin; LTG, lamotrigine; PB, phenobarbital; PHT, phenytoin; PRM, primidone; VPA, valproic acid; X, rarely used in combination; ↓, ↑, decreases and increases can occur; ↓, decreased level; ↑, increased level; ?, interaction not known; 0, no effect; PEMA, phenylethylmalonamide metabolite of primidone
Adapted from Brittan, J., & So, E. L. (1996). Symposium on epilepsy, part V: Selection of antiepileptic drugs: A practical approach to antiepileptic drug therapy. *Mayo Clinic Proceedings, 71*, 778–789.

of inappropriate diuretic hormone secretion (SIADH), rash (Stevens-Johnson syndrome), gastrointestinal (GI) upset, confusion, nystagmus, and seizures. (See **Table 39.2**.) Carbamazepine is not effective in the treatment of myoclonic seizures and may in fact exacerbate seizures in these patients. Asian patients should be screened for the variant HLA-B*1502 allele prior to initiating therapy because this variant is associated with a significantly increased risk of Stevens-Johnson syndrome and toxic epidermal necrosis. It can be neurotoxic at elevated serum concentrations. Therefore, when initiating therapy, slow titration to the desired dose is necessary.

Concentration-related adverse effects include dizziness, ataxia, drowsiness, nausea, vomiting, tremors, agitation, nystagmus, urinary retention, arrhythmias, coma, seizures, respiratory depression, and cardiac conduction disturbances. The suspension formulation is incompatible with chlorpromazine (Thorazine) solution and thioridazine (Mellaril) liquid. Carbamazepine suspension should be given at least 1 to 2 hours apart from that of other liquid medications.

Interactions

Carbamazepine is a significant inducer of numerous CYP450 enzymes, including CYP1A2, CYP2B6, CYP2C9, CYP2C19, and CYP3A4. Caution should be used when administering other medications metabolized via these pathways. **Table 39.4** and **Box 39.2** list drug interactions among carbamazepine, AEDs, and other drugs.

Oxcarbazepine

Indications/Uses

Oxcarbazepine (Trileptal) is indicated for monotherapy or as adjunctive therapy in treating partial seizures in adults or in children ages 4 to 16 and as adjunctive therapy for partial seizures in children younger than age 2.

BOX 39.2

Non-Antiepileptic Drugs That Interact with Carbamazepine

Non-AEDs Affected by Carbamazepine
Decreased Levels due to Carbamazepine
Benzodiazepines, corticosteroids, cyclosporine, doxycycline, folic acid, haloperidol, oral contraceptives, theophylline, warfarin

Non-AEDs Affecting Carbamazepine Levels
Increases Carbamazepine Level
Cimetidine, danazol, diltiazem, erythromycin, fluoxetine, imipramine, isoniazid, propoxyphene, verapamil, nicotinamide
Decreases Carbamazepine Level
Alcohol (long-term use), folic acid

Mechanism of Action

Oxcarbazepine's pharmacologic effect is exerted through oxcarbazepine and the 10-monohydroxy metabolite (MHD) of oxcarbazepine. The exact mechanism by which oxcarbazepine and MHD work is unknown. However, studies indicate that the drug blocks sodium channels, resulting in stabilization of hyper-excited neural membranes and inhibition of repetitive neuronal firing. Increased potassium conductance and modulation of high-voltage activated calcium channels may contribute to the anticonvulsant effect.

Dosage

The typical starting dosage is 300 mg twice daily, increasing by 600 mg/d at weekly intervals. The target maintenance dosage is 600 to 2,400 mg/d. There are no therapeutic levels established for this agent.

Contraindications

Oxcarbazepine is contraindicated in patients with a hypersensitivity to the drug or any of its components. Oxcarbazepine should be avoided in patients who have had a hypersensitivity reaction to carbamazepine because there is a cross reactivity of about 30% and in patients at risk for hyponatremia (2.5% of patients).

Adverse Events

Common adverse events include dizziness, somnolence, diplopia, fatigue, nausea, ataxia, vomiting, abnormal vision, abdominal pain, tremor, dyspepsia, and abnormal gait. (See **Table 39.2.**) Oxcarbazepine has been linked to fatal dermatologic reactions, including Stevens-Johnson syndrome, and patients with toxic epidermal necrolysis should be monitored for signs and symptoms.

Interactions

Oxcarbazepine is a strong inducer of CYP3A4 and a weak inhibitor of CYP2C19. This leads to interactions with numerous AEDs, including valproic acid, lamotrigine, carbamazepine, phenytoin, and phenobarbital. Strong inducers of CYP enzymes (carbamazepine, phenytoin, and phenobarbital) have been shown to decrease plasma levels of the metabolite MHD (29% to 40%). Oxcarbazepine also interacts with non-AEDs metabolized by CYP3A4, including dihydropyridine calcium antagonists and oral contraceptives, leading to decreased plasma concentrations.

Valproic Acid and Derivatives (Divalproex)

Indications/Uses

Valproic acid and its derivatives (divalproex) are approved as monotherapy and adjunctive therapy in complex partial and complex absence seizures and as adjunctive therapy in patients with multiple seizure types, including absence seizures. It is considered first-line therapy for generalized tonic-clonic, simple partial, complex partial, and absence seizures. It has also been used in the treatment of partial myoclonic seizures, atonic seizures, infantile spasms, and status epilepticus.

Mechanism of Action

The exact mechanism is not completely understood but is believed to work by affecting GABA. It has been postulated to affect GABA in numerous ways, including increasing GABA availability, enhancing the action of GABA, and mimicking its action at postsynaptic sites.

Dosage

There are three specific forms of valproic acid available in the United States. While the dosage forms and dosing intervals vary, the total daily starting dose is the same. (See **Table 39.2.**) The recommended initial dose is 15 mg/kg/d increasing at 1-week intervals by 5 to 10 mg/kg/d. The dose is titrated to a desired therapeutic effect or toxicity, whichever occurs first. Doses above 60 mg/kg/d are not recommended. The therapeutic range is 50 to 100 mg/L with some patients requiring levels higher than 100 mg/L to achieve seizure control.

Contraindications

Valproic acid is contraindicated in patients with significant hepatic disease and in those with urea cycle disorders.

Adverse Events

Principal adverse events include fatigue, tremor, GI upset, alopecia, behavioral changes, and weight gain. Severe adverse effects include thrombocytopenia, pancreatitis, hyperammonia/encephalopathy, and hepatotoxicity which may occur at various times in therapy. Severe hepatotoxicity has been reported, especially in children age 2 and younger who are also taking other anticonvulsants. Patients taking valproic acid should be monitored for symptoms of hepatotoxicity, including malaise, weakness, facial edema, anorexia, jaundice, and vomiting. Other adverse events include a change in the menstrual cycle, ataxia, drowsiness, impaired judgment, headache, erythema multiforme, prolonged bleeding time, transient increased liver enzymes, tremor, nystagmus, SIADH, and fever. Valproic acid is teratogenic and produces spina bifida in 1% to 2% of pregnancies. Levels above 100 mg/L are associated with increased adverse effects.

Interactions

Minor interactions may occur with drugs that affect the CYP2C19, CYP2C9, CYP2D6, and CYP3A3/4 enzyme systems. Valproic acid may increase free phenytoin levels through displacement from protein-binding sites. Carbamazepine, lamotrigine, and possibly clonazepam reduce serum concentrations of valproic acid (**Table 39.4**), while aspirin may increase valproic acid levels. Increased effects and possibly toxicity have been associated with the concomitant use of diazepam, CNS depressants, and alcohol.

Ethosuximide

Indications/Uses

Ethosuximide (Zarontin) is one of the drugs of choice for absence seizures. It should always be used in combination with another agent. It also is used for managing akinetic epilepsy and myoclonic seizures.

Mechanism of Action

The exact mechanism of ethosuximide is not completely understood, but it suppresses the paroxysmal spike-and-wave pattern in absence seizures and depresses nerve transmission in the motor cortex.

Dosage

The usual adult dosage is 500 mg daily adjusted by 250 mg every 4 to 7 days. The average daily maintenance dose is 20 to 30 mg/kg/d. The initial dose for children ages 3 to 6 is 250 mg daily with the same titration schedule and usual maintenance dose as adults. Doses greater than 1.5 g/d are not recommended. Serum concentrations should be monitored periodically with a therapeutic range of 40 to 100 mg/L. (See **Table 39.2.**)

Contraindications

Allergy is the only absolute contraindication to taking ethosuximide.

Adverse Events

Common adverse events are GI upset and fatigue. Ethosuximide has been associated with blood dyscrasias, CNS depression, SLE, and cutaneous reactions.

Interactions

Ethosuximide is a major substrate of CYP3A4 and, therefore, serum concentrations are affected by inducers and inhibitors of CYP3A4.

Barbiturates

Barbiturates have a relatively broad spectrum of antiepileptic activity and can be used as alternative monotherapy in generalized tonic-clonic seizures as well as in simple or complex partial seizures with or without secondary generalization. Barbiturates are usually sedating and have long-term cognitive, memory, and behavioral effects, and drug dependence may develop. Therefore, it is usually best to try exhausting other alternatives before initiating barbiturate therapy.

Phenobarbital

Indications/Uses

Phenobarbital is the most commonly used barbiturate-based anticonvulsant. In addition to the indications listed previously, phenobarbital is used for myoclonic epilepsies, status epilepticus, and neonatal and febrile seizures in children.

Mechanism of Action

Phenobarbital works by binding to the barbiturate-binding site at the GABA receptor complex, leading to enhanced GABA activity. It interferes with the transmission of impulses from the thalamus to the cerebral cortex, resulting in an imbalance in central inhibitory and facilitatory mechanisms.

Dosage

In status epilepticus, phenobarbital is commonly given as a 15 to 20 mg/kg loading dose to more rapidly achieve therapeutic levels. The loading dose should be given no faster than 1 mg/kg/minute with a maximum infusion of 30 mg/min for infants and children and 60 mg/minute for adults. The recommended adult maintenance dose is 2 to 3 mg/kg/d or 60 to 250 mg per day. The recommended maintenance dose in children is highly variable based on age and ranges from 1 to 5 mg/kg/d. Serum concentrations should be monitored periodically with the usual therapeutic range being 15 to 40 mg/L.

Contraindications

The drug should be administered cautiously to patients with severe liver disease because of increased side effects. It is also contraindicated in patients with porphyria, respiratory disease with dyspnea or obstruction, and those with a history of sedative or hypnotic addiction.

Adverse Events

The principal adverse events—drowsiness and fatigue—make phenobarbital difficult to use. (See **Table 39.2.**) It also may cause ataxia and blurred vision, nausea, vomiting, constipation and, over a long period, cognitive impairment and behavioral disturbances. Other major adverse events include cardiac arrhythmias, bradycardia, dizziness, lightheadedness, CNS excitation or depression, and gangrene with inadvertent intra-arterial injection. To a lesser extent, hypotension, hallucinations, hypothermia, Stevens-Johnson syndrome, rash, agranulocytosis, megaloblastic anemia, thrombocytopenia, laryngospasm, respiratory depression, and apnea (especially with rapid IV use) also may occur.

If an overdosage or toxicity occurs, the expected signs and symptoms include unsteady gait, slurred speech, confusion, jaundice, hypothermia, hypotension, respiratory depression, and coma. Patients may require an IV vasopressor to treat hypotension. Repeated doses of activated charcoal significantly reduce the half-life of phenobarbital; the usual dose is 0.1 to 1 g/kg every 4 to 6 hours for 3 to 4 days unless the patient has no bowel movement, causing the charcoal to remain in the GI tract. Urinary alkalinization with IV sodium bicarbonate helps promote elimination. Patients in stage 4 coma due to high serum barbiturate levels may require charcoal hemoperfusion.

Interactions

Phenobarbital is a CYP1A2, CYP2D6, and CYP3A3/4 enzyme inducer that interacts with many of the AEDs. (See **Table 39.4.**) Other drug interactions include increased toxicity of

Non-Antiepileptic Drugs That Interact with Phenobarbital

Non-AEDs Affected by Phenobarbital

Decreases Phenobarbital Level

Beta blockers, chloramphenicol, chlorpromazine cimetidine, corticosteroids, cyclosporine, desipramine, doxycycline, folic acid, griseofulvin, haloperidol, meperidine, methadone, nortriptyline, oral contraceptives, quinidine, theophylline, warfarin

Non-AEDs Affecting Phenobarbital Levels

Increases Phenobarbital Levels

Chloramphenicol, propoxyphene, quinine

Decreases Phenobarbital Levels

Chlorpromazine, folic acid, prochlorperazine

Increased Toxicity

Benzodiazepines, central nervous system depressants, methylphenidate

propoxyphene (Darvon), benzodiazepines, CNS depressants, and methylphenidate (**Box 39.3**).

Primidone

Indications/Uses

Primidone (Mysoline) is structurally related to the barbiturates. It is metabolized to phenobarbital and to phenylethylmalonamide (PEMA). PEMA may enhance the activity of phenobarbital. Primidone is used in the management of grand mal, complex partial, and focal seizures.

Mechanism of Action

Its mechanism of action is similar to phenobarbital and is thought to decrease neuronal excitability and raise the seizure threshold.

Dosage

The adult dose of primidone is 125 mg/d increased by increments of 125 mg every 3 days. The usual dose is 750 to 1,500 mg/d in 3 or 4 divided doses with a maximum recommended dose of 2,000 mg/d. The usual serum level for primidone is 5 to 12 mg/L; however, serum phenobarbital levels are typically used for monitoring purposes. (See **Table 39.2**.)

Contraindications

See the contraindications for phenobarbital.

Adverse Events

Primidone has an adverse event profile similar to phenobarbital. Dose-related adverse events include fatigue, cognitive impairment, and ataxia. Other adverse events include nausea, vomiting, hematologic abnormalities, and an SLE-like syndrome. A skin rash may develop, and over time further cognitive impairment and behavioral changes may develop. Patients who have GI upset while taking primidone may take the medication with food.

Interactions

Drug interactions with primidone are similar to those with phenobarbital. (See **Table 39.4**.)

Gabapentin

Indications/Uses

Gabapentin (Neurontin) is a safe and well-tolerated anticonvulsant with uncomplicated pharmacokinetics. However, it is uncommonly used in the treatment of epilepsy. It can be used as adjunct therapy in the treatment of complex partial seizures and possibly generalized tonic-clonic seizures. There are insufficient data to support its use as monotherapy.

Mechanism of Action

Gabapentin is structurally related to GABA and is thought to reduce presynaptic GABA release, but the precise mechanism of action in epilepsy is unknown.

Dosage

The mean dosage in adults is approximately 1,800 mg/day, with a maximum of 3,600 mg/d. The therapeutic range is not well defined. It may be given once or twice daily, and its half-life is 5 to 7 hours.

Contraindications

Gabapentin is contraindicated in patients who are hypersensitive to the drug or to any of its components.

Adverse Events

Principal adverse effects are fatigue, dizziness, and blurred vision. (See **Table 39.2**.) Many of the CNS-like symptoms resolve in a few weeks. There have also been reports of modest weight gain.

Interactions

Gabapentin does not have any major drug interactions (antacids decrease its bioavailability), and serum level monitoring is not required.

Pregabalin

Indications/Uses

Pregabalin (Lyrica) is a newer antiepileptic drug approved as adjunctive therapy for partial-onset seizures in adult patients.

Mechanism of Action

Pregabalin binds to the voltage-gated calcium channels in the brain, inhibiting excitatory neurotransmitter release.

Dosage

Pregabalin is typically started at a dose of 150 mg daily in two or three divided doses and should be titrated based on efficacy and side effects to a maximum dose of 600 mg/d. It requires dosage adjustment in patients with impaired renal function to avoid accumulation and increased adverse effects.

Contraindications

Hypersensitivity to pregabalin or any component of the formulation is a contraindication. Caution should be used in patients with a history of angioedema, heart failure, hypertension, or diabetes.

Adverse Events

Peripheral edema and weight gain are common adverse effects. Other common adverse events include dizziness, somnolence, ataxia, and blurred vision. Angioedema has also been reported.

Interactions

Pregabalin may enhance the sedative effects of other CNS depressants and may enhance the fluid-retaining effects of thiazolidinediones.

Lamotrigine

Indications/Uses

Lamotrigine (Lamictal) seems to be efficacious for generalized tonic-clonic, absence (especially atypical), and complex partial seizures. It also may be effective in Lennox-Gastaut's syndrome (not approved for use in children younger than age 2).

Mechanism of Action

Although its mechanism of action is not completely clear, lamotrigine stabilizes neuronal membranes by acting on excitatory amino acid release and inhibiting voltage-sensitive sodium channels.

Dosage

The starting dosage for lamotrigine is 25 mg daily, with a slow titration every 2 weeks to a maintenance dose of 300 to 400 mg per day. The titration may even be slower, such as 25 mg every other day, in patients taking valproic acid. This slower titration should help lower the risk for rash.

Contraindications

Lamotrigine is contraindicated in patients with a hypersensitivity to lamotrigine or any of its components.

Adverse Events

Overall, lamotrigine is well tolerated and does not appear to have any long-term cognitive side effects. The principal adverse events include nausea, fatigue, dizziness, diplopia, and ataxia. (See **Table 39.2.**) In approximately 5% to 10% of patients (most often in children), a rash may develop. If a rash develops, the drug should be discontinued immediately. Stevens-Johnson syndrome and toxic epidermal necrolysis have been reported with the majority of cases occur in the first 8 weeks of therapy. The risk may be increased by coadministration with valproic acid, higher than recommended starting doses, and rapid dose increases. However, isolated cases have been reported with prolonged therapy or without these risk factors. Other adverse events include angioedema, nystagmus, and hematuria.

Interactions

The combined use of lamotrigine and carbamazepine may result in increased serum concentrations of carbamazepine and carbamazepine 10/11 epoxide. Valproic acid inhibits lamotrigine metabolism, whereas carbamazepine and phenytoin induce its metabolism. These enzyme interactions may result in significant changes in the half-life of lamotrigine. When used with valproic acid, the half-life is extended to 48 hours (from 24 hours when used alone), and with carbamazepine or phenytoin, it is reduced to 12 hours. Phenobarbital and primidone tend to decrease lamotrigine levels by approximately 40%. (See **Table 39.4.**) Although acetaminophen (Tylenol) may decrease lamotrigine levels, caution must be used when giving lamotrigine concomitantly with a folate inhibitor because it is an inhibitor of dihydrofolate reductase.

Levetiracetam

Indications/Uses

Levetiracetam (Keppra) has shown efficacy in the adjunctive treatment of adults with partial-onset or primary generalized tonic-clonic seizures.

Mechanism of Action

The mechanism of action of levetiracetam is not known, but it is theorized to inhibit voltage-dependent N-type calcium channels, facilitate GABA-ergic inhibitory transmission, reduce delayed potassium currents, and bind to synaptic proteins that modulate neurotransmitter release.

Dosage

Levetiracetam is started at a dosage of 500 mg twice daily with immediate-release formulations (1,000 mg daily with extended release) and titrated up to 3,000 mg/day. Dosages of greater than 3,000 mg/d have been used in clinical trials with good tolerability but without evidence of additional benefit.

Contraindications

Levetiracetam is contraindicated in patients with a hypersensitivity to levetiracetam or any of its components.

Adverse Events

The primary adverse events associated with levetiracetam therapy include somnolence, asthenia, headache, and infection. Most of these occur within the first 4 weeks of therapy, with no dose-toxicity relationship seen. Another common adverse event is changes in behavior, including aggression, neurosis, and psychosis, which may require a dose reduction.

Interactions

Since levetiracetam does not undergo significant metabolism, there are no clinically relevant enzymatic drug interactions with this agent.

Tiagabine

Indications/Uses

Tiagabine (Gabitril) is used as adjunctive therapy in adults and children older than age 12 with partial seizures.

Mechanism of Action

Its mechanism of action is not known; however, in vitro experiments show that it enhances GABA activity.

Dosage

The starting dosage of tiagabine is 4 mg daily and is titrated 4 to 8 mg weekly to response or up to 56 mg daily in 2 to 4 divided doses. The maintenance dose typically ranges from 32 to 56 mg/d.

Contraindications

Avoid using tiagabine in patients with hypersensitivity to any components of the formulation. Caution should be used in patients with hepatic impairment.

Adverse Events

Adverse events of tiagabine include dizziness, headache, somnolence, CNS depression, memory disturbance, ataxia, confusion, tremors, weakness, and myalgia. (See **Table 39.2.**) Rarely, severe dermatologic reactions such as Stevens-Johnson syndrome may occur.

Interactions

Tiagabine is a CYP2D6 and CYP3A3/4 enzyme substrate and is cleared more rapidly when given with other hepatic enzyme-inducing AEDs (i.e., carbamazepine, phenytoin, primidone, and phenobarbital).

Topiramate

Indications/Uses

Topiramate (Topamax) is used as monotherapy or adjunctive therapy for partial-onset seizures and primary generalized tonic-clonic seizures. It is also used as adjunctive therapy for seizures associated with Lennox-Gastaut syndrome.

Mechanism of Action

It is thought to decrease seizure frequency by blocking sodium channels in neurons, by enhancing GABA activity, and by blocking glutamate activity.

Dosage

The dosage starts at 25 to 50 mg twice a day and is increased to 200 to 400 mg/d in weekly increases of 25 to 50 mg/d. In patients with a creatinine clearance of below 70 mL/min, the dosage should be lowered by 50%.

Contraindications

Caution must be used in patients with hepatic or renal impairment, during pregnancy, and in breast-feeding mothers.

Adverse Events

Prominent adverse events are fatigue, dizziness, ataxia, somnolence, psychomotor slowing, nervousness, memory difficulties, speech problems, nausea, paresthesia, tremor, nystagmus, and upper respiratory infections. (See **Table 39.2.**) These may occur more frequently in patients taking more than 600 mg/day of topiramate, or when titration occurs too rapidly (3 to 4 weeks to maintenance dose). Other adverse events include chest pain, edema, confusion, depression, difficulty concentrating, hot flashes, dyspepsia, abdominal pain, anorexia, xerostomia, gingivitis, myalgia, back pain, leg pain, rigors, nephrolithiasis, and epistaxis.

Therapy should never be withdrawn abruptly. Proper hydration is essential to decrease the risk of kidney stones.

Interactions

Topiramate is a CYP2C19 enzyme substrate inhibitor; thus, concurrent administration with phenytoin can decrease topiramate concentrations by as much as 48%, administration with carbamazepine reduces them by 40%, and administration with valproic acid reduces them by 14%. Digoxin (Lanoxin) and norethindrone (Aygestin) blood levels are decreased when given with topiramate, and concomitant administration with other CNS depressants increases topiramate's sedative effects. If used with carbonic anhydrase inhibitors, the risk of nephrolithiasis increases.

Zonisamide

Indications/Uses

Zonisamide is a broad-spectrum, sulfonamide-derivative AED with activity in partial-onset seizures in adults. This agent is indicated only for use as adjunctive therapy.

Mechanism of Action

Zonisamide appears to block sodium channels and select calcium channels.

Dosage

The dosage of zonisamide is 100 mg once daily, giving it a distinct compliance advantage over other agents requiring more frequent dosing. The titration to the daily maintenance dose of 400 to 600 mg is slow, at a rate of 100 mg daily every 2 weeks. There are no guidelines for dose adjustment in patients with renal or hepatic impairment, though it is not recommended for use in patients with creatinine clearance of less than 50 mL/min.

Contraindications

Use should be avoided in patients with a history of hypersensitivity to sulfonamide agents or any components of the zonisamide formulation.

Adverse Events

Potentially fatal reactions such as Stevens-Johnson syndrome, toxic epidermal necrolysis, and agranulocytosis have been reported. Other important adverse events include fatigue, dizziness, ataxia, and anorexia. In children, there have been reports of high fever secondary to hyperhidrosis; zonisamide is not approved for use in children.

Interactions

Zonisamide is a major substrate of CYP3A4. Concentrations may be decreased when using inducers, such as phenytoin, phenobarbital, and rifampin. Serum levels may be increased when used concomitantly with protease inhibitors, azole antifungals, and macrolide antibiotics.

Felbamate

Indications/Uses

Felbamate can be used as either monotherapy or adjunctive therapy in the treatment of partial seizures. It is also used as adjunctive therapy in the treatment of partial and generalized seizures associated with Lennox-Gastaut syndrome in children. Due to an increased risk of life-threatening adverse effects, the American Academy of Neurology has published a practice advisory directing use.

Mechanism of Action

The mechanism of action is unknown but is believed to have weak inhibitory effects on GABA and benzodiazepine receptor binding.

Dosage

The initial dose of felbamate is 1,200 mg/d in divided doses three or four times a day. The dose may be titrated in 600-mg increments every 2 weeks to 2,400 mg/d based on response and to 3,600 mg/d if clinically indicated. Prior to prescribing felbamate, an "informed consent" form needs to be signed by the patient and physician.

Contraindications

Avoid use in patients with hypersensitivity to felbamate or any component of the formulation or with a known sensitivity to other carbamates. In addition, its use should be avoided in patients with a history of blood dyscrasias or hepatic dysfunction.

Adverse Events

Common adverse effects of felbamate include somnolence, headache, dizziness, ataxia, skin rash, nausea, vomiting, anorexia, and miosis. Rarely, felbamate has been associated with cases of hepatic failure and therefore should not be used in patients with a history of liver disease. An increased risk of developing aplastic anemia is present as well, and routine hematologic monitoring should be performed to detect evidence of bone marrow suppression.

Interactions

Felbamate is a major substrate for CYP3A4 and may be affected by concomitant use of drugs such as phenytoin. In addition, felbamate may increase concentrations of valproic acid and phenobarbital and may decrease the effectiveness of oral contraceptives.

Vigabatrin

Indications/Uses

Vigabatrin (Sabril) is a new AED approved for the treatment of infantile spasms and refractory complex partial seizures not controlled with usual treatments. It is only available in the United States through a restricted distribution program called the SHARE program. Only prescribers and pharmacies registered with the program are able to prescribe and distribute the drug.

Mechanism of Action

Vigabatrin irreversibly inhibits GABA transaminase, increasing the levels of GABA in the brain.

Dosage

The adult dose of vigabatrin is 500 mg as an oral tablet twice daily. The dose should be titrated by increments of 500 mg weekly based on the patient's response and adverse effects. The recommended maintenance dose is 1,500 mg twice daily. Upon discontinuation, the drug should be tapered by 1,000 mg weekly. The dose for the treatment of infantile spasms is 50 mg/kg/day divided twice daily titrated by increments of 25 to 50 mg/kg/day every 3 days. The maximum dose for infants is 150 mg/day. Dose adjustments are necessary in renal impairment.

Contraindications

Hypersensitivity to vigabatrin or any component of the formulation contraindicates its use.

Adverse Events

Vigabatrin can cause permanent vision loss in patients receiving the drug. Patients who do not show substantial benefit within a short time after initiation (2 to 4 weeks for infantile spasms, <3 months for adults) should have the drug discontinued to avoid this adverse effect. Vision loss increases with larger doses and cumulative exposure and can affect more than 30% of patients. Vision should be assessed at baseline, at 4 weeks, and every 3 months thereafter. Other common adverse effects include somnolence, headache, dizziness, irritability, insomnia, weight gain, and diarrhea.

Interactions

Vigabatrin may increase the sedative effects of other drugs and alcohol.

Lacosamide

Indications/Uses

Lacosamide is approved for adjunctive therapy of partial-onset seizures.

Mechanism of Action

Lacosamide stabilizes neuronal membranes and enhances the slow inactivation of sodium channels.

Dosage

The initial dose of lacosamide is 50 mg twice daily and may be increased weekly by 100 mg/day to a maintenance dose of 200 to 400 mg/day. In patients with creatinine clearance of less than 30 mL/minute or mild to moderate hepatic impairment, the dose should not exceed 300 mg/day. Lacosamide should be avoided in patients with severe liver disease.

Contraindications

There are no contraindications to lacosamide according to the manufacturer.

Adverse Events

Common adverse events seen with lacosamide include dizziness, fatigue, somnolence, blurred vision, diplopia, nausea, and tremor. Syncope and atrial arrhythmias may occur, especially in patients with a history of cardiovascular disease.

Interactions

Phenytoin, carbamazepine, and phenobarbital may decrease the serum concentration of lacosamide.

Benzodiazepines

The benzodiazepine antianxiety agents are discussed in depth in Chapter 41.

Clonazepam

Indications/Uses

Clonazepam (Klonopin) is effective as an adjunctive drug in some patients with myoclonic, atonic, and generalized tonic-clonic seizures. It also is used for prophylaxis of absence, petit mal, variant (Lennox-Gastaut), akinetic, and myoclonic seizures.

Mechanism of Action

Clonazepam is thought to act at the GABA receptor to enhance GABA action, thereby depressing nerve transmission in the motor cortex area.

Dosage

Clonazepam is given in three divided doses with an initial daily starting dose of up to 1.5 mg in adults and 0.1 to 0.2 mg/kg/d in children. The dose may be increased by 0.5 to 1 mg every third day until seizures are controlled or adverse effects are evident (maximum: 20 mg/d). Tolerance to this drug is common.

Contraindications

Contraindications include hypersensitivity to clonazepam, any of its components, or other benzodiazepines; severe liver disease; and acute narrow-angle glaucoma. Caution must be used in patients with chronic respiratory disease or impaired renal function and in patients who are mentally challenged (may have more frequent drug-induced behavioral symptoms).

Adverse Events

Fatigue, sedation, and behavioral changes (e.g., aggressiveness and confusion) are the principal adverse reactions. Tachycardia, chest pain, headache, constipation, nausea, and decreased salivation are other adverse reactions.

Interactions

Medications that induce CYP3A4 enzyme substrates, such as phenytoin and barbiturates, may increase clonazepam clearance. Concomitant use of CNS depressants may increase the risk of sedation.

Lorazepam

Indications/Uses

Lorazepam (Ativan) is used intravenously to treat status epilepticus and has an unlabeled use for partial complex seizures.

Mechanism of Action

The drug is believed to depress all levels of the CNS, including the limbic system and reticular formation, probably through the increased action of GABA. Before IV use, the injection must be diluted with an equal volume of compatible diluent. If it is injected intra-arterially, arteriospasm and gangrene may occur. The injectable form contains benzyl alcohol 2%, polyethylene glycol, and propylene glycol, which may be toxic in high doses.

Dosage

In the treatment of status epilepticus, lorazepam may be given as a 4-mg slow IV bolus (maximum rate of 2 mg/min). Doses may be repeated every 10 to 15 minutes until seizures stop.

Contraindications

Lorazepam is contraindicated in patients with a hypersensitivity to lorazepam or to any of its components. There is also a risk of cross-sensitivity with other benzodiazepines. It should not be used in comatose patients; patients with preexisting CNS depression, narrow-angle glaucoma, severe, uncontrolled pain, and severe hypertension; and pregnant women. Caution must be used in patients with renal or hepatic impairment, organic brain syndrome, myasthenia gravis, or Parkinson's disease.

Adverse Events

Common adverse reactions include tachycardia, chest pain, drowsiness, confusion, ataxia, amnesia, slurred speech, paradoxical excitement, headache, and depression. Lightheadedness, rash, decreased libido, xerostomia, bradycardia, cardiovascular collapse, syncope, constipation, nausea, vomiting, decreased salivation, phlebitis, and blurred vision also may occur. Menstrual irregularities, increased salivation, blood dyscrasias, and physical and psychological dependence occur with prolonged use.

Interactions

Lorazepam has a decreased effect with oral contraceptives (combination products), cigarette smoking, and levodopa. Its effects are increased with morphine or other narcotic analgesics. An increased risk of toxicity occurs with the concomitant use of alcohol, CNS depressants, MAO inhibitors, loxapine (Loxitane), and tricyclic antidepressants.

Diazepam

Diazepam is used to treat status epilepticus and as an adjunct in convulsive disorders. Its mechanism of action is the same as that of lorazepam.

Dosage

Diazepam may be given intravenously 5 to 10 mg every 5 to 10 minutes 5 or less mg/min to treat status epilepticus (maximum dose of 30 mg). It may also be given as a rectal gel out-of-hospital as a 10-mg, one-time dose and may be repeated once if necessary.

Contraindications

Diazepam should not be used by patients with severe or acute liver disease. Contraindications include hypersensitivity to diazepam or to any of its components. Other contraindications are similar to those for lorazepam. Caution should be used in patients taking other CNS depressants, patients with low albumin levels or hepatic dysfunction, and elderly patients and infants. Because of its long-acting metabolite and the risk for falls in the elderly population, diazepam is not considered a drug of choice.

Adverse Events

Adverse drug effects resemble those of lorazepam.

Interactions

Diazepam is a CYP1A2 and CYP2C9 enzyme substrate. It is also a minor enzyme substrate for CYP3A3/4, and diazepam and desmethyldiazepam are CYP2C19 enzyme substrates. Enzyme inducers may increase the metabolism of diazepam, resulting in decreased efficacy. Increased toxicity, sedation, and respiratory depression may result when diazepam is given with CNS depressants (e.g., alcohol, barbiturates, and opioids). Cimetidine (Tagamet) may decrease the metabolism of diazepam. Valproic acid may displace diazepam from binding sites,

which may result in an increase in sedative effects. Selective serotonin reuptake inhibitors (e.g., fluoxetine [Prozac], sertraline [Zoloft], paroxetine [Paxil]) greatly increase diazepam levels by altering its clearance.

Selecting the Most Appropriate Agent

There are several excellent AEDs from which to choose for various seizure types. The goal of monotherapy is to promote patient compliance, minimize side effects and toxicity, and reduce cost. In general, first-line monotherapy drugs are tried before using second-line monotherapy drugs, and first-line drugs may be first combined before trying the various second-line, adjunctive agents. Whether the second-line, adjunctive agents will be effective in monotherapy is still to be determined. The choice of an AED is determined by ease of use (i.e., dosing regimen), pharmacokinetics, interactions, need for monitoring, and toxicity (which could be dose related, idiosyncratic, chronic, or teratogenic). Ultimately, the optimal treatment for a given patient can be established by a process of trial and error and by knowledge of prior AEDs used.

First-Line Therapy

Selecting the appropriate therapy for each patient is difficult, but there is a science to choosing the best treatment:

- Select the appropriate drug and dose for the type and severity of the seizure being treated.
- Consider the patient's characteristics. For example, does the patient have renal insufficiency, liver disease, hypoalbuminemia, burns, pregnancy, or malnutrition? What concomitant medications does the patient take? How old is the patient? Does the patient comply with the medication regimen? What adverse events are associated with the medication?
- Determine the patient's socioeconomic status.

If the initial AED fails, the practitioner should taper this drug's dosage while starting another first-line AED, if available. A list of commonly used first-line drugs for different seizure types can be found in **Table 39.1.**

Second-Line Therapy

Before switching to a second-line agent, the practitioner must optimize treatment with the selected first-line drug (unless the patient experiences intolerable adverse effects) and exhaust all possible first-line drug therapy choices. The practitioner at this point may, based on the patient's past medical history, initiate combination therapy with two or more first-line drugs or a first-line drug and a second-line drug. **Table 39.1** contains a list of second-line drugs.

Third-Line Therapy

If all medications fail and the patient experiences intractable seizures, surgery may be a third-line treatment option. Before recommending surgery, the practitioner should make sure drug treatment errors have been ruled out (**Box 39.4**).

<table>
<tr><td>

BOX 39.4

Common Drug Treatment Errors

- Incorrect or incomplete identification of seizure type(s), resulting in inappropriate choice of treatment (e.g., the practitioner may be confused between brief complex partial seizures and absence seizures, or may fail to recognize juvenile myoclonic epilepsy)
- Drug selection that is appropriate for the patient's seizure type(s) but not for the patient (e.g., phenytoin for an adolescent or valproate for a woman who is pregnant or likely to become pregnant in the near future)
- Correct diagnosis and drug choice, but incorrect dosage (e.g., the patient is given too low a dose, only the starting dose is tried, or the patient receives too high a dose too quickly)
- Insufficient follow-up (e.g., the patient is seen by a specialist and referred back to the general practitioner with an appropriate recommendation regarding treatment, but when this proves ineffective, further advice is not sought)

</td></tr>
</table>

Special Population Considerations

Pediatric

The most common seizure syndrome in childhood is Lennox-Gastaut syndrome. This usually is associated with mental retardation. Characteristically, multiple seizure types can occur, including atypical absence, atonic (drop attacks), secondarily generalized tonic-clonic, and myoclonic and tonic seizures. EEGs show considerable slow-wave and spike-wave activity. Although patients respond to valproic acid, benzodiazepines, and lamotrigine, there is a poor prognosis for seizure control.

Simple febrile seizures are another important category of seizures that affect children between ages 6 months and 5 years. Febrile seizures occur in 4% of all children and are preceded by high fevers, underlying the importance of controlling high fevers in children. The seizure is generalized and usually lasts under 15 minutes. Approximately 33% of children experience a recurrence, although almost never within the first 24 hours. These patients usually have no preceding neurologic abnormality or family history of epilepsy. Long-term anticonvulsant therapy is not indicated for this seizure type.

Geriatric

Understanding the basic pharmacologic principles involved in the administration of AEDs is the key to the optimal use of these drugs in older patients. Drug clearance and metabolism are significant issues in this population. Many older patients have decreased renal and liver function, which may have a profound effect on drug metabolism and excretion. Consequently, AED dosages may need to be adjusted.

AEDs are bound to different degrees by plasma proteins, particularly albumin. If a patient has a low albumin level (as elderly adults tend to have), higher free-drug concentrations are present in the blood, and may lead to an increased risk of adverse events.

In patients with liver disease, which is common in the geriatric population, the rates of hepatic biotransformation of drugs and of hepatic blood flow are decreased. Therefore, protein-binding of AEDs may also be affected by low protein and displacement by bilirubin or other substances. This has the net effect of increasing the serum concentration of free drug. In renal disease, there may be a decrease in the clearance of drugs eliminated entirely by the kidney. Renal failure also may complicate elimination of drugs principally cleared by the liver. Studies have shown that in the patients with uremia who are taking phenytoin, hepatic biotransformation processes continue or accelerate during the renal failure, but renal excretion of metabolites is decreased. Therefore, uremic patients tend to have lower total serum phenytoin concentrations but higher serum concentrations of the oxidized principal metabolite (hydroxyphenyl-phenylhydantoin).

Women

For women taking anticonvulsant therapy, a major point for discussion is the risk during pregnancy. Several anticonvulsants are listed as pregnancy category C or D (i.e., phenytoin, fosphenytoin, phenobarbital, primidone, valproic acid, ethosuximide, topiramate, and tiagabine), indicating a greater risk for fetal abnormalities. The practitioner must work closely with women who wish to become, or are, pregnant to assess the risks involved and to choose the most effective drug that's safest for the fetus. In order to minimize the risk of congenital malformations, valproic acid and polytherapy should be avoided during the first trimester of pregnancy.

MONITORING PATIENT RESPONSE

For patients taking an AED, the health care practitioner should monitor:

- frequency and severity of seizures
- adverse drug events
- plasma drug levels, if applicable.

Therapy is considered to be a failure if the AED dosage achieves and maintains optimal blood concentrations and seizures are still uncontrolled and/or adverse effects become intolerable. Some patients have good clinical responses at serum drug concentrations below the therapeutic range while others can exhibit toxicity within the therapeutic range. Some require serum concentrations above normal therapeutic values for seizure control, and these patients may tolerate very high levels without signs of toxicity.

Drugs should be added or subtracted as needed. Whenever a new AED is started or a dosage change is made, it takes five elimination half-lives (or the period over which a drug's plasma concentration falls to 50% of the peak level after a single dose) before the new steady-state serum concentration is achieved. It is at this point the full therapeutic impact of the new medication or dosage change can be assessed. Therefore, too much haste in changing an AED or discarding it as ineffective may have significant therapeutic implications.

When AEDs are administered in combination, it is important to note the types of drug interactions that may occur. (See **Table 39.4.**) Even when monotherapy is used, some AEDs alter their own biotransformation when they are administered chronically (e.g., carbamazepine and valproic acid). The existence of these interactions complicates the design of the therapeutic regimen when more than one AED is used, underscoring the desirability of using monotherapy whenever possible.

Phenytoin and Phenobarbital

For patients taking phenytoin, blood pressure, vital signs (with IV use), complete blood count (CBC), liver function tests, and plasma phenytoin levels should be monitored. Steady-state concentrations are reached in 5 to 10 days.

For patients taking phenobarbital, its concentration, mental status changes, CBC, liver function tests, seizure activity, and respiratory rate should be monitored. Prolonged use may result in vitamin D loss, and supplementation may be necessary.

Primidone and Valproic Acid

For patients taking primidone, serum primidone and phenobarbital concentrations, CBC (at 6-month intervals), neurologic status, excessive sedation, and CNS effects should be monitored. Monitoring for patients on valproic acid must include liver enzymes, CBC with platelets, and valproic acid levels. Patients should immediately report a sore throat, fever, fatigue, bleeding, or bruising that is severe or persists.

Lamotrigine and Tiagabine

During therapy with lamotrigine, the practitioner should monitor seizures (frequency and duration), serum levels of concurrent anticonvulsants, and signs of a rash. During therapy with tiagabine, periodic monitoring of the CBC, renal function tests, liver function tests, and routine blood chemistry are required.

PATIENT EDUCATION

More than 90% of patients with epilepsy lead normal lives. The patient should avoid sleep deprivation and excessive alcohol use, both of which can lower the seizure threshold and make recurrent seizure activity likely. The patient should avoid jobs that involve working at heights or near heavy machinery, flames, burners, or molten material, so there are some restrictions on careers (e.g., firefighter, commercial driver, or airline pilot). Patients should never swim alone. Most sports are permitted, but those with an increased risk of a sudden loss of consciousness, such as skydiving, hang gliding, mountain climbing, and scuba diving, could be deadly and should probably be avoided.

Drug Information

The American Academy of Neurology's practice guideline center (http://www.aan.com/professionals/practice/guide line/index .cfm) provides information about epilepsy and medications for practitioners. Other sources of information on AEDs include the American Epilepsy Society (http://www.aesnet.org/Visitors/ PatientsPractice/index.cfm) and the National Institute of Neurological Disorders and Stroke (http://www.ninds.nih.gov/).

Patient-Oriented Information Sources

Patients often have questions about epilepsy prognosis and treatment, first aid, educational needs, pregnancy, and driving and insurance. The American Epilepsy Foundation or the many epilepsy societies around the country can help answer those questions. These organizations provide both professional and lay support assistance, including counseling and psychotherapy, access to social workers, and financial assistance.

Nutrition/Lifestyle Changes

The ketogenic diet has been advocated as a means of treatment for patients with epilepsy. This diet, high in fat and low in carbohydrates, is usually used in children refractory to AEDs. However, there does not appear to be reliable evidence supporting the use of the ketogenic diet in people with epilepsy.

Driving is, of course, one of the most serious restrictions. Laws concerning driving vary from state to state, but in general driving is not advised for 6 months after the last seizure. Some exceptions are strictly nocturnal seizures or those related to the discontinuation of an anticonvulsant on a physician's advice. Individual state laws regarding the driving restriction need to be reviewed by the practitioner.

First-aid for seizure activity consists primarily of protecting the patient's head and body from injury. It usually is not advisable to try to open the patient's mouth or to put objects in the patient's mouth. This can result in injury to the patient's mouth and airway as well as to the bystander. However, removing dentures, excessive secretions, and foreign materials from the mouth after a tonic-clonic seizure phase is completed may be helpful. Turning the patient into a semiprone position in the postictal period helps to prevent aspiration.

Case Study

A ccompanied by his girlfriend, B. C., age 23, visits your office. His girlfriend states, "He hasn't been himself the last month. He has headaches and is completely confused and tired for no reason." B. C. denies using illicit drugs and any recent traumatic injuries. He thinks his problem started approximately a month ago when he and his girlfriend were at a club dancing. His friends told him that he became confused and began tugging at his clothes. Then he fell down and was unconscious for a few minutes. When he awoke, he felt extremely tired and did not know what was going on. He girlfriend recalls that he had been hit in the head with a softball during a game the day before they went dancing.

Past medical history discloses insulin use since early childhood (currently 10 units NPH in the morning and 10 units regular insulin before meals), Zantac at bedtime, and Advil (1 or 2 tablets twice a day) for headaches. The patient says he has no allergies.

Family history reveals healthy parents who died in a car crash when the patient was age 10. Social history discloses a love of dancing, an active sex life, and occasional alcohol use at social events. B. C. does not smoke cigarettes or use recreational drugs.

On physical examination, B. C. is 5-foot-10 and 155 lb. His temperature is 37°C, pulse rate 78, blood pressure 118/76, and glucose level 90. Skin appears normal. Head and neck are normal, chest is clear for anterior and posterior sounds, cardiovascular RRR and (2) r/m/g, and laboratory values are within normal limits. EEG findings include sharp-wave discharges.

At a follow-up visit 2 months later, B. C. and his girlfriend report that things have gotten worse. The girlfriend states that as B. C. was eating dinner one night, he had a seizure. He was completely stiff for a short time and then his arms and legs began moving. She believes that he was unconscious for a few minutes. B. C. says he could not remember what had happened when he woke up.

DIAGNOSIS: GENERALIZED TONIC-CLONIC SEIZURE

1. List specific goals of treatment for B. C.
2. What AED would you prescribe? Why?
3. What are the parameters for monitoring the success of this therapy?
4. Describe one or two drug–drug or drug–food interactions for the selected AED.
5. Discuss specific patient education based on the prescribed therapy.
6. List one of two adverse reactions to the selected AED that would cause you to change therapy.
7. If the above occurred, what would be your choice for the second-line therapy?
8. What over-the-counter and/or alternative medications would be appropriate for B. C.?
9. What dietary and lifestyle changes would you recommend for this patient?

BIBLIOGRAPHY

Berg, A. T., Shinnar, S., Levy, S. R., & Testa, F. M. (1999). Status epilepticus in children with newly diagnosed epilepsy. *Annals of Neurology, 45,* 618–623.

Bourgeois, B. (1998). New antiepileptic drugs. *Archives of Neurology, 55,* 1181–1183.

Brittan, J., & So, E. L. (1996). Symposium on epilepsy. Part V: Selection of antiepileptic drugs: A practical approach to antiepileptic drug therapy. *Mayo Clinic Proceedings, 71,* 778–789.

Browne, T. R., & Holmes, G. L. (2001). Epilepsy. *New England Journal of Medicine, 344*(15), 1145–1151.

De Silva, M., McArdle, B., McGowan, M., et al. (1996). Randomized comparative monotherapy trial of phenobarbitone, phenytoin, carbamazepine or sodium valproate for newly diagnosed childhood epilepsy. *Lancet, 347,* 709–713.

Dichter, M. A., & Brodie, M. J. (1996). Drug therapy: New antiepileptic drugs. *New England Journal of Medicine, 334,* 1583–1590.

Freely, M. (1999). Drug treatment of epilepsy: Fortnightly review. *British Medical Journal, 318,* 106–109.

French, J. A., Kanner, A. M., Bautista, J., et al. (2004a). Efficacy and tolerability of the new antiepileptic drugs, I: Treatment of new-onset epilepsy: Report of the therapeutics and technology assessment subcommittee and quality standards subcommittee of the American Academy of Neurology and the American Epilepsy Society. *Neurology, 62*(8), 1252–1260.

French, J. A., Kanner, A. M., Bautista, J., et al. (2004b). Efficacy and tolerability of the new antiepileptic drugs, II: Treatment of refractory epilepsy: Report of the therapeutics and technology assessment subcommittee and quality standards subcommittee of the American Academy of Neurology and the American Epilepsy Society. *Neurology, 62*(8), 1261–1273.

French, J., Smith, M., Faught, E., & Brown, L. (1999). Practice advisory: The use of felbamate in the treatment of patients with intractable epilepsy. *Neurology, 52,* 1540–1545.

Greenwood, R., & Tennison, M. (1999). When to start and stop anticonvulsant therapy in children. *Archives of Neurology, 56,* 1073–1077.

Harden, C. L., Meador, K. J., Pennell, P. B., et al. (2009). Practice Parameter update: Management issues for woment with epilepsy—Focus on pregnancy. *Neurology, 73,* 133–141.

Krumholz, A. (1999). Nonepileptic seizures: Diagnosis and management. *Neurology, 53*(Suppl. 2), S76–S83.

Krumholz, A., Wiebe, S., Gronseth, G., et al. (2007). Practice parameter: Evaluating an apparent unprovoked first seizure in adults (an evidence-based review): Report of the Quality Standards Subcommittee of the American Academy of Neurology and the American Epilepsy Society. *Neurology, 69,* 1996–2007.

Lacy, C., Armstrong, L., Goldman, M., & Lance, L. (2010–2011). *Drug information handbook* (19th ed.). Hudson, OH: Lexi-Comp, Inc.

LaRoche, S. M., & Helmers, S. L. (2004a). The new antiepileptic drugs: Clinical applications. *JAMA, 291*(5), 615–620.

LaRoche, S. M., & Helmers, S. L. (2004b). The new antiepileptic drugs: Scientific review. *JAMA, 291*(5), 605–614.

Mattson, R. H., Cramer, J. A., & Collins, J. F. (1992). A comparison of valproate with carbamazepine for the treatment of complex partial seizures and secondary generalized tonic-clonic seizures. *New England Journal of Medicine, 327,* 765–771.

Riviello, J. J., Ashwal, S., Hirtz, D., et al. (2006). Practice parameter: Diagnostic assessment of the child with status epilepticus (an evidence based review): Report of the Quality Standards Subcommittee of the American Academy of Neurology and the Practice Committee of the Child Neurology Society. *Neurology, 67,* 1542–1550.

Sillanpaa, M., et al. (1998). Long-term prognosis of seizures with onset in childhood. *New England Journal of Medicine, 338,* 1715–1722.

Sperling, M., et al. (1999). Seizure control and mortality in epilepsy. *Annals of Neurology, 46,* 45–50.

CHAPTER 40

Jennifer A. Reinhold

Major Depressive Disorder

Major depressive disorder (MDD) is a mood disorder characterized by alterations in cognition, behavior, and physical functioning. It is a constellation of symptoms that interfere with normal function and may render an individual unable to perform psychologically, emotionally, and cognitively at previously attainable levels. Among the cardinal symptoms associated with a depressive episode are depressed mood, sadness, hopelessness, sleep disturbance, changes in appetite and weight, loss of interest, guilt, difficulty concentrating, and suicidal ideation. Further delineated by its recurrence and chronicity, depression results in functional impairment in multiple life domains and is a leading predictor of worsened morbidity and mortality. The clinical course is further complicated by the strong correlation of depression to psychiatric and physical comorbidity.

It is estimated that MDD affects 151 million individuals worldwide, with 6.2% lifetime prevalence. In the United States alone, depression is associated with the loss of 225 million missed workdays and indirect productivity-related losses of $36.6 billion (Perry & Cassagnol, 2009). Initial onset of depression may occur at practically any time throughout life; however, the peak onset is considered to be during the fourth decade of life. Earlier onset of presentation is inversely associated with successful treatment outcome; younger patients with depression tend to have a more severe and complicated clinical course with less likelihood of remission and an increased likelihood of recurrence. Today, although 80% to 90% of those affected can be treated effectively, only one third seek treatment.

CAUSES

There has not been a single causative factor for the development of depression elucidated. Rather, the development of depression is thought to be a multifactorial, complicated interplay among numerous physiologic, social, genetic, environmental, and biochemical factors. First-degree relatives of an individual with MDD have a relative risk of developing MDD that is 2.8 times that of the general population. Though not confirmed in large randomized controlled trials, some studies suggest an overall heritability of 37% to 43% (Shyn & Hamilton, 2010). More than 50% of patients who have

experienced one episode of major depression will experience a second; over 80% of patients who experience a second episode will experience a third.

PATHOPHYSIOLOGY

Most current research focuses on neurochemical aspects of depression and has spurred several theories relating to the generation and maintenance of specific neurotransmitters in the central nervous system. The basis for these neurochemical theories is the hypothesis that abnormal neurotransmitter release or decreased postsynaptic receptor sensitivity is affected before and during a major depressive episode. At least four theories relate to this hypothesis (**Box 40.1**). Three of the four theories focus on a functional or absolute deficiency in the neurotransmitters serotonin, norepinephrine, or both. A functional

---

BOX 40.1

Pathophysiologic Hypotheses of Depression

Serotonin Hypothesis

A functional or an absolute deficiency in the neurotransmitter serotonin

Catecholamine Hypothesis

A functional or an absolute deficiency in the neurotransmitters norepinephrine, serotonin, or dopamine

Permissive Hypothesis

Diminished serotonin gives "permission" for a superimposed norepinephrine deficiency to manifest as depression

Beta-Adrenergic Receptor Hypothesis

Depression results from increased beta-adrenergic receptor sensitivity

deficiency suggests that neurotransmitters are produced but the postsynaptic receptors cannot fully transmit the neural impulse. This is in contrast to an absolute deficiency, in which no neurotransmitters are produced or the postsynaptic receptors cannot transmit the signal at all.

Similar to the theories associated with the monoamine catecholamines norepinephrine and serotonin, new evidence suggests that dopamine may play a significant role in the pathogenesis and symptomatology of MDD. Genetic polymorphisms in the genes associated with dopamine transmission may contribute to an increased susceptibility to depression. Deficits in dopamine release or transmission have been linked to dysphoria, one of the most prominent features of MDD (Opmeer, et al., 2010). The permissive hypothesis, a more contemporary theory, suggests that reduced serotonin activity sets the stage for a mood disorder, such as depression or mania, depending on the underlying norepinephrine level. A low serotonin level coupled with a low norepinephrine level suggests that depression results from an increased beta-adrenergic receptor sensitivity. This alteration in postsynaptic receptor sensitivity results in an imbalance between the effects of norepinephrine and serotonin and may create a functional deficiency in serotonin. Secondary to the interplay among the catecholamines within the monoaminergic network, any impact on one of the monoamines will likely impact the others. This is applicable to the predisposition and development of MDD as well as the therapeutics of MDD.

DIAGNOSTIC CRITERIA

Mildly depressed patients meet the minimum criteria for diagnosis, whereas moderately depressed patients display a greater degree of dysfunction. Severely depressed patients experience symptoms well in excess of the diagnostic criteria. Their symptoms often greatly interfere with social and occupational functioning. *The Diagnostic and Statistical Manual of Mental Disorders IV* (DSM-IV) has established criteria for the diagnosis of depression, which are listed in **Box 40.2.** A patient must exhibit at least five of these signs or symptoms in the same 2-week period along with symptoms of depressed mood or anhedonia, the inability to gain pleasure from normally pleasurable experiences (Snow, et al., 2000).

In addition to the DSM-IV diagnostic criteria, numerous rating scales are employed in clinical practice to assess the severity of depression as well as response to treatment. The 17-item Hamilton Depression Scale (HAM-D or HDS) and the Beck Depression Inventory (BDI) are clinician-rated scales that are frequently used for this purpose.

Subtypes of MDD delineate the etiology and severity of the illness or episode. These subtypes include mild, moderate, and severe depression. The descriptors (known as *specifiers*) refer to the severity of dysfunction and delineate comorbid or distinguishing features, such as melancholy, catatonia, and psychosis.

BOX 40.2

Diagnostic and Statistical Manual of Mental Disorders IV: Criteria for Diagnosing Major Depressive Episode

A. Five (or more) of the following symptoms have been present during the same 2-week period and represent a change from previous functioning. At least one of the symptoms must be #1 or #2.
   1. Depressed mood most of the day. In children or adolescents the mood can be irritable instead of depressed.
   2. Diminished interest or pleasure in all or almost all of usual activities
   3. Significant weight loss or weight gain, or decrease or increase in appetite
   4. Insomnia or hypersomnia
   5. Psychomotor agitation or retardation as observed by others
   6. Fatigue or loss of energy
   7. Feelings of worthlessness, or excessive or inappropriate guilt
   8. Diminished ability to think or concentrate, indecisiveness
   9. Recurrent thoughts of death, suicidal ideation, suicide attempt, or a specific plan for suicide
   10. The symptoms cause clinically significant distress or impairment in social, occupational, or other important areas of functioning.
B. The symptoms are not due to the direct physiologic effects of a substance or a medical condition.
C. Patient must not be purposefully altering diet to achieve weight loss or gain.

TYPES OF DEPRESSION

Postpartum Depression

The onset is usually within 6 weeks after childbirth, and symptoms last from 3 to 14 months. Prevalence of postpartum depression ranges from 3.5% to 33%. Women with a history of postpartum depression have a 50% risk of recurrence, and 30% of women with a history of depression not related to childbirth have postpartum depression (Evins, et al., 2000).

Seasonal Affective Disorder

Seasonal affective disorder (SAD) is a pattern of depressive or manic episodes that occurs with the onset of winter. As the days become shorter and the weather colder, there is an increase in depressive symptoms. SAD causes individuals to eat more, sleep more, experience chronic fatigue, and gain weight. In pronounced cases, significant social withdrawal may occur.

Dysthymia

Dysthymia is a chronic but less severe form of depression that is found in approximately 3% of the population (Snow, et al., 2000). It is characterized by functional impairment and at least 2 years of depressive symptoms. Common symptoms include appetite disturbances, insomnia or hypersomnia, fatigue, difficulty making decisions, and low self-esteem.

Major Depression with Melancholic Features

Melancholic depression is a severe form of depression characterized by a profoundly depressed mood, nonreactivity, and neurovegetative symptoms. This type of depression is markedly more difficult to treat; however, it tends to be highly responsive to drug therapy.

Major Depression with Psychotic Features

Patients suffering from psychotic depression, in addition to the typical depressive symptoms, will also experience mood-congruent delusions and hallucinations.

INITIATING DRUG THERAPY

When prescribing drug therapy, the practitioner considers many indicators, among them the severity of symptoms (e.g., mild, moderate, or severe), type of depression (major, acute episode, postpartum, seasonal, dysthymia), duration of therapy, the patient's age, sex, comorbid conditions, and concomitant medications. In addition, if the patient has experienced depressive episodes in the past, the choice of drug may depend on what drug or drug class the patient responded to previously. An abundance of evidence supports the relative efficacy equivalence among antidepressant drug classes. Therefore, selection of the initial drug is generally not based on efficacy but rather on the side effect profile, patient preference, and target symptoms.

Initial staging of depression severity and ongoing assessment of response to treatment is generally accomplished by utilizing patient- or clinician-rated scales. The 17-item clinician-rated HAM-D is traditionally considered the inventory of choice for monitoring response to therapy. Other tools used in assessing the severity or source of depression include a typical health and medication history. Also useful is a physical examination with documentation of the patient's height, weight, and pertinent laboratory test findings, such as a complete blood count with differential, electrolytes, and kidney and liver function. Caution must be exercised in diagnosing MDD since certain medications and illnesses can induce depression. These conditions must be ruled out prior to making the diagnosis (**Box 40.3**).

BOX **40.3**

Selected Conditions and Medications Associated with Depression

Endocrine disorders
  Addison's disease
  Cushing's syndrome
  Hypothyroidism

Gastrointestinal disease
  Irritable bowel syndrome
  Inflammatory bowel disease
  Cirrhosis

Infections
  AIDS
  Influenza
  Meningitis

Cardiovascular diseases
  Congestive heart failure
  Myocardial infarction

Neurologic disorders
  Alzheimer's disease
  Multiple sclerosis
  Parkinson's disease
  Stroke
  Chronic headache

Cancer

Alcoholism

Drug use
  Alcohol
  Antihypertensives
    reserpine
    methyldopa
    diuretics
    propranolol
    clonidine
  Oral contraceptives
  Steroids

Rheumatologic
  Systemic lupus erythematosus
  Chronic fatigue syndrome
  Fibromyalgia
  Rheumatoid arthritis

Nonpharmacologic therapy for depression includes several psychotherapeutic techniques such as cognitive-behavioral therapy and interpersonal therapy. Psychotherapy is traditionally reserved for patients with concurrent psychosocial stressors.

Although psychotherapy alone may be effective, patients meeting the criteria for major depression should be evaluated for medication therapy. Moderately depressed patients often need a combination of medication and psychotherapy. Severely depressed patients may be refractory to psychotherapy, and their risk for suicide should be assessed.

Goals of Drug Therapy

Although historically nearly unattainable secondary to poor tolerability of available drugs, the ultimate goal of therapy for depression is *remission* and resolution of residual symptoms. A *response* to therapy, defined as a 50% reduction in the HAM-D score from baseline, was previously accepted as an appropriate therapeutic outcome. However, with the advent of newer and more tolerable drug therapies, the paradigm has shifted such that full remission is considered the only acceptable goal of therapy. Remission represents a complete resolution of depressive symptoms and a full return to previous level of functioning. Patients who have remitted will no longer fulfill the *DSM-IV* diagnostic criteria for depression and will score 7 or above on the HAM-D (normal).

Residual symptoms refer to symptomatology suggestive of depression that persists after a response to treatment. Even upon a successful course of treatment and clinical remission, some patients may continue to experience cognitive depressive symptoms, such as forgetfulness or apathy, or physical symptoms like fatigue. Patients who do not remit or who continue to have residual symptoms are at a greater risk for relapse or recurrence, have a shorter duration between depressive episodes, and have a worsened overall mortality. Optimal drug therapy not only resolves the acute symptoms of depression but also reduces the risk of relapse (Shelton, 2009).

MONITORING PATIENT RESPONSE

Drug therapy for depression consists of three phases: acute, continuation, and maintenance. Usually the patient needs additional contact with the practitioner or other health care provider (psychologist, social worker) during all phases of drug therapy. Assessments of efficacy, side effects, and adherence to the drug regimen should be made weekly, if possible.

Acute Treatment Phase

The goal of drug therapy in the acute treatment phase is to treat the patient until full remission. The duration of this phase is 6 to 8 weeks and potentially up to 12 weeks with apparent improvements occurring within the first 1 to 2 weeks. Though some clinicians attribute early response to a placebo effect, there is a preponderance of evidence that supports a true therapeutic effect within the first 14 days. In fact, newer research suggests that improvement by week 2 of therapy is a highly sensitive predictor of eventual response and remission (Tadić, et al., 2010).

Patients should have frequent contact with their practitioner throughout therapy, but especially in the first few weeks. Lack of efficacy early on may negatively impact patient adherence and motivation. Early improvements tend to include sleep satisfaction, appetite normalization, and recovery of cognitive function. Eventually patients will experience an elevation in mood and resolution of anhedonia (Zajecka, 2003). Full assessment of the effects of the antidepressant should occur at the 4- to 6-week interval after drug therapy begins. At this point, the practitioner evaluates improvements in the target signs and symptoms, assesses adverse drug effects, and determines whether dosage increases or decreases are necessary. To assist the evaluation, several depression rating scales, such as the HAM-D, the Zung Self-Rating Scale for Depression, and the BDI, may again be used as an objective measure of the change, or lack thereof, in a depressive state.

Continuation Phase

The continuation phase represents the time after a treatment response is seen in the acute phase and usually lasts 9 months to 1 year. The practitioner should continue antidepressant therapy for 4 to 6 months after symptom resolution. Failure to continue medication beyond symptom resolution confers an increased risk of relapse. When therapy is eventually discontinued, the medication is typically tapered over a few weeks to avoid physical or psychological effects that occur with abrupt discontinuation of the medication (discontinuation syndrome). During this time, the patient should be monitored closely for reemergence of symptoms.

Maintenance Phase

For some patients, long-term or even indefinite therapy is indicated. Maintenance therapy should be considered in all patients with three or more prior episodes or any patient with two episodes within the past 5 years, a comorbid substance abuse or anxiety disorder, a family history of recurrent depression, or onset of depression earlier than age 20 or later than age 40. This phase of therapy uses the same effective antidepressant used during the acute and continuation phases for a minimum of 3 and up to 5 years or longer.

Elderly patients who had one episode of depression and those who had two or more previous episodes of depression have a risk of relapse of more than 80.5% (Breen & McCormac, 2002). These patients should receive antidepressant therapy indefinitely.

Modification of Drug Therapy

Despite the availability of pharmacologic therapies for depression and the relative equivalence in efficacy among the classes, approximately 50% of patients will not respond to the first trial of a first-line antidepressant (Zajecka, 2003). Subsequent trials of alternate medications after the initial failure yield success rates of 20% with a gradual decrease in rates of response and remission with each trial. Only about one third of patients will remit after the first trial, and almost 30% of patients will not remit even after a series of sequential therapies (Papakostas, 2009).

Initiation of an appropriate drug at an optimal dose, giving the drug an adequate trial (6 to 12 weeks), and educating the patient about the timeframe for response and the importance of adherence are critically essential therapeutic concepts. If the patient is started on an appropriate drug for an adequate period, has been compliant with therapy, and does not respond or remit in a reasonable amount of time, drug therapy may need to be adjusted.

There are four common strategies used to modify drug therapy in the depressed patient: dosage increase, switching to a different drug or class, augmenting the current drug, or combining medications. Increasing the dose of a drug is typically recommended if the patient has had a response or a partial response during the first few weeks. If an inadequate response or lack of response occurs within the first few weeks of therapy, a switch to a different drug may be warranted. Within-class and between-class switches are viable options depending upon the patient presentation. Lack of response to one drug within a class does not necessarily confer lack of response to all drugs within a class; therefore, switching within a class may be appropriate. Augmentation of the initial drug preserves any benefit experienced by the patient during the trial and also targets side effects or residual symptoms. The combination of two or more drugs with differing mechanisms of action has also been shown to be efficacious.

Antidepressant Drugs

Several drug classes are available for treating depression: selective serotonin reuptake inhibitors (SSRIs), serotonin-norepinephrine reuptake inhibitors (SNRIs), tricyclic antidepressants (TCAs), monoamine oxidase (MAO) inhibitors, and atypical agents. They all exert a pharmacologic effect by impacting one or more of the primary neurotransmitters theorized to contribute to depression. In theory, each of the antidepressants increases the amount of neurotransmitter available in the synapse, either by inhibiting its metabolic degradation or by decreasing the rate at which it is recycled (by the process called *reuptake*) back into the presynaptic neuron (**Figure 40-1**). For example, SSRIs inhibit the reuptake of select isoforms of serotonin, thereby increasing the functional availability of serotonin in the synaptic cleft. SNRIs increase the relative concentrations of both serotonin and norepinephrine, with more serotonergic or noradrenergic activity depending upon the dose. TCAs are thought to work by inhibiting the reuptake of norepinephrine from the synaptic cleft, thereby increasing the amount available to stimulate the postsynaptic neuron. Conversely, MAO inhibitors limit the metabolism of monoamines such as dopamine, serotonin, and norepinephrine. This nonselective inhibition also increases the relative amounts of each of these catecholamines available to stimulate the postsynaptic neurons. However, this nonselectivity may contribute to side effects.

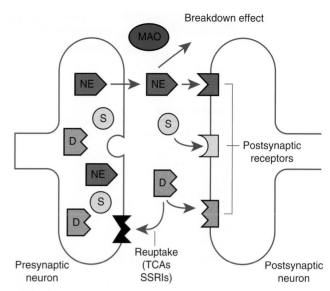

FIGURE 40–1 Schematic representation of the mechanism of action of antidepressant agents. Neurotransmitters (NE, S, D) are released from the presynaptic neuron into the synaptic space. They interact with the postsynaptic receptors and continue the neuronal transmission. After release from the postsynaptic neuron, these agents can be broken down by the enzyme monoamine oxidase (MAO) and the components recycled into the presynaptic neuron or they can be taken up again through the reuptake mechanism. Antidepressant agents can (1) block the MAO enzymes—MAO inhibitors; or (2) block the reuptake of the neurotransmitter. In effect, each mechanism increases the intrasynaptic concentration of the particular neurotransmitter.

Table 40.1 presents the antidepressants and the neurotransmitters primarily affected. Because all of these agents appear to have equal efficacy, the practitioner should select the most appropriate initial therapy based on side effect profiles, predicted patient compliance, and cost of therapy. The following discussion and accompanying tables and charts will help the practitioner in selecting the optimal initial agent for treating depression.

Selective Serotonin Reuptake Inhibitors

The development of SSRIs changed the landscape of depression pharmacotherapy. Just as effective as TCAs and older antidepressants, SSRIs boast improved tolerability and reduced lethality in overdose. The leading cause of death in the depressed patient population is suicide and therefore utilizing a drug class with minimal risk of successful overdose is paramount. The tolerability profile, relative safety in overdose, and the need for fewer titrations have resulted in SSRIs effectively replacing TCAs as the drug class of choice for treating depression. SSRIs work primarily by binding to the serotonin transporter and inhibiting the reuptake of this neurotransmitter into the presynaptic neurons. Relative efficacy is comparable within the class. **Table 40.2** identifies starting dosages and expected dosage ranges of SSRIs.

TABLE 40.1	Classification of Antidepressant Agents and Neurotransmitters Affected	Primary Neurotransmitters Affected		
Generic Name	Trade Name	NE	5-HT	D
Tricyclic Antidepressants				
amitriptyline	Elavil	+ + + +	+ + + +	0
desipramine	Norpramin	+	+ + +	0
doxepin	Sinequan	+	+ + +	0
imipramine	Tofranil	+ + +	+ +	0/+
nortriptyline	Pamelor	+ +	+ + +	0
protriptyline	Vivactil	+	+ + + +	0
trimipramine	Surmontil	+ +	+ +	0
Selective Serotonin Reuptake Inhibitors				
citalopram	Celexa	0	+ + + +	0
fluoxetine	Prozac	0	+ + + +	0
fluvoxamine	Luvox	0	+ + + +	
paroxetine	Paxil	0	+ + + +	0
sertraline	Zoloft	0	+ + + +	0
escitalopram	Lexapro	0	+ + + +	0
Serotonin-Norepinephrine Inhibitors				
venlafaxine	Effexor	+ + + +	+ + +	+
desvenlafaxine	Pristiq	+ + + +	+ + +	+
duloxetine	Cymbalta	+ + + +	+ + +	+
Monoamine Oxidase Inhibitors				
phenelzine	Nardil			
Atypicals				
amoxapine	Asendin	+ + +	+ + +	0
bupropion	Wellbutrin	+	0/+	+
maprotiline	Ludiomil	+ + + +	0	0
mirtazapine	Remeron	+	+ + + + +	0
nefazodone	Serzone	0/+	+ + +	0
trazodone	Desyrel	0	+ +	0
venlafaxine	Effexor	+ + + +	+ + + +	0/+

NE, norepinephrine; 5-HT, 5-hydroxytryptamine (serotonin); D, dopamine; + + + +, highly potent effect; +, minimally potent effect; 0, no effect

Time Frame for Response

The effects of these agents are apparent within 4 to 6 weeks of treatment. The length of therapy for first episodes of depression is 4 to 6 months after recovery. Continued treatment beyond the point of recovery drastically reduces the relapse potential over 1 to 3 years (Reid & Barbui, 2010). Measures of efficacy include improved scores in the initial rating scales, self-reported improvement in the target symptoms originally described by the patient, and improved affect observed by the practitioner.

Adverse Events

SSRIs are usually administered in the morning because of the potential to induce anxiety and insomnia. Insomnia is thought to be related to the suppression of rapid eye movement (REM) sleep and may be treated with a sedative–hypnotic drug such as the benzodiazepine temazepam (Restoril). Because long-term treatment of insomnia is not recommended, a gradual tapering of the sedative–hypnotic agent is advisable. If it appears necessary to continue a sedative–hypnotic, the practitioner should evaluate the reason for the sleep disturbance and treat accordingly. Some patients do, however, experience sedation with an SSRI, and these patients may be advised to take their medication at bedtime.

SSRIs have virtually no potential for inducing orthostatic hypotension or cardiac conduction abnormalities, which makes them ideal for elderly patients or those with a history of arrhythmias. They do have epileptogenic potential, so caution must be used in patients with a history of seizures.

A common side effect reported by patients taking SSRIs is sexual dysfunction. This is due to the increased serotonin activity

TABLE 40.2   Overview of Antidepressant Agents

Generic (Trade) Name and Dosage	Selected Adverse Events	Contraindications	Special Considerations
Tricyclic Antidepressants			
amitriptyline (Elavil) Start: 25 mg tid Range: 50–300 mg	Sedation, dry mouth	History of cardiovascular disease	Therapeutic plasma concentration range: 60–200 ng/mL
amoxapine (Asendin) Start: 50 mg tid Range: 100–600 mg	Anticholinergic, sedation	History of epilepsy or cardiac dysfunction	Therapeutic plasma concentration range: 180–600 ng/mL
clomipramine (Anafranil) Start: 25 mg hs Range: 150–200 mg	Sedation, orthostatic hypotension	History of cardiovascular disease	Blood levels not used clinically
desipramine (Norpramin) Start: 25 mg tid Range: 50–300 mg	Sedation, dry mouth	Same as above	Therapeutic plasma concentration range: 125–250 ng/mL
doxepin (Sinequan) Start: 25 mg tid Range: 75–300 mg	Sedation, orthostatic hypotension	Same as above	Therapeutic plasma concentration range: 110–250 ng/mL
imipramine (Tofranil) Start: 25 mg tid Range: 50–300 mg	Sedation, orthostatic hypotension	Risk of falling, history of cardiovascular disease	Therapeutic plasma concentration: 180 ng/mL
maprotiline (Ludiomil) Start: 25 mg tid Range: 50–300 mg	Anticholinergic, sedation, seizures	History of epilepsy or cardiac dysfunction	Therapeutic plasma concentration range: 200–400 ng/mL
nortriptyline (Pamelor) Start: 25 mg tid Range: 50–200 mg	Sedation	History of cardiovascular disease	Therapeutic plasma concentration range: 50–150 ng/mL
protriptyline (Vivactil) Start: 5 mg tid Range: 15–60 mg	Sedation, orthostatic hypotension	Same as above	Therapeutic plasma concentration range: 100–200 ng/mL
trimipramine (Surmontil) Start: 25 mg tid Range: 15–90 mg	Sedation, cardiac conduction disturbances	Same as above	
Selective Serotonin Reuptake Inhibitors			
citolapram (Celexa) Start: 20 mg qd Range: 20–40 mg qd	Nausea, dry mouth, increased sweating, somnolence, insomnia	MAO inhibitor therapy	In trials, approximately 6% of men experienced difficulty with ejaculation, and 3% reported impotence.
fluoxetine (Prozac) Start: 10–20 mg each morning Range: 10–80 mg	Insomnia	Same as above	Take in morning to avoid insomnia.
fluvoxamine (Luvox) Start: 75 mg bid Range: 100–300 mg	Increases in blood pressure	Same as above	Monitor blood pressure.
paroxetine (Paxil) Start: 20 mg qd Range: 10–50 mg	Mild sedation	Same as above	May be useful in patients displaying insomnia as depressive symptom
sertraline (Zoloft) Start: 50 mg qd Range: 50–200 mg	Insomnia	Same as above	Take in morning to avoid insomnia. May be agitating
escitalopram (Lexapro) Start: 10 mg qd Range: 10–20 mg qd	Nausea, diarrhea, increased sweating, somnolence, insomnia, fatigue	Same as above	Extensively metabolized in the liver The dose for hepatic impairment is 10 mg qd.

(continued)

TABLE 40.2 **Overview of Antidepressant Agents (*Continued*)**

Generic (Trade) Name and Dosage	Selected Adverse Events	Contraindications	Special Considerations
Serotonin-Norepinephrine Reuptake Inhibitors			
venlafaxine (Effexor) Start: 25 mg tid or 37.5 mg bid Range: 75–375 mg	Increases in blood pressure, sexual dysfunction	Do not use within 14 d of MAO inhibitor therapy; caution in narrow-angle glaucoma	Monitor blood pressure closely. Tachycardia and hypotension above 200 mg/day may occur.
desvenlafaxine (Pristiq) Start: 50 mg Range: 50–100 mg (no additional benefit above 50 mg)	Same as above	Same as above	May cause significant dose-related increases in total cholesterol, LDL, and triglycerides; nausea occurs in up to 30% of patients
duloxetine (Cymbalta) Start: 40–60 mg Range: 60–120 mg (no additional benefit above 60 mg)	Same as above	Same as above	May worsen psychosis in some patients or precipitate a shift to mania or hypomania in patients with bipolar disorder; nausea occurs in up to 30% of patients
Atypicals			
trazodone (Desyrel) Start: 50 mg tid Range: 50–600 mg	Orthostatic hypotension, priapism	Contraindicated in recovery phase of myocardial infarction	Therapeutic range: 800–1,600 ng/mL
bupropion (Wellbutrin, Wellbutrin SR, Wellbutrin XL) Start: 100 mg twice daily (IR); 150 mg daily (SR) Range: 300–450 mg	Headache, insomnia, xerostomia	Do not use within 14 d of MAO inhibitors; do not use during an abrupt cessation of sedatives or ethanol	Lowers seizure threshold at dose >450 mg; avoid concomitant alcohol ingestion

at the 5-HT2c receptor site. Sexual dysfunction is often a reason cited by patients for prematurely stopping their antidepressants (Breen & McCormac, 2002). All SSRIs have the potential to induce sexual dysfunction. The incidence varies from about 24% to 73%, depending on the individual drug. Paroxetine is comparatively associated with the highest rate of sexual side effects, and fluvoxamine may be the least likely in the class to cause sexual dysfunction (Schweitzer, et al., 2009). The manifestation is delayed or absent orgasm in both men and women along with loss of libido. Risk of this side effect must be communicated to the patient prior to starting therapy. Treatment of this dysfunction is available, but lowering the dose without compromising efficacy may be the first strategy. If the symptoms persist, cyproheptadine (Periactin), amantadine (Symmetrel), and yohimbine (Yohimex) may benefit some patients. In addition, sildenafil (Viagra), tadalafil (Cialis), or vardenafil (Levitra) may benefit some male patients who suffer from this sexual side effect.

Recently, the question of increased suicidality has been raised with respect to SSRIs and antidepressants in general. SSRIs specifically are associated with an increase in attempted and completed suicide in patients younger than age 25. They have no effect on suicidality in patients ages 25 to 64, and reduce suicidal behaviors in patients over age 65 (Reid & Barbui, 2010).

Interactions

The selection of an SSRI for an individual patient is determined by the drug interaction profile. SSRIs inhibit various components of the cytochrome P450 (CYP450) system, thus causing elevations in other medications that are metabolized by this system (Breen & McCormac, 2002). Before prescribing an SSRI, the practitioner must take a thorough medication history and identify the potential for altering the pharmacokinetics or pharmacodynamics of medications that the patient will be taking concomitantly. (**Table 40.3** offers a guide to the major drug–drug interactions with common SSRIs.)

Of special note, SSRIs are contraindicated with MAO inhibitors because the combination can lead to a sudden increase in systemic serotonin. The MAO inhibitor–mediated inhibition of the serotonin metabolism (thereby increasing its circulating availability) coupled with the action of the SSRI itself can result in serotonin excess. The manifestation of excessive serotonin, which is potentially life-threatening, is termed *serotonin syndrome*. Signs and symptoms include heat stroke, vascular collapse, fever, and tachycardia.

Serotonin-Norepinephrine Reuptake Inhibitors

The pharmacologic effect of SNRIs is primarily mediated through the potent inhibition of neuronal uptake of serotonin

TABLE 40.3   Selected Antidepressant Drug Interactions Involving the Cytochrome P450 System

Agent–Drug Interaction Potential	Isozyme Inhibited	Drugs Affected
Addition of this agent...	*will inhibit this isoenzyme...*	*resulting in increased levels of these drugs:*
fluoxetine—moderate	3A4	Type 1A antiarrhythmics
mirtazapine—low		Clozapine
nefazodone—high		Benzodiazepines (alprazolam, triazolam, clonazepam)
paroxetine—low		Calcium channel blockers
sertraline—low		Cannabinoids
venlafaxine—low		Carbamazepine
		Cyclosporine
		Estrogens
		Fentanyl
		HIV-1 protease inhibitors
		HMG-CoA reductase inhibitors
		Macrolide antibiotics
		Ondansetron
		Tricyclic antidepressants (amitriptyline, clomipramine, imipramine)
		R-warfarin
		Zolpidem
fluoxetine—high	2D6	Narcotic analgesics
mirtazapine—low		Chlorpromazine
paroxetine—high		Fluphenazine
sertraline—low		Haloperidol
venlafaxine—low		Perphenazine
		Risperidone
		Beta blockers (labetalol, metoprolol, pindolol, propranolol, timolol)
		Benztropine
		Cyclobenzaprine
		Dextromethorphan
		Donepezil
		Glimepiride
		Trazodone
		Tricyclic antidepressants
fluoxetine—low	1A2	Clozapine
fluvoxamine—high		Haloperidol
mirtazapine—low		Thioridazine
nefazodone—low		Olanzapine
paroxetine—low		Chlorpromazine
sertraline—low		Trifluoperazine
venlafaxine—low		Caffeine
		Diazepam
		Metoclopramide
		Ondansetron
		Propranolol
		Tacrine
		Theophylline
		Tricyclic antidepressants (amitriptyline, clomipramine, imipramine)
		Verapamil
		Warfarin
		Zolpidem

and norepinephrine and the weak inhibition of dopamine reuptake. SNRIs have no significant activity for muscarinic cholinergic, H_1-histaminergic, or alpha$_2$-adrenergic receptors and do not possess MAO inhibitor activity. Since the inception of SNRIs, there has been clinical debate regarding whether or not this newer class is superior to SSRIs because of its dual inhibition of serotonin and norepinephrine. It is postulated that this confers a broader antidepressant effect. Venlafaxine (Effexor), the first drug developed in this class, has been extensively studied in terms of its comparative efficacy to SSRIs. Numerous studies suggest that there may in fact be a slight but significant advantage in using venlafaxine over SSRIs with respect to remission rates. Literature also supports the use of SNRIs in more severe depression and in treatment-resistant depression (Bauer, et al., 2009). There are currently three SNRIs available in the United States: venlafaxine, desvenlafaxine (Pristiq), and duloxetine (Cymbalta). Desvenlafaxine, the R-isomer of venlafaxine, differs from its parent compound with respect to its simpler dosing regimen, greater bioavailability, and improved ability to inhibit norepinephrine reuptake. Duloxetine has a once-daily dosing schedule, reduced risk of treatment-emergent hypertension, and fewer discontinuation symptoms. Please see **Table 40.2.**

Time Frame for Response

Similar to SSRIs, SNRIs require approximately 4 to 6 weeks (and potentially up to 12 weeks) to exert a full pharmacologic effect. Some cognitive and physical symptoms of depression may begin to remit within the first week of therapy, but the full effect is slightly more protracted. As with any of the antidepressants, SNRIs should be taken through the continuation and maintenance phases to reduce the risk of relapse.

Adverse Events

SNRIs, though better tolerated than TCAs, have the potential to produce more adverse effects as compared to SSRIs secondary to the noradrenergic activity; there are higher rates of dry mouth, constipation, nausea, and insomnia. Treatment-emergent hypertension has occurred in patients taking venlafaxine, although the majority of cases occur in patients who are predisposed to developing hypertension. Increases in blood pressure of approximately 10 mm Hg have also been reported in patients who are hypertensive prior to starting venlafaxine therapy. Two dose-related side effects occur with venlafaxine: nausea and hypertension. Starting therapy with lower doses and gradually increasing the dose as tolerated minimizes the nausea. The prevalence of sexual dysfunction in patients taking venlafaxine, desvenlafaxine, or duloxetine approximates that of SSRIs.

Abrupt discontinuation of SNRI therapy is not recommended, especially venlafaxine. This can produce a discontinuation syndrome similar to that of SSRIs. Duloxetine has not been shown to elicit these types of symptoms to the extent that the other two members of this class have.

Interactions

SNRIs are metabolized by the CYP450 system, namely the CYP1A2, CYP3A4, and CYP2D6 isoenzymes. Coadminstration of SNRIs with other drugs that are substrates of or that otherwise impact those isoenzymes may result in drug interactions. Concomitant administration of MAO inhibitors with SNRIs is contraindicated because this may result in serotonin syndrome.

Tricyclic Antidepressants

Prior to the emergence of SSRIs, TCAs were the mainstay of therapy for years. There are no proven significant differences in terms of efficacy between TCAs and SSRIs (Mulrow, et al., 2000). TCAs are potent inhibitors of the reuptake of norepinephrine and exert fewer effects on serotonin. Clomipramine (Anafranil) is a potent serotonin reuptake blocker, and its metabolite is a potent norepinephrine reuptake blocker. (See **Table 40.2.**) Amitriptyline (Elavil), for example, significantly increases the amount of norepinephrine and serotonin available to the postsynaptic neuron. In contrast, nortriptyline (Pamelor) has a relatively low effect on both norepinephrine and serotonin. These agents, therefore, attempt to restore the balance of neurotransmitters and work in accord with several of the aforementioned theories.

TCAs are also active at acetylcholine and histamine receptors, which contribute to their side effect profile. This complex pharmacology, coupled with the cholinergic side effects, makes TCAs a second-line choice for treating depression.

Adverse Events

The selection of a TCA for treating depression is based on the side effect profile (**Table 40.4**) along with successful treatment in patients who received TCAs in the past. In varying degrees, all TCAs can cause sedation, which is an important consideration, especially if the depression is characterized by insomnia. Administering a TCA at bedtime may help alleviate this symptom.

In addition, the hypotensive effect of each agent varies and should be considered when selecting a particular agent. For example, nortriptyline and desipramine (Norpramin) have less potential for inducing orthostatic hypotension, making them advantageous in elderly patients. Moreover, the epileptogenic potential and life-threatening cardiac conduction abnormalities associated with various agents must be considered when selecting a TCA for a given patient. Preexisting epilepsy and cardiac conduction abnormalities are often considered contraindications to the use of TCAs.

Therapeutic Ranges

Because the pharmacokinetic properties of the individual agents may vary according to the patient and few TCAs have established therapeutic ranges, routine monitoring of drug levels is not common. However, establishing the drug level at which a patient has improved is reasonable. In this way, the practitioner has documentation of an effective drug concentration for that patient. Later, if needed, changes in drug therapy may be determined based on this baseline information. Otherwise, drug levels should be evaluated only if the practitioner suspects that the patient is not adhering to therapy or if drug toxicity becomes a concern.

Interactions

Drug interactions with TCAs tend to be pharmacodynamic, although some pharmacokinetic interactions do occur.

TABLE 40.4 Major Adverse Event Profile of Antidepressant Agents

Drug	Major Adverse Events				
	Anticholinergic	Cardiac Conduction	Seizures	Orthostatic Hypotension	Sedation
Selective Serotonin Reuptake Inhibitors					
citalopram	0	0	+	0	0
fluoxetine	0	0	+ +	0	0
fluvoxamine	0	0	+ +	0	0
paroxetine	+	0	+ +	0	+
sertraline	0	0	+ +	0	0
escitalopram	0	0	+ +	0	0
Serotonin-Norepinephrine Inhibitors					
venlafaxine	+	+	+ +	0	0
desvenlafaxine	+	+	+	0	0
duloxetine	+	0	0	0	0
Tricyclic Antidepressants					
amitriptyline	+ + + +	+ + +	+ + +	+ + +	+ + + +
desipramine	+ +	+ +	+ +	+ +	+ +
doxepin	+ + +	+ +	+ + +	+ +	+ + +
imipramine	+ + +	+ + +	+ + +	+ + + +	+ + +
nortriptyline	+ +	+ +	+ +	+	+ +
protriptyline	+ +	+ + +	+ +	+ +	+
trimipramine	+ + + +	+ + +	+ + +	+ + +	+ + + +
Monoamine Oxidase Inhibitors					
phenelzine	+ +	+	+ +	+ +	+ +
tranylcypromine	+ +	+	+ +	+ +	+ +
Atypical Antidepressants					
amoxapine	+ + +	+ +	+ + +	+ +	+ + +
bupropion	+	+	+ + + +	0	+ + + +
maprotiline	+ + +	+ +	+ + + +	+ + +	+ + + +
mirtazapine	+ +	+	+	+ + + +	+
nefazodone	0	+	+ +	+ + +	+ +
trazodone	0	+	+ +	+ + + +	+ +

+ + + + = highly potent effect; + = minimal effect; 0 = no effect

Pharmacokinetically, TCA drug levels may increase in combination with certain SSRIs (see **Table 40.3**) and other CYP450 enzyme inhibitors, such as cimetidine (Tagamet), human immunodeficiency virus protease inhibitors, and some antipsychotic agents. There are additive central nervous system effects with TCAs and anticholinergic drugs, such as diphenhydramine (Benadryl). In addition, TCA–MAO inhibitor interactions may significantly increase the level of circulating catecholamines and lead to a potentially fatal hypertensive crisis.

Monoamine Oxidase Inhibitors

MAO inhibitors were the first effective medications that were developed for the treatment of depression. They work by nonspecifically and irreversibly inhibiting type A and type B MAOs, leading to a decreased degradation of norepinephrine, serotonin, and dopamine in the synapse. However, the side effect profile and potential for life-threatening hypertensive crises have limited their use and relegated it a last-line treatment in clinical practice. Only skilled practitioners with extensive clinical expertise should prescribe MAO inhibitors. See **Table 40.2** for starting dosages and dosage ranges.

Adverse Events

Adverse reactions to MAO inhibitors are more common than any other class of antidepressant. Orthostatic hypotension occurring with high-dose therapy is probably the most common side effect. Attempts at preventing this reaction by applying support stockings, prescribing stimulants such as methylphenidate (Ritalin; 10 to 15 mg/d), or adding the mineralocorticoid fludrocortisone (Florinef; 0.025 to 0.05 mg/d) have met with reasonable success. However, caution must be used and the patient must be monitored carefully, especially when receiving the corticoid or the stimulant drug concomitantly. Hypertensive crisis can occur when MAO inhibitors are taken with medications that stimulate excessive release of the neurotransmitters dopamine, epinephrine, and norepinephrine. In addition, patients taking MAO inhibitors must be on a

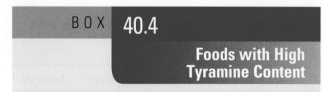

BOX 40.4

Foods with High Tyramine Content

- Aged cheese (cheddar, blue, Gouda, Swiss)
- Yeast products
- Aged meats, processed meats, nonfresh meat
- Beef liver or chicken liver
- Sauerkraut
- Licorice
- Tap beer

strict diet that eliminates tyramine-containing foods. **Box 40.4** identifies certain foods that have an extremely high tyramine content and, if ingested by patients taking MAO inhibitors, may cause a hypertensive crisis.

Concomitant use of TCAs and MAO inhibitors can lead to a hyperpyretic crisis resulting in seizures and death. Similarly, using SSRIs or SNRIs and MAO inhibitors together can lead to a serotonergic syndrome. Carefully monitored, these agents can be used together safely, but they should be prescribed and monitored only by experienced clinicians.

Atypical Antidepressants

The class of drugs labeled *atypical* represents compounds used to treat depression that elude the traditional classification schema. Their mechanisms of action are not consistent within the atypical group, but all impact one or more monoamines. These agents are generally considered alternatives to SSRIs, SNRIs, or TCAs; however, the utilization of bupropion has rivaled that of the SSRIs and SNRIs. See **Table 40.2** for starting dosages and dosage ranges.

Bupropion

Bupropion is a structurally distinct compound from the aminoketone class. It is a relatively weak inhibitor of neuronal uptake of norepinephrine and dopamine and its metabolite also inhibits the reuptake of norepinephrine. It does not inhibit the reuptake of MAO and, unlike all of the other available agents, it does not impact the serotonergic system. Buproprion is among the preferred pharmacologic agents, second only to SSRIs and SNRIs. Owing to its virtual absence of sexual side effects, buproprion is frequently used in patients who cannot tolerate the sexual side effects of SSRIs and SNRIs or may be used adjunctively with these drugs to diminish sexual dysfunction. Rates of somnolence, fatigue, and weight gain are markedly reduced compared to SSRIs, TCAs, and SNRIs (Papakostas, 2009). Bupropion has been implicated in lowering the seizure threshold, especially when combined with alcohol. This tends to occur when dosing exceeds 450 mg daily or more than 150 mg per dose, although the reported risk is less than 1%.

Trazodone

Trazodone (Desyrel) is a weak serotonin receptor antagonist that also blocks serotonin reuptake to a lesser degree. Trazodone is highly sedating at therapeutic doses secondary to its antihistamine properties. Patients whose target symptoms or residual symptoms include insomnia may benefit from the use of trazodone as adjunctive therapy. Antidepressant effects will be realized within a few weeks; however, the intended sedative effects occur several hours after the first dose. Also an anxiolytic drug, trazodone has a place in therapy for anxiety disorders as well as depression with comorbid anxiety. Important adverse effects include orthostatic hypotension, nausea, blurred vision, and priapism.

Nefazodone

Nefazodone (Serzone), structurally related to trazodone, acts similarly to trazodone but also inhibits the reuptake of norepinephrine and produces fewer side effects. Because it lacks significant anticholinergic and antihistamine effects, reports of blurred vision, urinary retention, and weight gain are relatively infrequent. Nefazodone interferes with the CYP3A4 subsystem, and caution should be used in patients taking drugs metabolized by this enzyme system. In addition, nefazodone increases the levels of agents such as alprazolam (Xanax) and triazolam (Halcion); practitioners should avoid prescribing these agents concomitantly. (See **Table 40.3**.) Prior to initiating nefazodone, the washout period after discontinuing an SSRI should generally be 4 to 5 days for paroxetine (Paxil) and sertraline (Zoloft) and several weeks for fluoxetine (Prozac).

Mirtazapine

Mirtazapine (Remeron) is a selective alpha$_2$-adrenergic receptor antagonist affecting both the norepinephrine and serotonergic systems. The role of mirtazapine in treating depression is similar to that of the TCAs. It has significant histamine-1 receptor blocking activity, thus causing sedation. In addition, because of its appetite stimulation, it may be a good choice for low-weight elderly or ill patients. This agent may be useful in combination therapy because there have been no reports of drug interactions. However, there have been rare cases of reversible agranulocytosis.

Selecting the Most Appropriate Agent

Selection of an initial pharmacotherapeutic treatment option involves numerous factors, the most important of which include the patient's target symptoms, comorbid medical or psychiatric conditions, concomitant medications, previous response to an antidepressant, and potential adverse effect and drug interaction profile. A patient's past experience with antidepressants should impact the decision regarding the choice of initial drug because past response tends to predict future response. Another consideration is the patient's perception about the efficacy and side effects she, he, or a family member has experienced. A negative perception of a drug may suggest potential for lack of adherence to drug therapy or an erosion of confidence in the therapy.

Scores of meta-analyses have evaluated the relative efficacy among antidepressants and assert that SSRIs consistently demonstrate relative efficacy as compared to SNRIs, TCAs, bupropion, trazodone, mirtazapine, and nefazodone. Patient-specific considerations will dictate the choice of drug as opposed to efficacy.

First-Line Therapy

SSRIs have replaced TCAs as first-line therapy for depression and are generally used initially in patients without contraindications. SNRIs, albeit newer compounds, are gaining some clinical momentum owing to mounting evidence of their efficacy compared to older products. In the absence of specific target symptoms, any of the available SSRIs are acceptable first choices. All SSRIs are available in generic formulations with the exception of escitalopram (Lexapro). Recent studies purport the superiority of escitalopram over other members of its class, although this claim has not been substantiated with large randomized, controlled trials. If insomnia is problematic in the patient, paroxetine (Paxil) may be the best choice within the SSRI class. If the patient is taking drugs metabolized by

CYP3A4, then avoiding fluoxetine (Prozac) is recommended. If the spectrum of depression-related symptoms includes sexual dysfunction, SSRIs should be avoided. If weight gain needs to be avoided, then bupropion is arguably a more appropriate option versus SSRIs (particularly paroxetine, which has the greatest potential to induce weight gain) or mirtazapine. See **Figure 40-2** and **Table 40.5** for an overview of treating a patient with depression.

Second-Line Therapy

When a patient fails an adequate trial of a first-line antidepressant and therapy needs to be modified, options include augmentation, switching, or combination therapy, as previously discussed. If a patient fails an SSRI, another member of the class could serve as the second choice since SSRIs are chemically distinct from one another. More commonly, however, when a patient is switched from an SSRI, it is likely a switch to a different class of medication. SNRIs or atypicals are generally chosen prior to attempting TCAs. The tolerability profiles of SNRIs and most of the atypicals make them more attractive than TCAs. The definitive selection should include

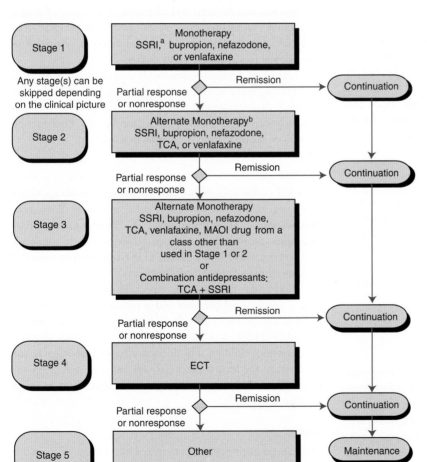

FIGURE 40–2 Texas Medication Algorithm Project (TMAP): Major depressive disorder without psychotic features. (Adapted from Crimson M. L., et al.: The Texas Medication Algorithm Project: Report of the Texas Consensus Conference Panel on Medication Treatment of Major Depressive Disorder. *Journal of Clinical Psychiatry* 60:145–156, 1999. The TMAP algorithms are in the public domain, and this figure may be reproduced without permission, but with the appropriate citation.)

Abbreviations: EC = electroconvulsive therapy, MAOI = monoamine oxidase inhibitor, SSRI = selective serotonin reuptake inhibitor, TCA = tricyclic antidepressant.
[a] SSRIs preferred.
[b] Consider TCA or venlafaxine if not tried.

TABLE 40.5	Recommended Order of Treatment in Antidepressant Therapy	
Order	**Agents**	**Comments**
First line	SSRIs	Fluoxetine and sertraline may be good for patients with somnolence. Paroxetine may be good for patients with insomnia. Selection of agent should be based on patient's past experiences with medications and drug interactions. Cost may be a consideration.
Second line	TCA (desipramine or nortriptyline) or atypical antidepressant	These agents have the better side effect profile of the class and should be considered as agents of choice for the TCA class.
Third line	Atypical antidepressant or TCA	Depending on past response to other agents and side effect profile

an assessment of the patient's underlying cardiac, neurologic, and comorbid conditions. For example, venlafaxine should be avoided in patients with uncontrolled hypertension because of its potential to increase blood pressure. Similarly, for an elderly man with a history of benign prostatic hyperplasia, TCAs and atypical agents with significant anticholinergic activity should be avoided because this action aggravates the condition.

Third-Line Therapy

If the first- and second-line agents fail, the clinician can try an agent from one of the remaining classes. Again, patient-specific indicators help the clinician decide on the next treatment regimen. For the most part, inexperienced general practitioners should not prescribe MAO inhibitors. The side effects and the potential for dangerous drug and food interactions suggest that only clinicians well versed in managing this kind of therapy prescribe these agents.

Special Population Considerations

Children and Adolescents

The risk for underdiagnosis and undertreatment is extremely prevalent in this patient population. Children of parents who have been diagnosed with serious depression are at risk for developing anxiety and MDD in childhood (Ainsworth, 2000). Early childhood depression may manifest as acting out, changes in eating or sleeping patterns, or social withdrawal. These patients can seldom communicate a feeling of sadness because of the early language development level. From ages 5 to 8, low self-esteem, underachievement at school, and aggressive or antisocial behaviors (including stealing and lying) may indicate depression.

Approximately 4% of adolescents experience depression in a given year (Ainsworth, 2000). Depressed adolescents experience symptoms similar to depressed adults such as sleep disturbances, irritability, difficulty concentrating, and loss of energy.

Currently, fluoxetine (Prozac) is the only SSRI approved by the U.S. Food and Drug Administration (FDA) for the treatment of depression in children age 8 and up. Escitalopram (Lexapro) is labeled for use in children age 12 and older. Caution has been recommended in using other agents, such as paroxetine (Paxil) or venlafaxine (Effexor), with depressed children and adolescents. Compared to adults, adolescents are more likely to become agitated or to develop a mania while they are taking an SSRI. The FDA has issued a black-box warning due to increased risk of suicide in children and adolescents taking SSRIs.

Geriatrics

Geriatric patients often have significant changes in physiologic function, including reduced renal and hepatic function, decreased muscle mass, decreased serum albumin, and dietary alterations. These changes may affect the absorption, distribution, metabolism, and excretion of a variety of drugs, particularly antidepressants. Most practitioners agree that antidepressant therapy should be prescribed at one-third to one-half the usual starting adult dosage.

Late-onset depression commonly occurs in elderly patients, with nursing home residents nearly three times more likely to be depressed than the general population. These patients may also have an underlying neurologic or vascular disorder. Determining the root of the depression is essential to resolution.

Women

As noted earlier, younger women are more likely to experience depression than older women or men in general. Women of childbearing age are at the greatest risk. The decision to initiate antidepressant medication in a pregnant woman is a difficult one, and the risk of fetal exposure to the drug must be balanced against the risk of continued depression.

Postpartum depression is especially prevalent in women with a history of depression and a previous episode of postpartum depression. The risk is increased with concomitant marital problems, lack of social support, and medical issues with newborn children. The decision about which agent to use depends on the factors previously discussed as well as on the issue of breast-feeding and the risk of transmission of drugs through breast milk.

Ethnic

There are genetic variations in the metabolism of drugs in patients with varying ethnicity. The CYP2D6 enzyme system, responsible for the metabolism of many psychotherapeutic agents, is influenced by age, gender, and ethnicity. Up to 10% of Whites and nearly 19% of African Americans are considered "poor metabolizers" of drugs via CYP2D6. Similarly, 33% of African Americans and 37% of

Asians are poor metabolizers of drugs metabolized by CYP2C19. The result of this poor metabolism can include quicker responses to drugs, greater than expected action of the agent, or even more pronounced side effects. As more data accrue on the effects of genetics on depression and CYP450 metabolism, the effects of race and ethnicity on treating depression and selecting antidepressants will play a more prominent role.

Emergencies

Suicide is the most feared consequence of inadequately treated (or unrecognized) depression. Up to two thirds of depressed patients have suicidal ideation, and 10% to 15% actually commit suicide (**Box 40.5**). The practitioner should be ever-vigilant for suicidal ideation and the potential for suicide. This is another reason for frequent contact between the practitioner and the patient. If the patient discloses thoughts of suicide, the practitioner and patient need to develop a plan for psychiatric referral or hospitalization. Contracting with the patient, such as by developing a written agreement to continue treatment without doing self-harm, may also be an effective means for minimizing the risk of suicide. All plans and actions should be documented in the patient's medical record.

PATIENT EDUCATION

Patients and caregivers should be instructed on the full range of issues surrounding depression and antidepressant therapy. Patients should be assured that depression is a biologic illness that occurs in a variety of people, and they should not feel ashamed of the disease. Moreover, the caregivers or significant others should also be counseled on the role they play in aiding in the patient's recovery. The more informed patients and significant others are of the illness, the more likely they will adhere to recommendations.

Expectations for a quick recovery can be detrimental to the healing process. Patients and caregivers should be informed that the antidepressant medication takes several (4 to 6) weeks to begin working and the patient might be required to continue taking the medication.

Teaching patients to recognize early signs and symptoms of behavior that may indicate a recurrence is crucial. Patients and family members should be instructed to contact the clinician if symptoms resume. A support group may also be a good resource for family and patients as a strategy for managing the illness.

Antidepressants and Suicide

Depression is the leading cause of suicide, and up to 80% of depressed patients experience suicidal impulses. Since 1990, whether antidepressant drugs are linked to suicide has been an acrimonious debate. Some argue that depressed adolescents who are suicidal and treated with antidepressants may regain initiative and energy before improvement in cognition and mood, thereby becoming mobilized to attempt suicide (Matthews & Fava, 2000). Others argue that the medication prescribed to treat depression is responsible for causing adolescents to attempt suicide. In 2003, British drug regulators warned that SSRIs, with the exception of fluoxetine, were unsuitable in minors experiencing depression. As a result, the FDA began public hearings in February 2004 to discuss this controversy. Currently, fluoxetine (Prozac) is the only FDA-approved antidepressant in patients as young as age 8. However, other antidepressants, such as sertraline (Zoloft), venlafaxine (Effexor), and paroxetine (Paxil), have been widely prescribed for adolescent depression. Current data suggest that the increase in suicidality impacts patients younger than age 25 to a greater extent than patients older than age 25. Therefore, a practitioner needs to be diligent in assessing the patient's risk of suicide.

Patient Information

The National Foundation for Depressive Illness, Inc. (NAFDI) (http://www.depression.org), was established in 1983 to educate the public and health care professionals about depression. This website contains useful information on the signs and symptoms of depression and provides public awareness on depression through a national "800" number.

The National Institute of Mental Health's website (http://www.nimh.nih.gov/publicat/depressionmenus.cfm), also available in Spanish, is an excellent resource for depression. It describes the different types of depression along with the causes and treatments. This website also offers valuable information on how family and friends may contribute and assist in therapy.

The National Mental Health Association (NMHA) (http://www.nmha.org) is a nonprofit organization that provides beneficial information to the public and practitioners on mental illness. This website contains news releases along with an online bookstore. A calendar notes coming events relating to mental health. This website provides access to comprehensive mental health care and increases public awareness of mental health issues.

BOX 40.5

Warning Signs of Suicidal Ideation

- Pacing, agitated behavior, frequent mood changes, and chronic episodes of sleeplessness
- Actions or threats of assault, physical harm, or violence
- Delusions or hallucinations
- Threats or talk of death (e.g., "I don't care anymore," or "You won't have to worry about me much longer")
- Putting affairs in order, such as giving possessions away or writing a new will
- Unusually risky behavior (e.g., unsafe driving, abuse of alcohol or other drugs)

The Depression and Bipolar Support Alliance (DBSA) (http://www.dbsalliance.org) is a nonprofit organization that provides a wide range of information and support on depression and bipolar disorders. Their mission, as stated on the website, is to improve the lives of those affected by depression and bipolar disorder. The DBSA is a patient-directed national organization focusing on the most prevalent mental illnesses, with a network of approximately 1,000 support groups. This website is updated regularly to provide up-to-date, scientifically based information. The DBSA is guided by a scientific advisory board comprising researchers and clinicians in the field of mood disorders.

Complementary and Alternative Medications

The use of herbal products in the United States has dramatically increased in the past few decades, resulting in consumer sales of $250 million in 2007. At its peak of popularity in 1998, more than $300 million was spent on the purchase of St. John's wort alone. Subsequent research with respect to drug–drug interactions and safety concerns made available to consumers caused a significant decrease in sales over the next decade. Depression is the most common diagnosis associated with complementary and alternative medication use. Despite the decline in popularity of St. John's wort, herbal sales continue to steadily rise. The FDA does not classify herbal products as drugs, and as such they are not regulated under the same scrutiny as other medications.

St. John's wort (*Hypericum perforatum*) has been used for centuries for a variety of illnesses, but it is currently used almost exclusively as an herbal antidepressant. Most clinical trials have studied 900 mg/d of standardized extract (usually standardized to 0.3% hypericin content) divided in three daily doses. The clinical effect is usually seen within 2 to 3 weeks of initiating therapy (Ernst, 2002). The mechanism of action is unknown, although it is theorized that it inhibits MAO and the synaptosomal uptake of serotonin, dopamine, and noradrenaline (Butterweck, 2003).

St. John's wort appears to be well tolerated, with the most frequent side effects reported as nausea, fatigue, restlessness, rash, and photosensitivity. There have been reported cases of increase in heart rate, but no significant effect was seen on the PR interval (Gupta & Moller, 2003).

St. John's wort may activate hepatic CYP450, so it has the potential to interact with medication that is metabolized by the CYP450 system. Therefore, it has been reported that St. John's wort decreases serum levels of theophylline, cyclosporine, warfarin, oral contraceptives, and indinavir. St. John's wort should not be taken in combination with any other antidepressant because of the risk of serotonin syndrome, especially in the elderly. Symptoms include changes in mental status, tremor, gastrointestinal disturbances, myalgia, restlessness, and headache.

Case Study

L. B. is a 55-year-old white female who presents to her family physician's office for a yearly routine physical. Her husband passed away 5 months ago after a 2-year battle with lung cancer. She has three children, two of whom are still in college. Her daughter accompanies her to the doctor's office and says she is concerned about her mother's recent behavior. She explains that her mother has been "sleeping all the time" and has lost 25 lb in the past 2 months without being on a diet. When the doctor examines L. B., she explains that she has become increasingly fatigued and "I have absolutely no energy." She no longer has any desire to participate in her lifelong hobbies of painting and photography because of frequent feelings of sadness. L. B.'s medical history is significant for hypothyroidism, hypercholesterolemia, and recently diagnosed hypertension. Her medications are levothyroxine (Synthroid) 0.075 mg daily, simvastatin (Zocor) 20 mg daily, hydrochlorothiazide (HydroDIURIL) 25 mg daily, lisinopril (Zestril) 10 mg daily, multivitamins 1 tab daily, and aspirin 81 mg daily.

DIAGNOSIS: MAJOR DEPRESSION

1. What are reasonable treatment goals for L. B.? How would you incorporate her activities of daily living into these goals?

2. What medications and disease states may be contributing to L. B.'s depression?

3. What would be the first agent you would consider prescribing for L. B.? What considerations did you take into account when making this choice?

4. How would you monitor for improvement in L. B., and in what time frame would you expect to see these improvements?

5. What are some adverse reactions that may occur in L. B. based on your selection? Which of these would cause you or L. B. to stop the therapy?

6. If the initial drug therapy failed or L. B. chose to stop therapy, what would be your choice for second-line therapy?

7. L. B. asks you if she should take St. John's wort. How do you respond?

8. How would you monitor for suicidal tendencies in this patient?

9. Describe one or two drug–drug or drug–food interactions for the selected agent.

BIBLIOGRAPHY

Starred items are cited in the text.

*Ainsworth, P. (2000). *Understanding depression* (Understanding Health and Sickness Series). Jackson, MS: University Press of Mississippi.

*Bauer, M., Tharmanathan, P., Volz, H., et al. (2009). The effect of venlafaxine compared with other antidepressants and placebo in the treatment of major depression: A meta-analysis. *European Archives of Psychiatry and Clinical Neuroscience, 259*(3), 172–185.

*Breen, R., & McCormac, R. J. (2002). A fresh look at management of depression. How to choose and use the newer antidepressant drugs. *Postgraduate Medicine, 112*(3), 28–40.

*Butterweck, V. (2003). Mechanism of action of St. John's Wort in depression. *CNS Drugs, 17*(8), 539–562.

*Ernst, E. (2002). The risk-benefit profile of commonly used herbal therapies: Gingko, St. John's wort, Ginseng, Echinacea, Saw Palmetto, and Kava. *Annals of Internal Medicine, 136*(1), 42–53.

*Evins, G. G., Theofrastous, J. P., & Galvin, S. L. (2000). Postpartum depression: A comparison of screening and routine clinical evaluation. *American Journal of Obstetrics & Gynecology, 182*(5), 1080–1082.

*Gupta, R. K., & Moller, H. J. (2003). St. John's wort. An option for the primary care treatment of depressive patients? *European Archives of Psychiatry & Clinical Neuroscience, 253*(3), 140–148.

Hamilton, M. (1967). Development of a rating scale for primary depressive illness. *British Journal of Social and Clinical Psychology, 6*, 278–296.

Harris, P. A. (2004). The impact of age, gender, race and ethnicity on the diagnosis and treatment of depression. *Journal of Managed Care Pharmacy, 10*(2, Suppl S-a), S2–S7.

Koenig, A., & Thase, M. (2009). First-line pharmacotherapies for depression—What is the best choice? *Polskie Archiwum Medycyny Wewnętrznej, 119*(7–8), 478–486.

*Matthews, J. D., & Fava, M. (2000). Risk of suicidality in depression with serotonergic antidepressants. *Annals of Clinical Psychiatry, 12*(1), 43–50.

Miller, L. J. (2002). Postpartum depression. *Journal of the American Medical Association, 287*(6), 762–765.

*Mulrow, C. D., Williams, J. W. Jr., Chiquette, E., et al. (2000). Efficacy of newer medications for treating depression in primary care patients. *American Journal of Medicine, 108*(1), 54–64.

*Opmeer, E. M., Kortekaas, R., & Aleman, A. (2010). Depression and the role of genes involved in dopamine metabolism and signalling. *Progress in Neurobiology, 92*(2), 112–133.

*Papakostas, G. (2009). Managing partial response or nonresponse: Switching, augmentation, and combination strategies for major depressive disorder. *Journal of Clinical Psychiatry, 70*(Suppl 6), 16–25.

*Perry, R., & Cassagnol, M. (2009). Desvenlafaxine: A new serotonin-norepinephrine reuptake inhibitor for the treatment of adults with major depressive disorder. *Clinical Therapeutics, 31*(Pt 1), 1374–1404.

*Reid, S., & Barbui, C. (2010). Long term treatment of depression with selective serotonin reuptake inhibitors and newer antidepressants. *British Medical Journal, 340*, 1468.

*Schweitzer, I., Maguire, K., & Ng, C. (2009). Sexual side-effects of contemporary antidepressants: Review. *The Australian and New Zealand Journal of Psychiatry, 43*(9), 795–808.

*Shelton, R. (2009). Long-term management of depression: Tips for adjusting the treatment plan as the patient's needs change. *Journal of Clinical Psychiatry, 70*(Suppl. 6), 32–37.

*Shyn, S. I., & Hamilton, S. P. (2010). The genetics of major depression: Moving beyond the monoamine hypothesis. *Psychiatric Clinics of North America, 33*(1), 125–140.

*Snow, V., Lascher, S., & Mottur-Pilson, C. (2000). Pharmacologic treatment of acute major depression and dysthymia. *Annals of Internal Medicine, 132*(9), 738–742.

*Tadić, A., Helmreich, I., Mergl, R., et al. (2010). Early improvement is a predictor of treatment outcome in patients with mild major, minor or subsyndromal depression. *Journal of Affective Disorders, 120*(1–3), 86–93.

Thase, M. (2009). Update on partial response in depression. *Journal of Clinical Psychiatry, 70*(Suppl. 6), 4–9.

Trivedi, M. (2009). Tools and strategies for ongoing assessment of depression: A measurement-based approach to remission. *Journal of Clinical Psychiatry, 70*(Suppl. 6), 26–31.

Trivedi, M., Rush, A., Wisniewski, S., et al. (2006). Evaluation of outcomes with citalopram for depression using measurement-based care in STAR*D: Implications for clinical practice. *American Journal of Psychiatry, 163*(1), 28–40.

Yesavage, J. A. (1988). Geriatric depression scale. *Psychopharmacology Bulletin, 24*, 709–711.

Young, S. A., Campbell, N., & Harper, A. (2002). Depression in women of reproductive age. Considerations in selecting safe, effective therapy. *Postgraduate Medicine, 112*(3), 45–50.

*Zajecka, J. (2003). Treating depression to remission. *Journal of Clinical Psychiatry, 64*(Suppl. 15), 7–12.

CHAPTER 41

Heather E. Fean
Andrea M. Heise
Andrew M. Peterson

Anxiety

Anxiety is defined as a vague, uneasy feeling with a source that often is nonspecific. People with anxiety frequently experience feelings of increased tension, apprehension, fear, restlessness, and worry along with physical symptoms such as increased heart rate, pupil dilation, trembling, and increased perspiration. With 14 different types, the anxiety disorders represent the largest group of psychiatric disorders (**Table 41.1**). The disorders discussed in this chapter are generalized anxiety disorder (GAD), panic disorder (PD), and obsessive-compulsive disorder (OCD). Anxiety often goes untreated in both children and adults, but millions of people seek help for what is broadly construed as anxiety or nervousness.

More than 30 million Americans have a lifetime history of anxiety, and anxiety disorders cost an estimated $42 billion per year in the United States, counting direct and indirect costs (Kroenke, et al., 2007). Epidemiologic studies report that 2% to 6% of adults and twice as many women as men have GAD (Kazdin, 2008). Approximately 1% of all patients have PD with resulting significant impairment, and 4% to 5% have agoraphobia. Approximately 12% of patients seen in anxiety disorder clinics present with GAD. Between 35% and 50% of individuals with major depression meet criteria for GAD. Coexisting GAD in depressed patients may worsen the outcome by increasing the suicide rate, worsening overall symptoms, conferring a poorer response to treatment, increasing the number of unexplained symptoms, and increasing functional disability. OCD has a lifetime prevalence of 2.5%; it was once thought to be a rare disorder, but it is now known to be twice as common as schizophrenia or PD in the general population.

Anxiety disorders most commonly begin in early adulthood. They tend to be chronic, with interspersed periods of remissions and relapses of varying degrees, and they frequently continue into old age. Late onset of an anxiety disorder is rare. In the elderly, anxiety disorders as a whole are the most common psychiatric disorders. It is unknown whether they are a continuation of an illness with an onset from a younger age or whether they appear for the first time in old age.

There is considerable variation in the expression of anxiety across cultures, so it is important to consider the patient's cultural context. Patients from one culture may express anxiety vocally and physically, while patients from a different culture may express anxiety with silence and withdrawal.

CAUSES

Physiologic Factors

Most patients with an anxiety disorder first come to the attention of primary health care providers. Although the etiology of anxiety disorders is largely unknown, a wide range of medical illnesses, such as cardiovascular disease, pulmonary disease, hyperthyroidism, hypothyroidism, hyperadrenocorticism, pheochromocytoma, hypoglycemia, vitamin B_{12} deficiency, and neurologic conditions, may cause symptoms of anxiety. In addition, alcohol, amphetamines, cannabis, caffeine, cocaine, hallucinogens, sedatives, hypnotics, phencyclidine, and inhalants may cause substance-induced anxiety.

Genetic Factors

A family history is seen frequently in people with anxiety disorders. Twin studies suggest that heredity accounts for 30% of the cases of various anxiety disorders; environmental factors seem to be responsible for the remaining cases. More than 50% of people with PD have relatives with the disorder. A twin study reported that anxiety disorder with panic attacks occurs five times more frequently in monozygotic twins than in heterozygotic twins. Reports estimate that 20% of patients who have OCD have a first-degree relative with OCD.

PATHOPHYSIOLOGY

Anxiety is a phenomenon that all people experience. One type of anxiety, fear, is a normal fight-or-flight response to an observable threat. In contrast, pathologic anxiety is a fight-or-flight response to an internal or external threat that is real or imagined and causes the person to experience an unpleasant emotional state. Walter B. Cannon (1963) was the first to describe the fight-or-flight response, which is associated with anxiety. During this response, the person's autonomic nervous system, which consists of the sympathetic and parasympathetic nervous systems, prepares the person to deal with a threat (**Box 41.1**).

A pediatric autoimmune neuropsychiatric disorder associated with streptococcal (group A beta-hemolytic streptococcal) infections is referred to as *PANDA*. In 1998, Swede et al. first

TABLE 41.1 Summary of Anxiety Disorders

Anxiety Disorder	Definition
Panic attack	A discrete period, in which there is a sudden onset of intense apprehension, fearfulness, or terror, often associated with feelings of impending doom. During these attacks, symptoms such as shortness of breath, palpitations, chest pain or discomfort, choking or smothering sensations, and fear of "going crazy" or losing control are present.
Agoraphobia	Anxiety about, or avoidance of, places or situations from which escape might be difficult (or embarrassing) or in which help may not be available in the event of having a panic attack or panic-like symptoms.
Panic disorder without agoraphobia	Recurrent unexpected panic attacks about which there is persistent concern.
Panic disorder with agoraphobia	Recurrent unexpected panic attacks and agoraphobia.
Agoraphobia without history of panic disorder	Agoraphobia and panic-like symptoms without a history of unexpected panic attacks.
Specific phobia	Clinically significant anxiety provoked by exposure to a specific feared object or situation, often leading to avoidance.
Social phobia	Clinically significant anxiety provoked by exposure to certain types of social or performance situations, often leading to avoidance behavior.
Obsessive-compulsive disorder	Characterized by obsessions (which cause marked anxiety or distress) and/or by compulsions (which serve to neutralize anxiety).
Posttraumatic stress disorder	Characterized by the reexperiencing of an extremely traumatic event accompanied by symptoms of increased arousal and by avoidance of stimuli associated with the trauma.
Acute stress disorder	Characterized by symptoms similar to those of posttraumatic stress disorder that occur immediately in the aftermath of an extremely traumatic event.
Generalized anxiety disorder	Characterized by at least 6 months of persistent and excessive anxiety and worry.
Anxiety disorder due to a general medical condition	Characterized by prominent symptoms of anxiety that are judged to be a direct physiological consequence of a general medical condition.
Substance-induced anxiety disorder	Characterized by prominent symptoms of anxiety that are judged to be a direct physiological consequence of a drug abuse, a medication, or toxin exposure.
Anxiety disorder not otherwise specified	Used for coding disorders with prominent anxiety or phobic avoidance that do not meet the criteria for any of the specific anxiety disorders defined in this list (or anxiety symptoms about which there is inadequate or contradictory information).

Source: American Psychiatric Association. (2000). *Diagnostic and statistical manual of mental disorders* (4th ed., text revision). Washington, DC: Author, with permission.

reported on children who developed neurologic abnormalities following a streptococcal infection known as *St. Vitus' dance*. It was thought to be a rare complication. Swede's group was the first to make the connection that this is a form of OCD caused by an immune response. Before treating a child for OCD, PANDA must be ruled out.

Response to Stress

The fight-or-flight response is associated with significant stress. In 1980, Hans Selye, the "father of stress research," developed a stress framework by which he defined stress as the rate of wear and tear on the body. Stressors may be physical, chemical, psychological, or developmental. The demands and challenges of life are stressful and are handled through adaptation to changes to limit damage. Selye (1991) proposed that although stress cannot be perceived, it can be measured by the chemical and structural changes produced in the body. Selye referred to these changes as *the general adaptation syndrome* (GAS), reflecting the entire body's need to adjust to the changes.

The GAS has three stages. First, the alarm reaction occurs when the person mobilizes the various defense mechanisms of the body or mind to cope with a stressful physical or emotional situation. The second stage, resistance, represents the opposite of the alarm reaction: the person stops feeling tense and anxious and may state that he or she has become used to the situation. Exhaustion, the third stage, occurs when the stress continues over a prolonged period or the person is exposed to multiple stressors simultaneously, thus leaving him or her too exhausted to maintain normal functioning.

Neurotransmitters

Norepinephrine, serotonin, and gamma-aminobutyric acid (GABA) are the major neurotransmitters studied in relation to the pharmacologic treatment of anxiety. People with anxiety disorders, especially PD, are found to have malfunctioning noradrenergic systems with a low threshold for arousal. This, coupled with an unpredictable increase in activity, causes the anxiety symptoms.

BOX 41.1

Physiologic Reactions to the Fight-or-Flight Response

The fight-or-flight response causes the following:

1. Epinephrine, norepinephrine, and cortisol are released into the blood.
2. The liver releases stored sugar into the blood to meet energy needs.
3. Digestion slows, allowing blood to be shifted to the brain and the muscles.
4. Breathing becomes rapid to allow for greater oxygen supply to the muscles.
5. The heart rate and blood pressure increase.
6. Perspiration increases to cool the body.
7. Muscles tense in preparation for action.
8. The pupils dilate.
9. All senses become more acute.
10. Blood flow to the extremities becomes constricted to protect the body from bleeding from injury.

This response is appropriate for extremely threatening situations, but the response would cause considerable damage to the body if people responded to all stressful situations in this manner.

The role of serotonin was identified by observing people with OCD who had favorable responses when treated with antidepressant medications such as the selective serotonin reuptake inhibitors (SSRIs). Drugs that release serotonin can precipitate anxiety in people with an anxiety disorder; selective reduction of serotonin levels restores normal functioning.

GABA and its associated receptors function as central nervous system (CNS) inhibitors. Although psychopharmacologic interventions support this role, the exact pharmacology of GABA receptors is still being examined.

DIAGNOSTIC CRITERIA

Anxiety disorders most commonly begin in early adulthood, tend to be chronic with interspersed periods of remission and relapse of varying degrees, and frequently continue into old age. In children, anxiety may develop, particularly in relation to school, and late onset of an anxiety disorder is rare but can occur. In the elderly, anxiety disorders are the most common psychiatric disorders seen.

Before a patient can be diagnosed with an anxiety disorder, he or she should undergo a thorough medical workup to rule out medical disease, neurologic problems, current medications that may cause anxiety symptoms, vitamin B_{12} deficiency, and drug or alcohol misuse. The history should focus on anxiety

disorders in family members, environmental factors, family dynamics, cognitive functioning, work or school situations, or exposure to chemical substances.

If the patient's anxiety is not linked to any of these possibilities, the practitioner should consult the American Psychiatric Association's (APA) *Diagnostic and Statistical Manual of Mental Disorders, IV, Text Revision* (2000) to review the diagnostic criteria before diagnosing a particular anxiety disorder. **Box 41.2** lists criteria for diagnosing GAD, **Box 41.3** lists the criteria for diagnosing PD, and **Box 41.4** lists the criteria for diagnosing OCD.

Comorbidity with major depression or a personality disorder is common in patients with anxiety. These patients may self-medicate with alcohol or other substances to relieve their symptoms.

INITIATING DRUG THERAPY

Many people with anxiety disorders are terrified of beginning treatment and worried about possible addiction to, and side effects of, the drugs used to treat these conditions. These people also worry about the social stigma associated with having a psychiatric condition. Both pharmacotherapy and psychotherapy may be necessary for satisfactory treatment of these disorders. Frequently, a patient's health insurance policy does not cover the psychiatric treatment that he or she needs.

Nonpharmacologic therapy includes several psychotherapeutic techniques such as supportive counseling, behavioral therapy, cognitive therapy, and psychoanalytic therapy. In the past, before drug therapy was widely available and effective for anxiety disorders, therapy consisted of psychoanalysis or behavioral or cognitive therapy, or a combination of these modalities. Today, in many cases, these therapies can be helpful and useful in conjunction with drug therapy. Therapeutic modalities may vary among the historic psychotherapies.

In the past, proponents of Freudian theory recommended psychoanalysis because they thought that anxiety was the response of the ego to unconscious, unacceptable thoughts, feelings, and impulses that threatened to emerge into the conscious mind. To remain intact, the ego used defense mechanisms to protect the self from becoming overwhelmed by anxiety. Followers of the interpersonal theorists, such as Sullivan, May, and Peplau, thought that the anxiety disorders developed and were maintained as a result of dysfunctional family relationships.

Behavioral therapists treat anxiety as a learned behavior, arguing that anxiety is an internal conditioned response to a perceived threat or stimulus in the environment. They propose that people with anxiety learn to avoid the stimulus in order to reduce anxiety; therefore, behavior modification is the vehicle for changing behavior. Systematic desensitization is used to control external stimuli and internal sensations as well as anticipation of fear of a panic attack.

BOX 41.2

APA Criteria for Diagnosing Generalized Anxiety Disorder

A. Excessive anxiety and worry (apprehensive expectation), occurring more days than not for at least 6 months, about a number of events or activities (such as work or school performance).
B. The person finds it difficult to control the worry.
C. The anxiety and worry are associated with three (or more) of the following six symptoms (with at least some symptoms present for more days than not for the past 6 months).
   Note: Only one item is required in children.
   1. Restlessness or feeling keyed up or on edge
   2. Being easily fatigued
   3. Difficulty concentrating or mind going blank
   4. Irritability
   5. Muscle tension
   6. Sleep disturbance (difficulty falling or staying asleep, or restless, unsatisfying sleep)
D. The focus of the anxiety and worry is not confined to features of an Axis I disorder, for example, the anxiety or worry is not about having a panic attack (as in Panic Disorder), being embarrassed in public (as in Social Phobia), being contaminated (as in Obsessive-Compulsive Disorder), being away from home or close relatives (as in Separation Anxiety Disorder), gaining weight (as in Anorexia Nervosa), having multiple physical complaints (as in Somatization Disorder), or having a serious illness (as in Hypochondriasis) and the anxiety and worry do not occur exclusively during Posttraumatic Stress Disorder.
E. The anxiety, worry, or physical symptoms cause clinically significant distress or impairment in social, occupational, or other important areas of functioning.
F. The disturbance is not due to the direct physiologic effects of a substance (e.g., a drug of abuse, a medication) or general medical condition (e.g., hyperthyroidism) and does not occur exclusively during a Mood Disorder, a Psychotic Disorder, or a Pervasive Development Disorder.

From the American Psychiatric Association. (2000). *Diagnostic and statistical manual of mental disorders* (4th ed., text revision). Washington, DC: Author, with permission.

BOX 41.3

APA Criteria for Diagnosing Panic Disorder without Agoraphobia

A. Both (1) and (2)
   1. Recurrent unexpected panic attacks
   2. At least one of the attacks has been followed by 1 month (or more) of one (or more) of the following:
      a. Persistent concern about having additional attacks
      b. Worry about the implications of the attack or its consequences (e.g., losing control, having a heart attack, "going crazy")
      c. A significant change in behavior related to the attacks
B. Absence of agoraphobia
C. The panic attacks are not due to the direct physiologic effects of a substance (e.g., a drug of abuse, a medication) or a general medical condition (e.g., hyperthyroidism).
D. The panic attacks are not better accounted for by another mental disorder, such as Social Phobia (e.g., occurring on exposure to feared social situations), Specific Phobia (e.g., on exposure to a specific phobic situation), Obsessive-Compulsive Disorder (e.g., on exposure to dirt in someone with an obsession about contamination), Posttraumatic Stress Disorder (e.g., in response to stimuli associated with a severe stressor), or Separation Anxiety Disorder (e.g., in response to being away from home or close relatives).

From the American Psychiatric Association. (2000). *Diagnostic and statistical manual of mental disorders* (4th ed., text revision). Washington, DC: Author, with permission.

therapy (CBT) and drug therapy complement each other and tend to produce a greater therapeutic response.

Goals of Drug Therapy

The goal of therapy is to reduce the patient's anxiety and any depressive symptoms, return the patient to a normal level of functioning with a minimum of side effects, and improve the patient's quality of life.

The primary use of sedative-hypnotic and anxiolytic drugs is to produce calmness or sleep. Many CNS depressants have some ability to relieve anxiety, but only at doses that produce noticeable sedation. Most anxiolytic and sedative-hypnotic drugs produce a dose-dependent depression of the CNS.

Cognitive therapists treat anxiety as a faulty thought pattern that evokes the physiologic symptoms of anxiety, feelings of loss of control, and fear of dying. Cognitive behavioral

BOX 41.4

APA Criteria for Diagnosing Obsessive-Compulsive Disorder

A. Either obsessions or compulsions
   Obsessions as defined by (1), (2), (3), and (4)
   1. Recurrent and persistent thoughts, impulses, or images that are experienced, at some time during the disturbance, as intrusive and inappropriate and that cause marked anxiety or distress.
   2. The thoughts, impulses, or images are not simply excessive worries about real-life problems.
   3. The person attempts to ignore or suppress such thoughts, impulses, or images, or to neutralize them with some other thought or action.
   4. The person recognizes that the obsessional thoughts, impulses, or images are a product of his or her own mind (not imposed from without, as in thought insertion).

   Compulsions as defined by (1) and (2)
   1. Repetitive behaviors (e.g., hand washing, ordering, checking) or mental acts (e.g., praying, counting, repeating words silently) that the person feels driven to perform in response to an obsession, or according to rules that must be applied rigidly.
   2. The behaviors or mental acts are aimed at preventing or reducing distress or preventing some dreaded event or situation; however, these behaviors or mental acts either are not connected in a realistic way with what they are designed to neutralize or prevent or are clearly excessive.

B. At some point during the course of the disorder, the person has recognized that the obsessions or compulsions are excessive or unreasonable.
   Note: This does not apply to children.
C. The obsessions or compulsions cause marked distress, are time-consuming (take more than 1 hour a day), or significantly interfere with the person's normal routine, occupational (or academic) functioning, or usual social activities or relationships.
D. If another Axis I disorder is present, the content of the obsessions or compulsions is not restricted to it (e.g., preoccupation with food in the presence of an Eating Disorder; hair pulling in the presence of Trichotillomania; concern with appearance in the presence of Body Dysmorphic Disorder; preoccupation with having a serious illness in the presence of Hypochondriasis; preoccupation with sexual urges or fantasies in the presence of Paraphilia; or guilty ruminations in the presence of Major Depressive Disorder).
E. The disturbance is not due to the direct physiologic effects of a substance (e.g., a drug of abuse, a medication) or a general medical condition.

Specify if:
With Poor Insight: if for most of the time during the current episode, the person does not recognize that the obsessions and compulsions are excessive or unreasonable

From the American Psychiatric Association. (2000). *Diagnostic and statistical manual of mental disorders* (4th ed., text revision). Washington, DC: Author, with permission.

The ideal anxiolytic drug should calm the patient without causing too much daytime sedation and drowsiness and without producing physical or psychological dependence. Pharmacologic agents used in the treatment of anxiety disorders can be classified into the following categories: antidepressants, benzodiazepines (BZDs), azapirones, other antianxiety agents, and beta-adrenergic blockers.

Benzodiazepines

BZDs are important and widely prescribed sedative-hypnotics. Their pharmacologic properties include reduction of anxiety, sedation, muscle relaxation, and anticonvulsant and amnestic effects. Among the prominent BZDs are alprazolam (Xanax), clonazepam (Klonopin), lorazepam (Ativan), oxazepam (Serax), diazepam (Valium), and chlordiazepoxide (Librium). They are best prescribed for motivated patients with acute exogenous anxiety to a time-limited stress.

Mechanism of Action

BZDs exert a therapeutic effect by binding to GABA-A receptors in the brain. They cause the GABA-A receptors to increase the opening of chloride channels along the cell membrane, leading to an inhibitory effect on cell firing. Other neurotransmitters, such as serotonin and norepinephrine, may play a role in the therapeutic effect of BZDs. The exact mechanism of BZDs' antianxiety effect is not yet fully understood. Most of the drugs in this class possess anxiolytic, sedative-hypnotic, and anticonvulsant properties.

BZDs can be used for treating GAD and PD. Approximately 75% of patients with GAD respond moderately or better to BZDs. At this time, there is no evidence that one BZD is superior to another for this disorder. The high-potency BZDs, alprazolam, clonazepam, and lorazepam, have been effective in controlling panic attacks and anticipatory anxiety in panic attacks. The clinical indications for a specific

BZD are not absolute, and considerable overlap in their use exists. Not only are they effective in pathologic anxiety, but also their calming effect is useful in nonpathologic anxiety states (temporary episodes of anxiety due to fear—such as of surgery or personal problems). BZDs have a wider therapeutic window than most other CNS depressants and are associated with fewer side effects.

The various BZDs differ little in their pharmacologic properties, but they differ significantly in their potency, their ability to cross the blood–brain barrier, and their half-lives. High-potency BZDs, such as alprazolam, clonazepam, and lorazepam, have a great affinity for the BZD receptor. The onset and intensity of action of an oral dose of a BZD is determined by the rate of absorption from the gastrointestinal (GI) tract. BZDs are highly bound to plasma proteins (70% to 90%) and are highly lipid soluble. The duration of action is related to their lipid solubility as well as hepatic biotransformation to active metabolites. Oxazepam and lorazepam are metabolized to inactive compounds and therefore have shorter half-lives and durations of activity than other BZDs. This one-step inactivation to an inactive compound makes them the preferred drugs for the treatment of anxiety in elderly patients and patients with liver disease.

Accumulation of BZDs with a long half-life (long-acting BZDs) occurs from one dose to another. Long-acting BZDs take a longer time to reach steady-state levels, are removed more slowly, and cause more pronounced side effects (e.g., sedation). However, use of these preparations reduces the likelihood and intensity of withdrawal symptoms when discontinued. Ultrashort-acting BZDs do not accumulate. High lipid solubility results in faster absorption, greater distribution in tissues, and faster entrance and exit from brain sites. Diazepam is a BZD with high lipid solubility used for anxiety. (See **Table 41.2** for more information.)

On discontinuation of BZD therapy, relapse rates are high (see "Monitoring Patient Response"). Longer-acting agents, such as clonazepam, can minimize dose-rebound anxiety. Similarly, rapid-onset agents, such as diazepam or alprazolam, can provide acute anxiolysis, whereas short-acting agents such as lorazepam can minimize accumulation and oversedation. In the elderly, use of long-acting BZDs is discouraged because impaired liver and kidney function may precipitate severe and prolonged adverse effects.

Tolerance and Dependence Issues

Tolerance to the sedative (but not anxiolytic) effects of BZDs develops at moderate doses. BZDs can cause dependence if used continuously for more than several weeks. If the patient's anxiety is episodic, episodic use of BZDs may control symptoms. If anxiety is prolonged, BZDs may control anxiety, but this therapeutic benefit must be weighed against their capacity to cause dependence. Abuse potential does not appear to be a problem in people who do not abuse alcohol or other substances. See "Monitoring Patient Response" for information on tapering technique and withdrawal issues.

Adverse Events

The major adverse events of BZDs are drowsiness and ataxia. Mild, transitory cognitive and memory impairments are seen occasionally. This is more significant in elderly people and those with high sensitivity to these drugs. Reactions of rage, excitement, and hostility, although rare, have been reported after overdoses of chlordiazepoxide. Other reported side effects include increased depression, confusion, headache, GI disturbances, menstrual irregularities, and changes in libido. Urticaria may occur in people with drug hypersensitivity, and drug interactions may occur with a variety of medications (**Table 41.3**).

Treatment of Benzodiazepine Overdose

Flumazenil (Mazicon) is a competitive BZD receptor antagonist that reverses the sedative effects of BZDs. Antagonism of BZD-induced respiratory depression is less predictable. Flumazenil is the only BZD receptor antagonist available for clinical use. It blocks many of the actions of BZDs but does not antagonize the CNS effects of other sedative-hypnotics such as ethanol, opioids, or general anesthetics. It is used for BZD overdose and after the use of drugs in anesthetic and diagnostic procedures. When given intravenously, it acts rapidly and has a short half-life (0.7 to 1.3 hours). Because all BZDs have a longer duration of action than flumazenil, sedation commonly recurs and repeated doses of flumazenil may be needed. Adverse effects of flumazenil include confusion, agitation, dizziness, and nausea.

Azapirones

An azapirone, buspirone (BuSpar) is an anxiolytic drug that inhibits the uptake of dopamine, serotonin, and norepinephrine. Buspirone is as effective in the treatment of GAD as BZDs and has minimal abuse potential. It is rapidly absorbed from the intestinal tract but undergoes extensive first-pass metabolism. People with liver dysfunction have a decreased clearance of buspirone. Buspirone has no hypnotic, anticonvulsant, or muscle-relaxant properties. Patients taking buspirone do not acquire a cross-tolerance for alcohol or BZDs. It is generally well tolerated, with only a few patients experiencing adverse effects. When adverse effects do occur, they include nausea, dizziness, headache, and nervousness. (See **Table 41.2.**) Doses over 70 mg have caused jitteriness and dysphoria.

In contrast to BZDs, buspirone's therapeutic effect may take 1 to 2 weeks. Because of its delayed effects, this drug is not useful in patients who need immediate relief from anxiety, and patient education is needed to enhance compliance with the medication regimen.

Other Antianxiety Medications

Hydroxyzines are sometimes used to relieve anxiety and tension associated with an anxiety state or as an adjunct in organic disease states with anxiety.

TABLE 41.2 Overview of Selected Drugs Used to Treat Anxiety

Generic (Trade) Name and Dosage	Selected Adverse Events	Contraindications	Special Considerations
Long-Acting Benzodiazepines			
Note: The use of long-acting benzodiazepines in the elderly is discouraged.			
clorazepate (Tranxene) Anxiety: 7.5–15 mg bid–qid. Adjust dose as needed within the range of 15–60 mg/d. Sustained-release forms may be given in a single dose of 11.25–22.5 mg hs in patients stabilized on 7.5 mg tid. Do not use to initiate therapy. Elderly or debilitated patients: initial dose 3.75–15 mg/d. May require adjustment of subsequent doses as needed. Children 9–12 y: 7.5 mg bid initially. May increase by 7.5 mg/wk but not to exceed 60 mg/d.	*CNS:* Drowsiness, dizziness, lethargy, mental depression, confusion, paradoxical excitement *EENT:* Blurred vision *Resp:* Respiratory depression *GI:* Constipation, diarrhea, nausea, vomiting *GU:* Urinary retention, incontinence *Derm:* Rashes *Misc:* Physical dependence, psychological dependence, tolerance	Hypersensitivity, cross-sensitivity with other benzodiazepines, preexisting CNS depression, severe, uncontrolled pain, narrow-angle glaucoma, pregnancy or lactation Use cautiously in preexisting hepatic disease, severe renal impairment, suicidal patients, past drug addiction, severe pulmonary disease, and geriatric or debilitated patients.	Half-life, including metabolites: 36–200 h Peak plasma level: 1–2 h Protein binding: 97%–98% Drowsiness may occur at initiation of treatment and with dosage increments. Avoid use of alcohol and other CNS depressants. Laboratory considerations: for patients on long-term therapy, check CBC and liver function studies periodically. May cause an increase in bilirubin, AST, and ALT. May cause decreased thyroid uptake of sodium iodide ^{123}I and ^{131}I.
chlordiazepoxide (Librium, Libritabs, Mitran, Reposans-10) Mild to moderate anxiety: 5–10 mg tid–qid Severe anxiety: 20–25 mg tid–qid Elderly or debilitated patients: 5 mg bid–qid Children: initial dose 5 mg bid–qid. A dose of 0.5 mg/kg/d q6–8h is also recommended for children >6 y. Not recommended for children <6 y.	*CNS:* drowsiness, dizziness, lethargy, mental depression, confusion, paradoxical excitement *EENT:* blurred vision *Resp:* respiratory depression *GI:* constipation, diarrhea, nausea, vomiting, dry mouth *GU:* urinary retention, incontinence *Derm:* rashes *Misc:* physical dependence, psychological dependence, tolerance	Hypersensitivity, cross-sensitivity with other benzodiazepines, preexisting CNS depression, severe, uncontrolled pain, narrow-angle glaucoma, pregnancy or lactation Some products contain tartrazine and should be avoided in patients who have intolerance. Use cautiously in preexisting hepatic disease, severe renal impairment, suicidal patients, past drug addiction, severe pulmonary disease, and geriatric or debilitated patients.	Half-life, including metabolites: 36–200 h Peak plasma level: 0.5–4 h Protein binding: 96% Avoid use of alcohol and other CNS depressants. Laboratory considerations: For patients on long-term therapy, check CBC and liver function studies periodically. May cause an increase in bilirubin, AST, and ALT. May cause decreased thyroid uptake of sodium iodide ^{123}I and ^{131}I. May alter 17-ketosteroids and 17-ketogenic steroids. May cause decreased response on metyrapone tests.
clonazepam (Klonopin) Panic disorder: 0.125 mg bid. Increase after 3 d toward a target dose of 1 mg/d. In some patients the dose may need to be increased to 4 mg/d.	*CNS:* Behavioral changes, drowsiness, slurred speech *EENT:* Abnormal eye movements, nystagmus, diplopia *Resp:* Respiratory distress, SOB, increased secretions, chest congestion	Hypersensitivity, cross-sensitivity with other benzodiazepines, and severe liver disease Use cautiously in chronic respiratory disease, narrow-angle glaucoma, pregnancy, lactation, children.	Rate of absorption: Intermediate Half-life, including metabolites: 18–50 h Peak plasma level PO: 1–2 h Protein binding: 97% Therapeutic serum levels: 20–80 ng/mL

diazepam (Valium, Valrelease, Vazepam; IV: Valium, Zetran; oral solution: Intensol) Anxiety: 2–10 mg bid–qid. Increase dosage cautiously to avoid adverse effects. Sustained-release 15- or 30-mg tablets may be used when the optimal daily oral dose of diazepam is 5 or 10 mg tid. Elderly or debilitated patients: Initial dose 2–2.5 mg qd–bid. Increase gradually as needed and tolerated. May also use 15-mg sustained-release tablets if this is the optimal established dose.
Children >6 mo: 1–2.5 mg PO tid–qid. Safety and efficacy have not been established in the neonate (≤30 d; injectable).

CV: Palpitations
GI: Constipation, diarrhea, hepatitis, changes in appetite
GU: Dysuria, nocturia, urinary retention
Neuro: Ataxia, hypotonia
Hemat: Anemia, eosinophilia, leukopenia, thrombocytopenia
Misc: Fever, physical dependence, psychological dependence, tolerance

Do not discontinue abruptly. Abrupt withdrawal may precipitate status epilepticus.
Withdrawal symptoms similar to those with barbiturates. Long-term use during pregnancy may result in withdrawal symptoms in the neonate.
Take with food to minimize gastric irritation.
Laboratory considerations: For patients on long-term therapy, check CBC and liver function studies periodically. May cause an increase in bilirubin, AST, and ALT. May cause decreased thyroid uptake of sodium iodide ^{123}I and [131]I.

CNS: Drowsiness, dizziness, lethargy, mental depression, paradoxical excitement, slurred speech, transient amnesia, hallucinations
EENT: Blurred vision
Resp: Respiratory depression
CV: Bradycardia, hypotension (IV only)
GI: Constipation, diarrhea, nausea, vomiting
GU: Urinary retention, incontinence
Derm: Rashes
Misc: Physical dependence, psychological dependence, tolerance

Hypersensitivity, cross-sensitivity with other benzodiazepines, preexisting CNS depression, severe, uncontrolled pain, narrow-angle glaucoma, and pregnancy or lactation
Some products contain tartrazine, alcohol, or propylene glycol and should be avoided in patients who have known intolerance.
Use cautiously in preexisting hepatic disease, severe renal impairment, suicidal patients, past drug addiction, children, and geriatric or debilitated patients.

Half-life, including metabolites: 20–100 h
Peak plasma level PO: 0.5–2 h
Protein binding: 98%
Avoid use of alcohol and other CNS depressants.
Laboratory considerations: For patients on long-term therapy, check CBC and liver function studies periodically.

Intermediate-Acting Benzodiazepines

alprazolam (Xanax) Initial dose: 0.25–0.5 mg tid. Titrate to maximal dose of 4 mg/d in divided doses. If side effects occur with starting dose, decrease dose.

CNS: Drowsiness, dizziness, lethargy, mental depression, paradoxical excitement
EENT: Blurred vision, nasal congestion
Resp: Respiratory depression

Hypersensitivity, cross-sensitivity with other benzodiazepines, preexisting CNS depression, severe, uncontrolled pain, narrow-angle glaucoma, and pregnancy or lactation

Half-life, including metabolites: 6–20 h
Peak plasma level: 1–2 h
Protein binding: 80%
May be administered with food if GI upset occurs. Avoid driving or other activities that require alertness.

(continued)

TABLE 41.2   Overview of Selected Drugs Used to Treat Anxiety (*Continued*)

Generic (Trade) Name and Dosage	Selected Adverse Events	Contraindications	Special Considerations
Elderly or debilitated patients: 0.25 mg bid–tid. Gradually increase as needed and tolerated. Panic disorder: Initial dose 0.5 mg tid. Depending on response, increase dose at intervals of 3–4 d in increments of 1 mg/d. Patients may require doses >4 mg/d. Do not exceed 10 mg/d. Children: Safety and efficacy for use in patients <18 y has not been established.	*GI:* Constipation, diarrhea, nausea, vomiting, dry mouth *Derm:* Rashes *Hemat:* Decreased hematocrit and neutropenia *Misc:* Physical dependence, psychological dependence, tolerance, weight gain, muscle rigidity	Use cautiously in hepatic dysfunction, suicidal patients, past drug addiction, and geriatric or debilitated patients.	Avoid use of alcohol and other CNS depressants. Patients on long-term or high-dosage therapy may experience withdrawal symptoms on abrupt cessation of therapy. Laboratory considerations: For patients on long-term therapy, check CBC and liver function studies periodically.
lorazepam (Ativan) Initial dose: 2–3 mg bid–tid (dose may vary from 1–10 mg/d). Elderly: initial dose: 1–2 mg/d in divided doses. Adjust dose based on need and tolerance. IM and IV routes are used for preoperative sedation. Children: Safety and efficacy for use in patients <12 y has not been established. Do not use injectable form in patients <18 y. May be used short term for insomnia due to anxiety, 2–4 mg/h.	*CNS:* Drowsiness, dizziness, lethargy, mental depression, paradoxical excitement, amnesia, disorientation *EENT:* Blurred vision *Resp:* Respiratory depression *CV:* Bradycardia, hypotension: with rapid IV infusion, apnea, cardiac arrest *GI:* Constipation, diarrhea, nausea, vomiting, change in appetite *Derm:* Rashes *Misc:* Physical dependence, psychological dependence, tolerance	Hypersensitivity, cross-sensitivity with other benzodiazepines, preexisting CNS depression, severe, uncontrolled pain, narrow-angle glaucoma, and pregnancy or lactation Use cautiously in hepatic, renal, or respiratory dysfunction, suicidal patients, past drug addiction, and geriatric or debilitated patients.	Half-life, including metabolites: 10–20 h Peak plasma level PO: 2–4 h Protein binding: 85% Avoid use of alcohol and other CNS depressants. Laboratory considerations: For patients on long-term or high-dose therapy, check CBC and renal and hepatic function periodically.
oxazepam (Serax) Mild to moderate anxiety: 10–15 mg tid–qid Severe anxiety syndromes or anxiety associated with depression: 15–30 mg tid–qid Older patients: initial dose 10 mg tid and if needed increase cautiously to 15 mg tid–qid Children: Dosage not established	*CNS:* Drowsiness, dizziness, lethargy, mental depression, paradoxical excitement, impaired memory, slurred speech *EENT:* Blurred vision *Resp:* Respiratory depression *CV:* Tachycardia *GI:* Drug-induced hepatitis, constipation, diarrhea, nausea, vomiting *Hemat:* Leukopenia (rare) *Derm:* Rashes *Misc:* Physical dependence, psychological dependence, tolerance, altered libido	Hypersensitivity, cross-sensitivity with other benzodiazepines, preexisting CNS depression, severe, uncontrolled pain, narrow-angle glaucoma, pregnancy or lactation Some products contain tartrazine and should be avoided in those patients who have intolerance. Use cautiously in preexisting hepatic disease, severe renal impairment, suicidal patients, past drug addiction, severe chronic pulmonary obstructive disease, and geriatric or debilitated patients.	Half-life, including metabolites: 10–20 h Peak plasma level: 2–4 h Protein binding: 85% Avoid use of alcohol and other CNS depressants. Laboratory considerations: In long-term therapy, monitor CBC and hepatic function periodically. May cause decreased thyroid uptake of sodium iodide [123] and [131].

buspirone (BuSpar)
Initial dose: 5 mg tid.
Increase dose 5 mg/d at intervals of 2–3 d as needed. Divided doses of 20–30 mg/d are common. Do not exceed 60 mg/d.

CNS: Drowsiness, dizziness, excitement, fatigue, headache, insomnia, nervousness, personality changes
EENT: Nasal congestion, blurred vision, sore throat, tinnitus, and altered taste and smell
GI: Nausea
CVP: Chest pain, chest congestion, palpitations, tachycardia, hyperventilation and shortness of breath
Neuro: Myalgia, incoordination, numbness, paresthesia
Derm: Hair loss, facial edema, clamminess, sweating, rashes
Sexual dysfunction: Irregular menses, decreased libido, delayed ejaculation, impotence
Other: Weight gain or loss, fever, roaring sensation in head, malaise

Hypersensitivity, pregnancy, lactation, children, severe liver dysfunction and concurrent use of antianxiety agents or other psychoactive drugs

Half-life: 2–3 h
Onset: 7–10 d
Peak plasma level: 3–4 wk
Optimal therapeutic results are usually after 3–4 wk. Some improvement will be seen in 7–10 d. Buspirone does not prevent withdrawal symptoms from other antianxiety agents, so gradual withdrawal from these medications is necessary.
Patient must inform caregiver if any chronic abnormal movements occur, such as motor restlessness, or involuntary repetitive movements of facial or neck muscles. Alcohol and other CNS depressant use must be avoided while on this medication.
Administration with food may decrease rate of GI absorption.

hydroxyzine HCl (Atarax)
hydroxyzine pamoate (Vistaril)
For mild to moderate anxiety: Begin with 25 mg tid. Optimum dose range is 75–150 mg/d in 3–4 divided doses. May increase to 300 mg/d.
For very mild symptoms: Patients may be maintained on 25 to 50 mg/d. Drugs may be given IM or PO.
Children: 50 mg/d in divided doses.

CNS: Drowsiness, dizziness, ataxia, headache, weakness
GI: Dry mouth
Hypersensitivity reactions
Infection at IM injection site

Hypersensitivity, pregnancy, and lactation
Use with caution in patients with hepatic dysfunction and geriatric patients.

Half-life: 3 h
Peak plasma level PO: 2–4 h
Additive CNS depression with other CNS depressants and alcohol.
Give deep IM in large muscles. May cause false-negative skin tests using allergen extracts. Discontinue medication 72 h before skin test.
Avoid driving or other activities that require alertness.
Also used as an antipruritic and an antiemetic.

meprobamate (Equanil, Miltown)
1.2–1.6 g/d in 3–4 divided doses
Sustained-release tabs: 400–800 mg AM and hs

CNS depression, nausea, vomiting, palpitations, tachycardia, dysrhythmias

Acute intermittent porphyria and allergy
Use with caution in patients with epilepsy and in pregnancy.

Use for <4 mo. With prolonged use, wean the patient off the medication. Drug dependence may develop.
This medication is rarely used now. It has been replaced by the benzodiazepines. Occasionally, elderly patients may have been on this medication for many years and continue to take the medication.

TABLE 41.3	Drug Interactions with Benzodiazepines	
Benzodiazepines	**Interacting Drugs**	**Interaction**
alprazolam (Xanax) chlordiazepoxide (Librium) clorazepate (Tranxene) diazepam (Valium) halazepam (Paxipam) lorazepam (Ativan) oxazepam (Serax)	cimetidine (Tagamet) ketoconazole (Nizoral) oral contraceptives metoprolol (Lopressor) disulfiram (Antabuse) propoxyphene (Darvon) fluoxetine (Prozac) propranolol (Inderal) isoniazid (Nydrazid)	Increased pharmacologic effect of BZDs and excessive sedation and impaired psychomotor function may occur because of decreased hepatic metabolism.
	valproic acid (Depakene)	Clearance rate of BZDs may be increased.
	alcohol and other CNS depressants, such as barbiturates and narcotics	May cause increased CNS effects such as sedation and impaired psychomotor dysfunction
	antacids	May alter rate of GI absorption but not extent of GI absorption. Do not administer at same time.
	digoxin (Lanoxin)	Serum concentrations of digoxin may be increased. Monitor digoxin serum levels and signs and symptoms of digoxin toxicity (GI and neuropsychiatric symptoms and cardiac dysrhythmias).
	levodopa (Dopar)	Antiparkinson efficacy may be reduced with concurrent use of BZDs.
	neuromuscular blocking agents	Concurrent use of BZDs may potentiate, counteract, or have no effect on the actions of these drugs.
	phenytoin (Dilantin)	Data are conflicting, but phenytoin serum levels may be increased, resulting in toxicity; oxazepam levels may be increased as well.
	probenecid (Benemid)	May interfere with BZD conjugation in the liver, resulting in a more rapid onset or prolonged effect
	ranitidine (Zantac)	GI absorption of diazepam may be reduced.
	rifampin (Rifadin)	May decrease the pharmacologic effects of some BZDs because it may increase the oxidative metabolism of these agents
	scopolamine (Hyoscine HBr)	Concomitant use with parenteral lorazepam may increase the incidence of sedation, hallucinations, and irrational behavior.
	theophylline (Slo-Phyllin)	May antagonize the sedative effects of BZDs

The use of hydroxyzines for long-term treatment of anxiety (more than 4 months) has not been assessed. Hydroxyzine hydrochloride (Atarax) and hydroxyzine pamoate (Vistaril) are drugs more commonly used for sedating patients before and after surgery and for managing pruritus, chronic urticaria, and atopic contact dermatitis. See **Table 41.2** for doses and adverse events.

Meprobamate (Equanil) has been used in anxiety disorders for short-term relief of symptoms. Long-term effectiveness (greater than 4 months) has not been assessed. Drug dependence and abuse can occur. This drug has been replaced by other antianxiety medications and is used infrequently today, but some elderly patients may have been on this drug for many years and have acquired drug dependence. See **Table 41.2** for dosages and adverse events.

Antidepressants

Antidepressants are thought of as specific for treating depression, but they are effective in many anxiety disorders. There

are three categories of antidepressants: tricyclic antidepressants (TCAs), nonselective serotonin reuptake inhibitors (NSRIs) and SSRIs, and monoamine oxidase (MAO) inhibitors (**Table 41.4**). Anxious patients often need long-term use of antidepressants to maintain benefit and prevent relapse. For further information on antidepressants, see Chapter 40.

Tricyclic Antidepressants

TCAs are effective in GAD and PD. Imipramine (Tofranil) is the prototypical TCA effective in controlling panic attacks in patients with PD and GAD. TCAs have largely been supplanted by SSRIs as first-line therapy for the treatment of anxiety disorders.

Mechanism of Action

TCAs block the reuptake of norepinephrine and serotonin into nerve endings, thus increasing the levels of norepinephrine and serotonin in the nerve cells. Imipramine does not have

TABLE 41.4	Antidepressants Used in Treating Anxiety Disorders	
Generic (Trade) Name	Initial Dose (mg)	Usual Dose (mg)
Tricyclic Antidepressants		
amitriptyline (Elavil)	10–50	150–300
amoxapine (Ascendin)	25–50	150–450
desipramine (Norpramin)	10–25	100–250
doxepin (Sinequan, Adapin)	10–25	150–300
imipramine (Tofranil)	10–50	150–300
maprotiline (Ludiomil)	25–50	150–200
nortriptyline (Pamelor)	25–50	150–200
protriptyline (Vivactil)	5–10	15–60
trimipramine (Surmontil)	25–50	150–300
Selective Serotonin Reuptake Inhibitors		
citalopram (Celexa)	20	20–40
escitalopram (Lexapro)	10	10–20
fluoxetine (Prozac)	10–20	10–80
fluoxetine (Prozac weekly)		
fluvoxamine (Luvox)	25–50	100–300
nefazodone (Serzone)	50–100	200–500
paroxetine (Paxil)	10–20	10–60
(Paxil CR)	12.5	12.5–75
sertraline (Zoloft)	25–50	75–200
venlafaxine (Effexor)	75 bid-tid	75–225
(Effexor XL)	37.5–75	75–225
Nonselective Serotonin Reuptake Inhibitors		
clomipramine (Anafranil)	20–50	150–450
Monoamine Oxidase Inhibitors		
phenelzine (Nardil)	15	45–90

any direct effects on anticipatory anxiety or phobic avoidance behavior. The response is gradual, over a period of weeks. Other TCAs are equally effective in treating patients with PD.

When a TCA is given for PD, approximately 33% of patients feel overstimulated when treatment begins. To reduce this problem, the patient may need to start with a lower dose and gradually increase the dose until a therapeutic dose response occurs. BZDs can be used on a short-term basis to lessen these initial symptoms.

Adverse Events

Because PD is episodic, it is considered a chronic condition that requires long-term management with TCAs. However, approximately 33% of patients on TCAs discontinue their treatment because they cannot tolerate the side effects of the drugs.

TCAs cause anticholinergic side effects such as dryness of the mouth and other mucosal surfaces, blurred vision, tachycardia, constipation, and urinary hesitancy. Other adverse effects are postural hypotension, carbohydrate craving, weight gain, excessive perspiration, and sexual dysfunction. They can also lower the seizure threshold and must be used cautiously in

patients with seizure disorders. These drugs are contraindicated in patients with narrow-angle glaucoma, urinary hesitancy, and heart conduction abnormalities. TCAs enhance the CNS effects of alcohol. Plasma measurements of TCAs should be done in selected situations as needed. See Chapter 40 for more information.

Selective Serotonin Reuptake Inhibitors

SSRIs have become the drugs of choice for treating most anxiety disorders. They have more benign side effects than TCAs, which makes them more acceptable to patients. They can be classified into NSRIs, such as clomipramine (Anafranil), which is structurally similar to cyclic antidepressants, and SSRIs such as escitalopram (Lexapro), fluoxetine (Prozac, weekly Prozac), fluvoxamine (Luvox), paroxetine (Paxil), and sertraline (Zoloft). Nefazodone (Serzone) blocks 5-hydroxytryptamine (serotonin; 5-HT) receptors as well as inhibiting serotonin transport. Venlafaxine (Effexor XL) causes strong inhibition of serotonin and norepinephrine and weak inhibition of dopamine reuptake. See **Table 41.4** and Chapter 40.

Medications indicated for treating OCD are the NSRI clomipramine (Anafranil) and the SSRIs fluoxetine (Prozac), fluvoxamine (Luvox), paroxetine (Paxil), sertraline (Zoloft), citalopram (Celexa), or escitalopram (Lexapro). More than 50% of patients treated with clomipramine have their symptoms controlled completely or controlled to subclinical levels; in other patients, the symptoms are reduced in intensity.

Dosage

The effective oral dosage of clomipramine for OCD is 150 to 250 mg/d. It takes approximately 4 to 6 weeks for the antiobsessional effects to become evident, and it may take up to 12 weeks for patients to attain full benefits. SSRIs and clomipramine are palliative only and not a cure for OCD; once patients discontinue drug therapy, most of them relapse. SSRIs are very effective in patients with PD and GAD. An advantage of sustained-release venlafaxine (Effexor XL) is that it is taken once daily, starting with a dose of 37.5 mg that is increased weekly to a maximum dose of 225 mg. (See **Table 41.4** and Chapter 40.)

Adverse Events

Common adverse events of SSRIs include nausea, headache, insomnia, drowsiness, nervous jitteriness, diarrhea, rash, urticaria, weight loss, and sexual dysfunction. Paroxetine (Paxil) and fluoxetine (Prozac) are associated with very significant inhibition of P410 IID6, which makes polypharmacy more difficult. Paroxetine (Paxil) may cause more weight gain and sexual inhibition than the other drugs. Approximately 15% of patients discontinue treatment because of side effects. The effects of an overdose of SSRIs are relatively benign, and death is rare. Caution should be used when SSRIs are given in combination with TCAs because SSRIs can inhibit one or more liver microsomal enzymes. The combination of SSRIs and MAO inhibitors has resulted in serious reactions such as hyperthermia, rigidity, and autonomic dysregulation that can be fatal. See Chapter 40 for more information.

Monoamine Oxidase Inhibitors

MAO inhibitors are effective in controlling panic attacks in most patients with PD. Their effectiveness in GAD has not been explored because of the necessary dietary restrictions and dangerous drug interactions that make their use cumbersome.

Mechanism of Action

MAO inhibitors inhibit the breakdown of 5-HT and norepinephrine in the synaptic cleft. The most commonly used MAO inhibitor is phenelzine (Nardil), which is given in a dose range of 45 to 90 mg/d.

Adverse Events

MAO inhibitors have anticholinergic side effects such as blurred vision, dry mouth and other mucosal surfaces, constipation, urinary hesitancy, and tachycardia. Weight gain, agitation, and sexual dysfunction frequently occur. Hypotension that is aggravated by postural changes may develop, but it usually diminishes in a few weeks. Palliative measures such as increased fluid intake, salt tablets, and low-dose fludrocortisone (Florinef) can be used to manage hypotension. The greatest danger with MAO inhibitors is hypertensive crisis, which can be caused by food or drug interaction and can result in cerebral hemorrhage and death. MAO inhibitors prevent the breakdown of monoamines, so the patient taking an MAO inhibitor must avoid sympathomimetic substances and foods that contain tyramine, such as cheese, liver, yogurt, yeast, soy sauce, red wine, and beer. For further information, see Chapter 40.

Beta-Adrenergic Blockers

Beta-adrenergic blockers neutralize the effects of epinephrine and norepinephrine on the beta-adrenergic receptors. The anxiolytic effects of all beta blockers are peripheral rather than central. Their main effect is to slow the heart rate and reduce tremors that decrease the perception of physical distress in anxiety-producing situations. They do not directly affect psychic anxiety, vigilance, or hyperalertness. Beta blockers are useful in the treatment of patients with palpitations, irregular heartbeat, or muscular tremor caused by anxiety. It is advantageous to combine beta blockers with a BZD when physical distress and anxiety symptoms coexist.

Selecting the Most Appropriate Agent

General Anxiety Disorder

First-Line Therapy

SSRIs have quickly become the drug of choice for GAD. No evidence has shown any one SSRI to be superior to another; however, the SSRIs have significant differences in side effects and drug interactions. Patients may have to try several SSRIs until they find one that best relieves their symptoms. TCAs may be used, but the side effect profiles of TCAs have tended to limit their use as first-line therapy agents since SSRIs have come into use. Antidepressants all require weeks to become effective, so BZDs may be given along with an antidepressant

until it begins to work. Once this occurs, the patient is slowly tapered off the BZD.

Second-Line Therapy

Buspirone may be considered a first-line therapy in newly diagnosed patients or for patients with chronic anxiety, but it is usually used in second-line therapy. Buspirone may be more appropriate if sedation or psychomotor impairment would be dangerous. Buspirone differs from the SSRIs in its efficacy spectrum and side effect profile. Buspirone is available in immediate and sustained-release formulations. It has fewer side effects than BZDs and minimal abuse potential. However, the therapeutic effect of the drug may take 1 to 4 weeks. Buspirone may be the most appropriate drug for patients with a history of substance abuse, personality disorder, or sleep apnea.

Third-Line Therapy

BZDs are considered first-line therapy only for exogenous anxiety related to a time-limited stress. The BZDs used most frequently are alprazolam, clorazepate (Tranxene), and diazepam. There is no evidence that one BZD is superior to another in this disorder. When choosing the specific BZD for treatment, the practitioner must consider the drug's onset of action and its half-life and the patient's metabolism (**Figure 41-1** and **Table 41.5**).

The drug dosage should be increased gradually to reach therapeutic response levels without producing unacceptable adverse effects. Use of BZDs with a long duration of action can be a problem because they may cause daytime sedation and motor impairment.

Drugs such as lorazepam or oxazepam are preferred because rebound and hangover effects may be avoided. Use of BZDs for more than 4 months may result in dependence, which can result in withdrawal symptoms and rebound effects. Concurrent psychotherapy may reduce the time needed for drug therapy as well as improving the patient's response rate. (See **Figure 41-1.**)

Panic Disorder

First-Line Therapy

Panic disorder is episodic, and patients with PD frequently do well with SSRIs. Alprazolam (Xanax) is the only BZD that is approved by the U.S. Food and Drug Administration (FDA) for PD, but clonazepam (Klonopin) is also used. These drugs are used along with an SSRI if rapid relief from anxiety is needed. The practitioner needs to monitor symptoms, assess for side effects, and gradually increase the dosages of SSRIs and alprazolam or clonazepam if needed (**Figure 41-2**).

Second-Line Therapy

Patients who do not respond to SSRIs may be changed to a TCA and monitored for effectiveness in decreasing panic attacks and controlling the severity of anxiety or panic symptoms while causing tolerable adverse events.

Third-Line Therapy

MAO inhibitors can be very effective in controlling panic attacks. Before the patient begins therapy, however, the

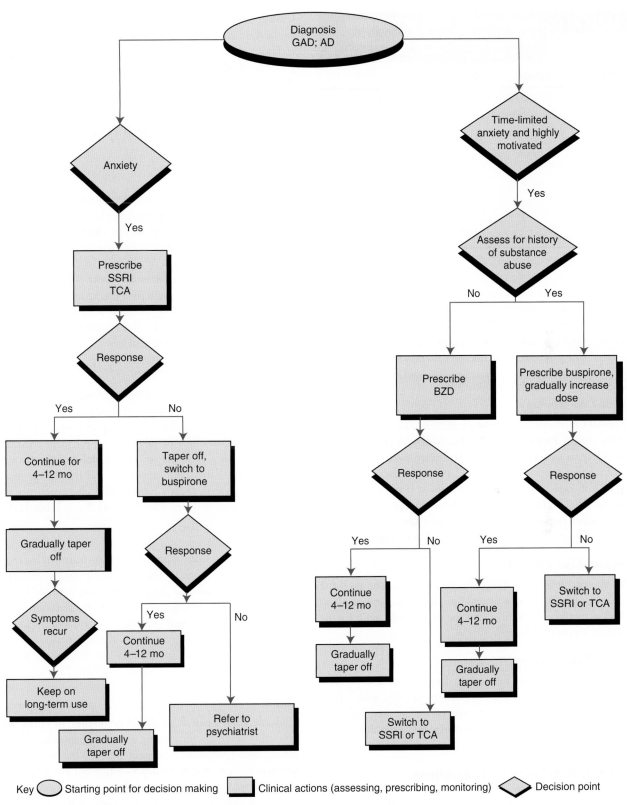

FIGURE 41–1 Treatment algorithm for GAD.

TABLE 41.5	Recommended Order of Treatment for Generalized Anxiety Disorder	
Order	**Agents**	**Comments**
First line	SSRI or TCA	Useful for anxiety disorder as well as a coexisting comorbidity
Second line	Buspirone	Takes 1–2 wk for effect
Third line		Select agent based on drug onset, half-life, and patient metabolism. Do not use if patient is alcohol or drug dependent. May be first-line drug in motivated patients with acute anxiety to a time-limited stress.

practitioner must assess his or her willingness to avoid the many tyramine-containing sympathomimetic drugs and foods, which can interact with MAO inhibitors to precipitate serious, life-threatening reactions. In addition, the patient should be referred to a psychiatrist for intensive therapy.

Obsessive-Compulsive Disorder
First-Line Therapy

The APA recommends the use of an SSRI as a first-line agent (APA, 2007). Patients with OCD do well with clomipramine, an NSRI, as well as with SSRIs. The practitioner must monitor for a decrease in symptoms and assess for adverse events. A gradual dosage increase may be employed if the patient does not see relief within the first 4 weeks of therapy. If the patient has a good response to therapy without uncomfortable side effects, therapy may continue for up to 1 year (**Figure 41-3**).

Second-Line Therapy

An alternative SSRI or buspirone (BuSpar) may be used for patients with OCD as a second-line drug. Response to drug therapy must be monitored and the patient referred for concurrent supportive therapy.

Third-Line Therapy

If the patient does not respond to drug therapy and psychotherapy and obsessions and compulsions interfere with activities of daily living, a psychiatric referral for intensive behavior therapy is indicated. **Table 41.6** summarizes drug therapy for GAD, PA, and OCD.

Special Population Considerations

Patients who have previously been treated for an anxiety disorder may have had drug treatment or psychotherapy that they found unsatisfactory. The practitioner should review with them what the treatments were, what adverse reactions they had, and the number of previous health care providers who treated them. Check with them for any history of drug withdrawal symptoms. If they report that a drug or treatment was

unacceptable, plan a different but effective treatment. Assess for adverse effects to the new program. Also assess for drug-seeking behavior to rule out BZD dependence. Sometimes patients "shop around" for new health care providers when their previous provider has advised withdrawing from BZDs.

Patients with a history of prescription medication abuse and substance or alcohol abuse can become drug dependent. Buspirone, a nonaddicting drug, is a choice for their treatment regimen.

Pediatric

Four BZDs—clorazepate, chlordiazepoxide, diazepam, and alprazolam—have been approved by the FDA for use in children. Doses vary according to the child's age and weight. Clomipramine (Anafranil) remains the drug of choice in the treatment of OCD. Onset of action is in 2 to 4 weeks, with a final improvement over 8 to 10 weeks. The dosage of clomipramine is up to 200 mg/d or 3 mg/kg for children or adolescents. SSRIs are effective in the treatment of OCD. Only sertraline (Zoloft) and fluvoxamine (Luvox) has been approved for the treatment of OCD in children.

Geriatric

Elderly patients may have decreased liver and renal function and metabolize and excrete drugs more slowly. They also may have neurologic disorders, cardiac disease, hypertension, hypotension, and glaucoma and may be taking drugs for these conditions. Elderly patients may be started on low doses of shorter-acting BZDs, TCAs, SSRIs, and buspirone, and the dosage may be gradually increased. Elderly patients may also experience paradoxical reactions to drugs. (See **Table 41.2** and **Table 41.3**.)

Women

Women are more likely than men to seek treatment for anxiety and depression. Women who are taking oral contraceptive drugs may have adverse drug interactions with BZDs. (See **Table 41.3**.) The practitioner needs to be alert for signs of anxiety disorders in men because they are not as likely as women to report these symptoms. Rather, men are likely to report physical signs of anxiety and not identify the problem as emotional in origin.

Ethnic

Understanding a patient's cultural orientation or ethnic background is necessary for making a correct diagnosis and establishing an appropriate treatment plan. What we view as a problem such as anxiety or depression is not always perceived the same way by patients from other cultures. Complaints of anxiety or depression may not be reported by some patients because this is considered to be a mental disorder that is to be kept secret from people outside the family.

Research findings indicate that people from various racial or ethnic groups may metabolize some drugs differently because of their genetic makeup. An example of a drug that is metabolized differently is the antitubercular drug isoniazid

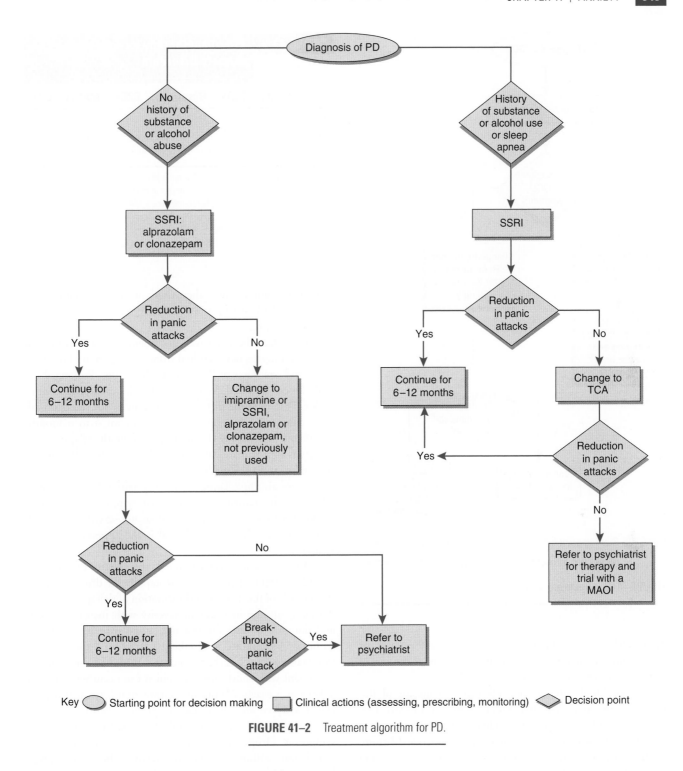

FIGURE 41–2 Treatment algorithm for PD.

(Laniazid). Researchers are beginning to examine other drug classifications for variations. Practitioners need to keep current with research that examines genetic differences in the metabolism of drugs. (See Chapters 2 and 3.)

Monitoring Patient Response

Patients need to be monitored for self-reports of decreased anxiety symptoms. The practitioner should monitor patients closely for compliance with the medication regimen as well as side effects.

Most side effects from SSRIs are transient. Dose-related sexual effects, such as decreased libido or delayed ejaculation in men and anorgasmia in women, are common and typically do not resolve without intervention. Management of treatment-related sexual dysfunction includes reducing the SSRI dosage reduction and adding or switching to an antidepressant not associated with sexual dysfunction, such as bupro-

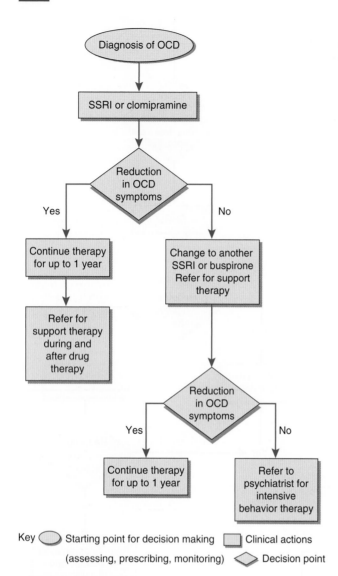

Key: ⬭ Starting point for decision making | ▢ Clinical actions
(assessing, prescribing, monitoring) | ◇ Decision point

FIGURE 41–3 Treatment algorithm for OCD.

TABLE 41.6	**Pharmacotherapy for Selected Anxiety Disorders**					
	SSRIs	**TCAs**	**Buspirone**	**BZDs**	**MAOIs**	**CBT**
GAD	+	+	+/−	+	+	+
PD	+	+	+	+	−	+
OCD	+	−	+/−	+/−	+	+

GAD, generalized anxiety disorder; PD, panic disorder; OCD, obsessive-compulsive disorder; SSRIs, selective serotonin reuptake inhibitors; TCAs, tricyclic antidepressants; BZDs, benzodiazepines; MAOIs, monoamine oxidase inhibitors; CBT, cognitive behavioral therapy
(Data from Liebowitz, N. R. [2004]. Anxiety disorders. In R. Rakel & E. Bope [Eds.], *Conn's current therapy* [56th ed.]. Philadelphia: Elsevier.)

pion (Wellbutrin, Wellbutrin SR), nefazodone (Serzone), or mirtazapine (Remeron). Another strategy includes the use of sildenafil (Viagra) or buspirone.

A non-life-threatening discontinuation syndrome of flu-like symptoms may occur after abrupt cessation of an SSRI. This syndrome can be minimized by gradually tapering the dose.

An overdose of TCAs can lead to anticholinergic delirium, ventricular arrhythmias, significant hypotension, seizures, and death. A TCA overdose is a medical emergency and requires close clinical and cardiac monitoring.

Many patients do not like buspirone because it takes 1 to 4 weeks to take effect. Frequently patients stop taking this medication because they think it is not helping their symptoms. Patient education and monitoring for compliance must be ongoing.

There have been no well-documented fatal overdoses of BZDs, but deaths have resulted from the ingestion of multiple drugs and overdoses of BZDs and other drugs. Prolonged use of BZDs can lead to dependence and withdrawal on discontinuation. Although the duration of therapy is not standardized, most clinicians prescribe the medication for 4 to 6 months and then try decreasing the dosage; however, the relapse rate of anxiety is approximately 60% to 80% within the first year that the patient is off the medication.

There are three components of a withdrawal syndrome: relapse is the return of the original symptoms of anxiety, rebound is a return of symptoms at greater severity than originally experienced, and withdrawal is the appearance of new symptoms.

When a BZD is discontinued, the severity of the withdrawal syndrome depends on how rapidly the drug is tapered, the half-life of the drug, and the duration of therapy. The withdrawal syndrome increases in severity with increased dosage and duration of use: for instance, more patients experience withdrawal symptoms after taking a BZD for 8 months than those taking it for less than 3 months. Withdrawal is relatively infrequent with short-term use, but it can occur with therapy as brief as 3 weeks. Abrupt discontinuation is frequently associated with withdrawal, usually of greater severity. Therefore, the rate of discontinuation should be slowed to moderate the symptoms. Drugs with shorter half-lives are also more associated with withdrawal phenomena than those with longer half-lives. The tapering period should be at least 4 weeks, and the rate of tapering should be approximately a 10% dosage decrease every 3 to 4 days. **Box 41.5** lists BZD withdrawal symptoms.

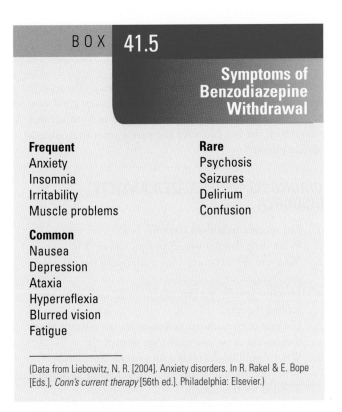

BOX 41.5

Symptoms of Benzodiazepine Withdrawal

Frequent
Anxiety
Insomnia
Irritability
Muscle problems

Rare
Psychosis
Seizures
Delirium
Confusion

Common
Nausea
Depression
Ataxia
Hyperreflexia
Blurred vision
Fatigue

(Data from Liebowitz, N. R. [2004]. Anxiety disorders. In R. Rakel & E. Bope [Eds.], *Conn's current therapy* [56th ed.]. Philadelphia: Elsevier.)

Patients on long-term (more than 4 months) BZD therapy need periodic blood counts and liver and thyroid function testing. BZDs can cause elevations in lactate dehydrogenase, alkaline phosphatase, alanine aminotransferase, and aspartate aminotransferase levels. Use of BZDs may cause leukopenia, blood dyscrasias, anemia, thrombocytopenia, eosinophilia, and decreased uptake of I^{125} and I^{131} sodium iodide. (See **Table 41.2;** see also Chapter 40 for a discussion of monitoring concerns related to antidepressant medications.)

PATIENT EDUCATION

Drug Information

The patient should know the name of the drug prescribed, dose, frequency of administration, expected outcome of therapy, drug interactions, adverse events, and the amount of time it will take for the drug to take effect. The patient should also know how to report adverse events to the primary caregiver. The patient should be taught to take the drug as ordered and not to increase the dose or stop the drug without first contacting the primary care provider.

The patient should know that the therapeutic effect of the drug needs to be monitored and that the dosage may need to be increased or another drug may be more helpful. If laboratory tests are needed, the patient should know the name of the laboratory test, what the test is, and the frequency of monitoring. The patient also needs to tell all health care providers what medications he or she is taking.

The National Institutes of Health's website (www.nih.gov/medlineplus/anxiety.html) provides useful patient information, as does the Anxiety Disorder Association of America's website (www.adaa.org).

Lifestyle Information

The patient should know that the physical symptoms of anxiety (e.g., increased heart rate, palpitations, pupil dilation, trembling, increased perspiration, muscle tension, and sleep disturbances) are not life threatening. The practitioner should instruct the patient about how combination treatment consisting of medications, psychotherapy, and relaxation therapy can control anxiety. Instruction on performing relaxation exercises is helpful. The practitioner should describe the various psychotherapeutic modalities so that the patient may select the one thought to be most appropriate. If the patient does not seek psychotherapy, the primary caregiver may need to provide emotional support. The patient who does not respond well to drug and relaxation therapy must be referred to a psychiatric specialist.

Providing written instructions is important because the patient may have trouble concentrating on or fully comprehending verbal instructions. After providing all instructions and materials, the practitioner should review the patient's comprehension of the instructions and willingness to comply with the medication regimen. This review should be part of each patient visit.

FUTURE DIRECTIONS IN ANXIOLYTIC PHARMACOLOGIC TREATMENT

Psychopharmacologists are developing new anxiolytic drugs that are fast-acting and free from the unwanted effects associated with BZDs. Drugs that are partial agonists at the BZD receptors have been studied in Europe, but no BZD partial agonists have been approved for anxiolytic use in the United States. Zolpidem, a structurally and pharmacologically similar agent, has been recently marketed as a hypnotic.

Neurosteroids are pharmacologic agents that target the BZD receptor. They now need to be tested in humans. Researchers are targeting various serotonin 5-HT receptor subtypes. Studies of neuropeptide receptor agonists and antagonists with anxiolytic properties have been conducted, but these agents need more clinical testing.

Case Study

L. P., age 23, is a white woman who graduated from college last year. She began working as an accountant 1 month after graduating. Approximately 2 months ago, she moved into a two-bedroom apartment with another woman who works at the same accounting firm. She states that her roommate recommended that she see a doctor to find out if she has anemia or "some sort of fatigue syndrome." She states that she has felt "restless" and "on edge" for most of the past 9 months. She becomes easily fatigued and irritable and has difficulty concentrating and falling asleep. She states that sometimes her mind "just goes blank," and she is worried that her work performance is no longer excellent. She reports that all her life she had good grades in school and was very successful in everything she attempted. Although she has been "a worrier from the day I was born," now she worries more than she ever has and feels nervous "all the time." L. P. reports that she has a good relationship with her boyfriend but they do not get to see each other very often because he is attending graduate school 100 miles away. She reports having a satisfying sexual relationship with him. She denies having any problems with relationships with her parents, roommate, or peers. She denies having any financial worries unless she is fired from her job for poor work performance. She reports that she has always been healthy and has taken good care of herself. The only medication she takes is birth control pills, which she has taken for the past 4 years without any adverse effects.

DIAGNOSIS: GENERALIZED ANXIETY DISORDER

1. List specific treatment goals for L. P.
2. What drug therapy would you prescribe? Why?
3. What are the parameters for monitoring the success of the therapy?
4. Describe specific patient monitoring based on the prescribed therapy.
5. List one or two adverse reactions for the selected agent that would cause you to change therapy.
6. What would be the choice for second-line therapy?
7. What dietary and lifestyle changes should be recommended for this patient?
8. Describe one or two drug–drug or drug–food interactions for the selected agent.

BIBLIOGRAPHY

*Starred references are cited in the text.

*American Psychiatric Association. (2000). *Diagnostic and statistical manual of mental disorders* (4th ed., text revision). Washington, DC: Author.

*American Psychiatric Association. (2007). *Practice guideline for the treatment of patients with obsessive-compulsive disorder.* Arlington, VA: Author.

American Psychiatric Association. (2009). *Practice guideline for the treatment of patients with panic disorder* (2nd ed.). Washington, DC: Author.

*Cannon, W. B. (1963). *Wisdom of the body.* New York: Norton.

Davis, R. D., & Winter, L. (2001). Antianxiety agents. In J. L. Jacobson, *Psychiatric secrets* (2nd ed.). New York: Hanley & Belfus.

DiPiro, J. T., Talbert, R. L., Yee, G. C., Matzke, G. R., Wells, B. G., & Posey, L. M. (Eds.). (1999). *Pharmacotherapy: A pathophysiologic approach* (4th ed.). Norwalk, CT: Appleton & Lange.

Ferri, F. (2004). *Practice guide to the care of the medical patient* (6th ed.). St. Louis: Mosby, Inc.

Goldstein, M. Z. (2002). Depression and anxiety in older women. *Primary Care Clinics in Office Practice, 29*(1).

Gutierez, K. (1999). *Pharmacotherapeutics: Clinical decision making in nursing.* Philadelphia: W. B. Saunders.

Herbert, F. B. (2001). Obsessive-compulsive disorder in children and adolescents. In J. L. Jacobson (Ed.), *Psychiatric disorders* (2nd ed.). New York: Hanley & Belfus.

Kaplan, H., & Sadock, B. (1999). *Comprehensive textbook of psychiatry* (7th ed.). Baltimore: Williams & Wilkins.

*Kazdin, A. E. (2008). Evidence-based treatment and practice: New opportunities to bridge clinical research and practice, enhance the knowledge base, and improve patient care. *American Psychology, 63,* 146.

Kercher, E. E. (2002). Anxiety disorders. In J. Marx, R. Hockenberger, & R. Walls (Eds.), *Rosen's emergency medicine: Concepts in clinical practice* (5th ed.). St Louis: Mosby, Inc.

*Kroenke, K., Spitzer, R., Williams, J., et al. (2007). Anxiety disorders in primary care: Prevalence, impairment, comorbidity, and detection. *American College of Physicians. 146,* 317–325.

Lauderdale, S. A., & Shiekh, J. I. (2003). Anxiety disorders in older adults. *Clinics in Geriatric Medicine, 19*(4).

Leichsenring, F., & Rabung, S. (2006). Effectiveness of long-term psychodynamic psychotherapy. *Nature Medicine, 12,* 1139.

Liebowitz, N. R. (2004). Anxiety disorders. In R. Rakel & E. Bope (Eds.), *Conn's current therapy* (56th ed.). Philadelphia: Elsevier.

Moore, D. P., & Jefferson, J. W. (2004). Secondary anxiety disorder due to a general medical condition, DSM-IV-TR #293.89; substance-induced anxiety disorder, DSM-IV TR #292.80. *Handbook of Medical Psychiatry* (2nd ed.). St. Louis: Mosby, Inc.

*Selye, H. (1991). History and present status of the stress concept. In A. Monat & R. S. Lazarus (Eds.), *Stress and coping* (3rd ed.). New York: Columbia University Press.

Semia, T. P., Beizer, J. L., & Higbee, M. D. (2003). *Geriatric dosage handbook* (9th ed.). Hudson, OH: Lexi-Comp.

Shader, R. I., & Greenblatt. (2000). Pharmacotherapy of acute anxiety: A mini update (Supported in part by a grant [MH-34223] from the Department of Health and Human Services) http://www.org/g4/GN401000128/CH126.html.

Sood, A. B., Weller, E., & Weller, R. (2004). SSRIs in children and adolescents. *Current Psychiatry, 3*(3), 83–89.

Stein, M. B., Roy-Bryne, P. P., Craske, M. G., et al. (2005). Functional impact and health utility of anxiety disorders in primary care outpatients. *Medical Care, 43,* 1164–1170.

*Swede, S. E., Leonard, H. L., Garvey, M., et al. (1998). Pediatric autoimmune neuropsychiatric disorders associated with streptococcal infections: Clinical descriptions of the first 50 cases. *American Journal of Psychiatry, 154*(1), 264–271.

Tancer, M. E., & Hussain, S. (2004). Panic disorder. In R. Rakel & E. Bope (Eds.), *Conn's current therapy* (56th ed.). Philadelphia: Elsevier.

Insomnia and Sleep Disorders

Sleep, a naturally recurring state of restfulness for the body, is a necessary element of our daily life and occurs in a daily rhythmic pattern. Sleep disorders can affect the quality of sleep and therefore how individuals function on a daily basis. A problem with sleep is a symptom of another underlying problem. Sleep disorders include insomnia, snoring and sleep apnea, narcolepsy, and chronic sleep deprivation. Pharmacologic therapy is not appropriate for snoring and sleep apnea but has a role in the management of the other diagnoses. The key to an appropriate treatment plan is to recognize the type of sleep disorder.

INSOMNIA

Although most people occasionally have problems falling or staying asleep, insomnia can be defined as persistent trouble sleeping. Some experts argue, however, that problems sleeping at any time may be referred to as *insomnia;* they define the condition as loss of sleep for a short period. The loss of sleep may be due to physiologic causes such as restless leg syndrome, gastroesophageal reflux, or fibromyalgia, or sleep loss may simply be due to ignoring sleep cues. Sleep that is not refreshing also can be classified as insomnia. According to the Sleep in America Poll (Sleep Facts and Stats, 2009), over 64% of respondents reported problems with sleep, but only 32% discussed their complaints with a healthcare professional. The 2010 Sleep Poll compared sleep complaints among African Americans, Whites, Asians, and Hispanics, finding variations in bedtime routines, meeting sleep needs, sleep partners, and general health related to sleep. Results show that Whites are more likely to be diagnosed with a sleep disorder (20%) compared to African Americans and Hispanics (19%); those least diagnosed are Asians (10%). Complaints are more prevalent in women and increase with age, especially in those over age 65: up to 67% of elderly people have frequent sleep problems, but only one in eight is diagnosed and treated (Sleep Facts and Stats, 2004).

Insomnia can have social and economic consequences, as measured through direct and indirect costs. The National Sleep Foundation (2004) estimated that the cost of sleep deprivation and sleep disorders equals $100 billion annually. This cost is seen in lost productivity, medical expenses, sick leave, and property and environmental damages (Rosekind, et al., 2010). Up to 40% of people medicate themselves, commonly treating their insomnia with a host of over-the-counter (OTC) drugs and other remedies before seeking the help of a health care provider. In the United States, more than $1 billion is spent yearly on sleep medications. According to a more recent Sleep America poll, little has changed regarding these demographics since the early 1990s.

CAUSES

Insomnia can be of physiologic or psychological origin, and it is important to rule out the physiologic causes before labeling insomnia as psychological. Changes in a patient's biological clock can contribute to insomnia (e.g., hyperarousal states, time zone and schedule changes), as can the sleep environment. Physiologic causes of insomnia have included restless leg syndrome, gastroesophageal reflux, and fibromyalgia; however, research has not been able to prove a direct cause and effect and should be considered comorbid insomnia (Dement & Vaughan, 1999; National Institutes of Health [NIH], 2005). Estimates are that up to half of all cases of insomnia are psychological in origin. In addition, 10% to 15% of cases result from drug or substance abuse. Medical causes are responsible for 10% of insomnia cases. Finally, primary or idiopathic sleep disorders account for 10% to 20% of all cases of insomnia (**Box 42.1**).

Insomnia can have both nocturnal symptoms and daytime consequences. This serious health care issue affects the quality of life, productivity, and safety of both the patient and society. Insomnia can be classified as *acute* or *transient*, lasting a few days; *short term,* lasting a few weeks; or *chronic* or *learned,* lasting months and years. It can also be classified as "difficulty falling asleep," "difficulty maintaining sleep," and "early morning awakening."

Acute insomnia is often related to environmental factors, such as sleeping in an unfamiliar place or excessive heat, noise, light, or movement of the bed partner. Transient insomnia often is related to stress or environmental changes. Usually, an acute emotional shock (either positive or negative) triggers

BOX 42.1

Causes of Insomnia

Medical

Endocrine problems (e.g., hypothyroidism, hyperthyroidism, degenerative disease)

Neurologic and cardiovascular problems that cause difficulties with breathing

Pain

Renal problems (e.g., urinary frequency)

Respiratory problems (e.g., COPD, asthma)

Sleep apnea

Psychiatric

Anxiety

Excess stress

Major depression

Drug and Alcohol Abuse

Sedatives and stimulants

Primary Sleep Disorders

Excessive arousal and wakefulness

Poor sleep hygiene: related to lifestyle

Sleep state misperception: achievement of adequate sleep but not perceived by patient

this type of insomnia. Chronic, or learned, insomnia has been defined as a condition lasting at least 3 weeks. Characteristics of chronic insomnia include somatized tension and acquired habits that prevent either the initiation or maintenance of sleep. Life stresses such as shift work, a family tragedy, or physical pain can exacerbate learned insomnia. As Regestein, et al., reported in 1993, learned insomnia also may be associated with a hyperarousable state. This study, which examined daytime alertness in patients with primary insomnia, concluded that the measurement of hyperarousal, as measured by alpha waves on the electroencephalogram (EEG), may be useful to refine the description of insomnia populations. Insomnia can start with an initially stressful event, but the hyperarousable state of chronic insomniacs extends well beyond the heightened levels of stress.

Whether insomnia is labeled as transient or chronic, Dement & Vaughan (1999) argued that insomnia is significant for any length of time and needs thoughtful evaluation and possible treatment.

Many adolescents have an increased need for sleep, but they may have difficulty getting to sleep, difficulty awakening in the morning, or both. Adolescents who lead very busy lives may not get enough sleep.

Older adults may report early-morning awakening or general sleep disturbances. Central nervous system (CNS) changes are also thought to affect the sleep of the elderly. Frequent nighttime awakenings may result from secondary changes in circadian rhythms and loss of effective circadian regulation of sleep. Such changes can affect the quality of life. Many elderly patients exhibit daytime sleepiness, which shows that age does not diminish the need for sleep but reduces the ability to sleep.

PATHOPHYSIOLOGY

To understand how insomnia develops, it is first necessary to understand the physiologic process of sleep. The brain seeks to balance alertness and sleepiness on a continuum between sleep debt, biological alerting, and environmental stimulation. Sleepiness is a function of the brain fighting to get enough sleep to cover the debt. This system of sleep debt versus sleep arousal is intricately linked to circadian rhythms and exposure to light. Additionally, various internally regulated biologic systems govern the circadian pattern of the sleep–wake cycle. The interaction of these biologic systems includes changes in body temperature, cardiac and renal functions, and hormone secretion throughout the day. The term *circadian* means "approximately 1 day" and refers to the fact that endogenous rhythms last approximately 24 hours.

Normal sleep is divided into two phases: rapid eye movement (REM) sleep and non-REM (NREM) sleep. During the REM stage, which accounts for approximately 20% of the sleep cycle, the brain is active and most dreaming occurs. NREM, which constitutes approximately 80% of the sleep cycle, is a phase of deep rest in which pulse, respiration, and brain activity all slow. NREM sleep can be divided into four phases. Stages I and II are called light NREM sleep. Stage I is the lightest sleep, and fleeting dreams often occur during the transition between the awake state and stage I. Stage II, which accounts for 50% of NREM sleep, lasts approximately 15 to 20 minutes and is characterized by fragmented thoughts with distinctive EEG changes. Hypnotics commonly increase stage II. Stages III and IV are called delta or deep NREM sleep. This stage begins after approximately 30 to 45 minutes and lasts 40 to 70 minutes. During stages III and IV, blood pressure, cerebral glucose metabolism, and heart and respiratory rates are at the lowest in the circadian cycle. The total sleep pattern begins with light NREM, followed by deep NREM, and then by REM. This cycle lasts approximately 90 to 100 minutes and occurs four to six times per night. **Box 42.2** summarizes the sleep stages.

Required amounts of sleep and of NREM sleep vary with age. Newborns sleep approximately 17 to 18 hours each day but have only two phases of sleep, NREM and REM. These two phases cycle every 60 minutes instead of every 90 minutes like adults. Children require 10 hours of sleep. In the early adult years, the total amount of sleep decreases to around 8 hours, which is normal for older adults as well as younger adults, with some variation among individuals. The total amount of REM sleep stays more constant at 15% to 20% throughout an adult's

BOX 42.2

Stages of Sleep

Stage I

Light NREM: dreamlike state, lasts a few minutes

Stage II

Relatively light NREM: fragmented thoughts, lasts 15–20 min

Stage III–IV

Deep NREM: lowering of blood pressure, cerebral glucose metabolism, heart rate, and respiratory rate, starts 35–40 min after falling asleep and lasts 40–70 min

REM Sleep

Starts after 90 min of sleep, lengthens toward the end of the night

This cycle alternates throughout the night at intervals of 90–100 min, four to six times per night

BOX 42.3

Selected Sleep History Questions

- What kind of work does the patient do? Is there shift work involved, and which shift?
- What time does the patient go to bed?
- What kind of bed partner does the patient have (restless, still, wakeful sleeper), if any?
- Does the patient regularly take any prescription or over-the-counter drugs?
- How many times during the night does the patient awaken?
- What does the patient do if he or she cannot go to sleep?
- Does the patient take daytime naps?

lifetime. Deep NREM sleep constitutes approximately 20% to 30% of total sleep in young children.

Insomnia is seen more often in people over age 65. The stages and architecture of sleep change, resulting in lighter stage II and decreases in stage III and IV sleep. This results in a decrease in deep NREM sleep. The circadian clock also becomes advanced, causing early-morning awakening in the elderly.

Light cues are important in the process of sleep. The absence of light cues tends to promote longer sleep–wake cycles. Two peaks in the daily need for sleep have been identified: the first at bedtime and the second in mid-afternoon. A study by Regestein et al. (1993) suggested that insomniacs have higher daytime alertness compared with normal subjects, which leads to higher hyperarousal states. Bonnet & Arand (1996) studied normal sleepers and found that sleep deprivation produces a primary hyperarousal state. They concluded insomniacs become more aware of small defects in the quality of sleep and daytime fatigue.

DIAGNOSTIC CRITERIA

Typical complaints of insomnia are malaise, fatigue, and too little sleep. These problems can lead to mild or moderate impairment in concentration and psychomotor abilities. The diagnosis is based on the patient's history, although a complete workup includes looking at all potential medical and psychological causes. The practitioner must determine the onset and duration of symptoms, along with the patient's regular sleeping schedule and general quality of sleep. The practitioner

should interview other family members and significant others regarding any psychiatric or substance abuse problems of the patient. If the patient does not sleep alone, the practitioner also should elicit information from the bed partner. Questions about sleep also should be included in the review of systems; **Box 42.3** lists suggested questions.

A complete physical examination is important to rule out medical causes of insomnia. Insomnia can be drug related (e.g., stimulating medications or alcohol). Finally, the practitioner should investigate psychiatric causes of insomnia.

The use of sleep questionnaires or diaries and screening tools for depression and anxiety can add to the evaluation of insomnia. Sleep patterns may be measured by using a special wristwatch that measures wrist movements, a process called *actigraphy*. In humans, movement of the wrist throughout the night is much less frequent than during the day, which enables the practitioner to estimate the patient's sleep and wake times. This tool, however, is not very accurate in assessing total sleep time of insomniacs. Polysomnography (all-night monitoring of EEG, respiration, muscle activity, and other physiologic parameters) may reveal shallow sleep that is fragmented by multiple arousals. If the patient is depressed, the polysomnogram manifests changes in the REM latency stage. Polysomnograms are indicated when the primary suspected cause of insomnia is sleep apnea. The American Sleep Disorders Association, however, does not recommend the routine use of polysomnography because a patient may not sleep normally at a sleep disorders center.

INITIATING DRUG THERAPY

In combination with behavioral management, the practitioner can consider using certain pharmacologic agents, but only with caution. In 1990, the NIH issued a consensus statement on the treatment of sleep disorders in older adults strongly recommending that hypnotic medications not become the mainstay of insomnia treatment because they are widely overused and have great potential to become habit-forming.

A wide range of therapies may be necessary to treat insomnia, because multiple causes of insomnia are the rule rather than the exception. Nonpharmacologic therapy includes evaluating for the key causes and treating with the appropriate intervention first: counseling, behavioral management, and lifestyle alterations for psychiatric problems. Patients with insomnia often have major depression, anxiety, obsessive disorders, or dysthymic disorders, and psychotherapy needs to focus on the specific psychiatric disorder.

In 1990, Everitt, et al., conducted a comparison study of the clinical decision making of physicians and nurse practitioners when evaluating sleep. Overall, 60% of the nurse practitioners elicited a sleep history, but only 17% prescribed medications as first-line intervention. In contrast, 47% of physicians elicited a comprehensive sleep history and 46% prescribed pharmacologic treatment as the initial therapy. This suggests that a detailed sleep history is crucial to help the practitioner promote effective nonpharmacologic therapy, such as relaxation techniques, meditation, and exercise.

Reviewing proper sleep hygiene can enhance the patient's sleep pattern. A thorough examination of sleep hygiene issues can help identify important lifestyle changes that may enhance sleep, and its importance should not be underestimated. The practitioner should implement only one or two behavioral changes at a time. Follow-up and a strong patient–provider relationship are key. Additional measures, such as exposure to bright light, may help those with circadian rhythm disturbances. Light therapy can retrain the light pacemaker and may be effective for night-shift workers, travelers, and those with delayed or advanced sleep phase disorders.

Goals of Drug Therapy

The goal of pharmacotherapy is to promote the patient's ability to fall asleep, maintain sleep, or awaken refreshed. Another goal is to use the agent for as short a time as possible. It is important to note that drugs to treat insomnia have not been studied and are not approved for long-term use. Each drug has a different onset and duration of action. Selection of a pharmacologic agent depends on the origin of the insomnia (e.g., pain, medical conditions), as previously discussed. If given in adequate doses, all hypnotics promote sleep; the key is to determine the *minimal* dose that will provide efficacy with few or no side effects.

Hypnotics, or sleeping pills, are the primary drugs used for insomnia, although other antidepressant agents also may be helpful. (See Chapter 40.) The practitioner should carefully consider selection of a hypnotic and prescribe use for as short a time as possible. Short-term use is defined as no more than 2 to 3 weeks combined with behavioral interventions; however, specific patients require occasional chronic hypnotic therapy. They may need to use a hypnotic agent two or three times

a week over longer periods than 2 to 3 weeks. Careless use of sedative-hypnotics can be dangerous in patients with sleep apnea or a history of substance abuse.

The sedative-hypnotic drugs act by exerting a calming or anxiolytic effect, causing drowsiness and aiding in the sleep process. This group of drugs includes a variety of barbiturate, nonbarbiturate (e.g., benzodiazepine agonists), and nonprescription drugs (e.g., antihistamines).

Barbiturates

Barbiturates are structurally related to compounds that act throughout the CNS. They act at the level of the presynaptic and postsynaptic membranes and also have a cellular component to their action. It is unclear at which level the sedative-hypnotic effects occur. As a class, barbiturates usually are no longer recommended for the treatment of insomnia. This category of drugs includes amobarbital sodium (Amytal Sodium), butabarbital (secbutabarbital), mephobarbital (Mebaral), and secobarbital sodium (Seconal Sodium). The only barbiturates still indicated for use with insomnia are amobarbital sodium and butabarbital. **Table 42.1** identifies starting doses and expected dosing ranges of the barbiturates still in use; however, with the advent of newer, safer agents, few reasons exist to use barbiturates to treat insomnia.

Adverse Events

The danger with barbiturates is that they can produce all levels of CNS depression, from mild sedation to coma to death. This is due to excessive sedation, short-term efficacy, and the potential for severe adverse reactions on withdrawal or overdose. Cardiac side effects include bradycardia, hypotension, and syncope. The respiratory system can experience hypoventilation, apnea, and respiratory depression. Barbiturate use rarely may cause Stevens-Johnson syndrome, which is sometimes fatal. Prolonged use of high doses in this class can lead to tolerance and physical or psychological dependence. Withdrawal syndrome can occur and is sometimes fatal.

Interactions

Serious side effects can result from drug–drug interactions with barbiturates. Alcohol may increase CNS depression. Barbiturates can decrease the effects of oral anticoagulants, corticosteroids, oral contraceptives and estrogens, beta-adrenergic blockers, theophylline (Slo-Phyllin), metronidazole (Flagyl), doxycycline (Vibramycin), griseofulvin (Grifulvin V), phenylbutazone, and quinidine (Cardioquin).

Benzodiazepines

Benzodiazepines are synthetically produced sedative-hypnotics. This group of structurally related chemicals selectively acts on polysynaptic neuronal pathways throughout the CNS. Benzodiazepines appear to enhance the effects of gamma-aminobutyric acid (GABA), an inhibitory neurotransmitter in the CNS. The subclass of benzodiazepines that is used to treat

TABLE 42.1   Overview of Selected Drugs Used to Treat Insomnia

Generic (Trade) Name and Dosage	Selected Adverse Events	Contraindications	Special Considerations
Barbiturates			
amobarbital sodium (Amytal Sodium, Navamobarb) Start: 50–100 mg PO Range: 100–200 mg PO qhs	Somnolence, confusion, residual sedation nightmares, nausea and vomiting, constipation, diarrhea, hypoventilation *Potentially fatal side effects:* apnea, respiratory depression, Stevens-Johnson syndrome	Hypersensitivity to barbiturates, marked liver impairment, nephritis, respiratory disease, previous addiction to sedative hypnotics, pregnancy	Use cautiously with acute or chronic pain, seizure disorder, lactation, fever, hyperthyroidism, diabetes mellitus, severe anemia, pulmonary or cardiac disease, asthma, impaired kidney function. For geriatric patients, reduce dosage and monitor carefully.
butabarbital (Secbutabarbital, Secbuto-arbiton) Start: 50 mg PO qhs Range: 50–100 mg PO qhs	Same as above plus circulatory collapse	Same as above	Same as above
Benzodiazepines			
alprazolam (Xanax) tablets 0.25, 0.5, 1, 2 mg Start: 0.25–0.5 mg PO tid; maximum 4 mg/d in divided doses Range: 0.25–2 mg tid–qd	*CNS:* transient mild drowsiness, sedation, depression, lethargy, apathy, fatigue, lightheadedness, disorientation, headache, mild paradoxical excitatory reaction in first 2 wk *GI:* constipation, diarrhea, dry mouth, nausea	Hypersensitivity to benzodiazepines, acute narrow-angle glaucoma, pregnancy, lactation	Use cautiously with impaired liver or kidney function, debilitation. Drug dependence and withdrawal result when abruptly discontinued, especially when used for longer than 4 mo. Use cautiously with elderly patients and gradually increase as tolerated.
estazolam (ProSom) tablets: 1, 2 mg Start: 0.5–1 mg qhs Range: 0.5–2 mg qhs	*CNS:* transient mild drowsiness, sedation lethargy, apathy, fatigue, lightheadedness, asthenia, mild paradoxical excitatory reaction in first 2 wk *GI:* constipation, diarrhea, dyspepsia *CV:* bradycardia, tachycardia *GU:* incontinence, urinary retention, changes in libido	Same as above	In addition to above: Drug–drug interactions: increased CNS depression with ethanol, omeprazole; increased effects of estazolam with cimetidine; increased sedative effects of estazolam with theophylline Drug dependence, withdrawal syndrome
flurazepam (Dalmane) 15–30 mg PO qhs Start: 15 mg PO qhs Range: 15–30 mg PO qhs	*CNS:* transient mild drowsiness, sedation lethargy, apathy, fatigue, lightheadedness, asthenia *GI:* constipation, diarrhea, dyspepsia *CV:* bradycardia, tachycardia *GU:* incontinence, urinary retention, changes in libido	Same as above	Same as above Has a long half-life
lorazepam (Ativan) 2–4 mg PO qhs	*CNS:* transient mild drowsiness, sedation, depression, lethargy, apathy, fatigue, lightheadedness, disorientation, headache, mild paradoxical excitatory reaction in first 2 wk *GI:* constipation, diarrhea, dry mouth, nausea	Same as above .	Use cautiously with patients with impaired liver or kidney function. Debilitation, drug dependence and withdrawal result when abruptly discontinued, especially when used for more than 4 mo. Use cautiously with elderly patients and gradually increase as tolerated.

(continued)

TABLE 42.1 Overview of Selected Drugs Used to Treat Insomnia (*Continued*)

Generic (Trade) Name and Dosage	Selected Adverse Events	Contraindications	Special Considerations
quazepam (Doral) 7.5–15 mg PO qhs	*CNS:* transient mild drowsiness, sedation, depression, lethargy, apathy, fatigue, lightheadedness, disorientation, restlessness, confusion *GI:* constipation, diarrhea *CV:* bradycardia, tachycardia *GU:* incontinence, urinary retention, changes in libido	Same as above	Drug–drug interactions: increased CNS depression with ethanol, quazepam; increased effects of cimetidine, disulfiram, oral contraceptives; increased sedative effects with theophylline
temazepam (Restoril) Start: 15 mg PO qhs Range: 15–30 mg PO qhs	Same as above	Same as above	Drug–drug interactions: increased CNS depression; increased sedative effects with theophylline
triazolam (Halcion) Start: 0.125 mg PO qhs Range: 0.125–0.5 mg PO qhs Elderly: 0.125–0.25 mg PO qhs	Same as above	Hypersensitivity to benzodiazepines, acute narrow-angle glaucoma, pregnancy, lactation	Same as above
Nonbenzodiazepines			
eszopiclone (Lunesta) Start: 1–2 mg PO qhs Range: 1–3mg Elderly: start at 1 mg	*CNS:* morning drowsiness, headache, dizziness *GI:* nausea	Hypersensitivity to eszopiclone	Caution in patients taking strong inhibitors or inducers of CYP3A4
zolpidem (Ambien) Start: 10 mg PO qhs Range: 5–10 mg PO qhs	*CNS:* morning drowsiness, hangover, headache, dizziness, suppression of REM sleep *GI:* nausea	Hypersensitivity to zolpidem	Use cautiously in patients with acute intermittent porphyria, impaired hepatic or renal function, in addiction-prone patients, and in pregnancy and lactation.
zaleplon (Sonata) Start: 10 mg PO qhs Range: 5–20 mg PO qhs	*General:* back pain, chest pain *CV:* migraine *GI:* constipation, dry mouth *MS:* arthritis *CNS:* depression, hypertonia, nervousness *Derm:* rash, pruritus	Pregnancy, lactation	Pregnancy category C Pregnancy category C Patient must use just before bedtime because of quick onset.
armodafinil (Nuvigil) Start: 150–250 mg q AM No maximum doses yet noted	*Serious:* arrhythmias, syncope, visual changes, abuse/dependency *Common:* headache, nausea/vomiting, rhinitis, diarrhea	Hypersensitivity to modafinil and armodafinil	Reduce dose in patients with severe hepatic dysfunction.
modafinil (Provigil) 200 mg q AM; maximum 400 mg daily	Same as above	Sensitivity to class, caution with coronary artery disease, mitral valve prolapse, impaired liver failure	Start at 100 mg daily in elderly.

insomnia is believed to facilitate the effects of GABA in the ascending reticular activating system, which increases inhibition and blocks thalamic, hypothalamic, and limbic arousal.

When choosing a benzodiazepine, the practitioner should select an agent with an onset of action that matches the patient's problem, yet has a short duration of effect, lacks rebound insomnia, and causes few or no mental problems (e.g., hangover, lack of motor coordination, or memory disturbance). (See **Table 42.1.**) The prescriber also should consider the patient's metabolic requirements. Agents with a short half-life, such as alprazolam (Xanax), lorazepam (Ativan), or oxazepam (Serax), may be best for patients with depressed renal or hepatic function.

The benzodiazepines most commonly used for treating sleep disorders are divided into short-, intermediate-, and long-acting agents; flurazepam (Dalmane) and quazepam (Doral) are examples of the latter. Agents with short-term effects and short-term onset are best for patients who have difficulty falling asleep. The only agent in this category is triazolam (Halcion). Chloral hydrate also has a short-term effect but is intermediate in duration. Agents with intermediate onsets and usually longer half-lives are useful for patients with problems staying asleep. These include temazepam (Restoril) and estazolam (ProSom). Two agents with a rapid onset of action, flurazepam and quazepam, assist with falling asleep and also have a longer duration of action, which can assist in maintaining sleep.

Researchers are looking at the three GABA receptor subtypes in the hope of developing a benzodiazepine that can target the receptors with an agonist or a partial agonist agent. This would ameliorate anxiety without causing corresponding sedation and motor impairment.

Adverse Events

Benzodiazepines have various actions, depending on their half-lives. Drugs of this class can produce drowsiness and impaired motor function, which may be persistent. Other side effects can include short-term memory loss, confusion, and shakiness. Prolonged use of benzodiazepines can lead to physical dependency; abrupt discontinuance can trigger withdrawal symptoms. The newer agents in the class have fewer side effects, but for optimal therapy the drug selected should address the patient's specific sleep problem.

Interactions

Patients taking benzodiazepines must be cautious with the concomitant use of alcohol. Use of low-dose contraceptives may slightly decrease clearance of lorazepam and temazepam; the patient may need to alter the dosage or switch to oxazepam. Use of erythromycin (E-mycin) can decrease triazolam clearance by 50%; thus, prescribers must consider reducing the dosage of triazolam in patients taking both drugs concomitantly.

Benzodiazepine Receptor Agonists

This class of hypnotic has been developed to improve the safety profile of the barbiturate-type compounds. The benzodiazepine

receptor agonists have one of the safest profiles in compounded medicines. They have a very short half-life with no development of tolerance after extended use. However, there is some question as to the potential for addiction to these drugs if used for longer than 4 weeks. All medications in this class have a half-life of 5 hours, therefore avoiding residual next-day effects. The drugs have greater receptor specificity of the GABAa BZ complex, which has been identified as being responsible for the sedative-hypnotic activity.

Eszopiclone

Eszopiclone (Lunesta) is a nonbenzodiazepine agent indicated for the treatment of insomnia.

Mechanism of Action

While the exact mechanism of action is unknown, eszopiclone is thought to work by interacting with GABA receptors located near benzodiazepine receptors and thus shares some of the same pharmacologic properties. It is classified as a Schedule IV controlled substance.

Dosage

For nonelderly adults, eszopiclone should be started at 2 mg immediately before retiring for bed. The dose may be started or increased to 3 mg to aid in sleep maintenance. For elderly patients, the doses should be started at 1 mg to help patients fall asleep and 2 mg if sleep maintenance is the issue.

Time Frame for Response

The onset of action is rapid, with a peak plasma concentration occurring within 1 hour of dosing. This peak concentration can be delayed if eszopiclone is taken with or shortly after a high-fat meal.

Contraindications

There are no known contraindications to eszopiclone. However, patients should be cautioned against the concomitant use of alcohol due to the sedative effects and the potential for enhancing anterograde amnesia.

Adverse Events

Headache, dry mouth, dizziness, respiratory system infections, and unpleasant taste have occurred in patients taking 2- to 3-mg doses of eszopiclone.

Interactions

Eszopiclone is metabolized by the cytochrome P (CYP) 3A4 enzyme system. Therefore, agents that inhibit (e.g., ketoconazole) or induce (e.g., rifampin) this system will affect eszopiclone metabolism.

Zolpidem

Another hypnotic agent that is a nonbenzodiazepine is zolpidem (Ambien). Zolpidem also modulates the GABA receptors to suppress neurons, causing sedation and relaxation. Zolpidem has a strong hypnotic component and improves the overall quality of sleep while producing less daytime impairment than other hypnotics. Onset of action is rapid and it peaks quickly, which limits the hangover effects. Zolpidem has no carryover anxiolytic effects, which makes it less desirable for patients with concomitant anxiety.

Zaleplon

Another nonbenzodiazepine is zaleplon (Sonata), which is chemically unrelated to benzodiazepines, barbiturates, and other drugs with hypnotic properties. Zaleplon is known to interact with the GABA-BZ omega 1 receptor, which causes sedation, muscle relaxation, and anticonvulsant activity. This interaction is also hypothesized to be responsible for the pharmacologic properties of benzodiazepines. Zaleplon works well for patients who have difficulty falling asleep. The onset of action is rapid, within 1 hour after oral administration, but the medication has a short half-life of 1 hour. Zaleplon can be taken as little as 5 hours before the scheduled wake-up time, with no lingering effects of daytime sedation. It may not be the agent of choice for patients who have difficulty maintaining sleep because of its short elimination half-life.

Antihistamines

Antihistamines are one of the most commonly used classes of OTC sleep-inducing agents. The most commonly used agent is diphenhydramine (Benadryl). The main mechanism of diphenhydramine is unknown, but it chiefly acts as a CNS depressant. No scientific evidence exists in the literature supporting the use of diphenhydramine to relieve insomnia or prolong sleep.

Some side effects of diphenhydramine include excessive daytime drowsiness, impaired psychomotor function, and increasing tolerance to the drug. A better approach may be to use one of the sedating antidepressants before using a trial of diphenhydramine. If a patient taking diphenhydramine is stopped while driving under the influence of antihistamines, in many states he or she can be charged with driving under the influence (DUI).

Antidepressants

Sedating antidepressants also may be used in the treatment of insomnia, especially for patients with a subcomponent of depression. The most commonly used antidepressants in this category are imipramine (Tofranil), amitriptyline hydrochloride (Elavil), and nortriptyline (Pamelor). If the patient has a panic or anxiety subcomponent as well, some newer agents may assist with sleep. These include nefazodone hydrochloride (Serzone) and venlafaxine (Effexor), which also have some sedating as well as antianxiety effects (see Chapter 40).

Selecting the Most Appropriate Agent

As emphasized earlier, sedative-hypnotics should be used on a short-term basis only. For treatment of acute insomnia, the suggested duration of hypnotic use is 1 week, but some patients may need a longer course. Practitioners should schedule follow-up

TABLE 42.2	Recommended Order of Treatment for Sleep Disorders	
Order	**Agents**	**Comments**
First line	Nonbenzodiazepine hypnotics (zolpidem, zaleplon)	Cleanest side effect profiles
Second line	Benzodiazepine hypnotics—Short half-lives: alprazolam, lorazepam, oxazepam. Rapid onset: triazolam, flurazepam, quazepam. Long half-lives: temazepam, estazolam.	Consider short-acting agents, especially with patients who have renal or hepatic problems.
Third line	Barbiturates, antidepressants	May have serious side effects Helpful when treating concomitant depression

visits to monitor the effectiveness of therapy. The time between follow-up visits can vary, but in general they should fall between every 1 and 2 weeks. Starting the medication at the lowest possible dosage should minimize side effects. The practitioner should ask the patient about the effects the drug is having on sleep and daytime functioning. Changes may exist with dreaming, learning, memory, and adaptation to stress. Having the patient complete and bring in a sleep log for review can help pinpoint initial management needs and can continue to assist with evaluation for signs of improvement (**Table 42.2** and **Figure 42-1**). Pharmacologic therapy along with cognitive therapy should be initiated for at least 7 to 8 weeks (Cochran, 2003).

First-Line Therapy

As stated previously, the key to pharmacologic therapy is identifying the sleep defect. The practitioner should match the patient's need for an agent to both the classification of insomnia and the aspect of sleep that is altered. In cases of acute/transient and short-term insomnia, it is important to look for underlying physical and behavioral causes. Medications are indicated based on the subset of insomnia. When the problem is difficulty falling asleep, the agent should have a quick onset. Zaleplon is the best choice, given its quick onset and clean side effect profile. Patients with difficulty maintaining sleep require a drug with an extended duration, so the practitioner should base the choice of agent on the half-life to decrease side effects. Temazepam has a shorter half-life than other benzodiazepines.

Chronic insomnia often has underlying psychological components, and the best drug choice here usually is in the sedating-antidepressant class. Amitriptyline is the first choice, but it should be used cautiously.

Diphenhydramine is the only agent available to treat any sleep defect in pregnant women. The practitioner must assess the potential side effects and benefits for both the fetus and mother before instituting therapy.

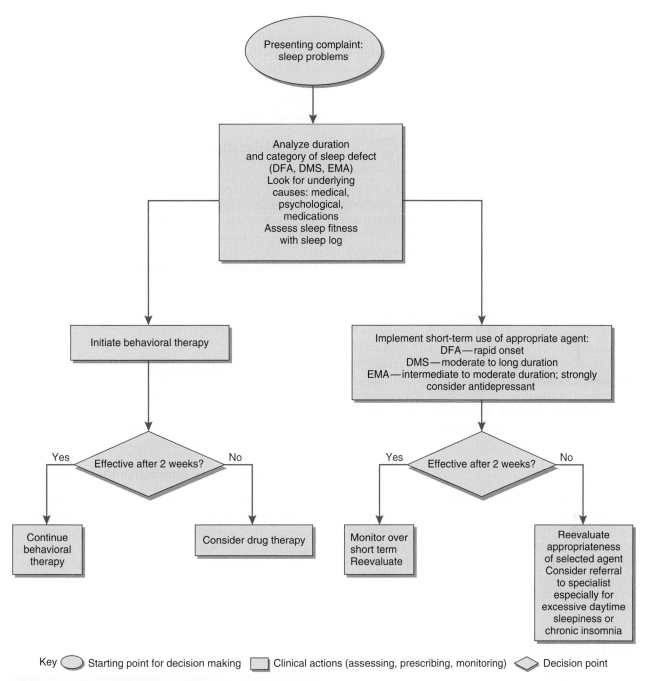

FIGURE 42–1 Treatment algorithm for insomnia (DFA: difficulty falling asleep; DMS: difficulty maintaining sleep; EMA: early morning awakening).

Second-Line Therapy

If the patient continues to have insomnia with first-line treatments, alternatives include switching to a benzodiazepine agent or using the other benzodiazepine receptor agonist, zolpidem. Again, the prescriber must consider the kind of sleep defect being treated and select a drug with the appropriate onset and half-life.

Third-Line Therapy

The practitioner should reassess the insomnia situation for patients who fail to respond to both first- and second-line

therapies. Insomnia that has become chronic benefits most from continual evaluation and behavioral therapy along with the smallest dose possible of hypnotic medication. An antidepressant may play a key role at this level.

Special Population Considerations

Pediatric

Use of barbiturates in the pediatric population is usually limited to those who have seizure disorders. In general, benzodiazepines are not indicated for children younger than age 15. Caution is necessary when very young patients use antihistamines because of potential delirium or paradoxical excitation. Melatonin may be considered as treatment for a limited time (Ivanenko, et al., 2003).

Geriatric

It is important to evaluate the geriatric patient for underlying comorbidities that contribute to insomnia. Treating the underlying illnesses is important and may assist with re-establishing good sleeping patterns. Extreme caution is essential when prescribing hypnotic medications to elderly patients because these drugs can increase the potential for delirium and subsequent falls. In 1996, Zisselman, et al., analyzed hospital costs for the elderly when sedative-hypnotics were used to promote sleep. They found a statistically significant increase in cost resulting from increased length of hospital stay for patients who took sedative-hypnotics. In 1990, Shorr, et al., analyzed the quantity of prescriptions given to elderly patients along with the number of refills. Their concern was the overuse of the agents and the risks at which they place elderly patients over time. They found that many different physician groups were overprescribing sedative-hypnotics.

Consistent monitoring of the elderly patient can be extremely important, especially when a long-acting hypnotic is prescribed. Antihistamines can cause delirium or paradoxical excitation.

Women

No sex differences exist in terms of the pharmacokinetics of the various agents used to treat sleep disorders. Caution is essential when prescribing all drugs to lactating women and women of childbearing age. Both antihistamines and zaleplon are pregnancy category C, whereas the barbiturates and benzodiazepines are pregnancy category D. Zolpidem, in category B, is in the lowest-risk pregnancy category.

MONITORING PATIENT RESPONSE

Sleep can be a reliable predictor of psychological and physical health. Differences in monitoring are related to whether the insomnia is an acute or chronic problem. Brief episodes of acute insomnia can warrant treatment, with the goal of preventing it from progressing and becoming chronic. A short course (up to 4 weeks) of sedative-hypnotic therapy is the current treatment of choice. Cognitive therapy can be included to improve the chance of an optimal response.

When insomnia becomes a chronic problem, consistent interaction between the patient and health care provider is important, as is the use of behavioral techniques. With chronic insomnia, issues of drug tolerance for the older benzodiazepines and rebound insomnia usually become paramount.

Current U.S. Food and Drug Administration guidelines allow only short-term prescription of hypnotic agents.

Tolerance and rebound insomnia have been cited as problems associated with these agents, but few studies have borne this out. In practice, many people take low-dose hypnotic agents for long periods with few side effects. Caution is warranted, however, if a patient requires escalation of a previously stable dosage. Careful analysis of changes in the patient's sleep patterns is necessary in this event.

Patient Education

Patient education plays a key role in the treatment of insomnia. A key side effect of most hypnotic agents is excessive drowsiness or hangover from the medication. The clinician must alert the patient to this possibility and monitor the side effects of each agent prescribed. (See **Table 42.1** and **Table 42.2**.)

Patient-Oriented Information Sources

Major sleep centers across the country have websites that are useful resources for patients and health care providers. These sites can provide information about diagnosis of sleep disorders and current research and therapies (**Box 42.4**).

Nutrition/Lifestyle Changes

Good sleep habits include setting a routine bedtime, getting regular exercise, using the bed for sleeping only, and getting in bed only when ready for sleep. Stimulants such as caffeine, alcohol, and excess fluids should be avoided before bedtime.

Complementary and Alternative Medications

Herbs and botanicals are often used as a "natural" way of promoting sleep. However, this is not without a certain danger, especially if these treatments are taken in conjunction with prescription drugs. Older patients are often likely to use herbal treatments: in 1997, it was reported that up to 3 million individuals over age 65 use such therapy (Desai & Grossberg, 2003).

Melatonin, an endogenous hormone, is synthesized by the pineal gland from tryptophan. It is mainly secreted at night and its level peaks during normal sleep hours. In

---

BOX 42.4

Sleep Websites

National Center on Sleep Disorders Research (NCSDR)
   http://www.nhlbi.nih.gov/about/ncsdr
National Heart, Lung, and Blood Institute (NHLBI)
Health Information Network
   http://www.nhlbi.nih.gov
Restless Legs Syndrome Foundation
   http://www.rls.org
Sleep Foundation
   http://sleepfoundation.org

1997, Lavie discovered that endogenous melatonin opens the nocturnal sleep gate and increases nocturnal melatonin secretion. Melatonin does not induce sleep but acts as a gatekeeper in the cascade of events that enables the CNS to favor sleep over wakefulness. Most studies have examined the use of melatonin to treat sleep disorders resulting from jet lag; few have looked at the use of melatonin in primary insomnia. A 1996 study by Attenburrow and Dowling on melatonin and primary insomnia examined healthy volunteers compared with the elderly. Through analysis of urine concentrations of endogenous melatonin, the study found that the elderly volunteers had a lower concentration of the melatonin metabolite and a delayed onset to peak secretion. These findings supported the possibility that some patients, especially those with delayed sleep phase insomnia, may benefit from the administration of exogenous melatonin; however, further study is necessary.

Valerian is a traditional sleep remedy that is derived from the perennial herb *Valeriana officinalis*. The direct physiologic activity is mediated by the active sesquiterpene components of the volatile oil. This creates a synergistic effect with neurotransmitters such as GABA and produces a direct sedative effect. Effective dosage ranges from 300 to 600 mg of the valerian root; 2 to 3 g of the dried root is soaked in a cup of hot water for 10 to 15 minutes, and the patient then drinks the tea. Administration can occur 30 minutes to 2 hours before bedtime. Significant herb or drug interactions have not been reported by the German E Commission.

RESTLESS LEG SYNDROME AND PERIODIC LIMB MOVEMENT DISORDER

Restless leg syndrome (RLS) and periodic limb movement disorder (PLMD) are neurologic disorders. RLS is characterized by an intense need to move the legs, accompanied by paresthesias and dysesthesias that worsen usually in the evening. Sometimes the sensations can occur in other large muscle groups, but most often the legs are involved. Moving around relieves the feeling, but only for a short time, as the sensation soon returns. These sensations interfere with sleep. PLMD is characterized by episodes of highly repetitive and stereotyped limb movements only during sleep.

Both disorders interfere with sleep and contribute to sleep deprivation and decreased alertness and daytime function. Indications are that 2% to 15% of the population may experience RLS, but the diagnosis is made rarely in primary care.

CAUSES

As a primary CNS disorder, RLS can be found in patients with end-stage renal disease, anemia, and sometimes in pregnancy (Gigli et al., 2004). RLS can also be hereditary or drug induced.

Allen (2004) argued that iron deficits may be a strong cause of RLS, altering the iron–dopamine linkage, but this hypothesis needs further study.

PATHOPHYSIOLOGY

RLS and PLMD are sensory-motor disorders that are not well understood. Primary RLS has a strong hereditary component, with 40% to 60% of patients having a familial association. Onset of familial RLS is before the age of 30 years, and studies have indicated the strong action of a single major gene (Zucconi & Ferini-Strambi, 2004). Secondary RLS can be associated with neuropathies from changes in axonal and small-fiber neural pathways. Patients with rheumatoid arthritis and diabetes also have shown a greater prevalence of RLS, again presumably from changes due to neuropathy. Parkinson's disease is frequently associated with RLS, pointing to a commonality in reduced dopaminergic functioning (Zucconi & Ferini-Strambi, 2004). A strong link has been established to the dopaminergic system by the positive response to the dopaminergic agonist classification of drugs (Allen, 2004).

DIAGNOSTIC CRITERIA

RLS is diagnosed primarily through the patient history. Clinical criteria have been established by the International Restless Legs Syndrome Study Group (**Box 42.5**).

PLMD is associated more with stereotyped repetitive movements of limbs (legs alone, or legs more than arms) that occur only during sleep. PLMD is generally diagnosed only through a sleep test.

The physical examination for RLS and PLMD should include a full neurologic examination with emphasis on the spinal cord and peripheral nerve function. A vascular examination is also necessary to rule out vascular disorders. Secondary causes of RLS should be evaluated by a serum ferritin level and serum

---

BOX **42.5**

Diagnostic Criteria for Restless Leg Syndrome

1. A compelling urge to move limbs associated with paresthesias/dysesthesias
2. Motor restlessness as evidenced by:
   - Floor pacing
   - Tossing and turning in bed
   - Rubbing legs
3. Symptoms worse or exclusively present at rest with variable and temporary relief by activity
4. Symptoms worse in the evening and at night

BOX 42.6

Differential Diagnoses for RLS and PLMD

1. Nocturnal leg cramps
   - Painful, palpable involuntary muscle contractions
   - Focal with sudden onset
   - Unilateral
2. Akathisia
   Excessive movement without accompanying sensory complaints
3. Peripheral neuropathy
   - Usually tingling, numbness, or pain sensations
   - Not associated with motor restlessness
   - Not helped by movement
   - Evening or nighttime worsening

chemistry to rule out uremia and diabetes. Polysomnography is not routinely indicated for RLS but can be helpful to establish the diagnosis. **Box 42.6** lists other possible diagnoses.

INITIATING DRUG THERAPY

Pharmacotherapy should be tailored for each patient. Patients with relatively mild symptoms may not need medications. Nonpharmacologic therapy should be instituted, including mental alerting activities and cessation of alcohol, nicotine, and caffeine. Any medications that may precipitate or worsen RLS symptoms, such as antidepressants and dopamine antagonists, should be avoided. Correction of underlying serum iron deficits may be helpful. Short-term studies have shown that drug therapy has significant benefits, but little is known about long-term treatment. A 3-year study of 70 patients by Clavadetscher et al. (2004) found that a good long-term response with drug therapy can be achieved in 80% of patients. This study helped to establish the benefit of pharmacologic therapy in RLS.

Goals of Drug Therapy

The goal of drug therapy is to calm the restless legs or periodic limb movements. Some patients can be refractory to pharmacologic treatment but still achieve partial relief of their symptoms. Pharmacologic agents for RLS include dopaminergic agents, dopamine agonists, opioids, benzodiazepines, anticonvulsants, and iron. (See **Table 42.1**.) Other than dopamine agonists, many of these drugs are being used in an "off-label" manner.

Dopaminergic Agents

These drugs are dopamine precursor combinations such as carbidopa–levodopa (Sinemet). These agents are useful for intermittent RLS because they have a quicker onset than dopamine agonists. This is useful for relief of sleep onset insomnia and RLS that occurs during long car or airplane journeys. Dosage of these agents is lower than used for Parkinson's disease.

Adverse Events

The carbidopa–levodopa agents may actually worsen RLS symptoms in up to 80% of patients. The therapeutic effect may be reduced if taken with high-protein food. Insomnia, sleepiness, and gastrointestinal problems are other adverse events.

Dopamine Agonists

The initial dopamine agonists used for RLS were bromocriptine and pergolide, which were prone to side effects. The newer dopamine agonists, such as pramipexole and ropinirole, are not ergot based; while they have fewer side effects, they can cause initial nausea and lightheadedness, nasal stuffiness, edema, and rarely daytime sleepiness. Increasing the dose slowly will help to mitigate these side effects.

Opioids

Opioids are reserved for the most severe cases of RLS or PLMD that are refractory to treatment with other pharmacologic agents. This class of medications can be used on a daily or intermittent basis. Clinical experience by sleep experts suggests that only a few patients will require opioids (Silber, 2004).

Benzodiazepines

Benzodiazepines (see **Table 42.1**) are used concomitantly with a dopamine agonist when use of a sole agent has failed. Clinical experience is particularly crucial with clonazepam and temazepam. These drugs may be helpful for patients who cannot tolerate the other medications. Caution is necessary when using these agents with the elderly, and they can cause daytime sleepiness and cognitive impairment.

Anticonvulsants

Anticonvulsants are considered when dopamine agonists have failed and in patients who describe the RLS discomfort as pain. Gabapentin is helpful in patients with RLS and peripheral neuropathy. It is useful in treatment of daily RLS. As with the dopamine agonists, lower dosages of gabapentin (100 to 600 mg one to three times daily) can be successful. The side effect of hypersomnia often limits the dosage. Other side effects can include nausea, sedation, and dizziness. See Chapter 39 for further discussion.

Selecting the Most Appropriate Agent

For treatment purposes, RLS can be classified as *intermittent* (not often enough to require drug therapy), *daily* (troublesome enough to require drug therapy), and *refractory* (not adequately treated by a dopamine agonist). The ideal agent will minimize or abate the symptoms of RLS. No one pharmacologic agent appears to help all patients, and often a combination of medications is needed. The severity of RLS can vary, and pharmacologic treatment needs to be individualized. See **Box 42.7** for considerations when selecting a pharmacologic agent (**Figure 42-2**).

Considerations in Pharmacologic Agent Selection in RLS

Age of patient	Benzodiazepines can cause cognitive impairment in elderly.
Severity of symptoms	Mild symptoms: no medication, or levodopa or dopamine agonist
	Severe symptoms: strong opioid
Frequency/regularity of symptoms	Patients with infrequent symptoms may benefit from prn medication.
Presence of pregnancy	No safety and efficacy clinical trials on treatment of RLS with medications in pregnancy
Renal failure	Need to decrease dosage if drugs are renally excreted

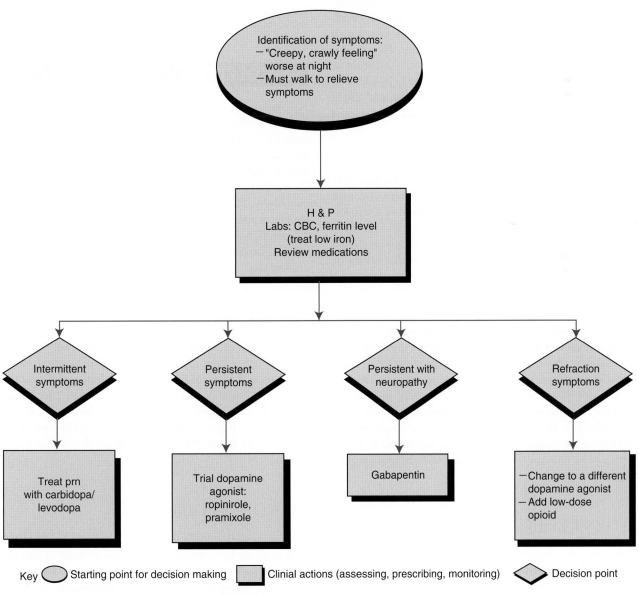

FIGURE 42–2   Algorithm for treatment for RLS.

First-Line Therapy

Dopaminergic antagonists such as low-dose carbidopa–levodopa should be reserved for patients with intermittent RLS. The first choice of therapy for daily RLS is one of the dopamine agonists. The largest placebo-controlled trial has been conducted on ropinirole (Requip) (Trenkwalder, et al., 2004). Other medications in this class include pramipexole (Mirapex). Nausea, dizziness, dyskinesia, and somnolence are potential side effects of both the dopaminergic antagonists and agonists.

Second-Line Therapy

Pharmacologic agents approved for neuropathic pain such as gabapentin (Neurontin) can be used alone or in conjunction with other agents. It is especially helpful for patients who describe RLS symptoms as painful. Other anticonvulsant agents such as carbamazepine (Tegretol) can be considered, but the older agents carry an increased risk of side effects such as dizziness, drowsiness, and lack of coordination. Patients also may experience nausea with these older agents. An opioid or opioid receptor agonist, tramadol (Ultram), may be added or used alone at low doses. If either the anticonvulsant or opioid fails, a repeat trial of dopamine agonists should be attempted (Silber, 2004).

Third-Line Therapy

Patients who continue to have symptoms may be refractory to treatment. Therapeutic doses may not have been obtained, or the patients could not tolerate the side effects of the medications. Substitution of different medications in the dopamine agonist class or adding higher-potency opioids should be considered. Consultation with a sleep specialist should be considered.

Monitoring Patient Response

Most patients will have remittance of symptoms with the first therapeutic dose of medication. This supports the theory that dopaminergic abnormality is a cause of this disorder. Another indicator of improvement is a decrease in excessive daytime sleepiness from lack of REM sleep. Patients need to be monitored for side effects of the pharmacologic agents. The long-term efficacy of these pharmacologic agents is uncertain, and monitoring for relapse of symptoms is important. It is also important to monitor for dependence when benzodiazepines or opioids are used.

PATIENT EDUCATION

Many patients who have RLS use OTC sleep medications, and poor sleep hygiene may contribute to the lack of sleep in RLS sufferers. Implementing cognitive sleep hygiene techniques may provide a modest improvement in short-term sleep symptoms (Edinger, 2003). Patients should inform all of their health care providers about their RLS diagnosis, and health care providers should be aware that the patient's inability to keep his or her limbs still is not due to lack of cooperation. Improper restraint of patients with this syndrome has resulted in mortality and morbidity.

Drug Information

A higher dosage of ropinirole (Requip) is needed compared to pramipexole (Mirapex) to achieve the same therapeutic effect. This may contribute to side effects and tolerability of the drug.

Patient-Oriented Information Sources

The Restless Legs' Syndrome Foundation supports research and provides information for patients and health care providers. Extensive international research is also being conducted on this serious sleep problem. (See **Box 42.4.**)

NARCOLEPSY

Narcolepsy is a sleep disorder caused by malfunctions in the primary brain mechanism that induces sleep. Individuals with narcolepsy achieve REM sleep in less than a minute, bypassing the other sleep stages. The other features of narcolepsy include excessive daytime sleepiness, cataplexy (attacks of muscle weakness), sleep paralysis, and hypnagogic hallucinations. Narcolepsy is the second leading cause of excessive daytime sleepiness and has an overall incidence in the world of 0.2 to 1.6 per thousand individuals (Stanford Center for Narcolepsy, 2004). Narcolepsy can have a dramatic impact on virtually all areas of life.

CAUSES

Narcolepsy usually starts in the second or third decade of life, but it has been identified in children as young as age 3. Excessive daytime sleepiness or cataplexy may be the first symptoms, but most often cataplexy is delayed 2 to 3 years. Cataplexy attacks are often precipitated by highly specific situations or triggers of strong emotions. Hypnagogic hallucinations can be present but are rarely the first manifestation of narcolepsy.

PATHOPHYSIOLOGY

The pathophysiology of narcolepsy is not well understood. It appears to be a disease where daily periods of internal clock-dependent alerting appear to be missing. Narcolepsy is sporadic and without a familial predisposition. Some evidence has shown a genetic component with specific human leukocyte antigens. It is possible that hypocretin-producing cells express toxins that provoke an autoimmune cascade that triggers narcolepsy.

DIAGNOSTIC CRITERIA

The International Classification of Sleep Disorders states that individuals with narcolepsy have excessive sleepiness, cataplexy, sleep paralysis, and hypnagogic hallucinations (the "narcoleptic tetrad"). Many narcolepsy patients also have disrupted nighttime sleep and automatic behaviors. Not all patients with narcolepsy have all symptoms of the narcoleptic tetrad, but excessive sleepiness is present in virtually every patient.

Silber et al. (2002) researched whether including human leukocyte antigen (HLA) typing provides a higher reliability of diagnosis. They used clinical and neurophysiologic data to evaluate 69 patients in four categories: definite narcolepsy, probable narcolepsy with two subgroups (confirmed by laboratory study), and probable narcolepsy (clinical). Seventy-four percent of patients had a positive HLA that helped to confirm the diagnosis of narcolepsy.

INITIATING DRUG THERAPY

There is no cure for narcolepsy, and pharmacologic therapy must be initiated to control the attacks. Evaluation for cataplexy, hypnagogic hallucinations, and sleep paralysis is important to identify the best agent for treatment. Most often antidepressants are used to block the REM paralysis of cataplexy. The mainstay of pharmacologic therapy until now has been amphetamines and amphetamine-like drugs such as methylphenidate (Ritalin). These are used to combat the abnormal sleepiness. Two newer pharmacologic agents that accomplish the same effect as amphetamines are modafinil (Provigil) and armodafinil (Nuvigil). These agents are nonamphetamines and are classified as Schedule IV controlled substances.

Goals of Drug Therapy

Pharmacologic therapy should be titrated to promote the optimal dose of stimulation. The health care provider needs to work with the patient to identify personal treatment goals such as staying awake in a classroom or social situation or while driving. The main goal is to achieve as normal a life as possible, staying awake in situations of normal daily living.

Psychostimulants

Modafinil and armodafinil (the R-enantiomer of modafinil) are psychostimulants with unique properties to promote wakefulness. The potential for abuse of these agents is much lower than with other stimulants, although it still needs to be monitored. The mechanism of action of modafinil and armodafinil is not well understood, but it appears to attenuate the central alpha-1 adrenergic system. The primary sites of action are the subregions of the hippocampus, the centrolateral nucleus of the thalamus, and the central nucleus of the amygdala. Modafinil can produce euphoria and psychoactive effects similar to other CNS stimulants. Absorption of the drug occurs rapidly, with peak plasma concentration in 2 to 4 hours and a half-life of 15 hours. Distribution of the drug is throughout the tissues, and it is moderately bound to plasma proteins. The drug is metabolized in the liver and excreted in the urine. In a recent study of the long-term efficacy of modafinil conducted by the Narcolepsy Multicenter Study Group (Mitler, et al., 2000), the most common adverse side effects of the drug were headache, nausea, nervousness, and anxiety. Most side effects are mild to moderate and transient. (See **Table 42.1.**)

SPECIAL POPULATIONS

Pediatrics

Modafinil has not been studied in children. The alternative drug of choice would be methylphenidate.

Geriatrics

Care must be taken when prescribing modafinil to the elderly population. The oral clearance of modafinil is reduced in the elderly by 20% to 50%. Renal failure does not influence the pharmacokinetics of the drug but does increase the inactive metabolite accumulation. Liver impairment can reduce the modafinil clearance and double serum concentrations.

MONITORING PATIENT RESPONSE

Narcolepsy is a life-long disease process, and patients must use the medications for their entire lives. Patient response is monitored by improvement in the disease's severity. Achieving the goals identified by the patient can help to improve compliance.

PATIENT EDUCATION

Patients and their families need to be aware of all available options to treat narcolepsy. Psychological distress is a consequence, not the cause, of the disease. Discussion of potential side effects of the drugs is important for compliance. Offering counseling and support groups when necessary is important.

Drug Information

Patients who are switched from amphetamine stimulants to modafinil may not experience the same euphoric effects, and this may make the switch undesirable to the patient. Amphetamines tend to produce a feeling of improved well-being and arousal, while modafinil increases arousal without a change in affect.

Patient-Oriented Sources

Health care providers and patients can find information about narcolepsy from a variety of sources. Online support groups exist. (See **Box 42.4.**)

Case Study 1

S. H., age 47, reports difficulty falling asleep and staying asleep. These problems have been ongoing for many years, but she has never mentioned them to her health care provider. She has generally "lived with it" and self-treated the problem with OTC Tylenol PM. Currently she is also experiencing perimenopausal symptoms of night sweats and mood swings. Current medical problems include hypertension controlled with medications. Past medical history includes childhood illnesses of measles, chickenpox, and mumps. Family history is positive for diabetes on the maternal side and hypertension on the paternal side. Her only medication is an angiotensin-converting enzyme inhibitor and diuretic combination for hypertension control. She generally does not like taking medication and does not take any other OTC products.

DIAGNOSIS: INSOMNIA

1. List specific goals of therapy for S. H.
2. What drug therapy would you prescribe? Why?
3. What are the parameters for monitoring the success of the therapy?
4. Discuss specific patient education based on the prescribed therapy.
5. List one or two adverse reactions for the selected agent that would cause you to change therapy.
6. What would be the choice for second-line therapy?
7. What OTC and/or alternative medicines might be appropriate for this patient?
8. What dietary and lifestyle changes might you recommend?
9. Describe one or two drug–drug or drug–food interactions for the selected agent.

Case Study 2

J. F., age 73, reports a "funny sensation in my legs at night." To get rid of this sensation, she has to move. She can sleep only 2 or 3 hours at a time before the sensation wakes her up. This problem has been ongoing from her early twenties but has steadily worsened with age. She finds herself walking around a lot in the early evening. She has tried to self-treat the problem with OTC Tylenol PM. Current medical problems include hypertension, hyperlipidemia, coronary artery disease, and depression. Family history is positive for coronary artery disease on the paternal side. Medications include Prinivil 10 mg qd, Zocor 40 mg qd, Lexapro 10 mg qd, and ASA 81 mg qd. She does not want to take any more medication but wants to help her legs stop moving at night.

DIAGNOSIS: RESTLESS LEG SYNDROME

1. List specific goals of therapy for J. F.
2. What drug therapy would you prescribe? Why?
3. What are the parameters for monitoring the success of the therapy?
4. Discuss specific patient education based on the prescribed therapy.
5. List one or two adverse reactions for the selected agent that would cause you to change therapy.
6. What would be the choice for second-line therapy?
7. What OTC and/or alternative medicines might be appropriate for this patient?
8. What dietary and lifestyle changes might you recommend?
9. Describe one or two drug–drug or drug–food interactions for the selected agent.

Case Study 3

D. W., age 35, mentions during a routine visit that he has been having horrible nightmares. He states that during the nightmares he is aware of his surroundings but just cannot seem to move. He also reports excessive daytime sleepiness, which he cannot understand since he is usually in bed by 10 PM and doesn't get up until 8 AM. This has been a problem for about the past 6 months. His family history is negative for any illnesses and sleep disorders. He does not take any medications or OTC products routinely.

DIAGNOSIS: POSSIBLE NARCOLEPSY

1. List specific goals of therapy for D. W.
2. What drug therapy would you prescribe? Why?
3. What are the parameters for monitoring the success of the therapy?
4. Discuss specific patient education based on the prescribed therapy.
5. List one or two adverse reactions for the selected agent that would cause you to change therapy.
6. What would be the choice for second-line therapy?
7. What OTC and/or alternative medicines might be appropriate for this patient?
8. What dietary and lifestyle changes might you recommend?
9. Describe one or two drug–drug or drug–food interactions for the selected agent.

BIBLIOGRAPHY

Starred references are cited in the text.

Ahmed, M. (2004). Circadian rhythm sleep disorders. [On-line.] Available: http://sleepmed.bsd.chicago.edu/circadianrhythm.html.

*Allen, R. (2004). Dopamine and iron in the pathophysiology of restless legs syndrome (RLS). *Sleep Medicine, 5,* 385–391.

Anacoli-Israel, S. (1997). Sleeping problems in older adults: Putting myths to bed. *Geriatrics, 52*(1), 20–28.

*Attenburrow, M., & Dowling, B. (1996). Case-control study of evening melatonin concentration in primary insomnia. *British Medical Journal, 312* [On-line], 1263. Available: http://gw5. epnet.com.

Bateson, A. (2004). The benzodiazepine site of the GABA$_A$ receptor: An old target with new potential? *Sleep Medicine, 5*(Suppl. 1), S9–S15.

Belinger, J., Fins, A., Goeke, J., et al. (1996). The empirical identification of insomnia subtypes: A cluster analytic approach. *Sleep, 19,* 398–411.

Boeve, B., Silber, M., & Ferman, T. (2003). Melatonin for treatment of REM sleep behavior disorders in neurologic disorders: Results in 14 patients. *Sleep Medicine, 4,* 281–284.

*Bonnet, M., & Arand, D. (1996). The consequences of a week of insomnia. *Sleep, 19,* 453.

Brostrom, A., Stromberg, A., Dahlstrom, U., & Fridlund, B. (2004). Sleep difficulties, daytime sleepiness, and health-related quality of life in patients with chronic heart failure. *Journal of Cardiovascular Nursing, 19*(4), 234–242.

Brown, D. (1999). Managing sleep disorders: Solutions in primary care. *Clinician Reviews, 9*(10), 51–69.

Bruck, D. (2001). The impact of narcolepsy on psychological health and role behaviours: Negative effects and comparisons with other illness groups. *Sleep Medicine, 2,* 437–446.

Buyssee, D. (2004). Insomnia, depression, and aging: Assessing sleep and mood interactions in older adults. *Geriatrics, 59*(2), 47–51.

*Clavadetscher, S., Gugger, M., & Bassetti, C. (2004). Restless legs syndrome: Clinical experience with long-term treatment. *Sleep Medicine, 5,* 495–500.

Clinical Pharmacology. (2004). *Melatonin.* [On-line]. Available: http://www.gsm.com.

Clinical Pharmacology. (2004) Available:. *Valerian, valeriana officinalis.* [On-line]. http://www.gsm.com.

*Cochran, H. (2003). Diagnose and treat primary insomnia. *Nurse Practitioner, 28*(9), 13–27.

Dato, C. (1999). Sleeping disorders. In J. Singleton, S. Sandowski, C. Green-Hernandez, et al. (Eds.), *Primary care* (pp. 686–691). Philadelphia: Lippincott Williams & Wilkins.

*Dement, W., & Vaughan, C. (1999). *The promise of sleep.* New York: Dell.

*Desai, A. K., & Grossberg, G. T. (2003). Herbals and botanicals in geriatric psychiatry. *American Journal of Geriatric Psychology, 11,* 498–506.

Drake, C., Roehers, T., & Roth, T. (2003). Insomnia cause, consequences, and therapeutics: An overview. *Depression and Anxiety, 18,* 163–176.

Dunn, S. (1998). Insomnia. In *Primary care consultant* (pp. 320–321). St. Louis: Mosby.

*Edinger, J. (2003). Cognitive and behavioral anomalies among insomnia patients with mixed restless legs and periodic limb movement disorder. *Behavioral Sleep Medicine, 1*(1), 37–53.

*Everitt, D. E., Avorn, J., & Baker, M. W. (1990). Clinical decision-making in the evaluation and treatment of insomnia. *American Journal of Medicine, 89,* 357–362.

*Gigli, G., Adorati, M., Dolso, P., et al. (2004). Restless legs syndrome in end-stage renal disease. *Sleep Medicine, 5,* 309–315.

Gillian, J. C., & Byerley, W. (1990). The diagnosis and management of insomnia. *New England Journal of Medicine, 322,* 239–248.

Hauri, P. (1987). Specific effects of sedative/hypnotic drugs in the treatment of incapacitating chronic insomnia. *American Journal of Medicine, 83,* 925–926.

Hauri, P. (1998). Sleep disorders: Insomnia. *Clinics in Chest Medicine, 19,* 157–168.

Hening, W., Walthers, A., Allen, R., et al. (2004). Impact, diagnosis and treatment of restless legs syndrome (RLS) in a primary care population: The REST (RLS Epidemiology, Symptoms, and Treatment) primary care study. *Sleep Medicine, 5,* 237–240.

*Ivanenko, A., Crabtree, V., Tauman, R., & Gozal, D. (Jan./Feb. 2003). Melatonin in children and adolescents with insomnia: A retrospective study. *Clinical Pediatrics,* 51–58.

Karch, A. (2000). *2001 Lippincott's nursing drug guide.* Philadelphia: Lippincott Williams & Wilkins.

Katz, D., & McHorney, C. (2002). The relationship between insomnia and health-related quality of life in patients with chronic illness. *Journal of Family Practice, 51*(3), 229. [On-line]. Available: http//www.jfponline.com/content/2002/03/jfp_0302_00229.asp.

Kryger, M., Monjan, A., Bliwise, D., & Ancoli-Israel, S. (2004). Sleep, health and aging: Bridging the gap between science and clinical practice. *Geriatrics, 59*(1), 24–30.

Late-life insomnia: Psychiatric and medical comorbidity common. (2004). *Geriatric Psychopharmacology Update, 8*(7), 1–7.

*Lavie, P. (1997). Melatonin: Role in gating nocturnal rise in sleep propensity. *Journal of Biological Rhythms, 12,* 657–668.

Leger, D., Guilleminault, C., Biol, D., et al. (2002). Medical and socioprofessional impact of insomnia. *Sleep, 25*(6), 625–629.

Lindberg, E., & Gisiason, T. (2000). Epidemiology of sleep-related obstructive breathing. *Sleep Medicine Reviews, 4*(5), 411–433.

Lustbader, A., Morgan, C., Pelayo, R. et al. (1997). Psychiatry: Insomnia. In L. Rucker (Ed.), *Essentials of adult ambulatory care* (pp. 607–615). Baltimore: Williams & Wilkins.

Lyznicki, J., Doege, T., Davis, R., & Williams, M. (1998). Sleepiness, driving, and motor vehicle crashes. *Journal of the American Medical Association, 279,* 1908–1913.

Medical Letter of Drugs and Therapeutics. (1995). (Issue 962). Melatonin: Therapeutic uses [On-line]. Available: http://gw5.epnet.com.

Mendelson, W., Thompson, C., & Firanko, T. (1996). Adverse reactions to sedative/hypnotics: Three years' experience. *Sleep, 19,* 702–706.

*Mitler, M., Harsh, J., Hirschowitz, M., & Guilleminault, C. (2000). Long-term efficacy and safety of modafinil (Provigil) for the treatment of excessive daytime sleepiness associated with narcolepsy. *Sleep Medicine, 1,* 231–243.

Morrish, E., King, M., Smith, I., & Shneerson, J. (2004). Factors associated with a delay in the diagnosis of narcolepsy. *Sleep Medicine, 5,* 37–41.

National Center on Sleep Disorders Research and Office of Prevention, Education, and Control. (1997a). *Problem sleepiness in your patient.* U.S. Department of Health and Human Services. NIH Publication No. 97-4073.

National Center on Sleep Disorders Research and Office of Prevention, Education, and Control. (1997b). *Working group report on problem sleepiness.* U.S. Department of Health and Human Services.

National Center on Sleep Disorders Research and Office of Prevention, Education, and Control. (2000). *Restless legs syndrome: Detection and management in primary care.* U.S. Department of Health and Human Services. NIH Publication No 00-3788.

National Heart, Lung, and Blood Institute Working Group on Insomnia. (1999). Insomnia: Assessment and management in primary care. *American Family Physician, 59,* 3029–3038.

National Institutes of Health Consensus Development Program. (1990). *The treatment of sleep disorders of older people.* NIH Consensus Statement. [On-line]. Available: http://home.mdconsult.com/das/article/body/jorg.

*National Institutes of Health State-of-the-Science. (2005). Conference on manifestation and management of chronic insomnia in adults. *NIH 22*(2), 1–30.

National Sleep Foundation. (1999). *Is melatonin a treatment for insomnia and jet lag?* [On-line]. Available: http://www.sleepfoundation.org/publications/melatonin.html.

National Sleep Foundation. (2002). Sleep in America poll. [On-line]. Available: http://www.sleepfoundation.org.

*National Sleep Foundation. (2004). *Melatonin: The basic facts.* [On-line]. Available http://www.sleepfoundation.org/publications/melatoninthefact.cfm.

Neubauer, D. (1999). Sleep problems in the elderly. *American Family Physician, 59,* 2551–2558.

Pagel, J., Zafralotifi, S., & Zammit, G. (1997). How to prescribe a good night's sleep. *Patient Care, 31*(4), 87.

Quan, S., & Zee, P. (2004). A sleep review of systems: Evaluating the effects of medical disorders on sleep in the older patient. *Geriatrics, 59*(3), 37–42.

*Regestein, Q., Dambrosia, J., Hallett, M., et al. (1993). Daytime alertness in patients with primary insomnia. *American Journal of Psychiatry, 150,* 1529–1534.

Requip improves symptoms of restless legs syndrome at 1 week, studies show. (July 5, 2004). *Health & Medicine Week, 952.*

*Rosekind, M., Gregory, K., Mallis, M., et al. (2010). The cost of poor sleep: Workplace productivity loss and associated costs. *Journal of Occupational & Environmental Medicine, 52*(1), 91–98.

Roth, T., & Drake, C. (2004). Evolution of insomnia: Current status and future directions. *Sleep Medicine, 5*(Suppl. 1), S23–S30.

Schwartz, J., Feldman, N., Fry, J., & Harsh, J. (2003). Efficacy of modafinil for improving daytime wakefulness in patients treated previously with psychostimulants. *Sleep Medicine, 4,* 43–49.

*Shorr, R., Bauwens, S., & Landefeld, C. S. (1990). Failure to limit quantities of benzodiazepine hypnotic drugs for outpatients: Placing the elderly at risk. *American Journal of Medicine, 89,* 725–732.

*Silber, M. (2004). Calming restless legs. *Sleep, 27*(5), 839–841.

*Silber, M., Krahn, L., & Olson, E. (2002). Diagnosing narcolepsy: Validity and reliability of a new diagnostic criteria. *Sleep Medicine, 3,* 109–113.

Silva, J., Chase, M., Sartorius, N., & Roth, T. (1996). Special report from a symposium held by the World Health Organization and the World Federation of Sleep Research Societies: An overview of insomnias and related disorders—recognition, epidemiology, and rational management. *Sleep, 19,* 412–416.

*Sleep Facts and Stats. (2004). 2004 Sleep in America Poll. [On-line]. Available: http://www.sleepfoundation.org/NSAW1/pk_sleepfacts.cfm.

*Sleep Facts and Stats. (2009). 2009 Sleep in America Poll [On-line]. Available: http://healthyliving.ocregister.com/files/2009/03/2009sleeppoll.pdf.

*Sleep Facts and Stats. (2010). 2010 Sleep in America Poll [On-line]. Available: http://www.sleepfoundation.org/sites/default/files/nsaw/NSF%20Sleep%20in%20%20America%20Poll%20-%20Summary%20of%20Findings%20.pdf.

Smith, D., Simonson, W., & Zammit, G. (1999, March). *New ideas for the management of sleep disorders.* Symposium conducted at the meeting of the American Medical Directors Association Annual Symposium, Orlando, Florida.

*Stanford Center for Narcolepsy. (2004). http://med.stanford.edu/school/Psychiatry/narcolepsy/symptoms.html.

Terzano, M., Rossi, M., Palomba, V., et al. (2003). New drugs for insomnia: Comparative tolerability of zopiclone, zolpidem and zaleplon. *Drug Safety, 26*(4), 261–282.

*Trenkwalder, C., Garcia-Borreguero, D., Montagna, P., et al. (2004). Therapy with ropinirole: Efficacy and tolerability in RLS 1 Study Group. *Journal of Neurological and Neurosurgical Psychiatry, 75*(1), 92–97.

Trevena, L. (2004). Practice corner: Sleepless in Sydney—Is valerian an effective alternative to benzodiazepines in the treatment of insomnia? *ACP Journal Club, 141*(1), 14.

Vitiello, M., Larsen, L., & Moe, K. (2004). Age-related sleep change: Gender and estrogen effects on the subjective-objective sleep quality relationships of healthy, noncomplaining older men and women. *Journal of Psychosomatic Research, 56,* 503–510.

Wagner, D. (1996). Sleep disorders I: Disorders of the circadian sleep–wake cycle. *Neurologic Clinics, 14,* 651–670.

Wallace, K., & Morbunas, A. (1997). Commonly abused prescription sedative-hypnotic drugs. *Topics in Emergency Medicine, 19*(4), 23–24.

What are the risks when elderly patients combine herbal and prescription medications? (2004). *Geriatric Psychopharmacology Update, 8*(1), 1–6.

*Zisselman, M., Rovner, B., Yuen, E., & Louis, D. (1996). Sedative-hypnotic use and increased hospital stay and costs in older people. *Journal of the American Geriatric Society, 44,* 1371–1374.

*Zucconi, M., & Ferini-Strambi, L. (2004). Epidemiology and clinical findings of restless legs syndrome. *Sleep Medicine, 5,* 293–299.

CHAPTER **43**

Andrew M. Peterson
Dharmi Patel

Attention-Deficit/Hyperactivity Disorder

Attention-deficit/hyperactivity disorder (ADHD) has become a commonly diagnosed condition among today's children. Hallmark symptoms include hyperactivity, impulsivity, and inattention. The American Psychiatric Association (APA) estimated in the *Diagnostic and Statistical Manual of Mental Disorders* (DSM-IV) that 3% to 5% of school-aged children had ADHD. The disorder is more common in boys than in girls, with a ratio ranging from 4:1 to 9:1 (APA, 2000; Spencer, et al., 2002). Research is increasingly revealing that ADHD also affects adults, with estimates of prevalence ranging from 2% to 7% (Wender, 1995). This realization is changing perceptions of ADHD because it is becoming imperative to understand the disorder as diagnosed in adulthood.

Researchers have found that many of the core symptoms of ADHD are treatable. Treatment should be individualized to the patient's symptoms. The treatment plan usually is multimodal. Even when treatment begins early in childhood, the patient may still show symptoms in adolescence or adulthood. The outcome of the childhood disorder is uncertain, as is determining which children will have the disorder.

CAUSES

Many causes of ADHD have been suggested, but none has yet to be accepted. Evidence suggests that the disorder may have a genetic link (Farone & Biederman, 1994). Estimates are that children who have a sibling with ADHD have a two to three times greater chance of being diagnosed with ADHD (Dulcan, et al., 1997). Growing evidence suggests that the principal cause of ADHD is genetic (Pliszka, 2007). ADHD has been associated with the dopamine transporter gene and the dopamine D_4 gene (Adler & Chua, 2002; Daley, 2004). Possible nongenetic causes are neurobiological, such as perinatal stress, low birth weight, traumatic brain injury, maternal smoking during pregnancy, and severe early deprivation (Pliszka, 2007). Other theories involve dietary intake of certain chemicals and sugars, but data are lacking.

PATHOPHYSIOLOGY

Neurotransmitter dysfunction is a proposed mechanism for ADHD, and several different pathways for this dysfunction have been studied. These include a baseline norepinephrine level that is too high, a central epinephrine level that is too high, a problem with the functioning of epinephrine in the peripheral system, or problems involving dopamine receptors or dopamine-mediated functions (Pliszka, et al., 1996). All these mechanisms may work together to cause ADHD symptoms. The complete pathophysiologic process of these mechanisms is not completely understood, but there appears to be a connection between the D_4 receptor and activity of the major neurotransmitters, epinephrine, norepinephrine and dopamine (Adler & Chua, 2002; Daley, 2004).

Risk factors may be involved in the development of ADHD, although many are only associations and do not indicate that ADHD is present. The practitioner must ascertain the patient's drug history and examine for visual disturbances and hearing dysfunction as possible causes of the child's behavior (Dulcan, et al., 1997). A rare genetic disorder, generalized resistance to thyroid hormone, has been associated with ADHD (Hauser, et al., 1993). Fragile X syndrome, fetal alcohol syndrome, glucose-6-phosphate dehydrogenase deficiency, and phenylketonuria are also associated risks for development of ADHD (Dulcan, et al., 1997). Limited numbers of cases have been associated with other risk factors, including such pregnancy variables as poor maternal health, young maternal age, maternal use of alcohol or cigarettes, toxemia or eclampsia, postmaturity, and extended labor (Dulcan, et al., 1997; Markussen, et al., 2003). Medical conditions and malnutrition in infancy may also play a role in ADHD, although this has not been proved (Dulcan, et al., 1997).

DIAGNOSTIC CRITERIA

The diagnostic criteria for ADHD are listed in **Box 43.1**. Children are required to show symptoms by age 7, and most children show symptoms for many years before the diagnosis is made (APA, 2000). For a definitive diagnosis, the child also must show symptoms in more than one setting, such as at home and in school. The adult with ADHD may display symptoms at home and at work. Adult patients also have trouble maintaining relationships as a result of their inattentiveness. In children and adults, the symptoms must interfere with

BOX 43.1

Criteria for Diagnosing Attention-Deficit/Hyperactivity Disorder

A. Either (1) or (2)
1. Six (or more) of the following symptoms of inattention have persisted for at least 6 months to a degree that is maladaptive and inconsistent with developmental level:

    Inattention
    a. often fails to give close attention to details or makes careless mistakes in schoolwork, work, or other activities
    b. often has difficulty sustaining attention in tasks or play activities
    c. often does not seem to listen when spoken to directly
    d. often does not follow through on instructions and fails to finish schoolwork, chores, or duties in the workplace (not due to oppositional behavior or failure to understand instructions)
    e. often has difficulty organizing tasks and activities
    f. often avoids, dislikes, or is reluctant to engage in tasks that require sustained mental effort (such as schoolwork or homework)
    g. often loses things necessary for tasks or activities (e.g., toys, school assignments, pencils, books, or tools)
    h. is often easily distracted by extraneous stimuli
    i. is often forgetful in daily activities
2. Six (or more) of the following symptoms of hyperactivity-impulsivity have persisted for at least 6 months to a degree that is maladaptive and inconsistent with developmental level:

    Hyperactivity
    a. often fidgets with hands or feet or squirms in seat
    b. often leaves seat in classroom or in other situations in which remaining seated is expected
    c. often runs about or climbs excessively in situations in which it is inappropriate (in adolescents or adults, may be limited to subjective feelings of restlessness)
    d. often has difficulty playing or engaging in leisure activities quietly
    e. is often "on the go" or often acts as if "driven by a motor"
    f. often talks excessively

    Impulsivity
    g. often blurts out answers before questions have been completed
    h. often has difficulty awaiting turn
    i. often interrupts or intrudes on others (e.g., butts into conversation or games)

B. Some hyperactive–impulsive or inattentive symptoms that caused impairment were present before age of 7 years.

C. Some impairment from the symptoms is present in two or more settings (e.g., at school [or work] and at home).

D. There must be clear evidence of clinically significant impairment in social, academic, or occupational functioning.

E. The symptoms do not occur exclusively during the course of a Pervasive Developmental Disorder, Schizophrenia, or other Psychotic Disorder and are not better accounted for by another mental disorder (e.g., Mood Disorder, Anxiety Disorder, Dissociative Disorder, or Personality Disorder).

From American Psychiatric Association. (2000). *Diagnostic and statistical manual of mental disorders* (4th ed., text revision). Washington, DC: Author, with permission.

---

the person's ability to function. The criteria are further broken into subtypes, and based on the symptoms, the patient's disorder is coded (**Box 43.2**).

Diagnosing ADHD in a child may be difficult because children often behave differently in the health care setting, therefore making it impossible for the provider to observe symptoms. For this reason, the practitioner must use other methods to evaluate behavior. Such methods include rating scales, which usually are administered by parents and teachers. All scales are similar, but each has its own criteria and rating system. Some commonly used scales include the parent-completed Child Behavior Checklist (Achenbach, 1991; Biederman, et al., 1993), the Teacher Report Form of the Child Behavior Checklist (Achenbach, 1991; Edelbrock, et al.,

1984), the Conners Parent and Teacher Rating Scale (Ullmann, et al., 1985), the Barkley Home Situations Questionnaire and School Situations Questionnaire (Barkley, 1990), and the Child Attention Problems Profile (Barkley, 1990; Barkley et al., 1989). These rating scales have been found to be accurate measures of ADHD behavior (Dulcan, et al., 1997). Practitioners may use these rating scales to follow a child's behavior after the initial diagnosis of ADHD.

Making the initial diagnosis also requires detailed parent interviews that focus on a family history of ADHD or other psychiatric disorders, psychosocial adversity (e.g., poverty, parental psychopathology or absence, family conflict), school behavior, learning, attendance and test reports, and medical evaluations (Dulcan, et al., 1997).

BOX 43.2

Diagnostic and Statistical Manual of Mental Disorders—IV: Coding Based on Type

314.01 Attention-Deficit/Hyperactivity Disorder, Combined Type: if both Criteria A1 and A2 are met for the past 6 months

314.00 Attention-Deficit/Hyperactivity Disorder, Predominantly Inattentive Type: if Criterion A1 is met but Criterion A2 is not met for the past 6 months

314.01 Attention-Deficit/Hyperactivity Disorder, Predominantly Hyperactive-Impulsive Type: if Criterion A2 is met but Criterion A1 is not met for the past 6 months

Coding note: For individuals (especially adolescents and adults) who currently have symptoms that no longer meet full criteria, "In Partial Remission" should be specified.

From American Psychiatric Association. (2000). *Diagnostic and statistical manual of mental disorders* (4th ed., text revision, p. 93). Washington, DC: Author, with permission.

A confounding factor in the diagnosis is the probability of comorbid disorders. Mood disorders, anxiety disorders, learning disorders, and communication disorders are more common in the child with ADHD (APA, 2000). Laboratory findings, physical examination, and evaluation of concurrent medical problems cannot be used to confirm the diagnosis. Minor physical anomalies such as hypertelorism, a highly arched palate, and low-set ears may be more common in this population (APA, 2000), but such characteristics do not mean that the child has ADHD. Many children diagnosed with ADHD can be expected to have some impaired social functioning in adult life.

The diagnosis of ADHD in the adolescent is less clear since as an ADHD child matures into adolescence, the symptoms change (Nahlik, 2004). Moodiness, laziness, boredom, or impatience may be common symptoms in the ADHD adolescent but may also be typical adolescent behavior or even another mood disorder.

Diagnosis in an adult consists of a complete psychiatric evaluation; childhood history; information from spouse or significant others, parents, or employers; and a review of school records. A medical history and physical examination can be used to rule out comorbid conditions. As with childhood diagnosis, rating scales and questionnaires may also be used (Weiss & Murray, 2003), such as the Conners Abbreviated Teacher's Rating Scale and the Wender Utah Rating Scale.

Practitioners cannot use a patient's response to stimulant therapy to determine ADHD status. A child not diagnosed with ADHD has the same response of reduced hyperactivity, impulsivity, and inattentiveness as a child diagnosed with ADHD (Goldman, et al., 1998).

INITIATING DRUG THERAPY

Many practitioners today follow a multimodal treatment plan. Multimodal treatment plans seem logical because different symptoms respond to different types of treatment. The Multimodal Treatment Study (MTA) showed that children receiving intensive behavioral management combined with medication fared better than those receiving intensive behavioral management alone (Anonymous, 1999). The core symptoms of the disorder (i.e., inattention, hyperactivity, and impulsivity) respond to medication, with or without the behavioral intervention. Behavioral symptoms seem to respond to environmental modification, while skills in sports, academics, and social situations may not respond to medication or behavior modification. Relationship problems usually can be treated through psychotherapy.

Nonpharmacologic aspects of a multimodal treatment plan consist of behavior modification, parent training, family therapy, social skills training, academic skills training, individual psychotherapy, cognitive behavior modification, and therapeutic recreation. These are discussed further in the Nutrition/Lifestyle section later in this chapter.

Goals of Drug Therapy

When a child is diagnosed with ADHD, questions arise regarding the outcome of this disorder. Parents want to know if there is a cure and, if so, what treatment will increase the chance for cure. However, the outcome of ADHD cannot be predicted, and the child will not always "grow out of it." Three outcomes have been identified. The first possible outcome is developmental delay, which occurs in approximately 30% of diagnosed children; this means that the child will outgrow the symptoms. The second possible outcome, which occurs in 40% of children, is continual display, which is marked by adult life with ADHD. Continual display may lead to social and emotional difficulties. The third possible outcome is developmental decay (30% of children with ADHD), which involves the continual display of core ADHD symptoms along with pathologic conditions such as substance abuse and antisocial personality disorder. Developmental decay is the most severe outcome (Sudak, 1998).

Medication therapy is usually one of the first options in treating patients newly diagnosed with ADHD. Pharmacotherapy offers several alternatives (**Table 43.1**). The medication class primarily used is stimulants, such as amphetamines and methylphenidate. Nonstimulant alternatives are atomoxetine (Strattera), buproprion (Wellbutrin), tricyclic antidepressants (TCAs), selective serotonin reuptake inhibitors (SSRIs), monoamine oxidase (MAO) inhibitors and alpha-adrenergic agonists (Pliszka, 2007). Although it is not clear how these medications actually affect the primary symptoms of ADHD, it is known which neurotransmitters they affect (**Table 43.2**).

TABLE 43.1	Recommended Order of Treatment for ADHD	
Order	Agents	Comments
First line	Stimulants	Methylphenidate or amphetamine works quickly with first dose, is available in extended release, and is easy to titrate. If patient does not respond, dextroamphetamine can be tried.
Second line	Nonstimulants	Nortriptyline works in 1–3 wk. Imipramine works in 2–4 wk. Similar side effect profiles.
Third line	Bupropion	Takes 4 wk to show effects. May impair cognitive skills.

TABLE 43.2	Neurotransmitters Affected by Pharmacotherapy			
	NE	DA	5-HT	Comments
methylphenidate		I		Blocks reuptake
dextroamphetamine	I, ↑	I		Blocks reuptake of NE, DA
				Causes release of NE
atomoxetine	↑			Blocks reuptake of NE
clonidine				Stimulates alpha$_2$ adrenoceptors
bupropion	I	I	I	Weak blocker of NE, 5-HT
nortriptyline	↑		↑	5-HT > NE
imipramine	↑		↑	5-HT > NE

NE, norepinephrine; DA, dopamine; 5-HT, serotonin; I, inhibits; ↑, increases concentrations in system

The long-term benefits of medication therapy have not been determined. It is clear that they work in the short term to improve symptoms, but there is a lack of long-term studies (Goldman, et al., 1998). The following information addresses concerns for the pediatric population using these medications.

Stimulants

A stimulant is usually the first-choice medication, based on 60 years of research and clinical experience (Dulcan, et al., 1997). Daley (2004) reported that nearly 70% of patients will respond to stimulant therapy. The most commonly used stimulants are methylphenidate (Ritalin, Concerta) and amphetamine salts (Adderall, Dexedrine). Either stimulant is appropriate; both are equally efficacious in the treatment of ADHD.

Dosage

Amphetamines should be started at the lowest dosage and titrated upward until the desired response is seen. Dosing is usually based on weight and titrated to a dosage that controls the symptoms of ADHD. **Table 43.3** lists medications and their dosages.

There is equal efficacy between long-acting and immediate-release formulations. Longer-acting formulations may provide improved convenience and compliance. A patient may be initially started on a long-acting form, but children (<16 kg) are often started on shorter-acting doses because long-acting forms are not manufactured in low doses (Pliszka, 2007). For immediate-release methylphenidate, the typical starting dose for children under age 6 is 5 mg before breakfast and 5 mg at lunch. The dose may be increased by 5 to 10 mg weekly, with a maximum recommended dose of 60 mg. Long-acting preparations are available if the immediate-release formulation is impossible or inconvenient to give, or if rebound is a problem. The long-acting methylphenidate Ritalin LA should be started after the patient is taking 20 mg of the immediate-release preparation. For patients taking 10 to 20 mg of immediate-release methylphenidate daily, Concerta

18 mg or Metadate ER 10 or 20 mg may also be used. Dose titrations occur every 1 to 3 weeks until the maximum allowed dose, symptom remission, or side effects prevent further titrations, whichever occurs first.

Mechanism of Action

As mentioned previously, it is not clear how stimulants help to reduce the core symptoms of ADHD. In addition to increasing levels of epinephrine and norepinephrine, these agents also can bind to central dopamine receptors and increase the systemic levels of dopamine.

Adverse Events

The primary adverse events related to stimulant therapy include palpitations, tachycardia, elevated blood pressure, and potentially arrhythmias. Changes in appetite, nausea, vomiting, and other gastrointestinal (GI) disturbances may occur. The neurologic adverse events range from headache and insomnia to seizure activity, particularly in patients predisposed to seizures.

In general, adverse events are manageable, results are quick and predictable with the first dose, and the medications are easy to titrate (Buitelaar, et al., 1995). The adverse events of the stimulants, such as headaches, dizziness, appetite suppression, tics, dyskinesias, sleep disturbances, abuse potential, and in particular growth retardation (below height or weight on normal growth charts), may be of concern. One study found a significant difference in growth between patients who took stimulants and those who did not. Other studies have shown a decrease in height or weight in patients taking stimulants. The clinician must assess the growth progress, need for continued treatment, and overall functioning of the ADHD patient every 1 to 3 months (Daley, 2004).

Determining the long-term effect of stimulants on children is difficult. To minimize these effects, it is reasonable for the patient to take drug-free periods, usually over the summer. These periods also allow for reassessment of ADHD. Because

TABLE 43.3 Overview of Agents Used to Treat ADHD

Generic (Trade) Name and Dosage	Selected Adverse Events	Contraindications	Special Considerations
atomoxetine (Strattera) Start: Children and adolescents <70 kg: 0.5 mg/kg/d for 4 d, then 1 mg/kg/d for 4 d, then 1.2 mg/kg/d	Increased heart rate and blood pressure, abdominal pain, decreased appetite, nausea, sedation Urinary retention in adults	Patients on MAO inhibitors, narrow- angle glaucoma	Atomoxetine does not appear to promote the development of new tics and therefore may be a good choice for patients unable to take stimulant medi- cations due to pre-existing tics.
bupropion (Wellbutrin) Children: Start: Children and adolescents <70 kg: 0.5 mg/kg/d for 4 d, then 1 mg/kg/d for 4 d, then 1.2 mg/kg/d Range: 3–6 mg/kg/d or 150–300 mg/d Adults: 100 mg BID, then 100 mg TID; max. 4.5 mg/d	Insomnia, anorexia, dizzi- ness, anxiety, confusion, xerostomia, constipation, nausea, agitation, fever, headache, vomiting, seizures	Seizure disorders, bulimia, anorexia nervosa Within 14 days of MAO inhibitors	Monitor weight.
clonidine (Catapres) Children: Start: <45 kg: 0.05 mg HS, then titrate in 0.05 mg increments BID >45 kg: 0.1 mg HS, then titrate in 0.1 mg increments BID to QID Range: 27–40.5 kg: 0.05 to 0.2 mg; 40.5–45 kg: 0.05 to 0.3 mg; >45 kg: 0.05–0.4 mg Adults: 0.1 mg BID; max. 2 to 4 mg/d	Dizziness, drowsiness, anxi- ety, confusion, xerostomia, constipation, impotence, nausea, hypotension	Hypersensitivity to clonidine	Monitor blood pressure (standing and supine), respiratory rate and depth, and heart rate.
imipramine (Tofranil) Children: Start: 1 mg/kg/d Range: 1–4 mg/kg/d or 200 mg Adults: 25 mg, tid–qid; max. 300/d	Dizziness, drowsiness, xerostomia, constipation, nausea, fever, headache, weight gain, skel- etal weakness, increased appetite	Same as above	Monitor blood pressure, pulse, ECG, CBC, mental status. May cause allergic reaction in patients with sulfa allergy Increases photosensitivity Lowers seizure threshold
nortriptyline (Pamelor) Children: Start: 0.5 mg/kg/d Range: 1–2 mg/kg/day or 100 mg Adults: 25 mg, tid–qid; max. 150 mg/d	Dizziness, drowsiness, xeros- tomia, constipation, nausea, fever, headache, weight gain, skeletal weakness, urinary retention	Acute post-myocardial infarction During or within 14 d of MAO inhibitors	Monitor blood pressure, pulse, mental status, weight. Increases risk of arrhythmia in patients receiving thyroid replacement therapy
Long acting: dexamphenidate (Focalin XR 5, 10, 15, 20, 30, 40 mg cap) 10 mg/d; max 40 mg/d dextroamphetamine (Dexedrine spansule 5,10,15 mg cap) 5 mg/d, titrate 5 mg/d weekly; max 40 mg/d dextroamphetamine/amphetamine (Adderall XR 5, 10, 15, 20, 25, 30 mg cap) 10 mg/d; max 30 mg/d lisdexamfetamine (Vyvanse 20, 30, 40, 50, 60, 70 mg cap) 30 mg QD; max 70 mg/d methylphenidate; max 60 mg/d: Concerta (18, 27, 36, 54 mg cap) 10 mg/d; titrate 18 mg/d weekly Daytrana (10, 15, 20, 30 mg/9 h patch) Metadate CD (10, 20, 30, 40, 50, 60 mg cap) 20 mg QAM Ritalin LA (10, 20, 30, 40 mg cap) 20 mg QAM	Nervousness, insomnia, arrhythmias, dry mouth, anorexia	Cardiovascular disease, hypertension, arterio- sclerosis, hyperthy- roidism, glaucoma, alcohol or drug abuse	Monitor growth and CNS activity. High abuse potential Not recommended for children <3 y Avoid late evening dosing.

(continued)

TABLE 43.3	**Overview of Agents Used to Treat ADHD (*Continued*)**			

Generic (Trade) Name and Dosage	Selected Adverse Events	Contraindications	Special Considerations

Short acting:
  dexamphenidate (Focalin 2.5, 5, 10 mg) 2.5 mg BID; max 20 mg/d
  dextroamphetamine (Dexedrine 5, 10, 15 mg cap): 5 mg/d, titrate 5 mg/d weekly; max 40 mg/d
  dextroamphetamine/amphetamine (Adderall 5, 7.5, 10, 12.5, 15, 20, 30 mg tab) 5 mg QD to BID; max 40 mg/d
  methylphenidate; > 6 y: 5 mg BID (before breakfast and lunch), titrate 5–10 mg/d weekly; max 60 mg/d
  methylphenidate (5, 10 mg tab)
  Methylin (5, 10, 20 mg tab)
  Ritalin (5, 10, 30 mg tab)
Intermediate acting:
  Methylphenidate; max 60 mg/d
    methylphenidate CR (10, 20 mg tab) 10 mg QAM
    Metadate ER (20 mg tab) 10 mg QAM
    Methylin ER (10, 20 mg cap) 10 mg QAM
    Ritalin SR (20 mg tab) 20 to 60 mg every 8h
	Tachycardia, nervousness, insomnia, anorexia, dizziness, drowsiness	Marked anxiety, tension, or agitation
		Glaucoma
		History of tics or Tourette syndrome in patient or family
			Monitor blood pressure, weight, height, heart rate, tics, sleep habits
			May potentiate effects of anticoagulants and anticonvulsants
			Abuse potential
			Not recommended for children <6 y

BID, twice daily; cap, capsule; CBC, comprehensive metabolic panel; CR, controlled release; ER, extended release; HS, at bedtime, max., maximum; QAM, every morning; QD, every day, QID, four times a day; tab, tablet; TID, three times a day; y, year

children frequently seem to show symptoms in structured settings such as school, weekend "drug holidays" are also reasonable, permitting dosage adjustments and disease assessment. Rebound hyperactivity may be more prominent. No studies have been done to compare the effectiveness of weekend holidays versus summer holidays.

While there is concern about the potential for addiction and future substance abuse, a review by Kollins (2003) suggested that the abuse potential for methylphenidate is less than that of other stimulants, such as cocaine. Other data indicate that there is less likelihood of substance abuse later in life when ADHD children take stimulant medication (Daley, 2004).

The stimulants are contraindicated in children with certain comorbid disorders. Practitioners should not prescribe methylphenidate to patients with marked anxiety, tension, or agitation; glaucoma; or a history of tics or Tourette syndrome. Dextroamphetamine is contraindicated in patients with cardiovascular disease, hypertension, arteriosclerosis, hyperthyroidism, glaucoma, or substance abuse.

Nonstimulant Medications

Atomoxetine

Atomoxetine (Strattera) is the first nonstimulant approved by the U.S. Food and Drug Administration (FDA) for treating ADHD. It is currently the only agent approved for adult ADHD. This agent also is not a controlled substance, and existing data suggest no real potential for abuse or diversion. While stimulants have greater treatment effect than atomoxetine, there are fewer adverse effects on appetite and sleep when compared to stimulants. However, there is more nausea and sedation, and it may be considered first-line therapy for ADHD treatment if the patient has an active substance abuse problem, comorbid anxiety, tics, or severe side effects to stimulants.

Mechanism of Action

Atomoxetine inhibits the reuptake of norepinephrine by inhibiting the presynaptic norepinephrine transporter (Christman et al., 2004). The agent has a relatively short half-life in normal metabolizers (5 hours) and an extended half-life in poor metabolizers (21 hours). The primary route of hepatic metabolism is the CYP2D6 pathway, and about 7% of Whites and less than 1% of Asians are considered poor CYP2D6 metabolizers (Christman, et al., 2004).

Dosage

In children and in adolescents who weigh <70 kg, the starting dose is 0.5 mg/kg/d for 4 days, then 1 mg/kg/d for 4 days, and then 1.2 mg/kg/day. For adolescents and adults over 70 kg, the starting dose is 40 mg; the dose is increased to an 80-mg target dose after a minimum of 3 days. The maximum recommended dose is 1.8 mg/kg/day for children and 100 mg for adolescents and adults; dosages should be adjusted only after 2 to 4 weeks of treatment at the lower dose. The medication is available in 10-, 18-, 25-, 40-, 60-, 80-, and

100-mg capsules. The agent can be given once or twice daily, with the second dose given in the evening.

Since this agent undergoes significant metabolism via the CYP2D6 system, slow metabolizers or patients taking agents with strong CYP2D6 effects (e.g., paroxetine, fluoxetine), the starting dose should be maintained for up to 4 weeks before dose adjustments are made. Patients with significant hepatic impairment should be started on a dose 50% of the usual starting dose.

Time Frame for Response

Atomoxetine is rapidly absorbed from the GI tract, leading to 63% bioavailability in extensive metabolizers and 94% bioavailability in poor metabolizers. The onset of action is quick, and dose adjustments are made in the first week. Despite the short half-life in extensive metabolizers, the duration of activity remains consistent throughout the day.

Contraindications

Atomoxetine should not be taken with MAO inhibitors because it increases synaptic norepinephrine concentrations. Further, due to the risk of angle closure, this agent should not be administered to patients with narrow-angle glaucoma.

Adverse Events

The increase in norepinephrine leads to an increase in blood pressure and heart rate, so this agent should be used cautiously in hypertensive patients or those with underlying cardiovascular disorders. In adults, there was a 3% rate of urinary retention or hesitation. Other common adverse effects include abdominal pain, vomiting, decreases in appetite, headache, irritability, and dermatitis. Atomoxetine dose not appear to promote the development of new tics and therefore may be a good choice for patients who cannot take stimulant medications due to pre-existing tics.

Interactions

This agent is a substrate of the CYP2D6 hepatic enzyme system, and levels of this agent can be increased when CYP2D6 inhibitors are administered.

Antidepressants

Efficacy of treatment with TCAs has been established, but not as substantially as with the stimulants (Spencer, et al., 1996). TCAs are most often used as second-line agents in patients who experience depression or other significant side effects with the stimulants, who do not respond to the stimulants, or who have tics or Tourette syndrome (Riddle, et al., 1988; Spencer, et al., 1993). They have a longer duration of action, so the patient does not need to take a dose during school hours. Also, no rebound effects are seen (Dulcan, et al., 1997).

TCAs also were effective in treating the core symptoms of ADHD. The sole controlled study that has been conducted using desipramine found that it was significantly more effective for treating core symptoms than a placebo (Wilens, et al., 1995). The rest of the drugs, including bupropion, fluoxetine

(Prozac), and venlafaxine (Effexor), have been studied only in open trials. Some clinicians have used them based on personal experience.

Dosage

Doses should be divided and the medication should be kept away from children because of the risk of overdose. Deaths have been reported in children taking desipramine (Norpramin); hence, imipramine (Tofranil) and nortriptyline (Pamelor) are the first-choice TCAs (Dulcan, et al., 1997).

Contraindications

Adequate monitoring is necessary, and practitioners must measure baseline vital signs and electrocardiograms (**Table 43.4**). Cardiac disease, a history of sudden death in the family, unexplained fainting, cardiomyopathy, or early cardiac disease may contraindicate the use of TCAs (Dulcan, et al., 1997).

Adverse Events

Toxicity manifests as irritability, mania, agitation, anger, aggression, forgetfulness, or confusion. Blood tests are necessary to determine whether the patient is experiencing toxicity (Dulcan, et al., 1997).

When discontinuing TCA therapy, the prescriber needs to taper the dose over 2 to 3 weeks to prevent anticholinergic withdrawal symptoms such as nausea, cramps, vomiting, headaches, and muscle pains. Of concern with TCAs is the potential for cardiac side effects, overdose, sedation, anticholinergic effects, and decreasing efficacy with continued use (Dulcan, et al., 1997).

Bupropion

Like the stimulants, bupropion (Wellbutrin) increases the reuptake of dopamine, but it also is a weak blocker of serotonin and norepinephrine. Again, it is unknown how these effects reduce ADHD symptoms. Studies show that the overall efficacy of bupropion does not differ from that of methylphenidate (Barrickman, et al., 1995). Adverse events are transient, lasting only for the first 2 weeks of treatment (Barrickman, et al., 1995), and include drowsiness, fatigue, nausea, anorexia, dizziness, "spaciness," anxiety, headache, and tremor. Rash and urticaria were also seen (Conners, et al., 1996). The most significant problem is a decrease in the seizure threshold, most often seen in patients with eating disorders (Dulcan, et al., 1997). Bupropion also may exacerbate tics and is contraindicated in patients with an active seizure disorder.

Table 43.3 lists the appropriate dose for bupropion. The dosage should not exceed 150 mg/day because of the increased risk for seizures with higher doses. Because of this increased risk, bupropion is contraindicated in patients with a history of seizure disorders.

Clonidine

Clonidine (Catapres) has been found to help with mood, activity level, cooperation, and tolerance of frustration. It is not effective in treating inattention but may be used to treat behavioral symptoms in children with tics (Steingard, et al., 1993) or in those who fail to respond to stimulants. In combination with stimulants, it may allow a lower dosage of stimulant medication.

Complications usually involve bradycardia, hypotension, and sedation. Sedation tends to decrease after several weeks and can be minimized with dose titration. The onset of action is slow, from 1 month to several months. When discontinuing clonidine, the prescriber needs to taper the dose to prevent withdrawal symptoms such as increased motor restlessness, headache, agitation, elevated blood pressure and pulse rate, and possible agitation of tics (Dulcan, et al., 1997).

Other adverse events include dry mouth, nausea, photophobia, hypotension, dizziness, and allergic skin reactions when the patch is used. Before prescribing the patch, the practitioner must determine the equivalent dose in tablets. (See **Table 43.3**.)

Guanfacine hydrochloride (Tenex), a longer-acting alpha-adrenergic agonist with a better side effect profile, has been studied only in open trials (Chappell, et al., 1995; Horrigan & Barnhill, 1995). Even though interest has been shown in using SSRIs to treat ADHD, no trials have supported their use for the core symptoms (Dulcan, et al., 1997). Because of their dietary restrictions and drug interaction profile, MAO inhibitors are not used to treat ADHD, even though efficacy has been shown (Dulcan, et al., 1997). Thioridazine (Mellaril) has been suggested as an alternative treatment of ADHD, but because of its limited effectiveness, sedation, cognitive dulling, and risk of tardive dyskinesia or neuroleptic malignant syndrome, it should be used only in unusual circumstances (Green, 1995). When discontinued, there should be a gradual taper over 1 to 2 weeks to avoid a sudden increase in blood pressure.

Special Population Considerations

Stimulants are also considered the best treatment option for adults. However, adults may have a difficult time because the frequency of dosing increases may lead to reduced compliance due to missed or forgotten doses. If ADHD is properly diagnosed, abuse of the drug usually is not a problem. In adults, tics and growth retardation are not a concern, but hypertension is. Methylphenidate is the stimulant most commonly used in adults because it is effective for nervousness, lack of concentration, anger, and fatigue (Wender, et al., 1981, 1985).

Selecting the Most Appropriate Agent

Because of the number of therapeutic options available, this section suggests only a general outline to follow. Nonpharmacologic therapy differs for children and adults. Nonpharmacologic therapy should be individualized for each patient. (See **Table 43.1**.) **Figure 43-1** outlines the therapeutic plan for a child, adolescent, and adult.

First-Line Therapy

Stimulants are the usual first-line therapy. It is possible to start with long- or short-acting amphetamines or methylphenidate, but methylphenidate is usually the first stimulant the practitioner tries because of its immediate action and ease of titration.

Second-Line Therapy

Most practitioners try atomoxetine or antidepressants, such as TCAs or buproprion, after a patient fails to respond to stimulant therapy. Currently, either nortriptyline or imipramine is used. Prescribers must consider the time frame of action for these agents. The longer onset of action and more extensive side effect profile make these agents less desirable than the stimulants.

Third-Line Therapy

After TCAs, bupropion is the next agent of choice. Again, prescribers must keep in mind the time it takes for the drug level to become therapeutic. This agent also may impair cognitive skills.

MONITORING PATIENT RESPONSE

To determine the efficacy of the drugs used to treat ADHD, practitioners must use the rating scales mentioned previously; no laboratory values or diagnostic tests can determine the patient's improvement.

Treatment is indicated for as long as the patient is showing core symptoms of ADHD. Practitioners can best determine the need to continue treatment by considering the patient's response during the "drug holidays." If symptoms are no longer present, treatment may not be needed. Continued assessment of the patient even when he or she is not using medication is essential. Monitoring parameters for the agents used to treat ADHD are summarized in **Table 43.4**. Medication should be given at the lowest effective dosage.

Studies show that stimulants' general side effects of insomnia, decreased appetite, dizziness, stomachache, and headache are usually mild and do not necessitate discontinuation of the drug (Ahmann, et al., 1993; Barkley, et al., 1990; Efron, et al., 1997). One study even suggested that these effects are more common in children with ADHD before

TABLE 43.4	Monitoring Parameters for Pharmacotherapy
Drug	**Monitoring Parameters**
atomoxetine	Blood pressure, pulse rate, mental status, weight periodically
bupropion	Weight monthly
clonidine	Blood pressure (standing and supine), respiratory rate and depth, heart rate monthly
dextroamphetamine	Growth, CNS activity monthly
imipramine	Blood pressure, pulse rate, ECG, CBC, mental status periodically
methylphenidate	Blood pressure, weight, height, heart rate, tics, sleep habits, drug use monthly
nortriptyline	Blood pressure, pulse rate, mental status, weight periodically

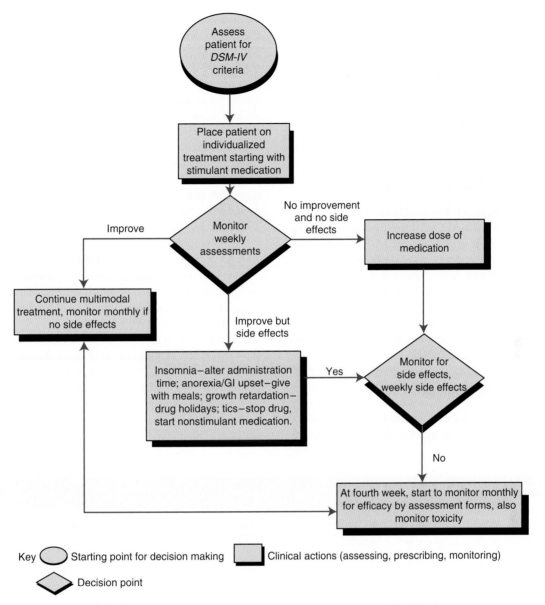

FIGURE 43–1   Treatment algorithm for attention-deficit/hyperactivity disorder.

treatment, although this has never been studied because of the difficulty of design (Efron, et al., 1997). In narrower studies involving sleep disturbances, the data are conflicting on whether treatment causes the child to have less satisfactory sleep and to take longer to fall asleep (Kent, et al., 1995; Tirosh, et al., 1993). Sleep difficulties may actually be related to the ADHD, which causes symptoms that prevent the child from sleeping. Because sleep disturbances cannot be generalized, it is reasonable to assess the patient and determine whether altered bedtimes or altered medication times are appropriate interventions.

In reviewing the complication of tics and dyskinesias, one study determined that transient tics develop in approximately 9% of children. The development of tics does not depend on prior personal or family history (Lipkin, et al., 1994). Even though this study showed that tics or dyskinesias are not

a contraindication, most health care professionals use stimulants cautiously in patients with prior histories.

Most of the other adverse events were discussed earlier. If any adverse event occurs that is disturbing to the patient, reasonable alternatives are to lower the dose or discontinue the medication. **Table 43.5** summarizes the most common adverse events. If the patient is using a stimulant and the outcome is poor, substituting another stimulant is reasonable before trying another medication class.

PATIENT EDUCATION

Medications prescribed for ADHD must be taken exactly as prescribed to get the full benefit. If any adverse events occur that are disturbing, the patient should contact the health care provider immediately. Parents and adult patients should be aware of adverse events to watch for, as previously discussed. Patients need to be evaluated on a regular basis to determine their treatment needs.

Drug Information

The FDA's website (www.fda.gov) is a good source of initial prescribing information. Sources such as Facts and Comparisons can also provide information about the use of these agents.

Patient-Oriented Information Sources

The National Institute of Mental Health (NIMH) has an excellent website related to ADHD (http://www.nimh.nih.gov/health/topics/attention-deficit-hyperactivity-disorder-adhd/index.shtml). This site provides access to booklets describing strategies for dealing with ADHD directed at parents of young children as well as adolescents. There are also links to local providers, clinical research trials, and other resources. CHADD (Children and Adults with Attention Deficit Disorder) at www.chadd.org is a great source of information and support for parents and patients with ADHD.

Nutrition/Lifestyle Changes

Dietary additives and supplements, such as dyes and preservatives, have long been implicated as a cause of ADHD symptoms.

Daley reviewed literature suggesting that removal of these from the diet in certain children may help, but the impact of the removal was less than that seen with stimulant medications (Daley, 2004).

Parent training involves teaching parents to recognize situations in which their child could learn or improve social skills. Parents must actively participate in the child's social life, using punishment effectively by clear instruction, positively reinforcing good behavior, ignoring some behaviors, and using negative reinforcement, such as time out, to decrease the child's stimulation. This method has been shown useful for the short term and is an alternative for parents who do not want to proceed directly to medication therapy (Anastopoulos, et al., 1993; Barkley, 1987, 1990).

As mentioned previously, the parents also may have ADHD (Dulcan, et al., 1997). Family therapy can help teach all members how to negotiate and solve problems together as a unit. Because family therapy may be expensive, parent support groups can promote effective problem-solving techniques and unity (Dulcan, et al., 1997).

Social skills training is based on the patient's deficits. Studies show that group training is more effective than individual training because self-observation usually is impossible for this patient population—both children and adults (Dulcan, et al., 1997).

Academic skills training helps to refine a child's ability to organize, take notes, improve study habits, and prioritize activities. This methodology has not been tested, but in clinical

TABLE 43.5	Summary of Adverse Events					
	MTH	**Dextro**	**Clon**	**Bupr**	**Imi**	**Nort**
Tachycardia	X					
Nervousness	X	X				
Insomnia	X	X		X		
Anorexia	X			X		
Dizziness	X		X	X	X	X
Drowsiness	X		X		X	X
Arrhythmias		X				
Anxiety			X	X		
Confusion			X	X		
Bradycardia						
Xerostomia			X	X	X	X
Constipation			X	X	X	X
Nausea			X	X	X	X
Agitation				X		
Fever, headache				X	X	X
Vomiting				X		
Seizures				X		
Tremor						
Increased appetite					X	
Weight gain					X	X
Skeletal weakness					X	X
Urinary retention						X

MTH, methylphenidate; Dextro, dextroamphetamine; Clon, clonidine; Bupr, bupropion; Imi, imipramine; Nort, nortriptyline

practice it has been found useful if academic deficiencies are present (Dulcan, et al., 1997).

Psychotherapy is not useful as treatment of ADHD but can help patients with moralization, self-esteem, and compliance problems. It may also be useful for patients with comorbid illnesses such as anxiety and depression. Psychotherapy may be needed only as difficulties arise (Dulcan, et al., 1997). Psychotherapy also can help adolescents become responsible for their own medication regimen (Dulcan, et al., 1997).

Cognitive behavior modification teaches stepwise problem solving and self-monitoring by using the reinforcement techniques of rewarding for good behavior and removing rewards for unwanted behavior. Although initially believed to be a good strategy, cognitive behavior modification was later found not to improve outcomes when added to medication therapy (Abikoff, 1985; Abikoff et al., 1988; Abikoff & Gittelman, 1985a, 1985b). Some adolescents and children may benefit, but young children are very unlikely to benefit (Abikoff & Hechtman, 1996). Practitioners of behavior modification try to determine how the child is responding to the environment and base interventions on the child's responses (Dulcan, et al., 1997).

Therapeutic recreation is based on the idea that development of sports skills or other recreational abilities can have a positive effect on a child or adolescent with ADHD. This can be accomplished through existing programs, such as those offered by the YMCA or the Big Brothers Big Sisters organizations, or even by promoting a role model relationship with a college or high-school student to build self-esteem (Dulcan, et al., 1997).

All these techniques offer different benefits, so individual assessment and reassessment are important to determine which techniques (if any) are making a difference for the patient. Some parents may want to try one or more of these methods before trying medication, and practitioners should permit the parents to try whatever methods they feel will be best for their child.

As with children, nonpharmacologic treatment also is beneficial for adults. "Coaching" involves daily encouragement to progress toward set goals. Educational programs help adults to identify their problem, understand it, and not blame themselves for it. Cognitive remediation also is used to teach attention enhancement, memory, problem solving, family relationships, time management, organization skills, and anger control (Kane, et al., 1990). Medication should not be used as a substitute for treating behaviors with behavior modification. Each patient's therapeutic plan should be assessed and reassessed for success and usefulness.

Complementary and Alternative Medications

There are several herbal medications that may have an impact on a person with ADHD. Gingko biloba, a plant-derived medication, has shown some efficacy in improving memory and improving concentration. This may prove useful in ADHD patients with inattention problems. Similarly, glutamine, a naturally occurring amino acid, may also improve concentration, alertness, and memory. However, neither of these agents has been proven in controlled clinical trials to improve these symptoms in patients with ADHD (Daley, 2004).

Case Study

Sam, age 8, is always interrupting his teacher, jumping out of his seat in class, fidgeting relentlessly, and butting into other children's games. At home, he runs around recklessly and is uncontrollable. His mother comes to you and wonders why he will not listen. She is concerned because his grades at school are dropping. After medical evaluation, you find nothing wrong with Sam physically, and he is taking no other medications. Through questioning, you determine that he has trouble concentrating on his homework, often forgets he has homework, loses pieces of games frequently, and hates to sit and read. His mother is unsure of the time frame over which these behaviors developed, but she thinks it has been since her second child was born 5 years ago. While in your office, Sam did not seem to be hyperactive or inattentive, but you notice he is easily distracted by people passing in the hallway because the door is slightly ajar.

DIAGNOSIS: ADHD

1. List specific goals of treatment for Sam.
2. What would be the first-line drug therapy for Sam? Why?
3. What monitoring parameters would you institute for Sam's parents? For his teachers?
4. Discuss specific patient education you would provide to Sam's parents based on the prescribed therapy.
5. Describe one or two drug–drug or drug–food interactions that you would be wary of when prescribing this agent.
6. List one or two adverse reactions to the agent you selected that would cause you to change therapy.
7. If the adverse reactions you described above occurred, what would be your second-line therapy for Sam? Why?
8. What over-the-counter and/or alternative medications would be appropriate for Sam?
9. What dietary and lifestyle changes would you recommend to Sam's parents?

BIBLIOGRAPHY

Starred references are cited in the text.

*Abikoff, H. (1985). Efficacy of cognitive training interventions in hyperactive children: A critical review. *Clinical Psychology Review, 5,* 479–512.

*Abikoff, H., Ganeles, D., Reiter, G., et al. (1988). Cognitive training in academically deficient ADHD boys receiving stimulant medication. *Journal of Abnormal Child Psychology, 16,* 411–432.

*Abikoff, H., & Gittelman, R. (1985a). Hyperactive children treated with stimulants: Is cognitive training a useful adjunct? *Archives of General Psychiatry, 42,* 953–961.

*Abikoff, H., & Gittelman, R. (1985b). The normalizing effects of methylphenidate on the classroom behavior of ADHD children. *Journal of Child Psychology, 13,* 334.

*Abikoff, H., & Hechtman, L. (1996). Multimodal therapy and stimulants in the treatment of children with ADHD. In P. Jensen & E. D. Hibbs (Eds.), *Psychosocial treatment for child and adolescent disorders: Empirically based approaches* (pp. 501–546). Washington, DC: American Psychological Association.

*Achenbach, T. M. (1991). *Manual for the Teacher's Report Form and 1991 Profile.* Burlington, VT: University of Vermont Department of Psychiatry.

*Adler, L. A., & Chua, H. C. (2002). Management of ADHD in adults. *Journal of Clinical Psychiatry, 63*(Suppl. 12), 29–35.

*American Psychiatric Association. (2000). *Diagnostic and statistical manual of mental disorders* (4th ed., text revision). Washington, DC: Author.

*Ahmann, P. A., Waltonen, S. J., Olson, K. A., et al. (1993). Placebo-controlled evaluation of Ritalin side effects. *Pediatrics, 91,* 1101–1106.

*Anastopoulos, A. D., Shelton, T. L., DuPaul, G. J., & Guevremont, D. C. (1993). Parent training for attention-deficit hyperactivity disorder: Its impact on parent functioning. *Journal of Abnormal Child Psychology, 21,* 581–596.

*Anonymous. (1999). A 14-month randomized clinical trial of treatment strategies for attention-deficit/hyperactivity disorder. The MTA Cooperative Group. Multimodal Treatment Study of Children with ADHD. *Archives of General Psychiatry, 56*(12), 1073–1086.

*Barkley, R. A. (1987). *Defiant children: A clinician's manual for parent training.* New York: Guilford.

*Barkley, R. A. (1990). *Attention deficit hyperactivity disorder: A handbook for diagnosis and treatment.* New York: Guilford.

*Barkley, R. A., McMurray, M. B., Edelbrock, C. S., & Robbins, K. (1989). The response of aggressive and nonaggressive children to two doses of methylphenidate. *Journal of the American Academy of Child and Adolescent Psychiatry, 28,* 873–881.

*Barkley, R. A., McMurray, M. B., Edelbrock, C. S., & Robbins, K. (1990). Side effects of methylphenidate in children with attention deficit hyperactivity disorder: A systemic, placebo-controlled evaluation. *Pediatrics, 86,* 184–192.

*Barrickman, L. L., Perry, P. F., Allen, A. J., et al. (1995). Bupropion versus methylphenidate in the treatment of attention-deficit hyperactivity disorder. *Journal of the American Academy of Child and Adolescent Psychiatry, 34,* 649–657.

*Biederman, J., Faraone, S. V., Doyle, A., et al. (1993). Convergence of the Child Behavior Checklist with structured interview-based psychiatric diagnoses of ADHD children with and without comorbidity. *Journal of Child Psychology and Psychiatry, 34,* 1241–1251.

*Buitelaar, J. K., Van der Gaag, R. J., Swaab-Barneveld, H., & Kuiper, M. (1995). Prediction of clinical response to methylphenidate in children with attention-deficit hyperactivity disorder. *Journal of the American Academy of Child and Adolescent Psychiatry, 8,* 1025–1032.

*Chappell, P. B., Riddle, M. A., Scahill, L., et al. (1995). Guanfacine treatment of comorbid attention-deficit hyperactivity disorder and Tourette's syndrome: Preliminary clinical experience. *Journal of the American Academy of Child and Adolescent Psychiatry, 34,* 1140–1146.

*Christman, A. K., Fermo, J. D., & Markowitz, J. S. (2004). Atomoxetine, a novel treatment for attention-deficit hyperactivity disorder. *Pharmacotherapy, 24*(8), 1020–1036.

Conners, C. K. (1969). A teacher rating scale for use in drug studies with children. *American Journal of Psychiatry, 126,* 884–888.

*Conners, C. K., Casat, C. D., Gualtieri, C. T., et al. (1996). Bupropion hydrochloride in attention deficit disorder with hyperactivity. *Journal of the American Academy of Child and Adolescent Psychiatry, 35,* 1314–1321.

*Daley, K. C. (2004). Update on attention-deficit/hyperactivity disorder. *Current Opinion in Pediatrics, 16,* 217–226.

*Dulcan, M. K., Dunne, J. E., Ayres, W., et al. (1997). Practice parameters for the assessment and treatment of children, adolescents, and adults with attention-deficit/hyperactivity disorder: AACAP Official Action. *Journal of the American Academy of Child and Adolescent Psychiatry, 36,* 85S–121S.

*Edelbrock, C., Costello, A. J., & Kessler, M. K. (1984). Empirical corroboration of attention deficit disorder. *Journal of the American Academy of Child Psychiatry, 23,* 285–290.

*Efron, D. E., Jarman, F., & Barker, M. (1997). Side effects of methylphenidate and dextroamphetamine in children with attention deficit hyperactivity disorder: A double-blind, crossover trial. *Pediatrics, 100,* 662–666.

*Farone, S. V., & Biederman, J. (1994). Genetics of attention-deficit hyperactivity disorder. *Child and Adolescent Psychiatry Clinics of North America, 3,* 285–301.

Gittelman, R. L., Mattes, J. A., & Klein, D. F. (1988). Methylphenidate and growth in hyperactive children. *Archives of General Psychiatry, 45,* 1127–1130.

*Goldman, L. S., Genel, M., Benzman, R. J., et al. (1998). Diagnosis and treatment of attention-deficit/hyperactivity disorder in children and adolescents. *Journal of the American Medical Association, 279,* 1100–1107.

*Green, W. H. (1995). The treatment of attention-deficit hyperactivity disorder with nonstimulant medications. *Child and Adolescent Psychiatry Clinics of North America, 4,* 169–195.

*Hauser, P., Zametkin, A. J., Martinez, P., et al. (1993). Attention deficit-hyperactivity disorder in people with generalized resistance to thyroid hormone. *New England Journal of Medicine, 328,* 997–1001.

Hechtman, L. (1993). Aims and methodological problems in multimodal treatment studies. *Canadian Journal of Psychiatry, 38,* 458–464.

*Horrigan, J. P., & Barnhill, L. J. (1995). Guanfacine for treatment of attention-deficit hyperactivity disorder in boys. *Journal of Child and Adolescent Psychopharmacology, 5,* 215–223.

Jensen, P. S. (1993). Development and implementation of multimodal and combined treatment studies in children and adolescents: NIMH perspectives. *Psychopharmacology Bulletin, 29,* 19–25.

*Kane, R., Mikalac, C., Benjamin, S., & Barkley, R. A. (1990). Assessment and treatment of adults with ADHD. In R. A. Barkley (Ed.). *Attention deficit hyperactivity disorder: A handbook for diagnosis and treatment* (pp. 613–654). New York: Guilford.

*Kent, J. D., Blader, J. C., Koplewics, H. S., et al. (1995). Effects of late-afternoon methylphenidate administration on behavior and sleep in attention-deficit hyperactivity disorder. *Pediatrics, 96,* 320–325.

Klein, R. G., Landa, B., Mattes, J. A., & Klein, D. F. (1988). Methylphenidate and growth in hyperactive children. *Archives of General Psychiatry, 45,* 1127–1130.

Klein, R. G., & Mannuzza, S. (1988). Hyperactive boys almost grown up: Methylphenidate effects on ultimate height. *Archives of General Psychiatry, 45,* 1131–1134.

*Kollins, S. H. (2003). Comparing the abuse potential of methylphenidate versus other stimulants: A review of available evidence and relevance to the ADHD patient. *Journal of Clinical Psychiatry, 64*(Suppl. 11), 14–18.

Levin, G. M. (1995). Attention-deficit/hyperactivity disorder: The pharmacist's role. *American Pharmacy, NS35,* 11–20.

*Lipkin, P. H., Goldstein, I. J., & Adesman, A. R. (1994). Tics and dyskinesias associated with stimulant treatment in attention-deficit hyperactivity disorder. *Archives of Pediatric and Adolescent Medicine, 148,* 859–861.

*Markussen, K., Dalsgaard, S., Obel, C., et al. (2003). Maternal lifestyle factors in pregnancy risk of attention deficit hyperactivity disorder and associated behaviors: Review of the current evidence. *American Journal of Psychiatry, 160,* 1028–1040.

*Nahlik, J. (2004). Issues in diagnosis of attention-deficit/hyperactivity disorder in adolescents. *Clinical Pediatrics, 43,* 1–10.

National Collaborating Centre for Mental Health. (2008). Attention deficit hyperactivity disorder. Diagnosis and management of ADHD in children, young people and adults. London: National Institute for Health and Clinical Excellence (NICE). (Clinical guideline; no. 72).

*Pliszka, S. (2007). AACAP Work Group on Quality Issues. Practice parameter for the assessment and treatment of children and adolescents with attention-deficit/hyperactivity disorder. *Journal of the American Academy of Child and Adolescent Psychiatry, 46*(7), 894–921.

*Pliszka, S. R., McCracken, J. T., & Maas, J. W. (1996). Catecholamines in attention-deficit hyperactivity disorder: Current perspectives. *Journal of the American Academy of Child and Adolescent Psychiatry, 35,* 264–272.

Richters, J. E., Arnold, L. E., Jensen, P. S., et al. (1995). NIMH collaborative multisite multimodal treatment study of children with ADHD: I. Background and rationale. *Journal of the American Academy of Child and Adolescent Psychiatry, 34,* 987–1000.

*Riddle, M. A., Hardin, M. T., Cho, S. C., et al. (1988). Desipramine treatment of boys with attention-deficit hyperactivity disorder and tics: Preliminary clinical experience. *Journal of the American Academy of Child and Adolescent Psychiatry, 27,* 811–813.

Rowe, K. S., & Rowe, K. J. (1994). Synthetic food coloring and behavior: A dose response effect in a double-blind, placebo-controlled, repeated-measures study. *Journal of Pediatrics, 125,* 691–698.

*Spencer, T., Biederman, J., Steingard, R., & Wilens, T. (1993). Bupropion exacerbates tics in children with attention-deficit hyperactivity disorder and Tourette's syndrome. *Journal of the American Academy of Child and Adolescent Psychiatry, 32,* 354–360.

*Spencer, T. J., Biederman, J., Wilens, T. E., & Faraone, S. V. (2002). Overview and neurobiology of attention-deficit/hyperactivity disorder. *Journal of Clinical Psychiatry, 63*(Suppl. 12), 3–9.

*Spencer, T., Biederman, J., Wilens, T., et al. (1996). Pharmacotherapy of attention-deficit hyperactivity disorder across the life cycle. *Journal of the American Academy of Child and Adolescent Psychiatry, 35,* 409–432.

*Steingard, R., Biederman, J., Spencer, T., Wilens, T., & Gonzales, A. (1993). Comparison of clonidine response in the treatment of attention-deficit hyperactivity disorder with and without comorbid tic disorders. *Journal of the American Academy of Child and Adolescent Psychiatry, 32,* 250–253.

*Sudak, H. S. (1998). Attending to attention deficit disorder: Diagnosis and treatment. *Notebook: Pennsylvania Hospital, 6*(1), 1–2.

*Tirosh, E., Saeh, A., Munvez, R., & Laurie, P. (1993). Effects of methylphenidate on sleep in children with attention-deficit hyperactivity disorder. *American Journal of Disorders in Children, 147,* 1313–1315.

*Ullmann, R. K., Sleator, E. K., & Sprague, R. L. (1985). Introduction to the use of ACTERS. *Psychopharmacology Bulletin, 21,* 915–919.

Ward, M. F., Wender, P. H., & Reimherr, F. W. (1993). The Wender Utah Rating Scale: An aid in the retrospective diagnosis of childhood attention deficit disorder. *American Journal of Psychiatry, 150,* 885–890.

*Weiss, M., & Murray, C. (2003). Assessment and management of attention-deficit hyperactivity disorder in adults. *Canadian Medical Association Journal, 168,* 715–722.

*Wender, P. H. (1995). *Attention-deficit hyperactivity disorder in adults.* New York: Oxford University Press.

*Wender, P. H., Reimherr, F. W., & Wood, D. R. (1981). Attention deficit disorder ("minimal brain dysfunction") in adults. *Archives of General Psychiatry, 38,* 449–456.

Wender, P. H., & Solanto, M. V. (1991). Effects of sugar on aggressive and inattentive behavior in children with attention deficit disorder with hyperactivity and normal children. *Pediatrics, 88,* 960–966.

*Wender, P. H., Wood, D. R., & Reimherr, F. W. (1985). Pharmacological treatment of attention deficit disorder, residual type (ADD, RT, "minimal brain dysfunction," "hyperactivity") in adults. *Psychopharmacology Bulletin, 212,* 222–231.

*Wilens, T. E., Biederman, J., Mick, E., & Spencer, T. J. (1995). A systematic assessment of tricyclic antidepressants in the treatment of adult attention-deficit hyperactivity disorder. *Journal of Nervous and Mental Disorders, 183,* 48–50.

CHAPTER 44

Angela Cafiero Moroney
Emily R. Hajjar

Alzheimer's Disease

Alzheimer's disease (AD), also known as *senile dementia of the Alzheimer's type,* is the most common cause of dementia accounting for approximately 60% to 80% of all dementias. AD is typified by a slow, progressive decline in cognition. Patients initially complain of short-term (recent) memory loss, forgetfulness, and a decreased ability to learn and retain new information.

Estimates suggest that approximately 5.5 million people in the United States and 35 million people worldwide have AD (Queforth & LaFerla, 2010). The number is expected to grow to 13.2 to 16 million in the United States by 2050 as the population continues to age (Queforth & LaFerla, 2010). A majority of individuals with AD are residing in the community, which represents a huge emotional and financial burden on the patient, friends, and family members, as well as on society as a whole. The cost of care (including general, medical, and long-term care at a facility outside of the home) per patient is estimated at approximately $40,000 to $60,000 a year, totaling approximately $150 billion each year in the United States. This number does not include the cost of unpaid care given by family members or loved ones.

Patients may have sporadic or familial AD. Sporadic AD is the classic form of AD, occurring most often in patients age 65 or older (late onset). Familial AD is less common and affects patients with genetic mutations of amyloid precursor protein (APP), presenilin-1, and presenilin-2. Familial AD may be of early onset (age 65) or of late onset (Lendon, et al., 1997). Genetic causes (e.g., apolipoprotein E4 allele, presenilin-1, and presenilin-2 gene mutations) have also been linked to sporadic or late-onset AD. Symptoms of AD can be divided between cognitive symptoms or noncognitive symptoms. Treatment is based on the particular domain of the symptoms. Cognitive symptoms, such as loss of short-term memory, usually present first in mild AD, whereas the noncognitive behavioral symptoms are seen in more moderate to severe AD. Currently, AD is incurable although pharmacologic agents have been used to modestly slow the progression of the disease. The average life span for patients with AD is reduced by as much as 70% and generally ranges from 4 to 6 years after diagnosis (Larson, et al., 2004). In the United States, AD is the sixth leading cause of death and the fifth leading cause of death for patients older than age 65. Women are at a slightly higher risk for developing AD than men. Prevalence increases with age, with AD affecting approximately 50% of those older than age 85. Patients commonly die from indirect causes of AD such as aspiration, infection, malnutrition, or pulmonary embolism (Morris, 1994).

CAUSES

Apolipoprotein E (ApoE), a protein involved in cholesterol transport, is linked to the development of AD. The E4 allele (homozygote E4/E4) is thought to increase the risk of AD, whereas the E2 allele may be protective, particularly for sporadic AD. Advanced age and family history are the most significant risk factors for AD. The risk factors and protective factors for AD are listed in **Box 44.1.**

PATHOPHYSIOLOGY

Pathologic changes in AD include formation of neurofibrillary tangles and senile plaques, cortical atrophy, and neuronal (cholinergic, glutamatergic) destruction and loss. In AD patients, acetylcholine levels are decreased and an excessive stimulation of glutamate causes neuronal toxicity. These changes affect several areas of the brain, including the hippocampus, amygdala, cerebral cortex, and ultimately the motor cortex. As a result of these changes, short- and long-term memory, learning, language, behavior, and eventually motor skills are impaired.

Neurofibrillary Tangles

Neurofibrillary tangles and senile (also known as *neuritic* or *β-amyloid*) plaques are the hallmark pathologic lesions in AD. Tau protein, the principal component of neurofibrillary tangles, becomes hyperphosphorylated in AD. The abnormal phosphorylation of tau protein leads to the formation of paired helical filaments and finally neurofibrillary tangles. As a result, microtubule assembly is inhibited and critical organelles may collapse, causing abnormal intracellular transport and neuronal cell death.

Senile Plaques

Senile plaques are brain lesions that contain a core of β-amyloid protein (BAP) and a shell of damaged neurites. APP is the parent protein of BAP. Proteases normally cleave APP through the BAP region, which prevents intact BAP from entering the extracellular fluid. When abnormal proteolysis occurs, leaving BAP intact, increased extracellular BAP becomes involved in senile plaque formation and neuronal degeneration. Senile plaques are also composed of protease inhibitors, tau protein, ApoE, and glial cells, which may be involved in the pathologic process of AD and are areas of interest to researchers. Neurofibrillary tangles and senile plaque density correlate with increased severity of AD.

Neuronal Destruction

The neuronal cell damage and death seen in AD results in impaired neurotransmitter function. The cholinergic and glutamatergic systems are significantly involved. In particular, cholinergic neurons in the nucleus basalis of Meynert are damaged. Destruction of cholinergic neurons leads to decreased levels of acetylcholine, a neurotransmitter that aids in learning and memory. The symptomatic presentation of AD (memory loss and cognitive impairment) appears to be associated with acetylcholine deficiency. The cholinergic system has been the subject of a vast amount of research and pharmacologic development (e.g., acetylcholinesterase inhibitors). Overstimulation or erratic stimulation of the glutamatergic system in the synapse causes neuronal toxicity leading to neuronal death. This disruption is thought to impair learning and memory.

The autoimmune system or inflammatory mediators may be linked to late-onset AD. Glial cells, complement cascade components, and cytokines are present in plaque areas. These cells and inflammatory mediators may contribute to neuronal cell damage and loss. Their role in AD is under investigation, as is the use of anti-inflammatory drugs and 3-hydroxy-3-methylglutaryl-coenzyme A (HMG CoA) reductase inhibitors to prevent cell damage.

DIAGNOSTIC CRITERIA

The clinical diagnosis of AD can be made using the National Institute of Neurological and Communicative Disorders, and Stroke and the Alzheimer's Disease and Related Disorders Association (NINCDS-ADRDA) criteria, or the *Diagnostic and Statistical Manual of Mental Disorders* (4th ed.), known as the *DSM-IV*. The diagnosis can be *confirmed* only by autopsy. Diagnostic criteria include MMSE, deficits in two or more areas of cognition, insidious onset, no loss of consciousness, and the absence of other diseases that may account for the symptoms of AD.

Patients and their caregivers should be intimately involved in the diagnostic process. A complete history and physical examination that includes a neurologic and mental status evaluation (**Table 44.1**) is essential. The Mini–Mental State Examination (MMSE) may be used to screen for cognitive impairment. The clock-drawing task (CDT) is another initial evaluation tool that is quick and can be performed by any health care professional (**Figure 44-1**). Additional tools that are useful for monitoring changes in function, behavior, and cognition are the Functional Activities Questionnaire and the Revised Memory and Behavior Problems Checklist.

INITIATING DRUG THERAPY

A careful assessment of baseline diagnostic findings is essential before initiating drug therapy. The patient, family, and caregiver should be informed of the severity of cognitive and functional impairment. Baseline scores on the MMSE, CDT, and Functional Activities Questionnaire can help guide decisions related to drug therapy. Reversible causes of dementia must also be considered and eliminated because several medications and medical conditions may cause or aggravate dementia (**Box 44.2**).

Before starting drug therapy for the cognitive symptoms of AD, the patient or family should demonstrate a clear under-

TABLE 44.1	**Mini–Mental State Examination for Cognitive Function**	
Function	**Test**	**Maximum Score**
Orientation	What is the year? season? date? month? day?	5
	Where are we—what state? county? town or city? hospital floor?	5
Registration	Repeat after me: "apple," "table," "penny." (*Physician names objects and asks the patient to repeat until accurate.*)	3
Attention and calculation	Spell "world" backwards.	5
Recall	What were the three words you named before? (*Patient should answer "apple," "table," "penny"*).	3
Language	What is this? (*Physician points to two common objects, e.g., a pencil and a watch.*)	2
	Repeat after me: "No ifs, ands, or buts."	1
	Take a piece of paper in your right hand, fold it in half, and put it on the floor.	3
	Close your eyes.	1
	Write a sentence.	1
	Copy this design:	1

Data from Folstein, M. F., Folstein, S. E., & McHugh, P. R. (1975). Mini–Mental State: A practical method for grading the cognitive state of patients for the clinician. *Journal of Psychiatric Research, 12*(3), 189–198.

standing of the efficacy and expected outcomes of treatment, as well as the potential adverse events, costs, and incurability of the disease. The choice not to initiate drug therapy is also a reasonable option as many patients only experience modest benefits from drug therapy.

Pharmacologic management of the noncognitive symptoms is tailored to the individual symptom. These medications are usually initiated when the patient progresses to the moderate to severe stages of AD. The use of both noncognitive and cognitive therapies may be necessary as the disease progresses.

Nonpharmacologic psychotherapies, such as behavior-oriented, emotion-oriented, cognition-oriented, and stimulation-oriented approaches, can be useful for some patients with AD. These treatments may have some initial benefit, but can be associated with an increase in patient frustration, agitation, and depression. The risks of these psychotherapies, especially cognition-oriented treatments, may outweigh the benefits.

Other nonpharmacologic interventions include using calendars, clocks, and written notes or instructions. The caregiver should attempt to maintain a predictable routine with the patient. Drastic changes in the environment, as well as confrontation and arguments, should be avoided. Recognition of

precipitants of agitation, psychosis, and anxiety can assist the caregiver and health care provider to best develop a patient-specific treatment plan.

The patient's ability to drive should be evaluated, and as AD progresses, the patient should be advised to stop driving because dementia may increase the risk of accidents. The patient's use of a stove should be evaluated because, if left on and unattended, it can be harmful. Families should be taught how to prevent falls and wandering. They should also be informed about the possibility of physical violence and suicide associated with more severe disease. Capable patients may want to discuss with their families advance directives, living wills, desires for nursing home placement, and powers of attorney.

Patient and family education are the most important nonpharmacologic interventions for AD. Depending on the stage of impairment, the patient requires some or full assistance with activities of daily living (ADL), such as dressing, toileting, and, particularly, driving. Support for patients and families is vitally important at any stage of AD (**Box 44.3**), and anyone involved with a patient with AD should be educated on the availability of support groups to deal with the wide variety of issues associated with AD. Other resources for the caregiver include the use of respite care centers and day care centers.

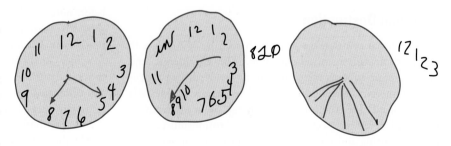

FIGURE 44–1 Clock drawing task completed by various elderly subjects. They were asked to draw a clock that represented 20 minutes after 8. The clock at left represents a normal result. The middle clock and the clock at right were drawn by elderly patients with dementia. (Adaptation based on a clock drawing test, courtesy of Pfizer Inc. and Ensai Inc.)

BOX 44.2

Potentially Reversible Causes of Dementia

Medications

Anticholinergics (e.g., benztropine, diphenhydramine)
Antidepressants (e.g., amitriptyline, imipramine)
Antipsychotics (e.g., thioridazine)
Anxiolytics (e.g., diazepam, lorazepam)
Cardiovascular agents (e.g., digoxin, propranolol)
Corticosteroids
Histamine (H_2) blockers (e.g., cimetidine)
Metoclopramide

Metabolic Disorders

Dehydration
Hyperthyroidism and hypothyroidism
Hyponatremia
Hypercalcemia

Intracranial Infection or Disease

Meningitis
Neurosyphilis
Normal-pressure hydrocephalus
Subdural hematoma
Tumor
Toxoplasmosis

Miscellaneous

Toxins (e.g., lead, mercury, alcohol)
Vitamin B_{12} deficiency
Depression
Psychoses

Data from Wiser, T. H. (1994). Alzheimer's disease. *US Pharmacist, 63.*

Goals of Drug Therapy

The optimal goal of drug therapy is to maintain and maximize the patient's functional ability, quality of life, and independence for as long as possible while minimizing adverse events and cost (Small, et al., 1997). A multidisciplinary approach to therapy, which includes the patient and family, a physician, a psychiatric specialist, a nurse, a social worker, and a pharmacist, is the ideal. Drug therapy choices for the cognitive symptoms include the cholinesterase inhibitors, memantine (Namenda), and selegiline (Eldepryl).

BOX 44.3

Alzheimer's Disease Support Groups and Resources

Alzheimer's Association

Phone: 1-800-272-3900
Web site: http://www.alz.org

Alzheimer's Disease Education and Referral (ADEAR) Center

Phone: 1-800-438-4380
Web site: http://www.nia.nih.gov/alzheimers

Eldercare Locator Service (ELS)

Phone: 1-800-677-1116
Web site: http://www.eldercare.gov

Selected Agents for Cognitive Symptoms

Cholinesterase Inhibitors

Cholinesterase inhibitors, also known as the *acetylcholinesterase inhibitors,* play a key role in the pharmacologic treatment of AD. This drug class includes tacrine (Cognex), donepezil (Aricept), rivastigmine (Exelon), and galantamine (Razadyne, Razadyne ER), which are indicated for mild to moderate dementia of the AD type. These agents are used to slow the progression of the cognitive, functional, and behavioral domains of AD. Patients and families may report improvement—or lack of continued decline—within 3 to 6 weeks of beginning treatment.

If no effect is seen within 3 to 6 months of treatment or the patient is experiencing an adverse effect, another agent from this class may be tried. They are not curative and the improvements correlate with approximately a 6-month symptom decline in untreated patients. It is unknown how long treatment with these agents should be continued. However, once a patient progresses to severe AD, these agents are no longer solely recommended. Additional pharmacologic therapy may be necessary once the disease progresses into the moderate to severe stages. Thoughtful discussions with caregivers or families may guide the decision to discontinue therapy.

Cholinesterase inhibitors inhibit one or both types of the cholinesterase enzymes, butyrylcholinesterase or acetylcholinesterase. Butyrylcholinesterase is primarily found in the periphery, and inhibition of this enzyme leads to many of the adverse effects of the cholinesterase agents. Acetylcholinesterase is found more centrally and thus is the primary focus of inhibition for the use in AD.

Tacrine was the first cholinesterase inhibitor approved by the U.S. Food and Drug Administration (FDA) for treating the cognitive symptoms of mild to moderate AD. This agent has fallen out of use due to the severe hepatotoxicity associated with it, 4-times-a-day dosing, and the approval of safer cholinesterase inhibitors. Donepezil is the second cholinesterase inhibitor approved and can be used for all stages of AD. Both agents are thought to improve cognitive symptoms by reversing cholinesterase inhibition to increase the concentrations of acetylcholinesterase in the cerebral cortex. The effects of tacrine and donepezil, however, depend on functioning cholinergic neurons, and their efficacy likely decreases as AD progresses.

Rivastigmine is the third cholinesterase inhibitor with its potential advantage of being pseudo-irreversible. It inhibits the enzyme for about 10 hours, making this an intermediate-acting agent. It is notable that rivastigmine is the only cholinesterase inhibitor that is approved to treat both mild to moderate AD as well as mild to moderate dementia associated with Parkinson's disease. Galantamine is the fourth approved cholinesterase inhibitor on the market and is indicated to treat mild to moderate AD. Besides inhibiting the cholinesterase enzyme, it also allosterically modulates the nicotinic receptor.

The cholinesterase inhibitors have been shown to slow the progression of AD. These medications have also had positive effects on the noncognitive or behavioral symptoms of AD. They have been shown to reduce apathy, psychosis, anxiety, depression, and agitation. Although these medications appear to improve the cognitive function of patients with AD, there is no evidence that they alter the course of the disease.

Dosage

The cholinesterase inhibitors may modestly improve cognitive function or delay decline in cognitive function. The observed delay in cognitive decline correlates with approximately a 6-month decline in patients treated with placebos. Clinical studies of these agents versus a placebo show that maximum efficacy by the maximum dose. Thus, it is necessary to titrate the cholinesterase inhibitor to the maximum tolerated dose.

Donepezil therapy is initiated at a dose of 5 mg daily. The dosage may be increased after 4 to 6 weeks to a maximum dose of 10 mg/d if tolerated. Donepezil 10 mg/d is slightly more effective than the 5-mg dose; therefore, increasing to 10 mg/d is appropriate for patients who do not respond within 6 weeks of treatment with the 5-mg dose. A 23-mg dose may be tried in moderate to severe patients that have been stable on 10 mg daily for at least 3 months. Donepezil is available as a tablet as well as an orally disintegrating tablet for patients who have trouble swallowing. Rivastigmine doses should be started at 1.5 mg twice a day and should increase to 3 mg twice a day after 2 weeks of treatment for the capsule and oral solution formulations. Further dose increases should be based on clinical response and can be attempted on a biweekly basis. The maximum dose is 6 mg twice a day for the capsule and oral solution formulations. If the patch formulation of rivastigmine is started, the dose should be 4.6 mg/24 hours and can be titrated to 9.5 mg/24 hours after 4 weeks, if tolerated. Galantamine is available as an immediate-release tablet and oral solution as well as in extended-release capsules. The immediate-release forms of galantamine are started at a dose of 4 mg twice a day and titrated up every 4 weeks as tolerated to a maximum dose of 24 mg/d (12 mg twice daily). The extended-release formulation of galantamine is started at 8 mg daily and can be titrated up to a dose of 24 mg/d in 4-week intervals.

Adverse Events

The major adverse effects of the cholinesterase inhibitors are cholinergic, most commonly nausea, vomiting, and diarrhea (5% to 47%). Oral formulations of rivastigmine have been associated with the highest incidence of these gastrointestinal (GI) disturbances (19% to 47%); the patch is associated with much lower rates (6% to 20%). These effects are dose dependent and can be minimized by slowly titrating to higher doses (**Table 44.2**).

A major adverse effect of tacrine, but not the other cholinesterase inhibitors, is the development of reversible hepatocellular damage. This occurs in approximately 30% of patients taking tacrine. As a result, strict hepatic enzyme monitoring is required with the medication. Tacrine has a limited use due to this adverse effect.

Bradycardia can occur with the use of the cholinesterase inhibitors, and they should be used with caution in patients with sick sinus syndrome. Hyperacidity can also occur with cholinesterase inhibitors, and they should be used with caution in patients with a history of peptic ulcer disease and who currently take nonsteroidal anti-inflammatory drugs (NSAIDs). Although these effects are not common, they are of concern and should be closely monitored in patients who are at risk. Donepezil is also associated with insomnia or nightmares. If these conditions occur, the dosing of donepezil before bed should be changed to a morning administration. Despite the GI effects associated with a rapid increase in dose, these agents appear to be well tolerated.

Interactions

Drug interactions with cholinesterase inhibitors include synergy with other cholinergic agents (e.g., succinylcholine [Quelicin]). Tacrine, donepezil, and galantamine are metabolized by the P450 enzyme system. Tacrine is a substrate for isoenzyme 1A2; donepezil and galantamine are substrates for 2D6 and 3A4. A potential advantage of rivastigmine is that it is metabolized by hydrolysis and thus is not susceptible to the drug interactions associated with the P450 enzyme system. Inhibitors of these isoenzymes would cause an increased drug concentration of the cholinesterase inhibitor and thus more susceptible to cholinergic adverse effects.

Memantine (Namenda)

Memantine is a new drug to a new class of agents, the *N*-methyl-D-aspartate (NMDA) receptor antagonists. This

TABLE 44.2   **Overview of Cholinesterase Inhibitors, Vitamin E, and Selegiline**

Generic (Trade) Name and Dosage	Selected Adverse Events	Contraindications	Special Considerations
donepezil (Aricept) Start: 5 mg every day Range: 5–23 mg/d Start 5 mg every day × 4 wk then 10 mg daily. If stable for 3 mo, may increase to 23 mg/d	*GI:* nausea, vomiting *CV:* bradycardia, syncope	Hypersensitivity to agent or piperidine derivatives	If nightmares occur, dose in the morning.
rivastigmine (Exelon) Oral: Start 1.5 mg bid for 2 wk, then increase by 1.5 mg bid; max. 6 mg bid Range: 3–6 mg bid Patch: Start one patch (4.6 mg/24 h) daily × 4 wk, then increase to one patch (9.5 mg/24 h) daily	Nausea, vomiting, anorexia, dyspepsia, fatigue, headache malaise	Hypersensitivity to agent or carbamate derivatives	Initial response seen within 12 wk of therapy
galantamine (Razadyne, Razadyne ER) IR: Start: 4 mg bid × 4 wk Range: 4–12 mg bid ER: Start 8 mg daily × 4 wk Range: 8–24 mg	Nausea, vomiting, diarrhea, anorexia, abdominal pain, dyspepsia, dizziness, sleep disturbances	Hypersensitivity to agent Severe hepatic, renal impairment	Moderate hepatic, renal impairment should not exceed a dose of 16 mg/d
tacrine (Cognex) Start: 10 mg qid Range: 10–40 mg qid	*GI:* nausea, vomiting *CV:* bradycardia, syncope Hepatic: elevated transaminases	Hypersensitivity to agent Prior history of jaundice with agent	Alanine aminotransferase monitoring required.
vitamin E Start: 1,000 IU bid	Falls, syncope, bleeding	Hypersensitivity to agent	May increase INR and risk of bleeding in vitamin K–deficient patients or those taking warfarin.
selegiline (Eldepryl) Start: 5 mg in AM and at lunchtime	Orthostatic hypotension, insomnia	Hypersensitivity to agent	Monitor blood pressure. Dose in morning and at lunchtime to minimize insomnia

ER, extended-release; INR, international normalized ratio; IR, immediate release.

drug was approved in 2003 for the treatment of moderate to severe AD. It has a novel mechanism of action, which focuses on the glutamatergic system as compared to the cholinesterase inhibitors' effect on the cholinergic system. Memantine blocks the activation of the NMDA receptor during an abundance of glutamate. Thus, this blocks overstimulation of the NMDA receptor, and neuronal degeneration is inhibited. It does not interfere with the pathologic activation of the NMDA receptor during learning and memory formation.

Clinical trials have shown that memantine used alone in patients with moderate to severe AD has produced reduced clinical deterioration over 28 weeks. When memantine was added to donepezil therapy, it resulted in significantly better cognition and activities of daily living compared to a placebo over 24 weeks. Memantine should be started at 5 mg once daily and titrated every week, if tolerated, to a maximum dose of 10 mg twice daily. Food has no effect on the onset or absorption of memantine. In general, memantine was well tolerated compared to a placebo. Memantine is minimally metabolized by the P450

enzyme system and thus not susceptible to P450 enzyme interactions. It is largely excreted renally via tubular secretion and, thus, there is the potential for decreased renal clearance with other drugs that undergo tubular secretion (e.g., amantadine, ranitidine).

Overall, clinical trials have been positive regarding the use of memantine for moderate to severe AD. With a different mechanism of action and indication for moderate to severe AD, memantine has a unique role for treatment of AD. In the past, once a cholinesterase inhibitor failed, no other viable option for therapy was available. Now, the addition of memantine to a cholinesterase inhibitor may be an option.

Selegiline

Selegiline (Eldepryl), a selective monoamine oxidase (MAO) type B inhibitor, is a potential treatment option for patients with moderate AD. The drug is thought to have antioxidant or neuroprotective properties. The evidence for the use of selegiline is still limited.

Selegiline may be tried for patients who cannot tolerate cholinesterase inhibitors because some evidence indicates that it not only delays disease progression, but it may improve cognition—although improvement in cognition was not observed in the study by Sano and colleagues (1997). There does not appear to be a combined role for the use of selegiline and vitamin E because their effects together may be worse than with either agent used alone. Again, patients and families should be educated about the potential risks and benefits of the use of these agents.

Based on efficacy data, a dosage of 5 mg orally twice a day is recommended. Orthostatic hypotension, hallucinations, agitation, and insomnia are possible adverse events, although selegiline is in general well tolerated at doses of 10 mg/d or less. Nonselective inhibition of MAO can occur at daily doses exceeding 10 mg. Doses greater than 10 mg/d increase the risk of hypertensive crisis with tyramine-containing foods (e.g., cheese, wine). For further discussion of tyramine and MAO inhibitors, refer to Chapter 40. Drug interactions with carbamazepine (Tegretol), selective serotonin reuptake inhibitors (SSRIs), tricyclic antidepressants (TCAs), venlafaxine (Effexor), or meperidine (Demerol) can cause increased toxicity (agitation, delirium, seizures, and death) as well.

Atypical Agents

Ergoloid mesylates (e.g., Hydergine) have been studied for treating cognitive impairment in dementia. Their use is not recommended because of lack of clear efficacy data.

Epidemiologic data also suggest that NSAIDs, cyclooxygenase inhibitors, and estrogen replacement therapy may protect patients against AD. The use of these agents, however, is not recommended because of the lack of well-designed efficacy trials, adverse effects, and the potential risks of therapy (American Psychiatric Association [APA], 1997).

The use of HMG CoA reductase inhibitors (statins) has been gaining notoriety for the use of preserving cognitive function in patients with cognitive impairment. The exact mechanism for preserving cognitive function is still unknown; however, it is postulated that reducing the cholesterol content in the brain could decrease the formation of the plaques. There are not enough data to support using a statin in all patients with cognitive impairment.

In patients older than age 60 using statins (lovastatin and pravastatin), one observational study showed up to a 73% lower risk of developing AD compared to those not taking one of these agents. Because it is not a true cause-and-effect relationship, it is not routinely recommended for use as AD prevention.

Selected Agents for Noncognitive Symptoms

Antipsychotic Agents

The noncognitive symptoms of AD include agitation, psychosis, anxiety, depression, and sleep disorders. Approximately one half of patients with dementia experience agitation. Many patients with AD also experience psychotic symptoms, such as delusions, hallucinations, and paranoia. Agitation and psychosis, which may be particularly frightening for families and caregivers, should be treated if the patient is causing harm to self or others.

The choice of an antipsychotic agent is based on cost and adverse events. Choosing an agent with a low degree of anticholinergic activity seems warranted in patients with AD. High-potency agents, such as haloperidol (Haldol), are associated with fewer anticholinergic effects as compared to low-potency agents, such as chlorpromazine (Thorazine). Atypical antipsychotics are associated with less extrapyramidal symptoms than the typical agents; thus, these agents are preferred.

Although atypical antipsychotics are preferred, none of the agents are approved to treat the noncognitive symptoms of dementia, and they all contain a black box warning alerting patients and caregivers to the fact that they are associated with an increased risk of death in patients with dementia-related psychosis. Risperidone (Risperdal) and olanzapine (Zyprexa) have also been associated with an increased risk of stroke in patients using these agents for behavioral disturbances associated with dementia. It is important for the practitioner to weigh the risks versus benefits of using these agents.

Cost may limit the use of atypical antipsychotics. The role of the newer atypical antipsychotic agents (e.g., quetiapine [Seroquel], ziprasidone [Geodon], aripiprazole [Abilify], iloperidone [Fanapt], asenapine [Saphris], and paliperidone [Invega]) remains to be determined. Regardless of the agent chosen, the lowest effective dose should be used. The practitioner should reassess the need for these medications periodically (every 3 to 6 months).

Benzodiazepines

Benzodiazepines have been prescribed to treat behavioral problems related to dementia. Because they do not appear to be as effective as the antipsychotics for treating behavioral problems, benzodiazepines are often reserved for treating symptoms of anxiety or for episodic agitation. These agents can be used as needed in situations that precipitate acute anxiety.

If a benzodiazepine is prescribed, lorazepam (Ativan) or oxazepam (Serax) are appropriate choices. They are inexpensive, have a short half-life, and hepatic metabolism is not significantly altered in the elderly. All benzodiazepines should be started at the lowest dose. The suggested starting dose for lorazepam is 0.5 to 1 mg orally every 4 to 6 hours, and the starting dose for oxazepam is 10 mg orally 3 times per day. The advantage of lorazepam is that it is available parenterally.

Adverse effects of benzodiazepines include falls, sedation, delirium, and loss of inhibition. Routine use is not recommended because of limited efficacy, adverse effects, and potential for worsening AD symptoms. The use of benzodiazepines for anxiety associated with dementia should be reevaluated periodically.

Data on using various other agents (trazodone [Desyrel], valproate [Depakene], carbamazepine [Tegretol], buspirone [BuSpar], SSRIs, and beta blockers) for treating anxiety associated with AD are limited. These agents may have a role in treating agitation in patients who do not tolerate or respond to antipsychotic agents or benzodiazepines.

Antidepressants

Because there is a high incidence of depression associated with dementia, pharmacologic treatment is often necessary. Patients may not meet explicit criteria for a depressive syndrome, but it is recommended that these patients still be offered treatment. Treatment may improve cognition, mood, apathy, function, behavior, appetite, sleep, and overall quality of life. Because there is no evidence that one class of antidepressants is superior to another in treating depression, the prescriber may base the choice of an agent on the individual patient, cost, side effect profile, and potential drug interactions.

In many clinical practices, SSRIs, such as sertraline (Zoloft) or citalopram (Celexa), have become a first-line therapy for depression in the elderly. The recommended starting dose of sertraline is 25 mg taken orally each morning. Patients who experience anxiety or insomnia with this agent can be given a trial of paroxetine, which is more sedating. Citalopram, in addition to its antidepressant effects, has proved beneficial in improving certain emotional symptoms of AD (panic, bluntness, depressed mood, confusion, irritability, anxiety, and restlessness) in patients with and without depression. SSRIs in general have fewer side effects (particularly anticholinergic) than TCAs or MAO inhibitors, but they may be more costly to the patient.

TCAs (e.g., nortriptyline [Pamelor]) may also have a beneficial role. However, TCAs have more anticholinergic side effects that have limited their use. Psychostimulants, such as methylphenidate (Ritalin), have been used for treating apathy, but they should be used with caution in patients with AD because they may worsen agitation and cause sleep disorders.

Selecting the Most Appropriate Agent for Cognitive Symptoms

First-Line Therapy

Once the decision has been made to initiate drug therapy, cholinesterase inhibitors may be tried (**Figure 44-2**). Donepezil is considered the first choice because fewer adverse events are associated with its use and the once-daily dosing schedule is easier to follow. These medications, however, are expensive and only modestly benefit cognitive function. Patients with severe AD may be offered memantine in conjunction with a cholinesterase inhibitor (**Table 44.3**). The combination therapy is expensive and could only provide moderate benefit.

Second-Line Therapy

Second-line therapy is a trial of a different cholinesterase inhibitor. In conjunction, some providers may add vitamin E. Vitamin E has a benign side effect profile and minimal cost and may be added to acetylcholinesterase inhibitor regimens in patients with mild to moderate AD.

Third-Line Therapy

Another trial of a different cholinesterase inhibitor is a third-line choice if the patient has mild to moderate AD. Selegiline may be considered for patients who experience adverse events (e.g., bleeding) with vitamin E and who are unable to tolerate acetylcholinesterase inhibitor therapy.

MONITORING PATIENT RESPONSE

Consensus guidelines suggest that the primary care provider should schedule appointments with patients with AD and families every 3 to 6 months to monitor cognitive and behavioral symptoms and to assess the patient's response to pharmacotherapy. If clinical improvement does not occur with a cholinesterase inhibitor after 3 to 6 months of treatment, the practitioner may consider switching to another cholinesterase inhibitor. After all cholinesterase inhibitors have been tried, the provider should assess whether the patient should stop the medication. The MMSE is a useful objective measure of cognitive response to therapy, but input from family and caregivers must also be recognized. Discontinuing the medication may be considered at any time during therapy if there is a perceived lack of efficacy. If a marked decline in cognitive function is noted within the first 3 to 6 weeks after discontinuing drug therapy, the practitioner may consider restarting the acetylcholinesterase inhibitor. When patients progress to severe impairment (i.e., MMSE score <10), addition of memantine may be an option.

Ability to perform ADLs, such as bathing, dressing, toileting, and feeding, and instrumental ADLs, such as transferring, housekeeping, shopping, and paying bills, should be assessed to help determine the functional status of the patient and response to treatment. Assessment of the noncognitive symptoms of AD could be a sign of disease progression.

In patients receiving antipsychotic medications, response is usually seen within the first day of therapy. If patients continue to have delusions, hallucinations, or agitation, doses can be gradually increased at 4- to 7-day intervals.

In contrast, response to antidepressant medications is seen within 4 to 6 weeks. The psychostimulants (e.g., methylphenidate) should be effective within 2 to 3 days of treatment and may be used while awaiting the onset of antidepressant effect with SSRIs or TCAs. Evidence of suicidal ideation should be taken seriously and immediately addressed by the practitioner.

If patients with sleep disorders continue to require regular pharmacotherapy, psychiatric referral is necessary to assist in determining the source of the insomnia. Nonpharmacologic interventions, such as limiting daytime napping, moderate daytime exercise, and avoiding large meals or beverages at bedtime, should be reinforced with the patient and family. If the insomnia is not disruptive or problematic for the family or patient, no treatment may be a viable option.

Treatment with any of these agents may be continued until the risk of pharmacotherapy outweighs the benefit to

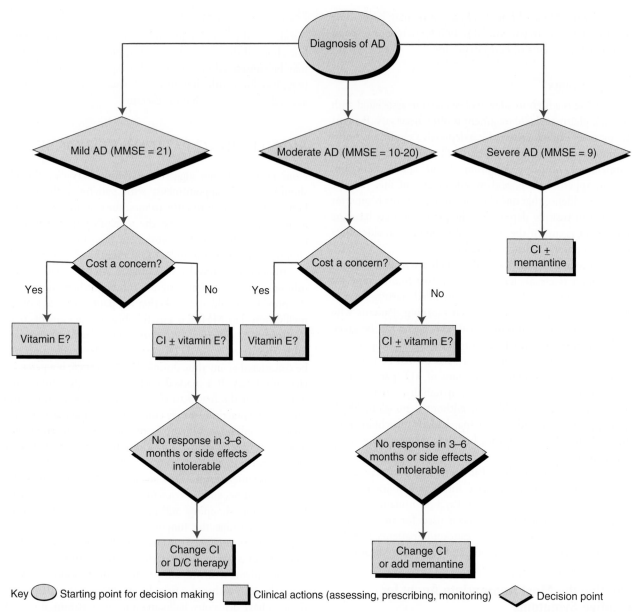

FIGURE 44–2   Treatment algorithm for the cognitive symptoms of Alzheimer's disease (AD). Initial treatment is determined by the severity of disease. An MMSE score of 21 suggests mild AD, whereas a score of 9 suggests severe disease.

the patient or family. Clear communication with the patient, family, and caregivers cannot be overemphasized because evaluation of pharmacotherapeutic efficacy and decisions to stop or continue treatment depend on this input.

PATIENT EDUCATION

Regardless of the agents chosen for AD treatment, patients, families, and caregivers must have realistic goals of drug therapy. Their goals should include increasing length of time of self-sufficiency, delaying the need for nursing home placement, and reducing the burden on the caregiver. It is important that

the family and patients understand the available agents are expected to slow the disease progression. They need to understand that no currently available agents are curative and only modest improvements can be expected.

Tacrine must be taken between meals for optimal absorption. Compliance with 4-times-daily dosing and liver function monitoring with tacrine must be emphasized. Patients taking donepezil should be instructed that if insomnia or nightmares occur, the drug may be given in the morning. Donepezil may be taken with or without food. Rivastigmine should be taken with food to have a slow dose titration to minimize the GI side effects. Galantamine can be taken without regard to food and should be slowly titrated to

TABLE 44.3	Recommended Order of Treatment of the Cognitive Symptoms Associated with Alzheimer's Disease	
Order	**Agents**	**Comments**
First line	Cholinesterase inhibitors (CIs)	Donepezil will be most likely the first-line CI for mild to moderate AD due to its convenient once-daily dosing and ability to achieve maximum dose rapidly.
	Memantine	Memantine is reserved for patients with moderate to severe AD; may be used in conjunction with a CI.
Second line	CIs	A trial of second CI is warranted.
	Vitamin E	Use of vitamin E may be added to the CI or used as monotherapy in patients who cannot afford CIs.
Third line	CI	Another trial of a different CI.
	Selegiline	Selegiline may be considered in a patient who cannot tolerate CIs or vitamin E.

minimize adverse effects. Memantine appears to be well tolerated. Because vitamin E may predispose certain patients (e.g., those with vitamin K deficiency) to bleeding, patients and families should be informed to report unusual bruising, blood in urine or stool, bleeding gums, and the like immediately to their health care provider. The practitioner should inform patients taking selegiline to take the first dose of the day in the morning and the second dose at lunchtime to minimize insomnia.

Patient-Oriented Information Sources

The various support resources available for patients and families of patients with AD are shown in **Box 44.3**.

Complementary and Alternative Medications

Vitamin E

Vitamin E, an antioxidant, has an emerging role in AD treatment. Due to its antioxidant effects, vitamin E can stabilize free radicals and the damage they produce. Patients with moderate AD started on vitamin E can expect approximately a 7-month delay in reaching a poor functional outcome or

end point (i.e., death, institutionalization, loss of the ability to perform basic ADLs, or severe dementia; Sano, et al., 1997). This difference is seen within 2 years of initiating treatment. Indefinite treatment with vitamin E is a reasonable approach.

Vitamin E may be effective because of its antioxidant effects. A starting dose of 1,000 international units given orally twice a day appears to be appropriate because this was the regimen used in the trial supporting its efficacy (Sano, et al., 1997). Vitamin E, because of its benign side effect profile, minimal cost, and lack of significant drug interactions, has become a good choice for treating AD. It has been suggested that vitamin E may also have a role in the treatment of mild AD and can be used in combination with a cholinesterase inhibitor (APA, 1997).

Minimal adverse effects are associated with vitamin E. Because vitamin E may worsen coagulation problems (causing bleeding) in patients with vitamin K deficiency or taking warfarin (Coumadin), it is suggested that these patients receive lower doses (200–800 international units/day; APA, 1997). An increase in syncope and falls was also noted for vitamin E (and selegiline) in the study by Sano and colleagues (1997). Patients should be monitored for an increase in such events if they are receiving either of these agents.

Herbal Agents

Ginkgo biloba extract, thought to have antioxidant properties, has been studied in a well-designed, controlled trial of patients with mild to severe AD or multi-infarct dementia. Modest improvement of cognition was recorded in results of the Alzheimer's Disease Assessment Scale. Caregivers also recognized improvement in function (Le Bars, et al., 1997).

Treatment was well tolerated, with some GI side effects reported. Additional well-designed studies should be conducted before routine use is recommended. Because this product is not regulated by the FDA as a medication, its safety remains unknown, and ginkgo biloba products may vary in extract concentrations and contents. Patients who choose to take this product should be cautioned that it may interact with warfarin or aspirin, increasing their risk of bleeding.

Huperzine A is another herbal product that reportedly benefits patients with AD. It appears to be a reversible cholinesterase inhibitor and may be more potent than either tacrine or donepezil. It has been used in China for treating dementia and appears to have fewer side effects and toxicities than tacrine or donepezil, as well as a longer half-life.

Case Study

M. W. is a 70-year-old white woman with a medical history of hypertension, osteoarthritis, irritable bowel syndrome, and total hysterectomy. She visits the primary care clinic with her daughter, who is concerned because M. W. has "bounced" a few checks and can no longer pay her bills without assistance. M. W. admits that she has been forgetful and appears anxious as she describes an incident in which she went shopping and could not remember where she parked her car. Her daughter states that her mother's memory has progressively worsened over the past year. M. W.'s medications include fosinopril (Monopril) 20 mg/d, raloxifene (Evista) 60 mg daily, calcium (Os-Cal 500) three times daily, and acetaminophen (Tylenol) 1,000 mg every 6 hours. A careful evaluation and work-up was ordered.

DIAGNOSIS: MILD AD WITH AN MMSE SCORE OF 22

1. List specific goals of treatment for M. W.
2. What over-the-counter or alternative medications would be appropriate for this patient?
3. What dietary and lifestyle changes should be recommended for this patient?
4. What drug therapy would you prescribe? Why?
5. How would you monitor for success with this therapy?
6. Discuss specific patient education based on the prescribed therapy.
7. Describe one or two drug–drug or drug–food interactions for the selected agent.
8. List one or two adverse reactions for the selected agent that would cause you to change therapy.
9. What would be the choice for the second-line therapy?

BIBLIOGRAPHY

Starred references are cited in the text.

American Psychiatric Association. (1994). *Diagnostic and statistical manual of mental disorders* (4th ed.). Washington, DC: Author.

*American Psychiatric Association. (1997). Practice guideline for the treatment of patients with Alzheimer's disease and other dementias in late life. *American Journal of Psychiatry, 154*(Suppl. 5), 1–39.

Brookmeyer, R., Corrada, M. M., Curriero, F. C., et al. (2002). Survival following a diagnosis of Alzheimer's disease. *Archives of Neurology, 59,* 1764–1767.

DeStrooper, B. (2010). Proteases and proteolysis in Alzheimer disease: A multifactorial view on the disease process. *Physiology Review, 90,* 465–494.

Farlow, M. R., & Cummings, J. L. (2007). Effective pharmacologic management of Alzheimer's disease. *American Journal of Medicine, 120,* 388–397.

*Folstein, M. F., Folstein, S. E., & McHugh, P. R. (1975). Mini–Mental State: A practical method for grading the cognitive state of patients for the clinician. *Journal of Psychiatric Research, 12,* 189–198.

In't Veld B. A., Ruitenberg A., Hofman A., et al. (2001). Nonsteroidal anti-inflammatory drugs and the risk of Alzheimer's disease. *New England Journal of Medicine, 345,* 1515–1521.

*Larson, E. B., Shadlen, M. F., Wang, L., et al. (2004). Survival after initial diagnosis of Alzheimer disease. *Annals of Internal Medicine, 140,* 501–509.

*Le Bars, P. L., Katz, M. M., Berman, N., et al. (1997). A placebo-controlled, double-blind, randomized trial of an extract of ginkgo biloba for dementia. *Journal of the American Medical Association, 278,* 1327–1332.

*Lendon, C. L., Ashall, F., & Goate, A. M. (1997). Exploring the etiology of Alzheimer's disease using molecular genetics. *Journal of the American Medical Association, 277,* 825–831.

McKhann, G., Drachman, D., Folstein, M., et al. (1984). Clinical diagnosis of Alzheimer's disease: Report of the NINCDS-ADRDA Work Group under the auspices of the Department of Health and Human Services Task Force on Alzheimer's Disease. *Neurology, 34,* 939–944.

*Morris, J. C. (1994). Differential diagnosis of Alzheimer's disease. *Clinics in Geriatric Medicine, 10,* 257–257.

National Advisory Council on Aging. (1995). *Report to Congress on the scientific opportunities for developing treatments for Alzheimer's disease.* Washington, DC: Author.

Nyth, A. L., & Gottfries, C. G. (1990). The clinical efficacy of citalopram in treatment of emotional disturbances in dementia disorders: A Nordic multicenter study. *British Journal of Psychiatry, 157,* 894–901.

Qaseem, A., Snow, V., & Cross Jr., T. (2008). Current pharmacologic treatment of dementia: A clinical practice guideline from the American college of physicians and the American academy of family physicians. *Annals of Internal Medicine, 148,* 370–378.

*Queforth, H. W., & LaFerla, F. M. (2010). Alzheimer's disease. *New England Journal of Medicine, 362,* 329–344.

Reisberg, B., Doody, R., Stoffler, A., et al. (2003). Memantine in moderate-to-severe Alzheimer's disease. *New England Journal of Medicine, 348,* 1333–1341.

*Sano, M., Ernesto, C., Thomas, R. G., et al. (1997). A controlled trial of selegiline, alpha-tocopherol, or both as treatment for Alzheimer's disease. *New England Journal of Medicine, 336,* 1216–1222.

Shah, S., & Reichman, W. E. (2006). Treatment of Alzheimer's disease across the spectrum of clinical activity. *Clinical Interventions in Aging, 1,* 131–142.

Skolnick, A. A. (1997). Old Chinese herbal medicine used for fever yields possible new Alzheimer disease therapy. *Journal of the American Medical Association, 277,* 776.

*Small, G. W., Rabins, P. V., Barry, P. P., et al. (1997). Diagnosis and treatment of Alzheimer's disease and related disorders: Consensus statement of the American Association for Geriatric Psychiatry, the Alzheimer's Association, and the American Geriatrics Society. *Journal of the American Medical Association, 278,* 1363–1371.

Talbot, C., Lendon, C., Craddock, N., et al. (1994). Protection against Alzheimer's disease with ApoE2. *Lancet, 343,* 1432–1433.

Tariot, P. N., Farlow, M. R., Grossberg, G. T., et al. (2004). Memantine treatment in patients with moderate to severe Alzheimer disease already receiving donepezil: A randomized controlled trial. *Journal of the American Medical Association, 291,* 317–324.

*Wiser, T. H. (1994). Alzheimer's cognitive disturbances: A case study. *US Pharmacist, 19,* 52–78.

Wolozin, B. K. W., Rousseau, P., Celesia, G. G., et al. (2000). Decreased prevalence of Alzheimer disease associated with 3-hydroxy-3-methylglutaryl coenzyme A reductase inhibitors. *Archives of Neurology, 57*(10), 1439–1443.

Yankner, B. A., & Mesulam, M. M. (1991). β-Amyloid and the pathogenesis of Alzheimer's disease. *New England Journal of Medicine, 325,* 1849–1857.

Pharmacotherapy for Endocrine Disorders

Diabetes Mellitus

Diabetes mellitus is the term used to represent a clinically and genetically heterogeneous group of disorders characterized by abnormally high blood glucose levels (hyperglycemia) as a result of either insulin deficiency or cellular resistance to the action of insulin. Four major classifications of diabetes have been defined: type 1 diabetes mellitus (formerly known as *insulin-dependent diabetes mellitus*), type 2 diabetes mellitus (formerly known as *non–insulin-dependent diabetes mellitus*), gestational diabetes mellitus, and diabetes secondary to other conditions (e.g., hormonal abnormalities and pancreatic diseases).

According to the Centers for Disease Control and Prevention (CDC, 2008), there are more than 24 million people with diabetes in the United States. Of this number, 90% to 95% have type 2 diabetes. Additionally, there is another 57 million who have a condition called *pre-diabetes* (CDC, 2008). The National Institute of Diabetes and Digestive and Kidney Diseases and the American Diabetes Association (ADA) found that diabetes was the seventh leading cause of death in the United States in 2006. Overall, the risk of death among people with diabetes is approximately twice that of people without diabetes. The annual medical costs for diabetes in the United States in 2007 were $174 billion in direct and indirect costs. This is a 32% increase in the overall dollar amount spent on all aspects of diabetes care (Diabetes Statistics, 2007).

CAUSES

Type 1 diabetes is thought to be an autoimmune disease in which pancreatic beta cells are destroyed. The beta cells are responsible for secreting insulin, a major hormone that promotes cellular uptake and use of glucose and maintains metabolic functions throughout the body. If the beta cells are destroyed, the pancreas produces no insulin, causing glucose levels in the blood to skyrocket. Onset can occur at any time, but most patients are younger than age 30.

Although type 1 diabetes is one of the most common chronic diseases in children, its etiology remains unclear. Suggested etiologies include genetic predisposition to the destruction of beta cells, infection, autoimmunity, and environmental factors. Viral agents are highly suspected in the pathogenesis of type 1 diabetes because mumps, rubella, varicella, measles, influenza, coxsackievirus, cytomegalovirus, and viral pneumonia have been reported to precede its onset. Furthermore, the incidence increases in the United States during the fall and winter, when viral infections are prevalent. Autoimmunity is evident because 80% of patients with type 1 diabetes test positive for specific human leukocyte antigen. It is likely that a combination of these factors contributes to the destruction of beta cells and the subsequent absence of insulin.

In type 2 diabetes, adipose and muscle cells become less sensitive to the actions of insulin or the pancreas produces less insulin than the body needs. In either situation, glucose levels in the blood escalate. Most patients with type 2 diabetes are older than age 30. **Box 45.1** lists risk factors for type 2 diabetes; the major risk factors are obesity and family history. Both beta cell defects and insulin resistance are found in patients with type 2 diabetes.

BOX 45.1

Major Risk Factors for Type 2 Diabetes Mellitus

- Family history of diabetes (i.e., parents or siblings with diabetes)
- Obesity (i.e., 20% over desired body weight or body mass index >27)
- Race/ethnicity (e.g., African Americans, Hispanic Americans, Native Americans, Asian Americans, Pacific Islanders have increased risk)
- Age older than 45 years
- Previously identified as having IFG (impaired fasting glucose)
- Hypertension
- High-density lipoprotein cholesterol level >35 mg/dL or triglyceride level >250 mg/dL
- History of gestational diabetes mellitus or delivery of babies weighing >9 lb
- Sedentary lifestyle
- Polycystic ovary syndrome

In gestational diabetes, pregnancy causes the woman to become intolerant to glucose. The causes are not fully clear, but they appear to be related to the anti-insulin effects created by progesterone, cortisol, and human placental lactogen. Usually, once the woman has delivered her infant, blood glucose levels return to normal; however, women who have had gestational diabetes have a 20% to 50% chance of developing diabetes in the next 5 to 10 years.

PATHOPHYSIOLOGY

In type 1 diabetes, the pancreatic beta cells are destroyed, causing a subsequent absence of insulin. In genetically susceptible people, an autoimmune attack occurs in which monocytes/macrophages and activated cytotoxic T cells infiltrate the islets. Multiple antibodies against beta cell antigens develop in the blood, and insulin reserve steadily decreases until the amount is insufficient to maintain a normal blood glucose level.

The pathogenesis of type 2 diabetes involves insulin resistance, impaired insulin secretion, elevated glucose production by the liver, or all these components. With insulin resistance, circulating insulin concentrations increase as compensation. Researchers have hypothesized that in type 2 diabetes, the ability of insulin to inhibit hepatic glucose production and to stimulate its uptake and use by adipose and muscle cells is diminished. In lean patients with type 2 diabetes, the primary defect appears to occur in the beta cells. In overweight patients, who represent most patients with type 2 diabetes, the most likely primary defect is impairment of the target cells. Although abnormal hepatic glucose metabolism plays an important role in maintaining the diabetic state, it is probably not the earliest development and most likely follows impaired insulin sensitivity in the muscle.

Insulin affects many body systems, and chronic hyperinsulinemia contributes to the pathogenesis and worsening of hypertension, dyslipidemia, and coronary heart disease. Hypertension, high plasma triglyceride levels, and low high-density lipoprotein (HDL) plasma levels correlate with hyperinsulinemia secondary to insulin resistance and a worsened cardiovascular risk profile. This collection of clinical markers or indicators associated with insulin resistance is referred to as *metabolic syndrome*.

Epidemiologic and interventional studies consistently point to the relationship between good glycemic control and the prevention or slowing of the progression of long-term complications of diabetes. The Diabetes Control and Complications Trial (DCCT) presented definitive evidence to support the hypothesis that diabetic complications are related to the degree of hyperglycemia. In this landmark study, patients with type 1 diabetes were randomized to two groups and followed for an average of 6.5 years. One group received conventional therapy (one or two daily insulin injections, daily self-monitoring of glucose, and diabetes education) to normalize blood glucose levels; the other group received intensive therapy (three or more daily administrations of insulin and glucose monitoring 4 times daily). The incidence of microvascular complications was 60% lower in the group that received intensive therapy than in the patients who received conventional therapy. Hence, intensive therapy delayed the onset of complications and slowed their progression. The United Kingdom Prospective Diabetes Study (UKPDS) Group answered the question as to whether the DCCT results could be extrapolated to include type 2 diabetes. In the UKPDS, patients with type 2 diabetes were randomized to intensive or conventional therapy and followed over a 10-year period. As in the DCCT, there was a significant (25%) risk reduction in microvascular end points with tight control.

DIAGNOSTIC CRITERIA

Patients with marked hyperglycemia present with the classic symptoms of polyuria (excessive urination), polydipsia (increased thirst), weight loss, polyphagia (increased hunger and caloric intake), and blurred vision. In type 1 diabetes, the onset of these symptoms usually is sudden and often preceded by ketoacidosis. In contrast, the course of development for type 2 diabetes is gradual, insidious, and frequently undiagnosed for years. The onset and sometimes the presence of symptoms often go unnoticed. Therefore, screening for diabetes as part of a routine medical examination is appropriate if a patient has one or more risk factors. (See **Box 45.1**.) The more risk factors that the individual has, the greater the chances are for him or her to develop or have diabetes. Because early detection and prompt treatment may reduce the impact of diabetes and its complications, screening is recommended for those at risk.

The new consensus for diagnosis includes use of hemoglobin A_{1c} (HbA_{1c}). Fasting plasma glucose (FPG) can also be used; less often the oral glucose tolerance test (OGTT) is employed. Diagnosis can also be made on presentation with classic overt signs and symptoms of diabetes. FPG and now the HbA_{1c} are generally the easiest and least expensive diagnostic tests. Fasting is defined as no intake of food or beverage other than water for at least 8 hours before testing. The OGTT is still the preferred test for pregnant women, and it can be performed in either a one-step or two-step method. The key with pregnant women is careful risk assessment in the early stages of pregnancy regarding their risk of diabetes.

Normal glucose is defined as an FPG level of <100 mg/dL and a 2-hour postload glucose (PG) value in the OGTT of less than 140 mg/dL. A normal HbA_{1c} is 4% to 6% and can be obtained regardless of the last oral intake. Those who test higher than or equal to 6.5% should have repeat testing to confirm the diagnosis. An FPG level of 126 mg/dL or more or a 2-hour PG value in the OGTT of 200 mg/dL or more warrants repeat testing on a different day to confirm the diagnosis. Patients with an FPG of at least 100 mg/dL but less than 126 mg/dL have impaired fasting glucose (IFG). Patients with a 2-hour PG value of at least 140 mg/dL but less than <200 mg/dL in the OGTT are considered as having impaired glucose tolerance (IGT). Patients with IFG or IGT are now referred

TABLE 45.1	Criteria for the Diagnosis of Diabetes Mellitus	
Normoglycemia	Impaired Glucose Metabolism	Diabetes Mellitus
FPG <100 mg/dL	FPG ≥100 and <126 mg/dL (IFG)	FPG ≥126 mg/dL
2-h PG <140 mg/dL	2-h PG ≥140 and <200 mg/dL (IGT)	2-h PG ≥200 mg/dL Random plasma glucose ≥200 mg/dL and symptoms of diabetes mellitus
HbA$_{1c}$ 4–6%	NA	HbA$_{1c}$ ≥ 6.5%

FPG, fasting plasma glucose; HbA$_{1c}$, hemoglobin A$_{1c}$; IFG, impaired fasting glucose; IGT, impaired glucose tolerance; PG, plasma glucose

to as having *pre-diabetes,* indicating the relatively high risk of developing diabetes. Diagnostic criteria are presented in **Table 45.1.**

Plasma glucose levels can be obtained from patients regardless of the time the patients last ate. Such levels are referred to as random plasma glucose levels. Any random plasma glucose level of 200 mg/dL or more is considered positive for diabetes and warrants additional testing, preferably by the FPG test on another day.

Certain drugs may cause hyperglycemia. These include glucocorticoids, furosemide, thiazide diuretics, products containing estrogen, beta blockers, and nicotinic acid.

INITIATING DRUG THERAPY

Effective treatment programs for diabetes mellitus require comprehensive training in self-management, ongoing support from the clinical care team, and, for many, intensive pharmacologic regimens. These programs must be individualized according to each patient's needs and should include the following features:

- Self-monitoring blood glucose (SMBG)
- Medical nutrition therapy
- Regular exercise
- Drug therapy individualized for each patient
- Oral glucose-lowering agents for some patients with type 2 diabetes
- Instruction in the prevention and treatment of acute and chronic complications, including hypoglycemia
- Continuing patient education and support
- Periodic assessment of treatment goals

Treatment of abnormal glucose levels consists of diet and exercise. The cornerstone of therapy for all patients with diabetes is diet, but the goals of therapy differ between types 1 and 2 diabetes. In general, patients with type 1 diabetes are usually thin and present at or below ideal body weight. Therefore, the goals of diet are directed toward regulation of caloric intake and proper spacing of meals and snacks. In the presence of

exogenously administered insulin, these patients require proper timing of meals and routine activities to prevent episodes of hypoglycemia. Patients taking insulin should carry a source of simple sugar at all times in the event of hypoglycemia.

Because most patients with type 2 diabetes are overweight, the goal of treatment is directed toward weight reduction. Weight loss leads to improved glucose tolerance by enhancing the sensitivity of peripheral glucose receptors. Patients with type 2 diabetes can control the condition through diet and exercise alone. If these interventions fail to achieve desirable glycemic control, practitioners should initiate drug therapy.

Goals of Drug Therapy

The major goals of drug therapy in diabetes mellitus are as follows:

GLYCEMIC CONTROL

- HbA$_{1c}$ level ≤6.9%, preferably ≤6.5%
- Preprandial plasma glucose level 90–130 mg/dL
- Postprandial plasma glucose level <180 mg/dL

BLOOD PRESSURE

- <130/80 mm Hg (125/75 for patients with proteinuria)

LIPIDS

- Low-density lipoprotein (LDL) level <100 mg/dL
- Triglyceride level <150 mg/dL
- HDL level >40 mg/dL

MICROALBUMIN (RANDOM COLLECTION)

- <30 μg/mL creatinine

In type 1 diabetes, insulin is the mainstay of drug therapy. When diet and exercise alone do not achieve glycemic control of type 2 diabetes, drug therapy is indicated. In type 2 diabetes, oral agents with glucose-lowering effects are used. The ADA suggests that pharmacologic therapy be selected with consideration to the following factors:

- Degree of hyperglycemia and the presence or absence of symptoms
- Presence of comorbidity
- Patient motivation
- Patient preference

Table 45.2 provides an overview of the various oral agents.

Sulfonylureas

Sulfonylureas are a major group of oral hypoglycemic agents used to treat type 2 diabetes. (See **Table 45.2.**) They correct derangements of carbohydrate, lipid, and protein metabolism.

Mechanism of Action

Sulfonylureas bind to specific receptors on beta cells, causing adenosine triphosphate (ATP)-dependent potassium channels

TABLE 45.2 Overview of Oral Antidiabetic Agents

Generic (Trade) Name and Dosage	Selected Adverse Events	Contraindications	Special Considerations
Sulfonylureas			
FIRST GENERATION			
tolbutamide (Orinase) 0.25–3 g in 1 or 2 divided doses	Hypoglycemia, increased risk of cardiovascular disease	Ketoacidosis, sulfa allergy	Onset occurs within 1 h, lasts 6–12 h. Give with morning meal. Effectiveness may decrease over time. Increased hypoglycemia may occur in elderly or debilitated patients. Signs and symptoms of hypoglycemia may be masked in patients taking beta blockers.
chlorpropamide (Diabinese) 100–750 mg qd	Hypoglycemia	Same as above	Onset is 1 h, lasts 72 h. Same as above
tolazamide (Tolinase) Initially 100–250 mg qd; increase weekly by 100–250 mg/d until desired blood glucose Maximum dose 1,000 mg/d	Hypoglycemia, increased risk of cardiovascular mortality	Same as above	Onset occurs within 4–6 h, lasts 10–14 h. Same as above
SECOND GENERATION			
glyburide (DiaBeta, Micronase) Initially 2.5–5 mg qd; increase by 2.5 mg/wk until desired blood glucose Elderly patients start at 1.25 mg/d Maximum dose 20 mg/d	Hypoglycemia	Same as above	Onset occurs within 1.5 h, lasts 18–24 h. Same as above
glyburide, micronized (Glynase) Initially 1.5–3 mg qd; 0.75 mg in elderly Maximum dose 12 mg/d	Same as above	Same as above	Onset occurs within 1.5 h, lasts 18–24 h. Same as above
glipizide (Glucotrol) Initially 5 mg qd (2.5 mg in elderly); increase weekly to a maximum of 40 mg/d to desired blood glucose	Same as above	Same as above	Patients should take medication 30 min before a meal. Onset occurs within 1 h, lasts for 10–24 h. Same as above
glimepiride (Amaryl) Initially 1–2 mg with breakfast; increase by 2 mg/wk until desired blood glucose Maximum dose 8 mg/d	Same as above	Same as above	Onset occurs within 2–4 h, lasts 24 h. Same as above
BIGUANIDE			
metformin (Glucophage) Initially 500 mg bid; increase by 500 mg/wk until desired blood glucose	GI distress: diarrhea, nausea, bloating, flatulence Rare lactic acidosis	Renal dysfunction, CHF, metabolic acidosis, ketoacidosis, impaired hepatic function, excess alcohol consumption, pregnancy	Patients should take with meals to minimize GI side effects. Medication must be temporarily held when patient is undergoing IV iodinated contrast study.

(continued)

TABLE 45.2 Overview of Oral Antidiabetic Agents (*Continued*)

Generic (Trade) Name and Dosage	Selected Adverse Events	Contraindications	Special Considerations
Maximum dose 2,550 mg/d in divided doses			Modest synergistic effect may occur when given with sulfonylurea. Medication should be held for patients undergoing surgery.
Thiazolidinediones			
rosiglitazone (Avandia) Initially 4 mg/d in single dose; if response is inadequate after 12 wk, increase to 8 mg/d in single dose	Anemia, edema, headache, reversible increase in ALT	Children, ketoacidosis	Monitor ALT at baseline, every 2 mo for the first 12 mo, and periodically thereafter. Discontinue medication if ALT is >3 times the upper limit of normal or if jaundice occurs. Medications may increase plasma volume; caution is necessary for patients with New York Heart Association class III and IV heart failure. Monitor for increased risk of myocardial infarction. Resumption of premenopausal ovulation may occur in anovulatory women. Unintended pregnancy may result. Use restricted for patients unable to take pioglitazone or to manage their blood sugar.
pioglitazone (Actos) 15–30 mg/d Maximum 45 mg/d as monotherapy and 30 mg/d as combined therapy	Same as above	Same as above	Same as above Increased risk of CHF but without myocardial infarction
α-Glucosidase Inhibitors			
acarbose (Precose) Initially 25 mg tid with the first bite of a meal; increase by 25 mg at 4- to 8-wk intervals to a maximum of 300 mg in three divided doses (150 mg if weight <60 kg)	Flatulence, diarrhea, abdominal pain/distention	Renal dysfunction, ketoacidosis, inflammatory bowel disease, colonic ulceration; predisposition to intestinal obstruction; disorders of digestion	Patient should take with first bite of each meal.
miglitol (Glyset): Same as above	Same as above	Same as above	Same as above
Meglitinide Analogs			
repaglinide (Prandin) Initially 0.5 mg with two to four meals daily if patient has never received other treatment for diabetes; if previous treatment, 1–2 mg with two to four meals daily Double dose weekly to a maximum of 16 mg/d	Hyperglycemia, upper respiratory tract infection, headache, diarrhea, constipation, arthralgia, back or chest pain	Type 1 diabetes, ketoacidosis	As monotherapy or in conjunction with metformin, medication is to be taken within 30 min of a meal. Patient should skip a dose if he or she skips a meal and add a dose if he or she adds a meal.
nateglinide (Starlix) Initially 120 mg before each meal to a maximum dose of 360 mg/d	Same as above	Same as above	Same as above

Combination drugs

	Side effects	Contraindications	Special considerations
SULFONYLUREA AND BIGUANIDE			
glyburide and metformin (Glucovance) 1.25 mg/250 mg; 2.5 mg/500 mg; 5 mg/500 mg; Maximum dose 20 mg/2000 mg/d	Hypoglycemia, GI distress, diarrhea, flatulence Rare lactic acidosis	Same as above	Same as above
glipizide and metformin (Metaglip) 2.5 mg/200 mg 2.5 mg/50 mg 5 mg/500 mg	Same as above	Same as above	Same as above
THIAZOLIDINEDIONE AND BIGUANIDE			
rosiglitazone and metformin (Avandamet) 1 mg/500 mg 2 mg/500 mg 4 mg/500 mg 2 mg/1,000 mg 4 mg/1,000 mg	GI distress, diarrhea, flatulence Rare lactic acidosis, edema, headache Reversible increase in ALT	Same as above	Same as above Restrict use to patients already on the medication or those who cannot tolerate pioglitazone combination.
DIPEPTIDYL PEPTIDASE-4 INHIBITORS			
sitagliptin (Januvia) 100 mg oral daily or 50 mg oral daily	Common to both acute upper respiratory infection, urinary tract infection, headache Must adjust dosage to mild renal insufficiency Increases tendency toward hypoglycemia when combined with sulfonylureas	Type 1 diabetes	Must check creatinine clearance prior to starting medication.
saxagliptin (Onglyza) 2.5 mg or 5 mg daily	Potential for acute pancreatitis, hypersensitivity to medication	History of pancreatitis	Only agent approved for use with insulin
DIPEPTIDYL PEPTIDASE-4 INHIBITORS & BIGUANIDE			
sitagliptin and metformin HCL (Janumet) 50 mg/500 mg 50 mg/1000 mg	Same as above Diarrhea Potential for serious acute lactoacidosis	Not approved for use in children	Do not exceed the maximum dose of 100 mg sitagliptin or 2,000 mg metformin.

ALT, alanine aminotransferase; CHF, congestive heart failure; GI, gastrointestinal.

to close. The calcium channels subsequently open, leading to increased cytoplasmic calcium, which stimulates the release of insulin. Theorists have hypothesized that these drugs also have extrapancreatic effects involving the liver, muscle, and adipose cells, but because these agents are ineffective in patients with type 1 diabetes, it appears that their predominant hypoglycemic action is on the beta cells. When used alone, these agents have the most significant effect on blood sugar, especially in patients who are lean and insulinopenic.

Sulfonylureas are divided into first- and second-generation agents. Second-generation drugs are more potent and more widely used than first-generation agents. Comparison of these drugs by potency and other pharmacologic properties is presented in **Table 45.3.**

Approximately one third of patients with type 2 diabetes fail to respond adequately to sulfonylureas, most often because of markedly impaired beta cell function, not adhering to diet, or stressful events such as infection. After 10 years of therapy, only 50% of initial responders have adequate glycemic control. For optimal response, careful patient selection should include the following criteria: duration of disease less than 5 years, no history of prior insulin therapy or good glycemic control on less than 40 units/day of insulin, close to normal body weight, and FPG less than 180 mg/dL.

Adverse Events/Contraindications/Interactions

The most important complication of the use of sulfonylureas is hypoglycemia. In the elderly population, this risk is greatest secondary to comorbidity, polypharmacy, or poor social situations (e.g., isolation, financial constraints). In younger patients, hypoglycemia may be associated with alcohol abuse or overexertion. Long-acting agents (e.g., chlorpropamide [Diabinese]) place elderly patients with other underlying disorders at risk for prolonged and sometimes fatal hypoglycemic episodes. Drugs with active metabolites also may increase the risk of hypoglycemia in patients with impaired renal function. Hence, patient education must include recognition of symptoms as well as prevention and treatment plans for hypoglycemia. Sulfonylureas can cause weight gain of about 2 to 3 kg. They cannot be used in patients with sulfa allergies.

Biguanides

Biguanides are oral hypoglycemics used in conjunction with diet as first-line monotherapy or in combination with other classes of diabetic drugs, including insulin, to treat type 2 diabetes. (See **Table 45.2.**) Their mechanisms of action and side effect profiles differ from those of sulfonylureas, offering notable advantages. Biguanides do not cause hypoglycemia (when used as monotherapy) and do not promote hyperinsulinemia or weight gain.

Mechanism of Action

This class inhibits hepatic glucose production and moderately improves peripheral sensitivity to insulin. Gluconeogenesis and glycogenolysis are inhibited in the liver. Glycemic control is achieved without stimulating insulin secretion, so hypoglycemia does not develop. Other advantages of biguanides over sulfonylureas include their tendency to induce weight loss and promote favorable effects on lipid profiles. In addition, in certain patients, biguanides can be combined effectively with sulfonylureas, thiazolidinediones (TZDs), or insulin because their mechanisms of action differ. Biguanides are the agents of choice in patients who exhibit secondary failure to sulfonylureas. In view of their many beneficial effects, biguanides appear to be a more rational choice than sulfonylureas for first-line therapy in patients with newly diagnosed type 2 diabetes. Metformin (Glucophage) is the only available biguanide. There is now a combination of glyburide and metformin (Glucovance) and glipizide and metformin (Metaglip) available. Metformin is also now available in liquid form (Riomet).

Dosage

The dose is started low and increased weekly as needed to the maximum. Patients usually take the medication before meals in the morning and evening. The dose is carefully titrated in elderly patients. With metformin, the starting dose is 500 mg twice a day with increases every 1 to 2 weeks to a maximum of 2,550 mg/day. Peak action is within 2 to 2.5 hours, and the effects last for 10 to 16 hours. Steady-state levels of the drug are achieved in 24 to 48 hours. Metformin also comes in an

TABLE 45.3	Comparison of Oral Sulfonylureas				
Drug	Equivalent Therapeutic Dose (mg)	Duration of Action (h)	Doses per Day	Adverse Events (%)	Hypoglycemic Reactions (%)
First Generation					
tolbutamide	1,000	6–12	2–3	3	<1
tolazamide	250	12–24	1–2	2	<1
acetohexamide	500	12–18	2	4	<1
chlorpropamide	250	24–72	1	8	<4–6
Second Generation					
long-acting glipizide	10	12–24	1–2	5	<2–4
long-acting glipizide	5–10	24	1	5	<1
long-acting glyburide	5	16–24	1–2	7	<4–6

extended-release formula. It is started at 500 mg daily with the evening meal and increased to a maximum of 2,000 mg daily.

Contraindications

Contraindications include renal dysfunction, serum creatinine level of 1.4 mg/dL or higher, heart failure, and pregnancy. This class also is contraindicated in children, alcoholics, binge drinkers, those over age 80, and those with dehydration. Patients must stop taking metformin when undergoing radiologic studies with iodinated contrast, when experiencing metabolic acidosis, and before surgery until they resume normal oral intake.

Adverse Events/Interactions

The most common side effect of metformin therapy is gastrointestinal (GI) upset, which includes diarrhea, nausea, vomiting, abdominal bloating, flatulence, anorexia, and a metallic taste in the mouth. Such problems occur in approximately 30% of patients during the initiation of therapy and usually resolve with continued treatment. To minimize these adverse effects, treatment is started with a low dose and increased slowly at no less than weekly intervals.

Because GI upset is rare late in therapy, any sudden onset of severe vomiting or diarrhea at that time should alert providers to the possibility of lactic acidosis, a rare but potentially fatal complication of metformin therapy. In such cases, patients should discontinue metformin immediately until they can be evaluated and stabilized. From data collected in Europe over 20 years, the reported worldwide incidence of metformin-induced lactic acidosis is 0.03 cases/1,000 patient-years. The risk of lactic acidosis increases with advancing age and worsening renal function. Therefore, metformin is contraindicated in patients with renal disease or dysfunction and acute or chronic metabolic acidosis. In addition, metformin should be temporarily withheld in patients undergoing radiologic studies requiring the use of iodinated contrast media because of their effects on renal excretion. Renal impairment is suggested in men with serum creatinine levels of 1.5 mg/dL or more and in women with levels of 1.4 mg/dL or more. Renal dysfunction may be secondary to a variety of comorbid conditions such as cardiopulmonary insufficiency, liver disease, alcoholism, and infection. These conditions predispose patients to impaired perfusion of tissues and decreased elimination of lactate and are therefore contraindications to the use of metformin. In addition, patients should temporarily discontinue metformin during any situation in which an acute decline in renal function may occur (e.g., aggressive diuresis, dehydration from gastroenteritis, surgery).

The concomitant use of metformin with cimetidine increases the risk of hypoglycemia. The concomitant use of metformin with glucocorticoids or alcohol increases the risk of lactic acidosis.

Thiazolidinediones

This class of antidiabetic agents (**Table 45.2**) reduces insulin resistance at sites of insulin action.

Mechanism of Action

TZDs bind to the nuclear steroid hormone receptor perixosome proliferator-activated receptor-gamma and increase insulin sensitivity in skeletal muscle and fat. Clinically, they decrease peripheral insulin resistance and at higher doses may decrease hepatic glucose production. Like biguanides, they improve the action of insulin without directly stimulating insulin secretion from the pancreatic beta cells. There is an improvement of endothelial function, preservation of beta cell function, and a decrease in albumin excretion.

The patient's alanine aminotransferase (ALT) levels are monitored for possible hepatic toxicity every 2 months for the first year after the patient starts the drug and periodically thereafter. The patient must stop taking the medication if ALT levels are greater than 3 times the upper limit of normal. Hypoglycemia may develop in patients taking this class of drug with insulin or sulfonylureas because TZDs are potent sensitizers of insulin. If this occurs, the drug should be discontinued or the dose of insulin or sulfonylurea should be reduced.

Pioglitazone (Actos) has been shown to increase HDL levels.

Adverse Events/Contraindications

Pioglitazone may cause reduced concentrations of combined oral contraceptives; therefore, patients using oral contraceptives should consider alternative contraception methods. The administration of rosiglitazone (Avandia) 4 mg twice daily had no clinically significant effects on the pharmacokinetics of combined oral contraceptives.

In premenopausal anovulatory women with insulin resistance, ovulation may resume when drugs of this class are used. Thus, the patient may be at risk of unintended pregnancy, and contraception should be considered. Because of increased plasma volume from this class of drugs, TZDs are not recommended for patients with New York Heart Association class III or class IV heart failure. Another contraindication is active liver disease. TZDs can stimulate weight gain from plasma volume expansion and generation and redistribution of fats into the subcutaneous compartments.

α-Glucosidase Inhibitors

Mechanism of Action

The enzyme α-glucosidase, found on the brush border of the intestine, is necessary for the absorption of starch and disaccharides. This class of drugs (**Table 45.2**) acts by slowing the absorption of carbohydrates from the intestines, minimizing the postprandial rise in blood sugar. The result of this delay is decreased levels of postprandial glucose and HbA$_{1c}$. The α-glucosidase inhibitors are most useful in patients with postprandial hyperglycemia and patients with very high HbA$_{1c}$ levels and poor dietary adherence. They are useful in patients from ethnic groups with high-carbohydrate diets, such as Asians and Hispanics.

Dosage

Agents from this class can be prescribed alone or with a sulfonylurea. Patients should take each dose with the first bite of each meal. Dosages are increased gradually (at 4- to 8-week intervals) to avoid GI side effects. The starting dose is 25 mg 3 times a day at the start of each meal. This regimen lasts for 4 to 8 weeks; then the dose may be increased to 50 mg 3 times a day. After 3 months at 50 mg, the dose can be increased to 100 mg 3 times a day. Peak concentration occurs in 2 to 3 hours.

Contraindications

Acarbose (Precose) is contraindicated in patients with diseases of the bowel (e.g., inflammatory bowel disease, absorptive disorders, history of bowel obstruction) or cirrhosis. Patients with motility disorders of the upper GI tract should not be treated with acarbose.

Adverse Events/Interactions

The most common side effects involve the GI tract. Increased fermentation secondary to the delay in carbohydrate absorption increases intestinal gas, causing flatulence, diarrhea, and abdominal distention.

A 1-hour postprandial glucose measurement is useful to assess the therapeutic response during the dosage titration period. Additional monitoring should include serum aminotransferases every 3 months during the first year of therapy. Intestinal adsorbents such as charcoal antagonize this class of drugs. The α-glucosidase inhibitors may decrease the levels of propranolol and ranitidine.

Meglitinide Analogs

Meglitinide analogs are rapid-acting insulin secretagogues that stimulate the release of insulin from the pancreas in response to a meal. (See **Table 45.2**.) Binding at characterized sites closes the ATP-dependent potassium channels in the membranes of the beta cells. This causes a depolarization of the beta cells and an opening of calcium channels. The resulting increased influx of calcium causes insulin secretion.

Meglitinide analogs are effective in patients who become hypoglycemic while taking sulfonylureas and have acceptable FPG readings but high postprandial blood glucose levels. They also are effective for patients with irregular meal schedules because patients take them at meals. Repaglinide (Prandin) and nateglinide (Starlix) are the two drugs available in this class. They lower postprandial blood glucose concentrations without any significant effects on FPG level.

Meglitinide analogs can be used as monotherapy or in combination with other oral agents. The starting dose of repaglinide is 0.5 mg before meals if the HbA_{1c} level is <8.0. If the HbA_{1c} concentration is greater than 8.0, the starting dose is 1 to 2 mg before meals. Patients must add a dose if they add another meal or skip a dose if they skip a meal. The dose may be doubled to 4 mg before meals to a maximum of 16 mg a day. Nateglinide is similarly administered with a starting dose of 60 to 120 mg before meals.

The peak level is achieved in 1 hour. In 96 hours, the body excretes 90% of the medication. Meglitinide analogs are contraindicated in patients with diabetic ketoacidosis.

Adverse Events

Adverse events include hypoglycemia, GI disturbances, upper respiratory infections, headache, diarrhea, constipation, arthralgias, and back or chest pain. Concomitant use with beta blockers or alcohol increases the risk of hypoglycemia. Ketoconazole, miconazole, erythromycin, and other cytochrome P450 (CYP450) 3A4 inhibitors may potentiate the drug, as may nonsteroidal anti-inflammatory drugs, aspirin, sulfonamides, and warfarin. Drugs such as rifampin, barbiturates, thiazides, phenothiazines, phenytoin, sympathomimetics, calcium channel blockers, and isoniazid may antagonize it.

Dipeptidyl Peptidase-4 Inhibitors

Physiologically in response to a glucose load, two incretin hormones, glucose-dependent insulinotropic polypeptide and glucagon-like peptide 1 (GLP-1), are released from the distal bowel. These hormones account for up to 50% of the response to postprandial glucose. However, dipeptidyl peptidase-4 (DPP-4), which is a surface enzyme, inactivates, GLP-1, therefore decreasing the levels of circulating GLP-1 and glucoregulatory functions. The class of agents called DPP-4 inhibitors acts to block the effect against GLP-1 and ultimately increase the amount of native active circulating incretins. (See **Table 45.2**.)

Currently there are only two DPP-4 inhibitors, sitagliptin (Januvia) and saxagliptin (Onglyza), on the market. Both medications are indicated for daily administration and co-administration with other oral antidiabetic agents. Sitagliptin is the only agent approved for use with insulin.

Dosage

Sitagliptin has one starting dose of 100 mg daily. Dosing should be decreased to 50 mg daily for patients with moderate renal insufficiency, defined by creatinine clearance greater than 30 mL/minute but less than 50 mL/minute. Sitagliptin has also been pre-combined with metformin. The sitagliptin dose is 50 mg with either 500 or 1,000 mg of metformin. It is also approved in combination therapy with sulfonylureas, TZDs, and insulin.

Saxagliptin has two doses, 2.5 mg or 5 mg, also prescribed daily. The starting dose of 2.5 mg is used for patients with mild renal insufficiency. Saxagliptin is a strong CYP3A4/5 inhibitor, which interacts with other drugs that use that pathway. Like sitagliptin, it is approved for combination therapy with sulfonylureas and TZDs but not insulin.

Contraindications

The contraindications for both medications are similar and include hypersensitivity to the agent and type 1 diabetes; caution should be used in patients with renal impairment. Only sitagliptin is contraindicated in the patient with a history of pancreatitis.

Adverse Events

The most common adverse effects are the same for sitagliptin and saxtagliptin and include upper respiratory infection, urinary tract infection, and headaches when compared to placebos. Both drugs have potential for hypoglycemia when given in combination therapy with sulfonylureas. Additional post marketing reports for sitagliptin include hypersensitivity reactions, such as anaphylaxis, angioedema, rash, urticaria, cutaneous vasculitis, and exfoliative skin conditions including Stevens-Johnson syndrome; hepatic enzyme elevations; and potentially fatal pancreatitis.

Interactions

Sitagliptin has no pharmacokinetic drug–drug interactions, but it pharmacodynamically potentiates the action of sulfonylureas and insulin. As a potent CYP3A4/5 inhibitor, saxtagliptin interacts with drugs such as ketoconazole, erythromycin, and diltiazem.

Incretins

This class is also called GLP-1. It is used as adjunctive therapy to diet and exercise in type 2 diabetes. The mechanism of action is to stimulate glucose-dependent secretion of insulin from pancreatic beta cells while suppressing the inappropriate release of glucagon from alpha cells. It slows gastric emptying, therefore increasing satiety. Fasting and postprandial glucose are reduced with the use of incretins. As euglycemia is approached, insulin secretion subsides, therefore avoiding hypoglycemia by the response of glucagon. Incretins are not a substitute for insulin, but augment the natural physiologic responses to elevated blood sugar levels.

Dosage

Exanitide (Byetta) is only available as an injectable and can be used as monotherapy or in conjunction with other oral agents, metformin, sulfonylureas, or TZDs. Exanitide is not approved for use with insulin. The starting dose is 5 mcg, injected over 60 minutes in the morning and evening or prior to the largest meals of the day and spaced more than 6 hours apart. Based on response, in 1 month the dose can be increased to 10 mcg twice a day. The onset of action is within 1 hour and peaks in 2 hours.

Contraindications

Exanitide is only contraindicated if the patient is allergic to known components of the drug. It should not be used in patients who have a history of pancreatitis or severe renal impairment. Caution should be exercised when using exanitide in those who have gastroparesis. There are a small number of cases in which patients develop antibodies or immunogenicity to the drug. Alternative therapy should be considered if this occurs.

Adverse Events

The most common adverse reactions to exanitide are GI-related, including nausea, vomiting, diarrhea, and dyspepsia.

Hypoglycemia is also a concern when exanitide is prescribed in combination with a sulfonylurea. Caution should be exercised with any dose increase to monitor for signs and symptoms of pancreatitis, especially severe abdominal pain with or without vomiting. Exanitide should be stopped immediately with any of these signs.

Interactions

Due to the decrease in gastric emptying, exanitide should not be administered close to drugs that have a narrow therapeutic window. Caution should be exercised when patients are taking warfarin, and the international normalized ratio should be monitored closely with drug initiation and dose changes. Exanitide can possibly decrease in the ethinyl estradiol component of oral contraceptives; therefore, exanitide and oral contraceptives should not be administered within 1 hour of each other.

Pramlintide Acetate

This is a new, injectable agent that is a synthetic of the pancreatic neurohormone amylin, which is co-secreted with insulin from beta cells in response to food. Pramlintide has three actions as an amylinomimetic agent. First, it helps to delay gastric emptying into the small intestine, which delays the rise in postprandial glucose release. This effect lasts for approximately 3 hours and does not alter nutrient absorption. Second, pramlintide alters the release of additional inappropriate glucagon by pancreatic alpha cells, which is abnormal in diabetes. Finally, there is an increase in satiety, which decreases the total calorie intake and promotes weight loss. Pramlintide can be used to treat type 1 or type 2 diabetes. Unlike exanitide, it is approved for use with insulin.

Dosage

The initiation and dosage of pramlintide differs for type 1 and type 2 diabetes; however, the management of changes in dosage, side effects, and monitoring blood sugar levels is the same for both. The starting dose for those with type 1 diabetes is 15 mcg just prior to any major meal. If tolerated, pramlintide is titrated by 15-mcg increments to a total dose of 30 to 60 mcg. Patients with type 2 diabetes also administer pramlintide just prior to any major meal at 60 mcg per injection. The dose is increased to 120 mcg in 3 to 7 days if there is no nausea. Both patients with type 1 and type 2 diabetes must reduce their current insulin regimen by 50%. The titration of pramlintide is based on blood glucose levels and the presence or absence of nausea. Close monitoring of blood glucose levels is very important to detect hypoglycemia. If significant nausea occurs, the dosage should be decreased until the drug is tolerated. If nausea persists even at the lowest dose, pramlintide should be discontinued.

Contraindications

Few physiologic contraindications exist for those whom pramlintide is appropriate; however, it is critical to select appropriate patients. Those with poor adherence to diabetic care regimens, those with HbA_{1c} >9%, those taking drugs that increase gastric motility gastroparesis, and pediatric patients should not take pramlintide. Additional precaution exists for anyone with known hypersensitivity to the product. Studies have shown no effects on the drug in those with renal or liver disease and are approved as safe.

Adverse Events

The most common side effects include nausea, vomiting, headache, and anorexia. The only serious side effect can be hypoglycemia.

Interactions

Delayed absorption of other medications can occur. Pramlintide should be administered at least 1 hour before or 2 hours after other medications. Pramlintide has not been officially studied with oral antidiabetic agents.

Insulin

Insulin is the drug therapy of choice for all patients with type 1 diabetes and those patients with type 2 diabetes who cannot control their condition with diet and exercise alone or in whom oral therapy fails. Other clinical situations in which insulin therapy is appropriate include newly diagnosed cases of type 2 diabetes presenting with severe, symptomatic hyperglycemia, pregnancy, and surgery.

Just like the insulin that the pancreas normally produces, insulin as drug therapy regulates glucose metabolism in the muscle and other tissues (except the brain). It causes the rapid transport of glucose and amino acids intracellularly, promotes anabolism, and inhibits protein catabolism. In the liver, it promotes the uptake and storage of glucose in the form of glycogen, inhibits gluconeogenesis, and promotes the conversion of excess glucose into fat.

The major characteristics of insulin preparations are onset of action and duration of action (**Table 45.4**). Semisynthetic insulin, which is produced by recombinant deoxyribonucleic acid technology, has the identical amino acid composition as human endogenous insulin and is therefore referred to as *human insulin*. Human insulin preparations lower the risk of local reactions. An insulin analog, lispro insulin, is a two-amino acid modification of regular human insulin. Aggregates do not form when lispro insulin is injected subcutaneously, allowing for a more rapid onset and shorter duration than regular insulin and minimizing the postprandial rise in blood sugar and the risk of late hypoglycemia. Another human insulin analog is insulin glargine.

Insulins are categorized as basal (NPH, lente, glargine, and detemir) or bolus (regular, lispro, and aspart). Initial insulin doses should be individualized in patients previously untreated with insulin. Preferably, a therapy with a basal insulin plus a bolus insulin 15 minutes before each meal is started. A minimum of two daily injections (split-dose regimen) should be

TABLE 45.4	Insulins				
Preparation	**Brand**	**Onset (h)**	**Peak (h)**	**Duration (h)**	
Very Rapid Acting					
Insulin analog	Humalog	<.5	0.5–3	3–5	
Short Acting					
Insulin injection	Novolog	0.5	1–5	8	
	Humulin R				
Regular (R)	Novolin R				
	Velosulin BR				
Intermediate Acting					
NPH	Humulin N	1–4	4–12	14–26	
	Novolin N				
Lente	Humulin L	1–4	4–15	16–26	
	Novolin L				
Long Acting					
Insulin extended zinc suspension (U)	Humulin U	4–6	8–20	24–36	
Insulin glargine	Lantus	1–2	None	24	
Insulin detemir	Levelin	1	6–8	20	
Combination					
NPH and Regular	70/30	0.5–3	Dual	12–14	
	51/50				
Humalog mix	75% insulin lisproprotamine/25% insulin Lispro	0.1–0.25	1–12	4–24	

considered to achieve regulation of blood glucose, especially in patients with type 1 diabetes.

A common regimen is injection of a mixture of an intermediate-acting insulin (NPH) and rapid or short-acting insulin twice a day, 15 minutes before breakfast and 15 minutes before dinner. Usually, patients take a 2:1 ratio of NPH to rapid/short-acting insulin before breakfast and a 1:1 ratio before dinner. Patients take two thirds of the total daily dose in the morning and one third in the evening. However, a more physiologic way to administer insulin is to inject a basal insulin (glargine or detemir) at least daily, but it can be twice a day. Additional bolus doses of short-acting insulin, preferably lispro, are administered just prior to each meal. This type of regimen can be used in patients with type 2 diabetes who require insulin and are not on oral antidiabetic agents. It is a preferred method for most patients with type 1 diabetes who require three to four injections a day for optimal control. **Table 45.5** lists various insulin regimens.

Dosage

To start insulin in patients with type 2 diabetes, an evening dose of 10 units of basal insulin is started. Additional doses are added based on the FBG as follows:

- 2 units if FBG >120 mg/dL
- 4 units if FBG >140 mg/dL
- 6 units if FBG >180 mg/dL

Insulin doses should be individualized and closely monitored. In lieu of empiric estimations, however, the following guidelines can be used for total daily dosing:

- Children and adults: 0.5 to 0.6 units/kg/day
- Adults during illness or adolescents: 0.5 to 0.75 units/kg/day
- Adolescents during a growth spurt: 1.25 to 1.5 units/kg/day
- Pregnancy: 0.7 units/kg/day

If two doses are given a day, it is recommended that two thirds of the total daily dose be given in the morning with a 2:1 ratio of intermediate- to short-acting insulin and one third of the total daily dose be given before dinner with a 1:1 ratio of short-acting insulin and intermediate-acting insulin.

Doses should be adjusted based on the patient's clinical response, as evidenced by blood glucose levels. Adjustments are made in 1- to 2-unit increments. Insulin must be decreased with hypoglycemia and increased with hyperglycemia. **Table 45.6** provides some suggestions on when dosages need adjusting. For information on time frame for response, see **Table 45.4**. Use of insulin is contraindicated with hypoglycemia.

Insulin glargine is given at bedtime and cannot be mixed with other insulins.

The 1,500 rule can be used to determine the change needed in the insulin dose. The insulin sensitivity factor (ISF) is determined by dividing a constant (1,500) by the total daily dose (TDD) of insulin. This determines the change in blood glucose from 1 unit of insulin. The formula is: $ISF = 1,500/TDD$. For example, if the patient takes 50 units of insulin in 24 hours, the ISF is $1,500/50 = 30$.

Therefore, each unit of insulin lowers the blood glucose level 30 mg/dL. If the SMBG at noon is 170, an addition of 2 units in the morning should lower the blood glucose level to 110 mg/dL.

Adverse Events

Hypoglycemia, hypokalemia, lipodystrophy, and local or systemic allergic reaction can occur with insulin. The dawn phenomenon, so-called for worsening hyperglycemia that occurs in the early morning hours, is caused by growth hormone surges that occur during sleep. The Somogyi effect, which also may be mistaken for inadequate control, is a rebound of hyperglycemia that occurs after an early morning episode

TABLE 45.5	Various Insulin Regimens	
No. of Daily Injections	**How Administered**	**Comments**
2	Two thirds of insulin 15–30 min before breakfast and $1/3$ 15–30 min before the evening meal In AM, $2/3$ intermediate, $1/3$ short or rapid acting In PM, $1/2$ intermediate, $1/2$ rapid or short acting	This regimen is the most commonly prescribed. It is the most desirable to patients. There may be too little coverage at noon and too much insulin during the night. There is less dawn phenomenon and Somogyi effect.
3	40% intermediate and 15% short or rapid acting 15–30 min before breakfast 15% short or rapid acting before dinner 30% intermediate at bedtime	There is too little coverage at noon.
4	20%–25% of daily dose with rapid or short acting before each meal 25%–40% intermediate or long acting at bedtime	Use of insulin glargine or detemir provides most predictable basal control.

TABLE 45.6	Adjusting Insulin Dosages Based on Clinical Response	
Problem	**Time Experienced**	**Possible Solutions**
Hyperglycemia	Fasting	If the patient is receiving a single dose of an intermediate-acting insulin, split into two doses: $^2/_3$ of total dose before breakfast, $^1/_3$ of total dose before supper. If the patient is receiving split-dose insulin, increase presupper dose or move to later in the evening.
	Midmorning	Add Regular to morning dose to achieve a ratio of 2:1 (intermediate to Regular).
	Midafternoon	Increase morning NPH or Lente dose. Add Regular at lunch.
	Bedtime	Add or increase Regular with presupper dose.
	Early morning (2:00–3:00 AM)	Give the presupper dose later in the evening. Give Regular at bedtime.
Hypoglycemia	Fasting	Decrease evening insulin dose.
	Midmorning	Decrease or omit prebreakfast dose of Regular.
	Midafternoon	Decrease morning NPH or Lente.
	Bedtime	Add a bedtime snack. Decrease presupper dose of Regular.
	Early morning (2:00–3:00 AM)	Consider Somogyi effect—decrease evening NPH.

Data from Francisco, G. E., & Brooks, P. J. (1999). Diabetes mellitus. In J. T. DiPiro, R. L. Talbert, G. C. Yee, et al. (Eds.), *Pharmacotherapy. A pathophysiologic approach* (4th ed., pp. 1219–1243). East Norwalk, CT: Appleton & Lange.

of insulin-induced hypoglycemia. The hypoglycemia goes unnoticed because it happens while the patient is sleeping, at approximately 3:00 AM. Assessment clues include night sweats, nightmares, sleep disturbances, and early morning headaches. Monitoring of blood glucose when hypoglycemia is thought to be occurring helps make the diagnosis.

Interactions

Salicylates, beta blockers, monoamine oxidase inhibitors, alcohol, and sulfa drugs potentiate insulin. Corticosteroids, isoniazid, niacin, estrogens, thyroid hormones, thiazides, phenothiazines, and sympathomimetics antagonize it.

Special Considerations

Pediatric/Adolescent

Until the mid-1990s, type 1 diabetes was the prevalent type of diabetes in children and adolescents. Recently, 40% of newly diagnosed cases of diabetes in children ages 10 to 19 have been type 2 diabetes. The greatest risk factor is childhood obesity. Diabetes is often discovered with glycosuria on a random urinalysis. A red flag for type 2 diabetes in adolescents is acanthosis nigricans, dark pigmentation in skin creases and flexural area. This is a sign of insulin resistance and is present in 60% to 90% of adolescents with type 2 diabetes. Hypertension is present in 20% to 30% of adolescents with type 2 diabetes. In type 1 diabetes, children present with inappropriate polyuria, dehydration, poor weight gain, and ketonuria.

Treatment for type 1 diabetes in children is insulin therapy. Doses are:

- 0.7 mg/kg before puberty
- 1.0 mg/kg midpuberty
- 1.2 mg/kg after puberty.

These children should be treated by a specialist.

Treatment for type 2 diabetes is weight loss, medical nutritional therapy, exercise, and in many cases, medication. The only drugs approved for adolescents are insulin and metformin.

Geriatric

Diabetes in the elderly is often complicated by coexisting conditions. Complications develop at an accelerated rate probably because poor glycemic control has been long standing. Also the elderly usually have a decrease in renal function. Exercise programs for the elderly have to be started carefully with comorbid conditions in mind.

Pregnancy

There are two types of diabetes during pregnancy. One is pregestational diabetes, present before the pregnancy. This is treated by a specialist during pregnancy and is considered very high risk. The most common is gestational diabetes, which is glucose intolerance detected during pregnancy and associated with probable resolution after pregnancy. Experts now believe that high-risk women found to have diabetes at pregnancy should be diagnosed with overt diabetes, not just gestational diabetes.

During pregnancy, human placental lactogen plays a pivotal role in triggering glucose intolerance. It has an anti-insulin and lipolytic effect. Peripheral insulin sensitivity decreases to 50% of the first trimester during the third trimester. Basal hepatic glucose output increases by 30%.

Screening is recommended between weeks 24 and 48. The recommended test is the 50-g 1-hour glucose screening test, although some women require a 3-hour glucose tolerance test.

TABLE 45.7	Capacity to Decrease HbA$_{1c}$ by Agent
Agent	**Decrease in HbA$_{1c}$**
insulin	>2%
sulfonylurea	1% to 2%
biguanide	1.5% to 2%
TZD	0.5% to 1.8%
α-glucosidase inhibitor	0.5% to 1%
meglitinide	0.6% to 1.8%
sitagliptin	1%
sitagliptin with biguanide	1.8%
saxagliptin	0.1% to .3%

In the gestational diabetic, multiple daily SMBG are required and it can often be controlled by diet and medical nutritional therapy. If this does not control glucose levels, insulin is required.

Potential neonatal complications include shoulder dystonia, hypoglycemia, polycythemia, and respiratory distress.

Selecting the Most Appropriate Agent

Insulin is necessary in all cases of type 1 diabetes. In patients with type 2 diabetes, various oral agents as monotherapy or in combination therapy can be prescribed, because the oral agents act in different ways. **Table 45.7** lists the potential decrease in HbA$_{1c}$ with each agent. **Table 45.8** shows first- and second-line for patients with type 1 diabetes. **Table 45.9** shows first-, second-, and third-line therapy for patients with type 2 diabetes (**Figure 45-1**).

First-Line Therapy

In type 1 diabetes, insulin is the first-line therapy. It usually is administered in a combination of intermediate- and short-acting insulin. The dosage is 0.5 to 0.6 units/kg/day. Several schedules can be used for administering insulin. (See **Table 45.5.**) The most common regimen is two injections a day, one in the morning and one in the evening. This promotes glycemic control during the day and while the patient sleeps. The insulin dose required is divided into two thirds of the dose in the morning and one third of the dose in the evening. The morning dose is divided into two-thirds intermediate insulin and one-third short- or rapid-acting insulin. The evening dose is one-half intermediate insulin and one-half short- or rapid-acting insulin.

First-line therapy for type 2 diabetes is monotherapy with an oral agent. The agents used for first-line therapy are sulfonylureas, biguanides, TZDs, α-glucosidase inhibitors, and meglitinides. They act in different ways. The rule for initiating therapy with any of these agents is to start slowly and increase the dose every 1 to 2 weeks as needed. If intensification of treatment is required to meet goals (i.e., HbA$_{1c}$ <7.0%), the addition of another drug from a different class is recommended.

Sulfonylureas are the best choice if the patient has a blood glucose level over 250 mg/dL and is thin. Biguanides and TZDs are the drugs of choice in patients with metabolic syndrome. The α-glucosidase inhibitors are most effective in patients with postprandial hyperglycemia but only mild fasting glucose elevations.

Second-Line Therapy

With failure to achieve optimal blood glucose levels in type 1 diabetes, practitioners must gradually increase the insulin dose, making adjustments 1 to 2 units at a time over 3 days. They must base adjustments on SMBG records. **Table 45.10** lists how to determine adjustments.

Failure to achieve optimal blood glucose levels in type 2 diabetes necessitates the addition of another oral agent. Combinations of sulfonylureas and biguanides, TZDs, or α-glucosidase inhibitors are effective. Insulin may be added to oral medication regimens for effective control. Insulin is started at the lowest dose and increased every 1 to 2 weeks as needed.

Third-Line Therapy

In patients with type 1 diabetes, clinicians should add a TZD or metformin to the regimen of insulin if control is still poor. They may add a α-glucosidase inhibitor if postprandial blood glucose is high. Patients with type 1 diabetes may be appropriate candidates for an insulin pump.

TABLE 45.8	Recommended Order of Treatment for Type 1 Diabetes Mellitus	
Order	**Agents**	**Comments**
First line	Insulin, usually a combined administration of intermediate and short acting; dose is 0.5–0.6 units/kg/d	Several schedules are used to administer insulin. (See **Table 45.5.**) The most commonly used regimen is two injections a day, one in the morning and one in the evening. This promotes glycemic control both during the day and while sleeping. The insulin dose required is divided into ⅔ of the dose in the morning and ⅓ of the dose in the evening. The morning dose is divided into ⅔ intermediate insulin and ⅓ short- or rapid-acting insulin. The evening dose is ½ intermediate insulin and ½ short- or rapid-acting insulin.
Second line	Insulin dose is gradually increased.	Adjustments are made at 1 to 2 units at a time over 3 days. Adjustments are based on SMBG records.

TABLE 45.9   **Recommended Order of Treatment for Type 2 Diabetes Mellitus**

Order	Agents	Comments
First line Tier 1 according to the ADA	Monotherapy with an oral agent: biguanides	The rule for initiating therapy with any of these agents is to start slowly and increase the dose every 1 to 2 wk as needed. The patient can be switched to another drug or class after 1 mo if the therapy is not effective in achieving glycemic control. Biguanides are the drugs of choice in the patient with metabolic syndrome X and when the blood glucose levels are <250 mg/dL. The α-glucosidase inhibitors are most effective in patients with postprandial hyperglycemia but only mild fasting glucose elevations.
Tier 2	Insulin or sulfonylureas	Sulfonylureas are the best choice if the patient is thin, older than age 40, has had diabetes for <5 y, and has a blood glucose >250 mg/dL. Glyburide is most effective in patients with fasting hypoglycemia, and glipizide is most effective in patients with postprandial hyperglycemia. Start with a single timed dose of 10 units of insulin with dose adjusted weekly (2 units if FPG >120 mg/dL; 4 units if FPG >140 mg/dL; 6 units if FPG >180 mg/dL).
Second line	Addition of another oral agent Combinations of sulfonylureas and biguanides, TZDs, or α-glucosidase inhibitors are effective. Also, metformin can be combined with a meglitinide or TZD for effective control. Consider pramlitidine injection	Again, the dose is started at the lowest level and increased every 1 to 2 wk as needed.
Third line	Triple oral therapy and consider additional basal insulin and short-acting boluses.	Oral medications at the same dose

In patients with type 2 diabetes, insulin is added if the addition of a second agent and third agent is unsuccessful. An intermediate or a basal insulin at bedtime added to the daytime oral regimen can be very effective in treating those with type 2 diabetes to goal.

Combination Therapy

The following are suggestions for combination therapy for type 2 diabetes mellitus:

- **A sulfonylurea and a biguanide** produces mealtime stimulation of endogenous insulin with the sulfonylurea and gluconeogenesis with the biguanide. This is recommended for a HbA_{1c} level above 8%.
- **A sulfonylurea and a TZD** improves insulin resistance and may enable a decrease in the sulfonylurea dose.
- **A biguanide and a TZD** combination provides a synergistic effect on glycemic reduction. Liver and renal function must be monitored with this regimen.
- **α-glucosidase inhibitor and another agent** are best used with an elevated postprandial blood glucose level.
- **Meglitinide and a TZD or biguanide** combination promotes a stimulation of insulin release and a decrease in peripheral insulin resistance and fasting hyperglycemia.

MONITORING PATIENT RESPONSE

Prolonged hyperglycemia of diabetes gives rise to long-term complications that involve lesions of the small (microvascular) and large (macrovascular) blood vessels. Microvascular complications include retinopathy, nephropathy, and neuropathy.

Control is measured using the patient's levels of blood glucose and HbA_{1c}. Patients use SMBG to keep a daily record of blood glucose. HbA_{1c} measures blood glucose over 3 months. **Table 45-10** lists the desired levels and levels that require changes in drug regimen.

PATIENT EDUCATION

Drug Information

Education is a hallmark of diabetes therapy. SMBG is essential for monitoring therapeutic response. Practitioners must educate patients about the signs and symptoms of hypoglycemia and instruct them to carry a source of glucose with them at all times. Possible sources are hard candy (not sugarless) or 4 oz of orange juice. All patients with diabetes should have

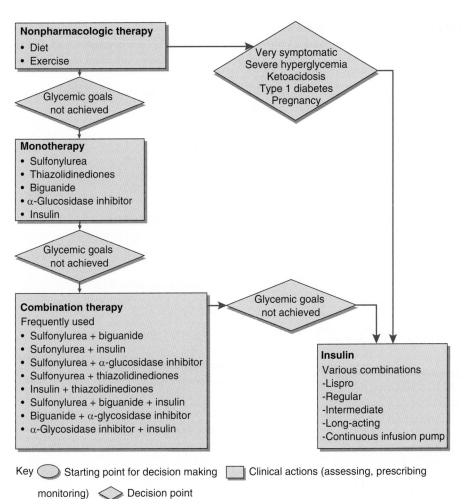

FIGURE 45–1 Algorithm for pharmacotherapy for Type 2 diabetes. (Adapted from the American Diabetes Association. [1995]. Algorithm for pharmacotherapy for NIDDM. *Diabetes Care, 18,* 1510–1518.)

medical identification in the form of a Medic Alert bracelet or necklace.

In patients taking insulin, meals are to be eaten on a regular basis. If a rapid-acting insulin is used, it is taken immediately before eating. The α-glucosidase inhibitors are only taken if a meal is eaten.

Here are some patient-oriented sources for information:

- www.diabetes.org is the site from the American Diabetes Association with information for managing the diabetic's life.
- www.niddk.nih.gov/health/diabetes.htm is a site from National Institutes of Health that serves as an information clearinghouse.

- www.diabetes.com provides information for the diabetic individual.

Nutritional and Lifestyle Changes

Diabetes management includes medical nutrition therapy, exercise, and, in most cases, drug therapy. Foods high in processed sugar and fat are to be avoided as is alcohol. Regular daily exercise helps to control blood sugar levels.

Patients with diabetes must follow "sick day guidelines" for the treatment of their condition when dealing with other illnesses. In general, practitioners should instruct people with diabetes not to stop their medication when they are ill. Infection, stress, and other variables increase plasma glucose levels, even though oral intake may be reduced. Practitioners should instruct patients to increase their fluid intake to approximately 8 oz of water or sugar-free beverage every hour, especially if they have a fever. Patients should monitor blood glucose levels at home more frequently, as often as every 4 hours. Urine also requires testing for ketones. If the blood glucose concentration is greater than 300 mg/dL on two consecutive readings, fever is persistently high, and symptoms of severe dehydration and ketonuria develop, the patient requires formal evaluation. Sick day plans should be developed with patients before illness occurs.

TABLE 45.10	Measures of Control of Fasting Blood Glucose	
Measure of Glucose	**Goal**	**Levels When Adjustment to Regimen Is Indicated**
Fasting glucose	90–130 mg/dL	<80 or >140 mg/dL
Bedtime glucose	110–150 mg/dL	<110 or >160 mg/dL
HbA$_{1c}$	<7	≥7

Complementary and Alternative Medicine

In a recent study conducted at the U.S. Department of Agriculture, cinnamon reduced serum glucose levels and improved lipid profiles in patients with type 2 diabetes. Patients were randomized into six groups that received 1, 2, or 3 g of cinnamon or a placebo. All groups receiving cinnamon had a decrease of 18% to 30% in fasting serum glucose values and a reduction of 23% to 30% in triglycerides and 7% to 27% reduction in LDL levels. Total cholesterol level declined 12% to 26%.

A daily vitamin is recommended if the patient is on a weight reduction plan.

Case Study

R. S. is a 55-year-old moderately obese Hispanic woman (body mass index is 29). She was referred to you when her gynecologist noted glucose on a routine urinalysis. She subsequently has an FPG of 190 and 200 mg/dL on two separate occasions. She is thirstier than usual and has more frequent urination. She also complains of decreased energy over the last several months.

- Family history: sister, mother, and maternal grandmother have diabetes
- Social history: nonsmoker, drinks alcohol socially (1 drink about 3 times a month), and does not exercise
- Review of systems: 20 lb weight gain over the past 2 years, has some blurred vision, has had two urinary tract infections in the past year and has frequent vaginal yeast infections
- Physical exam: unremarkable except blood pressure of 150/90
- Laboratory results: FPG 200 mg/dL, HbA_{1c} 10%, LDL 160 mg/dL, HDL 35 mg/dL, and triglycerides 266 mg/dL

DIAGNOSIS: TYPE 2 DIABETES MELLITUS

1. List specific goals for treatment for R. S.
2. What dietary and lifestyle changes would you recommend for R. S.?
3. What drug therapy would you prescribe? Why?
4. What is the goal for the FPG? Postprandial glucose? HbA_{1c}?
5. Discuss specific education for R. S. based on the prescribed therapy.
6. List one or two adverse reactions for the therapy selected that would cause you to change the therapy.
7. If the HbA_{1c} after 3 months on the prescribed therapy is 8.8%, what would be the next line of therapy?
8. What over-the-counter or herbal medicines might be appropriate for R. S.?
9. Describe one or two drug–drug or drug–food interactions for the selected agent.

BIBLIOGRAPHY

Starred entries are cited in the text.

Adler, A. I., Stratton, I. M., Neil, H. A., et al. (2000). Association of systolic blood pressure with macrovascular and microvascular complications of type 2 diabetes (UKPDS 36): Prospective observational study. *British Medical Journal, 321,* 412–419.

ALLHAT Collaborative Research Group. (2000). Major cardiovascular events in hypertensive patients randomized to doxazosin vs. chlorthalidone: The Antihypertensive and Lipid-Lowering Treatment to Prevent Heart Attack Trial (ALLHAT). *Journal of the American Medical Association, 283,* 1967–1975.

ALLHAT Study Group. (2002). Major outcomes in high-risk hypertensive patients randomized to angiotensin-converting enzyme inhibitor or calcium channel blocker vs. diuretic: The Antihypertensive and Lipid-Lowering Treatment to Prevent Heart Attack Trial (ALLHAT). *Journal of the American Medical Association, 288,* 2981–2997.

*American Diabetes Association. (1995). Algorithm for pharmacotherapy for NIDDM. *Diabetes Care, 18,* 1510–1518.

American Diabetes Association. (2000). Type 2 diabetes in children and doles-cents (Consensus Statement). *Diabetes Care, 23,* 381–389.

American Diabetes Association. (2004a). Aspirin therapy in diabetes (Position Statement). *Diabetes Care, 27*(Suppl. 1), S72–S73.

American Diabetes Association. (2004b). Gestational diabetes mellitus (Position Statement). *Diabetes Care, 27*(Suppl. 1), S88–S90.

American Diabetes Association. (2004c). Hyperglycemic crises in diabetes (Position Statement). *Diabetes Care, 27*(Suppl. 1), S94–S102.

American Diabetes Association. (2004d). Nephropathy in diabetes (Position Statement). *Diabetes Care, 27*(Suppl. 1), S79–S83.

American Diabetes Association. (2004e). Postprandial blood glucose (Consensus Statement). *Diabetes Care, 24,* 775–778.

American Diabetes Association. (2004f). Retinopathy in diabetes (Position Statement). *Diabetes Care, 27*(Suppl. 1), S84–S87.

American Diabetes Association. (2010a). Diagnosis and classification of diabetes mellitus (Position Statement). *Diabetes Care 33*(Suppl. 1), S62–S69.

American Diabetes Association. (2010b). Standards of medical care in diabetes – 2010 (Position Statement). *Diabetes Care, 33*(Suppl. 1), S11–S61.

Anderson, S., Tarnow, L., Rossing, P., et al. (2000). Renoprotective effects of angiotensin II receptor blockade in type 1 diabetic patients with diabetic nephropathy. *Kidney International, 57,* 601–606.

Arauz-Pacheco, C., Parrott, M. A., & Raskin, P. (2002). The treatment of hypertension in adult patients with diabetes mellitus [Technical Review]. *Diabetes Care, 25,* 134–147.

Bakris, G. L., Williams, M., Dworkin, L., et al. (2000). Preserving renal function in adults with hypertension and diabetes: A consensus approach: National Kidney Foundation Hypertension and Diabetes Executive Committees Working Group. *American Journal of Kidney Disease, 36,* 646–661.

Barteis, D. (2004). Adherence to oral therapy for type 2 diabetes: Opportunities for enhancing glycemic control. *Journal of the American Academy of Nurse Practitioners, 16*(1), 8–16.

Bartol, T. G. (2003). Treating type 2 diabetes to goal: The role of pharmacotherapy. *American Journal for Nurse Practitioners, 7*(11), 34–37.

Berl, T., Hunsicker, L. G., Lewis, J. B., et al. (2003). Cardiovascular outcomes in the Irbesartan Diabetic Nephropathy Trial of patients with type 2 diabetes and overt nephropathy. *Annals of Internal Medicine, 138,* 542–549.

Bode, B. W. (Ed.). (2004). *Medical management of type 1 diabetes* (4th ed). Alexandria, VA: American Diabetes Association, 2004.

Brenner, B. M., Cooper, M. E., de Zeeuw, D., et al. (2001). Effects of losartan on renal and cardiovascular outcomes in patients with type 2 diabetes and nephropathy. *New England Journal of Medicine, 345,* 861–869.

Buchanan, T. A., Xiang, A. H., Peters, R. K., et al. (2002). Preservation of pancreatic [beta]-cell function and prevention of type 2 diabetes by pharmacological treatment of insulin resistance in high-risk Hispanic women. *Diabetes, 51,* 2796–2803.

Bullock, B. A., & Henze, R. L. (2000). *Focus on pathophysiology.* Philadelphia: Lippincott Williams & Wilkins.

*Centers for Disease Control and Prevention (2008). *Estimates of diagnosed diabetes now available for all U.S. counties.* Atlanta, Georgia, Press Release June 24, 2008. Retrieved from http://www.cdc.gov/media/pressrel/2008/r080624.htm.

Chiasson, J. L., Josse, R. G., Gomis, R., et al. (2002). Acarbose for prevention of type 2 diabetes mellitus: The STOP-NIDDM randomized trial. *Lancet, 359,* 2072–2077.

Chobanian, A. V., Bakris, G. L., Black, H. R., et al., & the National Heart, Lung, and Blood Institute Joint National Committee on Prevention, Detection, Evaluation, and Treatment of High Blood Pressure, the National High Blood Pressure Education Program Coordinating Committee: The Seventh Report of the Joint National Committee on Prevention, Detection, Evaluation, and Treatment of High Blood Pressure. (2003). The JNC 7 report. *Journal of the American Medical Association, 289,* 2560–2572.

Chyan, Y., & Chuang, L. (2007). Dipeptidyl peptidase IV inhibitors: An evolving treatment for type 2 diabetes mellitus from the incretin concept. *Recent Patents on Endocrine, Metabolic & Immune Drug Discovery, 1*(1), 15–24.

Ciulla, T. A., Amador, A. G., & Zinman, B. (2003). Diabetic retinopathy and diabetic macular edema: Pathophysiology, screening, and novel therapies. *Diabetes Care, 26,* 2653–2664.

*DCCT Research Group. (1995). Effect of intensive therapy on the development and progression of diabetic nephropathy in the Diabetes Control and Complications Trial (DCCT). *Kidney International, 47,* 1703–1720.

DCCT/EDIC Research Group. (2000). Retinopathy and nephropathy in patients with type 1 diabetes four years after a trial of intensive therapy. *New England Journal of Medicine, 342,* 381–389.

Diabetes Control and Complications Trial Research Group. (1993). The effect of intensive treatment of diabetes on the development and progression of long-term complications in insulin-dependent diabetes mellitus. *New England Journal of Medicine, 329,* 977–986.

Diabetes Prevention Program Research Group. (2002). Reduction in the incidence of type 2 diabetes with lifestyle intervention or metformin. *New England Journal of Medicine, 346,* 393–403.

*Diabetes Statistics. (2007). National diabetes fact sheet. Retrieved from http://www.diabetes.org/diabetes-basics/diabetes statistics/?utm_source=WWW&utm_medium=DropDownDB&utm_content=Statistics&utm_campaign=CON.

Eknoyan, G., Hostetter, T., Bakris, G. L., et al. (2003). Proteinuria and other markers of chronic kidney disease: A position statement of the National Kidney Foundation (NKF) and the National Institute of Diabetes and Digestive and Kidney Diseases (NIDDK). *American Journal of Kidney Disease, 42,* 617–622.

Engelgau, M. E., Narayan, K. M. V., & Herman, W. H. (2000). Screening for type 2 diabetes [Technical Review]. *Diabetes Care, 23,* 1563–1580 [erratum appears in *Diabetes Care, 23,* 1868–1869, 2000].

Expert Committee on the Diagnosis and Classification of Diabetes Mellitus. (2003). Follow-up report on the diagnosis of diabetes mellitus. *Diabetes Care, 26,* 3160–3167.

Fagot-Campagna, A., Pettitt, D. J., Engelgau, M. M., et al. (2000). DM2 among North American children and adolescents: An epidemiologic review and a public health perspective. *Journal of Pediatrics, 136,* 664–672.

*Francisco, G. E., & Brooks, P. J. (1999). Diabetes mellitus. In J. T. DiPiro, R. L. Talbert, G. C. Yee, et al. (Eds.), *Pharmacotherapy: A pathophysiologic approach* (4th ed., pp. 1219–1243). East Norwalk, CT: Appleton & Lange.

Garg, J., & Bakris, G. L. (2002). Microalbuminuria: Marker of vascular dysfunction, risk factor for cardiovascular disease. *Journal of Vascular Medicine, 7,* 35–43.

Hayden, M., Pignone, M., & Phillips, C. (2002). Aspirin for the primary prevention of cardiovascular events: A summary of the evidence for the U.S. Preventive Services Task Force. *Annals of Internal Medicine, 136,* 161–171.

Heart Outcomes Prevention Evaluation (HOPE) Study Investigators. (2000). Effects of ramipril on cardiovascular and microvascular outcomes in people with diabetes mellitus: Results of the HOPE study and MICRO-HOPE study. *Lancet, 355,* 253–259.

Heart Protection Study Collaborative Group. (2003). MRC/BHF Heart Protection Study of cholesterol-lowering with simvastatin in 5963 people with diabetes: A randomized placebo-controlled trial. *Lancet, 361,* 2005–2016.

Janumet. (2010). *Janumet: Full prescribing information.* Whitehouse Station, N.J.: Mercke, Sharp, & Dohme.

Januvia. (2010). *Januvia: Full prescribing information.* Whitehouse Station, N.J.: Mercke, Sharpe & Dohme.

Jones, M., & Patel, M. (2006). Insulin detemir: A long acting insulin product. *American Journal of Health-System Pharmacy. 63*(24), 2466–2472.

Jovanovic, L. (Ed.). (2000). *Medical management of pregnancy complicated by diabetes* (3rd ed.). Alexandria, VA: American Diabetes Association.

Kilingensmith, G. (Ed.). (2003). *Intensive diabetes management* (3rd ed.). Alexandria, VA: American Diabetes Association.

Klein, R. (2003). Screening interval for retinopathy in type 2 diabetes. *Lancet, 361,* 190–191.

Nathan, D., Buse, J., Davidson, M., et al. (2009). Medical management of hyperglycemia in type 2 diabetes mellitus: A consensus algorithm for the initiation and adjustment of therapy. *Diabetes Care, 32,* 193–203.

National Cholesterol Education Program (NCEP) Expert Panel on Detection, Evaluation and Treatment of High Blood Cholesterol in Adults (Adult Treatment Panel III). (2001). Executive summary of the third report of the National Cholesterol Education Program (NCEP) Expert Panel on Detection, Evaluation and Treatment of High Blood Cholesterol in Adults (Adult Treatment Panel III). *Journal of the American Medical Association, 285,* 2486–2497.

National Institute of Diabetes and Digestive and Kidney Diseases. (2003/2004). National Diabetes Statistics fact sheet: General information and national estimates on diabetes in the United States, 2003. Bethesda, MD: U.S. Department of Health and Human Services, National Institutes of Health. 2004 Rev. ed. Bethesda, MD: U.S. Department of Health and Human Services, National Institutes of Health.

Ohkubo, Y., Kishikawa, H., Araki, E., et al. (1995). Intensive insulin therapy prevents the progression of diabetic microvascular complications in Japanese patients with non-insulin-dependent diabetes mellitus: A randomized prospective 6-year study. *Diabetes Research and Clinical Practice, 28,* 103–117.

Onglyza. (2009). *Onglyza: Full prescribing information.* Princeton, NJ: Bristol Myers Squibb.

Rohlfing, C. L., Wiedmeyer, H. M., Little, R. R., et al. (2002). Defining the relationship between plasma glucose and HbA^{1c}: Analysis of glucose profiles and HbA^{1c} in the Diabetes Control and Complications Trial. *Diabetes Care, 25,* 275–278.

Rosenstock, J. (2001). Insulin therapy: Optimizing control in type 1 and type 2 diabetes. *Clinical Cornerstone, 4*(2), 50–64.

Sacks, D. B., Bruns, D. E., Goldstein, D. E., et al. (2002). Guidelines and recommendations for laboratory analysis in the diagnosis and management of diabetes mellitus. *Diabetes Care, 25,* 750–786.

Smeltzer, S. C., & Bare, B. G. (2000). *Brunner & Suddarth's textbook of medical-surgical nursing* (9th ed.). Philadelphia, PA: Lippincott Williams & Wilkins.

Sullivan, M., & Mechcatie, E. (2010). Limits on rosiglitazone may effectively end use. *Clinical Endocrinology News, 5*(10), 1.

Tuomilehto, J., Lindstrom, J., Eriksson, J. G., et al. (2001). Prevention of type 2 diabetes mellitus by changes in lifestyle among subjects with impaired glucose tolerance. *New England Journal of Medicine, 344,* 1343–1350.

UK Prospective Diabetes Study Group. (1998). Effect of intensive blood-glucose control with metformin on complications in overweight patients with type 2 diabetes (UKPDS 34). *Lancet, 352,* 854–865.

UK Prospective Diabetes Study Group. (1998). Intensive blood-glucose control with sulphonylureas or insulin compared with conventional treatment and risk of complications in patients with type 2 diabetes (UKPDS 33). *Lancet, 352,* 837–853.

US Preventive Services Task Force. (2002). Aspirin for the primary prevention of cardiovascular events: Recommendation and rationale. *Annals of Internal Medicine, 136,* 157–160.

Vijan, S., Hofer, T. P., & Hayward, R. A. (2000). Cost-utility analysis of screening intervals for diabetic retinopathy in patients with type 2 diabetes mellitus. *Journal of the American Medical Association, 283,* 889–896.

Thyroid Disorders

Diseases of the thyroid gland are common clinical conditions, accounting for many office visits each year. Population-based studies have found that hypothyroidism exists to some degree in 4.6% to 9.5% of individuals, with higher rates occurring in the elderly (Canaris, et al., 2000; Hollowell, et al., 2002). These same studies found a 1.3% to 2.2% rate of hyperthyroidism. Both hypothyroidism and hyperthyroidism have been associated with adverse cardiovascular outcomes (Hak, et al., 2000; Sawin, et al., 1994). If these conditions are not treated properly, their morbidity can be high. Thyroid nodules are common, occurring clinically in approximately 5% of patients, but found using ultrasound studies in 22% of patients and in autopsy studies in 50% of patients. Although most thyroid nodules are nonmalignant and most thyroid cancers are not very aggressive, approximately 1,200 deaths per year are attributed to thyroid malignancy. Therefore, clinicians should understand the therapeutic options for these conditions.

To diagnose and treat thyroid disease, a basic understanding of thyroid anatomy and physiology is necessary (**Figures 46-1** and **46-2**). The gland is divided into two lobes that are separated by an isthmus. Histologically, the thyroid is composed of follicles that are made of cells that are cuboidal at rest but column shaped when activated by thyroid-stimulating hormone (TSH). These follicular cells encircle a mass of colloid that contains thyroglobulin, a glycoprotein that the follicular cells secrete. Iodine, which is consumed in the diet, is reduced to iodide in the gastrointestinal (GI) tract and readily absorbed. Iodide is then carried to the thyroid, where it is taken up by the follicular cells. In these cells, iodide is oxidized and incorporated into tyrosine residues of thyroglobulin to form monoiodothyronine (MIT). Two MITs are paired to make diiodothyronine (DIT), and combinations of MIT with DIT produce triiodothyronine (T_3) and thyroxine (T_4), respectively.

The pituitary gland secretes TSH, which controls the rate of release of T_3 and T_4. The hypothalamus secretes thyrotropin-releasing hormone (TRH), which modulates the release of TSH. All these hormones work in a negative-feedback system, in which low levels of thyroid hormones in the blood cause increased secretion of TSH and, subsequently, T_3 and T_4.

Once T_3 and T_4 are secreted into the bloodstream, proteins known as *thyroid-binding globulins* (TBGs) bind most of these hormones. Only a small amount of T_3 and T_4 is in the "free" or unbound state; the hormones in this state are the clinically significant ones. Free T_3 and free T_4 act at the cellular level to regulate metabolism by binding to nuclear receptors and affecting gene expression and protein synthesis. Any condition that can affect TBGs also can affect the level of free T_3 and free T_4. The thyroid produces only approximately 20% of circulating T_3, whereas monodeiodination of T_4 in the periphery produces the remainder.

Clinically, measurement of serum TSH and free T_4 are used most commonly to assess thyroid function. Given the availability of the free T_4 assay, total T_4 is used less frequently because actual thyroid function depends on the level of free T_4 rather than total T_4. **Table 46.1** depicts relative levels of TSH and free T_4 in disorders of thyroid function.

HYPOTHYROIDISM

Hypothyroidism is a relatively common clinical entity, occurring in up to 5.9% of women and 0.2% of men. Patients may complain of symptoms of fatigue, constipation, weight gain, or change in menstrual periods, among others. Physical examination may reveal thyromegaly, bradycardia, or peripheral edema (**Box 46.1**). Total cholesterol and low-density lipoprotein (LDL) levels may be elevated in 90% to 95% of patients.

CAUSES

Hypothyroidism has several causes (**Box 46.2**). In the United States and other developed countries, hypothyroidism nearly always results from a problem with the production or release (or both) of thyroid hormones. Worldwide, iodine deficiency is most commonly the cause. Hashimoto (or autoimmune) thyroiditis is the most common precipitant of hypothyroidism in the United States. It results from the infiltration of the thyroid gland by lymphocytes, which results in progressive fibrosis and decreased function of the gland. Patients may present with goiter and be euthyroid or hypothyroid initially; antithyroid antibodies are positive in high titers.

Post-therapeutic hypothyroidism is another common cause, whereas other entities such as subacute thyroiditis

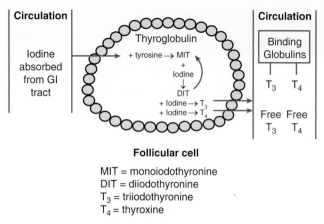

FIGURE 46–1 Thyroid hormone synthesis.

MIT = monoiodothyronine
DIT = diiodothyronine
T_3 = triiodothyronine
T_4 = thyroxine

TABLE 46.1	Thyroid Function Testing in Common Thyroid Disorders	
	TSH	**Free T_4**
Primary hypothyroidism	Increased	Decreased
Secondary or tertiary hypothyroidism	Decreased	Decreased
Mild thyroid failure	Increased	Normal
Hyperthyroidism	Decreased	Increased (or normal in T_3 thyrotoxicosis)
Subclinical hyperthyroidism	Decreased	Normal

or postpartum thyroiditis can produce brief periods of hypothyroidism. Subacute and postpartum thyroiditis are discussed at the end of this chapter.

Many drugs may interfere with thyroid function and induce hypothyroidism (**Box 46.3**). These include amiodarone (Cordarone) and lithium (Eskalith). If patients discontinue these drugs, thyroid function should return to normal; however, many patients taking these drugs have serious coexisting conditions and cannot stop using them. Therefore, clinicians should monitor these patients regularly for hypothyroidism and treat them with thyroid replacement if appropriate.

PATHOPHYSIOLOGY

Hypothyroidism results from a relative deficit of thyroid hormones, usually T_4. The deficit may result from failure of the thyroid gland itself (primary hypothyroidism) or, less commonly,

from failure of the pituitary gland or hypothalamus (secondary or tertiary hypothyroidism, respectively). Presenting symptoms of thyroid hormone deficiency are similar in all types of hypothyroidism.

DIAGNOSTIC CRITERIA

Primary hypothyroidism is confirmed, in the appropriate clinical setting, by the finding of an elevated TSH and a low free T_4 level. Secondary hypothyroidism, as a result of pituitary dysfunction, results in low free T_4 and low TSH levels. Tertiary hypothyroidism results from decreased production of TRH by the hypothalamus. Secondary hypothyroidism can be distinguished from tertiary hypothyroidism by imaging of the pituitary and hypothalamus. There is a TRH stimulation test in which exogenous TRH is administered and serum TSH response is measured, but this test is of limited value. Secondary hypothyroidism and tertiary hypothyroidism are not very common.

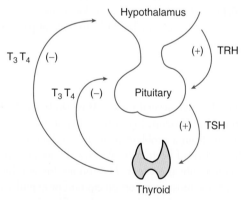

TRH = thyroid-releasing hormone
TSH = thyroid-stimulating hormone
T_3 = triiodothyronine
T_4 = thyroxine
(+) = positive effect
(−) = negative effect

FIGURE 46–2 Hypothalamic-pituitary-thyroid axis.

BOX 46.1 Symptoms and Signs of Hypothyroidism	
Fatigue	Bradycardia
Constipation	Delayed deep tendon reflexes
Menorrhagia	Hyperlipidemia
Weight gain	Goiter
Hair loss	Hypothermia
Cold intolerance	Periorbital swelling
Hoarseness	Jaundice
Depression	Ataxia
Dry skin	Edema
Infertility	Myalgias
Difficulty with memory and concentration	

BOX 46.2

Causes of Hypothyroidism

Primary Hypothyroidism (Elevated TSH)
Autoimmune (Hashimoto, lymphocytic) thyroiditis
Treated Graves disease
Subacute thyroiditis
Silent thyroiditis
Iodine excess, including iodine-containing
    medication
Lithium therapy
Inadequate thyroid hormone replacement

Secondary Hypothyroidism (Low TSH)
Hypopituitarism

Tertiary Hypothyroidism (Low TRH, TSH)
Hypothalamic dysfunction

Other Causes of Elevated TSH
Nonthyroid illness
Adrenal insufficiency
Drugs (e.g., metoclopramide and domperidone)
TSH-producing pituitary tumors
Thyroid hormone resistance syndromes

Data from Mazzaferri, E. L. (1997). Evaluation and management of common thyroid disorders in women. *American Journal of Obstetrics and Gynecology, 176,* 507–514.

BOX 46.3

Drug Interactions with T$_4$

Drugs That Decrease TSH Secretion
Dopamine
Glucocorticoids
Octreotide

Drugs That Alter Thyroid Hormone Secretion
Decreased Thyroid Hormone Secretion
Lithium
Iodide
Amiodarone
Aminoglutethimide
Increased Thyroid Hormone Secretion
Iodide
Amiodarone

Drugs That Decrease T$_4$ Absorption
Colestipol
Cholestyramine
Aluminum hydroxide
Ferrous sulfate
Sucralfate
Calcium carbonate

Drugs That Alter T$_4$ and T$_3$ Transport in Serum
Increased Serum TBG Concentration
Estrogens

Tamoxifen
Heroin
Methadone
Mitotane
Fluorouracil
Decreased Serum TBG Concentration
Androgens
Anabolic steroids (e.g., danazol)
Slow-release nicotinic acid
Glucocorticoids
Displacement from Protein-Binding Sites
Furosemide
Fenclofenac
Mefenamic acid
Salicylates

Drugs That Alter T$_4$ and T$_3$ Metabolism
Increased Hepatic Metabolism
Phenobarbital
Rifampin
Phenytoin
Carbamazepine
Decreased T$_4$ 5'-Deiodinase Activity
Propylthiouracil
Amiodarone
Beta blockers
Glucocorticoids

Data from Surks, M. I., & Sievert, R. (1995). Drugs and thyroid function. *New England Journal of Medicine, 333,* 1688–1694.

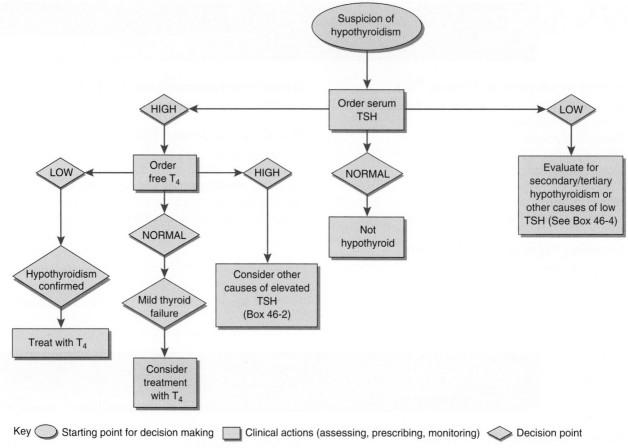

Key ⬭ Starting point for decision making   ▭ Clinical actions (assessing, prescribing, monitoring)   ◇ Decision point

FIGURE 46–3   Treatment algorithm for hypothyroidism.

INITIATING DRUG THERAPY

The only course of treatment for hypothyroidism is replacement with thyroid hormone. **Figure 46-3** shows an algorithm for the evaluation and treatment of hypothyroidism.

Goals of Drug Therapy

The goal of therapy is to return the patient to the euthyroid state with a TSH in the range of 0.5 to 4.0 mIU/mL. Clinicians should exercise caution not to overtreat hypothyroidism by suppressing the TSH to lower than normal levels because such overtreatment will put the patient at risk for hyperthyroidism and its attendant morbidities. Treatment of most cases of hypothyroidism usually is lifelong; exceptions include those cases that occur transiently in patients with postpartum or subacute thyroiditis (discussed later in this chapter).

Thyroid Hormone

Once they have made a diagnosis of hypothyroidism, practitioners should initiate treatment with thyroid hormone replacement in the form of levothyroxine (T_4). **Table 46.2** lists the various preparations available. Natural thyroid extract derives from porcine thyroid glands and is a combination of T_3 and T_4. This preparation is not used much because of variability in the amount of T_3. T_3 replacement alone is available (liothyronine [Cytomel]) but also is not prescribed frequently because of its association with an increased risk of iatrogenic hyperthyroidism. It is sometimes given for short-term use before radioactive iodine scanning. A combination product of T_3 and T_4 (liotrix [Klotrix]) exists but offers no advantage over T_4 alone. Furthermore, this product increases serum T_3 above physiologic levels within several hours, leading to palpitations.

Several branded preparations of T_4 are available, any one of which may be used. Historically, authorities have recommended against the use of generic T_4. A controversial study of the bioavailability of generic preparations compared with brand name T_4, however, found no significant difference between generic and nongeneric T_4 and concluded that generic drugs may be used safely. The drug is readily absorbed from the GI tract. Serum T_4 levels peak at 2 to 4 hours, although the rise in serum T_3 levels is slower because of the time needed for conversion from T_4. Synthetic T_4 has a half-life of 1 week and requires approximately 6 to 8 weeks of therapy to reach steady state; therefore, patients may not notice improvement in symptoms for 1 week or more.

TABLE 46.2	Overview of Drugs Used for Treatment of Hypothyroidism			

Generic (Trade) Name and Dosage	Selected Adverse Events	Contraindications	Special Considerations
levothyroxine (Synthroid, others) Start: 12.5–100 mcg/d Maintenance: 75–150 mcg/d	Only with excessive dosing: arrhythmias, palpitations, nervousness, tremor, weight loss	Untreated thyrotoxicosis, hypersensitivity to thyroid hormones, uncorrected adrenal cortical insufficiency	Goal TSH 0.5–4.0 milliunits/L
liothyronine (Cytomel) Start: 25 mcg/d Maintenance: 25–75 mcg/d	Only with excessive dosing	Same as above	Goal TSH 0.5–4.0 milliunits/L
liotrix (Thyrolar) (liothyronine and levothyroxine) Start: levothyroxine 50 mcg/d + liothyronine 12.5 mcg/d Maintenance: levothyroxine 100 mcg/d + liothyronine 25 mcg/d	Only with excessive dosing	Same as above	Goal TSH 0.5–4.0 milliunits/L
thyroid, dessicated (Armour) (liothyronine and levothyroxine) Start: 60 mcg/d Maintenance: 60–120 mcg/d	Only with excessive dosing	Same as above	Goal TSH 0.5–4.0 milliunits/L; not used much because of variability of T_3 content

Dosage

When initiating therapy, clinicians must consider the patient's age, the duration of hypothyroidism, and any concomitant conditions. For adolescents and young adults, treatment can begin with the full replacement dose (100–125 mcg/day, or 1.6 mcg/kg/day, or approximately 0.75 mcg/lb/day). Children require approximately 4 to 10 mcg/kg/day depending on age. In older adults or patients at risk for cardiac disease, thyroid hormone replacement should begin at 25 or even 12.5 mcg/day. Prescribers should increase the dosage incrementally (by 25 mcg/day every 4–6 weeks) until reaching the full replacement dose. Clinicians must monitor serum TSH levels and adjust the dose of T_4 accordingly. Many different dosage strengths (25–300 mcg) are available to allow titration to appropriate levels.

Interactions

Some drugs interfere with the absorption of thyroid hormone from the GI tract. (See **Box 46.3.**) These include cholestyramine (Questran), sucralfate (Carafate), aluminum-containing antacids, and calcium carbonate. Patients should not take T_4 several hours before or after ingesting these agents.

The concentration of total T_4 and T_3 depends on the concentration of serum TBGs. Any drug or condition that interferes with TBG levels can affect the interpretation of thyroid function tests. Furthermore, in patients who are taking T_4, the changing concentration of TBGs may necessitate adjustment of the dose. The most common causes of an increased serum TBG concentration are increased estrogen production (e.g., as in pregnancy) and the administration of estrogen, either in the form of an oral contraceptive or as estrogen replacement therapy. Patients receiving these therapies will likely need higher doses of T_4 to maintain the euthyroid state because the estrogen increases the level of TBGs, and more thyroid hormone is in the bound, inactive state rather than in the free, active state. Androgens and niacin can decrease TBG concentrations and have opposite effects on thyroid function tests; patients taking these drugs will likely need lower doses of T_4.

Several drugs decrease the affinity of T_4 and T_3 to TBGs, causing displacement of hormones and resulting in a transient increase in free T_4 and T_3 levels. Salicylates and high doses of furosemide (Lasix) can exert this effect.

Another concern is for the patient taking oral anticoagulants. When hypothyroid patients become euthyroid, metabolism of vitamin K–dependent clotting factors increases. Thus, the patient's prothrombin time may increase, as does the risk of bleeding. The opposite occurs in patients treated for hyperthyroidism. Thus, clinicians need to monitor carefully coagulation studies in patients taking warfarin (Coumadin) who are being treated for thyroid disease.

Drugs like phenytoin (Dilantin) and carbamazepine (Tegretol) alter the metabolism of thyroid hormones. Patients who use these agents require more frequent monitoring of thyroid function.

Special Population Considerations

Pediatric

In children, developmental defects like thyroid aplasia or hypoplasia or inborn errors in thyroid hormonogenesis may result in thyroid deficiency. Routine screening of newborns allows early identification and treatment of this potentially devastating condition. Children with congenital hypothyroidism require referral to a pediatric endocrinologist for treatment. Older children also may become hypothyroid as a result of lymphocytic

(Hashimoto) thyroiditis or secondary to irradiation or surgery on the thyroid. Treatment is similar to that for adults, but children may require doses of up to 4.0 mcg/kg/d of T_4 due to rapid metabolism (National Academy of Clinical Biochemistry website).

Geriatric

Clinicians need to maintain a high level of suspicion for thyroid disease in older adults because the presentation of illness may differ from that in younger patients. This difference is partly because of alterations in the rate of hormone secretion and clearance as well as increased nodularity and fibrosis of the thyroid gland. Furthermore, concomitant illnesses and medications can modify thyroid function in older adults. Symptoms of hypothyroidism may be subtle or nonexistent. Ataxia, paresthesias, and carpal tunnel syndrome may be the presenting symptoms of hypothyroidism in older adults. Psychiatric manifestations of thyroid disease (e.g., depression or change in sensorium) also are more common in this age group. Older adults also are more susceptible to complications of therapy. Treatment should be initiated at a lower dose for elderly patients.

Pregnancy

Hypothyroidism in pregnancy deserves special mention. Because of the increased amount of thyroglobulin during pregnancy, more T_4 is bound in the circulation. Total T_4 and T_3 increase early in the first trimester, even in women without hypothyroidism. The free T_4 consequently declines to such a degree that symptoms of hypothyroidism may develop in many pregnant women with previously controlled hypothyroidism treated with T_4, necessitating a dose increase by approximately 50 mcg until after delivery. Clinicians should evaluate thyroid function in pregnant women during every trimester by means of a TSH level. The serum total T_3 level returns to normal approximately 1 week after delivery, whereas the total T_4 level declines by 3 to 4 weeks if the patient is not using an oral contraceptive.

MONITORING PATIENT RESPONSE

Patients require clinical and laboratory evaluation with a serum TSH 6 to 8 weeks after initiating therapy or adjusting the dose of T_4. Because it takes this long for the TSH level to decline in response to T_4 replacement, a TSH test should not be ordered before this time. Clinicians should perform an interval history and physical examination, focusing on symptoms and signs of hyperthyroidism, which suggest overdosage, and residual symptoms of hypothyroidism to assess for underdosage.

Practitioners should check TSH levels 6 months after normalization to ensure stable metabolism of T_4, then annually unless new symptoms develop in the interim. Therapy is usually lifelong (although spontaneous recovery may occur in up to 20% of patients with hypothyroidism related to

Hashimoto thyroiditis), so clinicians must encourage patients to comply with their medication regimens. The finding of a very high TSH but a normal free T_4 level suggests intermittent compliance with T_4 therapy.

PATIENT EDUCATION

Patients with primary hypothyroidism most likely will require lifelong replacement with thyroid hormone. Patients should not expect to see a difference in their symptoms until 2 to 4 weeks after beginning therapy. Follow-up laboratory testing is necessary relatively frequently until a therapeutic dosage that results in a stable TSH is reached; at that point, testing should be done annually.

Drug Information

Patients are advised against taking excessive thyroid hormone replacement because of the increased risk of drug-induced hyperthyroidism, osteoporosis, and arrhythmias. Thyroid replacement should be taken on an empty stomach 30 minutes to 1 hour before ingestion of the first food of the day.

Patients on thyroid hormone replacement therapy should limit the use of adrenergic agents (e.g., nonprescription decongestants). Patients should not take thyroid hormone at the same time as iron or calcium supplements, antacids, bile acid sequestrants, or simethicone; these preparations require administration at least 2 hours before or after administration of thyroid hormone. Finally, clinicians should reassure patients that although hypothyroidism is a chronic condition, treatment is usually safe and effective.

HYPERTHYROIDISM

Hyperthyroidism results from an excess amount of thyroid hormone. It occurs in up to 2.2% of the population (Hollowell, et al., 2002), with a female-to-male ratio of 10:1 (Mulder, 1998).

CAUSES

Graves disease, an autoimmune disease that occurs most commonly in patients ages 20 to 50 with a female-to-male ratio of 4 to 8:1, is the most common cause of overt hyperthyroidism (**Box 46.4**). It develops as a result of stimulation of the thyroid gland by TSH receptor autoantibodies on the follicular cell surface. The autoantibodies act like TSH in stimulating thyroid gland function. The gland is not susceptible to the usual negative-feedback mechanism of the thyroid hormones; thus, levels of thyroid hormone escalate.

Toxic nodular goiter (Plummer disease) is another frequent cause of hyperthyroidism, especially in older adults. In this condition, one or more thyroid nodules begin to "hyperfunction" and are not dependent on the feedback mechanisms of the pituitary–thyroid axis. As a result of the increased systemic T_4 produced by the nodule, TSH is suppressed, and the remainder of the gland begins to atrophy. Eye findings (i.e., exophthalmos and lid lag sometimes found with Graves disease and thyrotoxicosis) are absent in this condition.

A less common cause of hyperthyroidism is thyrotoxicosis factitia, in which patients intentionally take T_4 in doses high enough to suppress their TSH. This finding is more common among those in the medical profession with access to prescription medications. These patients may want to use T_4 to help with weight loss or to treat fatigue or depression.

Several forms of thyroiditis may result in hyperthyroidism with a characteristically low radioactive iodine uptake. These are discussed in a later section.

Amiodarone and other drugs that contain iodine, including radiographic contrast agents, may induce hyperthyroidism in patients with autonomously functioning nodules. Clinicians must monitor such patients closely to see if they need to receive these agents.

DIAGNOSTIC CRITERIA

The patient with hyperthyroidism classically exhibits symptoms of enhanced metabolic activity (i.e., palpitations, sweating, heat intolerance, weight loss). Examination may reveal elevated blood pressure, tachycardia, a bruit over the thyroid gland, or exophthalmos in patients with Graves disease (**Box 46.5**). The diagnosis is confirmed by finding a low, or suppressed, TSH level with an elevated free T_4 level. A nuclear ^{123}I thyroid scan can confirm Graves disease, which causes a diffuse increase in uptake of radioactive iodine. Hyperthyroidism caused by a hyperfunctioning nodule appears as a localized area of increased radioiodine uptake (a "hot" nodule), with the remainder of the gland exhibiting generalized decreased uptake of the isotope.

INITIATING DRUG THERAPY

There are three main options to treat hyperthyroidism: (1) antithyroid drugs, (2) radioactive iodine ablation with ^{131}I, and (3) surgery (**Table 46.3** and **Figure 46-4**). In general, radioactive iodine is the treatment of choice for patients older than age 40; it often is used in younger patients as well. Because of the high rate of permanent hypothyroidism after treatment and the eventual need for lifelong thyroid replacement, as well as concerns about subsequent cancers after exposure to radioiodine at a young age, many clinicians initially attempt to treat younger patients with antithyroid medications. Data on this issue have been conflicting, but many investigators are now beginning to use radioactive iodine as first-line therapy in young patients. Radioactive iodine is contraindicated in pregnancy; however, it may be used in women of childbearing age and in children. Women should postpone pregnancy until 6 months after radioiodine therapy. Lactating women should not receive radioiodine because it passes into breast milk.

Practitioners should follow patients treated with ^{131}I every 4 to 6 weeks for 3 months after radioiodine treatment, then less frequently. Because most patients with Graves disease become hypothyroid after treatment, clinicians must screen for

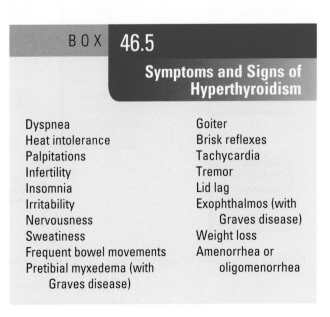

TABLE 46.3	Recommended Order of Treatment for Hyperthyroidism	
Order	**Agents**	**Comments**
First line	Radioactive iodine	Usually recommended in patients older than age 40, but may be used for younger patients High incidence of hypothyroidism when used to treat Graves disease; less when used for toxic nodules
Second line	Antithyroid drugs	Often used in younger patients to induce remission of Graves disease; also used to prepare some patients for treatment with radioiodine or surgery
Third line	Surgery	Usually reserved for patients with large goiters or suspected malignancy

symptoms and measure TSH and free T_4 levels intermittently. Conversely, when radioactive iodine is used to treat toxic nodules, the rate of post-therapeutic hypothyroidism is lower, likely related to the degree of suppression of the remainder of the gland by the nodule. If the free T_4 becomes low and the TSH elevated, patients should start T_4 supplementation with the goal of reaching the replacement dosage and maintaining euthyroidism. TSH levels should be done yearly or more frequently if the patient's clinical condition changes.

Surgery is reserved for patients with large goiters that compress vital structures or for those in whom there is a concern about a malignancy in the gland. It also may be used in pregnant women who are unable or unwilling to take antithyroid drugs. Before surgery, patients are often treated with antithyroid drugs until they are euthyroid, with inorganic iodide (discussed later) added 10 days after surgery.

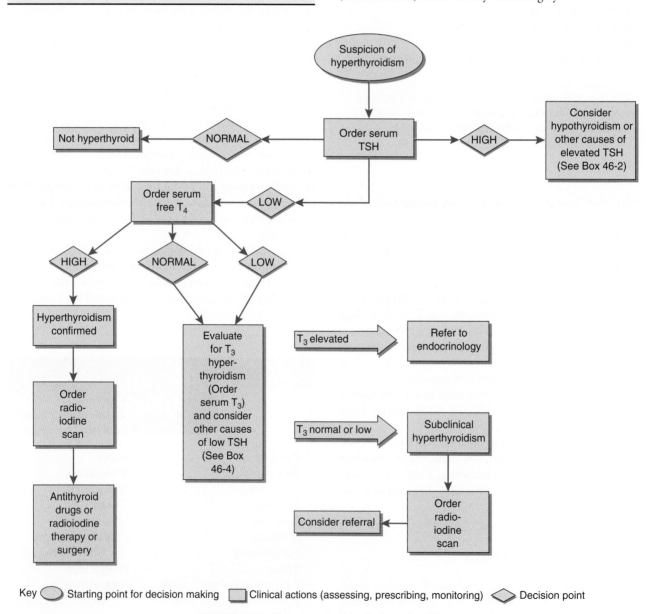

FIGURE 46–4 Treatment algorithm for hyperthyroidism.

Potential complications of surgery include hypoparathyroidism and injury to the recurrent laryngeal nerve, although in experienced hands these complications are rare. Hypothyroidism develops after thyroidectomy in up to 70% of cases depending on the extent of surgery, so postsurgical patients need regular follow-up and supplementation with T_4 as necessary.

Goals of Drug Therapy

The goals of therapy are to restore patients to the euthyroid state and eliminate the risks associated with chronic hyperthyroidism. Therapy usually is not lifelong. Patients usually stop taking antithyroid drugs after 1 to 2 years. If permanent hypothyroidism develops as a result of radioactive iodine treatment or surgery, however, then treatment of hypothyroidism (discussed previously) is lifelong.

Antithyroid Drugs

Antithyroid drugs commonly used are methimazole (Tapazole) and propylthiouracil (PTU [Propyl-Thyracil]; **Table 46.4**).

Mechanism of Action

These drugs act by inhibiting iodine organification. They also block the conversion of T_4 to T_3 in the periphery, although this mechanism has minimal clinical relevance. The drugs are rapidly absorbed and concentrated in the thyroid follicular cells. PTU has a short duration of action and thus requires multiple doses per day. Methimazole has a longer duration and may be dosed once a day, making it the drug of choice in most instances.

Dosage

The starting dose for PTU is 200 to 400 mg/day, whereas the initial dose of methimazole is 10 to 30 mg/day. Treatment usually continues for 12 to 24 months. Success rates for antithyroid drugs range from 10% to 75%, with remission rates inversely related to the duration of hyperthyroidism and the size of the goiter.

Antithyroid drugs also are used to prepare patients with severe hyperthyroidism for ablative therapy with either radioactive iodine or surgery, especially in those at risk for cardiac complications. The drugs usually are given for several weeks then stopped several days before definitive therapy, although patients sometimes may need to continue the drugs for several months after ^{131}I therapy to control persistent hyperthyroidism.

Adverse Events

Side effects are fairly minimal (**Table 46.5**), with the most common being rash, arthralgias, itching, and hepatic abnormalities.

TABLE 46.4 Overview of Drugs Used to Treat Hyperthyroidism

Generic (Trade) Name and Dosage	Adverse Effects	Contraindications	Special Considerations
Antithyroid Drugs			
propylthiouracil (PTU [Propyl-Thyracil]) Start: 100–600 mg/d Maintenance: 50–100 mg q8h	See Box 46-5	Hypersensitivity to drug	TSH 0.5–4.0 milliunits/L Monitor for fever, sore throat; check CBC.
methimazole (Tapazole) Start: 15–30 mg/d Maintenance: 5–15 mg/d		Same as above	Same as above
Beta Blockers			
propranolol (Inderal) Long acting: 80–160 mg/d	Fatigue, sexual dysfunction	Sinus bradycardia, heart block greater than first degree	For symptom control only Use with caution in asthma, diabetes, congestive heart failure, and depression.
atenolol (Tenormin) 50–200 mg/d	Same as above	Same as above	Same as above
Iodine-Containing Compounds			
SSKI (Lugol's solution) 0.1–0.3 mL tid sodium iodide (Iodopen) 0.5–1 g q12h	Rash, sialadenitis, vasculitis	Allergy to iodine	Administer after starting antithyroid drug.
Iodinated contrast agents: ipodate (Oragrafin) iopanoate (Telepaque) 0.5–2 g/d	Itching, skin rash, hives, diarrhea, nausea, vomiting; bruising/bleeding with iopanoate	Same as above	Reserved for severe thyrotoxicosis or thyroid storm Administer after starting antithyroid drug.
Other Agents			
lithium (Eskalith, others) Starting and maintenance: 900–1,200 mg/d in divided doses	May have multisystem effects		Monitor lithium levels.
Glucocorticoids dosage depends on agent selected	May have multisystem effects		Adjunctive therapy for thyroid storm

TABLE 46.5   **Side Effects of Antithyroid Drugs**

Side Effect	Estimated Frequency	Comments
Minor		
Skin reactions	4–6%	Urticarial or macular reactions
Arthralgias	1–5%	May be harbinger of more severe arthritis
Gastrointestinal effects	1–5%	Includes gastric distress and nausea
Abnormal sense of taste or smell	Rare	With methimazole only
Sialadenitis	Very rare	Methimazole
Major		
Polyarthritis	1–2%	So-called antithyroid arthritis syndrome
ANCA-positive vasculitis	Rare	ANCA positivity is seen in patients with untreated Graves disease and in asymptomatic persons who are taking antithyroid drugs, especially prophylthiouracil.
Agranulocytosis	0.1–0.5%	Mild granulocytopenia may be seen in patients with Graves disease; may be more common with propylthiouracil.
Other hematologic side effects	Vary rare	May include thrombocytopenia and aplastic anemia
Immunoallergic hepatitis	0.1–0.2%; 1% in some series.	Almost exclusively in patients taking propylthiouracil; a transient increase in aminotransferase levels is seen in 30% of patients taking propylthiouracil
Cholestasis	Rare	Exclusively with methimazole and carbimazole
Hypoprothrombinemia	Rare	No case reports since 1982; only with propylthiouracil.
Hypoglycemia	Rare	So-called insulin-autoimmune syndrome, which is seen mainly in Asian patients receiving sulfhydryl-containing drugs; only with methimazole.
Pancreatitis	Very rare	One case report.

From Cooper, D. S. (2005). Antithyroid drugs. *New England Journal of Medicine, 35,* 905–917. Copyright © 2005 Massachusetts Medical Society. All rights reserved.

Patients who have difficulty with one medication may be given a trial of another, although cross-sensitivity among the antithyroid drugs may occur. Rarely (0.3% of patients), a potentially fatal agranulocytosis may result, which occurs somewhat more often with PTU than with methimazole. Clinicians should consider routine monitoring of the complete blood count (CBC) during the first 3 months of therapy. They should warn patients who are taking these drugs to report symptoms of sore throat and fever immediately; they should obtain a CBC and stop the drug if the patient's white blood cell count is low.

Recently, the U.S. Food and Drug Administration (FDA) added a Black Box warning to PTU because of reports of severe liver injury, including some deaths, in pediatric and adult patients taking this medication. The FDA also recommends that PTU be reserved for patients who cannot tolerate other therapies for hyperthyroidism (http://www.fda.gov/Drugs/DrugSafety/PostmarketDrugSafetyInformationforPatientsandProviders/ucm209023.htm).

Interactions

Because these drugs decrease iodine uptake and organification, they can interfere with subsequent radioactive iodine therapy. Higher doses of ^{131}I may be needed to increase success rates in these patients.

A study from Japan (Hashizume, et al., 1991) demonstrated an increased remission rate in patients treated with high doses of antithyroid drugs combined with replacement doses of T_4 compared with those who received antithyroid drugs alone. The rationale was that by suppressing the TSH with T_4, there would be less stimulation of thyroid antigens. These results have not been confirmed in American and European studies; thus, most authorities in the United States recommend against this therapy for Graves disease.

Adjunctive Agents Used to Manage Hyperthyroidism

Beta Blockers

The beta blockers are used to treat the symptoms of hyperthyroidism. They do not affect thyroid hormone synthesis; rather, they act by decreasing the symptoms of adrenergic stimulation caused by the increased T_4 concentration. Practitioners should prescribe a nonselective beta blocker like long-acting propranolol starting at a dose of 80 mg/day. Alternatively, atenolol may be used. These drugs can help prevent hyperthyroid-induced atrial fibrillation or control the ventricular rate in patients with established atrial fibrillation. Clinicians should consider anticoagulation to reduce the risk of stroke in patients with atrial fibrillation; treatment of these patients should be in consultation with a cardiologist. Prescribers should taper beta blockers gradually and discontinue them as soon as the patient is euthyroid and asymptomatic. Patients in whom beta blockers are not tolerated or are contraindicated (e.g., those with asthma) may be treated with calcium channel blockers like diltiazem.

Iodine-Containing Compounds

Other agents used adjunctively in the treatment of hyperthyroidism are iodine-containing compounds like potassium iodide (in the form of saturated solution of potassium iodide [SSKI] 35 mg/drop or Lugol solution 7 mg/drop) and the iodinated contrast agents ipodate (Oragrafin) and iopanoate (Telepaque). These drugs are reserved for the treatment of severe thyrotoxicosis or thyroid storm. Such patients are usually treated in an intensive care unit under the care of an endocrinologist, intensivist, or both. Pharmacologic doses of iodine inhibit the release of thyroid hormones from the gland in the short term; however, because new hormone synthesis proceeds during treatment with iodine, iodine must be used in combination with antithyroid drugs, which are given 1 hour before the iodine compound.

Lithium

Lithium, which is chemically similar to iodine, is used rarely to block release of thyroid hormone from the gland in those patients who are intolerant of antithyroid drugs. The dose is 900 to 1,200 mg/day, divided, and clinicians should monitor lithium levels.

Glucocorticoids

Glucocorticoids are occasionally used in thyroid storm. They reduce peripheral conversion of T_4 to T_3.

Treatment of Ophthalmopathy of Graves Disease

None of the aforementioned therapies for hyperthyroidism affects the ophthalmopathy of Graves disease. Anti-inflammatory drugs, immunosuppressive drugs (e.g., prednisone and dexamethasone), and surgery are offered to patients as treatment for the ophthalmopathy. Sunglasses and artificial tears are used adjunctively for comfort.

Special Population Considerations

Geriatric

The term *apathetic hyperthyroidism* has been used to describe the atypical presentation of hyperthyroidism in some older patients. Rather than the usual symptoms of increased metabolic rate, these patients may present with weakness, dyspnea, anorexia, depression, or constipation. Physical examination may be unrevealing. Occasionally, new-onset atrial fibrillation or congestive heart failure is the initial presentation of hyperthyroidism in the older person.

Pregnancy

Radioactive iodine is contraindicated during pregnancy because it crosses the placenta and affects fetal thyroid development. PTU is the drug of choice for hyperthyroidism during both pregnancy and lactation because it crosses the placenta and

enters the breast milk less than methimazole. Furthermore, use of methimazole during pregnancy increases the risk of a rare congenital abnormality, aplasia cutis congenita. During pregnancy, practitioners should prescribe the lowest dosages possible of antithyroid drugs that still maintain euthyroidism. The dosage usually decreases as pregnancy progresses and the severity of Graves disease lessens, then increases again after delivery. Clinicians should treat pregnant patients who have hyperthyroidism in consultation with an endocrinologist.

MONITORING PATIENT RESPONSE

Patients usually become euthyroid within 6 to 12 weeks of beginning antithyroid drugs; however, permanent hypothyroidism may develop many years after a course of therapy, so long-term follow-up is necessary. Patients taking antithyroid drugs should be evaluated every 1 to 3 months after starting treatment depending on the degree of hyperthyroidism and comorbid conditions. Once euthyroidism is achieved, practitioners can decrease the dose of antithyroid drugs and reevaluate the patient in 3 to 4 months. Clinicians should order free T_4 levels to monitor the patient because the TSH level remains suppressed for several months after the patient becomes euthyroid. They should continue to reduce and eventually discontinue the antithyroid drugs, after which they should see patients every 4 to 6 weeks for 3 to 4 months, and less frequently thereafter.

PATIENT EDUCATION

Patients with hyperthyroidism may have very troublesome symptoms that resemble those of anxiety disorders, such as panic attacks. Clinicians should advise them that these symptoms (which can be severe) will resolve with treatment of their thyroid disease.

Practitioners should review all treatment options with patients. They should tell patients that antithyroid drugs will put their disease into remission, but that the relapse rate is high. They should discuss the high likelihood of permanent hypothyroidism after radioactive iodine therapy. Patients will likely gain weight after therapy for hyperthyroidism, even if they do not become hypothyroid. Clinicians should emphasize the chronic nature of the condition and the importance of long-term follow-up regardless of the chosen treatment.

Drug Information

There can be increased effects of digoxin, metoprolol, and propranolol when the patient becomes euthyroid. The effects of anticoagulants can be altered. Drugs should be taken at equal intervals.

Complementary and Alternative Medicine

Bugleweed has been shown to treat a mildly overactive thyroid. It decreases thyroid hormone activity and increases the absorption and storage of thyroid hormone, causing a decreased metabolism. This is not used in patients with hypothyroidism.

Lemon balm is used in hyperthyroidism for its sedative effects.

Special Populations

Women of childbearing age with Graves disease may want to consider definitive treatment (radioiodine or surgery) before conception. Although it is acceptable to prescribe PTU during pregnancy, clinicians must monitor thyroid function closely because of variations in the course of the disease in pregnancy.

THYROID NODULES

Thyroid nodules are encountered relatively often in clinical practice. The gland may have one or multiple nodules. Most are the result of adenomas, cysts, large collections of colloid, or focal areas of thyroiditis. Five percent of solitary nodules result from thyroid cancer, with higher rates in the very young and older age groups. Fine-needle aspiration biopsy (FNAB) is the initial diagnostic procedure to rule out carcinoma in a solitary nodule.

INITIATING DRUG THERAPY

Treatment of thyroid cancer is beyond the scope of this work; however, clinicians should be aware that high doses of T_4 are used in patients who have been treated for thyroid cancer in an effort to suppress the growth of any remaining cancer cells. Once a thyroid nodule is proved benign histologically, some clinicians previously attempted to reduce the size of the nodule medically (**Figure 46-5**). T_4 was given in higher than replacement doses (2.2 mcg/kg/day) in an attempt to turn off the secretion of TSH by the pituitary, with the presumption that growth of the nodule depends on TSH. With less circulating TSH, the nodule in theory will not increase in size and may decrease. The literature yields conflicting results in this regard, with some studies showing a significant effect on nodule size but most showing no effect. Therefore, this therapy is no longer utilized.

Radioactive iodine and surgery are appropriate for patients with large single nodules or multiple nodules.

MONITORING PATIENT RESPONSE

Patients with thyroid nodules should be monitored at least annually. If there are ongoing concerns about malignancy, practitioners should perform a repeat FNAB. Patients with hyperthyroidism as a result of toxic nodules respond to antithyroid drugs either in conjunction with or in lieu of ablative therapy.

PATIENT EDUCATION

Patients with thyroid nodules often are unaware of a problem. Therefore, practitioners need to emphasize the potential (although small) for malignancy and the need for further evaluation with FNAB.

If the nodule is found to be benign, clinicians must discuss treatment options. Patients need to follow up at least annually with a physical examination and an ultrasound to evaluate whether the existing nodule has enlarged or if new nodules have developed.

SUBCLINICAL THYROID DISEASE

The entity of mild thyroid failure, previously known as *subclinical hypothyroidism,* presents a therapeutic challenge. This condition is defined as an elevated TSH level with a normal free T_4 concentration, usually in a patient with no symptoms. Many authorities believe that mild thyroid failure requires the same treatment as overt hypothyroidism because both entities have been associated with adverse cardiovascular outcomes.

Proponents of therapy for mild thyroid failure cite studies showing higher levels of LDL cholesterol and lower levels of high-density lipoprotein cholesterol in these patients, as well as increased systolic time intervals and decreased cognitive function. After treatment with T_4, some of these problems show improvement. Patients who have coexisting cardiovascular disease or dysrhythmias probably should not be treated for mild thyroid failure because the risks of therapy outweigh the potential benefits. If treatment is attempted, it should be with T_4 at doses to lower the TSH level to the normal range. The incidence of mild thyroid failure is higher in older adults, occurring in up to 20% of people older than age 60.

A subclinical hyperthyroid entity has been defined by normal free T_4 and T_3 concentrations with a low TSH level in asymptomatic patients. This condition often results from overreplacement of T_4, autonomously functioning nodules, nonthyroid illness, or certain medications that decrease TSH. (See **Box 46.4.**) Risks of subclinical hyperthyroidism include increased bone turnover, which may predispose to osteoporosis and an increased risk of atrial fibrillation and other adverse cardiovascular outcomes. Antithyroid therapy similar to that of overt hyperthyroidism should be considered in consultation with an endocrinologist.

THYROIDITIS

After delivering a child up to 10% of women without previous thyroid disease have postpartum (also known as *painless* or *silent*) thyroiditis, a variant of Hashimoto thyroiditis. Patients present within 1 year after delivery with nonspecific symptoms of fatigue, palpitations, and depression. Tachycardia and goiter may be present on examination.

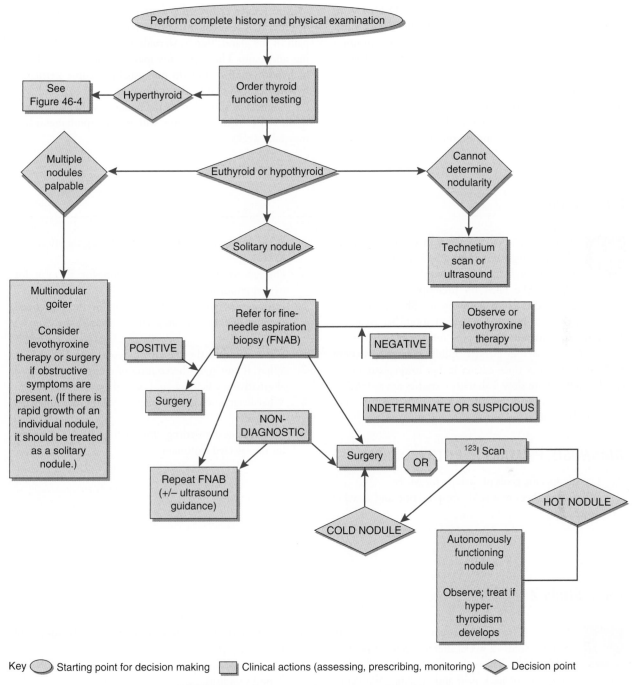

FIGURE 46–5 Evaluation and management of thyroid nodules.

Patients often go through a hyperthyroid phase that resolves in a few months. Some have transient hypothyroidism that can last from 2 to 6 months. This condition is usually self-limited, so treatment is indicated only to relieve the symptoms of hyperthyroidism. Beta blockers are the treatment of choice. Antithyroid drugs are not helpful because the hyperthyroidism that develops is a result of the gland's spilling of preformed thyroid hormone. Some patients require replacement doses of T_4 during the hypothyroid phase of their condition. Women with high titers of antithyroid peroxidase antibodies during or after the pregnancy are at increased risk for development of permanent hypothyroidism; these women should be followed closely.

Women with postpartum thyroiditis may experience symptoms similar to postpartum depression; therefore, practitioners should reassure these women that their symptoms will resolve once the condition subsides. Clinicians should encourage those women at higher risk for permanent hypothyroidism (those with a high titer of antithyroid peroxidase antibodies) to return for periodic follow-up.

Patients sometimes have subacute (DeQuervain) thyroiditis several weeks after an upper respiratory tract infection. They present with a painful, enlarged gland and symptoms and signs of hyperthyroidism, which is the result of leakage of thyroid hormones from the inflamed gland. If a radioiodine scan is performed, it shows diffusely decreased uptake of tracer (as opposed to the increased uptake seen in Graves disease).

This condition is self-limited and requires symptomatic treatment only. As in postpartum thyroiditis, beta blockers are used to reduce tachycardia, tremor, and nervousness. Aspirin or other nonsteroidal anti-inflammatory drugs can reduce the pain in the gland. Rarely, steroids are needed to reduce swelling and pain. These patients may experience a brief period of hypothyroidism but do not usually become permanently hypothyroid, so that vigilant follow-up is not required.

Clinicians should reassure patients with subacute thyroiditis that their condition will resolve spontaneously, but may take weeks.

Case Study 1

M. E. is a 29-year-old woman with a 7-month history of heavy, irregular menses, a 5-lb weight gain, constipation, and decreased energy. Her past history is unremarkable. She takes no prescription medications but uses iron and calcium supplements. She has a family history of thyroid disease. On examination, her weight is 152 lbs, her heart rate is 64 bpm, and her blood pressure is 138/86. Her thyroid gland is mildly enlarged, without nodularity. She has trace edema in her lower extremities, and her reflexes are slow. Laboratory studies are as follows: TSH is 15.3 mIU/mL (elevated), free T_4 is 0.3 mIU/mL (decreased), total cholesterol is 276 mg/mL.

DIAGNOSIS: PRIMARY HYPOTHYROIDISM

1. List the specific goals of therapy for M. E.
2. What drug therapy would you prescribe and at what dose?
3. What are the parameters for monitoring the success of M. E.'s therapy?
4. Discuss specific patient education for therapy for hypothyroidism.
5. List one or two adverse reactions for the prescribed therapy that would cause you to change the drug or dose.
6. What would be the choice for second-line therapy?
7. What, if any, over-the-counter or complementary and alternative medicine would be appropriate for M. E.?
8. What dietary and lifestyle changes would be recommended for M. E.
9. Describe one or two drug–drug or drug–food interactions for the selected treatment.

Case Study 2

J. C. is a 37-year-old woman who presents with "swollen glands" 2 weeks after an upper respiratory infection. She has no lingering respiratory symptoms but complains of neck pain and swelling. She denies palpitations, tremors and diarrhea, but has noted a weight loss of 4 pounds. Her blood pressure is 120/72, her pulse rate is 92, and her thyroid gland is tender to palpation and enlarged. Thyroid function testing reveals a TSH level less than 0.02 milliunits/L and a free T_4 of 3.0 ng/dL (elevated).

DIAGNOSIS: SUBACUTE (DEQUERVAIN) THYROIDITIS

1. List the specific goals of therapy for J. C.
2. What drug therapy would you prescribe and at what dose?
3. What are the parameters for monitoring the success of J. C.'s therapy?
4. Discuss specific patient education for therapy for hypothyroidism.
5. List one or two adverse reactions for the prescribed therapy that would cause you to change the drug or dose.
6. What would be the choice for second-line therapy?
7. What, if any, over-the-counter or complementary and alternative medicines would be appropriate for J. C.?
8. What dietary and lifestyle changes would be recommended for J. C.?
9. Describe one or two drug–drug or drug–food interactions for the selected treatment.

BIBLIOGRAPHY

*Starred references are cited in the text.

Brander, A., Viikinkoski, P., Nickels, J., et al. (1991). Thyroid gland: US screening in a random adult population. *Radiology, 181,* 683–687.

Bullock, B. A., & Henze, R. L. (2000). *Focus on pathophysiology.* Philadelphia: Lippincott Williams & Wilkins.

*Canaris, G. J., Manowitz, N. R., Mayor, G., et al. (2000). The Colorado thyroid disease prevalence study. *Archives of Internal Medicine, 160,* 526–534.

*Cooper, D. S. (2005). Antithyroid drugs. *New England Journal of Medicine, 35,* 905–917.

Cooper, D. S. (2003). Hyperthyroidism. *Lancet, 362,* 459–468.

Garcia, M., Baskin, H. J., & Feld, S. (1995). American Association of Clinical Endocrinologists (AACE) clinical practice guidelines for the management of hyperthyroidism and hypothyroidism. *Endocrine Practice, 1,* 54–62.

*Hak, A. E., Pols, H. A., Visser, T. J., et al. (2000). Subclinical hypothyroidism is an independent risk factor for atherosclerosis and myocardial infarction in elderly women: The Rotterdam Study. *Annals of Internal Medicine, 130,* 270–278.

*Hashizume, K., Ichikawa, K., Sakurai, A., et al. (1991). Administration of thyroxine in treated Graves' disease: Effects on the level of antibodies to thyroid stimulating hormone receptors and on the risk of recurrence of hyperthyroidism. *New England Journal of Medicine, 324,* 947–953.

*Hollowell, J. G., Staehling, N. W., Flanders, W. D., et al. (2002). Serum TSH, T_4, and thyroid antibodies in the United States Population (1988 to 1994): National Health and Nutrition Examination Survey (NHANES III). *Journal of Clinical Endocrinology and Metabolism, 87,* 489–499.

Kahaly, G. J. (2000). Cardiovascular and atherogenic aspects of subclinical hypothyroidism. *Thyroid, 10,* 665–679.

Mandel, S. J., Brent, G. A., & Larsen, P. R. (1993). Levothyroxine therapy in patients with thyroid disease. *Annals of Internal Medicine, 119,* 492–502.

Mokshagundam, S., & Barzel, U. S. (1993). Thyroid disease in the elderly. *Journal of the American Geriatric Society, 41,* 1361–1368.

*Mulder, J. E. (1998). Thyroid disorders in women. *Medical Clinics of North America, 82,* 103–125.

*National Academy of Clinical Biochemistry Website: NACB laboratory medicine practice guidelines. Available at: http://www.nacb.org/lmpg/main.stm. Accessed February 18, 2004.

Parle, J. V., Maisonneuve, P., Sheppard, M. C., et al. (2001). Prediction of all-cause and cardiovascular mortality in elderly people from one low serum thyrotropin result: A 10-year cohort study. *Lancet, 358,* 861–865.

Pearce, E. N., Farwell, A. P., & Braverman, L. E. (2003). Current concepts: Thyroiditis. *New England Journal of Medicine, 348,* 2646–2655.

*Sawin, C. T., Geller, A., Wolf, P. A., et al. (1994). Low serum thyrotropin concentrations as a risk factor for atrial fibrillation in older persons. *New England Journal of Medicine, 331,* 1249–1252.

Smeltzer, S. C., & Bare, B. G. (2000). *Brunner & Suddarth's textbook of medical-surgical nursing* (9th ed.). Philadelphia: Lippincott Williams & Wilkins.

Surks, M. I., Ortiz, E. O., Daniels, G. H., et al. (2004). Subclinical thyroid disease: Scientific review and guidelines for diagnosis and management. *Journal of the American Medical Association, 291,* 228–238.

Uzzan, B., Campos, J., Cucherat, M., et al. (1996). Effects on bone mass of long term treatment with thyroid hormones: A meta-analysis. *Journal of Clinical Endocrinology and Metabolism, 81,* 4278–4289.

UNIT 11

Pharmacotherapy for Immune Disorders

Lauren M. Czosnowski
Andrew M. Peterson

CHAPTER 47

Allergies and Allergic Reactions

The term *allergy* is derived from the Greek words *allos* (differing from the normal or usual) and *ergon* (work or energy). To describe it in simple, nonclinical terms, allergy is an abnormal release of energy in the body. In clinical or physiologic terms, allergy is an exaggerated immune response resulting from an antibody–antigen reaction.

Antibodies are soluble protein molecules made by B lymphocytes in response to foreign substances. Antibodies, also referred to as *immunoglobulins,* are tailored specifically and uniquely to bind to each foreign substance and remove it from the circulation. Invasion or contact with a foreign substance results in the production and secretion of antibodies. Therefore, the foreign substance is an *anti*body *gen*erator— hence the term *antigen*. Antigens also are referred to as *allergens;* the terms are interchangeable.

All people come in contact with the same antigens, yet not all people display allergic symptoms. Allergy symptoms appear when the immune response is exaggerated or inappropriate, causing inflammation and tissue damage. This exaggerated response to an antigen is referred to as *hypersensitivity*. Hypersensitivity is a characteristic of an individual. It is manifested on the second or a subsequent contact with a particular antigen.

Allergens can be food-based, chemical, or environmental. Typical food allergens include milk or egg protein, peanut, shellfish, and wheat or soy. Parabens and lanolin, commonly found in make-up and sunscreens; thimerosal, a preservative found in contact lens solutions; and fragrance enhancers found in perfumes are common chemical allergens. Drugs, such as the local anesthetics lidocaine and benzocaine, are also chemical allergens. Environmental allergens include mold, pollen, and dust.

In contrast to allergy, *anergy* is the term used to describe the unexpected failure of the immune system to respond to the challenge of a foreign substance (antigen or allergen). Several skin test antigens may be applied to the skin (an anergy panel) to determine the status of the immune system. The antigens selected are those to which a majority of the population would exhibit a reaction. Examples of these include *candida* species and histoplasmin. If the characteristic wheals do not appear in the prescribed period, it can be interpreted that the patient has not had prior exposure to the antigen or potentially has a compromised immune system.

CLASSIFICATION OF ALLERGIC REACTIONS

The medical literature describes four types of hypersensitivity reactions (Coombs and Gell classification) that are listed and described in **Box 47.1.** There are four types of reactions under this classification system. Type I reactions involve the interaction between an antigen and a specific immunoglobulin (Ig) E antibody. These antibodies are bound to member receptors on mast cells and basophils. When an antigen binds to these antibodies, the cell releases histamine, leukotrienes, and prostaglandins. These vasoactive substances produce vasodilation and increase capillary permeability, both of which allow for eosinophils and other inflammatory cells to infiltrate tissues, furthering the allergic

---

BOX 47.1

Coombs and Gell Classification of Hypersensitivity

- Type I (immediate hypersensitivity)—Immunoglobulin (Ig) E attached to mast cells binds with an antigen, inducing degranulation and release of histamine and other mediators of inflammation. (Asthma and allergic rhinitis are examples of type I hypersensitivity.)
- Type II—IgG attached to a T-lymphocyte killer cell is directed against antigens on target cell. This leads to direct cytotoxic action or complement-mediated lysis.
- Type III—Immune complexes of antibody and antigen are deposited in the tissue. Complement is activated, and polymorphonuclear leukocytes are attracted to the site of the complex. Local tissue damage occurs. (Autoimmune disease is an example of type III hypersensitivity.)
- Type IV (delayed hypersensitivity)—Antigen-sensitized T cells release inflammatory substances after a second contact with the same antigen. (Contact dermatitis, such as poison ivy, and the tuberculin skin test [PPD] are examples of delayed hypersensitivity.)

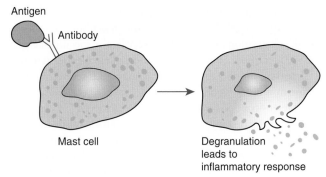

Antigen

Antibody

Mast cell

Degranulation leads to inflammatory response

FIGURE 47–1 Antibody–antigen reaction.

response. The first contact results in the formation of the antibody. Subsequent contact with the same antigen results in the antibody–antigen reaction, resulting in this type I hypersensitivity reaction. The antibody–antigen reaction triggers the immune response that results in allergy symptoms (**Figure 47-1**). Allergies can affect the airways, eyes, skin, or the entire body. Type I reactions are typically anaphylactic in nature and can be life-threatening.

Type II reactions, also known as *cytotoxic reactions,* occur when an antibody reacts with an antigenic component of a cell. This antibody–antigen reaction in turn activates killer T cells or macrophages to aid in the destruction of the antigenic cell. Complement activation is also involved in this process, furthering the cytotoxic process leading to tissue destruction. Transfusion reactions are typically type II allergic reactions.

Type III reactions result from immune complexes that activate the complement system. Activating this system promotes the migration and release of cells such as polymorphonuclear cells that can release proteolytic enzymes and factors that promote tissue permeability. Systemic lupus erythematosus is a form of a type III allergic reaction.

Type IV reactions are also called delayed-hypersensitivity reactions. These cell-mediated reactions are the result of sensitized T lymphocytes coming into contact with a specific antigen. The delay typically takes 2 to 3 days or up to a week. Allergic dermatitis is an example of a type IV reaction.

Immunologic Versus Nonimmunologic Reactions

Some cutaneous reactions, such as contact dermatitis, may appear to be allergic reactions, but they do not involve the immune system. Irritant contact dermatitis is the most common cutaneous reaction and is often caused by skin irritants such as powders or chemicals found in gloves.

Contact dermatitis differs from allergic dermatitis in that there is direct tissue insult from the skin irritant that causes the release of inflammatory mediators from skin cells. A common example of irritant contact dermatitis is a reaction to repeated hand washing with soap or other cleaners. In some instances, the cracked, dry skin occurring with contact dermatitis no longer can prevent allergens from entering the systemic circulation. With latex allergies, for example, the powder already present in the glove can give rise to a contact

dermatitis, thus allowing for the latex antigens to enter the circulation. This in turn increases the likelihood of an allergic reaction, resulting in allergic contact dermatitis. Because of this phenomenon, it is often difficult to distinguish allergic from nonallergic contact dermatitis. See Chapter 11 for more details on dermatitis.

General Treatment Overview of Allergic Reactions

The first step in treating an allergic reaction is to remove the allergen, if possible. This may involve removing the person from the environment causing the allergy, stopping the offending drug, or washing off the offending chemical. Most allergic reactions clear up within a few days of removing the cause. Symptomatic cutaneous reactions, such as pruritic rash, urticaria, or morbilliform eruptions as well as reactions involving multiple organs, should be treated.

Cutaneous Reactions

Cutaneous reactions such as urticaria, pruritus, and hives are often secondary to the release of histamine, making antihistamine therapy the mainstay of treatment. There are two types of antihistamines used in the general treatment of allergic reactions: first generation and second generation. The first-generation antihistamines include diphenhydramine, hydroxyzine, and chlorpheniramine, among others. These agents are typically very effective, but they may also be very sedating. The second-generation agents, such as loratadine and fexofenadine, are nonsedating antihistamines (NSAs) that work fairly well at controlling mild to moderate symptoms of cutaneous reactions. However, if the symptoms persist for more than a few days, or are not well controlled, a first-generation antihistamine may be substituted, or added to, the NSA. Close communication with the patient regarding resolution of the symptoms is necessary, along with balancing quality of life issues related to side effects, such as sedation, dry mouth, and urinary retention. If the reaction is moderate to severe or if there is no relief from antihistamine therapy, systemic glucocorticoids may be used. Short courses of treatment with oral prednisone or methylprednisolone are usually used. See Chapter 11 for more information on the use of oral steroids for treating cutaneous reactions.

Anaphylaxis and Anaphylactoid Reactions

Anaphylaxis is a type I hypersensitivity reaction involving IgE-mediated release of histamine, leukotrienes, and other mediators from already sensitized mast cells and basophils. The release of these mediators initiates a systemic chain of events that includes symptoms such as angioedema, flushing, pruritus, urticaria, nausea, vomiting, and wheezing. The onset of the reaction is quick, generally within 1 to 30 minutes. The histamine release causes a smooth muscle contraction and vasodilation. The wheezing resulting from smooth muscle contraction in the lungs decreases oxygenation, whereas vasodilation results in a release of fluids into the tissues, thus causing a lower effective plasma volume, leading to shock. Prolonged vasodilation, coupled with decreased oxygenation, can lead to arrhythmias, convulsions, and death.

Anaphylactoid reactions are similar in appearance to anaphylaxis, but may occur after the *first* injection of certain drugs and contrast media. They are non-IgE mediated and the agent causes a direct release of histamine and other inflammatory toxins. They have a dose-related, idiosyncratic mechanism rather than an immunologically mediated one. A classic example of an anaphylactoid reaction is the "red man syndrome" associated with vancomycin. Patients may experience itching, redness, and hives with rapid infusion of vancomycin due to histamine release; slowing the infusion rate usually improves the reaction.

Treatment

Immediate treatment with epinephrine is imperative. Epinephrine effectively increases the blood pressure and is antagonist to the effects of histamine on smooth muscle and other tissues.

For mild reactions, such as generalized pruritus, urticaria, angioedema, or mild wheezing, 0.01 mL/kg aqueous epinephrine 1:1000 (1 mg/mL) subcutaneously or intramuscularly (usual dose, 0.2 to 0.5 mL in adults; 0.3 mL maximum for children) should be given. This dose may be repeated every 15 minutes as necessary to control symptoms. If the reaction is caused by an injected antigen (e.g., a drug), then a tourniquet may be applied above the injection site and half the above dose of epinephrine also injected into the site to reduce systemic absorption of the antigen. If the reaction is severe but does not have cardiovascular involvement (e.g., collapse), then an injectable antihistamine such as diphenhydramine (usual dose for adults, 25 to 50 mg; children, 1 mg/kg) may be given in addition to epinephrine to prevent further complications from histamine release such as laryngeal edema.

If the reaction does involve the cardiovascular system, then intravenous fluids should be rapidly infused to maintain volume. Hypovolemia is usually the major cause of the hypotension. Colloid plasma expanders such as dextran are rarely necessary. Normal saline is an appropriate choice for most patients, and 1 to 2 L should be given as an initial bolus. Fluids may be continued as necessary to maintain hemodynamic stability. If fluid replacement is ineffective at restoring blood pressure, then dopamine or norepinephrine may be *cautiously* introduced. Alternatively, if the patient is experiencing bradycardia, atropine may be used to increase heart rate. Patients with severe reactions should be observed in the hospital for 24 hours after recovery in case of relapse.

Systemic corticosteroids are indicated for all patients experiencing moderate to severe anaphylaxis, although they will not have an effect for 4 to 6 hours. Typically, methylprednisolone 1 to 2 mg/kg/day divided every 6 to 8 hours for adults and 1 to 2 mg/kg/day divided every 8 to 12 hours for children is needed to prevent the onset of late-phase reactions. For milder attacks, oral prednisone dosed at 0.5 mg/kg/day may be administered.

Prophylaxis

The primary means of preventing an allergic reaction is avoidance. However, when this is not feasible or practical,

immunotherapy is an effective means of preventing reactions, particularly anaphylactic reactions from insect bites. This form of "desensitization" is only effective when a specific allergen can be identified. Some ragweed and pollen allergies respond well to immunotherapy, though it may take several months before immunity is conferred.

Desensitization may be rapidly achieved in patients requiring drug therapy to which they have an established allergy. For example, patients with anaphylactic reactions to penicillin may be desensitized by administering increasing concentrations of penicillin every 15 minutes. To ensure patient safety, desensitization is best done under constant supervision and in consultation with an experienced allergist. There are numerous protocols for penicillin desensitization and an increasing number for patients who are allergic to sulfa drugs.

ALLERGIC RHINITIS (HAY FEVER OR POLLEN ALLERGY)

Allergic rhinitis is an *airway allergy*. (Asthma, also an airway allergy, is discussed in Chapter 25.) Many people have hay fever. The National Institute of Allergy and Infectious Diseases states that pollen allergy may affect up to 35 million people in the United States, not including those with asthma.

CAUSES

Common inhaled allergens that cause allergic rhinitis in sensitized people include pollen (grass, trees, weeds), dust mites, mold spores, enzymes (in detergents), and insect body parts. The two most common types of allergic rhinitis are seasonal and perennial (**Table 47.1**). The incidence of seasonal rhinitis is approximately 10 times greater than that of perennial rhinitis.

In seasonal allergic rhinitis, symptoms correspond with seasonal peaks in tree, grass, and weed pollens. During the spring, tree pollens such as alder, birch, and oak cause problems for many people. In the summer, grass pollens, such as timothy grass, can cause allergies. Weeds, such as mugwort and ragweed, pollinate in late summer and autumn. Pollens usually

TABLE 47.1	Seasonal Versus Perennial Allergies
Causes of Seasonal Allergies	**Causes of Perennial Allergies**
Tree pollen (spring)	Mold (indoor)
Grass pollen (spring through fall)	Dust (dust mites)
Weeds (late summer)	Animal dander (skin flakes)
Leaf mold (early spring and late summer)	Animal fur
	Foods (nuts, shellfish, milk, eggs)

are windborne, and patients with seasonal allergic rhinitis often are said to have "hay fever." The most common cause of seasonal allergic rhinitis is ragweed pollen.

Patients with perennial allergic rhinitis have symptoms throughout the year, instead of only during certain months. They usually require chronic treatment. The most common causes of perennial rhinitis are animal dander and dust mites. In many cases, causative agents are difficult for patients to avoid because many such agents are indoor allergens. Perennial rhinitis may worsen when patients are exposed to non-natural irritants such as paint, cleaners, or tobacco smoke.

Genetic predisposition plays a major role in the development of allergic rhinitis. The genetically determined tendency to produce increased quantities of IgE expresses itself after prolonged exposure to an allergen. Consequently, allergic rhinitis is uncommon before age 3. Those in later childhood or young adulthood are at greatest risk for development of new symptoms. In general, neither sex exhibits more of a predilection for allergic rhinitis; however, some sources indicate that the perennial form is more common in women.

Patients with a family history of asthma or eczema are more likely to have an allergic basis for rhinitis. The incidence of allergic rhinitis increases by approximately 30% when one parent has a history and is even higher when both parents have allergic disorders. Studies of pediatric populations have uncovered certain factors that may increase the expression of allergy: maternal smoking during pregnancy, month of birth (e.g., being born during allergy season), and development of a viral infection in the upper respiratory tract.

PATHOPHYSIOLOGY

Initial exposure to the antigen/allergen stimulates the B lymphocytes (plasma cells) to produce an antigen-specific antibody (IgE) that binds to mast cell membranes (tissue-fixed antibody). The person is now sensitized to that specific antigen and susceptible to allergic reactions when re-exposed to it. On subsequent exposure, the antigen binds to the tissue-fixed IgE antibody and triggers breakdown of the mast cells (degranulation) and release of mediators (histamine, prostaglandins, leukotrienes, kinins, thromboxanes, and serotonin). Histamine, which is stored primarily in mast cells and basophils, is believed to be the mediator most responsible for the clinical signs and symptoms of allergic rhinitis.

Common symptoms in patients with allergic rhinitis are ocular pruritus (itching of the eyes) and conjunctival inflammation (inflammation of the membrane lining the eyelids). Other symptoms of allergic rhinitis are irritability, lethargy, fatigue, and loss of appetite. Once released into the nasal mucosa, the mediators cause vasodilation, increased capillary permeability, increased mucus production, and stimulation of nerve endings. The resulting symptoms are rhinorrhea (profuse, watery nasal discharge), nasal congestion (obstruction by mucus), and nasal pruritus. The most severe symptoms include violent episodes of sneezing (often a dozen or more times in a row) and total obstruction of nasal airflow resulting from copious amounts of mucus (**Figure 47-2**).

The specific IgE antibody made in response to the allergen also may attach to eosinophils. Antigen-provoked degranulation of eosinophils also causes allergic symptoms. The symptoms associated with eosinophils are related to a late-phase allergic response, occurring hours to days after the initial reaction.

DIAGNOSTIC CRITERIA

The diagnosis of allergic rhinitis begins with a thorough history determining the presence of classic signs and symptoms and the time, place, and circumstances under which they occur. A family history is also important because it may establish the familial predisposition to allergy.

Physical examination of the patient with suspected allergic rhinitis begins with assessment of facial appearance, which often includes teary eyes and a red, swollen nose with scaling and crusting from frequent blowing and rubbing with

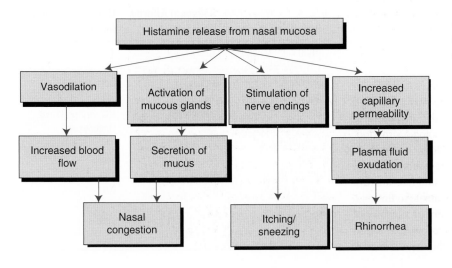

FIGURE 47-2 Results of histamine release in the nasal mucosa.

facial tissues. There also may be dark circles under the eyes (allergic shiners), pinched nostrils, and a gaping mouth (from mouth breathing). The nasal mucous membranes are typically pale, swollen, and coated with a clear, watery secretion. Some erythema and bleeding may be noted. Swelling, streaks of erythema, and mucus may be present in the posterior pharynx. Other positive physical findings include swelling around and watery discharge from the eyes.

Nasal Smears

Practitioners may use the Wright stain for nasal secretions to detect eosinophils. Although eosinophilia suggests an allergic etiology for rhinitis symptoms (in infectious rhinitis, neutrophils predominate), it is not diagnostic. Conversely, an absence of eosinophilia does not rule out allergy. Eosinophilia may be absent in patients who have superimposed infections or have not had a recent exposure to allergens.

Skin Testing

Skin testing with extracts of suspected allergens usually provides the most effective means of identifying specific sensitivities in patients with allergic rhinitis. In this test, a superficial scratch or prick is made in the skin and a diluted extract of antigen is applied. If the patient has allergen-specific IgE antibodies bound to tissue mast cells, a classic wheal-and-flare reaction appears over the next 15 to 30 minutes. To avoid false-negative results, patients should discontinue the use of antihistamines before they undergo skin testing. Clinicians should individualize this time frame based on the pharmacokinetics of the specific antihistamine that the patient is taking. In most cases, it is adequate to stop taking antihistamines 48 to 72 hours before testing. If patients do not stop taking antihistamines before skin testing, practitioners may mistakenly exclude a diagnosis of allergic rhinitis and subject patients to unnecessary further evaluations.

If the results of the scratch test are negative or unclear, practitioners may administer a more dilute extract of antigen intradermally. Clinicians should not use the intradermal test in patients with a positive response to scratch testing because of the risk of significant allergic reaction, including anaphylaxis.

Radioallergosorbent Testing

Radioallergosorbent testing (RAST) permits in vitro detection of serum IgE antibodies to allergens. Because only 1% of IgE molecules circulate in the blood (the remainder are bound to tissue), RAST results may not reflect the biologic situation. Although RAST is more specific, skin testing is less costly, more sensitive, and simpler to perform. Despite these shortcomings, RAST is helpful when the results of skin testing are unclear. The test is likewise useful when patients are unable to undergo skin testing because of dermatologic conditions or a history of anaphylactic reaction to the suspected allergen. RAST is also indicated for evaluating children younger than age 2 as well

as for patients unable to discontinue using antihistamines, as required before skin testing.

Differential Diagnosis

Symptoms similar to those of allergic rhinitis may result from *mechanical nasal obstruction* (foreign body or anatomic factors); as a *side effect of medications* (oral contraceptives, hormone replacement therapy, tricyclic antidepressants, propranolol [Inderal], reserpine [Serpasil], methyldopa [Aldomet], and aspirin-containing compounds); or from *medical conditions associated with increased vasodilation* (e.g., hypothyroidism, cystic fibrosis, tumors, alcoholism, or pregnancy). **Table 47.2** compares the symptoms of seasonal rhinitis with common cold symptoms to illustrate the similarities and differences between these conditions.

Although seasonal rhinitis usually is relatively easy to diagnose, identification of perennial rhinitis may be more elusive. Other nonallergic conditions could cause similar symptoms. *Vasomotor rhinitis* (congestion of the nasal mucosa without infection or allergy) could be difficult to differentiate from perennial rhinitis. In vasomotor rhinitis, however, irritants (e.g., fumes, cold air, high humidity, alcoholic beverages, or emotional stress) rather than allergens usually trigger symptoms. Moreover, vasomotor rhinitis is associated with an absence of nasal, palatal, or conjunctival pruritus. In *nonallergic rhinitis with eosinophilia,* testing likewise fails to indicate a specific allergen.

INITIATING DRUG THERAPY

Allergic rhinitis may be treated through avoidance of the allergen, pharmacologic agents, and immunotherapy. The basic approach to pharmacologic management of allergic rhinitis is the use of antihistamines, nasal decongestants, and intranasal corticosteroids (**Figure 47-3**).

TABLE 47.2	Symptoms of Seasonal Allergies Versus Respiratory Infections	
Symptoms	**Seasonal Allergy (Hay Fever)**	**Upper Respiratory Infection**
Head congestion/ runny nose	Yes	Yes
Sneezing	Yes	Sometimes
Itchy, watery eyes	Yes	No
Cough	Usually dry	Dry or productive
Predictable seasonal patterns	Yes	Uncommon
Fever	No	Yes
Short duration (3–7 d)	No	Yes
Long duration (weeks)	Yes	No
Productive cough	Uncommon (except in asthma)	Yes

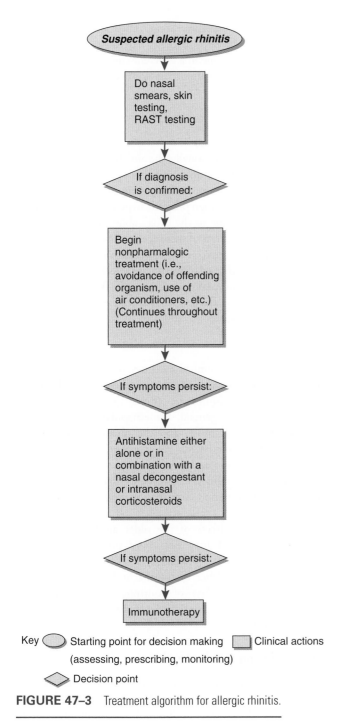

FIGURE 47–3   Treatment algorithm for allergic rhinitis.

and upholstered furniture. They can use high-efficiency particulate air (HEPA) cleaners to help filter out dust molds and pollen. Ideally, pets should be removed from the home; however, many patients and their families find doing so unacceptable. At a minimum, families should keep pets out of the allergic person's bedroom, as well as away from heating and cooling systems.

Immunotherapy, also known as *desensitization, hyposensitization,* or *allergy shots,* has been used for decades for the treatment of allergic rhinitis and asthma. It consists of repeated subcutaneous injections of gradually increasing concentrations of the allergens considered to be specifically responsible for the patient's allergy symptoms. However, patients must have documented IgE antibodies to these allergens. The injections are purified extracts of the "trigger" substances, such as ragweed, grass, dust mite, and animal dander. Clinical benefits are related to the administration of high doses of allergens weekly or every other week. The duration of treatment is typically 3 to 5 years, but if there is no improvement after 1 year, consider discontinuing immunotherapy. Treatment is discontinued based on minimal symptoms over two consecutive seasons of exposure. The benefit is derived from a reduction in the percentage of histamine released after immunotherapy compared with before treatment. The result is milder or no symptoms of allergy. Immunotherapy is not first-line treatment. It is usually initiated when avoidance of the triggers and drug therapy fail to control the symptoms of hay fever and other allergies.

Goals of Drug Therapy

The goal of drug therapy for patients with allergies is to alleviate the symptoms with a little to no adverse effects from medications. This is accomplished primarily through decreasing the release or inhibiting the effect of histamine release and other mediators of inflammation from mast cells. Mast cells are distributed throughout the body; however, the greatest concentration of histamine occurs in the skin, respiratory system, and gastrointestinal (GI) mucosa. Relief of symptoms with minimal drug side effects should lead to an improved quality of life.

Histamine released in the GI tract does not cause allergy symptoms. It may result in hyperacidity by stimulating histamine type 2 (H_2) receptors and lead to peptic ulcer disease or gastroesophageal reflux disease. Treatment of these conditions is with H_2 blockers. It is the histamine released in the skin and respiratory tract (H_1 receptors) that causes classic allergy symptoms. The medications used to treat these symptoms are antihistamines (H_1 blockers), nasal decongestants, intranasal corticosteroids, and intranasal cromolyn. Suggestions for their selection are outlined in the following sections. The decision to treat with medications will depend on the severity of symptoms and patient tolerance of symptoms. If drug treatment is chosen by the patient, it will be required as long as exposure to the triggers continues or until the patient becomes desensitized to the trigger, either naturally ("outgrowing the allergy") or through immunotherapy (described earlier).

The ideal treatment for allergic rhinitis is avoidance of the offending allergen. Complete avoidance often is not feasible, but most patients usually can reduce exposure. Basic strategies include the use of air conditioners in homes and automobiles to lessen exposure to pollen by keeping windows closed and use of dehumidifiers to discourage the growth of molds and mites. If possible, humidity should be maintained at 30% to 40% throughout the year. Patients can lessen exposure to mites by encasing mattresses in plastic, washing all bedding in very hot water each week, and removing carpeting

Antihistamines

Antihistamines are classified according to their sedative effects or as first generation (older) and second generation (newer) depending on when they were marketed. The older antihistamines cross the blood–brain barrier, causing the greatest degree of sedation as well as other central nervous system (CNS) effects. These agents can be subclassified on the basis of chemical structure. The main groupings include the ethanolamines, alkylamines, phenothiazines, piperazines, and piperidines.

First-Generation Antihistamines

The first-generation antihistamines, such as diphenhydramine, chlorpheniramine, and brompheniramine, are the older antihistamines. As noted earlier, these tend to be more sedating than newer, second-generation agents such as loratadine or cetirizine.

Mechanism of Action

Antihistamines are drugs that exert their effect in the body primarily by blocking the actions of histamine at receptor sites. They are classified as pharmacologic antagonists of histamine. They do not prevent histamine release, but act by competitive inhibition. Most antihistamines can be classified as either H_1-receptor blockers, which block the smooth muscle response, or H_2-receptor blockers, which block the histaminic stimulation of gastric acid. In general, H_2-receptor blockers are not used for patients with allergies. If the concentration of antihistamine drug at the receptor site exceeds the concentration of histamine, then the effects of histamine are blocked. Antihistamines usually ameliorate itching, sneezing, ocular symptoms, and nasal discharge but do not always reduce nasal congestion.

Dosage

The dosage varies depending on the age and weight of the patient. The frequency of dosing is typically every 4 to 6 hours as needed, but can be upwards of every 12 hours depending on the half-life of the drug and the formulation. For example, diphenhydramine (Benadryl) is given every 4 to 6 hours, but brompheniramine is dosed every 12 to 24 hours. These are often over-the-counter (OTC) agents and are supplied as tablets, capsules, elixirs, or suspensions. Further, these formulations come in a variety of flavors, and some are even free of dye.

Time Frame for Response

The onset of action of these agents typically ranges from 15 to 30 minutes and lasts nearly as long as the dosing interval. Those agents with a longer half-life will take longer to get to steady state, but the initial effect is often seen fairly rapidly.

Some regular users of antihistamines find that tolerance, or drug failure, develops after several weeks or months. One reason for this decreased effectiveness is that some antihistamines are capable of hepatic enzyme induction, resulting in increased metabolism in the liver. Essentially, the antihistamine drug hastens its own destruction and removal from circulation. The various antihistamine classes differ in their capacity to induce hepatic enzymes. Some practitioners have found that if tolerance develops, patients may benefit by switching to another antihistamine in a different chemical category. The effectiveness of this technique has not been evaluated by controlled studies.

Contraindications

First-generation antihistamine therapy is contraindicated in lactating mothers. Additionally, the anticholinergic side effects of the first-generation antihistamines put patients with narrow-angle glaucoma at risk for an increase in intraocular pressure. Similarly, men with benign prostatic hyperplasia (BPH) should avoid these agents due to the drug's ability to decrease urine flow. The sedating effects of these agents should also be considered when patients are required to perform hazardous tasks or drive. Because of the sedating and anticholinergic properties, first-generation antihistamines are on the Beers list, a list of drugs that should be avoided or used with extreme caution in elderly patients (Fick, et al., 2003).

Adverse Events

Knowledge of the chemical category to which an antihistamine belongs can help determine the relative degree of sedation and anticholinergic effects associated with the particular agent. In general, the ethanolamine derivatives, such as diphenhydramine, and the phenothiazine derivatives, such as promethazine (Phenergan), cause the greatest degree of sedation and anticholinergic effects. The most problematic anticholinergic effects are dry mouth, blurred vision, urinary hesitancy, constipation, confusion, and mental cloudiness.

The sedative effects of the older antihistamines vary among patients and may not cause problems for some. Tolerance to the sedative effect develops, and many patients find that sedation either disappears or becomes less bothersome after several days of continued use. Nonetheless, sedation may affect the patient's acceptance of the older antihistamine drugs.

Less Sedating Antihistamines

More recently, antihistamines have been developed that do not cross the blood–brain barrier to the extent exhibited by the older agents. These newer antihistamines, commonly referred to as *NSAs,* are considered to act peripherally and do not produce sedation or cause clinically important changes in mental status. In general, the anticholinergic effects of these agents are also minimal. Cetirizine, a metabolite of the antipruritic hydroxyzine (Atarax), is not always accepted as an NSA because it is reported to have a higher incidence of sedation than the other newer antihistamines. It is generally classified as a peripherally acting antihistamine and is often still listed in the same category. Nonetheless, it is an effective antihistamine approved by the U.S. Food and Drug Administration (FDA) for seasonal and perennial rhinitis. The NSAs are listed and compared in **Table 47.3**.

TABLE 47.3   Overview of Selected Antihistamines and Decongestants

Generic (Trade) Name and Dosage	Selected Adverse Events	Contraindications	Special Considerations
Nonsedating Antihistamines			
certirizine (Zyrtec) 　5–10 mg PO daily 　Children 2–6 y: 2.5 mg daily 　6–11 y: 5–10 mg daily	Somnolence, dry mouth, pharyngitis, dizziness	Known hypersensitivity to certirizine or hydroxyzine	Renal or hepatic impairment: Adults—5 mg qd; Children—not recommended Pregnancy category B
levocetirizine (Xyzal) 　2.5–5 mg PO daily 　Children 2–5 y: 1.25 mg daily 　6–11 y: 2.5 mg PO daily	Same as cetirizine	Known hypersensitivity to levocetirizine or cetirizine, end stage renal disease, renal impairment in children	Use with caution in patients with renal impairment. Pregnancy category B
fexofenadine (Allegra) 　60 mg PO bid 　180 mg tablet PO daily 　Children 2–11 y: 30 mg BID	Viral infection (cold, influenza), nausea, dysmenorrhea, drowsiness, dyspepsia, fatigue	Known hypersensitivity to any of its ingredients	Erythromycin and ketoconazole may increase plasma levels of fexofenadine. Pregnancy category C
loratadine (Claritin) 　10 mg PO qd 　Children 2–5 y: 5 mg daily	Headache, somnolence, fatigue, dry mouth	Known hypersensitivity to any of its ingredients	Give same dose every other day in renal or hepatic impairment. Pregnancy category B
desloratadine (Clarinex) 　5 mg PO daily 　Children 2–5 y: 1.25 mg daily 　6–11 y: 2.5 mg daily	Same as loratadine	Known hypersensitivity to any ingredients or loratadine	Give same dose every other day in renal or hepatic impairment. Pregnancy category C
Intranasal Antihistamines			
olopatadine (Patanase) Two sprays per nostril twice daily 　Children 6–11 y: One spray per nostril twice daily	Headache, somnolence, cough, epistaxis, throat irritation, bitter taste, dry mouth	None	Amount of drug per actuation (spray): 127 mcg
azelastine (Astelin or Astepro Nasal Spray) 　1–2 sprays in each nostril BID; 100 doses per bottle	Bitter taste, headache, somnolence, nasal burning, pharyngitis, dry mouth, paroxysmal sneezing, nausea, rhinitis, fatigue, dizziness	Known hypersensitivity	Amount of drug per spray: 137 mcg (Astelin), 205.5 mcg (Astepro) Astepro may be dosed 2 sprays once daily rather than BID. Not recommended in children 6–12 y
Oral Nasal Decongestants			
pseudoephedrine 　60 mg q6h (240 mg); extended release, 120 mg q12h; controlled release 240 mg q24h 　Children 6–12 y: 30 mg q6h (120 mg) 　Children 2–6 y: 15 mg q6h (60 mg)	Headache, insomnia, dry mouth, somnolence, nervousness, dizziness, fatigue, dyspepsia, nausea, pharyngitis, anorexia, thirst	Hypersensitivity to drug or its components, use within 14 days of an MAO inhibitor	Extended release should not be recommended for children <12 y. Pregnancy category C
phenylephrine 　10–20 mg q4h 　Children 6–12 y: 10 mg q4h	Same as pseudoephedrine	Same as pseudoephedrine	Pregnancy category C
Intranasal Cromolyn			
cromolyn (Nasalcrom Nasal Solution) 　Patients ≥2y: one spray in each nostril 3–6 times a day until symptom relief, then every 8–12 h	Common: burning, stinging, or irritation inside nose, increase in sneezing Rare: cough, headache, unpleasant taste, bloody nose	Hypersensitivity to cromolyn or the formula; acute asthma attacks	Comes in 13-mL bottle and 26-mL bottle—13-mL bottle = 100 sprays, 26-mL bottle = 200 sprays Not recommended in children <2 y

Dosage

Loratadine (Claritin) is dosed as 10 mg once daily for adults and children age 6 and older. For children ages 2 to 5, the dose is 5 mg once daily. Cetirizine (Zyrtec) is given 5 to 10 mg once daily for children older than age 6 and adults. The lower dosage can be used for younger children or for patients with less severe symptoms. Children ages 2 to 5 should be started on 2.5 mg once daily. Levocetirizine and desloratadine are generally half the dose of cetirizine and loratadine. Fexofenadine (Allegra) doses are for adults and children age 12 and older. The starting dose is 60 mg twice daily or 180 mg once daily for the extended-release formulation. Children ages 6 to 11 should start at 30 mg twice a day.

Time Frame for Response

This class of agents has a rapid onset of action, with a time to maximum effect ranging from 1 to 2.5 hours. The half-life of these drugs is 8 to 28 hours, leading to a 1- to 3-day delay in reaching a steady state. Food can delay the time to peak of cetirizine and loratadine, but not fexofenadine.

Contraindications

The lower propensity for anticholinergic effects allows for wider use of NSAs in the elderly, patients with glaucoma, and men with BPH because they do not share the same contraindications. NSAs are contraindicated in patients with previous hypersensitivity to these drugs and are not recommended in lactating mothers.

Adverse Events

Overall, this class of drugs is well tolerated in patients. Common adverse events include headache, dry mouth, dyspepsia, nausea, and fatigue. See **Table 47.3** for specific agents. It is important to note that cetirizine and levocetirizine are known to be more sedating than the other drugs in this class. More serious but rare side effects include dizziness, myalgia, somnolence, and dysmenorrhea.

Interactions

While loratadine and desloratadine do not have any significant drug interactions, fexofenadine does have some interactions that should be clinically considered. Fexofenadine concentrations may be increased by azole antifungals and erythromycin. Antacids and grapefruit juice administered with fexofenadine may decrease the absorption of fexofenadine. There is also a remote possibility that fexofenadine may prolong the QT interval on an electrocardiogram when administered with other drugs that concurrently prolong the QT interval. Cetirizine or levocetirizine administered with sedating drugs may increase sedation.

Intranasal Antihistamines

Azelastine (Astelin) and olopatadine (Patanase) intranasal antihistamines are also available to treat allergic rhinitis.

In placebo-controlled trials, they significantly improved the symptoms of rhinorrhea, sneezing, and nasal pruritus. The adverse events that occurred more frequently than in the patients treated with placebos were bitter taste (19.7% versus 0.6% for placebo) and somnolence (11.5% vs. 5.4%). These agents still have some systemic absorption, so it is important to remember that they may cause side effects and interact with allergy skin tests. Intranasal prescribing information is noted in **Table 47.3**.

Nasal Decongestants

Mechanism of Action

Nasal decongestants are sympathomimetic amines chemically related to norepinephrine, a major neurotransmitter of the sympathetic nervous system. These drugs are vasoconstrictors. They offer relief from nasal congestion by constricting the blood vessels of the nasal mucosa that have been dilated by histamine and are available in either oral or topical nasal formulations. The results are a shrinking of swollen nasal passages and more air movement to make breathing easier. However, just as norepinephrine is a CNS stimulant, so are the synthetic oral and topical (nasal) decongestants, which is an important clinical consideration.

Dosage

Dosing for common nasal decongestant products is noted in **Table 47.3**. Many decongestants are available in combination with antihistamines. Fixed combination products containing antihistamines and sympathomimetic amines are convenient, but the effective dose of oral decongestants varies among patients. If use of a fixed combination causes side effects or does not relieve symptoms, then clinicians should titrate with single agents to achieve the required dosage.

Because these agents are available OTC, counsel patients to read all labels carefully in order to select a product with only the components that they need to treat symptoms. Many of these combination products may also contain pain relievers or caffeine in addition to antihistamines and decongestants. If patients are also taking separate doses of pain relievers, they could be in danger of overdose.

Time Frame for Response

The onset of action for these agents, in immediate-release form, is typically 15 to 30 minutes with a peak response within 30 to 60 minutes. The half-life of pseudoephedrine is 9 to 16 hours, but the effect of the decongestant activity wears off within 4 to 6 hours after administration.

Contraindications

Caution should be used when recommending OTC oral decongestants. Patients with high blood pressure, heart disease, hyperthyroidism, narrow-angle glaucoma, seizure disorders, and BPH may see exacerbation of their disease. In addition, use of oral decongestants is contraindicated in patients taking monoamine oxidase (MAO) inhibitors within 14 days of the administration of pseudoephedrine. Pseudoephedrine and phenylephrine cause the release of norepinephrine into the synapse, and MAO inhibitors inhibit the enzymatic degradation of norepinephrine. As such, the concomitant use of these agents increases the sympathetic activity of the nervous system and can lead to hypertensive crisis.

Adverse Events

Oral decongestants constrict blood vessels throughout the body and also act as CNS stimulants, thus increasing blood pressure and heart rate and causing palpitations. Stimulation of the CNS can lead to insomnia, irritability, restlessness, and headache. Many patients find that they can use oral decongestants only during the daytime because the stimulatory effects of these drugs can cause nervousness, agitation, and insomnia.

Topical (Intranasal) Decongestants

Intranasal application (sprays or drops) of sympathomimetic amines provides a prompt and dramatic decrease of nasal congestion. A rebound phenomenon (rhinitis medicamentosa), however, often follows topical application of these drugs. In this scenario, the nasal mucous membrane becomes even more congested and edematous as the drug's vasoconstrictor effect wears off. This secondary congestion is believed to result from ischemia caused by the drug's intensive local vasoconstriction and local irritation of the agent itself. If the use of a topical decongestant is limited to 3 or 4 days, rebound congestion is minimal. With chronic use or overuse of these drugs, rebound nasal stuffiness may become quite pronounced. This phenomenon may begin a vicious cycle, leading to more frequent use of the drug that causes the problem. Should this occur, patients should discontinue topical decongestant therapy. They may use an oral decongestant, isotonic saline drops or spray, or both instead (**Table 47.4**). Side effects from topically administered agents include local irritation and rebound congestion.

Intranasal Corticosteroids

Nasal-inhaled corticosteroids are the most effective forms of therapy for allergic rhinitis. They help to relieve congestion and rhinorrhea by limiting the late-phase response and reducing inflammation. Corticosteroids have a wide range of inhibitory activities against multiple cell types (e.g., mast cells, eosinophils, neutrophils, macrophages, and lymphocytes) and mediators of inflammation (e.g., histamine, eicosanoids, leukotrienes, and cytokines).

Mechanism of Action

Corticosteroids exert their anti-inflammatory effect by disabling the cells that present antigen to antibody. Interfering with the antigen–antibody reaction reduces the stimulus for mast cell degranulation. With reduced mast cell degranulation, secretion of cytokines is diminished. The result is a weaker inflammatory reaction with milder or no symptoms of runny nose, nasal congestion, itching, and sneezing.

Dosage

The dosage of the individual intranasal steroids is listed in **Table 47.5**. In general, mometasone furoate, fluticasone propionate, and budesonide have been rated as most potent in vitro. However, these differences have not been shown to translate into meaningful clinical differences in patients. Intranasal corticosteroids must be primed before initial use. Clinicians should counsel patients to squeeze the pump a few times until a fine spray appears. If patients do not use the pump for more than 1 week, they should re-prime it.

Time Frame for Response

The therapeutic effects of intranasal corticosteroids are not immediate, but will begin working within 3 to 12 hours. Clinicians must counsel patients that they may not experience maximal effects for 1 to 2 weeks if they are using intranasal steroids continuously. Although continuous use is more efficacious, as-needed dosing has also been shown to be useful in

TABLE 47.4	**Topical Nasal Decongestants**						
				Patient Age			
Generic	Trade	Concentration (%)	>6 mo	2–6 y	6–12 y	>12 y
phenylephrine	Neo-Synephrine	0.125	Yes	Yes	Yes	Yes
	Neo-Synephrine	0.25	No	No	Yes	Yes
	Neo-Synephrine	0.5	No	No	No	Yes
naphazoline	Privine	0.05	No	No	No	Yes
oxymetazoline	Afrin	0.05	No	Yes	Yes	Yes
tetrahydrozoline	Tyzine Pediatric	0.05	No	Yes	Yes	Yes
	Tyzine	0.1	No	No	Yes	Yes
xylometazoline	Triaminic Nasal and Sinus Congestion	0.05	No	Yes	Yes	Yes

TABLE 47.5	Intranasal Corticosteroid Prescribing Information				
Drug	**Brand Name (Manufacturer)**	**Amount of Drug per Spray/Doses per Bottle**	**How Supplied**	**Suggested Dose**	
				Adult	**Pediatric (6–12 y)**
beclomethasone	Beconase AQ (Glaxo SmithKline)	42 mcg/200	25-g amber glass bottle with spray pump	One or 2 sprays in each nostril bid spray pump	Same as adult
budesonide	Rhinocort Aqua (Astra)	32 mcg/120	8.6-g bottle with spray pump	One to 4 sprays in each nostril daily	Same as adult
ciclesonide	Omnaris (Sepracor)	50 mcg/120	12.5-g bottle with spray pump	Two sprays in each nostril daily	Same as adult
flunisolide	N/A	25 μg/200	25-mL bottle with spray pump	Two sprays in each nostril bid	Same as adult
fluticasone	Flonase (Glaxo SmithKline)	50 mcg/120	16-g bottle with spray pump	Two sprays in each nostril daily	Not recommended
	Veramyst (Glaxo SmithKline)	27.5 mcg/120	10-g bottle with spray pump	Two sprays in each nostril daily	One spray in each nostril daily.
mometasone	Nasonex (Schering)	50 mcg/120	17-g bottle with spray pump	Two sprays in each nostril daily	One spray in each nostril daily
triamcinolone	Nasacort AQ (Aventis)	55 mcg/100	10-g aerosol canister	One spray up to 4 sprays in each nostril daily	One spray up to 2 sprays in each nostril qd

patients with seasonal allergic rhinitis. Intranasal corticosteroids should be initiated 2 to 4 weeks before the start of allergy season in patients with recurrent seasonal allergic rhinitis for maximal benefit.

If nasal blockage is severe, patients should use a topical nasal decongestant for the first 2 to 3 days to reduce the swelling and increase the delivery of corticosteroid to the nasal mucosa. Use of nasal corticosteroids should not continue beyond 3 weeks in the absence of significant symptomatic improvement, according to the manufacturers' professional product information.

Contraindications

All intranasal corticosteroids are designated as pregnancy category C. This means that either animal reproduction studies have shown adverse effects on the fetus and there are no controlled studies in women, or there are no studies in women or animals. The drug should be given only if potential benefit justifies potential risk.

Adverse Events

These agents are supplied as aqueous solutions in manually activated metered-dose nasal spray pumps, with separate patient instructions for use with every package. Some of these formulations have a flowery odor that some patients may find annoying. Local side effects such as irritation, bleeding, and septal perforation may occur but are rare; ensure that patients are using these products correctly in order to minimize these side effects.

Overall, intranasal steroids do not achieve significant systemic concentrations, although the effects of long-term systemic absorption could be concerning. Probably the most concerning adverse effects of intranasal steroids are the possibility of decreasing the rate of growth and suppressing the hypothalamic-pituitary-adrenal axis. Transient effects on growth in children have been noted, but the studies looking at this end point have varied widely. At normal recommended doses, fluticasone, mometasone, and budesonide have not shown growth suppression. The only study to show growth suppression used higher than recommended doses for long periods, so this should not be a serious concern in clinical practice.

All aqueous preparations contain preservatives. Benzalkonium chloride, which may cause ciliary dysfunction, is the preservative in the beclomethasone, flunisolide, fluticasone, mometasone, and triamcinolone products, whereas budesonide contains potassium sorbate as the preservative.

Interactions

Interactions with other drugs are generally not a concern due to low systemic absorption of intranasal corticosteroids.

Intranasal Cromolyn

Cromolyn is classified as a mast cell stabilizer. It prevents antigen-induced degranulation, thereby inhibiting the release of histamine and other cytokines that mediate inflammatory cell function. Cromolyn is of no value in treating acute allergic rhinitis. It is helpful only in preventing the nasal symptoms of allergic rhinitis. Treatment is more effective if it begins 2 to 4 weeks before exposure and continues throughout the exposure period. Intranasal cromolyn is available to patients as Nasalcrom 4% Nasal Solution. It does not require a prescription. Patient use information is noted in **Table 47.3.**

Selecting the Most Appropriate Agent

Nasal symptoms of allergic rhinitis include watery rhinorrhea (runny nose), paroxysmal sneezing (sudden fits of sneezing), nasal congestion (stuffy nose, sinus headache, or both), and postnasal drip that may cause coughing. Allergic rhinitis also may involve the conjunctiva (allergic conjunctivitis). The resulting symptoms are ocular pruritus (itching eyes), lacrimation (watery eyes), conjunctival hyperemia (bloodshot eyes), and chemosis (swollen eyelids). Drug treatment must be tailored to address the most bothersome symptoms. See **Box 47.2** and **Figure 47-3** for a stepwise approach to treating allergic rhinitis. **Table 47.6** lists the recommended treatment order for allergies.

First-Line Therapy

Intranasal corticosteroids are the most potent agents available for the relief of *established* seasonal or perennial rhinitis. They provide efficacy with substantially reduced side effects compared with oral corticosteroids. Selection of the best agent mostly depends on the patient's insurance formulary.

However, due to the long time frame for response and that they may not be as effective for systemic symptoms, these agents are often given in combination with antihistamines. First-generation antihistamines were considered first-line agents for the prevention and treatment of allergic symptoms. However, the sedative side effects of the traditional antihistamines limit

TABLE 47.6	Recommended Order of Treatment for Allergies	
Order	**Agents**	**Comments**
First line	Intranasal corticosteroids	Intranasal corticosteroids are the most potent agents available for relief of established seasonal or perennial rhinitis.
Second line	Antihistamines/ nasal decongestants	Either first- or second-generation agent can be used. Product selection is based on dosing frequency, potential for adverse effects, and cost. Second-generation antihistamines may be given only once or twice a day, and they are relatively nonsedating. First-generation antihistamines are given 3–4 times a day. Pseudoephedrine and phenylephrine are the most popular oral nasal decongestants.
Third line	Intranasal cromolyn	Must be used prophylactically.

their usefulness in patients who must remain awake and alert. Fortunately, NSAs, also known as *newer* or *second-generation antihistamines,* cause minimal sedation because they do not cross the blood–brain barrier into the CNS.

The various first- and second-generation antihistamines are equally effective in treating symptoms of allergic rhinitis. Product selection is based on dosing frequency (i.e., duration of action), potential for adverse effects, and cost. Second-generation antihistamines may be given only once or twice a day, and they are relatively nonsedating. First-generation antihistamines are given 3 to 4 times a day. Some products are available in long-acting dosage forms that may be given only twice a day. While more sedating, first-generation antihistamines are also significantly less expensive than the second-generation drugs. These agents have the best results when patients take them before exposure to a known allergen. During seasonal attack, patients may need to take antihistamines around-the-clock for maximal effectiveness.

Second-Line Therapy

Because antihistamines do not reduce nasal congestion, they are often used in combination with nasal decongestants. Pseudoephedrine and phenylephrine are the most popular oral nasal decongestants. Nasal decongestants are α-adrenergic receptor agonists. As such, they stimulate α-adrenergic receptors, causing vasoconstriction in the nasal mucosa, decreasing congestion, and opening nasal passages. Side effects include CNS and cardiovascular stimulation. Elevation in blood pressure may also occur. Many prescription and nonprescription drugs

BOX **47.2**

A Stepwise Approach Is Used to Manage the Symptoms of Allergic Rhinitis

1. Identify the offending allergens by history with confirmation of the allergy by skin test.
2. Teach the patient to avoid the offending allergens.
3. For mild symptoms, prophylactic treatment with cromolyn nasal spray (Nasalcrom) or treatment with an antihistamine/decongestant combination may be necessary.
4. For prominent symptoms, begin with topical corticosteroid nasal spray.
5. For treatment failures despite avoidance and pharmacotherapy, progress to immunotherapy.

contain a combined antihistamine and nasal decongestant. Some examples are given in **Table 47.3**.

Topical (intranasal) decongestants avoid systemic adverse effects. Prolonged use leads to rebound nasal congestion, however, so they are impractical for seasonal or perennial allergies. Their use should be limited to short periods (a few days).

Third-Line Therapy

Cromolyn, in the form of a metered-dose nasal spray, could be considered a first-line treatment for allergic rhinitis, but it is a prophylactic measure only. It is classified as a mast cell stabilizer in that it prevents or attenuates the allergen activation of nasal mast cells. To be efficacious, cromolyn must be administered continuously (usually 4 times a day) during seasonal allergen exposure or immediately before an anticipated exposure such as animal dander.

Intranasal cromolyn is an alternative to antihistamines and nasal decongestants for allergic rhinitis. It generally is considered less effective than intranasal corticosteroids, but it is virtually free of side effects.

Special Population Considerations

Pediatric

If one parent has allergies, the child has a 50% chance of having allergies. Allergies may also be more common in children who were formula fed, of low birth weight, or exposed to dogs, cats, or tobacco smoke early in life. In childhood, more boys have allergic rhinitis than do girls, but this difference begins to disappear after adolescence. No sex differences are found in adults.

To determine the dose of allergy medication for a child, practitioners should use weight if possible. Otherwise, they may base according to age. The official product literature usually provides child dosage recommendations by age and weight. Parents should also be counseled to look at package labeling carefully and use dose recommendations for their child's weight if the directions specify. Also, parents should use appropriate teaspoon or tablespoon measurements rather than kitchen utensils. Counsel patients to ask the pharmacist at their local pharmacy if they are not sure if they have an accurate measuring tool.

In determining the dose of medication for a child, practitioners must recognize that infants and small children are not merely "scaled-down" adults. Organs such as the GI tract, liver, and kidneys are not developed enough in children for them to handle medications. Estimating a child's dose based on the adult dose is not always safe. Most pharmaceutical manufacturers do not provide such comprehensive pediatric dosing guidelines. Usually, an age range for children's doses is stated in the official package insert or on the commercial package. If not, prescribers should contact the manufacturer or consult with a specialist who is experienced with the treatment. The *Physicians' Desk Reference* contains a Manufacturers' Index of addresses and telephone numbers.

As noted earlier, a major consideration in prescribing intranasal steroids in children is the impact on growth. The FDA has approved the use of mometasone and fluticasone furoate for children older than age 2, fluticasone propionate for children older than age 4, and ciclesonide, budesonide, and flunisolide for children age 6 and older. The other agents are approved for use in children older than age 6.

Geriatric

Although few factors provoke rhinitis in older adults, treatments need to be more tailored because of slower metabolism and the potential for side effects, especially in the CNS. Also, this population is more likely to be taking multiple medications, and therefore runs a greater risk of drug interactions than most other patients.

Women

In women, allergic rhinitis symptoms may worsen during pregnancy. The antihistamines diphenhydramine, loratadine, and cetirizine are pregnancy category B agents, whereas desloratadine and fexofenadine are category C agents. All intranasal steroids are category C agents.

MONITORING PATIENT RESPONSE

Assessing the efficacy of treatment requires monitoring the patient's adherence to the drug therapy plan, quality of life, and degree of satisfaction with the care provided. **Box 47.3** could be a useful office tool for this purpose.

PATIENT EDUCATION

Patient education is extremely important in the prevention and management of allergy symptoms. Teaching each patient about the causes of allergic reactions, how triggers evoke symptoms, the various medications available and their use, when to self-treat and when to seek medical help, and how to assess whether treatment is working is highly desirable and appropriate during an office visit. But comprehensive teaching may not be practical because of time constraints. It may be more efficient to determine what the patient *does not* understand and fill in the gaps at that time. For example, at the end of the visit, practitioners could ask the patient three very basic questions about treatment:

- What is the name of the medication you are taking for allergy symptoms?
- What beneficial effects do you expect, and what side effects may occur?
- How do you take the medication (i.e., dose, time of day, with meals, and what to avoid taking with it)?

BOX 47.3

Questions to Ask the Allergy Patient at Every Office Visit

MONITORING SIGNS, SYMPTOMS, AND FUNCTIONAL STATUS

- Has your allergy been better or worse since your last visit?
- In the past 2 weeks, how many days have you had: *(Ask the patient to tell you how symptoms developed, what they were like, and how long they lasted.)*
    A runny, stuffy or itchy nose?
    Any wheezing or coughing?
    Any hives or swelling?
    Eczema or other skin rashes?
    Reactions to foods?
    Reactions to insects?
- Since your last visit, how many days has your allergy caused you to:
    Miss work or school?
    Reduce your activities?
    (For caregivers) change your activity because of your child's allergies?
- Since your last visit, have you had any unscheduled or emergency department visits or hospital stays?
- Since your last visit, have you had any times when your allergy symptoms were a lot worse than usual?
    If yes, what do you think caused the symptoms to get worse?
    If yes, what did you do to control the symptoms?
- Have there been any changes in your home, school, or work environment (e.g., new smokers or pets)? Any new hobbies or recreational activities?
- Has there been difficulty sleeping at night due to symptoms of allergy?

MONITORING PHARMACOTHERAPY

- What medications are you taking?
- How often do you take each medication? How much do you take each time?
- Have you had any unusual reactions to your medications?
- Have you missed or stopped taking any regular doses of your medications for any reason?
- Have you had trouble filling your prescriptions (e.g., for financial reasons, not on formulary)?
- Have you tried any other medications?
- Has your allergy medicine caused you any problems (e.g., sleepiness, bad taste, sore throat)?
- Have you had any nighttime awakenings?

MONITORING PATIENT–PROVIDER COMMUNICATION AND PATIENT SATISFACTION

- What questions do you have about your allergy management?
- What problems have you had in following your allergy management plan, such as taking your medications or reducing your exposure to allergens?
- Has anything prevented you from getting the treatment you need for your allergies?
- Have the costs of your allergy treatment interfered with your ability to get appropriate care?
- How can we improve your allergy care?

This information is provided by the Asthma and Allergy Foundation of America (AAFA) as part of its educational outreach to patients and their caregivers. The information was adapted from the 2007 National Asthma Education and Prevention Program's Guidelines for the Diagnosis and Treatment of Asthma published by the National Heart, Lung, and Blood Institute.

If the patient can articulate the correct answers to these questions, little more needs to be discussed about treatment. Practitioners could provide verbally or in writing those things that the patient does not know or understand. Also, they should encourage patients to accept written materials that pharmacists provide when they fill prescriptions and to question any ambiguous or contradictory information.

Drug Information

A variety of sources provide information regarding the treatment of allergic rhinitis. The American Association of Allergies,

Asthma, and Immunology provides practice parameters for the treatment of allergic rhinitis (www.aaaai.org). Further, the FDA provides drug information specific to the product, particularly in relation to children or pregnant women.

Patient-Oriented Information Sources

The American Association of Allergies, Asthma, and Immunology provides patient-directed information (http://www.aaaai.org/patients/resources/fastfacts/rhinitis.stm). Similarly, the FDA has information regarding medications in an easy to use format for patients.

TABLE 47.7	Selected Ophthalmic Drugs for Allergic Conjunctivitis by Drug Class			
Class	**Generic (Trade) Name**	**Strength (Potency)**	**How Supplied**	**Dose**
Corticosteroid	prednisolone (Pred-Mild)	0.12%	5- and 10-mL ophthalmic suspension	One drop in each affected eye BID–QID
Antihistamine	emedastine (Emadine)	0.05%	5-mL ophthalmic solution	One drop in each affected eye QID
Antihistamine	olopatadine (Patanol)	0.1%	5-mL ophthalmic solution	One to 2 drops in each affected eye BID at 6- to 8-h intervals
Mast cell stabilizer	lodoxamide (Alomide)	0.1%	10-mL ophthalmic solution	One to 2 drops in each affected eye QID up to 3 mo
Mast cell stabilizer	cromolyn (Crolom)	4%	10-mL ophthalmic solution a day at regular intervals	One to 2 drops in each affected eye 4–6 times
NSAID	ketorolac (Acular)	0.5%	3-, 5-, 10-mL ophthalmic solution	One drop in each affected eye QID

Complementary and Alternative Medications

There is some suggestion that acupuncture and biofeedback may be effective means of treating allergic rhinitis. However, controlled studies evaluating the effectiveness of these treatment modalities are lacking. Further, although few studies have examined the effectiveness of specific homeopathic therapies, *nux vomica* has been used to help in the treatment of nasal congestion and discharge.

ALLERGIC CONJUNCTIVITIS

The signs and symptoms of allergic conjunctivitis result from the same allergens that cause allergic rhinitis. Mast cells are abundant in the eyelid and conjunctiva, but are infrequently found in the eye. This limits allergic ocular inflammation to the lining of the eyelid and the ocular surface (the conjunctiva).

Histamine and arachidonic acid derivatives are the mediators that probably cause most ocular signs and symptoms. Mast cell activation, however, also leads to recruitment of eosinophils, which can be found in the conjunctiva 3 to 5 hours after mast cell degranulation.

Many patients experience ocular symptoms only when allergens directly contact the eyes. For example, patients with sensitivity to cat dander may not have reactions in a room with cats but experience symptoms if they bring their hands to their face. Patients who have symptoms even without direct contact need to be particularly rigorous in their efforts to eliminate or avoid allergens in their homes, workplaces, or schools. Eye rubbing not only introduces allergens into the eye but may degranulate mast cells mechanically.

Practitioners should encourage patients to apply cool compresses to their eyelids rather than rubbing their eyes to alleviate symptoms. Artificial tears also may reduce symptoms and wash away allergens and inflammatory mediators from the conjunctiva. Often, however, these approaches are inadequate. In such cases, patients require pharmacologic intervention. The types of eye drop medications used to treat allergic conjunctivitis are corticosteroids, antihistamines, vasoconstrictor/antihistamine combinations, mast cell stabilizers, and nonsteroidal anti-inflammatory drugs (NSAIDs).

Topical corticosteroids are effective, but the use of these drugs is limited because they can induce cataracts and glaucoma. If topical corticosteroids are required, a lower-potency agent is preferred. Primary care practitioners should refer any patient who requires topical corticosteroids for more than 2 weeks to an ophthalmologist.

First-generation oral antihistamines, which can help reduce ocular itching, may cause more problems by decreasing tear production due to anticholinergic effects. NSAIDs provide temporary relief of ocular itching due to seasonal allergic conjunctivitis. They work by inhibiting biosynthesis of prostaglandin, a mediator of pain and inflammation. Prescribing information for the ophthalmic drops used to treat allergic conjunctivitis is noted in **Table 47.7**.

Case Study

G. B., an 18-year-old African American female college student, lives on campus with three other students. Her home is approximately 100 miles away. She has been at college since the beginning of the fall semester, approximately 2 weeks. She presents today with a chief complaint of fits of sneezing (sometimes 10 in a row); a runny, itchy, stuffy nose; and red, tearing eyes. Her temperature is 99°F; blood pressure is 118/78. She denies cough and headache. Her chest is clear. Her past medical history is unremarkable, except for "hay fever" when she was younger, which she "outgrew" during high school. These symptoms are the same. She is having difficulty studying because of the sneezing and itching nose, and she is embarrassed to be in class with these symptoms. She was nervous about meeting the challenges of college and making new friends. Her local physician prescribed lorazepam (Ativan) 1.0 mg as needed for stress, anxiety, or both. So far, she has taken two doses of a prescription for 30 tablets.

DIAGNOSIS: ALLERGIC RHINITIS/ CONJUNCTIVITIS

1. List two specific goals of treatment of G. B.
2. What would be your first class of agents to prescribe? Why? Within that class, which agent would you choose?
3. What OTC and/or alternative medications would be appropriate for G. B.?
4. How would you monitor for the success of your selected treatment?
5. What adverse events would you monitor for and what would you do if they occurred?
6. Describe one or two drug–drug or drug–food interactions for the selected agent.
7. What aspects of the drug would you emphasize in your patient education discussion with G. B.?
8. What would you do if your first-line therapy was ineffective?
9. What dietary and lifestyle changes should be recommended for G. B.?
10. What would be the choice for the second-line therapy?

BIBLIOGRAPHY

Starred references are cited in the text.

Conner, S. J. (2002). Evaluation and treatment of the patient with allergic rhinitis. *Journal of Family Practice, 51,* 883–890.

Dipiro, J. (2008). Allergic and pseudoallergic drug reactions. In J. T. Dipiro (Ed.), *Pharmacotherapy: A pathophysiologic approach* (7th ed.). New York: McGraw-Hill Medical.

Dykewicz, M. S., Fineman, S., Nicklas, R., et al. (1998). Joint Task Force Algorithm and Annotations for Diagnosis and Management of Rhinitis. *Annals of Allergy, Asthma & Immunology, 81,* 469–473.

*Fick, D. M., Cooper, J. W., Wade, W. E., et al. (2003). Updating the Beers criteria for potentially inappropriate medication use in older adults: Results of a U.S. consensus panel of experts. *Archives of Internal Medicine, 163,* 2716–2724.

Gendo, K., & Larson, E. B. (2004). Evidence-based diagnostic strategies for evaluating suspected allergic rhinitis. *Annals of Internal Medicine, 140,* 278–289.

Lichtenstein, L., & Fauci, A. (1996). *Current therapy in allergy, immunology, and rheumatology* (5th ed.). St. Louis: Mosby-Year Book.

Lieberman, P., Kemp, S. F., Oppenheimer, J., et al. (2005). The diagnosis and management of anaphylaxis: An updated practice parameter. *Journal of Allergy and Clinical Immunology, 115,* S483–S523.

Medical Economics Company. (2004). *Physicians' desk reference* (54th ed.). Montvale, NJ: Author.

Middleton, E., Reed, C., Ellis, E., et al. (Eds.). (1998). *Allergy: Principles and practice* (5th ed., Vols. I and II). St. Louis: Mosby-Year Book.

National Institute of Allergy and Infectious Disease. (1997). *Disease state management sourcebook.* New York: Faulkner and Gray.

Patterson, R., Grammar, L., & Greenberg, P. (1997). *Allergic diseases: Diagnosis and management* (5th ed.). Philadelphia: Lippincott-Raven.

Wallace, D. V., Dykewicz, M. S., Bernstein, D. I., et al. (2008). The diagnosis and management of rhinitis: An updated practice parameter. *Journal of Allergy and Clinical Immunology, 122,* S1–S84.

Wingard, L., Brody, T., Larner, J., et al. (1991). *Human pharmacology: Molecular to clinical.* St. Louis: Mosby-Year Book.

Yanez, A., & Rodrigo, G. J. (2002). Intranasal corticosteroids versus topical H$_1$ receptor antagonists for the treatment of allergic rhinitis: A systematic review with meta-analysis. *Annals of Allergy, Asthma & Immunology, 89,* 479–484.

CHAPTER 48

Linda M. Spooner

Human Immunodeficiency Virus

The first known case of human immunodeficiency virus (HIV) infection was documented in 1959 in a man from Kinshasa, Congo. How he became infected with the virus is unknown. Furthermore, how the disease grew to epidemic proportions also is unclear. In the United States, HIV infection was first recognized in 1981 after it was discovered that young homosexual men were contracting unusual cases of pneumonia and rare cancers that typically were not seen in immunocompetent patients.

HIV is the virus that causes acquired immunodeficiency syndrome (AIDS). A diagnosis of AIDS is based on the presence of an AIDS-defining condition (**Box 48.1**) or a CD4$^+$ T-cell count of less than 200/mm^3 (Centers for Disease Control and Prevention [CDC], 1992). Although rates of progression from HIV infection to AIDS vary greatly among individuals, the median is approximately 10 years in patients not receiving antiretroviral medications.

The two types of HIV that have been identified are HIV-1 and HIV-2. HIV-1 accounts for the majority of cases worldwide, including in the United States, whereas HIV-2 is primarily found in West Africa. HIV-2 is less efficiently transmitted and results in a slower disease progression than HIV-1. Unfortunately, since there are no randomized clinical trials that have assessed the efficacy of antiretroviral medications for treatment of HIV-2 infection, the ideal initial treatment regimen is unknown. It appears reasonable to base a regimen on a protease inhibitor boosted with ritonavir for patients with HIV-2 infection (Panel on Antiretroviral Guidelines, 2009).

Over the past 25 years, HIV infection has reached epidemic proportions. The World Health Organization (WHO) estimates that approximately 33 million people worldwide are infected with HIV, with two thirds of cases occurring in sub-Saharan Africa (WHO, 2009). Of these, 2 million children younger than age 15 are infected. In 2007, 2.7 million people were newly infected with HIV, and there were 2 million deaths attributed to HIV throughout the world. Explanations for these overwhelming numbers include limited access to health care and antiretroviral medications as well as lack of education about prevention and transmission of HIV.

According to the most recent estimates, 1,106,400 adults and adolescents were infected with HIV in the United States at the end of 2006, representing an 11% increase compared to 2003 data (CDC, 2010). This phenomenon may be a result of more people seeking potent combination antiretroviral therapy (ART) as well as a larger number of people becoming infected and a smaller number of people dying from the disease every year. The number of new infections occurring annually has remained stable for the past 10 years.

The management of patients infected with HIV is challenging for several reasons. First, ART regimens can be complex, requiring a large pill burden as well as specific food and timing requirements. Second, adverse effects of the medications may affect a patient's ability to tolerate and comply with therapy. Third, nonadherence to ART results in treatment failure as well as the development of resistance due to suboptimal serum concentrations of antiretroviral drugs. The health care practitioner should collaborate with the individual patient to select a regimen that the patient can take successfully and still manage the potential adverse effects.

CAUSES

HIV is transmitted through four types of contact: sexual intercourse, bloodborne contact, perinatal transmission, and breast-feeding. *Prevention is the key to avoiding transmission* (**Box 48.2**). The most common route of transmission worldwide is through sexual contact with an infected person's genital fluids. The virus is also transmitted via intravenous (IV) transfer of infected blood through transfusions, IV drug use and needle sharing, or occupational exposure. An infected mother may transmit the virus to her baby prior to or during birth as well as during breast-feeding. It is important to note that HIV is *not* transmitted through casual contact (e.g., contact with tears, saliva, toilet facilities).

Effective treatment with ART may reduce the risk of transmission, as lower concentrations of HIV ribonucleic acid (RNA) in plasma are associated with decreased levels of HIV in genital secretions. Therefore, consistent use of ART leading to sustained reductions in HIV viral loads should be combined with safer sexual and drug use practices to prevent HIV transmission.

BOX 48.1
AIDS-Defining Conditions

Candidiasis, pulmonary or esophageal

Cervical cancer

Coccidioidomycosis

Cryptococcosis

Cryptosporidiosis

Cytomegalovirus

Herpes simplex virus

Histoplasmosis (microscopy [histology or cytology], culture, or detection of antigen in a specimen obtained directly from the tissues affected or a fluid from those tissues)

HIV-associated dementia

HIV-associated wasting

Isosporiasis

Kaposi sarcoma

Lymphoma

Mycobacterium avium infection

Pneumocystis jiroveci pneumonia

Other pneumonias, recurrent (more than one episode in a 1-year period)

Progressive multifocal leukoencephalopathy

Salmonella septicemia

Toxoplasmosis

Tuberculosis

Adapted from Centers for Disease Control and Prevention. (1992). 1993 revised classification system for HIV infection and expanded surveillance case definition for AIDS among adolescents and adults. *Morbidity and Mortality Weekly Report, 41*(RR-17), 1–19.

PATHOPHYSIOLOGY

HIV is a retrovirus; each viral particle contains two single-stranded molecules of RNA rather than deoxyribonucleic acid (DNA). Following infection of host cells, the viral enzyme reverse transcriptase allows synthesis of a DNA molecule that is then inserted into the DNA of the host cell, allowing the virus to replicate. In the case of HIV, the host cells are $CD4^+$ T lymphocytes, a white blood cell involved in cell-mediated immunity. As the virus replicates, it destroys the $CD4^+$ T lymphocytes, thereby leading to immune deficiency.

HIV incorporates itself into the host cell through a number of steps. A viral envelope surrounding the HIV RNA contains proteins on its outer surface that react specifically with the $CD4^+$ receptor on the T lymphocyte ($CD4^+$ T cell). Additionally, the viral membrane uses co-receptors (CCR5 or CXCR4) to attach to the $CD4^+$ T cell. Once this is completed, the viral envelope fuses to the host cell and allows the HIV RNA to enter the host cell. Next, reverse transcriptase catalyzes the formation of a single-stranded DNA intermediate from the viral RNA. This step is followed by duplication of the single-stranded DNA to form a double-stranded DNA. Catalyzed by the enzyme integrase, viral DNA is integrated into the host cell's nucleus. After the DNA is transcribed and translated back to RNA, the virus then makes long chains of polyproteins that are split by the enzyme protease to form new copies of HIV RNA. To protect the viral RNA, a protective core protein called a *capsid* surrounds the genetic material. This process is rapidly repeated, producing an estimated 10 billion new particles each day. The average half-life of a viral particle is 6 hours. The largest concentration of viral particles can be found in lymph node tissue and genital secretions.

DIAGNOSTIC CRITERIA

The signs and symptoms of HIV disease vary among patients. The acute retroviral syndrome occurs 2 to 3 weeks following exposure to the virus. During this time, the number of $CD4^+$ T lymphocytes ($CD4^+$ count) declines dramatically and the number of HIV RNA particles in the plasma (viral load)

BOX 48.2
Preventing HIV Transmission

Preventing Sexual Transmission

Abstinence, safer sexual practices, use of latex condoms, risk factor modification, notification of sexual partners, education (especially to adolescents), treating sexually transmitted infections, and consistent and effective use of antiretroviral therapy may be used to prevent sexual transmission of HIV.

Preventing Blood Exposure Transmission

Since 1985, all donated blood is tested for the presence of HIV. Implementation of universal precautions training programs has decreased transmission among health care workers. Needle exchange and drug treatment programs are available throughout the United States.

Preventing Perinatal Transmission

Lowering antepartum viral load in the mother with combination antiretroviral therapy, combined with pre- and postexposure prophylaxis of the infant with antiretroviral therapy, aggressive family planning services (e.g., HIV testing, counseling), and recommending against breast-feeding for infected women.

increases greatly. Clinically, the patient may experience fever, swollen lymph nodes, sore throat, skin rash, muscle soreness, headache, nausea, vomiting, and diarrhea. The specific symptoms and their duration vary among patients, and their presence alone does not constitute a diagnosis. Diagnosis of HIV is based on the presence of virus in the plasma, often with a negative or indeterminate HIV antibody test (Panel on Antiretroviral Guidelines, 2011).

The currently used method for diagnosing HIV-1 infection is the enzyme-linked immunosorbent assay (ELISA), which detects circulating antibodies to the virus. This assay is highly sensitive and specific (99% sensitivity and specificity), but false-positive results may occur in patients who recently received hepatitis B or rabies vaccines, have acute infections, or have autoantibody formation. False-negative results may occur in newly infected patients whose antibody titer has not risen to detectable levels. Antibodies develop within 6 months after infection in 95% of patients, and the median time for antibody development is 2 months. If the ELISA test is positive, a Western blot test is used to confirm the diagnosis. Other confirmatory tests include an indirect immunofluorescence assay and a radioimmunoprecipitation assay.

Laboratory Parameters

Once the diagnosis of HIV has been confirmed using the above tests, initiation of therapy should be guided by the patient's clinical status as well as two main laboratory parameters, the CD4+ T-cell count and the plasma HIV RNA (viral load). Determination of these results allows the clinician to understand the patient's risk of opportunistic infections and risk for disease progression and to monitor response to drug therapy.

CD4+ T-Cell Count

The CD4+ T-cell count indicates the extent to which HIV has damaged the immune system. Normally, the CD4+ T-cell count ranges between 500 and 1,600/mm^3. As the viral infection progresses, the CD4+ count declines, correlating with increasing immunosuppression. CD4+ T-cell counts of less than 200/mm^3 are associated with an increased risk of AIDS malignancies, such as Kaposi sarcoma, and opportunistic infections, such as *Pneumocystis jiroveci* pneumonia, toxoplasmosis, and cytomegalovirus infection.

Plasma HIV RNA (Viral Load)

Quantification of HIV replication is determined by measuring the viral load in number of copies per milliliter of plasma. The primary assay used is the HIV-1 reverse transcriptase-polymerase chain reaction assay, which has a lower limit of detection of 40 to 70 copies/mL. Clinical trials demonstrate that viral loads that are undetectable (e.g., <40 to 70 copies/mL) are associated with longer duration of suppression of viral replication as compared with detectable levels. The viral load is a useful tool to monitor a patient's virologic status, disease progression, and ART regimen.

HIV Drug-Resistance Testing

Because of the significant association between the presence of drug-resistant HIV and failure of antiretroviral treatment regimens, HIV resistance assays have become useful mechanisms for guiding the selection of appropriate therapy. When used in combination with medication histories and patient counseling, these assays have assisted in attainment of more efficient and sustained viral suppression. Drug resistance testing is recommended for all patients in the initial laboratory testing they receive as they enter into care.

The two methods used to assess resistance include genotypic and phenotypic assays. Genotypic assays detect genetic mutations that may confer viral resistance. Interpretation of these genotypes requires an understanding of the mutations and their correlation with resistance to specific classes of antiretroviral medications. Results are typically available within 1 to 2 weeks. Phenotypic assays calculate the concentrations of antiretroviral drugs required to inhibit HIV replication by 50%. This value is known as the *median inhibitory concentration* and is abbreviated as the IC_{50}. The ratio of the IC_{50} of the patient's and reference virus is noted as the -fold increase in IC_{50} for a variety of antiretroviral medications. Results of phenotypic assays are available within 2 to 3 weeks due to automation techniques, but they are more expensive to perform than genotypic assays and more complicated to interpret. Both assays may be unsuccessful in patients with low viral loads (<500 to 1,000) due to inadequate presence of the virus.

Several limitations exist with HIV drug-resistance testing. First, there is no standardized method for quality assurance for the available genotypic and phenotypic assays. Second, they are expensive to perform. Lastly, if drug-resistant virus comprises less than 10% to 20% of a patient's total virus population, the assays will not detect the resistant virus. Overall, these assays provide a method for making decisions on initiating ART, changing ART in patients experiencing virologic failure or suboptimal response, and selecting ART in pregnant women.

INITIATING DRUG THERAPY

When discussing treatment of patients with HIV infection, it is helpful to classify them into three clinical categories: those with a history of an AIDS-defining illness or CD4+ count less than 350/mm^3; those with a CD4+ count of 350 to 500/mm^3; and those with a CD4+ count greater than 500/mm^3 (Panel on Antiretroviral Guidelines, 2011). All patients in the first category should be offered treatment with ART. Although the ideal time to initiate ART for asymptomatic patients with CD4+ T-cell counts of 350 to 500/mm^3 is unknown, it is recommended to initiate treatment in this population. For those individuals with CD4+ T-cell counts above 500/mm^3, the Panel members who authored the DHHS treatment guidelines are divided on their recommendations for initial therapy; 50% of the members suggest initiating treatment because the benefit outweighs the risk. The other 50% consider therapy as optional for this population because there are less data to support the benefits of treatment and the risks of long-term adverse effects. The clinician must make an individualized decision for each patient who falls into this category. Current recommendations also note that ART should be initiated in all patients who have any of the following conditions, regardless of CD4+ count: pregnancy, HIV-associated nephropathy, and hepatitis B coinfection requiring treatment.

If treatment is deferred in the patient with a CD4+ count greater than 500/mm³, as in cases where adherence may be suboptimal or comorbidities that complicate or prevent initiation of ART may be present, CD4+ count and viral load should be monitored closely. Depending on the values of these tests, discussion regarding initiation of therapy should be revisited, as clinical trials have shown that suppression of the virus delays or prevents complications, such as HIV-associated nephropathy, cardiovascular disease, malignancies, and liver disease. Before therapy is started for any patient, a thorough history and physical examination should be performed, in addition to a complete blood count, basic chemistry profile, liver function tests, fasting lipid profile and glucose, urinalysis, CD4+ T-cell count, viral load, genotypic resistance testing, and additional evaluation of various serologies (e.g., hepatitis B and C).

Goals of Therapy

Because currently available antiretroviral regimens cannot achieve eradication of HIV, goals of therapy primarily focus on sustained suppression of viral replication to undetectable levels. There are five main goals of antiretroviral therapy (Panel on Antiretroviral Guidelines, 2011). These include maximal and sustained suppression of viral load, restoration and preservation of immune system function, enhancement of quality of life, reduction in morbidity and mortality from HIV-related complications, and prevention of HIV transmission. Patients' responses to ART are variable, although successful regimens initiated in treatment-naïve patients can decrease viral loads to undetectable levels within 12 to 24 weeks. Virologic success is improved with high-potency ART, excellent treatment adherence, low baseline viral load, higher baseline CD4+ T-cell count, and rapid reduction of viral load in response to treatment.

To maximize the benefits of ART, it is important to select drug regimens carefully based on drug-resistance testing, adverse effects, convenience, drug interaction profile, and comorbidities. There are several preferred and alternative regimens that may be used as initial therapy for HIV infection, as they have comparable efficacy. These include nonnucleoside reverse transcriptase inhibitor-based regimens, protease inhibitor-based regimens, and integrase inhibitor-based regimens. **Table 48.1** lists characteristics of all of the currently available antiretroviral medications.

Reverse Transcriptase Inhibitors

There are two subclasses of reverse transcriptase inhibitors (RTIs): the nucleoside reverse transcriptase inhibitors (NRTIs) and the nonnucleoside reverse transcriptase inhibitors (NNRTIs).

Nucleoside Reverse Transcriptase Inhibitors

There are six NRTIs marketed in the United States. These include abacavir (Ziagen), didanosine (Videx), emtricitabine (Emtriva), lamivudine (Epivir), stavudine (Zerit), and zidovudine (Retrovir). There is one nucleotide RTI, tenofovir disoproxil fumarate (Viread), which is similar in mechanism of action but is slightly different in structure than the nucleoside analogs. In addition, several combination products are available for dosing convenience; these are listed in **Table 48.1**.

The NRTIs must be phosphorylated in the target cells before becoming active. This intracellular phosphorylation results in an active triphosphorylated form that interferes with the transcription of viral RNA to DNA. This interference can occur through two mechanisms: chain termination and competitive inhibition.

The *chain termination* process results in the reverse transcriptase enzyme adding the NRTI to the growing chain of HIV viral DNA instead of the needed DNA nucleoside. The NRTI acts as a nucleoside analog in the DNA production, and its addition is relatively simple. Once this is accomplished, no more DNA nucleosides can be added to the chain, thus terminating its growth and halting the production of viral DNA.

Competitive inhibition occurs when the active (phosphorylated) NRTI competes with the cell's own nucleoside building block. By competing for the cell's building block, these agents also halt the production of viral DNA.

With the exception of abacavir, all NRTIs require elimination by the kidneys and therefore must be dose-adjusted for patients with renal insufficiency. This is an important concept because it helps to minimize the incidence of adverse effects.

The first NRTI that received U.S. Food and Drug Administration (FDA) approval in the United States was zidovudine. It has been studied extensively as a component of ART and has proven to be effective in delaying progression of the disease, reducing the incidence of opportunistic infections, and prolonging survival. Significant adverse effects of zidovudine include bone marrow suppression, which can lead to clinically significant anemia and neutropenia, gastrointestinal (GI) toxicity, fatigue, and lactic acidosis with hepatic steatosis. This has resulted in this agent's classification as an alternative component of a dual NRTI regimen with lamivudine.

Lamivudine is one of the better-tolerated NRTIs and was the second NRTI to receive FDA approval. Because it is effective for treatment of chronic hepatitis B, it should be considered as a component of ART in patients co-infected with HIV and hepatitis B.

Other NRTIs have been available for many years, including didanosine and stavudine. The bioavailability of didanosine is decreased in the presence of gastric acidity. Therefore it is formulated as an enteric-coated capsule or as a solution that is reconstituted with liquid antacid to allow for improved absorption. Dosing of didanosine and stavudine should be based on weight. (See **Table 48.1**.) Both of these NRTIs have

TABLE 48.1 **Overview of Drugs Used to Treat HIV Infection**

Generic (Trade) Name and Adult Dosage in Treatment-Naïve Patients	Selected Adverse Effects	Contraindications	Special Considerations
Nucleoside Reverse Transcriptase Inhibitors			
abacavir (Ziagen) 300 mg PO bid or 600 mg PO daily	Hypersensitivity reaction (fever, rash, malaise, fatigue, nausea, vomiting, respiratory symptoms), possible increased risk of myocardial infarction	Hypersensitivity to any component Moderate to severe hepatic impairment Rechallenge following the hypersensitivity reaction	Take without regard to meals. Hypersensitivity reaction can be fatal (black box warning). Discontinue immediately. Do not rechallenge. Requires HLA-B*5701 screening prior to use. Available in combination with lamivudine (Epzicom) and zidovudine and lamivudine (Trizivir)
didanosine (Videx) ≥60 kg: 400 mg PO daily; with tenofovir, 250 mg PO daily <60 kg: 250 mg PO daily; with tenofovir, 200 mg PO daily	Pancreatitis, peripheral neuropathy, lactic acidosis with hepatic steatosis, noncirrhotic portal hypertension	Concomitant use of allopurinol or ribavirin	Take 30 min before or 2 h after a meal. Dose adjustment is required for renal insufficiency.
emtricitabine (Emtriva) 200 mg PO daily	Skin hyperpigmentation, severe acute exacerbation of hepatitis B in co-infected patients who discontinue treatment	Hypersensitivity to any component	Take without regard to meals. Dose adjustment is required for renal insufficiency. Available in combination with tenofovir (Truvada) and with tenofovir and efavirenz (Atripla)
lamivudine (Epivir) 150 mg PO bid or 300 mg PO daily	Severe acute exacerbation of hepatitis B in co-infected patients who discontinue treatment	Hypersensitivity to any component	Take without regard to meals. Dose adjustment is required for renal insufficiency. Available in combination with zidovudine (Combivir); with abacavir (Epzicom); and with zidovudine and abacavir (Trizivir)
stavudine (Zerit) ≥60 kg: 40 mg PO bid <60 kg: 30 mg PO bid	Peripheral neuropathy, pancreatitis, lactic acidosis with hepatic steatosis, lipoatrophy, hyperlipidemia	Hypersensitivity to any component	Take without regard to meals. Do not use with zidovudine. Dose adjustment is required for renal insufficiency.
tenofovir disoproxil fumarate (Viread) 300 mg PO daily	Nausea, vomiting, diarrhea, headache, asthenia, renal insufficiency, decreased bone mineral density, severe acute exacerbation of hepatitis B in co-infected patients who discontinue treatment	Hypersensitivity to any component	Take without regard to meals. Dose adjustment is required for renal insufficiency. Available in combination with emtricitabine (Truvada) and with emtricitabine and efavirenz (Atripla)
zidovudine (Retrovir) 200 mg PO tid or 300 mg PO bid	Nausea, headache, malaise, bone marrow suppression, lactic acidosis with hepatic steatosis, nail pigmentation	Hypersensitivity to any component	Take without regard to meals. Do not use with ribavirin. Dose adjustment is required for renal insufficiency. Available in combination with lamivudine (Combivir) and with lamivudine and abacavir (Trizivir)
Nonnucleoside Reverse Transcriptase Inhibitors			
delavirdine (Rescriptor) 400 mg PO tid	Headache, rash, elevated liver function tests	Hypersensitivity to any component	Take without regard to meals. Antacids decrease absorption; separate dosing by at least 1 h.

TABLE 48.1   Overview of Drugs Used to Treat HIV Infection (*Continued*)

Generic (Trade) Name and Adult Dosage in Treatment-Naïve Patients	Selected Adverse Effects	Contraindications	Special Considerations
efavirenz (Sustiva) 600 mg PO hs	Central nervous system effects (hallucinations, abnormal dreams, dizziness, impaired concentration, euphoria, confusion), rash, elevated liver function tests, false positive cannabinoid and benzodiazepine screening tests, teratogenic	Hypersensitivity to any component Avoid in pregnancy. Numerous drug interactions; see Table 48.2 for contraindicated combinations.	Take on empty stomach at bedtime. Available in combination with emtricitabine and tenofovir (Atripla)
Protease Inhibitors	Class adverse effects: lipodystrophy, GI intolerance, hepatotoxicity, hyperlipidemia (except unboosted atazanavir), hyperglycemia, increased risk of bleeding in hemophiliacs		
amprenavir (Agenerase) 1,200 mg capsules PO bid	Rash, headache, perioral paresthesia	Hypersensitivity to any component Oral solution contains propylene glycol; avoid use in pregnant women, children <4 y, hepatic or renal failure patients, concomitant use with disulfiram or metronidazole Numerous drug interactions; see Table 48.2 for contraindicated combinations.	Avoid high-fat meals. Dose adjustment is required for hepatic insufficiency
atazanavir (Reyataz) 400 mg PO daily or 300 mg PO daily plus ritonavir 100 mg PO daily	Prolonged PR interval, hyperbilirubinemia, nephrolithiasis	Hypersensitivity to any component Avoid concomitant use with proton pump inhibitors in protease inhibitor–experienced patients. Numerous drug interactions; see Table 48.2 for contraindicated combinations.	Take with food. Must use ritonavir-boosted regimens if using concomitant tenofovir. Use caution when dosing with acid-reducing agents. Dosage adjustment is required in hepatic insufficiency.
darunavir (Prezista) 800 mg PO daily plus ritonavir 100 mg PO daily	Rash, headache	Numerous drug interactions; see Table 48.2 for contraindicated combinations.	Take with food. Must be boosted with ritonavir.
fosamprenavir (Lexiva) 1400 mg PO bid **or** 1,400 mg PO daily plus ritonavir 100–200 mg PO daily **or** 700 mg PO bid plus ritonavir 100 mg PO bid	Rash, headache, nephrolithiasis	Hypersensitivity to any component Numerous drug interactions; see Table 48.2 for contraindicated combinations.	Take without regard to meals. Prodrug of amprenavir Dosage adjustment is required for hepatic insufficiency.
indinavir (Crixivan) 800 mg po q8h or 800 mg PO bid plus ritonavir 100–200 mg PO bid	Nephrolithiasis, hyperbilirubinemia, headache, dizziness, metallic taste, rash	Same as above	Should be taken 1 h before or 2 h after meals when unboosted. Take without regard to meals when boosted with ritonavir. Drink 1.5 L fluid daily to avoid renal stones. Dosage adjustment is required for hepatic insufficiency.

(*continued*)

| TABLE 48.1 | Overview of Drugs Used to Treat HIV Infection (*Continued*) | | |

Generic (Trade) Name and Adult Dosage in Treatment-Naïve Patients	Selected Adverse Effects	Contraindications	Special Considerations
lopinavir/ritonavir (Kaletra) 400/100 mg PO bid or 800/ 200 mg PO daily	Prolonged PR interval or QT interval, asthenia	Same as above	Take with food. Alternative dosing is required in patients taking concomitant efavirenz or nevirapine.
nelfinavir (Viracept) 1,250 mg PO bid or 750 mg PO tid	Diarrhea	Same as above	Take with food.
ritonavir (Norvir) Use only as a booster with other protease inhibitors; 100–400 mg PO daily in 1–2 divided doses	Circumoral and peripheral paresthesias, taste perversion, asthenia	Same as above	Take with food. Numerous drug interactions; check references carefully.
saquinavir (Invirase) 1,000 mg PO bid plus ritonavir 100 mg PO bid	Headache	Same as above, plus severe hepatic impairment	Take with large meal. Must be boosted with ritonavir.
tipranavir (Aptivus) 500 mg PO bid plus ritonavir 100 mg PO bid	Hepatotoxicity (including hepatic decompensation and fatal hepatitis) rash, fatal and nonfatal intracranial hemorrhage	Same as above, plus moderate to severe hepatic impairment	Take without regard to meals. Must be boosted with ritonavir.
Fusion Inhibitors enfuvirtide (Fuzeon) 90 mg subcutaneously bid	Local injection site reactions, increased rate of bacterial pneumonias, hypersensitivity reaction (<1%)	Hypersensitivity to any component	Store reconstituted solution in refrigerator and use within 24 h.
Integrase Inhibitors raltegravir (Isentress) 400 mg PO bid	Nausea, diarrhea, headache, creatine kinase elevation, fever	Hypersensitivity to any component	Take without regard to meals. When dosed with rifampin, administer raltegravir 800 mg PO bid. Use caution with concomitant agents that cause myopathy.
CCR5 Antagonists maraviroc (Selzentry) 150 mg PO bid with strong CYP450 3A inhibitors (including protease inhibitors other than tipranavir/ritonavir); 300 mg PO bid with non-strong CYP450 3A inhibitors or inducers; 600 mg PO bid with CYP450 3A inducers (efavirenz, etravirine)	Hepatotoxicity, cough, dizziness, rash, orthostatic hypotension	Severe renal impairment or end stage renal disease with concomitant use of potent CYP450 3A inhibitors or inducers Numerous drug interactions; see Table 48.2 for contraindicated combinations.	Take without regard to meals.

similar toxicities, including pancreatitis, peripheral neuropathy, and GI disturbances. Didanosine also has been associated with noncirrhotic portal hypertension. Neither of these agents is recommended as preferred or alternative initial treatment for treatment-naïve patients.

Abacavir is an effective component of ART. Patients who initiate treatment with this agent must be cautioned about the hypersensitivity reaction that occurs in 5% to 8% of patients. Symptoms of the hypersensitivity reaction include fever, rash,

GI disturbances, lethargy, and malaise. These can occur at any time after initiating therapy (median, 9 days), although the majority of reactions occur within the first 6 weeks of therapy. Symptoms resolve after discontinuation of the drug but may recur and result in death if abacavir is restarted. The risk of this reaction is correlated with the presence of the HLA-B*5701 allele. As a result, pretreatment screening for this allele should be performed before initiating therapy. Abacavir should not be used in those individuals who test positive for the HLA-B*5701 allele on the screening test, and they should be considered allergic to abacavir. Patients who test negative for the allele should still be counseled about the signs and symptoms of the hypersensitivity reaction. Additionally, there is controversy over an association between abacavir and cardiovascular disease, as some analyses have demonstrated increased risk of myocardial infarction, while others have not. At this time, it is recommended to use caution when considering initiation of abacavir in patients with risk factors for cardiovascular disease.

Tenofovir and emtricitabine are the two newest NRTIs available for use as a part of an ART regimen. Both are well tolerated, dosed once daily, and can be taken without regard to meals. These two NRTIs, which are also available in a coformulated tablet (Truvada), are the preferred dual NRTI combination for treatment-naïve patients, as they are very potent in suppressing viral replication and are superior to zidovudine plus lamivudine in virologic efficacy and adverse effect profile. Also, since both tenofovir and emtricitabine exhibit activity against hepatitis B virus, they are the agents of choice for management of patients who are co-infected with HIV and hepatitis B.

Dual NRTIs are used as part of ART in combination with either a boosted protease inhibitor, an NNRTI, or an integrase inhibitor. Preferred dual NRTIs include tenofovir/emtricitabine, while alternatives include abacavir/lamivudine and zidovudine/lamivudine. Triple-NRTI regimens are less effective than protease inhibitor– or NNRTI-based regimens; therefore, they should not be used in routine clinical practice.

A class adverse effect observed with all NRTIs includes lactic acidosis with hepatic steatosis. Although this adverse effect is rare, it results in a high risk of death. This may be due to mitochondrial dysfunction that occurs on administration of NRTIs. The clinical presentation of lactic acidosis varies greatly among patients but often includes nonspecific GI symptoms (nausea, vomiting, abdominal pain) as well as generalized weakness, myalgias, and paresthesias that can progress to tachycardia, tachypnea, mental status changes, and multiorgan failure. Hepatic steatosis may manifest as an enlarged fatty liver on computed tomography scan as well as increased liver transaminases.

Risk factors for development of this syndrome include female gender, pregnancy, obesity, regimen components (stavudine, didanosine, zidovudine), and prolonged use of NRTIs. If this syndrome develops, the NRTIs should be discontinued immediately, and supportive care should be initiated. Because other clinical interventions such as administration of thiamine, riboflavin, and levocarnitine have not been adequately assessed in clinical trials, their efficacy cannot be determined at this time. Patients taking NRTIs should be cautioned about the signs and symptoms of lactic acidosis, and if these are observed, the patient should notify the practitioner immediately. It is optimal to use NRTIs with less risk of mitochondrial toxicity, such as tenofovir, emtricitabine, lamivudine, or abacavir, instead.

Nonnucleoside Reverse Transcriptase Inhibitors

By binding to reverse transcriptase, NNRTIs also interfere with the conversion of RNA to DNA. The four available NNRTIs are delavirdine (Rescriptor), efavirenz (Sustiva), etravirine (Intelence), and nevirapine (Viramune). Delavirdine is the least potent NNRTI and therefore is not recommended as part of initial ART. Trials have shown that efavirenz-based regimens have similar virologic efficacy as compared with atazanavir-, raltegravir-, and nevirapine-based regimens. Nevirapine has a higher incidence of rash and hepatotoxicity than efavirenz, making it an alternative NNRTI option in treatment-naïve patients. Etravirine has only been studied in treatment-experienced patients, and its use is reserved for this purpose. Thus, the DHHS Panel recommends efavirenz as the preferred agent for NNRTI-based regimens.

The most frequently reported adverse effects of NNRTIs include GI disturbances, rash, and elevations in hepatic transaminases. Efavirenz commonly causes central nervous system adverse effects, including dizziness, impaired concentration, abnormal dreams, and hallucinations. These events occur within the first few days of initiating therapy but resolve over 2 to 4 weeks with continued treatment. Dosing at bedtime is helpful in minimizing these adverse effects. Congenital defects have been observed in offspring of both animals and humans exposed to efavirenz during pregnancy; therefore, this agent must be avoided in pregnant women in their first trimester of pregnancy or those of childbearing potential who are not using consistent and effective contraception.

Nevirapine has been associated with severe, life-threatening hepatotoxicity, including hepatic necrosis and hepatic failure, primarily occurring within the first few weeks of initiation. This may also occur along with a hypersensitivity reaction that includes rash and fever. A black box warning in the nevirapine labeling notes women with CD4+ counts greater than 250 cells/mm^3 and men with CD4+ counts greater than 400 cells/mm^3 have a considerably higher risk of hepatotoxicity. Therefore, all patients who initiate therapy with nevirapine should initiate dosing once daily for 14 days followed by twice daily, and they should receive close monitoring of liver function tests and clinical symptoms throughout the treatment course. If hepatotoxicity occurs, nevirapine should be discontinued permanently.

Etravirine is the newest NNRTI on the market; it demonstrates activity against some HIV viruses that express mutations conferring resistance to the other three NNRTIs. Its adverse effects include nausea, rash, and hypersensitivity reactions associated with organ dysfunction.

All of the NNRTIs are metabolized by the cytochrome P450 (CYP450) 3A4 isoenzyme system in the liver. Each NNRTI also has variable effects on inhibiting or inducing this enzyme system. Therefore, caution should be used when administering NNRTIs with drugs dependent on CYP450 3A4 for metabolism, including protease inhibitors, phenytoin, phenobarbital, and clarithromycin. Concomitant use of rifampin with etravirine is contraindicated because of increased metabolism of etravirine that results in reduced serum concentrations and reduced efficacy. Rifampin may be used with caution with nevirapine. Rifampin must be used with an increased dose of efavirenz (800 mg daily). Concomitant use of St. John's wort is contraindicated with all NNRTIs due to risk of virologic failure secondary to the resulting suboptimal NNRTI concentrations. Additional contraindicated concomitant medications can be found in **Table 48.2**.

Protease Inhibitors

Introduced in the mid-1990s, protease inhibitors (PIs) have demonstrated potent virologic efficacy, durable effects, and high barriers to resistance. They act near the final stage of HIV viral replication through inhibiting the protease-mediated cleavage of the polyproteins. These polyproteins are responsible for creating new HIV RNA copies. Inhibiting this final stage by use of PIs decreases the production of HIV RNA copies.

Ten PIs are available: amprenavir (Agenerase), atazanavir (Reyataz), darunavir (Prezista), fosamprenavir (Lexiva), indinavir (Crixivan), lopinavir/ritonavir (Kaletra), nelfinavir (Viracept), ritonavir (Norvir), saquinavir (Invirase), and tipranavir (Aptivus). These agents vary greatly in terms of their potency, adverse effects, and pharmacokinetic characteristics.

PI-based regimens provide excellent efficacy in virologic suppression. Ritonavir, a potent CYP450 3A4 isoenzyme inhibitor, can be used to increase the concentrations of other PIs, allowing greater exposure of the virus to the PI. These ritonavir "boosted" regimens demonstrate more potent virologic activity while reducing pill burden and adverse effects. However, it is important to note that there is an increased risk of hyperlipidemia as well as drug interactions due to the presence of ritonavir. Despite these risks, boosting regimens with low-dose ritonavir is now the standard of care in PI-based ART regimens.

The pharmacokinetic characteristics of the PIs vary greatly across the class. Food affects the bioavailability of many of the PIs. (See **Table 48.1**.) For example, administration of atazanavir with food increases its bioavailability substantially and therefore should be administered with a meal. In contrast, concentrations of indinavir decrease by 77% with food, resulting in the requirement that this drug be taken on an empty stomach or with a small, low-fat snack (e.g., pretzels) when used without ritonavir booster doses.

The adverse effects of all PIs include GI disturbances, such as nausea, vomiting, and diarrhea, occurring upon treatment initiation. Diarrhea is especially problematic with nelfinavir and some ritonavir-boosted PIs, and it can be managed with over-the-counter antidiarrheals such as loperamide. All PIs can cause increases in levels of hepatic transaminases. Clinical hepatitis and hepatic decompensation are more common in patients receiving regimens containing tipranavir/ritonavir. Risk factors for hepatotoxicity with PIs include hepatitis B or C coinfection, alcohol abuse, underlying liver disease,

TABLE 48.2	Non-Antiretroviral Medications That Are Contraindicated for Concomitant Use with NNRTIs, PIs, or Maraviroc	
Class/Drug	**Contraindicated Medications and/or Classes**	**Comments**
All NNRTIs	St. John's wort	Results in virologic failure
	rifapentine	Results in tuberculosis treatment failure
Efavirenz	cisapride, pimozide, midazolam, triazolam	Results in concomitant medication toxicity
Etravirine	rifampin, carbamazepine, phenytoin, phenobarbital	Results in decreased etravirine concentrations
All PIs	simvastatin, lovastatin	Results in increased risk of rhabdomyolysis
	cisapride, pimozide, midazolam, triazolam, ergot alkaloids, alfuzosin, salmeterol, fluticasone, sildenafil (when used for pulmonary arterial hypertension)	Results in concomitant medication toxicity
	rifampin	Results in virologic failure
	rifapentine	Results in tuberculosis treatment failure
	St. John's wort	Results in virologic failure
Atazanavir	proton pump inhibitors	When used with unboosted atazanavir, results in decreased atazanavir concentrations
	irinotecan	Results in concomitant medication toxicity
Darunavir	carbamazepine phenytoin, phenobarbital	Results in concomitant medication toxicity
		Results in decreased concentrations of phenytoin and phenobarbital
Fosamprenavir	oral contraceptives	Results in oral contraceptive failure
Saquinavir	garlic supplements	May result in virologic failure
Maraviroc	rifapentine	Results in tuberculosis treatment failure
	St. John's wort	Results in virologic failure

and concomitant use of hepatotoxic agents. This should be monitored carefully.

A class effect of the PIs includes fat maldistribution, also known as *lipodystrophy*. This results in accumulation of fat in the abdomen, breasts, and dorsocervical fat pad ("buffalo hump"). This occurs in a large percentage of patients receiving ART, depending upon the regimen used and the duration of treatment. Fat maldistribution may be accompanied by metabolic abnormalities such as hyperlipidemia and hyperglycemia. Management of lipodystrophy includes use of diet and exercise as well as administration of tesamorelin, a growth hormone releasing factor. Improvements have been demonstrated in clinical trials of patients changed from lopinavir/ritonavir to atazanavir.

All of the PIs, with the exception of unboosted atazanavir, have been associated with hyperlipidemia, including increased levels of triglycerides, total serum cholesterol, and low-density lipoproteins. Lopinavir/ritonavir and fosamprenavir/ritonavir cause a substantial increase in triglycerides when compared to atazanavir/ritonavir or darunavir/ritonavir. These lipid abnormalities may be associated with accelerated coronary artery disease in HIV patients. Management includes dietary modifications, exercise, smoking cessation, and changing to agents with a lower likelihood of lipid abnormalities, as well as the addition of lipid-lowering treatments, such as 3-hydroxy-3-methylglutaryl-coenzyme A (HMG-CoA) reductase inhibitors (statins). However, it is important to note that most statins cause drug interactions with the PIs, and some are contraindicated (**Table 48.2**). Therefore, pravastatin is the preferred agent because it does not have as many interaction concerns.

Another class effect of PIs includes hyperglycemia, which may lead to new-onset diabetes mellitus as a result of insulin resistance in approximately 3% to 5% of patients. Patients should be cautioned about warning signs of hyperglycemia, including polydipsia, polyphagia, and polyuria. Management of hyperglycemia includes lifestyle modifications (diet and exercise), consideration of NNRTI use as an alternative, and pharmacologic management according to the American Diabetes Association.

Based upon virologic efficacy and durability data, dosing convenience and low pill burden, and good tolerability, the guidelines published by the Panel on Antiretroviral Guidelines (2011) list atazanavir/ritonavir and darunavir/ritonavir as the preferred components of a PI-based regimen (**Table 48.3**). Atazanavir/ritonavir has fewer adverse effects on lipids when compared to other PI-based regimens. Its primary adverse effect is hyperbilirubinemia with or without jaundice or icteric sclerae. Since it requires an acidic GI environment for dissolution, acid-reducing agents such as antacids, histamine$_2$ receptor antagonists, and proton pump inhibitors may inhibit the absorption of atazanavir, requiring staggered dosing and limitations on the use of these agents. Clinical trials comparing darunavir/ritonavir to lopinavir/ritonavir demonstrated superior virologic efficacy with darunavir/ritonavir after 96 weeks of treatment. Darunavir contains a sulfa moiety and therefore can cause a rash.

TABLE 48.3	**Recommended Regimens for Treatment of HIV Infection in Treatment-Naïve Patients**
NNRTI-Based Regimens	
Preferred regimen:	efavirenz* + tenofovir + emtricitabine^
Alternative regimens:	efavirenz* + (abacavir or zidovudine) + lamivudine^
	nevirapine# + zidovudine + lamivudine^
PI-Based Regimens	
Preferred regimen:	atazanavir/ritonavir + tenofovir + emtricitabine^
	darunavir/ritonavir tenofovir + emtricitabine^
Alternative regimens:	atazanavir/ritonavir + (abacavir or zidovudine) + lamivudine^
	fosamprenavir/ritonavir + either [(abacavir or zidovudine) + lamivudine^] or [tenofovir + emtricitabine^]
	lopinavir/ritonavir + either [(abacavir or zidovudine) + lamivudine^] or [tenofovir + emtricitabine^]
Integrase Inhibitor–Based Regimen	
Preferred regimen:	raltegravir + tenofovir + emtricitabine^
Regimen for Pregnant Patients	
Preferred regimen:	Lopinavir/ritonavir (twice daily) + zidovudine + lamivudine^

*Cannot be used in first trimester of pregnancy or in those women not using consistent and effective contraception who may become pregnant.
^May substitute lamivudine for emtricitabine or vice versa.
#Should not be used in women with pre-ART CD4+ T cell count > 250 or men with pre-ART CD4+ T cell count > 400.
Panel on Antiretroviral Guidelines for Adults and Adolescents. (2011). *Guidelines for use of antiretroviral agents in HIV-1-infected adults and adolescents. Department of Health and Human Services* [On-line]. Available: http://www.aidsinfo. nih.gov/ContentFiles/AdultandAdolescentGL.pdf.

All PIs are metabolized by the CYP450 3A4 isoenzyme system in the liver. Each of the PIs has a different effect on inducing or inhibiting the efficiency of this isoenzyme system. Therefore, caution must be used when combining PIs with any medications that are metabolized by CYP450 3A4 or that induce or inhibit this system. Concurrent use of PIs with ergot alkaloids, simvastatin, lovastatin, rifampin, and St. John's wort is contraindicated. A summary of these contraindicated medications is provided in **Table 48.2**.

Fusion Inhibitors

Enfuvirtide (Fuzeon) is the only available agent in this class of antiretroviral drugs. It inhibits fusion of the virus to the cell membrane of the CD4+ T cell, thereby preventing HIV from entering the cell. Because its mechanism of action is distinct from the intracellular agents previously discussed, it may be useful for highly treatment-experienced patients with the virus that is resistant to other currently available antiretroviral agents.

Enfuvirtide must be injected subcutaneously twice daily. Adverse effects include local injection site reactions, such as erythema, induration, and pain, which occur in almost all patients. Less than 1% of patients experience hypersensitivity reactions, including rash and fever. Enfuvirtide significantly increases tipranavir/ritonavir concentrations, resulting in an increased risk of adverse effects.

Integrase Inhibitors

Raltegravir is the first and only integrase inhibitor that is available for use in the management of HIV infection. It prevents integration of viral DNA into the host cell's genome. Initially, it was only approved for use in treatment-experienced patients with multiple resistance mutations. Currently, it is also approved for use in treatment-naïve patients, as it has demonstrated comparable efficacy and safety to efavirenz-based regimens. As a result, the guidelines published by the Panel (2011) recommend raltegravir in combination with tenofovir and emtricitabine (or lamivudine) as a preferred regimen in the treatment-naïve population.

Raltegravir is metabolized via UGT1A1-mediated glucuronidation and therefore exhibits minimal drug–drug interaction risk. This agent can cause elevations in creatine kinase and should be used with caution in patients receiving concomitant medications that have similar adverse effects.

CCR5 Antagonists

Maraviroc is the only available agent in this class of antiretrovirals. It blocks the CCR5 receptor on the membrane of CD4+ T cells, preventing entry of the HIV virus. Prior to use, a coreceptor tropism assay (e.g., Trofile) must be performed to determine if the patient's virus utilizes the CCR5 receptor, since not all HIV strains do. Maraviroc has a black box warning in its package insert describing hepatotoxicity that may be preceded by a systemic allergic reaction. This agent may also cause cough, orthostatic hypotension, rash, and fever. It also has a multitude of drug–drug interactions associated with its use, requiring dose adjustment (**Table 48.1**). At this time, the Panel (2011) recommends maraviroc-based regimens as acceptable for treatment-naïve patients.

Selecting the Most Appropriate Regimen

Although guidelines exist for the combinations of agents to be used in antiretroviral therapy, each patient must have a highly individualized regimen. Although current regimens are effective at keeping the viral load at undetectable levels, eradication of the virus is not yet attainable. This is due to the early development of latently infected CD4+ T cells with a long half-life that, even with prolonged therapy, persist.

Previously Untreated Patients

One of the most important therapeutic interventions in the care of the patient with HIV infection is the initial treatment regimen (**Tables 48.1** and **48.3**). It is essential to select the most potent and appropriate therapy possible, keeping in mind adverse effects and adherence issues. Discontinuing pre-

ferred therapy due to nonadherence increases the risk of drug resistance and failure with alternate regimens.

"Preferred regimens" have been selected by the DHHS Panel based on optimal efficacy and durability demonstrated in clinical trials as well as tolerability and convenience of use. "Alternative regimens" demonstrate efficacy but have disadvantages in terms of virologic activity, durability of effect, tolerance, and pill burden. An alternative regimen may actually be preferred in some patients, depending on the individual situation. "Acceptable regimens" have either less virologic activity, less supportive data from clinical trials, or increased risk of toxicities compared to the preferred and alternative options.

There are three main regimens recommended for treatment-naïve patients: NNRTI-based, PI-based, and integrase inhibitor–based regimens (**Table 48.3**). The preferred NNRTI-based regimen is efavirenz plus tenofovir plus emtricitabine; it is potent and convenient with a low pill burden (available co-formulated as Atripla, dosed as 1 tablet daily at bedtime) but cannot be used in pregnant patients due to concerns of teratogenicity. Nevirapine can be used as an alternative for pregnant patients or in women who wish to conceive. Both have many drug interactions due to their effects on the CYP450 system, and they have a low genetic barrier to resistance, in that one mutation confers resistance by the virus. These regimens demonstrate far less lipodystrophy and dyslipidemia than PI-based regimens, and they allow the PIs and raltegravir to be spared for future use in the event of resistance development.

PI-based regimens contain a PI with a booster dose of ritonavir in combination with two NRTIs. These combinations have proven to be effective in numerous clinical trials. Preferred PI-based regimens include atazanavir/ritonavir or darunavir/ritonavir in combination with tenofovir/emtricitabine due to their virologic potency, tolerability profile, and low pill burden. Alternative PI options include fosamprenavir with or without ritonavir and lopinavir/ritonavir. The PI class has a higher genetic barrier to resistance than NNRTIs. All of the PI-based regimens are associated with metabolic complications, including lipodystrophy, dyslipidemia, hyperglycemia, and hepatotoxicity as well as numerous drug–drug interactions (**Table 48.2**).

The integrase inhibitor–based regimen of raltegravir plus tenofovir and emtricitabine is also a preferred initial regimen in treatment-naïve patients. Its advantages include comparable virologic efficacy to efavirenz with fewer adverse effects and lipid abnormalities. It also has far fewer drug interactions than PI- or NNRTI-based regimens. Its disadvantages include fewer data on long-term use, a lower genetic resistance barrier than boosted PIs, and twice daily dosing.

Treatment-Experienced Patients

When antiretroviral treatment failure occurs, it is necessary to assess why this occurred to determine the appropriate therapy change. Antiretroviral treatment failure is a term that encompasses all potential reasons for suboptimal response to therapy that must be assessed, including incomplete medication adherence, drug toxicities, suboptimal pharmacokinetic issues, resistance, and suboptimal ART potency (Panel on Antiretroviral Guidelines, 2011). Treatment regimen failure often results in virologic, immunologic, and/or clinical failure. *Virologic failure* is defined as the failure to achieve nondetectable HIV RNA plasma levels within 48 weeks of initiating therapy or a rebound in viral load after prior virologic suppression. *Immunologic failure* results when CD4+ T-cell counts do not increase to more than 350 to 500 cells/mm^3 while on therapy or if there is a failure to increase by 50 to 100 cells/mm^3 above baseline. *Clinical progression* results if an HIV-related event occurs or recurs after receiving at least 3 months of ART. These three responses may occur independently of each other or simultaneously.

After the practitioner considers the causes and types of treatment failure, the drug regimen should be changed accordingly. The patient's previous treatment experience and current drug resistance pattern must be considered because there may be cross-resistance between agents within the same therapeutic class. In addition, if an adverse effect or unacceptable toxicity caused a cessation of therapy, the practitioner should avoid alternative agents likely to cause that adverse effect. Furthermore, agents with complicated dosing schedules and strict diet and fluid requirements should be avoided if that is what caused the first treatment failure. Selecting agents that are free of side effects and strict dosing, diet, and fluid requirements is not easy, but each patient must be given the regimen to which he or she will most likely adhere.

When changing therapy, one or more of the agents in the regimen may need to be replaced. This will vary depending on the individual patient's situation. Expert advice from an HIV clinician is crucial to selecting the most appropriate option.

Special Population Considerations

Pediatric

Guidelines exist for treating HIV infection in the pediatric patient (Working Group on Antiretroviral Therapy and Medical Management of HIV-Infected Children, 2010). Although the principles remain the same in all HIV-infected individuals, unique considerations in subsets of the pediatric population need brief discussion. These include diagnosis of disease, differences in CD4+ T-cell counts and viral loads, changes in pharmacokinetic parameters, and adherence issues.

Diagnostic testing on suspected HIV-infected infants can be performed as early as at birth and by age 4 months in almost all infants. Testing in suspected infants should occur by 48 hours of life because in nearly 30% to 40% of infected infants the diagnosis can be made within this time frame. If the initial test is negative, repeat testing should be performed at age 1 to 2 months and age 4 to 6 months. HIV DNA polymerase chain reaction or RNA assays are the preferred virologic methods for diagnosing HIV in infants. Antibody testing is not accurate due to the transfer of maternal HIV antibodies to the infant.

The CD4+ T-cell counts in children younger than age 5 are typically higher than adult counts. Therefore, monitoring absolute CD4+ counts may not be as reliable as measuring the percentage change in CD4+ counts as disease progresses. Pediatric patients with a positive virologic test should have CD4+ T-cell counts and viral loads monitored every 3 to 4 months or more frequently in infants less than age 6 months; in children with clinical, immunologic, or virologic failure; and in those initiating or changing ART. Similarly, because of immunologic differences, particularly in those patients acquiring the disease perinatally, viral loads may be difficult to interpret during the first year of life. Using CD4+ T-cell count and viral load together can more accurately predict prognosis and survival.

Pharmacokinetic variables, particularly volume of distribution and clearance, change as a person ages. These changes should be considered when designing drug therapy regimens for children. Similarly, the issue of medication adherence in this population is crucial. Some of the solution formulations for these agents may be unpalatable, depending on the child's preferences. Also, absorption of drugs can be affected by food, and timing of drug administration around food schedules can be extremely difficult. Mixing medications in bottles with formula may increase palatability but may create compatibility issues. Additionally, children depend upon their caregivers to administer ART; therefore, the complexity and convenience of the regimen must be considered. It is preferable for an HIV expert to manage these patients in order to select optimal treatment and monitor short- and long-term adverse effects and quality of life.

Women/Pregnancy

Thresholds for initiation of ART in HIV-infected women are the same as those for HIV-infected men. Selection of antiretrovirals in women of childbearing potential should reflect regimen efficacy as well as its potential for teratogenicity if the woman becomes pregnant. For example, efavirenz should be avoided in women considering pregnancy or who are not using reliable contraception. It is also important to note that the efficacy of many oral contraceptives is reduced by ART.

When considering the use of ART in pregnant women with HIV infection, practitioners must consider two main issues: antiretroviral therapy of HIV in the mother and prophylaxis to reduce the risk of perinatal HIV infection (Panel on Treatment of HIV-Infected Pregnant Women and Prevention of Perinatal Transmission, 2010). The benefits and risks of using antiretroviral therapy must be assessed prior to initiating therapy in a pregnant patient as well as special considerations for medication counseling.

The acquisition of disease through exposure in utero is a major source of HIV infection in infants. Therefore, early identification of HIV-infected women is crucial before or during pregnancy. Preconception HIV prevention counseling and testing for all pregnant women have been advocated by national organizations, including the American College of Obstetricians and Gynecologists and the CDC.

One of the more remarkable aspects of zidovudine therapy was the discovery that this agent reduced the maternal–fetal transmission of HIV. The pivotal study by Connor and colleagues showed a maternal–fetal transmission rate of 8.3% with zidovudine versus 25.5% with placebo in expectant mothers between 14 and 34 weeks of gestation (Connor, et al., 1994). Therefore, antiretroviral chemoprophylaxis antepartum and intrapartum is recommended for all pregnant women as well as postnatally in the infant in an effort to reduce perinatal transmission. Additionally, breast-feeding is not recommended for any HIV-positive woman in the United States, regardless of ART regimen.

Health Care Workers/Occupational Exposure

The primary means of transmission of HIV in the health care worker population is through an accidental needle stick. However, transmission can occur through exposure of HIV-infected blood or other infected body fluids to a health care worker's non-intact skin or mucous membranes. The risk of HIV transmission after a percutaneous exposure to infected blood is approximately 0.3%; the risk decreases to approximately 0.09% for a mucous membrane exposure.

In theory, initiation of antiretroviral postexposure prophylaxis (PEP) within hours after exposure may prevent or inhibit systemic infection by limiting the replication of virus in the lymphocytes and lymph nodes. As such, the CDC has published recommendations regarding the initiation and continuation of PEP in health care personnel (CDC, 2005). The primary role of PEP is to prevent HIV infection after an accidental occupational exposure.

Current guidelines suggest a two- or three-drug approach to PEP, depending upon the type of exposure and infection status of the source. The basic two-drug approach consists of two NRTIs including zidovudine plus either lamivudine or emtricitabine or tenofovir plus either lamivudine or emtricitabine. These basic regimens are used for the majority of occupational exposures, and the specific choice is based upon adverse effects and dosing convenience. An expanded,

three-drug regimen is used for an exposure with an increased risk of transmission or suspected resistance. These regimens include the two drugs used in the basic regimen plus one of the following PIs: lopinavir/ritonavir (preferred), atazanavir, fosamprenavir, indinavir/ritonavir, saquinavir/ritonavir, or nelfinavir (acceptable). PEP should be initiated within hours after exposure, and a regimen should be started while awaiting results of source identification, resistance profile, or both. Therapy should be continued for 4 weeks, and HIV antibody testing should be performed at baseline, 6 weeks, 12 weeks, and 6 months after exposure. **Tables 48.4** and **48.5** outline the current recommendations for PEP (CDC, 2005).

MONITORING PATIENT RESPONSE

The CD4+ T-cell counts are important not only because they indicate the risk of development of opportunistic infections, but also because they help the health care provider initiate therapy or evaluate the effectiveness of current therapy. If CD4+ counts decline, a change in therapy may be warranted. Therefore, it is important to measure CD4+ counts at diagnosis and recheck them every 3 to 6 months in order to determine when ART should be started, to assess response to ART, and to determine the necessity of opportunistic infection prophylaxis. CD4+ counts may be obtained every 6 to 12 months in those individuals who are receiving suppressive ART and have CD4+ counts well above the threshold for risk of opportunistic infections. More frequent monitoring would be required in patients with changes in clinical status or in those initiating treatment with interferon, steroids, or cancer chemotherapeutic agents.

Viral load should be measured at baseline for all patients. Once therapy has been initiated or changed, viral load should

TABLE 48.4	Recommended HIV PEP for Percutaneous Injuries				
Exposure Type	HIV-Positive Class 1*	HIV-Positive Class 2†	Unknown HIV Statusª	Unknown Source‡	HIV-Negative
Less severe (solid needle or superficial injury)	Recommend basic 2-drug PEP	Recommend expanded ≥3-drug PEP	No PEP warranted; may consider basic 2-drug PEP for source with HIV risk factors	No PEP warranted; may consider basic 2-drug PEP in settings with likely exposure to HIV-infected patients	No PEP warranted
More severe (hollow needle, deep puncture, visible blood on needle)	Recommend expanded 3-drug PEP	Recommend expanded ≥3-drug PEP	No PEP warranted; may consider basic 2-drug PEP for source with HIV risk factors	No PEP warranted; may consider basic 2-drug PEP in settings with likely exposure to HIV-infected patients	No PEP warranted

*HIV-positive class 1: asymptomatic HIV or viral load <1,500 copies/mL
†HIV-positive class 2: symptomatic HIV, AIDS, acute seroconversion, or viral load >1,500 copies/mL
ªUnknown HIV status: e.g., a deceased source person without a sample that can be HIV tested
‡Unknown source: e.g., a discarded needle from a sharps disposal container
Adapted from Centers for Disease Control and Prevention (2005). Updated U.S. public health service guidelines for the management of occupational exposures to HIV and recommendations for postexposure prophylaxis. *Morbidity and Mortality Weekly Report, 54* (RR-9), 3.

TABLE 48.5	Recommended HIV PEP for Mucous Membrane Exposures and Nonintact Skin Exposures				
Exposure Type	**HIV-Positive Class 1***	**HIV-Positive Class 2†**	**Unknown HIV Status[a]**	**Unknown Source‡**	**HIV Negative**
Small volume (few drops)	Consider basic 2-drug PEP	Recommend basic 2-drug PEP	No PEP warranted	No PEP warranted	No PEP warranted
Large volume (splash)	Recommend basic 2-drug PEP	Recommend expanded ≥3-drug PEP	No PEP warranted; may consider basic 2-drug PEP for source with HIV risk factors	No PEP warranted; may consider basic 2-drug PEP in settings with likely exposure to HIV-infected patients	No PEP warranted

*HIV-positive class 1: asymptomatic HIV or viral load <1,500 copies/mL
†HIV-positive class 2: symptomatic HIV, AIDS, acute seroconversion, or viral load >1,500 copies/mL
[a]Unknown HIV status: e.g., a deceased source person without a sample that can be HIV tested
‡Unknown source: e.g., a splash from blood disposed inappropriately
Adapted from Centers for Disease Control and Prevention (2005). Updated U.S. public health service guidelines for the management of occupational exposures to HIV and recommendations for postexposure prophylaxis. *Morbidity and Mortality Weekly Report, 54* (RR-9), 3.

be assessed immediately at that time and again 2 to 8 weeks later. The viral load should be repeated every 4 to 8 weeks until it becomes undetectable. Subsequent testing should reveal an undetectable viral load by 12 to 24 weeks in those patients adherent to ART. At that point, viral load testing should be repeated every 3 to 4 months to determine continuing effectiveness of the regimen. This duration can be extended to 6 months in those patients who are stable and have fully suppressed viral loads for at least 2 years. If a patient exhibits a suboptimal response, it is important to review medication adherence, drug interactions, and resistance mutations to permit consideration of regimen changes.

Genotypic resistance testing is recommended for all patients at baseline, regardless of when treatment is initiated, in order to optimize regimen selection by determining which drugs still retain activity. It is also useful for patients with suboptimal viral load reduction and virologic failure. Resistance testing is not recommended for patients with viral loads of fewer than 500 copies/mL because the assays cannot consistently determine resistance patterns with such low level viremia. Recommendations for genotypic resistance testing in pregnant patients include baseline testing prior to therapy as well as testing those with detectable viral loads while taking ART.

PATIENT EDUCATION

To minimize the likelihood of treatment regimen failure and development of drug resistance, the health care professional must be aware of who is at high risk for adherence issues as well as the most common reasons for poor adherence. Risk factors for poor adherence to antiretroviral regimens include active substance abuse, active mental illness, lack of disease and medication education, low levels of literacy, and stigma. Several treatment factors affect adherence, such as pill burden,

frequency of dosing, food requirements, adverse effects, and treatment fatigue.

Strategies the practitioner can use to minimize the risk of failure due to nonadherence include encouraging the patient to develop a strong relationship with the health care team, taking an active role in his or her therapy, and involving the patient's family, friends, and peers in the therapy. In addition, counseling on HIV and the consequences of poor adherence may encourage an otherwise indifferent patient to adhere to a regimen.

Another strategy the practitioner should use to promote drug adherence is preparing the patient for adverse events. The patient needs to know which adverse events are likely to occur, how to minimize the risk of experiencing adverse events, and which adverse events demand discontinuation of therapy. The patient also needs to understand the importance of following the dosing schedule in addition to the food requirements for each agent (Panel, 2011). **Table 48.1** provides information on dosing, diet, and fluid requirements of each agent.

Developing a plan for scheduling medications and carefully explaining to the patient how each medication should be taken is imperative. This plan should focus on daily pill taking as well as future events in a patient's life that threaten to interrupt the established schedule (e.g., holidays or vacations). This plan must consider lifestyle factors such as work schedule and privacy issues (e.g., taking medication at work or storage of medication at work). Regardless of how much or little assistance the patient needs in developing strategies for ensuring adherence, success is often determined by the patient's outlook. If the patient perceives that therapy will lead to an improved quality of life or increased length of life, chances for adherence are greater (Reynolds, 1998). Therefore, before attacking the logistics of a medication schedule, the health care provider must convince the patient of the benefits of continuing therapy.

Once the daily plan is developed, it should evolve into a long-term plan that allows the patient to adhere to therapy and allows the health care provider to monitor adherence. Aids for adherence include pill boxes that separate doses per day, alarms to remind patients of their doses, or something as simple as a calendar that lists dosing schedules. Whatever method is used, the patient must remain adherent and be checked for adherence. The simplest way to check for adherence is to ask the patient. However, a patient may not confess to missed doses or may not be aware of missed doses. Pill counting is another option, but patients may remove missed doses to appear adherent. Testing the viral load may reveal adherence information, but if levels increase because of resistance, not nonadherence, the results will be misleading.

Case Study

A. P. is a 36-year-old woman who was diagnosed with HIV infection 2 years ago. She has been feeling well for the past 2 years, and she maintains a healthy, active lifestyle by exercising three to four times a week and eating a balanced diet. Her medications include a multiple vitamin and occasional omeprazole for heartburn. She has never received antiretroviral therapy. She comes to your office for a routine physical exam and blood work. The physical examination is unremarkable, and the laboratory results are as follows:

Electrolytes, serum creatinine, liver function tests: within normal limits

Complete blood count with differential: within normal limits

CD4+ T-cell count: 210 cells/mm^3

Viral load: 10,000 copies/mL

Genotype: No resistance mutations detected

DIAGNOSIS: ASYMPTOMATIC HIV INFECTION

1. List specific goals for treatment for this patient.
2. What drug therapy would you prescribe? Why?
3. What are the parameters for monitoring success of the therapy?
4. Discuss specific patient education based on the prescribed therapy.
5. List one or two adverse reactions for the selected agents that would cause you to change therapy.
6. What would be the choice for the second-line therapy?
7. What dietary and lifestyle changes should be recommended for this patient?
8. Describe one or two drug–drug or drug–food interactions for the selected agents.

BIBLIOGRAPHY

*Starred references are cited in the text.

Anonymous. (2009). Drugs for HIV infection. *Treatment Guidelines from the Medical Letter, 7*(78), 11–22.

*Centers for Disease Control and Prevention. (1992). 1993 revised classification system for HIV infection and expanded surveillance case definition for AIDS among adolescents and adults. *Morbidity and Mortality Weekly Report, 41*(RR-17), 1–19.

*Centers for Disease Control and Prevention. (2005). Updated U.S. public health service guidelines for the management of occupational exposures to HIV and recommendations for postexposure prophylaxis. *Morbidity and Mortality Weekly Report, 54*(RR-9), 1–17.

*Centers for Disease Control and Prevention. (2010). *HIV in the United States: An Overview. June 2010.* [On-line]. Available: http://www.cdc.gov/hiv/topics/surveillance/resources/factsheets/pdf/us_overview.pdf.

*Connor, E. M., Sperling, R. S., Gelber, R., et al. (1994). Reduction of maternal-infant transmission of human immunodeficiency virus type 1 with zidovudine treatment. Pediatric AIDS Clinical Trials Group Protocol 076 Study Group. *New England Journal of Medicine, 331,* 1173–1180.

Elsayed, R. K., & Cladwell, D. J. (2010). Etravirine: A novel nonnucleoside reverse transcriptase inhibitor for managing human immunodeficiency virus infection. *American Journal of Health-System Pharmacy, 67,* 193–205.

Lacy, C. F., Armstrong, L. L., Goldman, M. P., & Lance L.L. (2010). *Drug information handbook* (19th ed.). Hudson, OH: Lexi-Comp.

*Panel on Antiretroviral Guidelines for Adults and Adolescents. (2011). *Guidelines for use of antiretroviral agents in HIV-1-infected adults and adolescents. Department of Health and Human Services* [On-line]. Available: http://www.aidsinfo.nih.gov/ContentFiles/AdultandAdolescentGL.pdf.

*Panel on Treatment of HIV-Infected Pregnant Women and Prevention of Perinatal Transmission. (2010). *Recommendations for use of antiretroviral drugs in pregnant HIV-1-infected women for maternal health and interventions to reduce perinatal HIV transmission in the United States.* [On-line]. Available: http://www.aidsinfo.nih.gov/ContentFiles/PerinatalGL.pdf.

*Reynolds, N. R. (1998). Initiatives to get HIV-infected patients to adhere to their treatment regimens. *Drug Benefit, 10*(11), 23–25, 29–30, 32.

Schafer, J. J., & Squires, K. E. (2010). Integrase inhibitors: A novel class of antiretroviral agents. *The Annals of Pharmacotherapy, 44,* 145–156.

Spooner, L. M., & Olin, J. L. (2007). Upcoming therapies for HIV infection. *U.S. Pharmacist, 32,* HS14–HS23.

Thompson, M. A., Aberg, J. A., Cahn, P., et al. (2010). Antiretroviral treatment of adult HIV infection: 2010 recommendations of the international AIDS Society USA Panel. *Journal of the American Medical Association, 304,* 321–333.

*World Health Organization (WHO). (2009). *Towards universal access. Scaling up priority HIV/AIDS interventions in the health sector. Progress report September 2009.* [On-line]. Available: http://www.who.int/hiv/pub/2009progressreport/en/.

*Working Group on Antiretroviral Therapy and Medical Management of HIV-Infected Children. (2010). *Guidelines for the use of antiretroviral agents in pediatric HIV infection.* [On-line]. Available: http://www.aidsinfo.nih.gov/contentfiles/PediatricGuidelines.pdf.

UNIT 12

Pharmacotherapy for Hematologic Disorders

CHAPTER 49

Angela A. Allerman
Ellen Boxer Goldfarb

Anticoagulation Disturbances

VENOUS THROMBOEMBOLIC DISEASE STATES AND ANTITHROMBOTIC THERAPY

Thromboembolic disease and patients with risk factors for thromboemboli are frequently encountered in the ambulatory population, and an understanding of the pathogenesis of these conditions and underlying patient risk factors, along with the clotting cascade, is essential for determining appropriate treatment. The indications for anticoagulation continue to expand, and treatment for some conditions has now shifted to the outpatient setting. Several disorders warrant anticoagulant therapy, including venous thromboembolism (VTE), atrial fibrillation, ischemic stroke, prosthetic cardiac valves, coronary and peripheral vascular disease, and hypercoagulable conditions. Recognizing when prophylaxis for clotting events is appropriate is also important, including during orthopedic surgery or periods of prolonged immobility. An increased awareness of thromboembolic disease has been prompted by regulatory agencies focusing on patient safety. The mainstays of therapy include anticoagulants, which prevent clot extension and formation; antiplatelet agents, which interfere with platelet activity; and thrombolytic agents, which dissolve existing thrombi. Several investigational anticoagulants nearing Food and Drug Administration (FDA) approval are likely to challenge the role of traditional therapies. For all patients requiring anticoagulation, balancing the benefits of treatment versus bleeding risk is essential when choosing the most appropriate therapy. Anticoagulants and antiplatelet drugs are discussed in this chapter, whereas thrombolytics and anticoagulants, whose use is confined to the inpatient setting, are not. Coronary and peripheral arterial diseases are not discussed here, but they are included in the chapters discussing atherosclerotic conditions of hyperlipidemia and angina.

DISORDERS REQUIRING ANTICOAGULATION AND THEIR CAUSES

Venous Thromboembolism

VTE is a thromboembolic event occurring in the venous system, and it is manifested as either deep vein thrombosis (DVT) or pulmonary embolism (PE). VTE contributes significantly to patient morbidity and mortality and is considered a major public health concern (U.S. Department of Health and Human Services, 2008). Venous thrombus formation occurs in the setting of venous stasis (sluggish blood flow), vascular endothelial wall injury, and hypercoagulability (propensity for increased blood clotting); these three features are classically referred to as *Virchow's triad* (Merli, 2008).

The components of Virchow's triad can assist with categorizing the most common causes and risk factors for VTE. Venous stasis, which results in pooling of blood in the lower extremity veins, is precipitated by prolonged immobility occurring during hospitalization, surgery, spinal cord injury, or paralyzing stroke; in conditions that increase venous pressure, including varicose veins or venous insufficiency from the postthrombotic syndrome; or less frequently, in obesity or pregnancy. Vascular intimal injury is often related to recent surgery, especially abdominal and orthopedic surgery, recent trauma or fracture to the pelvis or lower extremities, childbirth, and previous venous thrombosis. Imbalances between the body's regulatory mechanisms of procoagulant and anticoagulant proteins can result in hypercoagulable conditions. Hypercoagulability may be present secondary to inherited abnormalities of coagulation (thrombophilia), malignancy, oral contraceptive use, and estrogen therapy (Merli, 2008). In addition, central venous catheters and age older than 40 years also increase the risk of venous thromboembolic disease (Ortel, 2010). Risk factors for VTE should be identified and corrected, if possible (Heit, 2006). See **Box 49.1** for more information on predisposing risk factors for VTE.

In DVT, the characteristic symptom of lower extremity swelling is due to the thrombus partially or completely occluding the vein. Proximal DVT develops in the popliteal, femoral, or iliac veins above the knee, while calf vein DVT is isolated below the knee. Calf vein DVT may extend proximally in 40% to 50% of patients.

The major complication of proximal DVT is thrombus dislodgment and extension into the pulmonary circulation. PE is a life-threatening emergency, with an associated mortality rate of 25%. Lower extremity DVTs are the source of 90% of PEs (Piazza & Goldhaber, 2006). Distal DVT isolated to the calf veins has a lower risk of long-term complications. In hospitalized patients, proximal DVT accounts for 80% of cases, with distal DVT comprising 20% (Righini & Bounameaux, 2008).

Reversible

Trauma,[§] surgery,[*] pregnancy, estrogen therapy,[±] chemotherapy, prolonged or transient immobility, fractures, central venous catheters, obesity, long-haul air travel[~]

Acquired

Increasing age >40 y, malignancy,[†] previous venous thromboembolism, hematologic disease, heart failure, paralytic stroke, inflammatory bowel disease, nephrotic syndrome, spinal cord injury, varicose veins, antiphospholipid antibodies, lupus anticoagulant[~]

Inherited Disorders

Activated protein C resistance, antithrombin III deficiency, protein C deficiency, protein S deficiency, anticardiolipin antibodies,[‡] factor V Leiden, prothrombin gene mutation

---

[*]Especially orthopedic, gynecologic, neurosurgical, or urologic procedures
[§]Especially major or lower-extremity injury
[±]Oral contraceptives or hormone replacement therapy
[†]Especially of the lung, breast, or viscera
[‡]May also be acquired
[~]Considered weak factor
Data from Geerts, W. H., Bergqvist, D., Pineo, G. F., et al. (2008). Prevention of venous thromboembolism: American College of Chest Physicians Evidence-Based Clinical Practice Guidelines (8th Edition). *Chest, 133*(6 Suppl.), 381S–453S; and Osinbowale, O., Ali, L., & Chi, Y. W. (2010). Venous thromboembolism: A clinical review. *Postgraduate Medicine, 122*(2), 54–65.

Nearly 50% of patients experiencing DVT develop chronic venous insufficiency or postphlebitic (postthrombotic) syndrome. The acute thrombus and accompanying inflammation lead to valvular incompetence and venous stasis, with resultant chronic lower extremity edema, ulceration, and chronic pain (Vazquez, et al., 2009). These symptoms are frequently debilitating to the patient's quality of life. The lower extremities should be assessed for edema, skin pigmentation changes, spider veins, varicosities, and scarring from previous ulcers to assist with recognizing chronic venous insufficiency and implementing preventive measures (Kelechi & Bonham,

2008). Whether varicose veins contribute to the development of VTE is controversial, and varicose veins are not included as a risk factor in the most recent evidence-based guidelines on antithrombotic therapy from the American College of Chest Physicians (ACCP) (Geerts, et al., 2008).

Atrial Fibrillation

Atrial fibrillation is a cardiac arrhythmia characterized by loss of coordination of electrical and mechanical activity in the atria. Thrombi can form in the left atrial appendage due to impaired ventricular filling and incomplete emptying of the atria. Atrial fibrillation may initially present with the embolic complication of stroke, when atrial thrombi dislodge and travel through the bloodstream. Other major complications of atrial fibrillation include heart failure and death. Patients with atrial fibrillation caused by conditions other than valvular problems (e.g., nonvalvular atrial fibrillation) have a fivefold risk of ischemic stroke compared with those in sinus rhythm (Garcia & Hylek, 2008).

Atrial fibrillation is the most common cardiac rhythm disturbance seen in clinical practice. Hospitalization for this arrhythmia is increasing, accounted for by the aging of the population and an increased incidence of chronic heart disease (Fuster, et al., 2006). The incidence increases with advancing age and is highest in those older than age 65 or in younger patients with comorbidities of hypertension or underlying heart disease. Other underlying cardiovascular conditions that can cause atrial fibrillation include hypertension with left ventricular hypertrophy, coronary artery disease, chronic heart failure (CHF), and rheumatic valvular disease, especially mitral valve disease. Additional cardiac causes include atrial enlargement, atrial septal defect, and coronary artery bypass graft surgery. Noncardiac etiologies include thyrotoxicosis, hypothermia, fever, stroke, chronic pulmonary disease, electrolyte disorders, PE, alcohol intoxication, obesity, and genetic predisposition (Fuster, et al., 2006; McCabe, 2005).

The three key components to managing atrial fibrillation include preventing stroke with anticoagulant drugs, restoring and maintaining sinus rhythm, and controlling the ventricular heart rate. The patient's risk of stroke determines the need for anticoagulation. Patients with a history of stroke or transient ischemic attack (TIA) have the highest risk of a recurrent event. Other independent risk factors for stroke in atrial fibrillation are increasing age, hypertension, heart failure with impaired systolic function, and diabetes mellitus. Patients older than age 75 comprise over half of atrial fibrillation–associated strokes; thus, the elderly represent a population in which stroke prophylaxis is essential (Fuster, et al., 2006). Anticoagulation therapy is the cornerstone for prevention of stroke in atrial fibrillation.

Ischemic Stroke

An ischemic stroke, or cerebral infarction, results from obstructed cerebral blood supply due to underlying vascular disease or an embolic event. If neurological symptoms last more than 24 hours, the episode is called a stroke. Episodes of brief ischemia causing neurological symptoms that resolve within 24 hours (usually lasting less than 1 hour) are TIAs, which are usually caused by an embolus. Distinguishing between stroke and TIA is not as important today as in previous years because treatments and preventive measures are similar (Sacco, et al., 2006). Stroke is the third leading cause of death in the United States, and it causes significant disability, functional impairment, and decreased quality of life (Goldstein, et al., 2011).

Strokes are categorized into two types; ischemic strokes occur in 85% of patients, while hemorrhagic strokes account for the remaining 15%. Ischemic strokes are further classified by their etiology. The most common cause of ischemic stroke is atherosclerosis in the cerebral arteries (occurring in half of all cases), 25% of ischemic strokes are attributable to cerebral small-vessel disease (lacunar infarcts), and 20% occur from cardioembolic sources (Albers, et al., 2008). Cardioembolic sources include atrial fibrillation, especially with left atrial appendage thrombus or precipitated by rheumatic heart disease; heart failure with left ventricular thrombus; mitral stenosis; prosthetic mechanical valves; recent myocardial infarction (MI) with left ventricular thrombosis; aortic atheroma; patent foramen ovale; atrial myxoma; infective endocarditis; and dilated cardiomyopathies. The remaining ischemic strokes are due to unusual etiologies, including hypercoagulable conditions, drug abuse, or unknown causes (Sacco, et al., 2006).

Stroke prevention is divided into primary prevention (preventing a first episode) or secondary prevention (preventing a recurrent event), and corresponding professional guidelines and approaches to treatment vary, depending on the patient's presentation. There are several well-documented and modifiable risk factors for primary prevention of ischemic stroke, including cardiovascular disease, dyslipidemia, hypertension, diabetes, cigarette smoking, nonvalvular atrial fibrillation, asymptomatic carotid stenosis, sickle cell disease, obesity, and high dietary sodium intake (>2,300 mg/d). Stroke risk can be reduced with appropriate management of these factors (e.g., antihypertensive therapy, statins, smoking cessation, surgical endarterectomy) (Sacco, et al., 2006). For secondary stroke prophylaxis, controlling the risk factors previously mentioned, as well as instituting antiplatelet or anticoagulant therapy, remains the focus of treatment (Goldstein, et al., 2011).

Native and Prosthetic Valvular Heart Disease

Prosthetic heart valves confer a high risk of systemic embolism, and anticoagulation therapy is warranted in most patients. Valvular heart disease is most commonly caused by degenerative valve disease due to increasing life spans and rheumatic heart disease. Indications for prosthetic heart valve replacement include mitral stenosis, mitral regurgitation, aortic stenosis, and aortic regurgitation, as progressive deterioration of the native valve can lead to syncope, dyspnea, angina, and heart failure. There are two main types of prosthetic heart valves: mechanical, made from synthetic materials, or bioprosthetic, of porcine origin. Prosthetic valves are more thrombogenic than bioprosthetic valves and require lifelong anticoagulation, but they are more durable. Factors contributing to thrombus formation with mechanical valve replacement include disruption of the vessel wall during surgery, leading to altered blood flow and activation of hemostasis, or exposure of circulating blood to the artificial surfaces of the valve prosthesis (Sun, et al., 2010).

Prosthetic valves in the mitral position are more thrombogenic than those in the aortic position. In the mitral position, shear stress is low, blood flow is stagnant, and stasis occurs. In the aortic position, blood flow is rapid and shear stress is high, which causes red blood cell hemolysis and activation of platelets and coagulation factors (Sun, et al., 2010).

The risk of thromboembolism in native valvular heart disease is influenced by the position of the valve; for example, mitral versus aortic, heart chamber dimension, ventricular performance, and concomitant risk factors such as prior thromboembolism and atrial fibrillation. In native valvular disease, individuals with rheumatic mitral valve disease have the greatest incidence of systemic embolism. Thromboembolism in aortic valve disease has been noted but is uncommon. Without the coexistence of mitral valve disease or atrial fibrillation, anticoagulation is not indicated in these patients (Salem, et al., 2008).

Anticoagulant therapy for thromboprophylaxis is recommended in all patients having prosthetic valve replacement. The rate of embolism reported with mechanical valves (St. Jude bileaflet valve) when antithrombotic prophylaxis was not administered ranged from 12%/year with aortic valves to 22%/year with mitral valves (Salem, et al., 2008). Bioprosthetic tissue valves present a much lower risk of thromboembolism, averaging 1%/year; the risk of thromboembolic events is highest in the first 3 months following surgery, after which anticoagulant therapy is usually discontinued (Sun, et al., 2010).

PATHOPHYSIOLOGY

Disrupting the body's normal system of checks and balances for hemostasis will lead to either excessive bleeding or inappropriate clotting. The three major components of the coagulation system—endothelial cells, platelets, and coagulation proteins—preserve hemostasis by promoting clot formation in response to vascular injury. The intact vessel wall of the vascular endothelium maintains blood fluidity by inhibiting blood coagulation and platelet aggregation while promoting fibrinolysis. When the vessel wall is injured, substances in the endothelial cell lining stimulate formation of a hemostatic plug by promoting platelet adhesion and aggregation and by activating blood coagulation, resulting in a fibrin clot (Colman, et al., 2006).

Role of Clotting Cascade

In response to tissue injury, a series of complex enzymatic reactions (the clotting cascade, **Figure 49-1**) is initiated that leads to the formation of a stable fibrin clot. Circulating inactive coagulation factors are sequentially converted into activated

COAGULATION PATHWAY

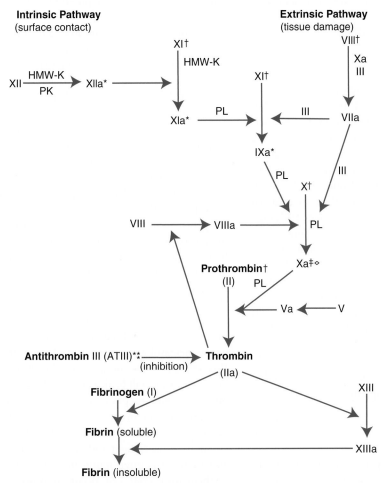

* Major site of activity for unfractionated heparin
† Site of activity for warfarin
‡ Major site of activity for fractionated heparin
⁑ Minor site of activity for fractionated heparin
◇ Minor site of activity for unfractionated heparin

HMW-K: high molecular weight kininogen; PK: prekallekrein; PL: phospholipids from activated platelets

FIGURE 49–1 The coagulation system.

coagulation factor complexes. The final step in the cascade is the formation of thrombin (factor II), which leads to the conversion of fibrinogen to fibrin and the formation of a fibrin clot (Colman, et al., 2006).

Platelets also participate in repairing tissue injury by adhering to the site of injured blood vessels, attracting other platelets to the site, and forming large platelet aggregates that help stabilize the platelet–fibrin clot. When platelets are activated, receptors for clotting factors are exposed. This also provides a stable environment for the initiation of the clotting cascade (Colman, et al., 2006).

The coagulation system is traditionally divided into the intrinsic and extrinsic pathways. Activity through the extrinsic pathway is initiated by components from the blood and vasculature, with factor VII as the major initiating factor.

Activation occurs when procoagulant components migrate to sites of vascular damage or when blood is exposed to substances released as a result of vascular wall damage. In contrast, activity through the intrinsic coagulation pathway is initiated by activation of factor XII when blood comes in contact with a foreign surface (such as a prosthetic device) or damaged endothelial blood vessels. Once factor X is activated in either the extrinsic or intrinsic pathways, the two pathways merge to form a final common pathway for clot formation by converting prothrombin to thrombin (Colman, et al., 2006). (See **Figure 49-1**.)

Several inhibitory processes limit the clotting process. One of the main regulatory proteins of the clotting cascade is antithrombin III, which inhibits factors IX, X, XI, XII, and II (thrombin). Two other regulatory proteins, proteins C and

S, must be present in sufficient amounts because they prevent excessive clot formation by inhibiting factors V and VII. Deficiency in any of these proteins creates a predisposition to pathologic thrombosis (Colman, et al., 2006).

Thrombotic Process

Thrombi can form in any part of the cardiovascular system—the veins and arteries (including those of the brain) as well as the heart. Thrombi can cause local complications by obstructing vessels or by breaking off and traveling to a distant site (embolization). Arterial thrombi often form in the setting of preexisting atherosclerosis or other vascular disease, especially at the sites of ruptured atherosclerotic plaques. In the heart, thrombi can develop on damaged cardiac valves, in a dilated or dyskinetic heart chamber, or on prosthetic valves. Although most intracardiac thrombi cause no symptoms, serious consequences can arise if the thrombi migrate to the systemic circulation, especially the brain. In the venous system, thrombi usually occur in the lower extremities as DVT or in the pulmonary circulation as PE. Venous thrombi form in areas of sluggish blood flow (venous stasis) and contain primarily red cells held together with fibrin, with only small amounts of platelets. In contrast, arterial thrombi form in areas of high blood flow and are composed primarily of platelets bound with fibrin strands (Colman, et al., 2006). The type of thrombus will dictate whether treatment is most appropriate with anticoagulant drugs or antiplatelet drugs.

Hypercoagulable States

Patients with thrombophilia, or hypercoagulable conditions, have an increased tendency to develop thrombosis, most often venous thrombosis. Hypercoagulability may be inherited or acquired. The two most common genetic risk factors for VTE are factor V Leiden mutation and the prothrombin gene mutation 20210. The antiphospholipid antibody syndrome is the most common nongenetic acquired thrombophilia. Genetic risk factors increase the likelihood of an initial VTE but don't impact the risk of a recurrent event (Goldhaber, 2010).

A mutation in coagulation factor V, one of the key proteins in the coagulation cascade, occurs with factor V Leiden. Normally, activated protein C and S will inactivate factor V; in individuals with factor V Leiden, activated factor V is not degraded as efficiently, resulting in increased coagulability (Varga, 2008). Factor V Leiden occurs in 2% to 10% of Whites in the U.S. and increases the risk of VTE two- to fivefold (Coppola, et al., 2009).

Another genetic mutation that causes an increased risk of thrombosis is prothrombin gene mutation 20210 or 20210A. Some patients will have increased prothrombin activity, which is thought to contribute to thrombosis. The incidence in the population and the risk of VTE is similar to factor V Leiden. Both the factor V Leiden and prothrombin gene mutation are uncommon in Blacks and Asians (Merli, 2008).

Antithrombin III, activated protein C, and activated protein S are natural anticoagulants, so deficiencies in

these clotting factors, although very rare, will also induce a prothrombotic state, corresponding to a 5- to 10-fold increase in VTE risk.

Homocysteine is an amino acid formed when the essential amino acid methionine is metabolized. Genetic defects (polymorphism) in the enzymes that regulate homocysteine metabolism can lead to elevated levels (hyperhomocysteinemia), but the exact association between this defect and resultant VTE is still uncertain. Hyperhomocysteinemia has been linked to an increased risk of stroke (Goldstein, et al., 2011). Hyperhomocysteinemia is likely due to genetic and acquired causes (e.g., dietary deficiencies of folate, vitamin B_6, or vitamin B_{12}) (Coppola, et al., 2009).

The presence of a genetic risk factor superimposed with an acquired risk factor significantly increases the risk of VTE (Coppola, et al., 2009). Clues that a patient with VTE has an underlying inherited hypercoagulable condition include thrombosis in patients younger than age 50, a positive family history of VTE, idiopathic or unprovoked thrombosis, recurrent thrombosis, and thrombosis in unusual locations, such as the adrenal glands, renal veins, or upper extremities (Merli, 2008).

A wide spectrum of acquired hypercoagulable states exist, including antiphospholipid (aPL) antibody syndrome, malignancy, hematologic disorders, and nephrotic syndrome. (See **Box 49.1**.) For the purposes of this chapter, only aPL antibody syndrome will be discussed. aPLs are autoantibodies that bind to membrane phospholipid proteins, which are thought to cause the proteins to be antigenic and initiate thrombosis. Several aPLs have been identified, but the two most common are lupus anticoagulant and anticardiolipin antibodies. Lupus anticoagulant is often found in patients with systemic lupus erythematosus, but can occur in other diseases, including syphilis. Lupus anticoagulant is a strong predictor of thrombotic risk for arterial and venous thrombosis. The hallmark characteristics of aPL antibody syndrome are recurrent arterial or venous thrombosis, unexplained fetal loss, and thrombocytopenia with the presence of circulating aPLs. Ischemic stroke is a well-established criterion for diagnosis of aPL antibody syndrome (Dafer & Biler, 2008).

A work-up for thrombophilia is usually deferred until after the acute thrombosis phase because diagnosis does not impact treatment (Goldhaber, 2010). Widespread screening for inherited disorders is not recommended unless it is expected to change clinical management. A hematologist referral is required to determine what, if any, laboratory testing is required and whether wider testing of family members is warranted. The presence of drug therapy, in particular warfarin, will dictate the best timing for laboratory testing because warfarin treatment will affect protein C and S levels (Merli, 2008).

Although inherited thrombophilia increases the risk of VTE, prophylaxis with long-term anticoagulation is not necessary because the risk of bleeding, including fatal bleeding, outweighs the benefits of prophylaxis. However, in the setting of a potential triggering risk factor (e.g., surgery), anticoagulation prophylaxis is beneficial during the period of exposure (Coppola, et al., 2009).

DIAGNOSTIC CRITERIA

Venous Thromboembolism

Erythema, pain, swelling, venous distention, and warmth in the affected leg are common presenting symptoms of DVT. Other conditions, such as muscle strain, cellulitis, and postphlebitic syndrome, may mimic symptoms of DVT. Approximately 50% of patients with DVT have no symptoms. Diagnosing VTE based on clinical factors is often unreliable because only 20% of patients who present with suspected VTE actually have a thrombosis. Therefore, objective confirmatory tests are required (Merli, 2008).

The methods used for detecting DVT are contrast-enhanced venography, compression ultrasonography (CUS), and magnetic resonance imaging (MRI). Contrast-enhanced venography is the gold standard for confirming DVT because it is nearly 100% sensitive and specific and can visualize the distal and proximal venous system. However, it is no longer used in the initial diagnosis of DVT due to high cost, invasiveness, and risk of contrast dye–induced allergic reactions and renal impairment. CUS measures the rate and direction of blood flow and can visualize clot formation in the proximal leg veins. CUS is the diagnostic method of choice because it is noninvasive, can be conducted at the bedside, and is relatively easy to perform. In CUS, DVT is diagnosed if the common femoral or popliteal veins cannot be compressed. For CUS, the sensitivity is 95% and specificity is 96% with a first episode of symptomatic proximal DVT. Disadvantages of CUS include decreased accuracy for detecting calf vein thrombi (73% sensitivity), operator variability, and limitations caused by obesity, casts, and immobilization devices. Although MRI is useful for examining pelvic veins, it has limited usefulness for diagnosing DVT because it is expensive and requires the presence of an experienced radiologist (Merli, 2008).

PE is the most serious complication of DVT. The PE mortality rate is related to the size of the thrombus. A massive PE obstructs 50% of the pulmonary vasculature. The term *submassive* is used when less than 50% of the pulmonary circulation is affected. Death occurs from acute right-sided heart failure in untreated patients. The diagnosis of PE is difficult when based on symptoms because presenting symptoms are not specific. For patients presenting with PE, shortness of breath with or without leg pain may be the first symptom. Other physical findings include sudden onset of dyspnea, pleuritic chest pain, cough, tachycardia, and tachypnea; these symptoms also occur in heart failure, interstitial lung disease, and pneumonia, so thorough examination and further testing is important. Suspicion of PE is based on symptoms along with such risk factors as immobility, recent trauma or surgery, underlying malignancy, and oral contraceptive use. Baseline tests for evaluating PE include a chest x-ray, an electrocardiogram (ECG) to differentiate between PE and MI, and arterial blood gas evaluations (to assess the severity of hypoxemia). Chest x-ray is often normal, so it is most useful in excluding the diagnosis of other conditions with similar symptoms of PE, including pneumothorax (Merli, 2008).

For PE, ventilation/perfusion (V/Q) lung scanning is used to measure the distribution of blood and air flow in the lungs. The results are reported as high, intermediate, or low probability or normal. A normal scan excludes clinically important PE and is sufficient evidence to withhold anticoagulant therapy. An abnormal scan, even though it might suggest PE, can result from other disease states. V/Q lung scanning previously was the major test for diagnosing PE. However, the combination of clinical suspicion and V/Q scan results is nondiagnostic in 72% of patients. Thus, additional confirmatory testing is required. Pulmonary angiography is the gold standard for confirming PE, but it is invasive, expensive, uses contrast dye, and is not always readily available. It is reserved for patients when noninvasive tests are inconclusive (Merli, 2008).

Computed tomography pulmonary angiography (CTPA) has replaced the pulmonary angiogram as the preferred test for diagnosing PE, and it has largely replaced V/Q lung scanning due to higher sensitivity. With CTPA, the sensitivity is 92%, and its specificity is 94%. Disadvantages to CTPA include radiation exposure and the need for injected contrast agent and subsequent risk of renal impairment; V/Q lung scanning is preferred in this setting. CTPA and V/Q lung scanning can reliably exclude the diagnosis of PE (Weitz, 2009).

Imaging of the chest and vascular structures is possible with MRI. In magnetic resonance angiography (MRA), the contrast agent gadolinium is used, which has a lower risk of renal toxicity than the contrast agents used in computed tomography (CT) scans. Disadvantages to MRA include cost and patient physical limitations (e.g., implanted metallic devices and cardiac pacemakers, claustrophobia, obesity) (Merli, 2008).

As discussed previously, the diagnosis of VTE is shifting away from invasive tests to less invasive measures. A laboratory test is now available that measures d-dimer, the major degradation product released into the circulation when cross-linked fibrin undergoes fibrinolysis. Levels of d-dimer are elevated (>500 µg/L) in most patients with ongoing thrombosis. Current assays for d-dimer are over 95% sensitive but not specific. Therefore, a negative d-dimer (<500 µg/L) test helps to rule out DVT or PE. Clinical prediction models that divide patients into low-, moderate-, or high-risk categories for DVT/PE have been validated. Using clinical judgment along with d-dimer assays may decrease the need for unnecessary testing and patient exposure to radiation and contrast dye (Merli, 2008).

Atrial Fibrillation

Symptoms associated with atrial fibrillation include palpitations, chest discomfort, shortness of breath, weakness, hypotension, dizziness, and syncope. Clinical signs of atrial fibrillation include pulmonary edema, dyspnea, and possibly hemodynamic instability (Fuster, et al., 2006). On physical examination, findings of an irregular pulse, irregular jugular venous pulsations, or variations in the intensity of the first heart sound (S_1) can guide the practitioner in suspecting atrial fibrillation (Bentz, 2006). The ECG is used to confirm the diagnosis; an irregularly irregular rhythm is the hallmark of atrial fibrillation.

Other ECG characteristics include the absence of P waves and ventricular response rates of 100 to 180 beats/minute. A thorough history and physical examination is needed to rule out underlying causes of atrial fibrillation. Other baseline assessments include evaluation of electrolytes, thyroid function tests, complete blood count (CBC), and chest x-ray. The diagnostic workup also includes a transthoracic echocardiogram, which can detect left ventricular dysfunction, left ventricular hypertrophy, valvular heart disease, and atrial enlargement. In some cases, a stress test is ordered to rule out the presence of ischemic heart disease. Transesophageal echocardiography (TEE) is frequently used to identify left atrial thrombi in preparation for electrical cardioversion, which attempts to restore normal sinus rhythm (Fuster, et al., 2006).

Nurses and physician assistants can assist with the initial management of atrial fibrillation by remembering the mnemonic *SALTE*—stabilize (monitor heart rate, blood pressure, respiratory status, and medication), assess (fluid and electrolyte status, medication management, risk factor identification and modification), label/treat (arrhythmia management, reducing anxiety, anticoagulation management), and educate (disease process, anticoagulation teaching, prescribed medications) (McCabe, 2005).

Ischemic Stroke

Ischemic stroke is characterized by a sudden or progressive onset of focal neurologic signs due to an inadequate blood supply to the brain. The resulting neurologic deficits depend on the location of cerebral infarction. Most often, the deficits are confined to one side of the body, right or left. The most common presenting stroke symptom is tingling, numbness, and weakness or paralysis on one side of the body. Incoordination, aphasia, dysarthria, and visual disturbances also can occur. Other manifestations include changes in mental status or loss of consciousness. The time of onset of symptoms is a key piece of historical information to determine from the patient or family members because it will dictate treatment. Neurologic signs or symptoms may progress in approximately 25% of patients in the first 24 to 48 hours. Approximately 50% of patients are left with a permanent disability (Adams, et al., 2007).

The physical examination may show signs of trauma or seizures (e.g., contusions, tongue lacerations), or carotid disease (bruits). A comprehensive neurological exam is necessary to determine the extent of neurologic deficit, identify the possible location of the thrombus, and help determine the most appropriate intervention (Adams, et al., 2007).

All patients presenting with suspected ischemic stroke require several diagnostic tests, including blood glucose, electrolytes, CBC with platelets, ECG, cardiac enzymes, prothrombin time (PT), international normalized ratio (INR), activated partial thromboplastin time (aPTT), and oxygen saturation (Adams, et al., 2007).

Brain imaging studies, including noncontrast CT scan and MRI, are used to detect the presence, extent, and progression of a cerebral infarction and if there is intracranial bleeding.

Several tests can help detect the source of a presumed thromboembolic ischemic stroke. Noninvasive carotid ultrasound will show occlusion or stenosis. An ECG differentiates between atrial fibrillation and MI. Transthoracic and transesophageal echocardiograms visualize cardiac function and the presence of an atrial thrombus. Carotid-cerebral angiography can be performed to examine the arteries and veins of the brain and neck. This provides the most accurate visualization to detect abnormalities such as stenosis or occlusion that may have caused the ischemic event (Adams, et al., 2007).

Native and Prosthetic Valvular Heart Disease

Signs and symptoms of valvular heart disease vary depending on the valve that is affected. In aortic stenosis, the cardinal symptoms are dyspnea, angina, syncope, and heart failure. Aortic regurgitation is often asymptomatic. Dyspnea is the hallmark symptom of mitral stenosis, although this usually is present with exertion and has a gradual onset over approximately 20 years. Mitral regurgitation also progresses slowly and may be asymptomatic for many years. The initial symptoms may be fatigue, dyspnea on exertion, and palpitations that, in severe cases, may lead to pulmonary edema. Each valvular disorder is associated with a characteristic murmur, but the intensity of the murmur does not always correlate with the severity of the valvular disorder (Maganti, et al., 2010).

Findings on physical examination also vary with the severity of the valve calcification, severity of stenosis, and left ventricular dysfunction. The chest x-ray will show cardiomegaly, which can occur with aortic stenosis. An ECG is used to determine the possible cardiac effects of valve incompetence or stenosis such as left ventricular hypertrophy in mitral and aortic regurgitation. Confirmation of the diagnosis of valvular disease is best accomplished by an echocardiogram, which will also give an estimate of disease severity. Cardiac catheterization is used when noninvasive tests are inconclusive. When physical symptoms of valvular disease lead to limitations in daily activities or if cardiac decompensation occurs despite medical treatment, surgical intervention, frequently with prosthetic valve replacements, is recommended (Maganti, et al., 2010).

INITIATING DRUG THERAPY

Anticoagulants

Anticoagulants include vitamin K antagonists, direct thrombin inhibitors, unfractionated heparin (UFH), low-molecular-weight heparins (LMWHs), and factor Xa inhibitors. A valid indication for anticoagulation is essential before starting anticoagulant therapy. Several patient factors also warrant consideration to determine if the risk of hemorrhage outweighs the benefit of therapy.

Vitamin K Antagonists

Currently, warfarin (Coumadin) is the most widely used oral vitamin K antagonist in the United States. However, it has a very narrow therapeutic index and requires routine laboratory monitoring. Patient education is essential because patients must comply with laboratory follow-up and accurately follow dosing instructions. An assessment of any contraindications to therapy, including active bleeding and pregnancy, is necessary before starting therapy. The risk of bleeding may exceed the benefits of taking warfarin in patients with a previous history of medication nonadherence, falls, significant alcohol consumption, memory impairment, and lack of adequate support from family members or caregivers. Patients and caregivers must agree with the decision to initiate therapy (Witt, 2010).

Baseline laboratory values including PT, INR, aPTT, urinalysis, CBC, and a liver profile are recommended before initiating warfarin therapy (**Box 49.2**). In women of childbearing age, laboratory testing for β-human chorionic gonadotropin is strongly encouraged to rule out pregnancy. Obtaining the patient's telephone number and an alternative contact, such as a responsible family member or neighbor (obtain consent to contact others per HIPAA guidelines), is also advised. A detailed medical, surgical, and medication history, including over-the-counter (OTC) medications and dietary supplements, is needed to assess the patient's risk of bleeding events or inadequate anticoagulation. It is also important to document the indication for anticoagulation, which determines the duration of therapy, and to define the corresponding target INR, which defines the intensity of anticoagulation. When all these issues are addressed, an initial warfarin-dosing regimen is selected (Witt, 2010).

Direct Thrombin Inhibitors

Dabigatran (Pradaxa) is the first oral direct thrombin inhibitor to receive FDA approval (in October 2010). It is indicated for reducing the risk of stroke in patients with atrial fibrillation (**Box 49.3** and **Table 49.2**). Ximelagatran, another oral direct thrombin inhibitor, was never marketed due to hepatotoxicity. Dabigatran is an alternative anticoagulant to warfarin that does not require routine laboratory monitoring to determine response to therapy. In contrast to warfarin, dabigatran has fixed dosing and a predictable anticoagulant response; therefore, dosing adjustments are not necessary. As a result, baseline laboratory values for aPTT, PT, and INR are not required with dabigatran unless a patient is switching therapy from one anticoagulant to the other. Before initiating therapy, it is appropriate to check the CBC and renal panel because 80% of the drug is renally eliminated. The patient's bleeding risk and medical, surgical, and medication history also should be assessed (Wood, 2010). Determining a patient's past history of medication compliance is also recommended because dabigatran requires twice-daily dosing, and anticoagulant efficacy will be decreased if a patient misses one dose. Dabigatran cannot be

---

BOX 49.2

International Normalized Ratio: Sensitive Test for Clotting Time

The international normalized ratio (INR) is the universally accepted laboratory test for monitoring anticoagulation therapy with the vitamin K antagonists. The INR has replaced the previously used prothrombin time (PT) ratio.

PT is the time in seconds for a blood sample to clot after the addition of laboratory reagents, including specific plasma proteins (tissue thromboplastins) that aid in coagulation. PT measures the reduction in three of the four vitamin K–dependent clotting factors (II, VII, and X) of the extrinsic coagulation cascade. The PT ratio is simply the patient's individual PT divided by a laboratory's control PT. A change in the tissue thromboplastin source from human brain to rabbit brain 40 years ago resulted in a reduced sensitivity in the PT test, leading to lower PT values, and accordingly higher PT ratio goals, with subsequent increased bleeding risk. The international sensitivity index (ISI) was developed by the World Health Organization (WHO) as a reference standard to correct this problem.

Mathematically, the INR is the PT ratio raised to the power of the ISI, or $INR = PT\ ratio^{ISI}$. The ISI for

commercially available tissue thromboplastins vary between individual lots and manufacturers. The WHO reference standard was assigned an ISI of 1.0, although most commercial laboratories use tissue thromboplastins with ISIs ranging from 1.0 to 2.88. The ISI for a particular reagent is identified in the package insert. The INR can be determined using a calculator, if needed.

Most laboratories commonly report PT and INR. However, only the INR should be used for dosing changes. Relying on the INR minimizes variability in reported results if different laboratories, with different thromboplastin preparations, are used (**Table 49.1**). The INR represents the best method for standardizing results from different thromboplastin reagents. The American College of Chest Physicians has standardized the desired target INR goal for anticoagulation therapy for each clinical indication. Current guidelines recommend an INR range of 2 to 3 for most indications of anticoagulation. INRs of 2.5 to 3.5 are reserved for patients with prosthetic heart valves or hypercoagulable conditions.

Data from Ansell, J., Hirsh, J., Hylek, E., et al. (2008). Pharmacology and management of the vitamin K antagonists. American College of Chest Physicians Evidence-Based Clinical Practice Guidelines (8th Edition). *Chest, 133*(6 Suppl.), 160S–198S.

TABLE 49.1	Relationship Between the Prothrombin Time Ratio and the International Normalized Ratio for Thromboplastins with Varying International Sensitivity Index Values				
Hospital	**ISI**	**Control PT (s)**	**PT (s)**	**PT ratio**	**INR**
A	1.3	14.8	33.9	2.3	2.9
B	2.3	11.4	18.2	1.6	2.9

PT, prothrombin time; PT ratio, observed PT divided by control PT; ISI, international sensitivity index; INR, international normalized ratio (INR = PT ratio^{ISI}).

The INR takes into account the differences in thromboplastin sensitivity, thus giving a more accurate reflection of the level of anticoagulation.

put in weekly pillboxes to help with compliance because it is packaged in moisture-proof containers (Boehringer Ingelheim, 2010). Several oral direct thrombin inhibitors and factor Xa inhibitors are under investigation (**Box 49.3** and **Table 49.2**).

Unfractionated Heparin

When using UFH, obtain a baseline aPTT, PT/INR, and a CBC before starting therapy. In addition, rule out any active major bleeding from the central nervous system (CNS) or gastrointestinal (GI) tract. A digital rectal examination or guaiac test to detect blood in the stool is recommended. As with warfarin therapy, a detailed medical, surgical, and medication history is needed to assess the patient's risk of bleeding. Before initiating UFH therapy, define the target aPTT, establish the frequency of aPTT monitoring, and determine the duration of therapy.

Low-Molecular-Weight Heparin and Factor Xa Inhibitors

Subcutaneously administered LMWHs and the factor Xa inhibitor fondaparinux (Arixtra) are increasingly replacing UFH, especially in the outpatient management of VTE. Enoxaparin (Lovenox) is the most widely used LMWHs. Baseline tests should include PT/INR, aPTT, and serum creatinine. As with UFH, perform baseline and periodic CBC and stool occult blood tests and determine the length of therapy. Consider the risks and benefits of therapy when using LMWHs or fondaparinux in patients who have medical

---

BOX 49.3

New Oral Anticoagulants

Since the 1950s, when warfarin was first used in humans, there has been no other comparable oral anticoagulant for the treatment of venous thromboembolism (VTE) and VTE prophylaxis. The U.S. Food and Drug Administration's approval of dabigatran has now changed that, and a variety of oral anticoagulants are currently under development and investigation. The traditional anticoagulants unfractionated heparin (UFH) and low-molecular-weight heparin (LMWH) inhibit both thrombin and activated factor Xa by binding to antithrombin. These newer anticoagulants target the propagation part of the coagulation cascade by inhibiting factor Xa, either directly or indirectly through antithrombin (rivaroxaban or apixaban) or by direct inhibition of thrombin (dabigatran or the now-abandoned ximelagatran). (See **Figure 49-1**.)

The goal for these new drugs is to have an oral anticoagulant that is administered in a fixed dose that does not require monitoring to evaluate anticoagulant effect. Effects of the factor Xa inhibitors are limited to the coagulation cascade because they decrease the formation of thrombin from prothrombin. The direct thrombin inhibitors have other actions, including prevention of fibrin formation, prevention of platelet aggregation, and inhibition of thrombin-induced activation of factors V, VIII, XI, and XIII. Direct thrombin inhibitors can act on thrombin that is bound to fibrin, in contrast to heparin, which can only affect free thrombin (Spyropoulos, 2008; Schirmer, et al., 2010). Intravenous direct thrombin inhibitors are available (bivalirudin, hirudin, and argatroban) and are administered via infusion in the hospital and used primarily for heparin-induced thrombocytopenia. The oral factor Xa inhibitors furthest along in development are rivaroxaban and apixaban. Both drugs are currently undergoing large comparative trials with warfarin for atrial fibrillation. Phase III clinical trials have been conducted in the areas of both treatment and prophylaxis of VTE and for stroke prevention in atrial fibrillation. **Table 49.2** provides a summary of the phase III testing with the pipeline oral anticoagulants.

TABLE 49.2	New Oral Anticoagulants: Direct Thrombin Inhibitors and Factor Xa Inhibitors		
	Dabigatran	**Rivaroxaban**	**Apixaban**
Coagulation target	Thrombin	Factor Xa	Factor Xa
FDA status	Approved	Investigational	Investigational
Proposed/actual brand name	Pradaxa	Xarelto	Not yet established
Manufacturer	Boehringer Ingelheim	Bayer/Johnson & Johnson	Pfizer/Bristol Myers Squibb
Dosing	Fixed, QD-BID, depending on indication	Fixed, QD	Fixed, BID
Coagulation monitoring required?	No	No	No
Metabolism	Conjugation; no role of CYP450	CYP3A4	CYP3A4
Clinical trials	Atrial fibrillation	Atrial fibrillation	Atrial fibrillation
	VTE prophylaxis in orthopedic surgery	VTE prophylaxis in orthopedic surgery	VTE prophylaxis in orthopedic surgery
	VTE treatment	VTE treatment	VTE treatment
		VTE prophylaxis in medical patients	VTE prophylaxis in medical patients
		Acute coronary syndromes	Acute coronary syndromes
Reversibility	No specific antidote	No specific antidote	No specific antidote

conditions or who are taking concomitant medications that increase bleeding risk. Since dosing is based on patient weight, laboratory monitoring is usually not necessary. However, anti-factor Xa levels may be useful in some circumstances, including patients with renal impairment, pregnant patients, or obese patients (Hirsh, et al., 2008). When LMWHs or fondaparinux are used in the outpatient setting, patient education regarding subcutaneous injection is necessary. Establish that the patient or their caregiver can reliably and accurately administer the subcutaneous injection or consider arranging for home health care visits.

Antiplatelet Agents

Antiplatelet agents include aspirin and the platelet aggregation inhibitors aspirin/dipyridamole (Aggrenox), clopidogrel (Plavix), and ticlopidine (Ticlid). Prasugrel (Effient) is an antiplatelet agent used to reduce arterial thrombosis in patients with acute coronary syndrome undergoing percutaneous coronary intervention and is not discussed here. A detailed medication history is needed before initiating therapy with antiplatelet agents. For aspirin and aspirin/dipyridamole, a medication history will help to determine if any concomitant medications will increase the risk of gastric ulcerations/erosions, such as nonsteroidal anti-inflammatory drugs (NSAIDs). Patients receiving aspirin should be questioned carefully regarding any medication allergies because antiplatelet agents are contraindicated in patients with a history of aspirin allergy or hypersensitivity to NSAIDs or

salicylates. Pay particular attention to a history of nasal polyps and asthma due to an increased risk of aspirin allergy in these patients. Patients with severe anemia or a history of coagulation defects also should not receive aspirin. Before initiating therapy with clopidogrel or ticlopidine, a baseline CBC with differential and liver function tests should be performed. Patients also need to be assessed for any active major bleeding (Lexi-Comp Online, 2010).

Goals of Drug Therapy

Preventing the development of a stroke is the primary goal of anticoagulant therapy in patients with atrial fibrillation, prosthetic heart valves, and in those with a history of cardioembolic stroke. Anticoagulation treatment in patients with existing DVT/PE is initiated to prevent extension of the thrombus; thromboembolic complications, including postthrombotic syndrome; and development of a new thrombus. Anticoagulation prophylaxis after orthopedic surgery is initiated to decrease the risk of DVT or PE. The goals of antiplatelet therapy are to prevent and treat ischemic strokes from noncardioembolic sources.

Warfarin

Warfarin is the most widely used oral vitamin K antagonist in North America because of its good absorption (bioavailability), relatively predictable onset of action, long duration of action, and proven efficacy (Ansell, et al., 2008) (**Table 49.3**).

TABLE 49.3 **Overview of Drugs Used to Treat Coagulation Disorders**

Generic (Trade) Name and Dosage	Selected Adverse Events	Contraindications	Special Considerations
Anticoagulants			
warfarin (Coumadin) Start: 2.5–5 mg qd PO Range: 1–15 mg qd PO—must individualize dose	Bleeding	Contraindicated in pregnancy or in active major bleeding; for other contraindications, see text.	Used for prophylaxis and treatment of DVT, PE, and prophylaxis and treatment of stroke in atrial fibrillation and for prosthetic heart valves Monitored with the PT/INR Vitamin K will reverse effects. See text for drug interactions and dietary restrictions.
dabigatran (Pradaxa) CrCl >30 mL/min: 150 mg bid PO CrCl 15–30 mL/min: 75 mg bid PO	Bleeding	Contraindicated in active major bleeding (GI or intracranial); see text for considerations in renal impairment	Approved for prevention of stroke in atrial fibrillation Routine coagulation monitoring not required Fixed dosing No antidote to reverse effects
Heparin SC: 8,000–10,000 units q8h SC: 15,000–20,000 units q12h IV: 20,000–40,000 units/d continuous infusion	Bleeding, thrombocytopenia	Contraindicated in active major bleeding (GI or intracranial), or in patients with thrombocytopenia	Used for prophylaxis and treatment of DVT, PE, atrial fibrillation with embolization, peripheral artery embolism, and surgical procedures Monitored with the aPTT Monitor CBC with platelets periodically for thrombocytopenia. Protamine will reverse effects.
dalteparin (Fragmin) abdominal surgery: 2,500 IU/d SC or 5,000 IU/d SC hip replacement: 5,000 IU/d SC medical patients: 5,000 IU/d SC cancer patients with DVT/PE: month 1: 200 IU/kg qd months 2–6: 150 IU/kg qd	Bleeding, local irritation at the injection site	Active major bleeding (GI or intracranial); thrombocytopenia in association with positive *in vitro* testing for antiplatelet antibodies	LMWH used for prophylaxis of DVT in patients undergoing abdominal surgery, hip replacement surgery, or in medical patients. Also for extended treatment/prevention of DVT in patients with cancer Evaluate CBC periodically for bleeding effects. Weight-based fixed dosing Routine coagulation monitoring not required
enoxaparin (Lovenox) orthopedic surgery: 30 mg SC bid	Bleeding, local irritation at the injection site, transient elevated liver function test values	Active major bleeding (GI or intracranial); thrombocytopenia in association with positive *in vitro* testing for antiplatelet antibodies Hypersensitivity to heparin, LMWH Patients with severe renal insufficiency	LMWH used for prophylaxis of DVT/PE after total hip replacement, total knee replacement, and abdominal surgeries and in immobilized medical patients; DVT/PE treatment in hospitalized or inpatient setting
abdominal surgery or medical patients: 40 mg SC qd DVT treatment with or without PE: 1 mg/kg or 1.5 mg/kg qd			Evaluate CBC periodically for bleeding effects. Weight-based fixed dosing Routine coagulation monitoring not required
fondaparinux (Arixtra) prophylaxis of DVT: 2.5 mg SC qd treatment of DVT/PE: body weight <50 kg: 5 mg SC qd body weight 50–100 kg: 7.5 mg SC qd body weight >100 kg: 10 mg SC qd	Bleeding, injection site bleeding and LFT elevation, thrombocytopenia and irritation	Active major bleeding, body weight <50 kg thrombocytopenia, severe hepatic impairment	Pentasaccharide factor Xa inhibitor used for DVT prophylaxis in patients following hip fracture, hip and knee replacement surgery, and abdominal surgery; also for treatment of DVT or PE Weight-based, fixed dosing Routine coagulation monitoring not required

TABLE 49.3	Overview of Drugs Used to Treat Coagulation Disorders *(Continued)*		
Generic (Trade) Name and Dosage	**Selected Adverse Events**	**Contraindications**	**Special Considerations**
tinzaparin (Innohep) 175 anti–ka IU/kg SC qd	Bleeding, local irritation at injection site	Hypersensitivity to sulfites, benzyl alcohol, or LMWH History of heparin-induced thrombocytopenia	LMWH used for treatment of DVT with and without PE; may affect PT/INR—check PT/INR just prior to a dose when using with warfarin. Weight-based, fixed dosing
Antiplatelet Agents			
aspirin (Ascriptin, Bufferin, Bayer Aspirin) 30–1,500 mg/d PO	Bleeding, gastric ulceration, allergic reactions	Active stroke or stroke in progress; active GI bleeding, or aspirin allergy or hypersensitivity	Decreases the risk of death/nonfatal MI in patients with previous MI or unstable angina Decreases the risk of recurrent ischemic stroke Text discusses controversies with dosing.
aspirin/dipyridamole (Aggrenox) 25 mg aspirin/200 mg dipyridamole bid PO	Headache, diarrhea, abdominal pain LFT elevations	Hypersensitivity, aspirin or NSAID allergy Active peptic ulcer disease	Combination product used to reduce the risk of stroke in patients with previous thrombotic stroke Swallow whole capsules; do not crush or chew.
clopidogrel (Plavix) 75 mg qd PO	Bleeding, GI effects, rash (rare)	Active major bleeding (peptic ulcer or intracranial hemorrhage)	Reduces risk of MI, stroke, or vascular death in patients with atherosclerosis documented by recent stroke, MI, or established peripheral artery disease Decreased risk of neutropenia compared with risk of neutropenia from ticlopidine
ticlopidine (Ticlid) 250 mg bid PO	Neutropenia, thrombocytopenia, rash, GI effects, hepatic impairment	Neutropenia or thrombocytopenia; active bleeding (GI or intracranial hemorrhage); severe hepatic impairment	Decreases the risk of thrombotic stroke in patients with a history of stroke or transient ischemic attack Must monitor CBC and platelets every 2 wk for the first 3 mo of therapy because of neutropenia Discontinue if the ANC drops below 1,200, or if the platelet count falls below 80,000 Reserved for patients allergic to or intolerant to aspirin because of neutropenia

aPTT, activated partial thromboplastin time; CBC, complete blood count; CrCl, creatinine clearance; DVT, deep vein thrombosis; GI, gastrointestinal; INR, international normalized ratio; IU, international units; IV, intravenous; LFT, liver function test; LMWH, low-molecular-weight heparin; MI, myocardial infarction; NSAID, nonsteroidal anti-inflammatory agent; PE, pulmonary embolism; PT, prothrombin time; SC, subcutaneous; UFH, unfractionated heparin.

Mechanism of Action and Time Frame for Response

Oral anticoagulants produce their clinical effects through the extrinsic pathway of the clotting cascade. In contrast, heparin, a parenteral anticoagulant, influences the intrinsic coagulation cascade. Warfarin inhibits activation of the clotting factors in the liver that depend on vitamin K for synthesis—factors II, VII, IX, and X and the coagulation inhibitor proteins C and S. Warfarin interferes with the conversion of vitamin K from its inactive form to active vitamin K. Vitamin K is depleted, and the rate of clotting factor formation is decreased, which ultimately prevents clot formation and extension. Warfarin does not affect the function of existing clotting factors and has no effect on an existing thrombus (Ansell, et al., 2008).

The half-lives of clotting factors range from 6 hours (factor VII) to 60 hours (factor II) as indicated in **Table 49.4** (Tran & Ginsberg, 2006). The average half-life of warfarin is 36 to 42 hours. The onset of anticoagulant effect depends on both the half-life of warfarin and the time required to deplete the vitamin K–dependent clotting factors. The anticoagulant effect of warfarin is monitored with PT and INR, with the INR being the gold standard. The PT/INR will show an initial prolongation 1 to 3 days after warfarin is first administered, which is due to the rapid depletion of factor VII. However, the full antithrombotic effect of warfarin won't be seen for 8 to 14 days, when factor II (prothrombin) is depleted. In cases of acute DVT or PE, UFH, LMWHs, or fondaparinux is often given with warfarin when rapid anticoagulation is needed or in hypercoagulable patients

TABLE 49.4	Normal Half-Lives of the Vitamin K–Dependent Clotting Factors and Proteins C and S	
Activity	**Vitamin K–Dependent Factor**	**Half-Life (h)**
Anticoagulant	Protein C	8–10
Anticoagulant	Protein S	40–60
Coagulant	Factor II (Prothrombin)	60–100
Coagulant	Factor VII	6–8
Coagulant	Factor IX	20–30
Coagulant	Factor X	24–40

(protein C or S deficiency). Warfarin causes a quick fall in protein C (half-life of 8 to 10 hours), which can induce a temporary hypercoagulable state, putting patients at risk for thrombosis. The injectable anticoagulant is continued until the INR is stable for at least 2 days, which allows for additional reductions in the levels of factors X and II (Ansell, et al., 2008).

Dosage

Because of its long half-life, warfarin is administered once daily. Warfarin is completely absorbed after oral administration and is metabolized to inactive metabolites by the liver. Warfarin has a narrow therapeutic window; therefore, the dose needed to exert clinical efficacy is similar to the dose that causes adverse effects (Ansell, et al., 2008). Individual patients vary widely in their ability to absorb and eliminate warfarin (pharmacokinetic variations) and in their rate of clinical response and dosage requirements (pharmacodynamic variations). Patient variability in the dose response to warfarin is not related to weight or sex but is influenced by age, comorbid disease states, concomitant medications, and one's genetically predetermined rate of metabolism. Warfarin binds extensively to plasma proteins and is metabolized by the cytochrome P450-2C9 (CYP2C9) system of the liver. Genetic variation in the CYP2C9 genotype can influence warfarin-dose requirements and lead to an enhanced thrombotic effect (Garcia, et al., 2008; Ansell, et al., 2008). **Box 49.4** provides more information on warfarin genomics.

An increased warfarin response can occur in patients with hepatic dysfunction, in which there is impaired synthesis of clotting factors and decreased warfarin metabolism. Likewise, lower warfarin doses may be needed in patients with low serum albumin or those with significant congestive heart failure (Jacobs, 2008). Other pharmacodynamic factors that may potentiate warfarin response include hypermetabolic states, such as hyperthyroidism, and febrile states when there is an increased catabolic rate of vitamin K–dependent clotting factors. The elderly also seem to be more sensitive to warfarin, possibly because of altered pharmacodynamic parameters, but the etiology is unknown (Jacobs, 2008).

If the patient receives a prescription for warfarin, the prescriber needs to choose among nine different dosage strengths

BOX 49.4

Warfarin Genomics

Genetic factors are now identified that cause certain patients to need lower or higher-than-anticipated warfarin doses. Warfarin's metabolism is influenced by the proteins cytochrome P450-2C9 enzyme (CYP2C9) and vitamin K epoxide reductase complex 1 (VKORC1), which is involved in the conversion of the vitamin K from active to inactive forms. Genetic mutations in CYP2C9 (affecting the rate of warfarin metabolism) and VKORC1 (affecting the body's sensitivity to warfarin) account for some of the variation in warfarin doses needed to maintain a stable INR. Some studies have found that the presence of CYP2C9 polymorphisms predicts low warfarin dose requirements due to slowed metabolism and that VKORC1 mutations cause warfarin resistance.

Knowing a patient's genotype has been proposed to assist with determining a patient's initial and maintenance warfarin requirements. Patients with widely fluctuating international normalized ratio test results may benefit from genetic-guided warfarin dosing. A commercial test is now marketed that identifies these genetic polymorphisms, and the Coumadin package insert includes information on using genotype status to guide warfarin dosing. One disadvantage to knowing a patient's genotype is that it will not help patients who are noncompliant. Additionally, multiple factors, not just genetics, influence warfarin requirements. Whether pharmacogenetic testing will improve patient care has not been firmly established in randomized trials, and the most recent American College of Chest Physicians guidelines do not advocate use of genetic testing to individualize warfarin dosing.

Data from Garcia, D. A., Witt, D. M., Hylek, E., et al. (2008). Delivery of optimized anticoagulant therapy: Consensus statement from the anticoagulation forum. *Annals of Pharmacotherapy, 42*(9), 79–88, and Ansell, J., Hirsh, J., Hylek, E., et al. (2008). Pharmacology and management of the vitamin K antagonists. American College of Chest Physicians Evidence-Based Clinical Practice Guidelines (8th Edition). *Chest, 133*(6 Suppl.), 160S–198S.

and colors (e.g., a 1-mg tablet is pink, whereas a 5-mg tablet is peach). For safety's sake and to avoid confusing the patient, prescribe only one warfarin tablet strength (e.g., 2.5- or 5-mg tablets, but not both). Patients also need to be taught to remember the tablet color, shape, and tablet strength with each new prescription and refill. There are several manufacturers of warfarin, and although differences in bioequivalence between products were initially a concern, this has not been shown to significantly impact patient response (Jacobs, 2008). It is appropriate to monitor the INR more frequently in patients when one warfarin product is switched to another to identify patients who would experience a change in anticoagulation response (Witt, et al., 2003).

Initial Dose

It is difficult to predict an individual's warfarin requirement needed to reach the INR range that is considered therapeutic for the disease state. The common practice of administering a warfarin "loading" dose of 10 mg for 3 days is no longer recommended because the target INR is often exceeded in 20% to 50% of patients, which increases the risk of bleeding, causes an interruption in therapy, and delays attainment of a stable dose. Large warfarin loading doses do not reach a therapeutic INR faster than starting a usual maintenance dose (Ansell, et al., 2008).

Several dosing nomograms are available that assist in rapidly achieving therapeutic INR values when warfarin is started, and computer software programs are also used (Jacobs, 2008; Witt, 2010). Warfarin is usually started at an average maintenance dose of 4 to 5 mg daily; the dose is adjusted based on daily INR values. Certain patient populations, such as the elderly, patients with congestive heart failure, those with underlying malignancy, those with severely impaired renal or hepatic function, or those taking interacting drugs that increase warfarin's effect, are at high risk for bleeding and should receive a lower initial dose of 2 to 4 mg daily. Larger starting doses, such as 7.5 to 10 mg, may be used if rapid effect is urgently needed, but this is unnecessary for most patients. During the initial titration phase, daily dosage increases or decreases are commonly made in 2- to 2.5-mg increments based on INR values. If rapid anticoagulation is not necessary and the patient's risk of thrombosis and bleeding are not high, warfarin can be started on an outpatient basis with INR evaluations every 2 to 3 days. Administering warfarin at the same time daily is recommended to reduce variability in effects (Ansell, et al., 2008). In patients who don't require rapid anticoagulation, as in chronic atrial fibrillation, warfarin can be started without concurrent heparin or LMWHs. In patients needing rapid anticoagulation who are at risk for recurrent VTE, concurrent treatment with parenteral anticoagulants is needed (Jacobs, 2008). (See the **Mechanism of Action** section.)

Maintenance Dose

The relationship between the warfarin dosage and the INR is not linear. Therefore, minor changes in dose can result in greater than expected changes in the INR. The maintenance warfarin dose varies widely among individuals, and there are no widely accepted patient characteristics that reliably predict the necessary maintenance dose. Warfarin-dosing algorithms can also assist with determining maintenance warfarin doses (Witt, 2010). Calculating the total weekly warfarin dose and then increasing or decreasing the weekly regimen by only 10% to 20%, spread over the course of the week, can cause measurable changes in the INR. Some clinicians advocate administering the same dosage daily, whereas others agree that giving varying doses on alternate days is rational. Patients with low education levels, cognitive impairments, or those receiving several other medications may benefit from a simple dosing schedule. If an alternating-day regimen is chosen, defining the actual dosage for each day of the week is recommended (e.g., 5 mg administered on Tuesdays, Thursdays, Saturdays, and Sundays and 7.5 mg on Mondays, Wednesday, and Fridays, rather than 5 mg alternating with 7.5 mg every other day). This helps to reduce patient confusion and avoid fluctuations in the INR. Sensitive patients with reduced requirements should receive warfarin daily rather than alternating between drug and drug-free days; for example, 1.5 mg given every day, rather than 2 mg alternating with 1 mg every other day (Ansell, et al., 2008). Once a patient has reached a therapeutic INR with a consistent warfarin dose, INR monitoring should continue at least every 4 weeks (Witt, 2010).

Patients with frequent INR fluctuations not due to the usual known causes may benefit if low doses (100 to 200 mcg) of daily vitamin K are added to their diet. Daily vitamin K supplementation is thought to override variations in day-to-day dietary vitamin K intake, eventually resulting in stable INR values (Witt, 2010). Patients using vitamin K supplementation will require frequent INR value checks to avoid the INR dropping below the therapeutic range. Patients also need to be cautioned to not abruptly discontinue the vitamin K supplement due to the risk of excessive anticoagulation (Ansell, et al., 2008).

Contraindications

Absolute contraindications to warfarin include pregnancy, recent hemorrhagic stroke, risk of or active major bleeding, recent trauma or traumatic surgery, use in the immediate postoperative period after CNS or ocular surgery, or the presence of spinal catheters and aneurysms or CNS tumors with a high bleeding risk (Bristol-Myers Squibb, 2010). Refer to the section on initiating anticoagulation therapy for some important relative contraindications to consider with warfarin.

Adverse Events

Bleeding is the most worrisome adverse event associated with warfarin therapy. As the intensity of anticoagulation increases, so does the bleeding risk. The highest risk of bleeding, especially intracranial hemorrhage, occurs when the INR exceeds a 4 to 5 range. The frequency of major bleeding in patients with a target INR of 2 to 3 is half of that seen in patients with a target INR above 3. Refer to the section on monitoring warfarin therapy for a discussion of INR testing. In addition to the intensity of anticoagulation, the other major factors that determine bleeding risk include individual patient characteristics; concurrent use of other drugs that affect hemostasis, such as aspirin, clopidogrel, cyclooxygenase (COX)-2 inhibitors, or NSAIDs; and the duration of therapy (Schulman, et al., 2008).

Minor bleeding occurring from the oral or nasal mucosa, urine, stool, or soft tissues is the most common adverse effect of anticoagulation therapy. Bleeding complications in order of frequency are epistaxis, purpura, hematuria, GI bleeding, and hemoptysis (Jacobs, 2008). Women are more likely to experience minor bleeding than men (Schulman, et al., 2008). Minor bleeding is usually managed by temporarily discontinuing warfarin therapy for 1 to 2 days, and then restarting warfarin at a reduced dosage or reducing the target INR range.

Major bleeding is commonly defined as any bleeding resulting in hospitalization, requiring transfusion, occurring in the intracranial or retroperitoneal areas, or causing death. Risk factors for major bleeding episodes include patients older than age 65, previous history of GI bleeding, and history of ischemic stroke, treated and untreated hypertension, severe cardiac disease, cerebrovascular disease, diabetes, alcoholism, or renal insufficiency. As the number of patient risk factors increases, the risk of major bleeding also increases (Schulman, et al., 2008). Although controversial, most studies show that elderly patients have a higher frequency of bleeding. The greatest risk of bleeding occurs within the first months of warfarin therapy (Ansell, et al., 2008). In studies in which patients had close monitoring of warfarin therapy, the risk of major bleeding was increased by 0.3% to 0.5% per year, and the risk of intracranial hemorrhage was increased by approximately 0.2% per year compared to control patients (Schulman, et al., 2008). The rate of hemorrhage seen in actual use may differ from the rates reported in clinical trials because high-risk patients are frequently excluded from participating in trials. Although intracranial bleeding is a rare complication, it is the most frequent cause of fatal events, and patients often do not fully recover (Jacobs, 2008).

Patients with a history of falling are commonly thought to have an increased risk of intracranial hemorrhage. One researcher evaluated the risk of elderly patients falling and subsequent development of a subdural hematoma, compared to the benefits of warfarin for stroke prevention in atrial fibrillation. Their conclusion was the risk of stroke if the patient did not receive warfarin (5% per year) was much larger than the risk of developing a subdural hematoma (0.0004 per patient-year). An elderly patient with atrial fibrillation would need to fall 300 times a year for the risk of subdural hematoma to outweigh the benefits of warfarin therapy (Man-Son-Hing, et al., 1999).

When the INR is elevated, management depends on the patient's potential risk of bleeding, whether the patient is actively bleeding, and the INR level. Treatment options include simply omitting one or more warfarin doses with more frequent INR testing or administering vitamin K. In the inpatient setting, administering fresh frozen plasma or prothrombin concentrates can also be considered (Ansell, et al., 2008). Management of major bleeding focuses on reversing the anticoagulation effects of warfarin (**Box 49.5**). Any bleeding event should be adequately investigated because an underlying comorbidity, such as malignancy, may be the cause.

Interactions

The list of medications that increase or inhibit the anticoagulant effect of warfarin is extensive. The potential pharmacokinetic mechanisms of drug interactions with warfarin include alterations in absorption; CYP2C9 enzyme induction leading to increased warfarin hepatic clearance (which would reduce antithrombotic activity) or CYP2C9 inhibition, causing reduced hepatic clearance and increased antithrombotic effect; or altered protein binding with warfarin. Reduced clotting factor synthesis, which occurs in liver disease, can potentiate warfarin response. An increased risk of bleeding without alterations in the INR can occur when medications that inhibit platelet function (e.g., NSAIDs, aspirin, or clopidogrel) are given concomitantly with warfarin. Medications that commonly affect warfarin include but are not limited to amiodarone; antibiotics such as erythromycin, metronidazole, and trimethoprim–sulfamethoxazole; antifungals; salicylates; NSAIDs; histamine-2 (H_2) antagonists; sucralfate; lipid-lowering medications; thyroid hormones; anticonvulsants; steroids; influenza vaccine; and vitamin E (Jacobs, 2008). Many of the reports of drug interactions with warfarin are from single patient cases, so determining the likelihood that a drug will clinically impact warfarin response is difficult to predict. **Table 49.5** provides a list of drug interactions with warfarin; a more extensive list is found in Holbrook, et al. (2005). There is much patient variability when interacting drugs are added to or discontinued from warfarin therapy. Close laboratory monitoring and warfarin dosage adjustment is needed to prevent either supratherapeutic or subtherapeutic INRs, resulting in hemorrhagic effects or thromboembolic complications. Extended INR monitoring for several weeks or months is often needed when drugs with a prolonged effect, such as amiodarone or rifampin, are administered (Witt, 2010).

Nutritional Supplement/Over-the-Counter Drug Interactions

Several herbal preparations can potentially interfere with the anticoagulant effect of warfarin. Although stringently performed clinical trials are lacking, bilberry, feverfew, garlic, and ginger have limited data that show an increased anticoagulant effect when used with warfarin (Nutescu, et al., 2006). Fish oil has been noted to increase the INR (Jacobs, 2008). Garlic has platelet-inhibitory effects that can increase bleeding risk, and there are anecdotal reports of increases in the PT/INR in patients receiving warfarin. Herbal products that can decrease the effect of warfarin include ginseng and green tea, due to its vitamin K content (Holbrook, et al., 2005). Literature and regulatory actions on herbal

BOX 49.5

Reversing the Anticoagulant Effects of Warfarin

Managing patients with elevated international normalized ratio (INR) test results is essential for safe and effective anticoagulation therapy.

MODERATELY ELEVATED INRS

INRs <5. For patients with INRs above the therapeutic range but <5 who are not experiencing significant bleeding, simply decreasing the warfarin dose and monitoring the INR more frequently is a rational approach. The dose may be held for 24 hours and then therapy restarted in a reduced regimen, which can bring the INR to within the target range. If the INR is only slightly above the target range, it may not be necessary to reduce the dose.

INRs 5 and <9. For patients with INRs above 5 but less than 9 who are not experiencing significant bleeding, omitting the next one to two doses, monitoring the INR more frequently, and resuming therapy at a lower dose is one approach. The alternative is to administer 1 to 2.5 mg of oral vitamin K, which should cause the INR to decrease in 24 hours.

HIGHLY ELEVATED INRS

Patients with INRs above 9 who are not experiencing significant bleeding should have their warfarin held and receive a higher dose of oral vitamin K (2.5 to 5 mg). The INR will fall substantially in 24 to 48 hours. Frequent INR checks are necessary, and additional doses of oral vitamin K can be given if the INR is still elevated. Once the INR falls within the target range, warfarin can be resumed at a lower dose.

SIGNIFICANT BLEEDING

Patients experiencing significant bleeding, regardless of how high the INR is elevated, or patients with life-threatening bleeding need immediate reversal of the INR and should have their warfarin temporarily discontinued

and vitamin K 10 mg should be administered via slow intravenous (IV) infusion. Depending on the INR, repeat doses of vitamin K can be given every 12 hours. If necessary, fresh frozen plasma, prothrombin complex concentrate, or recombinant factor VIIa can be given if the situation is urgent.

VITAMIN K

Patients with highly elevated INRs or patients with active bleeding may need vitamin K in addition to temporary discontinuance of warfarin therapy. An initial drop in the INR occurs within 6 hours after vitamin K administration. However, the full effect does not occur for 24 hours. Doses of vitamin K larger than 1 mg may induce a state of warfarin resistance that can last for up to 2 weeks until the vitamin K–dependent clotting factors are depleted. The goals of vitamin K therapy are to reduce the INR to within the therapeutic range, without dropping below the target INR, and to prevent inducing a state of temporary warfarin resistance.

Administering oral vitamin K in doses of 1 to 2.5 mg for INRs between 5 and 9 and in doses of 2.5 to 5 mg for INRs greater than 9 is now advocated rather than the former practice of giving 10 mg. Oral vitamin K has also replaced the use of subcutaneous vitamin K due to a more predictable response, faster onset of effect, and improved safety and convenience. IV vitamin K is reserved for use in patients with severe bleeding who are hospitalized because of the risk of anaphylaxis.

Oral vitamin K (Mephyton) is available in 5-mg tablets. Parenteral vitamin K (AquaMEPHYTON) is available in concentrations of 2 mg/mL in 0.5-mL ampules, 10 mg/mL in 1-mL ampules, or 2.5- and 5-mL vials. Oral vitamin K tablets in 100-μg strength can be purchased at health food stores without a prescription, or the parenteral preparation can be taken orally.

Data from Ansell, J., Hirsh, J., Hylek, E., et al. (2008). Pharmacology and management of the vitamin K antagonists. American College of Chest Physicians Evidence-Based Clinical Practice Guidelines (8th Edition). *Chest, 133*(6 Suppl.), 160S–198S.

supplements can be accessed through the U.S. Department of Agriculture Food and Nutrition Information Center website at http://fnic.nal.usda.gov. Supplements containing multiple ingredients are a concern because there may be variations in the amount and purity of the substances comprising the product (Wittkowsky, 2008). Providers may forget to ask patients about nutritional supplements, so it is important

to educate patients that they must notify the prescriber of any changes, additions, or deletions in their medications or herbal supplements.

Dietary Interactions

Dietary habits can cause alterations in warfarin's antithrombotic response. Excessive dietary vitamin K interacts with

TABLE 49.5	Drug and Food Interactions with Warfarin and Direction of Interaction	
Likelihood of Interaction	**Potentiation**	**Inhibition**
Highly likely	Alcohol (if concomitant liver disease), amiodarone, anabolic steroids, cimetidine, citalopram, ciprofloxacin, cotrimoxazole, diltiazem, erythromycin, fenofibrate, fluconazole, isoniazid, metronidazole, miconazole, omeprazole, phenylbutazone, piroxicam, propafenone, sertraline	Barbiturates, carbamazepine, cholestyramine, griseofulvin, mesalamine, nafcillin, rifampin, high vitamin K–content foods/enteral feeds, large amounts of avocado
Probable	Acetaminophen, amoxicillin/clavulanate, aspirin, azithromycin, celecoxib, clarithromycin, chloral hydrate, disulfiram, itraconazole, levofloxacin, quinidine, phenytoin (biphasic with later inhibition), simvastatin, tamoxifen, tetracycline, tolterodine, grapefruit	Azathioprine, dicloxacillin, ritonavir, sucralfate, influenza vaccine, soy milk
Possible	Amoxicillin, fluorouracil, gatifloxacin, gemfibrozil, metozalone, nalidixic acid, norfloxacin, ofloxacin, propoxyphene, sulindac, tolmetin, topical salicylates	Cyclosporine, sulfasalazine, telmisartan
Not likely	Cefamandole, cefazolin, fluoxetine/diazepam, heparin, levonorgestrel, sulfisoxazole	Cloxacillin, furosemide, propofol

warfarin by antagonizing its clinical effect. The practitioner should discuss diet when prescribing warfarin to avoid subtherapeutic INR values. (See the **Patient Education** section.)

Direct Thrombin Inhibitor—Dabigatran

Dabigatran is the first new oral anticoagulant therapy available for use since the 1950s, when warfarin was introduced, and it may permanently alter the way providers manage anticoagulation therapy. Several oral direct thrombin inhibitors and factor Xa inhibitors are under investigation, but whether these new agents and dabigatran will eventually replace warfarin remains to be determined. The cost of dabigatran is likely to impact the popularity of the drug. Estimates are that dabigatran will cost more ($5 to $6/day) than generic warfarin combined with INR testing (Anonymous [FDA Pink Sheet], 2010). (See **Box 49.3** and **Table 49.2**.) **Table 49.6** contrasts warfarin with dabigatran.

The Randomized Evaluation of Long-Term Anticoagulation Therapy (RE-LY) trial enrolled over 18,000 patients with atrial fibrillation and compared two doses of dabigatran (150 mg twice daily or 110 mg twice daily) with warfarin. The primary endpoint was the occurrence of ischemic or hemorrhagic stroke. After 2 years, the 150-mg dose was superior to warfarin at preventing stroke; the 110-mg dose showed similar efficacy as warfarin (Connolly, et al., 2009).

Mechanism of Action

Direct thrombin inhibitors, including dabigatran, bind to the active site of thrombin to prevent the generation of additional thrombin, decrease platelet activation stimulated by thrombin, and prevent the conversion of fibrinogen to fibrin. (See **Figure 49-1**.) Blocking thrombin is an effective method of inhibiting coagulation since thrombin is needed for fibrin formation and to activate factors V, VII, VIII, IX, and XIII. Dabigatran directly inhibits free and clot-bound thrombin. The anticoagulant response with dabigatran is more predictable than warfarin because it acts directly on thrombin, rather than working higher up in the clotting cascade (Spyropoulos, 2008).

Dabigatran has poor oral bioavailability (about 6%), so it is formulated as the pro-drug dabigatran etexilate to increase absorption. After administration, dabigatran etexilate is rapidly converted by esterases to active dabigatran (Boehringer Ingelheim, 2010). Dabigatran requires an acidic environment for absorption, and the capsules contain pellets with a tartaric acid core, which controls the pH to help increase the absorption rate (Eriksson, et al., 2009).

Dosage and Time Frame for Response

The predictable anticoagulation response with dabigatran allows for fixed dosing and does not require laboratory monitoring for adjusting doses. Dabigatran is approved in the United States for stroke prevention in atrial fibrillation. (See

TABLE 49.6	Characteristics of Warfarin and Dabigatran
Warfarin (Coumadin)	**Dabigatran (Pradaxa)**
Long history of use (60+ years)	
Slow onset of action (days)	Fast onset of action (hours)
Once-daily dosing	Twice-daily dosing
Narrow therapeutic window	Wide therapeutic window
Large number of FDA-approved indications	One indication—stroke prevention in atrial fibrillation
Variable dose response	More predictable dose response
Frequent adjustments	No dosage adjustments
Routine INR monitoring	No laboratory monitoring required for efficacy
Can assess adherence based on INR	No lab test to assess adherence
Multiple food and drug interactions	Limited drug interactions; no food interactions
Reliable antidote (vitamin K)	No antidote
Inexpensive (generic availability)	High cost
Patient inconvenience due to laboratory monitoring	Convenient to patient

Warfarin, a vitamin K antagonist, and dabigatran, a direct thrombin inhibitor, have different properties. When determining the most appropriate therapy for an individual patient, these different characteristics will translate into advantages and disadvantages.

Table 49.3.) The clearance of dabigatran occurs via the kidneys. Therefore, for atrial fibrillation in patients with normal renal function, a dose of 150 mg twice daily is recommended. A dosage of 75 mg twice daily is recommended for patients with severe renal impairment and creatinine clearance (CrCl) ranging from 15 to 30 mL/min. The clinical trial in patients with atrial fibrillation used to gain FDA approval (RE-LY) (Connolly, et al., 2009) used a 150-mg or 110-mg dosage regimen, but 110-mg tablets are not available in the United States. The manufacturer submitted pharmacokinetic data to the FDA to obtain approval of the 75-mg twice-daily dose (Wood, 2010). Because of the novelty of dabigatran, providers are likely to switch patients from other anticoagulants to the direct thrombin inhibitor. **Box 49.6** provides more information on switching anticoagulants.

A twice-daily dosage regimen is required with dabigatran because it has a half-life of about 14 to 17 hours. The time to maximal plasma concentrations occurs in 1.5 to 3 hours, and steady state occurs within 2 to 3 days; thus, the onset of anticoagulation is faster than with warfarin. Dabigatran can be given with or without meals (Eriksson, et al., 2009).

If a patient misses a dose of dabigatran and it is more than 6 hours until the next dose is due, the skipped dose can be taken at any time. If the next dabigatran dose is due in less than 6 hours, the patient should resume dosing at the appointed time and omit the skipped dose (Wood, 2010). If a patient requires surgery or an invasive procedure, dabigatran should be stopped either 1 to 2 days (in patients with CrCl ≥50 mL/min) or 3 to

5 days (in patients with CrCl <50 mL/minute) before the procedure (Boehringer Ingelheim, 2010).

Although the indication for dabigatran is currently limited to stroke prevention in atrial fibrillation, clinical trials have shown benefit for the prevention of VTE in hip and knee replacement surgery and for treatment of DVT. (See **Table 49.2.**) As dabigatran becomes more popular, it is likely to be used off-label for uses other than atrial fibrillation.

Contraindications

Contraindications to dabigatran listed in the package insert include active serious bleeding or hypersensitivity to the drug (e.g., anaphylaxis). Other reasonable contraindications include a CrCl less than 15 mL/minute or dialysis because no dosing instructions are provided by the manufacturer. Patients with prosthetic heart valves should not receive dabigatran because they were not included in the major clinical trial used to gain FDA approval (Wood, 2010).

Adverse Events

The major adverse effect reported with dabigatran is bleeding, and fatal bleeding has been reported. In the RE-LY trial, although the rate of major bleeding was similar for dabigatran 150 mg and warfarin (3.3% vs. 3.6%), the rate of major GI bleeding was higher with dabigatran (1.6% with dabigatran vs. 1.1% with warfarin), while warfarin had a higher rate of intracranial hemorrhage (0.8% with warfarin vs. 0.3% with dabigatran). The risk of bleeding was higher with the 150-mg twice-daily regimen than the 110-mg twice-daily regimen. (The 110-mg formulation is not available in the United States.) The risk of bleeding with dabigatran is increased if the patient is receiving concomitant therapy with other anticoagulant or antiplatelet drugs. A medication guide outlining the bleeding risks is supplied to the patient when the drug is dispensed.

Patients with active bleeding will require dabigatran to be discontinued. Fresh frozen plasma can be given if bleeding is severe. Unlike warfarin, which is reversed by vitamin K, there is no agent that will reverse dabigatran's effect, but hemodialysis is an option in overdoses (Boehringer Ingelheim, 2010).

Dabigatran has a low pH, and dyspepsia occurred in 10% of patients enrolled in the RE-LY trial with the 150-mg dose. If GI distress is a problem, taking the drug with food or acid-suppressing drugs (H$_2$ blockers or proton pump inhibitors) may be an option (Anonymous [*Pharmacist's Letter*], 2010). Despite these measures, some patients may not be able to tolerate therapy due to GI adverse effects. The potential for adverse events has previously been limited to the controlled setting of clinical trials, so the true safety profile of dabigatran won't be known until it gains more widespread use in patients who were not candidates for inclusion in the original trial.

Drug Interactions

Since dabigatran is cleared renally and is not metabolized by the hepatic CYP450 enzyme system, drug interactions via this route are not a concern, but interactions can occur through other

---

BOX 49.6

Switching Between Anticoagulant Drugs

Since dabigatran is a novel oral therapy, patients are likely to be switched from other anticoagulants to the direct thrombin inhibitor. Likewise, patients receiving dabigatran may require a change to another anticoagulant. In the RE-LY trial, after 2 years, 20% of patients receiving dabigatran discontinued therapy due to adverse events. There are several factors to consider when deciding whether to change to dabigatran in a patient who is currently taking warfarin, including the stability of international normalized ratio (INR) control, and whether the patient has been able to comply with laboratory visits. Patients who are well stabilized on warfarin should not have therapy changed to dabigatran unless there is a compelling reason. The dabigatran package insert provides guidance on how to switch between therapies.

Switching from warfarin to dabigatran. To reduce the risk of bleeding, discontinue warfarin first, and wait until the INR drops below 2 before starting the direct thrombin inhibitor.

Switching from dabigatran to warfarin. The patient's renal function will influence the time frame for starting warfarin.

Creatinine clearance (CrCl) >50 mL/min: warfarin therapy is initiated 3 days before discontinuing dabigatran.

Creatinine clearance (CrCl) 31 to 50 mL/min: warfarin therapy is initiated 2 days before discontinuing dabigatran.

Creatinine clearance (CrCl) 15–30 mL/min: warfarin therapy is initiated 1 day before discontinuing dabigatran.

Creatinine clearance (CrCl) <15 mL/min: no recommendations are provided in the package insert. However, severe renal dysfunction and dialysis can be considered relative contraindications to dabigatran therapy.

Converting from a parenteral anticoagulant to dabigatran. Dabigatran should be started within 2 hours before the next dose of subcutaneous unfractionated heparin (UFH) or low-molecular-weight heparin (LMWH) was due to be administered. For patients receiving intravenous (IV) UFH, start dabigatran when the IV UFH infusion is stopped.

Converting from dabigatran to a parenteral anticoagulant. If the CrCl is >30 mL/min, wait 12 hours after the last dose of dabigatran is administered before initiating treatment with subcutaneous UFH, LMWH, or IV UFH. If the CrCl is <30 mL/min, the waiting interval is 24 hours after the last dose of dabigatran is administered before initiating treatment with subcutaneous UFH, LMWH, or IV UFH.

Data from Boehringer Ingelheim. (2010). Product information for Pradaxa. Ridgefield, CT: Author.

---

mechanisms (Eriksson, et al, 2009). Dabigatran is a substrate for the P-glycoprotein (P-gp) transporter. Quinidine, a potent P-gp inhibitor, causes a 100% increase in dabigatran plasma concentrations due to reduced clearance of the drug. Amiodarone is a weak P-gp inhibitor and can increase dabigatran levels by 50%. Increased dabigatran plasma levels may potentially increase the risk of adverse events. However, in the RE-LY trial, patients receiving concomitant amiodarone did not experience problems due to this interaction (Eikelboom & Connolly, 2010). According to the dabigatran package insert, dosage adjustments are not required when dabigatran is administered with verapamil, amiodarone, or quinidine. Rifampin is a P-gp inducer and can reduce dabigatran plasma concentrations.

Dabigatran requires the acid pH found in the intestines and stomach for absorption, so an interaction with proton pump inhibitors (PPIs) and antacids is a potential concern. When dabigatran is administered with PPIs, absorption is reduced 2% to 25%, but this has not translated into clinically relevant effects (Eriksson, et al., 2009).

Unfractionated Heparin

UFH has been available since the 1940s, and although in several cases it has been replaced by LMWHs, it remains the preferred anticoagulant in selected patients due to its short half-life, established safety in patients with renal failure, and reversal of effects with protamine. UFH augments the inhibitory effects of antithrombin III, thus disrupting the clotting cascade. It is indicated for the prevention of VTE and the treatment of DVT and PE. UFH may also be used in the early treatment of unstable angina and acute MI and for those undergoing cardiac bypass, catheterization, and stenting.

Mechanism of Action

UFH inhibits reactions that lead to clotting, but it does not alter the concentration of the normal clotting factors of the blood. When UFH binds to antithrombin III, the shape of the structure changes, which increases the inactivation rate of the intrinsic clotting cascade pathway, including factors XII,

XI, X, IX, and thrombin (factor II). Once active thrombosis has developed, UFH inhibits further coagulation by inactivating thrombin and preventing the conversion of fibrinogen to fibrin. UFH is a very large molecule (i.e., it has an average molecular weight of 15,000 Da with chains of 18 to 50 saccharide units), but only a small portion of the entire structure is necessary for binding with antithrombin III. Because the structure is so large, UFH can bind to both factor Xa and thrombin. Heparin derivatives with smaller structures cannot bind to thrombin, but can bind to and inhibit factor Xa (Hirsh, et al., 2008). One disadvantage of heparin's large size is that it cannot inactivate clot-bound thrombin or activated factor X that is bound to platelets. Clot-bound thrombin can continue to generate more thrombin, activate platelets, and convert fibrinogen into fibrin, promoting clotting. In contrast to UFH, direct thrombin inhibitors do not activate platelets (Spyropoulos, 2008).

Heparin is not absorbed from the GI tract, so it must be administered parenterally. UFH has an immediate onset of action and is administered by intravenous (IV) infusion when rapid anticoagulation is needed, as in acute DVT, PE, or unstable angina. UFH may also be administered subcutaneously with peak levels occurring 2 to 4 hours after administration, depending on the dose. Subcutaneous dosing must be at a sufficient amount to overcome the lower bioavailability, approximately 30%, associated with this route of administration. The duration of action and half-life are dose-dependent. The average half-life is 30 to 180 minutes, which may be significantly prolonged at high doses. UFH is metabolized by liver heparinase and the reticuloendothelial system and possibly secondarily in the kidneys. It is then excreted in urine as unchanged drug (Lexi-Comp Online, 2010).

Limitations of UFH include variability in its size, anticoagulant activity, and pharmacokinetic profile. UFH can range in size from 5,000 to 30,000 Da. Agents with higher molecular weights are cleared from the circulation more rapidly than agents with lower molecular weights. UFH is highly bound to plasma proteins and cellular components, including endothelial cells and macrophages, which reduces its therapeutic effect and increases the incidence of immunologic reactions (e.g., heparin-induced thrombocytopenia [HIT]). Furthermore, some patients exhibit heparin resistance. This is characterized by no measurable change in anticoagulant effect despite receiving large doses (35,000 units) of heparin daily. UFH also has a nonlinear dose response, so that small changes in dosage can result in large changes in anticoagulant effect (Hirsh, et al., 2008).

Dosage and Time Frame for Response

UFH dosing is based on weight. Initial dosing should be 80 units/kg as an IV bolus and then 18 units/kg/hour as a continuous IV infusion. UFH's effect is monitored by aPTT. Dosage changes should be made based on aPTT levels monitored every 6 hours until the patient is stable and then every 12 hours. For DVT or PE treatment, a therapeutic aPTT of 1.5 to 2.5 times control must be achieved within the first 24 hours of therapy to reduce the rate of recurrent thrombotic

TABLE 49.7	Weight-Based Heparin-Dosing Nomogram
Activated Partial Thromboplastin Time	**Rate Change**
Initial dose	80 U/kg bolus, then 18 U/kg/h
<35 (<1.2 × control)	80 U/kg bolus, then increase infusion by 4 U/kg/h
35–45 (1.2–1.5 × control)	40 U/kg/h bolus, then increase infusion by 2 U/kg/h
46–70 (1.5–2.3 × control)	No change
71–90 (2.3–3 × control)	Decrease infusion rate by 2 U/kg/h
>90 (>3 × control)	Hold infusion for 1 h, then decrease infusion rate by 3 U/kg/h

Adapted from Hirsh., J., Bauer, K. A., Donati, M. B., et al. (2008). Parenteral anticoagulants. American College of Chest Physicians Evidence-Based Clinical Practical Guidelines (8th Edition). *Chest, 133*(6 Suppl.), 141S–159S.

events and decrease mortality. Several dosing nomograms are available to assist clinicians in rapidly attaining a therapeutic aPTT within the first day of therapy. One popular method is the weight-based nomogram (Hirsh, et al., 2008) shown in **Table 49.7**. Anticoagulation may be subtherapeutic with UFH despite the use of validated dosing protocols.

Adjusted-dose subcutaneous heparin has been used in patients with limited IV access or in those with contraindications to warfarin (e.g., pregnancy). Intramuscular injections are not recommended because of the increased risk of bleeding and bruising. UFH in a fixed low dose of 5,000 units subcutaneously every 8 to 12 hours is used for VTE prophylaxis and reduces the risk of VTE by 60% to 70%. This regimen may be used in postoperative patients and medical patients with decreased mobility (Hirsh, et al., 2008).

Contraindications

Contraindications to heparin use are hypersensitivity to heparin products, active bleeding, severe thrombocytopenia, and history of HIT.

Adverse Events

Adverse effects associated with UFH include bleeding, osteoporosis, and thrombocytopenia. (See **Table 49.3**.) Other non-hemorrhagic adverse events (skin reactions, alopecia, and hypersensitivity) are uncommon (Hirsh, et al., 2008). The risk of bleeding increases in patients who have preexisting renal failure, hepatic disease, or cardiovascular disease; who have sustained recent trauma or surgery; who have had recent CNS procedures, such as surgery or spinal anesthesia; who have a history of or current GI lesions or bleeding; who have a hematologic disorder; and who are using aspirin concurrently. Risk of bleeding with heparin is enhanced with increasing heparin doses and when concomitantly used with other anticoagulants, antiplatelets, or fibrinolytics. Excessive anticoagulation with UFH can be reversed with IV protamine sulfate, which rapidly binds to heparin, forming a stable salt (Hirsh, et al., 2008).

The mechanism causing heparin-induced osteoporosis is not fully understood. UFH is thought to impair bone deposition and accelerate bone resorption. This is a concern in those requiring long-term treatment with UFH, especially with heparin doses of more than 20,000 units/d administered for more than 3 months or UFH doses less than 20,000 units/d given for longer than 12 months. Pregnant women receiving UFH are particularly at risk for osteoporosis since they may receive heparin for the duration of gestation. A baseline bone density scan and supplementation with calcium can be considered here.

Thrombocytopenia during heparin therapy may be mild, remain stable, and possibly reverse itself during therapy. However, platelet counts should be closely monitored during heparin therapy because a drop in platelet count below 150×10^9/L or greater than 50% of baseline necessitates discontinuation of heparin therapy. This may be related to HIT, an antibody-mediated reaction. The clinical effects can result in DVT, PE, MI, limb ischemia, gangrene requiring limb amputation, cerebral thrombosis, and death. Discontinuation of all heparin sources such as heparin flushes and heparin-coated catheters is required for platelet counts to normalize. In patients in which HIT is strongly suspected or confirmed, factor Xa inhibitors given subcutaneously (fondaparinux) or intravenously (danaparoid) or intravenously administered direct thrombin inhibitors (recombinant hirudin, argatroban, and bivalirudin) are preferred over further use of LMWHs or UFH. Note that danaparoid is not available in the United States and that fondaparinux and bivalirudin are used off-label for HIT and are not approved by the FDA for this use (Warkentin, 2010).

Low-Molecular-Weight Heparins

LMWHs are fragments of UFH, prepared by the depolymerization of porcine heparin. Like UFH, LMWHs produce their major anticoagulant effect via thrombin and factor Xa. LMWHs are used for prophylaxis of VTE in patients after orthopedic and abdominal surgery, in medical patients with decreased mobility or increased risk of VTE, and for treatment of DVT/PE. As with UFH, most patients need subsequent treatment with warfarin, depending on the indication for anticoagulation. Other uses that will not be discussed in this chapter include the treatment of unstable angina and MI.

Three LMWHs are available in the United States: dalteparin (Fragmin), enoxaparin (Lovenox), and tinzaparin (Innohep).

Mechanism of Action

LMWHs preferentially inhibit the activation of factor X but have minimal effects on thrombin (factor II) because of their small size. The average molecular weight of LMWHs ranges from 4,000 to 6,500 Da with 13 to 22 saccharide units. (UFH has a mean molecular weight of 12,000 to 15,000 Da with 18 to 50 saccharide units.) Only the LMWHs with saccharide chains having 18 or more units can bind to and inhibit thrombin. UFH has a ratio of anti-Xa to anti-IIa activity of 1:1, and the anti-Xa to anti-IIa activity of LMWHs ranges from 2:1 to 4:1 (Hirsh, et al., 2008). Refer to **Table 49.3** and **Table 49.8** for comparisons of the LMWHs and the factor Xa inhibitor fondaparinux.

LMWHs given by the subcutaneous route have a bioavailability of greater than 90% of the given dose. In contrast to UFH, LMWHs have minimal binding to cells or plasma proteins, which results in the persistence of free drug in the circulation and a longer half-life of activity. The half-lives of LMWHs range from 108 to 252 minutes. Dosing is fixed in prophylaxis, but is based on weight for treatment.

As previously noted, the major antithrombotic and bleeding effects of LMWHs arise through their ability to inactivate factor Xa. UFH is monitored using aPTT, which primarily reflects anti–activated factor II (IIa) activity, but LMWHs have minimal effects on the aPTT. Theoretically, LMWHs may be monitored by anti–factor Xa activity, with a target range for treatment regimens of 0.5 to 1.2 units/mL 3 to 4 hours after a subcutaneous dose. Studies have demonstrated that the anti-Xa effect of LMWHs is linearly related to the dose administered. Therefore, plasma levels are predictable, and anti-Xa activity monitoring is not routinely performed. Monitoring may be considered in selected patients, such as those with renal dysfunction because LMWHs are cleared primarily by the renal route, morbidly obese patients (150 kg) because weight-adjusted dosing has not been evaluated in patients with severe obesity, and pregnant patients because their weight changes, volume shifts occur, and clearance changes as pregnancy progresses. In addition to the recommendation for monitoring anti-Xa levels in patients with renal dysfunction, dosing reductions of 50% are

TABLE 49.8	Pharmacokinetic Profiles of SC Low-Molecular-Weight Heparins and Factor Xa Inhibitors			
Product	**Trade Name**	**Molecular Weight (Da)**	**Half-Life (h)**	**Anti-Xa/IIa Ratio**
dalteparin	Fragmin	5,000	3	2.7:1
enoxaparin	Lovenox	4,500	4.5	3.8:1
tinzaparin	Innohep	4,500	3–4	1.9:1
fondaparinux	Arixtra	1,728	17–21	Not applicable –does not inactivate factor IIa

recommended when using LMWHs in patients with a CrCl of less than 30 mL/min. UFH can be used in these patients instead of LMWHs (Hirsh, et al., 2008).

Advantages of LMWHs over UFH include greater bio-availability with subcutaneous administration; longer duration of anticoagulant effect, allowing for once-daily or twice-daily dosing; high degree of correlation between anti-Xa and body weight, allowing for fixed dosing; less intensive nursing care; and less intensive laboratory monitoring and more predictable anticoagulant response, permitting use in the outpatient setting (Hull & Pineo, 2004). The treatment of DVT and PE can now occur in the home, reducing hospital lengths of stay and costs.

Dosage and Time Frame for Response

Each LMWH has a unique dosing regimen because of its unique chemical properties and the relative proportions of anti-Xa to anti-IIa activity. (See **Table 49.8**.) Because of differences in the manufacturing process, molecular weight, half-life, ratio of anti-Xa to anti-IIa activity, and dose, the FDA does not consider these agents therapeutically interchangeable (Hirsh, et al., 2008). Enoxaparin at 30 mg every 12 hours or 40 mg daily is currently approved for prophylaxis in medical inpatients and patients after hip, knee, and abdominal surgery. Dalteparin at 2,500 units every 12 hours or 5,000 units daily is approved for prophylaxis in patients after hip and abdominal surgery. For VTE treatment, current FDA-approved dosing for enoxaparin is 1 mg/kg every 12 hours or 1.5 mg/kg daily for inpatients with acute DVT with and without PE when administered in conjunction with warfarin and for outpatients with acute DVT without PE when administered in conjunction with warfarin. Tinzaparin 175 international units/kg daily is FDA approved for inpatient treatment of acute DVT with and without PE when administered in conjunction with warfarin.

Contraindications

Contraindications to LMWH use are active major bleeding, indwelling epidural catheters, hypersensitivity to LMWHs or pork products, and history of HIT associated with LMWHs (Sanofi Aventis, 2010).

Adverse Effects

Adverse effects associated with LMWHs include bleeding, thrombocytopenia, and elevations in liver function test results. Less common effects are injection-site reactions, fever, nausea, wound hematoma, and hypochromic anemia. Hemorrhage is the most common complication of LMWH therapy, along with hematoma at the injection or surgical site. The incidence of hemorrhage is similar to or slightly lower than that of UFH. The aPTT is not used to monitor therapeutic efficacy, and a patient receiving LMWHs should have periodic CBC and platelet monitoring and Hemoccult testing to assess for bleeding. There is no proven method for reversing excessive anticoagulation occurring with LMWHs, although consensus guidelines provide dosing recommendations for using

protamine. The incidence of thrombocytopenia is much lower than with UFH. Transient, benign thrombocytopenia is seen in approximately 5% of patients treated with LMWHs. The immune-mediated thrombocytopenia, HIT, has been reported in less than 1% of patients. In patients with active or previous HIT, thrombocytopenia may be reproduced during the use of LMWHs with a reported cross-reactivity in HIT of more than 90%. Asymptomatic elevations in aspartate aminotransferase and alanine aminotransferase levels have been reported with LMWHs; elevations are reversible when the drug is discontinued. As previously described, patients with renal insufficiency may have reduced LMWH elimination. Therefore, careful use is recommended, including dosage reduction or monitoring of anti-Xa concentrations. LMWHs are less likely to cause osteoporosis than UFH (Hirsh, et al., 2008).

Factor Xa Inhibitor—Fondaparinux

Fondaparinux (Arixtra) is an injectable product similar to LMWHs; it is an indirect factor Xa inhibitor—it reversibly binds to antithrombin, but has little effect on platelet aggregation (Spyropoulos, 2008). The structure contains a 5-saccharide chain that has a smaller molecular weight than LMWHs. (See **Table 49.8**.) Unlike LMWHs or UFH, which are derived from porcine sources, fondaparinux is synthetic.

Fondaparinux is rapidly absorbed after subcutaneous administration, and the half-life is 17 hours. It produces a predictable anticoagulant response and is dosed once daily. As with LMWHs, anticoagulation monitoring is not necessary with fondaparinux (Hirsh, et al., 2008).

FDA-approved indications for fondaparinux include prophylaxis of DVT/PE in patients after hip fracture and hip or knee replacement surgery, after abdominal surgery, and for the treatment of DVT and PE when administered with warfarin. For VTE prophylaxis, the dose is 2.5 mg subcutaneously daily. VTE treatment doses vary based on patient weight, ranging from 5 mg (for patients weighing <50 kg), 7.5 mg (for patients weighing 75 to 100 kg), and 10 mg (for patients >100 kg). In studies for orthopedic surgery prophylaxis of VTE, fondaparinux was more effective than the LMWH enoxaparin when given in a daily subcutaneous dose of 2.5 mg, but it had a higher rate of bleeding. One advantage of this drug is that there is no interaction with platelets. Fondaparinux has been found to be safe and effective for the prevention and treatment of VTE in patients with a prior history of HIT. Consensus guidelines recommend fondaparinux over LMWHs or UFH in patients with HIT. The clearance of fondaparinux is decreased in renal impairment, so a 50% reduction in dose is required (Hirsh, et al., 2008).

Aspirin

Aspirin is the oldest and most frequently used antiplatelet drug. Antiplatelet agents, such as aspirin, decrease platelet aggregation and decrease the formation of arterial thrombi. Aspirin is commonly used in patients for primary prevention of atherosclerotic heart disease to reduce the risk of subsequent

MI, stroke, and vascular death. It is also used in patients to prevent TIAs and acute ischemic stroke secondary to cerebral vascular disease. Aspirin has also been used as an alternative therapy for patients with atrial fibrillation who are considered poor candidates for anticoagulation and who have no high or moderate risk factors and no clinical or echocardiographic evidence of cardiovascular disease (Patrono, et al., 2008). Aspirin use in atherosclerotic heart disease will not be discussed in this chapter.

Mechanism of Action

Aspirin prevents prostaglandin synthesis in platelets and other tissues by irreversibly modifying and inhibiting the enzyme COX, which catalyzes the conversion of arachidonic acid to thromboxane A_2, a prostaglandin derivative, which is a potent vasoconstrictor and promoter of platelet aggregation. After discontinuing aspirin, platelets are impaired for their normal life span of 7 to 10 days because of the irreversible inhibition of COX. Every 24 hours, 10% of platelets are replaced; 5 to 6 days after aspirin ingestion, approximately 50% of platelets function normally (Patrono, et al., 2008).

Aspirin is rapidly absorbed in the stomach and upper intestine with peak levels occurring 30 to 40 minutes after ingestion. Inhibition of platelet function is evident by 1 hour after ingestion. The half-life of aspirin is 15 to 20 minutes and salicylic acid, to which aspirin is hydrolyzed during absorption, has a half-life of 2 to 3 hours at low doses and may exceed 20 hours at higher doses. Aspirin is eliminated by renal excretion (Lexi-Comp Online, 2010).

Dosage and Time Frame for Response

The optimal aspirin dosage for thrombotic disorders is still controversial because doses ranging from 30 to 1,500 mg/d are effective (Albers, et al., 2008; Adams, et al., 2008). Inhibition of platelet aggregation can be shown at doses as low as 20 mg/d given over several days. Maximal inhibition of platelet aggregation occurs at doses of 80 to 100 mg/d. Higher doses of aspirin have other effects such as acetylation of fibrinogen, which results in a diminished capacity for fibrinogen to form fibrin and formation of a fibrin product that is more susceptible to lysis. It is not yet known how these nonplatelet effects of aspirin contribute to its overall antithrombotic properties. Randomized trials have found lower aspirin doses ranging between 50 and 100 mg/d effective as an antithrombotic agent (Patrono, et al., 2008).

Efficacy of aspirin is well established for secondary prevention of noncardioembolic stroke; its use in primary prevention is less well established. The largest trial of antiplatelet agents, the Antiplatelet Trialists' Collaboration, evaluated over 100,000 patients in 145 trials. The study concluded that antiplatelet agents were beneficial in patients with a history of ischemic stroke or TIA (25% reduction in stroke) and that larger aspirin doses were no more effective than smaller doses. This analysis showed that aspirin doses of 75 to 325 mg/d were as effective as higher doses in secondary prevention in high-risk patients. However, aspirin doses lower than 300 mg/d produced fewer GI adverse events than doses of 1,200 mg/d (Antithrombic Trialists' Collaboration, 2002). Gastric erosions and hemorrhage can occur even with short courses of aspirin therapy, and enteric-coated preparations do not always prevent GI complications. As a result, the lowest effective aspirin dose should be used. Because of its low cost and relatively good safety profile, aspirin is the standard therapy for patients experiencing a first episode of acute, noncardioembolic, ischemic stroke (**Table 49.9**). When used for stroke prevention in low-risk patients with atrial fibrillation who have a contraindication to anticoagulation therapy with warfarin, an aspirin dose of 75 to 325 mg/d is recommended (Singer, et al. 2008; Fuster, et al., 2006).

Contraindications and Adverse Effects

Aspirin's contraindications are active stroke or stroke in progress, active GI bleeding, or aspirin allergy or hypersensitivity. The most common adverse effects of aspirin are GI upset, such as nausea, dyspepsia, heartburn, epigastric discomfort, anorexia, and bleeding. These effects are dose related and are more likely to occur at doses greater than 325 mg/d. Although lower aspirin doses cause fewer GI symptoms, they still can cause significant GI bleeding. Aspirin may also potentiate peptic ulcer disease. Caution should be exercised when using aspirin with other drugs that affect platelet function (e.g., NSAIDs, clopidogrel, ticlopidine) or anticoagulants because the bleeding potential will be increased. Chronic therapy may cause persistent iron deficiency anemia. Although modest and unpredictable, aspirin can also prolong bleeding time, and some studies suggest it may increase postoperative bleeding. Other possible adverse effects are leukopenia, thrombocytopenia, purpura, shortened erythrocyte survival time, hives, rash, and angioedema (Lexi-Comp Online, 2010).

Aspirin/Dipyridamole

A combination product containing 25 mg aspirin and 200 mg extended-release dipyridamole (Aggrenox) administered twice daily is available for preventing recurrent stroke in patients who have experienced a TIA or previous ischemic stroke. Dipyridamole inhibits platelet adhesion, but its full mechanism of action is unknown. A European trial conducted in 6,000 patients (ESPS2) was the basis for FDA approval of this agent. Efficacy was also confirmed in a second trial (ESPRIT). The most common adverse effects include GI complaints, diarrhea, and headache. Elevations in hepatic enzymes have also been reported. Contraindications for aspirin with dipyridamole include hypersensitivity or allergy to aspirin or NSAIDs and active peptic ulcer disease. The drug is now considered an initial choice for preventing noncardioembolic stroke along with aspirin or clopidogrel, but clinically it is usually used as an alternative to aspirin (Adams, et al., 2008; Albers et al., 2008). The section "Selecting the Most Appropriate Agent" provides more information.

TABLE 49.9	Recommended Order of Treatment for Coagulation Disturbances	
Order	**Agent**	**Comments**
DVT/PE		
Initial therapy	Heparin, LMWH, or fondaparinux	Can now treat with LMWH in the outpatient setting
Long term	Warfarin	Consider patient risk factors for duration of therapy.
Orthopedic Surgery Prophylaxis		
First line	LMWH, fondaparinux, or warfarin	LMWH is more effective than warfarin but bleeding risk is increased. Duration of warfarin therapy is controversial.
Second line	UFH or IPC	UFH is a more complex option. IPC recommended in patients at high risk for bleeding
Third line	ASA, UFH, dextran	Refer to American College of Chest Physicians Guidelines for more information. Sole therapy with these agents is not recommended.
Secondary Prevention of Noncardioembolic Ischemic Stroke		
First line	ASA, ASA/dipyridamole, or clopidogrel	ASA is inexpensive, relatively safe; use clopidogrel in ASA-sensitive patients.
Second line	ASA/dipyridamole or clopidogrel	Clopidogrel is an option for patients with ASA allergy. Refer to the text for further information on characteristics to consider for first- vs. second-line therapy.
Third line	Ticlopidine	Risk of neutropenia
Atrial Fibrillation Prevention of Cardioembolic Stroke		
First line	Warfarin or dabigatran	Choice is based on patient risk factors and cost.
Second line	ASA	Choice is based on patient risk factors.
Third line	ASA with clopidogrel	The combination of aspirin with clopidogrel might be considered in patients when anticoagulation with warfarin is unsuitable, but warfarin is superior at preventing strokes. Refer to professional guidelines from the American Stroke Society/American Heart Association and the American College of Chest Physicians for more details.

ASA, aspirin; IPC, intermittent pneumatic compression; LMWH, low-molecular-weight heparin; UFH, unfractionated heparin

Clopidogrel

Dosage and Time Frame for Response

Clopidogrel and ticlopidine are structurally related antiplatelet agents that differ mechanistically from aspirin. These agents do not affect COX but prevent platelet aggregation by inhibiting adenosine diphosphate (ADP), a promoter of platelet receptor binding (Patrono, et al., 2008). A clopidogrel dose of 75 mg/d irreversibly inhibits ADP-mediated platelet aggregation. (See **Table 49.3**.) Dose-dependent inhibition of platelet aggregation is seen 2 hours after a single oral dose, and platelet aggregation and bleeding time return to baseline approximately 5 days after discontinuing clopidogrel. Clopidogrel is a pro-drug and must be activated (biotransformed) to inhibit platelet aggregation. Clopidogrel is extensively metabolized by the liver (Lexi-Comp Online, 2010).

Clopidogrel received FDA approval based on one major study, the CAPRIE (Clopidogrel Versus Aspirin in Patients at Risk of Ischemic Events) trial. A clopidogrel dosage of 75 mg/d was compared with aspirin 325 mg/d in more than 6,000 patients. The effects of clopidogrel were similar to those of aspirin in decreasing the risk of stroke, but clopidogrel was superior to aspirin when ischemic stroke, MI, and vascular death were considered together; the relative risk reduction in favor of clopidogrel over aspirin was 8.7% (Patrono, et al.,

2008; Albers, et al., 2008). Current FDA-labeled indications for clopidogrel are prophylaxis against thrombotic events in patients with recent MI, recent stroke, and peripheral arterial disease. Clopidogrel is also frequently used for prophylaxis against thrombosis in acute coronary syndrome in patients undergoing percutaneous coronary intervention (Bristol-Myers Squibb/Sanofi Aventis, 2010). It is now recommended that clopidogrel plus aspirin be given prior to coronary intervention and continued for 9 months to 1 year or longer for patients with coronary artery stents. Dual antiplatelet therapy with clopidogrel and aspirin has not proven successful to prevent recurrent stroke in patients after a previous noncardioembolic stroke or TIA. When clopidogrel was given with aspirin for stroke prevention in patients with atrial fibrillation who were unable to take warfarin, there was a higher risk of bleeding with the combination versus aspirin alone, although the rate of major vascular events was decreased (ACTIVE-A).

Contraindications and Adverse Events

Bleeding is the primary risk of clopidogrel therapy, and the risk is increased in the setting of dual antiplatelet therapy with aspirin. In the CAPRIE trial, there was no major difference between clopidogrel and aspirin in terms of safety, although there was a slightly higher rate of serious hemorrhage in the patients receiving aspirin. Clopidogrel is considered to have a safety profile similar to that of 325 mg/d dose of aspirin (Patrono, et al., 2008). Contraindications to clopidogrel are active major bleeding, including from peptic ulcer or intracranial hemorrhage. Other possible adverse effects of clopidogrel, occurring in more than 3% of patients, include dyspepsia, abdominal pain, diarrhea, and nausea. Rash occurs rarely (Lexi-Comp Online, 2010). Neutropenia is not a concern with clopidogrel, as it is with ticlopidine.

Drug Interactions

Bioactivation of clopidogrel occurs via cytochrome P450 isoenzymes, with the CYP2C19 isoenzyme being the most important. Patients vary in their ability to biotransform clopidogrel because the activity of CYP2C19 is controlled genetically. An early communication from the FDA in January 2009 acknowledged that clopidogrel was less effective in some patients and that genetic differences in drug metabolism likely accounted for the reduced effectiveness. Another mechanism for reduced clopidogrel activity is via inhibition of CYP2C19 by interacting drugs. PPIs are frequently given with clopidogrel to protect against GI bleeding. Omeprazole is a strong inhibitor of CYP2C19 and reduces the conversion of clopidogrel to the active form. Reduced antiplatelet activity occurs to a lesser extent when pantoprazole is given with clopidogrel, based on pharmacokinetic data. An FDA public health advisory in November 2009 recommended against using clopidogrel with any PPI except pantoprazole. Several retrospective reviews of pharmacy claims databases reported that patients receiving a PPI, most commonly omeprazole, with clopidogrel had reduced effectiveness of the antiplatelet drug, shown by an increase in cardiovascular events, including MI, hospitalization for acute coronary syndrome, and all-cause mortality (Abraham, et al., 2010). Only one randomized trial has prospectively examined cardiovascular event rates in patients receiving clopidogrel 75 mg/d with omeprazole 20 mg/d (Bhatt, et al., 2010). The study was terminated early due to the manufacturer going into bankruptcy, but an interim analysis showed no significant difference in the incidence of cardiovascular death, MI, or stroke in patients receiving clopidogrel with omeprazole compared to a placebo. The combination did protect against GI bleeding; the number of GI events was similar between a placebo and the antiplatelet/PPI combination. Limitations to the trial include that it was not powered to detect differences in cardiovascular events and it was terminated early after a median duration of 133 days, which may not have been long enough to show a difference in outcomes. There is ongoing controversy regarding the clinical impact of this drug interaction. Current joint consensus from leading cardiology and gastroenterology groups is that PPIs are appropriate in patients with multiple risk factors for GI bleeding (e.g., history of ulcer disease, dual antiplatelet therapy, concomitant anticoagulant therapy, advanced age) who require antiplatelet therapy (Abraham, et al., 2010). Omeprazole is available OTC, so its cost is significantly lower than the prescription PPIs, which may be of importance to patients on limited incomes.

Ticlopidine

Ticlopidine is a prodrug that is hepatically metabolized to its active form. The usual dose is 250 mg administered twice daily. The full antiplatelet effect requires 3 to 5 days of oral administration. Although the drug's half-life is 24 to 36 hours, antiplatelet effects persist for up to 10 days after ticlopidine discontinuation, paralleling the platelet life span. The FDA-approved indications for ticlopidine include the secondary prevention of TIAs and ischemic stroke in patients who have had a stroke despite receiving aspirin therapy and coronary artery stenting. Currently, clopidogrel is primarily used after coronary stent placement (Patrono, et al., 2008). Neutropenia is the most serious adverse effect of ticlopidine, affecting approximately 2% of patients. The greatest risk of neutropenia occurs within the first 3 months of therapy; neutropenia is reversible within 1 to 3 weeks of drug discontinuation. The FDA requires CBC monitoring every 2 weeks for the first 3 months of therapy. Ticlopidine must be discontinued if the absolute neutrophil count (ANC) falls below 1,200/mm^3 or if the platelet count drops lower than 80,000/mm^3. Patients need to inform the clinician of any symptoms of neutropenia, such as fever, chills, or sore throat. Due to the risk of life-threatening blood dyscrasias such as neutropenia, agranulocytosis, and thrombotic thrombocytopenic purpura, ticlopidine is reserved for patients who are intolerant or allergic to aspirin or in whom aspirin therapy has failed and who are not candidates for clopidogrel. Hepatotoxicity is another rare complication of ticlopidine, and baseline liver function tests along with a CBC should be ordered and results reviewed before therapy is initiated. These effects include GI toxicity, rash, and bleeding complications such as ecchymosis, epistaxis, hematuria, conjunctival hemorrhage, GI bleeding, and posttraumatic and preoperative bleeding. (See **Table 49.3.**) Adverse effects are relatively common with at least one being reported in more than 50% of patients (Lexi-Comp Online, 2010). Use of ticlopidine has largely fallen into disfavor because of the adverse event profile.

Selecting the Most Appropriate Agent

In cases of DVT or PE, all patients receive LMWHs, fondaparinux, or heparin first. Then, drug therapy switches over to oral drug therapy with warfarin. Warfarin is also commonly used in thromboembolism prevention in atrial fibrillation and native or prosthetic heart valvular disease. For more information, see **Table 49.9** and **Figure 49-2**.

Deep Vein Thrombosis or Pulmonary Embolism
First-Line Therapy

All patients with a diagnostically confirmed DVT of the proximal leg veins or diagnostically confirmed PE should receive a bolus of IV UFH followed by a continuous IV infusion of UFH, adjusted-dose subcutaneous heparin, subcutaneous LMWHs, or subcutaneous fondaparinux as initial therapy. A UFH IV bolus followed by continuous IV UFH, LMWH, or

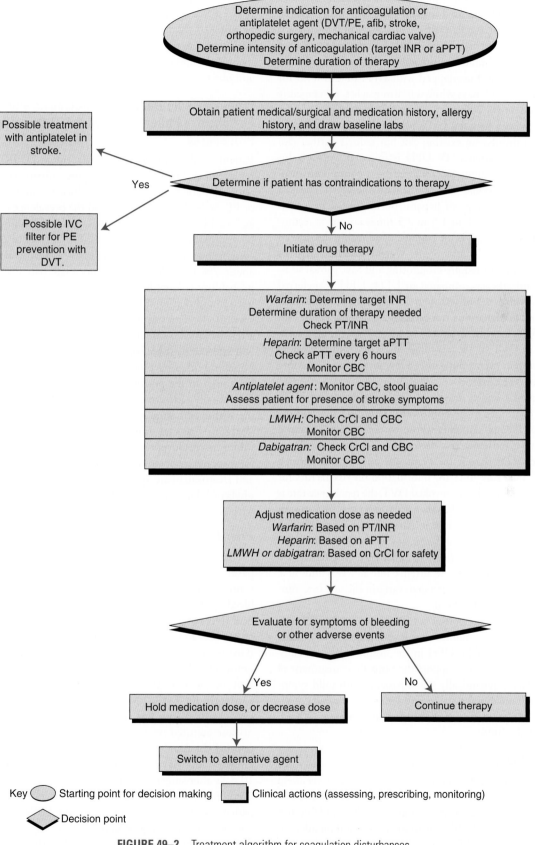

FIGURE 49–2 Treatment algorithm for coagulation disturbances.

fondaparinux therapy may also be started before a definitive diagnosis in patients with a high clinical suspicion of VTE. UFH and LMWHs are used initially for DVT or PE because of their rapid anticoagulant effect. However, oral anticoagulation with warfarin is recommended for the remainder of therapy. Warfarin should be initiated on day 1 after confirmation of DVT/PE and overlapped with UFH or LMWHs for approximately 4 to 5 days while warfarin reaches a therapeutic level (Kearon, et al., 2008).

Therapy with heparin, LMWHs, fondaparinux, or warfarin does dissolve an existing clot but reduces further clot extension and recurrence. IV UFH is initiated with a bolus of 80 international units/kg, followed by a continuous infusion at 18 international units/kg/h, with the aPTT checked every 6 hours. A dosage of heparin during initial treatment that prolongs the aPTT to 1.5 to 2.5 times normal is recommended. **Table 49.7** gives an example of adjusting the dose of UFH based on weight and aPTT. Weight-based LMWH or fondaparinux do not require monitoring and have shown similar safety and efficacy compared to UFH. UFH is preferred in patients with CrCl of less than 30 mL/min. Subcutaneous LMWH and fondaparinux can accumulate in renal failure and require a 50% decrease in dose. The target INR for long-term treatment of DVT or PE is a range of 2 to 3, which protects against recurrent events but causes a low incidence of bleeding complications (Kearon, et al., 2008).

Warfarin is widely used to prevent recurrence of VTE, but there continues to be controversy regarding the optimal duration of therapy. Patients whose thrombus can be traced to reversible (transient) risk factors have a lower incidence of recurrent VTE than if the event was unprovoked (termed *idiopathic*). (See **Box 49.1** for information on risk factors for VTE.) For patients with a provoked DVT, the recurrence rate is less than 5% at year 1 and less than 15% at 5 years. A 3-month course of warfarin is sufficient in patients with reversible risk factors, if the provoking risk factor has resolved. Patients with idiopathic VTE are more likely to experience recurrent DVT than provoked events (10% recurrence rate at 1 year and 30% recurrence rate at 5 years); extended warfarin therapy is recommended (Kearon, et al., 2008).

As mentioned previously, an advantage of LMWHs is that anticoagulation monitoring is not necessary. Studies comparing the use of IV UFH in the hospital with subcutaneous LMWHs at home support the outpatient treatment of LMWHs. Hemodynamically stable patients with mild symptoms, normal renal function, and no serious co-morbid conditions may be candidates for the outpatient treatment of VTE (Kearon, et al., 2008).

Nondrug Therapy

An inferior vena cava (IVC) filter or umbrella filter (Greenfield filter) is inserted percutaneously into the IVC and traps thrombi in the leg veins to prevent migration to the lungs (Anderson & Bussey, 2006). IVC filter placement is recommended in patients with proximal DVT or PE in which anticoagulants are contraindicated due to risk of bleeding. However, the routine use of IVC filters in addition to anticoagulation is not recommended for patients with DVT or PE. If the patient's bleeding risk resolves, a conventional course of anticoagulation should be initiated (Kearon, et al., 2008). Vena cava filters have not been shown to decrease mortality. Complications of IVC filters include thrombosis, migration of the filter (rarely to the heart), and obstruction of the vena cava.

Prophylaxis for Deep Vein Thrombosis and Pulmonary Embolism in Patients Undergoing Orthopedic Procedures

Patients undergoing total hip replacement (THR), total knee replacement (TKR), or hip fracture surgery should receive anticoagulation prophylaxis to reduce the high risk of DVT or PE. Several studies have found the prevalence of total DVT at 7 to 14 days after THR, TKR, and hip fracture surgery to be approximately 50% to 60%. The incidence of PE is less certain, but in studies in which a V/Q scan was performed, about 7% to 11% of THR and TKR patients had a high probability scan within 7 to 14 days after surgery. It has also been found that total DVT rate is greater in TKR than THR. Overall, the data suggest that asymptomatic VTE is common after orthopedic surgery and, in the absence of prophylaxis, will affect at least half of these patients (Geerts, et al., 2008). Numerous pharmacologic and nonpharmacologic agents have been used in the postoperative setting to decrease the risk of DVT or PE. Effective drugs for prophylaxis of VTE following orthopedic surgery include LMWHs, fondaparinux, and warfarin. The oral direct thrombin inhibitors and factor Xa inhibitors could potentially be added as therapeutic options for prophylaxis pending approval by the FDA. Dabigatran and rivaroxaban are approved in Europe and Canada for prophylaxis following THR and TKR based on comparative trials with enoxaparin.

First-Line Therapy

For patients undergoing THR or TKR, LMWHs and fondaparinux are considered more effective than warfarin in preventing VTE, but they do have a higher risk of surgical site bleeding and hematoma. However, warfarin therapy with a goal INR range of 2 to 3 is effective prophylaxis in this group of patients and causes less bleeding risk if monitored properly (Geerts, et al., 2008). Therefore, the consensus guidelines recommend that a decision between the use of LMWHs and warfarin be made on an institutional level (Geerts, et al., 2008). Currently, for THR, LMWH therapy or adjusted-dose warfarin is recommended as first-line therapy. For TKR, LMWH or dose-adjusted warfarin therapy is also recommended. The optimal duration of prophylaxis after THR and TKR is not known. Prophylactic therapy is recommended for at least 7 to 10 days after surgery (Geerts, et al., 2008). However, warfarin is commonly administered for 3 to 6 weeks after surgery. In patients having surgery for hip fracture, LMWHs or adjusted-dose warfarin with a goal range of 2 to 3 is recommended as first-line therapy, but the bleeding risk with these agents must be considered.

Second-Line Therapy

Second-line therapy recommended for THR in patients with increased risk of bleeding is the use of adjusted-dose UFH started preoperatively, but this is a more complex option and not favored by most surgeons. Additional prophylaxis with intermittent pneumatic compression (IPC) devices is thought to improve efficacy, but it must be applied intraoperatively or immediately postoperatively and worn continuously (at least 23 hours a day) until the patient is fully ambulatory. For TKR, UFH is not recommended, but an alternative therapy is the optimal use of IPC devices. For hip fracture surgery, a second-line, alternative treatment is low-dose UFH therapy (Geerts, et al., 2008).

Third-Line Therapy

Third-line therapies for prophylaxis after orthopedic surgery include aspirin, low-dose UFH, and dextran because of their decreased effectiveness compared with warfarin or LMWHs. Sole therapy with any of the above agents is not recommended by the consensus guidelines (Geerts, et al. 2008).

The most recent consensus guidelines should be consulted for more detailed information. Recommendations for VTE prophylaxis in general, gynecologic, urologic, and neurologic surgeries as well as neurologic trauma and spinal cord injury can be found in the ACCP consensus guidelines for antithrombotic therapy (Geerts, et al. 2008).

Nondrug Therapy

Nondrug therapies help prevent or treat the complications of DVT, including venous stasis ulcers and the post-thrombotic syndrome. Mechanical measures, including IPC devices and graduated compression stockings, offer the advantage of carrying no risk of bleeding compared to anticoagulants. IPC sleeves applied to the lower extremities periodically inflate and deflate, to squeeze the calf and prevent venous stasis and pooling of blood in the leg veins. Nonambulatory patients can have IPC devices applied to reduce the risk of VTE. Current guidelines recommend the use of IPC therapy in addition to traditional anticoagulants to prevent VTE in high-risk patients following orthopedic or general surgery. Use of IPC alone is recommended in patients with a high risk of bleeding following general orthopedic or general surgery, until the bleeding risk resolves (Geerts, et al., 2008). IPC therapy is also effective in patients with post-thrombotic syndrome or nonhealing venous stasis ulcers (Kearon, et al., 2008).

Elastic graduated compression stockings (e.g., JOBST hose) are used to prevent venous incompetence following DVT. The stockings provide graduated compression, with the highest pressure at the ankle and decreasing pressure up the length of the leg, which reduces blood pooling. Stockings providing pressure of 30 to 40 mm Hg have demonstrated efficacy in clinical trials at preventing post-thrombotic syndrome and are recommended in the most recent ACCP guidelines (Geerts, et al., 2008), but other strengths are available, depending on the individual patient's needs (Vazquez, et al., 2009). In an acute DVT, compression stockings should be instituted only after therapeutic anticoagulation is achieved. A disadvantage of these mechanical measures is that compliance is often poor by both the patient and the hospital staff.

Ischemic Stroke

Treatment of Acute Ischemic Stroke

Treatment of acute ischemic stroke is typically managed in the hospital setting with thrombolytics. This chapter focuses on chronic treatment and prevention. Refer to consensus guidelines for additional information.

Secondary Prevention of Noncardioembolic Ischemic Stroke

First-Line Therapy

In contrast to venous disease in which anticoagulants are the preferred drugs, antiplatelet agents are recommended in arterial disease since platelet aggregation contributes to clot formation. The three drugs used most commonly to prevent cardioembolic stroke include aspirin, clopidogrel, or aspirin/dipyridamole (the fixed-dose combination product Aggrenox); see **Table 49.9**. Oral anticoagulants, such as warfarin, are not recommended because they increase the risk of brain hemorrhage and outweigh the possible benefits. For primary prevention of cardiovascular disease (which includes stroke), aspirin in doses of 81 mg a day or 100 mg every other day is recommended in high-risk individuals. Aspirin is not useful for preventing a first stroke in low-risk patients (Goldstein, et al., 2011). The remainder of this section focuses on the use of antiplatelet agents for the secondary prevention of a stroke in patients who have a history of stroke or TIA.

To prevent noncardioembolic ischemic stroke or TIA in patients with a history of noncardioembolic stroke or TIA, aspirin 50 to 325 mg/d is recommended because of its low cost, safety profile, and proven effectiveness in several clinical trials with thousands of patients. In several studies, aspirin was found to reduce the odds of stroke by approximately 23% (Antithrombic Trialists' Collaboration, 2002). Therefore, aspirin is used as a first-line agent by many practitioners to prevent noncardioembolic stroke in high-risk patients (Adams, et al., 2008; Albers, et al., 2008). The ACCP recommends an aspirin dose ranging from 50 to 100 mg, compared to the higher dosage range recommended by the American Heart Association and American Stroke Association (50 to 325 mg/d). In addition to aspirin, clopidogrel at a dose of 75 mg/d and aspirin/dipyridamole 25/200 mg twice daily are also considered as first-line therapy by both professional groups, but clopidogrel and the combination of aspirin and dipyridamole are usually considered second-line therapy by practitioners.

Second-Line Therapy

The combination of aspirin and dipyridamole in comparison to placebo reduced the risk of stroke in those with prior events by 37% to 38% in two trials (ESPS2 and ESPRIT). Although aspirin/dipyridamole 25/200 mg twice daily is more effective than aspirin alone and is an acceptable option as an initial therapy, it is viewed as an alternative treatment to aspirin therapy in the prevention of stroke due to its higher cost, less convenient dosing schedule (twice-daily dosing), and decreased tolerability due to GI distress and headache (Albers, et al., 2008).

Clopidogrel 75 mg/d is also acceptable as an option for initial therapy in the prevention of noncardioembolic stroke, but it is regarded as an alternative to aspirin therapy, primarily due to cost. In the CAPRIE trial, clopidogrel conferred a risk reduction of about 9% over aspirin for the combined outcomes of stroke, MI, and vascular death. There were no major differences between safety profiles, and adverse experiences with both clopidogrel and aspirin were minimal. Therefore, clopidogrel should be used as a first-line treatment in patients unable to take aspirin due to allergy (Albers, et al., 2008).

The combination of low-dose aspirin (75 to 160 mg/d) and clopidogrel compared to aspirin monotherapy was studied in one trial (CHARISMA) (Albers, et al., 2008). There was no difference in the efficacy endpoint of MI, stroke, or death. However, the combined use of clopidogrel with aspirin is not recommended, as the MATCH trial found that an increased risk of life-threatening or major bleeding offset any benefit in reduction of stroke or other vascular events. The combination of aspirin with clopidogrel is reserved for patients with other compelling reasons, including following coronary stenting or acute coronary syndromes (Albers, et al., 2008).

Third-Line Therapy

Ticlopidine reduces the risk of stroke in patients with cerebrovascular disease. However, because it is associated with an approximately 1% risk of severe adverse effects such as neutropenia, it is considered a third-line or last-choice treatment. Most clinicians have completely abandoned its use because of the associated risks (Albers, et al., 2008).

Cardioembolic Stroke Prevention—Atrial Fibrillation

The risk of thromboembolic stroke in patients with atrial fibrillation who are not receiving anticoagulation is approximately 5%/year, and this risk increases rapidly after age 65. In the Framingham Heart Study, the risk of stroke in patients with atrial fibrillation rose from 1.5% in those ages 50 to 59 to 23.5% in those ages 80 to 89. In patients older than age 80, atrial fibrillation was the only cardiovascular condition associated with increased risk of stroke (Singer, et al., 2008; Fuster, et al., 2006).

First-Line Therapy

To prevent the future risk of stroke in patients with atrial fibrillation, long-term anticoagulation with warfarin at a target INR of 2 to 3 is recommended by two professional guidelines (Singer, et al., 2008; Fuster, et al., 2006). The highest risk of stroke is in patients with prior thromboembolic stroke or TIA or those with mitral stenosis caused by rheumatic heart disease. Other patient factors (moderate risk factors) that increase the risk of stroke include patients older than age 75, hypertension, heart failure, impaired left ventricular systolic function, and diabetes mellitus (**Table 49.10**).

TABLE 49.10	Risk Stratification for Treating Atrial Fibrillation
Risk Factor Status	**Recommendation**
No high or moderate risk factors	Aspirin
One moderate risk factor	Aspirin or warfarin
High-risk factor or two moderate-risk factors	Warfarin with a target INR of 2–3, or dabigatran.

Six major, well-conducted trials have documented the benefits of warfarin in reducing the risk of stroke in patients with atrial fibrillation. The 5% annual risk of stroke in non–anticoagulated patients was reduced to 1.4% with warfarin, a risk reduction of 68%. Anticoagulation therapy did not significantly increase the incidence of major bleeding events. In contrast, the benefits provided by aspirin alone contributed to a 21% risk reduction, much less than the effects provided by warfarin (Singer, et al., 2008).

The Stroke Prevention in Atrial Fibrillation-II Study results suggested that warfarin is more effective in those older than age 75 compared to their younger counterparts, but the over 75-year-old age group has a substantial risk of intracerebral bleeding, which negated the benefit of warfarin. However, four other pooled trials did not support these findings. These studies found that most major bleeding occurred at INRs higher than 4. Therefore, warfarin therapy is not withheld in those over age 75. The decision to choose warfarin versus aspirin therapy is based on patient risk factors, but warfarin is viewed as first-line therapy in patients with any high-risk factor (Singer, et al., 2008).

The current recommendations for anticoagulation in atrial fibrillation include warfarin with a goal INR range of 2 to 3 for patients with any high-risk factor, such as previous TIA, systemic embolism, stroke, or rheumatic mitral valve disease. Warfarin is preferred over aspirin in patients with two or more moderate risk factors. Patients with prosthetic heart valves and atrial fibrillation require a higher intensity or anticoagulation, with an INR of at least 2.5 recommended. Aspirin therapy should be offered to patients with contraindications to warfarin therapy or to those who refuse warfarin therapy. Aspirin in addition to low, fixed-dose warfarin therapy is not recommended.

Although warfarin has been the drug of choice for stroke prevention in atrial fibrillation for several years, dabigatran can also be considered a first-line therapy for stroke prevention in atrial fibrillation. Updated guidelines from U.S. professional groups (Wann, et al., 2011) consider dabigatran as an alternative to warfarin in preventing stroke in patients with atrial fibrillation who do not have a prosthetic heart valve, significant valvular disease, severe renal failure, or advanced liver disease. The results of the RE-LY trial reported that the risk of stroke was significantly lower with dabigatran 150 mg twice daily than warfarin adjusted to an INR of 2 to 3 (Connolly, et al., 2009). The benefit of dabigatran in particular exceeded warfarin in patients who had poor INR control (INR range of 2 to 3 maintained only 40% of the time). Keep in mind that patients with atrial fibrillation are likely to have conditions that were excluded in the RE-LY trial, including severe renal impairment and prosthetic heart valves.

Second-Line Therapy

Aspirin therapy has shown a 21% to 22% risk reduction in stroke as compared to a placebo. Warfarin therapy is clearly superior to aspirin in risk reduction for stroke, but it does have a higher risk of hemorrhage. The rate of intracranial hemorrhage in one primary prevention study was found to be 1.8% in those older than age 75 treated with warfarin as compared to 0.8% in those treated with aspirin. Therefore, the risk intensity for stroke versus that of hemorrhage must be considered when choosing between warfarin and aspirin therapy (Singer, et al., 2008; Fuster, et al., 2006).

Consensus guidelines state that warfarin with a target INR of 2 to 3 or aspirin can be used in patients with atrial fibrillation and one risk factor. Those who are younger than age 65 and with no high or moderate risk factors and no clinical or echocardiographic evidence of cardiovascular disease may receive aspirin 75 to 325 mg/d. **Table 49.10** summarizes recent recommendations.

Third-Line Therapy

A 2011 update to the American Heart Association/American Stroke Society guidelines for atrial fibrillation now mention the combination of aspirin with clopidogrel. In situations in which warfarin is unsuitable either due to patient preference or physician assessment, the combination of aspirin with clopidogrel might be considered. The ACTIVE-W and ACTIVE-A trials were the basis for this recommendation. In the ACTIVE-W trial, clopidogrel with aspirin was inferior to warfarin at preventing stroke, but the bleeding risk was similar for both groups. The ACTIVE-A trial compared clopidogrel with aspirin vs. aspirin with a placebo in patients who were deemed unsuitable for warfarin therapy. There were fewer vascular events with the dual-antiplatelet therapy group (6.7%/year) compared to aspirin plus a placebo (7.6%/year), but a higher rate of major bleeding (2.0%/year vs. 1.3%/year) (Wann, et al., 2011).

Anticoagulation for Elective Cardioversion

Patients with atrial fibrillation undergoing electrical or pharmacologic cardioversion should also receive anticoagulation therapy. The risk of systemic embolization after direct current cardioversion is 5% in patients not receiving anticoagulation compared with 1% in those receiving anticoagulation. Once a thrombus is formed in the heart, 2 to 3 weeks is required for clot organization and adherence to the atrial wall. Therefore, patients with atrial fibrillation should receive warfarin for 3 weeks before cardioversion, which is then continued for 4 or more weeks after the procedure or until normal sinus rhythm has been maintained for 4 or more weeks. Although electrical activity of the atria resumes quickly after successful cardioversion, normal atrial contraction (mechanical activity) may not resume for 3 to 4 weeks, thus supporting continued anticoagulation. Patients may also be offered anticoagulation therapy and then undergo TEE followed by immediate cardioversion if no thrombi are detected, with warfarin continued for at least 4 weeks (Singer, et al., 2008).

Prophylaxis Against Systemic Embolism in Patients with Native and Prosthetic Mechanical Heart Valves

Long-term anticoagulation with warfarin alone or in combination with aspirin is required in patients with mechanical heart valves because the valve itself is thrombogenic and because of the high risk of thromboembolism (Sun, et al., 2010). The rate of major thrombotic events in patients who have mechanical heart valves and who are not receiving anticoagulation is 8%; anticoagulation therapy decreases this risk by 75% (Carnetiger, et al., 1995). Refer to the professional guidelines for information on anticoagulation in patients with native valvular disease (rheumatic mitral valve disease, mitral stenosis) and other conditions.

Both the position and type of the mechanical valve influence the risk of embolism. The prevalence of thromboembolism is higher with a valve in the mitral position than in the aortic position. Caged-ball valves like the Starr Edwards valves, which are rarely seen today, have the highest risk of thromboembolism, followed by tilting-disk valves (Bjork-Shiley valves) and then bileaflet valves (St. Jude Medical valves, which are most commonly used today, or Medtronic Hall valves). Patients with double mechanical valves (i.e., aortic and mitral valve replacement) have a higher risk of thromboembolism compared with those with only one prosthetic valve. The risk of thromboembolism is highest in the 3 months following valve replacement surgery, until the valve becomes covered with endothelial tissue. Immediately after surgery, LMWH or UFH is used short term until the INR with warfarin is therapeutic (Sun, et al., 2010). Individual patient risk factors that increase the risk of embolic events include atrial fibrillation, previous thromboembolic event, impaired left ventricular systolic function, and concomitant hypercoagulable conditions.

First-Line Therapy

Guidelines for antithrombotic therapy in patients with heart valve replacement are available from two professional groups (Bonow, et al., 2006; Salem, et al., 2008). There are some slight differences in the recommended INR values and whether aspirin co-administration with warfarin is necessary. Patients with mechanical valves in the mitral position or patients with aortic valves that are a caged ball or tilting disk require life-long therapy with warfarin maintained at a target INR of 2.5 to 3.5. A lower target INR of 2 to 3 can be considered for patients with bileaflet or Medtronic hall valves in the aortic position because studies show there is not an increased risk of thromboembolism and the bleeding risk is lower than with a higher target INR (Sun, et al., 2010).

Adding 100 mg/day of aspirin to warfarin therapy reduces mortality and thromboembolic events without increasing the risk of bleeding. The American College of Cardiology/American Heart Association guidelines recommend that all patients with mechanical prosthetic valves receive aspirin 75 to 100 mg/day in addition to warfarin. The ACCP only recommends adding aspirin to warfarin if the patient has additional risk factors or a compelling need for antiplatelet therapy, such as coronary or peripheral artery disease (Sun, et al., 2010).

For bioprosthetic porcine heart valves, the two professional guidelines recommend warfarin with an INR of 2 to 3 for 3 months for aortic valves and warfarin with an INR of 2.5 to 3.5 for 3 months for mitral valves. Only 3 months of anticoagulation is warranted because after that time frame, the risk of bleeding outweighs the risk of thrombosis. Aspirin monotherapy in doses ranging from 75 to 100 mg/day for 3 months is also an option for either mitral or aortic valves. Following the initial 3-month period, life-long therapy with aspirin 100 mg/day is recommended regardless of the valve position (Bonow, et al., 2006; Salem, et al., 2008).

Patients with mechanical heart valves can experience thromboembolic events even if antithrombotic therapy is administered appropriately; the risk is 0.5% to 1.7%/patient-year. Options in these cases from expert consensus are to increase the target INR for patients on warfarin, to add aspirin to patients not already receiving warfarin, or to add warfarin if the patient is receiving aspirin (Sun, et al., 2010).

Second-Line Therapy

For patients with mechanical heart valves in either the mitral or aortic position who cannot take warfarin, the American College of Cardiology/American Heart Association guidelines list aspirin in a dosage of 75 to 325 mg as an option. In a patient with a prosthetic valve who has risk factors for thromboembolism and who can't use aspirin, clopidogrel 75 mg/day or warfarin with the INR adjusted to 3.5 to 4.5 are alternatives.

Special Population Considerations

When considering anticoagulation therapy, special populations are those who pose more difficult issues when it comes to diagnosis and treatment. Those with renal impairment or obesity and pregnant patients are considered special population groups when addressing anticoagulation for various disease states. Obesity and renal impairment were briefly discussed in anticoagulant dosing in the appropriate sections of this chapter. The following section will discuss special considerations in other groups.

Pregnancy

Pregnancy is an independent risk factor for VTE, and the incidence of VTE is estimated at 0.5 to 2 per 1,000 pregnancies. The increased risk is secondary to changes in procoagulant and anticoagulant proteins, blood stasis related to reduced venous return from the legs, and vascular injury. In one study, women with known prepregnancy thrombophilia states were found to have an 8-fold risk of VTE. Thrombophilia also puts women at risk for pregnancy loss and pregnancy complications associated with placental infarction, such as intrauterine growth retardation, preeclampsia, placental abruption, and intrauterine death. Women with a history of VTE have an increased risk of recurrence during pregnancy (Chunilal & Bates, 2009).

Diagnosis of VTE in pregnant women is difficult by clinical evaluation because many nonthrombotic symptoms of pregnancy mimic DVT and PE. In addition, tests used to diagnose DVT can be altered by the compressive effects of the gravid uterus. Concerns of fetal radiation exposure from diagnostic tests have not been confirmed clinically. Clinical suspicion of VTE in a pregnant woman should be investigated. Treatment and prophylaxis of VTE in pregnancy are based primarily on clinical experience because there are no major clinical studies to support evidence-based practice (Chunilal & Bates, 2009).

Warfarin crosses the placenta and is a known teratogen, with the highest risk occurring between 6 and 12 weeks' gestation. Bleeding risk is highest close to delivery. Warfarin therapy should be discontinued immediately and an alternative agent selected in women who are attempting pregnancy or who become pregnant (Bates, et al., 2008).

Heparin is the treatment of choice in pregnant patients requiring anticoagulation therapy, and an extensive body of literature supports the efficacy and safety of heparin. However, heparin is a pregnancy category C medication and maternal risks include bleeding, osteoporosis, HIT, and allergic skin reactions. LMWHs, which may potentially decrease the risk of osteoporosis and HIT, are an option and are pregnancy category B medications. UFH and LMWHs do not cross the placenta and therefore are unlikely to cause hemorrhage or be teratogenic (Lexi-Comp Online, 2010).

In lactation, warfarin appears in an inactive form in breast milk and has not been found to change the PT in nursing infants of women taking warfarin. UFH is not secreted into breast milk. It is not known if LMWHs are secreted into breast milk; however, in practice they are used in nursing mothers when necessary (Lexi-Comp Online, 2010).

For prophylaxis in pregnant patients with previous VTE associated with a transient risk factor, surveillance and postpartum anticoagulation is recommended. Those who have had an idiopathic VTE or a prior VTE and the presence of thrombophilia but who are not on long-term anticoagulation, surveillance, low-dose (5,000 international units subcutaneously every 12 hours) or moderate-dose (adjusted doses every 12 hours to a target anti-Xa level of 0.1 to 0.3 international units/mL) UFH, or prophylactic LMWHs in addition to postpartum anticoagulation is recommended. Pregnant patients with no prior VTE but with confirmed thrombophilia and not on long-term anticoagulation therapy are recommended to be offered surveillance, low-dose UFH, or prophylactic LMWHs in addition to postpartum anticoagulation. When patients have had two or more episodes of VTE or are currently on long-term anticoagulation, adjusted-dose UFH, prophylactic LMWHs, or adjusted-dose LMWHs in addition to long-term postpartum anticoagulation is recommended (Bates, et al., 2008).

For treatment of VTE in pregnancy, those with an average risk of recurrence should be offered adjusted-dose LMWHs throughout pregnancy or an IV UFH bolus followed by continuous infusion for 5 or more days and then adjusted-dose UFH until delivery. LMWHs and UFH should be discontinued 24 hours before elective induction of labor. For those at very high risk for VTE recurrence (i.e., proximal DVT within the prior 2-week period), IV UFH, discontinued 4 to 6 hours before expected delivery and anticoagulation for 6 or more weeks postpartum or 3 or more months after VTE occurrence is recommended (Bates, et al., 2008).

Pregnant women with mechanical heart valves require assessment of the valve type and position and other risk factors for thromboembolism, along with patient preference. Anticoagulation should be given throughout pregnancy. Options here include LMWHs administered twice daily with anti-factor Xa monitoring to determine efficacy; UFH administered every 12 hours with aPTT monitoring; or LMWHs or UFH administered up until week 13 of gestation, and then warfarin given until close to delivery. Patients with a very high risk of thromboembolism (mitral valve, previous thromboembolism) should consider warfarin throughout pregnancy after a full discussion of the risks and benefits (Bates, et al., 2008).

Consult the ACCP consensus guidelines for prophylaxis in pregnant women with increased risk of pregnancy loss related to thrombophilia states.

Malignancy

Malignancy is known to confer an increased risk of developing VTE. The incidence of VTE in the general population is estimated at 0.1% per year, compared to 0.5% per year in cancer. Individual patient factors will determine whether anticoagulation prophylaxis is needed. For hospitalized medical oncology or surgical oncology patients requiring prophylaxis, UFH, LMWHs, or fondaparinux are recommended in the guidelines from the National Comprehensive Cancer Center Network. Patients with contraindications to anticoagulation treatment can use an IPC device or graduated compression stockings. Chemotherapy with lenalidomide or thalidomide is associated with VTE; therefore, outpatient VTE prophylaxis is recommended for patients receiving these two drugs. Anticoagulation prophylaxis in patients with central venous catheters is not recommended (Streiff, 2010). Treatment of VTE consists of UFH, LMWHs, or fondaparinux, with the ultimate selection based on factors such as drug half-life, cost, and the individual's renal function (Weitz, 2009).

Maintaining a therapeutic INR with warfarin in patients with cancer can be challenging. Warfarin efficacy can be decreased due to nausea and vomiting from chemotherapy and poor nutritional intake. Warfarin therapy may need to be temporarily disrupted if an invasive procedure is required. LMWHs are preferred over warfarin for initial and chronic therapy because clinical trials have shown a lower recurrence

rate of VTE and reduced bleeding. LMWHs should be continued 3 to 6 months for DVT and PE, respectively. One trial compared warfarin with dalteparin for 6 months in patients with cancer. Treatment with dalteparin was associated with a 50% reduction in the risk of VTE, with no significant increase in bleeding events (Weitz, 2009). Dalteparin is approved for extended treatment of VTE in patients with cancer.

The newer factor Xa inhibitors apixaban and rivaroxaban are currently being studied for extended VTE prophylaxis in medically ill patients, and patients with cancer are included in the trials. More data are required before definitive recommendations can be made regarding the use of these investigational agents in patients with cancer.

Deep Vein Thrombosis/Pulmonary Embolism Risk and Airline Travel

Media attention has been given to the risk of developing DVT and PE with long airline flights, but VTE due to air travel is a rare event. The risk of VTE is greatest with flights lasting more than 8 to 10 hours, and most events have occurred in patients with other contributing risk factors (prior VTE, malignancy, recent trauma, thrombophilia). Graduated compression stockings or a one-time dose of LMWHs administered before departure are advocated only in high-risk travelers, and a patient's individual risk versus benefit should be determined. All passengers can reduce venous stasis by staying hydrated, avoiding wearing constrictive clothing, and performing periodic calf stretches during flight (Goldhaber, 2010; Geerts, et al., 2008).

MONITORING PATIENT RESPONSE

Warfarin

Outpatient management of VTE and other conditions is now common, so anticoagulation therapy is often not stabilized before a patient is discharged from the hospital. Subcutaneous LMWH injections, when overlapped with warfarin, allow patients to be discharged before a therapeutic INR is achieved. UFH or LMWHs can be discontinued when the INR is within therapeutic range on two measurements taken 24 or more hours apart. Regardless of whether UFH or LMWHs are overlapped with warfarin, patients receiving warfarin require evaluation within 3 to 5 days after discharge to avoid increasing the risk of either thromboembolic or bleeding events. The INR is then monitored weekly until a stable INR is reached, which is often defined as two consecutive INRs within the target range measured at least 72 hours apart (Ansell, et al., 2008).

Maintaining a stable INR is important since patients with fluctuating INRs have an increased risk of complications compared to patients with stable INR control (Witt, 2010). How frequently to monitor a patient's INR during chronic therapy is determined by patient compliance and changes in clinical status (e.g., heart failure exacerbations), medications, and diet (Ansell, et al., 2008). In patients newly started on warfarin, the INR is checked weekly for 1 to 2 weeks. Once the INR is stable for 2 weeks, the interval of laboratory monitoring can be increased to once every 2 weeks and then every 3 weeks (Jacobs, 2008). For patients on a stable warfarin dose, the interval between INR checks should be no longer than every 4 weeks (Ansell, et al., 2008). More frequent INR checks are needed in patients who develop bleeding complications or those experiencing the factors noted above that can affect warfarin requirements.

When unexpected INR results are obtained, several questions should be addressed (**Box 49.7**). If highly elevated INR results are reported, the practitioner needs to rule out laboratory error and perform the INR test again if necessary before adjusting the warfarin dose. An increased warfarin effect leading to elevated INRs can occur with exacerbation of congestive heart failure, hepatic disease, fever, hyperthyroidism, and diarrhea (Jacobs, 2008). INRs that fluctuate widely without apparent cause should raise the question of medication noncompliance. Instructing patients to bring in all prescription and OTC medications and conducting tablet counts can help determine patient reliability.

Identifying trends in the INR rather than reacting to an individual laboratory result is also important. For patients with an INR slightly out of range, frequent warfarin-dosing changes can cause a cycle of unnecessary dosing adjustments. Some experts recommend to not adjust the warfarin dose unless the INR is less than 1.7 or above 3.3 in patients with a target INR of 2 to 3 (Witt, 2010). Another option is to adjust the dose up or down by 5% to 20% based on the total weekly warfarin dose (Ansell, et al., 2008). See **Box 49.8** for information on point-of-care testing devices for INR monitoring.

Dabigatran

One major advantage of the direct thrombin inhibitors is that routine laboratory monitoring is not needed to determine response to therapy. Phase III clinical trial testing with dabigatran did not include coagulation monitoring. Smaller trials assessing pharmacodynamic properties have evaluated the effect of dabigatran on traditional coagulation tests. There is a minimal effect of the drug on the PT/INR at clinically relevant plasma concentrations. The aPTT is prolonged with dabigatran etexilate, but the effect is not linear, and the aPTT reaches a plateau with high doses. The ecarin clotting time (ECT; an anticoagulation test originating from snake venom, which is used to monitor the effects of the IV direct thrombin hirudin) will be prolonged in a linear fashion with therapeutic concentrations of dabigatran (Eriksson, et al., 2009). The package insert for dabigatran does mention that the ECT is a better marker of anticoagulant activity than the aPTT in bleeding situations, but it does not provide detailed guidance on how to use these tests clinically to guide treatment decisions in patients who experience bleeding complications. Some may view the lack of monitoring as a disadvantage for the direct thrombin inhibitors because there is not an objective way to determine if a patient has been compliant with dabigatran or if the anticoagulation effect is adequate.

Due to the risk of GI and other bleeding with dabigatran, patients should be assessed routinely for signs of overt or occult bleeding, including bleeding from the soft tissues (gums and nose), genitourinary tract (hematuria), and GI tract (black tarry stools). Laboratory testing for bleeding, including hematocrit and Hemoccult, is warranted if bleeding is suspected. It is also important to look for bleeding if a patient experiences a drop in blood pressure.

Inform patients on the storage and packaging requirements for dabigatran. The drug is degraded if it is exposed to moisture, so it should only be kept in the original container, which contains 60 capsules. Once a bottle of dabigatran is opened, it must be used within 30 days. Crushing or chewing the capsules is not recommended because the bioavailability can increase up to 75% (Boehringer Ingelheim, 2010).

Unfractionated Heparin

The aPTT is used to monitor the effect of UFH and is sensitive to thrombin, factor Xa, and factor IXa. A target ratio range of 1.5 to 2.5 (observed aPTT/mean laboratory aPTT) is considered a therapeutic aPTT, which is equivalent to an anti-Xa level of 0.35 to 0.7 international units/mL for most aPTT reagents, and is multiplied by the control aPTT. Blood should be drawn for an aPTT evaluation every 6 hours until the aPTT is stable and within the therapeutic range.

Regular assessment for occult or overt bleeding is necessary with all anticoagulants, including UFH. Refer to the section on initiating therapy and adverse events for more information.

BOX **49.7**

Questions to Ask When INR Results Are Unexpected

- Have any warfarin doses been missed in the past 3 to 5 days?
- Have extra warfarin tablets been ingested?
- Is the patient taking a warfarin regimen other than prescribed?
- Is the patient experiencing bleeding problems?
- Is the patient experiencing thromboembolic complications?
- Have any new medications (prescription, over-the-counter, herbal) been started, deleted, or changed from the patient's medication regimen?
- Has the patient's underlying condition changed, as in acute congestive heart failure exacerbation or worsening renal or hepatic impairment?
- Has the patient had a recent acute febrile or GI illness?
- Has thyroid status changed or has a malignancy been diagnosed?

BOX 49.8

Patient Self-Testing and Patient Self-Management for Warfarin

The blood specimen necessary to obtain an international normalized ratio (INR) value may be retrieved via venipuncture and processed in the laboratory or by fingerstick and processed immediately by a point-of-care (POC) monitor. POC monitors measure a thromboplastin-mediated clotting time that is converted to a prothrombin time (PT) equivalent by a microprocessor and expressed as a PT and INR. The thromboplastin is impregnated into the testing strips to which a sample of the patient's blood is applied. The international sensitivity index and precision of the testing procedure determine the accuracy of the result, and although results are typically comparable to that of the laboratory, variability in INR results has been reported (Ansell, et al., 2008). Each device must be calibrated to evaluate accuracy, and the POC devices cannot be used interchangeably (Spinler, et al., 2005). If possible, patients should use the same setting and device (home vs. office or lab, POC vs. venipuncture) for INR monitoring. POC INR testing can simplify management of warfarin in physician offices or anticoagulation clinics and has moved into the home setting. POC testing provides immediate INR results, allowing for immediate decisions on warfarin dosing (Jacobson, 2008).

Several POC devices are also approved for home use, although they are expensive. CoaguChek and ProTime are two of the commonly used POC monitors. POC testing in the home falls into two models: patient self-testing, in which the patient tests his own INR and then calls the results into the physician or anticoagulation clinic to obtain dosing instructions; and patient self-management, where patients are trained to manage their own warfarin therapy, based on INR results. Studies have shown that patient self-testing and self-management can result in a higher percentage of INRs maintained in the therapeutic range than traditional physician office settings. Advantages of patient self-testing and self-management include patient convenience, more frequent testing with resultant improved anticoagulation control, quick results, and potentially better compliance due to immediate feedback. Careful patient selection is crucial when deciding if an individual is a candidate for patient self-testing or self-management (Spinler, et al.,2005).

Data from Jacobson, A. K. (2008). Warfarin monitoring: Point-of-care INR testing limitations and interpretation of the prothrombin time. *Journal of Thrombosis and Thrombolysis, 25*, 10–11, and Spinler, S. A., Nutescu, E. A., Smythe, M. A., et al. (2005). Anticoagulation monitoring part 1: Warfarin and parenteral direct thrombin inhibitors. *Annals of Pharmacotherapy, 39*, 1049–1055.

A drop in blood pressure or decreased hematocrit can signal bleeding (Palatnik, 2007). Hypersensitivity reactions can manifest as chills, fever, and urticaria. Clinical symptoms of recurrent thrombosis, such as unilateral leg edema for DVT or increased shortness of breath for PE, are clues that the intensity of anticoagulation is inadequate.

Low-Molecular-Weight Heparins

As stated earlier, one of the major advantages of LMWHs compared with heparin administered by continuous infusion or subcutaneously is that the aPTT does not need to be monitored because LMWHs have a minimal effect on the aPTT. Theoretically, anti-Xa activity can be used to monitor LMWH therapy, but this is not routine and is reserved for morbidly obese patients or those with renal dysfunction and women who are pregnant. Minimal therapeutic anti-Xa levels have not been definitively established. A conservative therapeutic range for twice daily dosing and an anti-Xa level 4 hours after subcutaneous administration is 0.6 to 1.0 international units/mL. For once-daily dosing, the target range 4 hours after dosing is not as clear, but a range of 1.0 to 2.0 international units/mL is deemed reasonable.

LMWH treatment has the same concerns for bleeding, hypersensitivity reactions, and inadequate anticoagulation

as with UFH, and similar monitoring procedures should be followed.

Antiplatelet Agents

As with dabigatran, there are no laboratory tests to monitor the therapeutic efficacy of the antiplatelet agents aspirin, clopidogrel, aspirin/dipyridamole, or ticlopidine. Adverse events of these agents, especially bleeding or neutropenia, can be monitored by CBC or guaiac testing to detect blood in the stools. The patient may also be assessed for bruises and petechiae. Therapeutic efficacy is most commonly assessed by the absence of new thromboembolic or stroke symptoms.

PATIENT EDUCATION

Patient education regarding anticoagulation therapy is started at the initiation of therapy and reinforced at every encounter. Explain the rationale for anticoagulation and the risks and benefits of therapy. Extensive discussion of the potential for drug interactions, the need for frequent laboratory monitoring (**Box 49.9**), and the importance of stable dietary habits also is

BOX 49.9

Teaching about Therapeutic Ranges for Anticoagulant Therapy

Not only do patients receiving anticoagulant therapy need to know why they are taking medication, they need to know why they must have their blood tested frequently. In taking time to explain the rationale for testing as well as for treatment, the practitioner can help enhance the chances that patients will comply with the therapeutic plan.

INR GOAL 2 TO 3

Prophylaxis of venous thrombosis

Treatment of venous thrombosis

Treatment of pulmonary embolism

Prevention of systemic embolism

Stroke prevention in atrial fibrillation

Tissue heart valves

Mechanical prosthetic heart valves (bileaflet valves; St. Jude Medical, Medtronic Hall)

Valvular heart disease

Hypercoagulable conditions (antiphospholipid antibodies with lupus anticoagulant)—if no history of thrombotic events

NR GOAL 2.5 TO 3.5

Mechanical prosthetic heart valves (caged ball, tilting disk)

Hypercoagulable conditions (antiphospholipid antibodies with lupus anticoagulant)—if a history of thromboembolic events with INR of 2 to 3

in occupations that pose a risk of injury should use extra caution in the workplace and always wear shoes and gloves, as appropriate. Review the signs and symptoms of bleeding, such as excessive or unexplained bruising, red or amber urine, and black stools, at patient visits.

Drug Information

Patients receiving warfarin therapy should know their dosage, tablet size, and tablet color so that they maintain the prescribed regimen and will be able to know if they are given the correct medication from their pharmacy. Caution patients against switching between tablets from different manufacturers. It is important that patients are instructed to inform all health care practitioners (physicians, nurse practitioners, pharmacists, podiatrists, and dentists) that they are receiving anticoagulation therapy. In addition, because the list of potentially interacting substances with warfarin is exhaustive, the practitioner should encourage patients to report any new prescribed or OTC drug, any herbal medicines, or changes in drug dosages. Patients should also be alerted to OTC medications they should avoid such as NSAIDs. Patients also must be instructed to notify the practitioner of any changes in health status, such as fever, diarrhea, viral syndromes, weight changes, and increased fluid retention secondary to congestive heart failure. Patients must also be advised to notify the practitioner monitoring their anticoagulation therapy if they will be having any invasive procedures, such as colonoscopy, tooth extraction, and surgery. If this occurs, a decision is needed as to whether or not warfarin will need to be stopped before the procedure, for how long, and if therapy with a shorter-acting agent such as LMWHs will be needed while the patient is off warfarin. See **Box 49.10** for discussion of bridging therapy with LMWHs while holding warfarin in preparation for an invasive procedure.

In addition, counsel patients receiving ticlopidine regarding the signs and symptoms of neutropenia (including fever, chills, or sore throat). Those taking ticlopidine and clopidogrel must be aware of the symptoms of thrombocytopenia (fever, weakness, difficulty speaking, seizures, yellowing of the skin or eyes, dark or bloody urine, or petechiae). Discussing what to do about symptoms of liver dysfunction, such as yellow skin or sclera, dark urine, or light-colored stools, is also recommended.

Patient-Oriented Information Sources

The amount of patient-centered information on the Internet is vast and sometimes of suspect quality. Reputable sites include the National Library of Medicine and National Institutes of Health-sponsored Medline plus http://www.nlm.nih.gov/medlineplus/, which provides patient information on a wide range of diseases and treatments, and http://www.clot.care.com, which has articles and videos pertaining to all areas of anticoagulation, including INR testing.

For warfarin, several types of educational materials are available in several languages (including Spanish) from drug manufacturers, such as Bristol-Myers Squibb (1-800-268-6234 or 1-800-COUMADIN). Products include pillboxes,

essential for patients receiving warfarin. Active participation by the patient is necessary for successful warfarin therapy.

Patients receiving antiplatelet agents must recognize the signs and symptoms of bleeding, particularly from the GI tract. Aspirin can cause GI upset, so mealtime administration is crucial. Crushing or chewing sustained-release aspirin products is not advocated because this destroys their delayed-absorption properties. Advise the patient to report large bruises or unusual bleeding to the practitioner. Patients receiving aspirin/dipyridamole should understand that the combination product contains aspirin and should be cautioned to check the labels of OTC products to prevent inadvertent ingestion of aspirin from other sources.

Contact sports and dangerous activities, such as motorcycle riding, should be discouraged. Simple measures to reduce minor bleeding include the use of soft-bristled toothbrushes, and electric razors can replace razor blades. Patients engaged

BOX 49.10

Management of Anticoagulation in Preparation for Invasive Procedures

When a patient receiving warfarin therapy is scheduled for an invasive diagnostic or treatment procedure, warfarin must be held 4 to 5 days prior to allow the international normalized ratio (INR) to fall to an acceptable level to decrease the risk of bleeding. The type of procedure and the risk of bleeding involved will determine if warfarin therapy must be held. For most dermatologic procedures, such as Mohs surgery, it is not necessary to hold anticoagulation because the risk of bleeding while on anticoagulants is less than the risk of thromboembolic complications when anticoagulation is interrupted. Also, many dental procedures do not require anticoagulation interruption. Routine cleaning, cavity fillings, and root canals can be performed while the patient is receiving therapeutic anticoagulation. Gum scraping and tooth extractions may require warfarin to be held so that the INR can fall to ≤2.0. Cataract removal, because it is not a very vascular procedure, can also be performed without anticoagulation interruption. Most major surgeries, endoscopic procedures, and urologic procedures require warfarin cessation to reach an INR ≤1.5. The practitioner performing the procedure, regardless of the type of procedure, should always be contacted to discuss the risks of the procedure and to determine the need to interrupt warfarin therapy because each case is unique.

If warfarin cessation is required, the length of interruption required for the INR to fall sufficiently must be determined. For those maintained at an INR of 2 to 3, stopping warfarin 4 to 5 days prior to the procedure should allow the INR to return to near a normal level. For those maintained at an INR of 2.5 to 3.5, stopping warfarin for 5 to 6 days may be required.

Based on the patient's thromboembolic risk, it must then be determined if a fast-acting anticoagulant, such as unfractionated heparin (UFH) or low-molecular-weight heparin (LMWH), should be given as a bridge therapy during the period of warfarin cessation. LMWH is frequently chosen for bridge therapy because it can be administered on an outpatient basis without frequent monitoring, can be given once or twice a day, and only needs to be held 12 to 24 hours prior to the procedure to decrease the risk of bleeding. For patients with a low risk of thromboembolism, such as patients without venous thromboembolism (VTE) for more than 3 months and patients with atrial fibrillation without a history of stroke and only one moderate risk factor, warfarin may be stopped without the use of UFH or LMWH. Prophylaxis may be given after the procedure, whereas warfarin is restarted if the procedure creates a higher risk of thrombosis. Patients with intermediate risk of VTE should be given low-dose UFH or prophylactic dose LMWH. High-risk patients, such as those with a recent VTE (>3 months) and those with a mechanical cardiac valve, should be given full-dose UFH or full-dose LMWH starting 1 to 2 days after warfarin is stopped, stopped 24 hours before the procedure, and restarted after the procedure along with warfarin and continued until the INR is at a therapeutic level. UFH or LMWH should be resumed at the same dose after the procedure while warfarin is resumed and continued until the INR reaches a therapeutic level. INR testing should be checked at least every 2 to 3 days to determine if the INR is therapeutic and the UFH or LMWH can be stopped. The risk of bleeding after the procedure with the addition of UFH and LMWH must be discussed with the practitioner performing the procedure and a plan to minimize both the bleeding and thrombotic risk must be arranged. Refer to the latest guidelines from the American College of Chest Physicians for more detailed information (Douketis, et al., 2008).

---

information booklets, audiotapes, videotapes, DVDs, CDs, and Coumadin wallet-sized identification cards. MedicAlert bracelets or pendants are encouraged for patients who need lifelong anticoagulation therapy. Instructional aides to assist with patient self-administration of subcutaneous injections are available from the manufacturers of enoxaparin and fondaparinux. Patient assistance programs for low-income individuals are also available from the manufacturers of LMWHs. Local American Heart Association branches have several pamphlets discussing atrial fibrillation and stroke.

Nutrition

Education concerning food restrictions for patients taking warfarin is essential. Vitamin K_1, the antidote to warfarin, is naturally found in several plant foods. In contrast, vitamin K_2 is primarily synthesized by normal intestinal flora. The estimated necessary dietary intake of vitamin K_1 is 80 µg/day for men older than age 25 and 65 µg/day for women older than age 25. In the United States, typical American dietary vitamin K_1 intake is 300 to 500 µg (Suttie, 1992). Excessive amounts of dietary vitamin K_1 may antagonize warfarin's clinical effect and decrease the INR. Khan and coworkers (2004) found that for every 100-µg increase in vitamin K_1 intake in the 4 days before an INR measurement, the INR fell by 0.2. In another study, it was found that higher warfarin doses at 5.7 ± 1.7 mg/day were needed by those consuming 250 µg or more of vitamin K daily compared to that of 3.5 ± 1.0 mg/day by those consuming less than 250 µg of vitamin K daily (Khan, et al., 2004).

Dark green leafy vegetables (spinach and turnip, collard, and mustard greens), broccoli, Brussels sprouts, and cabbage are the primary sources of vitamin K and contain high amounts, greater than 100 mg/100-g serving. Herbal and green teas may also contain large quantities of vitamin K_1 (1,400 mg/100 g), and high levels of vitamin K_1 (50 mg/100 g) are found in soybean and soy products and olive oils, whereas peanut and corn oils contain minimal amounts. Vitamin K is also found in certain plant oils and prepared foods containing these oils, such as baked goods, margarine, and salad dressings. Food preparation with oils rich in vitamin K may also contribute to total vitamin K intake and affect warfarin action. The *Coumadin Cookbook* (available from amazon.com) is a great resource for patients taking warfarin because it provides tips for monitoring and maintaining a consistent vitamin K intake and provides many recipes with a low vitamin K content. Patients should be encouraged to eat a healthy diet, maintain consistency in their choice of foods, and avoid large fluctuations in dietary vitamin K_1 intake. Instructing patients to maintain a consistent intake of vitamin K–containing foods, rather than trying to eliminate all sources of dietary vitamin K_1, is essential. Patients must also be educated on portion sizes and their vitamin K content so that they are not only consistent with the frequency of intake of vitamin K foods, but are also consistent with the number of servings of vitamin K they consume. Fad diets, such as the "cabbage soup" diet, are discouraged, and if diets such as the Atkins diet or low-carbohydrate diets are to be started, the patient must notify the practitioner so that INRs can be monitored more often. These diets, when strictly followed, frequently lead to a change in the intake amount of vitamin K foods. **Table 49.11** lists examples of vitamin K food content and serving sizes.

Hidden sources of excess vitamin K include enteral supplements, which can cause resistance to warfarin. Checking the amount of vitamin K in any nutritional supplement is advised because several of these preparations are now marketed directly to patients through the lay press. In addition, many OTC vitamin preparations contain vitamin K, and patients should be counseled to read the label or bring in all medication bottles to the practitioner. For example, one Viactiv calcium chew contains 40 mcg of vitamin K; this translates to 80 mcg of vitamin K daily if the recommended dose of two chews is ingested. Questioning patients regarding any changes in dietary habits may provide clues when the INR varies. Extensive lists of the vitamin K content of common foods are now widely available on the Internet.

Complementary and Alternative Medications

There are no complementary and alternative medications available for treating VTE or preventing stroke in patients with atrial fibrillation or prosthetic heart valves. Refer to the section on nutritional supplements and OTC drug interac-

tions for information on how these types of medications can affect warfarin response. Alternative medications have been used, however, for treatment of edema and venous ulcers occurring due to post-thrombotic syndrome, although the supporting clinical evidence is weak. Horse chestnut has anti-inflammatory and vasoconstrictive properties. One small clinical trial found horse chestnut was as effective as graduated compression stockings in patients with venous insufficiency, and a systematic review has also reported benefit (Vazquez, et al, 2009). Rutosides are a class of flavonoids produced from plant glycosides that improve symptoms of venous insufficiency by reducing capillary permeability and decreasing inflammation. Rutosides in the form of a micronized purified flavonoid fraction were reported in one meta-analysis to induce complete healing of venous ulcers in 61% of patients, compared to 48% of control patients (Kearon, et al., 2008). Consensus guidelines from the ACCP recom-

TABLE 49.11	**Vitamin K Content of Selected Foods**
Food	**Amount of Vitamin K in mg per 100-g Portion**
Abalone	23
Asparagus, raw	40
Avocado, raw	40
Broccoli, raw	205
Brussels sprouts, raw	177
Cabbage, raw	145
Canola oil	141
Chinese green tea (dry)	1428
Coleslaw	57
Coriander leaf, cooked	1510
Cucumber peel, raw	360
Endive, raw	231
Green beans, snap	47
Kale, raw	817
Lettuce, raw	210
Margarine, stick*	51
Mayonnaise	81
Mustard greens, raw	170
Nightshade leaf, raw	620
Parsley, raw	540
Purslane, raw	381
Seaweed, purple	1385
Soybean oil	193
Soybeans, raw	47
Spinach leaf, raw	400
Swiss chard, raw	830
Tofu, raw	2
Turnip greens, raw	251
Watercress, raw	250

*1 stick of margarine is equivalent to 113 g.
From Spandorfer, J., Konkle, B. A., & Merli, G. J. (2001). *Management and prevention of thrombosis in primary care*. London: Arnold; New York: Oxford University Press. By permission of Oxford University Press, Inc.

mend the addition of rutosides to compression measures in patients with persistent venous ulcers; however, a specific commercial product is not mentioned. A rutoside product with the brand name Daflon is marketed in Europe in a 500-mg dosage administered twice daily, but this product is not available in the United States, and there is wide variation in the constituents of the supplements available in this country.

Case Study

D. G. is a 74-year-old woman who arrives at the emergency center complaining of shortness of breath, palpitations, nausea, and vomiting for the past 4 days. Her medical history includes diabetes mellitus, hypertension, CHF, cataract in the left eye, and osteoarthritis. She ambulates with a cane and is considered legally blind. The patient's current medications are losartan 100 mg/d, metoprolol succinate 50 mg/d, metformin 500 mg twice daily, ibuprofen 800 mg 3 times daily with food, and omeprazole magnesium 10 mg PRN heartburn.

Vital signs are as follows: blood pressure of 160/95, respiratory rate of 30, and heart rate of 140 bpm. ECG shows an irregular rhythm with a rapid ventricular response. Echocardiography reveals a moderately dilated left atrium, moderately depressed left ventricular systolic function, moderate mitral stenosis, and a thrombus in the apex of the left atrium.

Pertinent laboratory values include the following: hemoglobin 11 g/dL, hematocrit 35%, platelets 300,000/ microliter, and serum creatinine 1.7 g/dL. Her weight is 60 kg, and height is 5 ft 3 inches. She does not smoke and does not drink alcohol. Dietary habits include one can of Ensure daily, with other meals provided by a social service agency (Meals on Wheels). Social concerns include the fact she lives alone, but a son visits every 1 to 2 weeks and transports her to physician appointments. She is living on a limited budget. With regard to her medication compliance, her son states that she occasionally forgets to take her afternoon medications, but overall she is considered to be reasonably compliant with her drug regimens.

DIAGNOSIS: ATRIAL FIBRILLATION, ACUTE ONSET

1. List specific goals of treatment for D. G.
2. What drug therapy would you prescribe? Why?
3. What are the parameters for monitoring success of the therapy?
4. Discuss specific patient education based on the prescribed therapy.
5. List one or two adverse reactions for the selected agent that would cause you to change therapy.
6. What would be the choice for the second-line therapy?
7. What OTC or alternative medications would be appropriate for D. G.?
8. What lifestyle changes would you recommend to D. G.?
9. Describe one or two drug–drug or drug–food interactions for the selected agent.

BIBLIOGRAPHY

Starred references are cited in the text.

*Abraham, N. S., Hlatky, M. A., Antman, E. M., et al. (2010). ACCF/ACG/ AHA 2010 expert consensus document on the concomitant use of proton pump inhibitors and thienopyridines. *Journal of the American College of Cardiology, 56,* 2051–2066.

*Adams, H. P., del Zoppo, G., Albers, M. J., et al. (2007). Guidelines for the early management of adults with ischemic stroke: A guideline from the American Heart Association/American Stroke Association Stroke Council, Clinical Cardiology Council, Cardiovascular Radiology and Intervention Council, and the Atherosclerotic Peripheral Vascular Disease and Quality of Care Outcomes in Research Interdisciplinary Working Groups: The American Academy of Neurology affirms the value of this guideline as an educational tool for neurologists. *Stroke, 38,* 1655–1711.

*Adams, R. J., Albers, G., Alberts, M. J., et al. (2008). Update to the AHA/ ASA recommendations for prevention of stroke in patients with ischemic stroke or transient ischemic attack. *Stroke, 39,* 1647–1652.

*Albers, G. W., Amarenco, P., Easton, J. D., et al. (2008). Antithrombotic and thrombolytic therapy for ischemic stroke: American College of Chest Physicians evidence-based clinical practice guidelines (8th edition). *Chest, 133*(6 Suppl.), 630S–669S.

*Anderson, R. C., & Bussey, H. I. (2006). Retrievable and permanent inferior vena cava filters: Selected considerations. *Pharmacotherapy, 26*(11), 1595–1600.

*Anonymous. (2010). FDA Pradaxa approval balances efficacy and bleeding risk. *The Pink Sheet.* http://ThePink Sheet.ElsevierBI.com. Accessed March 5, 2011.

*Anonymous. (2010). New drug: Pradaxa (dabigatran). *Pharmacist's Letter/ Prescriber's Letter, 26*(11), 261101.

*Ansell, J., Hirsh, J., Hylek, E., et al. (2008). Pharmacology and management of the vitamin K antagonists. American College of Chest Physicians Evidence-Based Clinical Practice Guidelines (8th Edition). *Chest, 133* (6 Suppl.), 160S–198S.

*Antithrombotic Trialists' Collaboration. (2002). Collaborative meta-analysis of randomised trials of antiplatelet therapy for prevention of death, myocardial infarction, and stroke in high risk patients. *British Medical Journal, 324*(7), 1–86.

*Bates, S. M., Greer, A. N., Pabinger, I., et al. (2008). Venous thromboembolism, thrombophilia, antithrombotic therapy and pregnancy. American College of Chest Physicians Evidence-Based Clinical Practice Guidelines (8th Edition). *Chest, 133*(6 Suppl.), 844S–886S.

*Bentz, B.A. (2006). Gaining control over atrial fibrillation. *RN, 69*(12), 35–38.

*Bhatt, D. L., Cryer, B. L., & Contant, C. F. (2010). Clopidogrel with or without omeprazole in coronary artery disease. *New England Journal of Medicine, 363*, 1909–1917.

Boehringer Ingelheim. (2009). Product information for Aggrenox. Ridgefield, CT: Author.

*Boehringer Ingelheim. (2010). Product information for Pradaxa. Ridgefield, CT: Author.

*Bonow, R. O., Carabello, B. A., Chaterfee, K., et al. (2006). ACC/AHA 2006 practice guidelines for the management of patients with valvular heart disease: Executive summary. *Journal of the American College of Cardiology, 48*, 598–675.

*Bristol-Myers Squibb. (2010). Product information for Coumadin. Princeton, NJ: Author.

*Bristol-Myers Squibb/Sanofi Aventis. (2010). Product information for Plavix. Bridgewater, NJ: Author.

Cantrell, H. W., Ward, K. S., & Van Wicklin, H. A. (2007). Translating research on venous thromboembolism into clinical practice. *AORN Journal, 86*(4), 590–606.

*Carnetiger, S. C., Rosendaal, F. R., Wintzen, A. R., et al. (1995). Optimal anticoagulant therapy in patients with mechanical heart valves. *New England Journal of Medicine, 333*, 11–17.

*Chunilal, S. D., & Bates, S. M. (2009). Venous thromboembolism in pregnancy: Diagnosis, management and prevention. *Thrombosis and Haemostasis, 101*, 428–438.

*Colman, R. W., Clowes, A. W., George, J. N., et al. (2006). Overview of hemostasis. In R. W. Colman (ed.). *Hemostasis and thrombosis: Basic principles and clinical practice* (5th ed., pp. 13–17). Philadelphia: J. B. Lippincott.

Connolly, S., Pogue, J., Hart, R., et al. (2006). Clopidogrel plus aspirin versus oral anticoagulation for atrial fibrillation in the Atrial fibrillation Clopidogrel Trial with Irbesartan for prevention of Vascular Events (ACTIVE W): A randomized controlled trial. *Lancet, 367*, 1903–1912.

*Connolly, S. J., Ezekowitz, M. D., Yusuf, S., et al. (2009). Dabigatran versus warfarin in patients with atrial fibrillation. *New England Journal of Medicine, 361*, 1139–1151.

*Coppola, A., Tufano, A., Cerbone, A. M., et al. (2009). Inherited thrombophilia: Implications for prevention and treatment of venous thromboembolism. *Seminars in Thrombosis and Hemostasis, 35*, 683–694.

*Dafer, R. M., & Biler, J. (2008). Antiphospholipid syndrome: Role of antiphospholipid antibodies in neurology. *Hematology/Oncology Clinics of North America, 22*, 95–105.

*Douketis, J. D., Berger, P. B., Dunn, A. S., et al. (2008). The perioperative management of antithrombotic therapy. American College of Chest Physicians Evidence-Based Clinical Practice Guidelines (8th Edition). *Chest, 133*(6 Suppl.), 299S–339S.

*Eikelboom, J. W., & Connolly, S. J. (2010). Explaining the RE-LY trial. *Canadian Journal of Hospital Pharmacy, 63*(4), 334.

Eisai. (2009). Product information for Fragmin. Woodcliff Lake, NJ: Author.

Eli Lilly. (2010). Product information for Effient. Indianapolis: Author.

*Eriksson, B. I., Quinlan, D. J., & Weitz, J. (2009). Comparative pharmacodynamics and pharmacokinetics of oral direct thrombin and factor Xa inhibitors in development. *Clinical Pharmacokinetics, 48*(1), 1–22.

*Fuster, V., Ryden, L. E., Cannon, D. S., et al. (2006). American College of Cardiology/American Heart Association/European Society of Cardiology 2006 Guidelines for the management of patients with atrial fibrillation. *Circulation, 114*, e-257–354.

*Garcia, D. A., & Hylek, E. (2008). Reducing the risk of stroke for patients who have atrial fibrillation. *Clinical Cardiology, 26*, 267–275.

*Garcia, D. A., Witt, D. M., Hylek, E., et al. (2008). Delivery of optimized anticoagulant therapy: Consensus statement from the anticoagulation forum. *Annals of Pharmacotherapy, 42*(9), 79–88.

*Geerts, W. H., Bergqvist, D., Pineo, G. F., et al. (2008). Prevention of venous thromboembolism: American College of Chest Physicians Evidence-Based Clinical Practice Guidelines (8th Edition). *Chest, 133*(6 Suppl.), 381S–453S.

GlaxoSmithKline. (2010). Product information for Arixtra. Research Triangle Park, NC: Author.

*Goldhaber, S. Z. (2010). Risk factors for venous thromboembolism. *Journal of the American College of Cardiology, 56*(1), 1–7.

*Goldstein, L. B., Adams, R., Bushnell, C. D., et al. (2011). Guidelines for the primary prevention of ischemic stroke: A Guideline for Healthcare Professionals from the American Heart Association/American Stroke Association. *Stroke. 42*, 517–584.

Granitto, M., & Galitz, D. (2008). Update on stroke: The latest guidelines. *The Nurse Practitioner, 33*, 39–46.

Hardin, S. R. (2008). Atrial fibrillation among older adults: Pathophysiology, symptoms, and treatment. *Journal of Gerontological Nursing, 34*, 26–32.

*Heit, J. A. (2006). Epidemiology of venous thromboembolism. In R. W. Colman (Ed.). *Hemostasis and thrombosis: Basic principles and clinical practice* (5th ed., pp. 1227–1233). Philadelphia: J. B. Lippincott.

*Hirsh, J., Bauer, K. A., Donati, M. B., et al. (2008). Parenteral anticoagulants. American College of Chest Physicians Evidence-Based Clinical Practical Guidelines (8th Edition). *Chest, 133*(6 Suppl.), 141S–159S.

*Holbrook, A. M., Pereira, J. A., Labiris, R., et al. (2005). Systematic overview of warfarin and its drug and food interactions. *Archives of Internal Medicine, 165*, 1095–1106.

*Hull, R. D., & Pineo, G. F. (2004). Heparin and low molecular-weight heparin therapy for venous thromboembolism: Will unfractionated heparin survive? *Seminars in Thrombosis and Hemostasis, 30*(Suppl. 1), 11–23.

*Jacobs, L. G. (2008). Warfarin pharmacology, clinical management, and evaluation of hemorrhagic risk for the elderly. *Cardiology Clinics, 26*, 157–167.

*Jacobson, A. K. (2008). Warfarin monitoring: Point-of-care INR testing limitations and interpretation of the prothrombin time. *Journal of Thrombosis and Thrombolysis, 25*, 10–11.

*Kearon, C., Kahn, S. R., Agnelli, G., et al. (2008). Antithrombotic therapy for venous thromboembolic disease: American College of Chest Physicians Evidence-Based Clinical Practical Guidelines (8th Edition). *Chest, 133* (6 Suppl.), 454S–545S.

*Kelechi, T., & Bonham, P. A. (2008). Lower extremity venous disorders: Implications for nursing practice. *Journal of Cardiovascular Nursing, 23*(2), 132–143.

*Khan, T., Wynne, H., Wood, P., et al. (2004). Dietary vitamin K influences intra-individual variability in anticoagulant response to warfarin. *British Journal of Haematology, 124*(3), 348–354.

Lambing, A. (2005). Clearing the way: Treating venous thromboembolism and deep venous thrombosis. *Advance for Nurse Practitioner, 14*(6), 24–30.

Leo Pharma. (2010). Product information for Innohep. Parsippany, NJ: Author.

*Lexi-Comp Online. (2010). Lexi-Comp, Inc. Retrieved November 24, 2010, from www.lexi.com.

Madden, S. (2009). Treatment of older patients with aortic valve stenosis. *Nursing Standard, 24*(12), 42–48.

*Maganti, K., Rigolin, V. H., Enriquez Sarano, M., et al. (2010). Valvular heart disease: Diagnosis and management. *Mayo Clinic Proceedings, 85*, 483–500.

*Man-Son-Hing, M., Nichol, G., Lau, A., et al. (1999). Choosing antithrombotic therapy for elderly patients with atrial fibrillation who are at risk for falls. *Archives of Internal Medicine, 159*, 677–685.

Marsh, J. D., & Keyrouz, S. G. (2010). Stroke prevention and treatment. *Journal of the American College of Cardiology, 56*(9), 683–691.

*McCabe, P. J. (2005). Spheres of clinical nurse specialist practice influence evidence-based care for patients with atrial fibrillation. *Clinical Nurse Specialist, 19*(6), 308–317.

*Merli, G. J. (2008). Pathophysiology of venous thrombosis and the diagnosis of deep venous thrombosis-pulmonary embolism in the elderly. *Cardiology Clinics, 26*, 203–219.

Merrill, J. (2010). Oral anticoagulants: Big bucks, but payers are on guard. *The Pink Sheet*, October 25.

National Institutes of Health Drug-Nutrient Interaction Task Force. Important drug and food information. http://ods.od.nih.gov/factsheets/cc/coumadin1.pdf.

*Nutescu, E. A., Shapiro, N. L., Ibrahim, S., et al. (2006). Warfarin and its interactions with foods, herbs and other dietary supplements. *Expert Opinion on Drug Safety, 5*(3), 433–451.

*Ortel, T. L. (2010). Acquired thrombotic risk factors in the critical care setting. *Critical Care Medicine, 28*(Suppl.), S43–S50.

*Osinbowale, O., Ali, L., & Chi, Y. W. (2010). Venous thromboembolism: A clinical review. *Postgraduate Medicine, 122*(2), 54–65.

*Palatnik, A. (2007). Putting a stop to thrombi. *Nursing, 37*(Suppl.), 2–6.

*Patrono, C., Baigent, C., Hirsh, J., et al. (2008). Antiplatelet drugs: American College of Chest Physicians Evidence-Based Clinical Practice Guidelines (8th Edition). *Chest, 133*(6 Suppl.), 199S–233S.

*Piazza, G., & Goldhaber, S. Z. (2006). Acute pulmonary embolism. Part 1: Epidemiology and diagnosis. *Circulation, 114*, e28–e32.

Ridings, H. G., Holt, L., Cook, R., et al. (2009). Genetic susceptibility to VTE: A primary care approach. *Journal of the American Academy of Physician Assistants, 22*(7), 20–25.

*Righini, M., & Bounameaux, H. (2008). Clinical relevance of distal deep vein thrombosis. *Current Opinion in Pulmonary Medicine, 14*, 408–413.

Rincon, F., & Sacco, R. L. (2008). Secondary stroke prevention. *Journal of Cardiovascular Nursing, 23*, 34–41.

Roche. (2001). Product information for Ticlid. Nutley, NJ: Author.

*Sacco, R. L., Adams, R., Albers, G., et al. (2006). Guidelines for prevention of stroke in patients with ischemic stroke or transient ischemic attack: A statement for health care professionals from the American Heart Association/American Stroke Association Council on Stroke. *Stroke, 37*, 577–617.

*Salem, D. V., O'Gara, P. T., Madias, C., et al. (2008). Valvular and structural heart disease: American College of Chest Physicians Evidence-Based Clinical Practice Guidelines (8th Edition). *Chest, 133*(6 Suppl.), 593S–626S.

*Sanofi Aventis. (2010). Product information for Lovenox. Bridgewater, NJ: Author.

Sawyer, N. A. (2010). Lower extremity edema: To maintain a balance, treat the underlying disease. *Advance for Physician Assistants, 6*(8), 16–20.

*Schirmer, S. H., Baumhakel, M., Neuberger, H. R., et al. (2010). Novel anticoagulants for stroke prevention in atrial fibrillation. *Journal of the American College of Cardiology, 56*(25), 2067–2076.

*Schulman, S., Beyth, R. J., Kearon, C., et al. (2008). Hemorrhagic complications of anticoagulant and thrombolytic treatment. American College of Chest Physicians Evidence-Based Clinical Practice Guidelines (8th Edition). *Chest, 133*(6 Suppl.), 257S–298S.

Simmons, B. B., Yeo, A., & Fung, K. (2010). Current guidelines on antiplatelet agents for secondary prevention of noncardiogenic stroke. *Postgraduate Medicine, 122*(2), 49–53.

*Singer, D. A., Albers, G. A., & Dalen, J. E. (2008). Antithrombotic therapy in atrial fibrillation: American College of Chest Physicians Evidence-Based Clinical Practice Guidelines (8th Edition). *Chest, 133*(6 Suppl.), 546S–592S.

Slusher, K. B. (2010). Factor V Leiden: A case study and review. *Dimensions of Critical Care Nursing, 29*(1), 6–10.

Somarouthu, B., Abbara, S., & Kalva, S. (2010). Diagnosing deep vein thrombosis. *Postgraduate Medicine, 122*(2), 66–73.

*Spandorfer, J., Konkle, B. A., & Merli, G. J. (2001). *Management and prevention of thrombosis in primary care*. London: Arnold.

*Spinler, S. A., Nutescu, E. A., Smythe, M. A., et al. (2005). Anticoagulation monitoring part 1: Warfarin and parenteral direct thrombin inhibitors. *Annals of Pharmacotherapy, 39*, 1049–1055.

*Spyropoulos, A. C. (2008). Brave new world: The current and future use of novel anticoagulants. *Thrombosis Research, 123*, S29–S35.

*Streiff, M. B. (2010). The National Comprehensive Cancer Network (NCCN) guidelines on the management of venous thromboembolism in cancer patients. *Thrombosis Research, 125*(Suppl. 2) S128–S133.

*Sun, J. C., Davidson, M. J., Lamy, A., et al. (2010). Antithrombotic management of patients with prosthetic heart valves: Current evidence and future trends. *Lancet, 374*, 565–576.

*Suttie, J. W. (1992). Vitamin K and human nutrition. *Journal of the American Dietetic Association, 92*, 585–590.

*Tran, H. A., & Ginsberg, J. S. (2006). Anticoagulant therapy for major arterial and venous thromboembolism. In R. W. Colman (ed.). *Hemostasis and thrombosis: Basic principles and clinical practice* (5th ed., pp. 1676–1680). Philadelphia: J. B. Lippincott.

Turka, J. (2005). Understanding the INR. *Nursing, 35*(8), 18–19.

*U.S. Department of Health and Human Services (2008). The Surgeon General's call to action to prevent deep vein thrombosis and pulmonary embolism. Accessed September 2010 at http://www.surgeongeneral.gov/topics/deepvein/calltoaction/call-to-action-on-dvt-2008.pdf.

*Varga, E. A. (2008). Genetics in the context of thrombophilia. *Journal of Thrombosis and Thrombolysis, 25*, 2–5.

*Vazquez, S. R., Freeman, A., Van Woerkom, et al. (2009). Contemporary issues in the postthrombotic syndrome. *Annals of Pharmacotherapy, 23*, 1824–1835.

*Wann, L. S., Curtis, A. B., January, C. T., et al. (2011). 2011 ACC/AHA/HRS focused update on the management of patients with atrial fibrillation (updating the 2006 guidelines). *Circulation, 123*, 104–123.

*Wann, L. S., Curtis, A. B., Ellenbogen K. A., et al. (2011). 2011 ACCF/AHA/HRS Focused update on the management of patients with atrial fibrillation (update on dabigatran): A report of the American College of Cardiology Foundation/American Heart Association Task Force on Practice Guidelines. *Circulation, 123*, 1144–1150.

*Warkentin, T. E. (2010). Agents for the treatment of heparin-induced thrombocytopenia. *Hematology and Oncology Clinics of North America, 24*, 755–775.

*Weitz, J. I. (2009). Unanswered questions in venous thromboembolism. *Thrombosis Research 123*(4 Suppl.), S2–S10.

Welch, E. (2006). The assessment and management of venous thromboembolism. *Nursing Standard, 20*(28), 24–30.

Weyland, P. (2009). Warfarin management: Tap into new ways to slow the clot. *The Nurse Practitioner, 34*(3), 22–28.

*Witt, D. M., Tillman, D. J., Evans, C. M., et al. (2003). Evaluation of the clinical and economic impact of a brand name-to-generic warfarin sodium conversion program. *Pharmacotherapy, 23*(3), 360–368.

*Witt, D. (2010). Optimizing use of current anticoagulants. *Hematology Oncology Clinics of North America, 24*, 717–726.

*Wittkowsky, A. K. (2008). Dietary supplements, herbs and oral anticoagulants: The nature of the evidence. *Journal of Thrombosis and Thrombolysis, 25*, 72–77.

*Wood, S. (2010). Dabigatran Q+A: The who, when, and how for switching, starting and stopping the new oral anticoagulant. *Heartwire*, November 3, 2010. Retrieved November 24, 2010, from http:www.theheart.org/article/1161057.do#socialcomments.

Anemias

Anemia is a condition in which the number of red blood cells (RBCs) or their oxygen-carrying capacity is insufficient to meet physiologic needs, which vary by age, sex, altitude, and pregnancy status (**Table 50.1**). There is not one set of "normal ranges" for hemoglobin, hematocrit, and RBCs. In general, anemia can be defined as values that are more than two standard deviations below the mean. For example, a hemoglobin <13.5 g/dL or a hematocrit <41% represents anemia in men; in women, <12.0 g/dL or <36%.

CAUSES

Anemia may develop through blood loss, nutritional deficiency, or malabsorption syndromes, or concurrently with inflammation or malignancy, or be inherited as in sickle cell disease, thalassemia, or hemoglobinopathy. Anemia may also occur from the treatment of diseases such as cancer, human immunodeficiency virus (HIV)/acquired immunodeficiency syndrome, or hepatitis C.

PATHOPHYSIOLOGY

RBCs, also known as *erythrocytes,* are formed in the marrow of ribs, sternum, clavicle, vertebrae, pelvis, and proximal epiphyses of the humerus and femur. RBCs play a vital role in the support of tissue metabolism by transporting oxygen to and removing carbon dioxide from tissue. To maintain proper tissue oxygenation and sustain a normal acid–base balance, an adequate number of RBCs must be available and they must be a specific shape and size.

The production of RBCs involves a series of maturational steps beginning with a pluripotent cell that differentiates into erythroid precursors. As the cells undergo maturational changes, they lose their nuclei and acquire hemoglobin as a component. The production of RBCs is initiated by the hormone erythropoietin (EPO), which is produced by the kidneys in response to a decrease in tissue oxygen concentration. Decreased tissue oxygen then signals the kidneys to increase production and release EPO. This EPO stimulates the stem cell to differentiate into proerythroblasts; EPO also increases the rate of mitosis and increases the release of reticulocytes from the marrow and induces hemoglobin formation. When hemoglobin synthesis is accelerated, the critical hemoglobin concentration necessary for maturity is reached more rapidly, causing an earlier release of reticulocytes. The appearance of reticulocytes in peripheral circulation indicates that RBC production is being stimulated. The maturation process takes about 1 week. Several days are then required for the reticulocyte to become an erythrocyte. The normal RBC survival time is 120 days. The survival time can be decreased to 18 to 20 days before occurrence of an anemia if the bone marrow functions at maximal capacity. When hemolytic destruction of RBCs exceeds marrow production, anemia will develop, causing the hemoglobin value to decrease.

DIAGNOSTIC CRITERIA

Anemia is a reduction in the number of circulating RBCs (the hemoglobin concentration) or the volume of packed RBCs (hematocrit) in the blood. Anemias are classified according to their pathophysiologic basis and occur due to decreased production or increased destruction of RBCs (**Box 50.1**). They are also classified according to cell size using the mean corpuscular volume (MCV). Microcytic anemias are those anemias due to RBCs with a lower than normal size. These include iron deficiency anemia, thalassemia, and anemia of chronic disease. In contrast, macrocytic anemia may be megaloblastic such as folate or vitamin B_{12} deficiency or nonmegaloblastic causes such as myelodysplasia, liver disease, or reticulocytosis.

TABLE 50.1	Hemoglobin Thresholds
Age or Gender Group	**Hemoglobin Thresholds (g/L)**
Children (0.5–4.99 y)	110
Children (5.00–11.99 y)	115
Children (12.0–14.99 y)	120
Nonpregnant women (15.00 y)	120
Pregnant women	110
Men (15.00 y)	130

BOX **50.1**

Classification of Anemias by Pathophysiology

Increased destruction
  Blood loss
  Hemolysis
  Sickle cell disease
  G6PD deficiency
  Thrombotic thrombocytopenic purpura
  Hemolytic-uremic syndrome
  Clostridial infection
  Hypersplenism
Decreased production
  Iron deficiency
  Thalassemia
  Anemia of chronic disease
  Aplastic anemia
  Myeloproliferative leukemia
G6PD, glucose-6-phosphate dehydrogenase.

The signs and symptoms of anemia depend on the rate of development, age, and cardiovascular status of the patient. Rapid onset of anemia is most likely to present with cardio-respiratory symptoms (tachycardia, lightheadedness, breathlessness). Anemia of a chronic nature may present with symptoms including fatigue, weakness, headache, vertigo, faintness, sensitivity to cold, pallor, and loss of skin tone.

ANEMIAS CAUSED BY INCREASED DESTRUCTION

ACUTE POSTHEMORRHAGIC ANEMIA/CHRONIC BLOOD LOSS

Posthemorrhagic anemia results from massive hemorrhage associated with spontaneous or traumatic rupture or incision of a large blood vessel, erosion of an artery by lesion (peptic ulcer, neoplasm), or failure of normal hemostasis. The sudden loss of one third of blood volume may be fatal, whereas a two-thirds loss of blood volume slowly over 24 hours is without immediate risk. During and immediately after hemorrhage, the RBC count, hemoglobin value, and hematocrit may be high due to vasoconstriction. Within a few hours, fluid from tissue enters the circulation resulting in hemodilution causing a drop in the RBC count and hemoglobin value. This result is proportional to the severity of bleeding. Signs of vascular instability appear with acute losses of 10% to 15% of the total blood volume. Signs of vascular instability are hypotension and decreased organ perfusion. When more than 30% of blood volume is

lost, suddenly hypotension and tachycardia occurs. When the volume of blood lost is greater than 40%, signs of hypovolemic shock, including confusion, dyspnea, diaphoresis, hypotension, and tachycardia, appear.

Diagnostic Criteria

Initial evaluation of anemia includes a careful history and physical examination. Laboratory evaluation includes complete blood count (CBC), reticulocyte index, iron studies, examination of the peripheral blood smear, and a stool sample for occult blood. Further studies are indicated based on the results of the preliminary evaluation.

Initiating Therapy

Immediate therapy consists of hemostasis, restoration of blood volume, and treatment of shock. In many cases, the blood lost needs to be replaced promptly. Blood transfusion is the only means of rapidly restoring blood volume.

SICKLE CELL ANEMIA

Sickle cell anemia is an autosomal recessive disorder in which abnormal hemoglobin leads to chronic hemolytic anemia with numerous clinical consequences. It most commonly affects African Americans and, to a lesser extent, Hispanics.

Pathophysiology

Patients with sickle cell disease (SCD) predominantly make hemoglobin S. Hemoglobin S differs from normal hemoglobin A by the substitution of a single amino acid within one of the two polypeptide chains. Deoxygenation causes RBCs to sickle and leads to vaso-occlusion and blockage of microvasculature, which can cause sickle cell crisis. This blockage causes significant damage to the endothelium of the arterial and venous circulation. Crisis occurs when patients are physically stressed (exercise), exposed to high altitude or cold temperatures, or have a high fever or infection. The underlying cause includes hypoxia, dehydration, and acidosis. Sickle cell crises last about a week but may not resolve for several weeks to months. Pain typically occurs in the back, ribs, and limbs. Patients with sickle cell anemia are susceptible to infection, particularly *Streptococcus pneumoniae* and *Haemophilus influenzae,* and are prone to gallstones and renal failure. Other complications include chronic leg ulcer, priapism, aseptic necrosis of the humoral and femoral heads, and chronic osteomyelitis. Long-term effects include stroke, heart failure, and death.

Therapeutic transfusion therapy is reserved for individuals with acute stroke, acute chest syndrome, acute multi-organ failure, and acute symptomatic anemia. A lifelong cure for SCD is available through an HLA-matched sibling donor hematopoietic stem cell transplant. However, this treatment is limited to individuals who are younger than age 16 due to toxicities and death among individuals older than age 16.

Diagnostic Criteria

Examination of a peripheral blood smear for sickling and checking a reticulocyte count can provide supportive data for the diagnosis of SCD. Hemoglobin electrophoresis or a sickle cell preparation can also be useful in the diagnosis of SCD. Laboratory findings also show reduced hemoglobin and a RBC count between 2 and 3 million/μL.

For those at risk, techniques such as chorionic biopsy have been used during early gestation (6–8 weeks of pregnancy) to identify SCD. Genetic counseling and education must also be offered. Risk of the procedure to mother and fetus, risks of false-positive and false-negative results, and the acceptability of therapeutic abortion should also be discussed.

Initiating Drug Therapy

No specific treatment is available for patients with sickle cell anemia. The management of SCD focuses on primary prevention and treatment of the complication as well as a potential cure. Children with SCD should be immunized against *S. pneumoniae*, *H. influenzae* type B, hepatitis B virus, and influenza. The pneumococcal conjugate vaccine (Pneumovax) is given at age 2 months followed by two more doses 6 to 8 weeks apart and a booster at age 12 months. This is followed by the pneumococcal polysaccharide vaccine at ages 2 and 5. In adults, the Centers for Disease Control and Prevention recommends that the Pneumovax be readministered every 5 years. Patients are maintained on folic acid supplementation, 1 mg/day, because of accelerated erythropoiesis.

Hydroxyurea

In selected patients, hydroxyurea is used for prophylaxis treatment to reduce the number of crises (acute chest syndrome or >3 crises per year). The effects of hydroxyurea on RBCs include increasing hemoglobin F levels, increasing water content of RBCs, increasing deformability of sickled cells, and altering the adhesion of RBCs to endothelium. Evidence suggests that hydroxyurea reduces the number of chest syndromes and transfusions and may reverse organ dysfunction.

The optimal regimen of hydroxyurea has not been determined. Doses start at 15 mg/kg/day and are increased by 5 mg/kg/day every 12 weeks until marrow suppression is present. The suggested maximum dose is 35 mg/kg/day. The goal of hydroxyurea is to achieve a white blood cell (WBC) count between 5,000 and 8,000 WBCs/mm^3 and suppression of the granulocyte and reticulocyte counts. Hydroxyurea is a cytotoxic agent and has the potential to cause life-threatening cytopenia. This drug should not be used in patients likely to become pregnant or those unwilling or unable to follow instructions regarding treatment. Patients should be monitored for myelotoxicity. Serious adverse reactions include myelosuppression and the risk of cancer. Side effects include cutaneous hyperpigmentation, alopecia, xerosis, nail pigmentation, and leg ulcers. A long-term study of the use of hydroxyurea showed that it is safe and might decrease mortality.

Pain Management

Management of acute painful episodes consists of exclusion of causes (infection), hydration by oral or intravenous (IV) fluid resuscitation, and aggressive pain relief, including analgesics and opiates. Acetaminophen has analgesic and antipyretic effects. The daily total adult dose must not exceed 4 g in four to six divided doses. High dosages damage the liver and could be fatal. In the presence of liver disease, the daily dose should be decreased.

Nonsteroidal anti-inflammatory agents (NSAIDs) have anti-inflammatory effects in addition to analgesic and antipyretic proprieties. NSAIDs act primarily at the level of nociceptors where pain impulses originate. They exert their analgesic effect by inhibiting cyclo-oxygenase enzymes and decreasing prostaglandin synthesis. NSAIDs have potentially serious adverse effects, including gastropathy, neuropathy, and homeostatic defects. NSAIDs should not be administered to patients with renal disease or a history of peptic ulcer disease.

Ketorolac 0.5 mg/kg IV (maximum dose, 30 mg) followed by 0.5 mg/kg IV should be given every 6 hours (maximum dose, 15 mg). Ketorolac is contraindicated in patients with advanced renal impairment. Patients with moderately elevated serum creatinine should use half the recommended dose. Caution should be used in patients with hepatic impairment. Side effects include headache, gastrointestinal (GI) pain, diarrhea, dyspepsia, nausea, edema, hypertension, dizziness, drowsiness, anemia, and increased bleeding time and liver enzymes.

Tramadol is a synthetic centrally acting analgesic that binds to opiate receptors in the central nervous system and inhibits the pain pathway and alters the perception of pain. Tramadol also inhibits serotonin and norepinephrine, which also modifies pain pathways. Tramadol requires dose adjustment in patients with hepatic and renal impairment. Side effects include nausea, vomiting, dyspepsia, flushing, dizziness, headache, somnolence, insomnia, pruritus, and constipation.

The management of acute painful crisis includes aggressive narcotic analgesia, such as meperidine, morphine, or hydromorphone. (See Chapter 7.) Adverse effects of opioid analgesics include severe sedation and respiratory depression. Side effects include itching, nausea, and vomiting. Opioid analgesics should be used carefully in patients with asthma, impaired ventilation, liver failure, renal failure. and increased intracranial pressure.

Meperidine should be used with caution in the treatment of acute SCD because multiple doses are associated with the accumulation of its major metabolite, normeperidine, and central toxicity, including twitching, multifocal clonus, and seizures. Coadministration with antipsychotics may cause neuromuscular disorders, including dystonia, tardive dyskinesia, akathisia, and neuroleptic malignant syndrome. Meperidine in combination with monoamine oxidase inhibitors may cause severe adverse reactions, including excitation, hyperpyrexia, convulsions, and death.

Patients with chronic sickle cell pain are managed with a combination of long-acting and short-acting opioids for breakthrough pain.

ANEMIAS CAUSED BY DIMINISHED PRODUCTION OF RED BLOOD CELLS

IRON DEFICIENCY ANEMIA

Iron deficiency anemia is the most common nutritional deficiency worldwide. Iron demands are increased in menstrual blood loss, pregnancy, and lactation. Iron deficiency has been implicated as a cause of perinatal complications such as low birth weight and premature delivery in affected mothers. In children, long-term findings include increased susceptibility to infection, poor growth, developmental and behavioral delays, and low mental and motor test scores.

Causes

Iron deficiency is related to insufficient iron intake, inadequate absorption from the GI tract, and increased iron demands; it is exacerbated by chronic intestinal blood loss due to parasitic and malarial infections. Dietary deficiencies result from decreased consumption of animal protein and ascorbic acid as a consequence of chronic alcoholism, food faddism, prolonged illness with anorexia, or poor nutrition (**Box 50.2**).

Inadequate absorption from the GI tract is usually related to malabsorption syndromes, postgastrectomy, and the presence of certain foods or drugs or unrelenting diarrhea. The prevalence of iron deficiency anemia in the United States is declining as a result of food and formula supplementation. However, it remains of concern in toddlers, adolescents, and women of childbearing age.

Pathophysiology

The predominant use of iron is for the creation of heme groups that are incorporated into hemoglobin and myoglobin. Additionally, iron is involved in the production of cytochromes and other enzymes. Immediately bioavailable, iron is bound in the bloodstream to a specific carrier protein, transferrin. Excess of immediate iron needs are stored in the liver, spleen, and bone marrow as ferritin. Patients with iron deficiency anemia may be asymptomatic or have vague symptoms. Other manifestations include koilonychia (spoon nail), angular stomatitis, glossitis, and pica (eating dirt, paint, clay, ice, or cornstarch).

Diagnostic Criteria

Laboratory findings are critical for the diagnosis. The classic criteria for iron deficiency anemia include low serum iron and ferritin concentrations and a high total iron-binding capacity (TIBC). In mild iron deficiency, the hemoglobin, hematocrit, and RBC indices remain normal. In the later stages, the hemoglobin and hematocrit levels fall below normal values.

A low concentration of ferritin (<0–12 g/L) is the earliest and most sensitive indication of iron deficiency. However, patients with renal or liver disease, malignancies, or infectious or inflammatory processes may have elevated ferritin levels that may not correlate with iron stores in the bone marrow. Transferrin saturation (serum iron divided by TIBC) is also used to assess iron deficiency anemia. Low values (<15%) indicate iron deficiency anemia, although low serum transferrin saturation values may also be present in inflammatory disorders. In this case, TIBC helps to differentiate the diagnosis. A TIBC over 400 mcg/dL suggests iron deficiency anemia, whereas values below 200 mcg/dL usually represent inflammatory disease. Free erythrocyte protoporphyrin (FEP) can also be used to distinguish between iron deficiency anemia and thalassemia minor. Iron binds with protoporphyrin to form heme. The serum concentration of protoporphyrin not bound to iron is elevated when iron levels are low. Thus, FEP is elevated in patients with iron deficiency anemia, inflammatory disorders, and lead poisoning. Rarely, a bone marrow examination is performed to assess iron stores.

Initiating Drug Therapy

The treatment of iron deficiency anemia consists of dietary supplementation and iron preparations (**Table 50.2**). Iron is best absorbed from red meat, fish, and poultry. Plant-based foods are good sources of iron, although they are less easily absorbed. Whole-grain or iron-fortified cereals, breads, and pastas are among the best. Beverages such as tea or milk will reduce the absorption of iron and should be consumed

---

BOX 50.2

Causes of Iron Deficiency

Deficient diet
Decreased absorption
Increased requirements
  Pregnancy
  Lactation
Blood loss
  GI
  Menstrual
  Blood donation
Hemoglobinuria
Iron sequestration

TABLE 50.2   Elemental Iron Content of Various Iron Salts

Iron Salt	% Iron
Ferrous fumarate	33
Ferrous gluconate	11.6
Ferrous sulfate	20
Ferrous sulfate, anhydrous	30

in moderation between meals. Medications such as antacids, proton pump inhibitors, and histamine-2 (H_2) antagonists reduce absorption and should be avoided if possible. Vitamin C (500 mg daily), as well as orange juice, increases the absorption of iron due to increased stomach acidity. They should be given together and are recommended with meals. Transfusion should be considered for patients with iron deficiency anemia complaining of fatigue or dyspnea on exertion.

Indications for the use of IV iron include chronic uncorrectable bleeding, intestinal malabsorption, intolerance to oral iron, nonadherence, or hemoglobin of less than 6 g/dL with signs of poor perfusion.

Goals of Drug Therapy

Goals are specific to the patient and include an evaluation of the impact the anemia has on quality of life, activities of daily living, and general well-being. Minimization of the impact chronic iron deficiency anemia has on adequate iron replacement has typically occurred when the serum ferritin level reaches 50 mcg/L and when the hemoglobin and hematocrit have returned to normal levels.

Iron Replacement Therapy

Dosage

Treatment of adult iron deficiency anemia should start with 2 to 3 mg/kg oral elemental iron daily in three divided doses. Infants (ages 0 to 6 months) should receive 10 to 25 mg/kg/day, also in divided doses. Children ages 6 months to 2 years should receive 6 mg/kg/day. Oral iron therapy with soluble ferrous iron salts is the preferred therapy due to the improved bioavailability of the ferrous ion. Non–enteric-coated ferrous salts containing ferrous sulfate are the least expensive and provide adequate elemental iron. Typically, a dose of 325 mg ferrous sulfate three times daily provides sufficient iron replacement (195 mg elemental iron or about 2.7 mg/kg for a 70-kg adult). Slow-release or sustained-release iron preparations do not dissolve until reaching the small intestines, significantly reducing iron absorption. Iron should be administered daily in divided doses preferably 1 hour before meals.

Iron dextran is administered intravenously in one large dose of 200 to 500 mg. Safer alternatives include sodium ferric gluconate and iron sucrose. Sodium ferric gluconate is administered intravenously in eight weekly 125-mg doses for a total of 1,000 mg, and iron sucrose is administered intravenously five times over 2 weeks in 200-mg doses.

Time Frame for Response

Therapeutic doses of iron should increase hemoglobin value by 0.7 to 1 g/week. Reticulocytosis occurs within 7 to 10 days after initiation of iron therapy. Iron therapy should be continued for at least 3 to 6 months. Common causes of treatment failure include noncompliance with therapy, malabsorption, and blood loss equal to the rate of production. Malabsorption can be ruled out by the iron test in which plasma iron levels are determined at half-hour intervals for 2 hours following administration of 50 mg of ferrous sulfate. Absorption is satisfactory if iron plasma levels increase by more than 50 ng/dL.

Adverse Events

Adverse reactions to iron are primarily GI difficulties, consisting of discolored feces, anorexia, constipation or diarrhea, nausea, and vomiting. To minimize the GI side effects, iron supplements should be taken with food. However, the impact of this on bioavailability of agents may be as high as a 66% decrease in iron absorption. Changing to a different iron salt or to a controlled-release preparation may also reduce side effects.

A major adverse reaction of iron dextran is the risk of anaphylaxis, which can be fatal. Delayed reactions include myalgias, headache, and arthralgias.

Interactions

There is a host of drug–drug interactions with iron preparations. Many antibiotics, such as tetracyclines and fluoroquinolones, have a decrease in absorption due to the formation of a chelation product with the ferrous ions. The absorption of iron may be decreased when it is given with products containing aluminum, calcium, or magnesium. This effect may be as much as 30% to 40% reduction in absorption. The theory is that the reduced stomach acidity secondary to the antacid-like properties of products reduces the iron absorption. Similarly, patients taking proton pump inhibitors or H_2 antagonists may also have decreased iron absorption due to the lowered stomach acid. If the patient is taking both medications, space them at least 1 to 2 hours apart. In contrast, acidifying agents such as ascorbic acid (vitamin C) may enhance the absorption of iron-containing salts.

ANEMIA OF CHRONIC RENAL FAILURE

Anemia is a common complication of chronic renal failure and is primarily due to reduced EPO production by the kidney. Anemia occurs when the glomerular filtration rate (GFR) declines below 60 mL/minute. Stages of chronic kidney disease (CKD) are defined according to the estimated GFR (**Table 50.3**) based on National Kidney Foundation guidelines

TABLE 50.3	Classification of Chronic Kidney Disease
Stage	**GFR, mL/minute/1.73 m^2**
0	>90[a]
1	>90[b]
2	60–89
3	30–59
4	15–29
5	<15

[a] With risk factors for CKD
[b] With demonstrated kidney damage (e.g., persistent proteinuria, abnormal urine sediments, abnormal blood and urine chemistry, and abnormal imaging studies)

(Kidney Dialysis Outcomes Quality Initiative [KDOQI]). Risk factors that increase the risk of CKD include hypertension, diabetes mellitus, autoimmune disease, older age, African ancestry, a family history of renal disease, a previous episode of acute renal failure, and the presence of proteinuria, abnormal urinary sediment, or structural abnormalities of the urinary tract. Measurement of albuminuria is a good test for early detection of renal disease; a 24-hour urine collection is the "gold standard." A first-morning urine sample is often more practical and correlates well, but not perfectly. Persistence in the urine of greater than 17 mg of albumin per gram of creatinine in adult males and 25 mg of albumin per gram of creatinine in adult females usually signifies chronic renal damage.

With advanced renal impairment, metabolic and endocrine functions are impaired and result in anemia, malnutrition, and the abnormal metabolism of carbohydrates, fats, and proteins. Plasma levels of hormones, including parathyroid hormone (PTH), insulin, glucagon, sex hormones, and prolactin, change with renal failure as a result of urinary retention, decreased degradation, and abnormal regulation. Progressive renal impairment is associated with worsening systemic inflammation as seen with elevated levels of C-reactive protein, which contributes to the acceleration of vascular disease and comorbidity associated with advanced renal disease. Calciphylaxis is a devastating condition seen in patients with advanced kidney disease. It is heralded by livedo reticularis and advances to patches of ischemic necrosis, especially on the legs, thighs, abdomen, and breasts.

Pathophysiology

CKD is characterized by the progressive loss of functioning nephrons. With a reduction in nephron mass, renal vasodilation occurs and leads to hyperperfusion of the remaining glomeruli. Nephrons exposed to prolonged hyperperfusion begin to leak protein, become sclerotic, and eventually are destroyed. Substances that are filtered that are neither secreted nor resorbed by the tubule, such as urea, begin to rise early in the course of renal impairment.

Serum concentration of phosphorus, which is under the influence of PTH, is kept within the normal range until more than 80% of real function is lost. This is because increased PTH reduces the amount of phosphorus resorbed by the tubule. Failure of the kidney to fulfill its excretory, endocrine, and metabolic function results in inadequate quantities of EPO and 1,25-dihydroxy-vitamin D_3. Other hormones, such as PTH, insulin, and prolactin, are present in excess. The primary cause of anemia in patients with CKD is insufficient EPO production by the diseased kidneys. The mechanisms impairing renal EPO production are not well understood.

Initiating Drug Therapy

Patients should be placed on a multivitamin to replace the vitamins lacking in restrictive diets. Adequate bone marrow iron stores should be available before EPO treatment is initiated. Iron supplementation is usually essential to ensure an adequate response to EPO because the demand for iron by the marrow frequently exceeds the amount of iron immediately available for erythropoiesis (measured by percentage of transferring saturation) as well as the amount of iron stores (measured by serum ferritin). Current practice is to target a hemoglobin concentration of 110 to 120 g/L.

The treatment of anemia caused by chronic renal failure begins with treating reversible causes of deteriorating renal function. Disorders of mineral metabolism (calcium, phosphorus, and bone) are common in CKD. Oral phosphorus-binding agents, calcium carbonate, and calcium acetate are used to treat hyperphosphatemia. Phosphorus-binding agents that do not contain calcium are sevelamer and lanthanum. Vitamin D or vitamin D analogs (calcitriol, paricalcitol) are given to treat secondary hyperparathyroidism.

Many of the immunologically mediated renal diseases (e.g., membranous nephropathy, Wegener disease, Goodpasture syndrome, lupus nephritis) respond to treatment with corticosteroids, cytotoxic agents, or plasmapheresis. This will not be discussed here. These patients should be under the care of a rheumatologist and/or a nephrologist.

When renal disease is associated with a metabolic disorder such as diabetes (Chapter 45) or gout (not discussed here), the treatment is directed at metabolic control to slow the course of renal deterioration.

When a drug (methicillin, indomethacin, NSAID, metformin, meperidine, and oral hypoglycemics) or other toxic substance is identified as the cause of renal failure, the offending agent should be withheld or avoided. Many antibiotics, antihypertensives, and antiarrhythmics require a reduced dosage or a change in the dose interval in patients with kidney disease.

Goals of Drug Therapy

The goals of therapy are to (1) treat the underlying renal disease; (2) slow the progression of renal deterioration by modifying the known or suspected factors that are thought to aggravate the primary process and avoid factors that may aggravate existing renal failure; and (3) treat the specific complications of renal disease and prevent long-term complications of uremia. Correction of anemia decreases morbidity and reduces hospitalization and mortality among patients with CKD. Benefits of correcting anemia include improvements in quality of life, exercise capacity, cognitive function, and sexual function.

Epoetin and Darbepoetin

Recombinant EPO (epoetin, Epogen, Procrit) is indicated for the treatment of anemia due to chronic renal failure, zidovudine administration (in HIV-infected patients), and chemotherapy administration. Epoetin is used in patients whose hematocrits are less than 30% to 35%. Other indications include a reduction in blood transfusions in anemic patients undergoing elective, noncardiac, nonvascular surgery. Similarly, darbepoetin is indicated for patients with chronic renal failure and patients receiving chemotherapy.

Mechanism of Action

Epoetin and darbepoetin are recombinant hormones that stimulate the production of RBCs from the erythroid tissues in the bone marrow. Epoetin also stimulates the division and differentiation of erythroid progenitors in bone marrow. Darbepoetin is a longer-acting erythropoietic agent than epoetin (serum half-life of 25 hours versus 8.5 hours).

Dosage

The starting dose of epoetin is 50 to 100 units/kg given subcutaneously or intravenously 3 times a week until the hematocrit approaches 30% to 36% or increases greater than 4 points in a 2-week period. The dosing is the same whether it is given subcutaneously or intravenously. The subcutaneous route provides sustained serum levels compared to the IV route.

The recommended starting dose for darbepoetin is 0.45 mcg/kg body weight, administered as a single IV or subcutaneous injection once weekly. Dosing is the same whether it is given subcutaneously or intravenously. A target hemoglobin concentration of 12 g/dL should not be exceeded. After initiating therapy, the hemoglobin level should be monitored weekly for at least 4 weeks until the hemoglobin value has stabilized.

All patients receiving erythropoietic stimulation should receive iron supplementation unless iron stores are already in excess. Iron supplementation should be initiated no later than the beginning of treatment and continue throughout the course of therapy. Oral therapy with ferrous sulfate 325 mg once to 3 times daily is adequate. Monitor the patient's hematocrit, blood pressure, clotting times, platelet counts, blood urea nitrogen level, and serum creatinine concentration.

Time Frame for Response

Two to 6 weeks may be required to evaluate the effectiveness of epoetin. If the response is not satisfactory in terms of reduced transfusion requirements or increased hematocrit after 8 weeks of therapy, the dose may be increased up to 300 units/kg 3 times a week. If patients do not respond, it is unlikely that they will respond to higher doses. Maintenance doses are individualized for each patient.

With once-weekly dosing, steady-state serum levels are achieved within 4 weeks with darbepoetin. Dose adjustment should not be increased more frequently than once a month. If the hemoglobin is increasing and approaching 12 g/dL, the dose should be reduced by 25%. If the hemoglobin continues to increase, the dose is withheld temporarily until the hemoglobin begins to stabilize.

Contraindications

Epoetin and darbepoetin are contraindicated in patients with uncontrolled hypertension or hypersensitivity to mammalian cell-derived products or human albumin. They are not intended for patients with chronic renal failure who require correction of severe anemia or in patients with iron folate deficiencies or GI bleeding.

Adverse Events

Epoetin and darbepoetin are generally well tolerated. Adverse reactions may include hypertension, headache, seizure, arthralgia, nausea, edema, fatigue, diarrhea, vomiting, chest pain, asthenia, and dizziness. Other adverse reactions include infection, hypertension, hypotension, and myalgia. Serious adverse reactions include vascular access thrombosis, heart failure, sepsis, and cardiac arrhythmia. There are no significant drug interactions.

Calcitriol

Calcitriol is indicated in patients with secondary hyperparathyroidism and hypocalcemia as a result of CKD. Calcitriol suppresses PTH secretion by increasing serum calcium concentrations through enhanced gut absorption of calcium as well as by directly decreasing PTH synthesis and parathyroid cell secretion. The size of the largest parathyroid gland may be a critical marker for response to calcitriol therapy. It is difficult to suppress PTH in patients with a gland larger than 0.5 cm^3. Larger glands are more likely to be composed of nodular tissue, which has a lesser density of vitamin D receptors and therefore is less responsive to calcitriol therapy. Patients are initially started on calcitriol 0.25 mcg daily. Dosage may increase by 0.25 mcg daily at 2- to 4-week intervals. The maintenance dose is 0.5 to 2 mcg daily. The KDOQI recommends a target PTH level of 150 to 300 pg/mL. A very low PTH level is associated with adynamic bone disease and possible consequences of fracture and ectopic calcification.

Contraindications

Calcitriol should not be used in patients with hypercalcemia.

Adverse Events

Calcitriol enhances phosphorus absorption from the gut and frequently leads to hyperphosphatemia.

ANEMIA OF CHRONIC DISEASE

Anemia of chronic disease is a hypoproliferative anemia and is associated with infection, organ failure, trauma, inflammation, and neoplasia (**Box 50.3**) and accounts for approximately 75% of all cases.

Pathophysiology

Anemia of chronic disease typically occurs despite adequate reticuloendothelial iron stores and is characterized by reduced concentrations of serum iron, transferrin, and TIBC; normal or raised ferritin levels; and high erythrocyte sedimentation rate. EPO production has also been implicated in the pathogenesis. It can mimic or coexist with other types of anemia (Fitzsimons & Brock, 2001). RBCs are often normochromic and normocytic. In patients with rheumatoid arthritis and Crohn's disease, RBCs are similar to the effects of iron deficiency, with hypochromic and microcytic indices.

BOX 50.3

Causes of Anemia of Chronic Disease

Common Causes
Chronic infections
  Tuberculosis
  Subacute bacterial endocarditis
  Osteomyelitis
Chronic inflammation
  Rheumatoid arthritis and inflammatory osteoarthritis
  Systemic lupus erythematosus
  Collagen-vascular diseases
  Gout
Malignancies
Less Common Causes
Alcoholic liver disease
Heart failure
Thrombophlebitis
Chronic obstructive lung disease
Ischemic heart disease

Diagnostic Criteria

In anemia of chronic disease, the hematocrit rarely falls below 60% of baseline. The MCV is usually normal or slightly reduced. Serum iron values may be unmeasurable, and transferrin saturation may be extremely low. Serum ferritin values should be normal or increased. A serum ferritin value lower than 30 mcg/L suggests coexistent iron deficiency.

Initiating Drug Therapy

Treatment is directed at the underlying cause and at eliminating exacerbating factors such as nutritional deficiencies and marrow-suppressive drugs. Other causes of anemia should be treated before initiating therapy.

Doses of recombinant epoetin are higher than those in renal anemia. Epoetin is administered subcutaneously and doses may vary from 150 to 1,500 units/kg/week.

Goals of Drug Therapy

A good response is likely if, after 2 weeks of therapy, the hemoglobin increases more than 0.5 g/dL. If no response has been observed at 900 units/kg/week, further escalation is unlikely to be effective. Iron supplements are required to ensure an adequate epoetin response.

THALASSEMIA

The thalassemias are hereditary disorders of hemoglobin synthesis, which are considered among the hypoproliferative

anemias. The α-thalassemia syndromes are seen primarily in persons from India and China and are less commonly seen in African Americans. The β-thalassemia syndrome affects primarily persons of Mediterranean origin (Italian, Greek). Every year, more than 200,000 babies are born with thalassemia major. They have a life expectancy of less than 30 years and are dependent on blood transfusions. Repeated transfusions result in cirrhosis of the liver, cardiomyopathy, endocrinopathies, and death due to hemosiderosis (Savulescu, 2004).

Pathophysiology

Normal adult hemoglobin is primarily hemoglobin A. Hemoglobin A consists of equal quantities of α- and β-globin chains. Thalassemia is present when a hemoglobinopathy is associated with a decreased production of either the α or β globins or a structurally abnormal globin chain. In α-thalassemia, the production of α-globin chains is controlled by four genes. Mutation of all four genes is incompatible with life (hydrops fetalis). Mutation of only one of the four is considered a silent carrier. Mutations of two of the four genes results in both microcytosis and mild anemia. Mutations of three of the four genes allow excess β chains to form tetramers (hemoglobin H) and results in severe anemia in addition to microcytosis. Physical examination will reveal pallor and splenomegaly. β-thalassemia is commonly classified by the severity of anemia; many genotypes exist for each phenotype. In β-thalassemia, β-globin chain is controlled by two genes. Mutations of one of two genes results in β-thalassemia trait (β-thalassemia minor). Thalassemia intermedia is associated with dysfunction of both β-globin genes. Clinical severity is intermediate (hemoglobin level of 7–10 g/dL) and patients are usually not dependent on transfusions. Thalassemia major (Cooley anemia) results from mutations of both genes and reveals a majority of hemoglobin F, which results in severe anemia and RBC transfusions are required to sustain life. Clinical problems include growth failure, bony deformities (abnormal facial structure, pathologic fractures), hepatosplenomegaly, jaundice, leg ulcers, and cholelithiasis. As a result of transfusion dependency, iron overload results because of the body's inability to excrete iron from the transfused RBCs. This results in hemochromatosis, heart failure, cirrhosis, and endocrinopathies typically after more than 100 units.

Diagnostic Criteria

α-Thalassemia Trait

Patients with mild anemia have a hematocrit between 28% and 40%. The MCV is low despite modest anemia, and the RBC bound is normal or increased. Peripheral blood smear shows microcytic, hypochromia, target cell and acanthocytes (cell with irregularly spaced bulbous projections). The reticulocyte and iron parameters are normal.

Hemoglobin H

Patients have marked hemolytic anemia with a hematocrit between 22% and 32%. The MCV is low. The peripheral blood smear reveals hypochromia, microcytosis, target cells, and poikilocytosis. The reticulocyte count is elevated. A peripheral blood smear demonstrates the presence of hemoglobin.

β-Thalassemia Minor

Patients have modest anemia with a hematocrit between 28% and 40%. The MCV ranges from 50 to 75 fL, and the RBC count is normal or increased. The peripheral blood smear reveals hypochromia, microcytosis, and target cells and basophilic stippling may be present. The reticulocyte count is normal or slightly elevated.

β-Thalassemia Major

Patients have severe anemia, and the hematocrit may fall to less than 10%. The peripheral blood smear is bizarre, revealing severe poikilocytosis, hypochromia, microcytosis, target cells, basophilic stippling, and nucleated RBCs.

Initiating Drug Therapy

Patients with mild thalassemia (α-thalassemia trait or β-thalassemia minor) require no treatment. Patients should be identified so that they will not be subjected to repeated evaluation and treatment for iron deficiency. Patients with hemoglobin H should take folate supplements and avoid iron and oxidative drugs such as sulfonamides. Patients with severe thalassemia are maintained on a regular transfusion schedule and receive folate supplementation. Iron chelation therapy with deferoxamine mesylate may be used when transfusions result in tissue iron overload. Deferoxamine is administered by continuous subcutaneous infusion for 10 to 24 hours/day. Adverse reactions include local irritation at the injection site, pruritus, hypotension, tachycardia, abdominal discomfort, diarrhea, nausea, and vomiting. Ocular and auditory disturbances may occur and patients should have baseline and annual vision and hearing examinations.

VITAMIN B$_{12}$ DEFICIENCY

Vitamin B$_{12}$ (cyanocobalamin) deficiency, or pernicious anemia, is a disorder of impaired DNA synthesis. Vitamin B$_{12}$ deficiency is considered a macrocytic anemia and may arise because of genetic or acquired abnormalities. Special populations, such as older adults, alcoholics, patients with malnutrition, and strict vegans, are at high risk for developing vitamin B$_{12}$ deficiency. Vitamin B$_{12}$ is essential in maintaining the integrity of the neurologic system.

Pathophysiology

Vitamin B$_{12}$ deficiency has several causes, including lack of intrinsic factor, inadequate intake, decreased absorption, and inadequate utilization. Other causes include fish tapeworm infestation, *Helicobacter pylori* infection, malignancy,

---

BOX 50.4

Causes of Vitamin B$_{12}$ Deficiency

Dietary deficiency
Decreased production of intrinsic factor
    Pernicious anemia
    Gastrectomy
Helicobacter pylori infection
Fish tapeworm
Pancreatic insufficiency
Surgical resection of ileum
Crohn's disease

---

pancreatitis, gluten enteropathy, sprue, and small bowel bacterial overgrowth (**Box 50.4**). More recently, the increased incidence of obesity and the option of gastric bypass surgery raise greater concerns about vitamin B$_{12}$ deficiency. Vitamin B$_{12}$ is water soluble and obtained by ingestion of fish, meat (beef, pork, organ meat), and dairy products. Its absorption occurs in the terminal ileum and requires intrinsic factor (found in gastric mucosa) for transport across the intestinal mucosa. Ileal absorptive sites may be congenitally absent or destroyed by inflammation or surgical resection. Other causes of decreased absorption include chronic pancreatitis, malabsorption syndromes, and drugs (oral calcium-chelating drugs, aminosalicylic acid, and biguanides).

Vitamin B$_{12}$ deficiency can present with gastric mucosal atrophy, neuropsychiatric abnormalities (paranoia, delirium, confusion), and yellow-blue color blindness. GI manifestations include anorexia, intermittent constipation and diarrhea, and poorly localized abdominal pain. An early symptom may be glossitis or weight loss. In the early stages, neurologic symptoms include peripheral loss of position and vibratory sensation in the extremities, weakness, and loss of reflexes. Later stages include spasticity, Babinski responses, and ataxia. Early diagnosis is important because neurologic defects, if left untreated, are irreversible.

Diagnostic Criteria

Serum vitamin B$_{12}$ assay is the most commonly used method for establishing B$_{12}$ deficiency. A normal level of vitamin B$_{12}$ is greater than 300 pg/mL. A level between 200 and 300 pg/mL is a borderline result, and a <200 pg/mL is consistent with vitamin B$_{12}$ deficiency. Serum concentrations of homocysteine as well as serum and urinary concentrations of methylmalonic acid are elevated in vitamin B$_{12}$ deficiency due to a decreased metabolism rate. In patients with an intrinsic factor deficiency, the Schilling test can confirm the diagnosis.

Initiating Drug Therapy

Pernicious anemia, malabsorption syndromes, or surgical removal of the stomach causes absence of intrinsic factor. Therefore, dietary vitamin B_{12} cannot be absorbed. In this case, therapy consists of parenteral administration of vitamin B_{12}. In the case of inadequate intake, dietary allowance and supplementation can be recommended.

Goals of Drug Therapy

Clinical improvement is evidenced by increased alertness, appetite, and cooperation. Reticulocytosis occurs within 2 to 3 days and peaks within 5 to 8 days. The hematocrit begins to rise within 2 weeks and reaches normal values within 2 months. The MCV will increase initially due to increased reticulocytes and then will gradually decrease to normal.

Vitamin B_{12} (Cyanocobalamin)

Pernicious anemia is typically treated with parenteral (i.e., intramuscular or deep subcutaneous) cyanocobalamin in a dose of 1,000 mcg (1,000 mcg, 1 mg) every day for 1 week followed by 1 mg every week for 4 weeks. Then, if the underlying disorder persists (e.g., pernicious anemia, surgical removal of the terminal ileum), 1 mg is administered every month for the remainder of the patient's life.

Vitamin B_{12} therapy is not usually recommended for pernicious anemia because of insufficient absorption due to lack of intrinsic factor.

For dietary insufficiency, the recommended daily doses of vitamin B_{12} are 0.4 mcg for patients ages 0 to 6 months; 0.5 mcg, ages 7 to 12 months; 0.9 mcg, ages 1 to 3; 1.2 mcg, ages 4 to 8; 1.8 mcg, ages 9 to 13; 2.4 mcg, age 14 and older; 2.6 mcg in pregnant patients; and 2.8 mcg in breast-feeding women.

FOLATE DEFICIENCY

Pathophysiology

Folic acid is necessary for the production of nucleic proteins, amino acids, purines, and thymine. Humans are unable to synthesize total daily folate requirements and depend on a dietary source. Major sources of folate include fresh vegetables and fruits, yeast, mushrooms, and animal organs such as liver and kidney. The minimum daily requirement is 50 to 100 mcg. Folic acid deficiency results in the development of large functionally immature erythrocytes (megaloblasts). Major causes of folic acid deficiency include inadequate intake, inadequate absorption, inadequate utilization, increased requirement (pregnancy, lactation, infancy, malignancy, increased metabolism), and increased excretion (renal dialysis; **Box 50.5**). Folic acid deficiency is associated with poor eating habits as seen in the elderly, alcoholics, food

BOX **50.5**

Causes of Folate Deficiency

Dietary deficiency
Decreased absorption due to
  Phenytoin
  Sulfasalazine
  Trimethoprim–sulfamethoxazole
Increased requirements
  Chronic hemolytic anemia
  Pregnancy
Exfoliative skin disease

faddists, and those who are chronically ill. It is also seen in patients with malabsorption syndromes, Crohn's disease, and celiac disease. Several drugs reported to cause folic acid deficiency include co-trimoxazole, primidone, phenytoin, and phenobarbital.

Symptoms associated with folate deficiency are similar to those in patients with vitamin B_{12} deficiency. However, the major difference is the absence of neurologic manifestations.

Diagnostic Criteria

Laboratory assessment of folate status includes a serum folic acid level. Serum folic acid levels less than 4 ng/mL suggest deficiency. A low RBC folate level identifies tissue deficiency; however, the values depend on the laboratory method used. Serum homocysteine measurement provides the best evidence of tissue deficiency. Both methylmalonic acid and homocysteine must be measured because B_{12} uses the same pathway. A normal methylmalonic acid level with an elevated homocysteine level confirms the diagnosis of folate deficiency.

Initiating Drug Therapy

Folic acid 1 mg daily replenishes tissues.

Goals of Drug Therapy

The evaluation of symptomatic improvement is the same as those with vitamin B_{12} deficiency.

Folate Replacement

Folic acid is present in most fruits and vegetables (citrus fruits and green leafy vegetables). The recommended dietary allowances for adult men is 0.15 to 0.2 mg; for women, 0.15 to 0.18 mg. Total body stores are approximately 5 mg and supply requirements for up to 2 to 3 months. Folate deficiency is

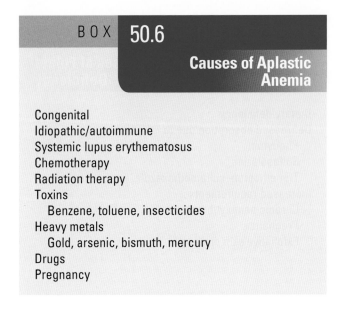

BOX 50.6

Causes of Aplastic Anemia

Congenital
Idiopathic/autoimmune
Systemic lupus erythematosus
Chemotherapy
Radiation therapy
Toxins
   Benzene, toluene, insecticides
Heavy metals
   Gold, arsenic, bismuth, mercury
Drugs
Pregnancy

treated by oral replacement therapy. The usual dose of folate is 1 mg daily. Higher doses up to 5 mg daily may be required for folate deficiency due to malabsorption. The duration of therapy depends on the cause of deficiency. Patients with hemolytic anemia or those with malabsorption or chronic malnutrition should receive oral folic acid indefinitely. Side effects include erythema, skin rash, nausea, abdominal distention, altered sleep patterns, irritability, mental depression, confusion, and impaired judgment.

APLASTIC ANEMIA

Aplastic anemia is a condition of bone marrow failure that can be hereditary or arise from injury to or abnormal expression of the stem cell. Aplastic anemia is defined as pancytopenia with a hypocellular bone marrow in the absence of an abnormal infiltrate and with no increase in reticulin (Marsh, et al., 2009). There are several causes of aplastic anemia (**Box 50.6**). One cause is direct stem cell injury from radiation, chemotherapy (alkylating agents), antimetabolites, antimitotics, toxins (benzenes), or pharmacologic agents (**Box 50.7**).

Pathophysiology

Erythrocytes, granulocytes, and platelets, which are normally produced in the bone narrow, decrease to dangerously low levels. The bone marrow becomes hypoplastic with replacement of normal marrow hemopoietic cells by fat cells, and pancytopenia develops. This results in bleeding and increased risk of infection. Patients most commonly present with fatigue, dyspnea, weakness, and skin or mucosal hemorrhage or visual disturbance due to retinal hemorrhage. Physical examination may reveal signs of pallor, purpura, and petechiae.

Diagnostic Criteria

A CBC typically shows pancytopenia. In most cases, the hemoglobin level and neutrophil, reticulocyte, and platelet counts are depressed with a preserved lymphocyte count. The bone marrow aspirate and bone marrow biopsy appear hypocellular with scant amounts of normal hematopoietic progenitors. Magnetic resonance imaging of the vertebrae shows uniform replacement of marrow with fat.

Initiating Drug Therapy

Mild cases of aplastic anemia may be treated with supportive care. RBC transfusions and platelets are given as necessary. Antibiotics are given to treat infections. Treatment for severe acquired aplastic anemia includes hematopoietic stem cell transplantation and immunosuppression therapy. When the cause of aplastic anemia is related to drugs or chemicals, these should be discontinued. Patients presenting with aplastic anemia should be referred to a hematologist/oncologist.

BOX 50.7

Drugs Associated with Aplastic Anemia

Antiprotozoals (quinacrine and chloroquine, mepacrine)
NSAIDs (phenylbutazone, indomethacin, ibuprofen, sulindac, aspirin)
Anticonvulsants (hydantoins, carbamazepine, phenacemide, felbamate)
Sulfonamides
   Antithyroid drugs (methimazole, methylthiouracil, propylthiouracil)
   Antidiabetes drugs (tolbutamide, chlorpropamide)
   Carbonic anhydrase inhibitors (acetazolamide, methazolamide)
Antihistamines (cimetidine, chlorpheniramine)
D-penicillamine
Estrogens
Sedatives and tranquilizers (chlorpromazine, prochlorperazine, piperacetazine, chlordiazepoxide, meprobamate, methyprylon)
Allopurinol
Methyldopa
Quinidine
Lithium
Guanidine
Potassium perchlorate
Thiocyanate
Carbimazole

SPECIAL POPULATION CONSIDERATIONS

Pediatric

Iron deficiency anemia significantly impairs mental and psychomotor development in infants and children. Iron deficiency can be reversed with treatment; however, the reversibility of the mental and psychomotor effects is unclear. Furthermore, iron deficiency increases a child's susceptibility to lead toxicity as lead replaces iron in the absorptive pathway when iron is unavailable.

Young children are at greatest risk of iron deficiency anemia due to rapid growth, increased iron requirements, and lack of iron in the diet. Poverty, abuse, and living in a home with poor household conditions also place children at risk for iron deficiency anemia. Iron deficiency anemia is seen most commonly in children ages 6 months to 3 years. Those at highest risk are low-birth-weight infants after age 2 months, breast-fed term infants who receive no iron-fortified food or supplemental iron after age 4 months, and formula-fed term infants who are not consuming iron-fortified formula. During the first months of life, the newborn rapidly uses iron stores due to an accelerated growth rate and increased blood volume. Maternally derived iron stores are generally sufficient for the first 4 to 6 months; however, sustained growth demands an increased iron supply. By the end of the second year of life, the growth rate decreases and accompanying iron needs level off. During adolescence, growth accelerates and iron needs increase. Adolescent girls are at increased risk and need additional iron to compensate for menstrual loss. Patients with iron deficiency who are responding poorly to the usual dietary supplementation regimens should be screened for lead poisoning. Heavy metal poisoning, as with lead and bismuth, is often overlooked.

Geriatric

Anemia should not be accepted as an inevitable consequence of aging. The most common causes of anemia in elderly patients are chronic disease (CKD, infections, malignancies, inflammatory disorders), iron deficiency, and nutritional and metabolic disorders. Anemia resulting from blood loss due to surgery, injury, and GI and genitourinary bleeding is more common in hospitalized patients. Untreated geriatric anemia has been associated with increased mortality, increased prevalence of various comorbid conditions, and decreased function.

Women

Pregnant women and women who are 4 to 6 weeks postpartum are at increased risk for anemia. Pregnant women who are iron deficient are at increased risk for a preterm delivery and delivering a low-birth-weight baby. However, two to three times more iron is required in pregnancy and in childhood. In pregnant women who had a previous pregnancy with a fetus or infant with a neural tube defect, the recommended dose is 5 mg daily. Also, women who may become pregnant and have seizure disorders should take folate supplementation.

MONITORING PATIENT RESPONSE

In almost all cases of anemia, evaluation should proceed in an orderly manner and therapy withheld until a specific diagnosis can be made. Patients with significant cardiopulmonary disease, who may be compromised by a decreased oxygen capacity, require immediate correction of anemia. This may require inpatient evaluation and consideration of transfusion therapy when they are experiencing dyspnea, angina, or marked fatigue related to anemia. Once treatment has been initiated, patient response should be evaluated on at least a monthly basis. Correction of anemia decreases morbidity and reduces hospitalization and mortality among patients with CKD. Benefits of correcting anemia include improvements in the patient's quality of life, exercise capacity, cognitive function, and sexual function.

PATIENT EDUCATION

Patients need to be told to what extent the anemia accounts for symptoms, what the possible causes are, and what the appropriate workup will be. Patient education and the importance of adherence to therapy are integral to successful management. Because some cases of anemia require the need for medication, the patient needs to be informed about possible side effects and when to report dangerous side effects.

Nutrition

All patients are encouraged to limit the use of alcohol, to avoid tobacco, to exercise, and to consume a diet of meat, poultry, fish, and fresh fruits and vegetables. To prevent deficiency, all patients are encouraged to eat fortified foods (fortified cereals, dairy products) or take supplements as prescribed by their physician. Patients with specific problems, such as pica, may need additional counseling.

Complementary and Alternative Medications

Herbal medicine to supply iron, iodine, and calcium include yellow dock root, Irish moss, and horsetail in equal parts made into a tea. Other herbal medicine for the treatment of iron deficiency include burdock, devil's bit, meadow sweet, mullein leaves, restharrow, salep, silver weed, stinging nettle, strawberry leaves, and toad flax. Patients should be educated that herbs are not regulated by the U.S. Food and Drug Administration and may interact with prescription medications. Patients must also understand that they should report any adverse reactions and stop the herbal medication immediately.

Case Study

. W. is a 69-year-old African-American man and was referred to clinic for evaluation of increasing shortness of breath.

Past medical history

Pulmonary hypertension

Hypertension

Congestive heart failure

Diabetes mellitus type 2, poor control

Deep vein thrombosis

Alcohol abuse

Chronic obstructive pulmonary disease with respiratory failure

Family history

Noncontributory

Physical examination

Height 69 in., weight 205 lb

Blood pressure: 138/88

Pulse 86 bpm, regular

Lungs clear, neck supple negative for jugular venous distention

Lower extremities +1 edema

Laboratory findings

Scr = 1.7	K^+ = 4.2
BUN = 24	Na^+ = 141
WBC = 3.0	Hb = 9.8
Hct = 29.4	

Serum ferritin 189 mg/dL

Social history

Tobacco: 52 pack-years

Alcohol: distant past

DIAGNOSIS: ANEMIA OF CKD

1. List specific goals of treatment for this patient.
2. What drug therapy would you prescribe? Why?
3. What are the parameters for monitoring success of the therapy?
4. Discuss specific patient education based on the prescribed therapy.
5. List one or two adverse reactions for the selected agent that would cause you to change therapy.
6. What dietary and lifestyle changes should be recommended for this patient?
7. What over-the-counter or alternative medications would be appropriate for this patient?
8. What dietary and lifestyle changes should be recommended for this patient?
9. Describe one or two drug–drug or drug–food interactions for the selected agent.

BIBLIOGRAPHY

Starred references are cited in the text.

Abramson, J., Jurkovitz, C., Vaccarino, V., et al. (2003). Chronic kidney disease, anemia, and incident stroke in a middle-aged, community-based population: The ARIC study. *Kidney International, 64,* 610–615.

Alleyne, M., Horne, M., & Miller, J. (2008). Individualized treatment for iron-deficiency anemia in adults. *The American Journal of Medicine, 121,* 943–948.

Amgen. (2001). ARANESP (darbepoetin alfa) package insert. Thousand Oaks, CA: Amgen.

Andrews, N. (2008). Forging a field: The golden age of iron biology. *Blood, 112,* 219–230.

Angerio, A., & Lee, N. (2003). Sickle cell crisis and endothelin antagonists. *Critical Care Nursing Quarterly, 26,* 225–229.

Argyriadou S., Vlachonikolis, I., Melisopoulou, H., et al. (2001). In what extent anemia coexists with cognitive impairment in elderly: A cross-sectional study in Greece. *BMC Family Practice, 2*(1), 5.

Bacigalupo, A. (2008). Treatment strategies for patients with severe aplastic anemia. *Bone Marrow Transplantation, 42,* S42–S44.

Benoist, B., McLean, E., Egli, I., & Cogswell, M. (2008). *Worldwide prevalence of anaemia 1993–2005.* WHO global database on anaemia. Geneva: World Health Organization.

Borgna-Pignatti, C. (2009). Modern treatment of thalassaemia intermedia. *British Journal of Haematology, 138,* 291–304.

Brawley, O., Cornelius, L., Edwards, L., et al. (2008). National Institutes of Health Consensus Development Conference statement: Hydroxyurea treatment for sickle cell disease. *Annals of Internal Medicine, 148,* 932.

Butler, C., Vidal-Alaball, J., Cannings-John, R., et al. (2006). Oral vitamin B_{12} versus intramuscular vitamin B_{12} for vitamin B_{12} deficiency: A systematic review of randomized controlled trails. *Family Practice, 23,* 279–285.

Cao, A., & Galanello, R. (2002). Effect of consanguinity on screening for thalassemia. *New England Journal of Medicine, 347,* 1200–1202.

Carley, A. (2003). Anemia: When is it iron deficiency? *Pediatric Nursing, 29,* 127–133.

Claster, S., & Vichinsky, E. (2003). Managing sickle cell disease. *British Medical Journal, 327,* 1151–1160.

*Fitzsimons, E., & Brock, J. (2001). The anaemia of chronic disease: Remains hard to distinguish from iron deficiency anaemia in some cases. *British Medical Journal, 322,* 811–812.

Guidi, G., & Santonastaso, C. (2010). Advancements in anemias related to chronic conditions. *Clinical Chemistry & Laboratory Medicine, 48,* 1217–1226.

Kaptan, K., Beyan, C., Ugur, A., et al. (2000). *Helicobacter pylori:* Is it a novel causative agent in vitamin B-12 deficiency? *Archives of Internal Medicine, 160,* 1349–1353.

Kikuchi, M., Inagaki, T., & Sinagawa, N. (2001). Five-year survival of older people with anemia: Variation with hemoglobin concentration. *Journal of American Geriatric Society, 49*(9), 1226–1228.

Killip, S., Bennett, J., & Chambers, M. (2007). Iron deficiency anemia. *American Family Physician, 75,* 671–678.

Kopecky, E., Jacobson, S., Joshi, P., & Koren, G. (2004). Systemic exposure to morphine and the risk of acute chest syndrome in sickle cell disease. *Clinical Pharmacology and Therapeutics, 75,* 140–146.

Lanzkron, S., Strouse, J., Wilson, R., et al. (2008). Systematic review: Hydroxyurea for the treatment of adults with sickle cell disease. *Annals of Internal Medicine, 12,* 939–950.

*Marsh, J., Ball, S., Cavenagh, J., et al. (2009). Guidelines for the diagnosis and management of aplastic anaemia. *British Journal of Haematology, 147,* 43–70.

Marsh, J., Ball, W., Darbyshire, P., et al. (2003). Guidelines for the diagnosis and management of acquired aplastic anaemia. *British Journal of Haematology, 123,* 782–801.

Miller, H., Hu, J., Valentine, J., & Gable, P. (2010). Efficacy and tolerability of intravenous ferric gluconate in the treatment of iron deficiency anemia in patients without kidney disease. *Archives of Internal Medicine, 167,* 1327–1328.

*National Kidney Foundation. KDOQI clinical practice guidelines and clinical practice recommendations for anemia in chronic kidney disease. (2006). http://www.kidney.org/professionals/KDOQI/guidelines_anemia/index.htm, accessed October 18, 2010.

National Kidney Foundation. KDOQI clinical practice guideline and clinical practice recommendations for anemia in chronic kidney disease: 2007 update of hemoglobin target. http://www.kidney.org/professionals/KDOQI/guidelines_anemiaUP/index.htm, accessed October 14, 2010.

Poskitt, E. (2003). Early history of iron deficiency. *British Journal of Haematology, 122,* 504–562.

Robinson, A., & Mladenovic, J. (2001). Lack of clinical utility of folate levels in the evaluation of macrocytosis or anemia. *American Journal of Medicine, 110,* 88–90.

*Savulescu, J. (2004). Thalassaemia major: The murky story of deferiprone. *British Medical Journal, 328,* 358–359.

Spivak, J. (2000). The blood in systemic disorders. *Lancet, 350,* 1707–1712.

Steinberg, M., McCathy, W., & Castro, O. (2010). The risks and benefits of long term use of hydroxyurea in sickle cell anemia: A 17.5 yr follow-up. *American Journal of Hematology, 6,* 403–408.

Tefferi, A. (2003). Anemia in adults: A contemporary approach to diagnosis. *Mayo Clinic Proceedings, 78,* 1274–280.

U.S. Renal Data System. (2001). USRDS 2001 Annual Data Report. Bethesda, MD: National Institute of Diabetes and Digestive and Kidney Diseases, National Institutes of Health.

Yen, P. (2000). Nutritional anemia. *Geriatric Nursing, 21,* 111–112.

Young, N. (2002). Acquired aplastic anemia. *Annals of Internal Medicine, 136,* 534–546.

Pharmacotherapy in Health Promotion

Immunizations

Although the tendency is to place the primary focus of immunization efforts on infants and preschool children, immunization prophylaxis is important for all age groups—infants through older adults. This is particularly true when the potential loss of time from work, additional cost of health care, the possible need for additional caretakers, and potential side effects are considered. The dollar amount of these effects may be monumental. Relocation, change in job status or field of employment, travel, assumption of caretaker responsibilities, and the like may place a person into a different risk category, requiring a review of immunization status. The challenge faced by practitioners is to develop a system that facilitates review of immunization status at all health care visits so that no opportunity is missed to update immunizations for those who are not adequately vaccinated and thus inadequately protected against preventable diseases.

Immunization prophylaxis offers an opportunity to prevent disease, improve clinical outcomes for those at high risk, and realize significant savings to the person in terms of cost, time, and resources. The plan to eradicate transmissible communicable diseases by the year 2000 and the reduced number of reported cases of communicable diseases have had a significant impact on preventing communicable diseases, reducing preventable complications, and improving clinical outcomes. In the United States, immunization has sharply curtailed or practically eliminated diphtheria, measles, mumps, pertussis, congenital and acquired rubella, tetanus, and *Haemophilus influenzae* type B disease. However, because these diseases persist in the United States and other countries, immunization prophylaxis needs to be continued. Recommendations for immunization prophylaxis come from multiple sources, including:

Advisory Committee on Immunization Practices (ACIP)
American Academy of Pediatrics (AAP)
American Academy of Family Physicians
Canadian Task Force on the Periodic Health Examination
U.S. Preventive Task Force and the Centers for Disease Control and Prevention (CDC)

The CDC is responsible for providing vaccine management, technical assistance, information, epidemiology, and assessment. In January of each year, the immunization schedule is reviewed and revised as indicated.

CHARACTERISTICS OF IMMUNIZATIONS

Many infectious diseases can be prevented by immunoprophylaxis, which is accomplished either through active or passive immunization. Active immunization involves giving a person either live or attenuated (live but killed; inactivated) vaccine to stimulate the development of immune system defenses against future natural exposure.

Active immunization involves administration of all or part of a microorganism or a modified product of that microorganism (e.g., toxoid, a purified antigen, or an antigen produced by genetic engineering) to evoke an immune response that mimics the response of the body to natural infection but that usually presents little or no risk to the recipient. Protection may be afforded for a limited time or for a lifetime. If protection is for a limited time, the vaccine must be readministered at specified intervals.

Passive immunization is used for those people who have already been exposed or who have the potential to be exposed to certain infectious agents. Passive immunization involves the administration of a preformed antibody when the recipient has a congenitally acquired defect or immunodeficiency, when exposure is likely to result in high-risk complications, or when time does not permit adequate protection by active immunization (e.g., immunizations against rabies or hepatitis B). In addition, passive immunity can be used therapeutically during active disease states to help suppress the effects of a toxin or the inflammatory response.

VACCINES

Vaccines are the pharmacologic substances used to provide or boost immunity to disease. The major constituents of vaccines include active immunizing antigens (toxoid, live virus, or killed bacteria), suspending fluid, preservatives, stabilizers, antibiotics, and adjuvants. The differences depend on the manufacturer, and the person prescribing or administering the vaccine should check the package insert for the active and inert ingredients for each product. Potential allergic reactions may result from one or more of the preservatives, stabilizers, adjuvants, or antibiotics in the vaccine, and the recipient's sensitivity to one or more of the additives should be anticipated as a hypersensitivity. Current vaccines licensed in the United States are identified in **Box 51.1**.

RECOMMENDED CHILDHOOD AND ADOLESCENT IMMUNIZATION SCHEDULES

The recommended childhood immunization schedule for the United States is listed in **Figure 51.1**. **Figure 51.2** presents the recommended immunizations for children who are behind in immunizations.

Recommendations for hepatitis B; rotavirus; diphtheria, tetanus, and pertussis (DTaP); *H. influenzae* type B; pneumococcus; poliomyelitis; influenza; measles, mumps, and rubella (MMR); varicella; hepatitis A; and meningococcus are included for birth to age 18. Additionally, human papillomavirus (HPV) immunization is recommended for males and females ages 11 to 18.

Combination vaccines are available that assist in reducing the number of injections a child must receive at any one time. In addition, recommended acceptable ranges for administration provide some flexibility regarding the number of injections administered at any one time as recommendations for catch-up vaccinations. A consideration for flexible scheduling should include parental or guardian compliance with appointments as well as office follow-up methods used for those patients who do not keep scheduled appointments for immunizations.

Special Circumstances

Preterm infants and children who are immunocompromised, infected with human immunodeficiency virus (HIV), lack a spleen, or have a personal or family history of seizures require special consideration when immunization prophylaxis is reviewed and administered.

BOX 51.1

Vaccines Licensed in the United States

Anthrax
BCG (live)
Cholera
Diphtheria and tetanus toxoid adsorbed
Diphtheria and tetanus toxoids and acellular pertussis vaccine adsorbed
Diphtheria and tetanus toxoids and acellular pertussis vaccine adsorbed and inactivated polio
Diphtheria and tetanus toxoids and acellular pertussis adsorbed, inactivated polio, and *H. influenzae* B conjugate
H. influenzae B conjugate
H. influenzae B conjugate and hepatitis B
Hepatitis A
Hepatitis B
Hepatitis A and hepatitis B
Human papillomavirus quadrivalent (types 6, 11, 16, 18)
Human papillomavirus bivalent (types 16, 18)
Influenza A (H1N1)
Influenza (H5N1)
Influenza virus types A and B
Influenza vaccine (live—intranasal)
Japanese encephalitis
Measles (live)
Measles and mumps (live)
Measles, mumps and rubella (live)
Measles, mumps, rubella and varicella (live)

Meningococcal (groups A, C, Y, and W-135) Oligosaccharide diphtheria CRM197 Conjugate
Meningococcal polysaccharide (serogroups A, C, Y and W-135) diphtheria toxoid conjugate
Meningococcal polysaccharide groups A, C, Y and W-135 combined
Mumps (live)
Plague
Pneumococcal polyvalent
Pneumococcal 7-valent conjugate
Pneumococcal 13-valent conjugate
Poliovirus, inactivated
Rabies
Rotavirus (live, oral)
Rubella (live)
Smallpox (live)
Smallpox (dried)
Tetanus and diphtheria toxoids adsorbed for adults
Tetanus toxoid
Tetanus toxoid adsorbed
Tetanus toxoid, reduced diphtheria toxoid, and acellular pertussis, adsorbed
Typhoid (live, oral)
Typhoid Vi polysaccharide
Varicella virus (live)
Yellow fever
Zoster (live)

Recommended Immunization Schedule for Persons Aged 0 Through 6 Years—United States • 2010
For those who fall behind or start late, see the catch-up schedule

Vaccine ▼ Age ▶	Birth	1 month	2 months	4 months	6 months	12 months	15 months	18 months	19–23 months	2–3 years	4–6 years
Hepatitis B[1]	HepB	HepB				HepB					
Rotavirus[2]			RV	RV	RV[2]						
Diphtheria, Tetanus, Pertussis[3]			DTaP	DTaP	DTaP	see footnote[3]	DTaP				DTaP
Haemophilus influenzae type b[4]			Hib	Hib	Hib[4]	Hib					
Pneumococcal[5]			PCV	PCV	PCV	PCV					PPSV
Inactivated Poliovirus[6]			IPV	IPV		IPV					IPV
Influenza[7]						Influenza (Yearly)					
Measles, Mumps, Rubella[8]						MMR		see footnote[8]			MMR
Varicella[9]						Varicella		see footnote[9]			Varicella
Hepatitis A[10]						HepA (2 doses)				HepA Series	
Meningococcal[11]										MCV	

Range of recommended ages for all children except certain high-risk groups

Range of recommended ages for certain high-risk groups

This schedule includes recommendations in effect as of December 15, 2009. Any dose not administered at the recommended age should be administered at a subsequent visit, when indicated and feasible. The use of a combination vaccine generally is preferred over separate injections of its equivalent component vaccines. Considerations should include provider assessment, patient preference, and the potential for adverse events. Providers should consult the relevant Advisory Committee on Immunization Practices statement for detailed recommendations: **http://www.cdc.gov/vaccines/pubs/acip-list.htm**. Clinically significant adverse events that follow immunization should be reported to the Vaccine Adverse Event Reporting System (VAERS) at **http://www.vaers.hhs.gov** or by telephone, **800-822-7967.**

1. **Hepatitis B vaccine (HepB).** (Minimum age: birth)
   At birth:
   - Administer monovalent HepB to all newborns before hospital discharge.
   - If mother is hepatitis B surface antigen (HBsAg)-positive, administer HepB and 0.5 mL of hepatitis B immune globulin (HBIG) within 12 hours of birth.
   - If mother's HBsAg status is unknown, administer HepB within 12 hours of birth. Determine mother's HBsAg status as soon as possible and, if HBsAg-positive, administer HBIG (no later than age 1 week).
   After the birth dose:
   - The HepB series should be completed with either monovalent HepB or a combination vaccine containing HepB. The second dose should be administered at age 1 or 2 months. Monovalent HepB vaccine should be used for doses administered before age 6 weeks. The final dose should be administered no earlier than age 24 weeks.
   - Infants born to HBsAg-positive mothers should be tested for HBsAg and antibody to HBsAg 1 to 2 months after completion of at least 3 doses of the HepB series, at age 9 through 18 months (generally at the next well-child visit).
   - Administration of 4 doses of HepB to infants is permissible when a combination vaccine containing HepB is administered after the birth dose. The fourth dose should be administered no earlier than age 24 weeks.
2. **Rotavirus vaccine (RV).** (Minimum age: 6 weeks)
   - Administer the first dose at age 6 through 14 weeks (maximum age: 14 weeks 6 days). Vaccination should not be initiated for infants aged 15 weeks 0 days or older.
   - The maximum age for the final dose in the series is 8 months 0 days
   - If Rotarix is administered at ages 2 and 4 months, a dose at 6 months is not indicated.
3. **Diphtheria and tetanus toxoids and acellular pertussis vaccine (DTaP).** (Minimum age: 6 weeks)
   - The fourth dose may be administered as early as age 12 months, provided at least 6 months have elapsed since the third dose.
   - Administer the final dose in the series at age 4 through 6 years.
4. ***Haemophilus influenzae* type b conjugate vaccine (Hib).** (Minimum age: 6 weeks)
   - If PRP-OMP (PedvaxHIB or Comvax [HepB-Hib]) is administered at ages 2 and 4 months, a dose at age 6 months is not indicated.
   - TriHiBit (DTaP/Hib) and Hiberix (PRP-T) should not be used for doses at ages 2, 4, or 6 months for the primary series but can be used as the final dose in children aged 12 months through 4 years.
5. **Pneumococcal vaccine.** (Minimum age: 6 weeks for pneumococcal conjugate vaccine [PCV]; 2 years for pneumococcal polysaccharide vaccine [PPSV])
   - PCV is recommended for all children aged younger than 5 years. Administer 1 dose of PCV to all healthy children aged 24 through 59 months who are not completely vaccinated for their age.
   - Administer PPSV 2 or more months after last dose of PCV to children aged 2 years or older with certain underlying medical conditions, including a cochlear implant. See *MMWR* 1997;46(No. RR-8).

6. **Inactivated poliovirus vaccine (IPV)** (Minimum age: 6 weeks)
   - The final dose in the series should be administered on or after the fourth birthday and at least 6 months following the previous dose.
   - If 4 doses are administered prior to age 4 years a fifth dose should be administered at age 4 through 6 years. See *MMWR* 2009;58(30):829–30.
7. **Influenza vaccine (seasonal).** (Minimum age: 6 months for trivalent inactivated influenza vaccine [TIV]; 2 years for live, attenuated influenza vaccine [LAIV])
   - Administer annually to children aged 6 months through 18 years.
   - For healthy children aged 2 through 6 years (i.e., those who do not have underlying medical conditions that predispose them to influenza complications), either LAIV or TIV may be used, except LAIV should not be given to children aged 2 through 4 years who have had wheezing in the past 12 months.
   - Children receiving TIV should receive 0.25 mL if aged 6 through 35 months or 0.5 mL if aged 3 years or older.
   - Administer 2 doses (separated by at least 4 weeks) to children aged younger than 9 years who are receiving influenza vaccine for the first time or who were vaccinated for the first time during the previous influenza season but only received 1 dose.
   - For recommendations for use of influenza A (H1N1) 2009 monovalent vaccine see *MMWR* 2009;58(No. RR-10).
8. **Measles, mumps, and rubella vaccine (MMR).** (Minimum age: 12 months)
   - Administer the second dose routinely at age 4 through 6 years. However, the second dose may be administered before age 4, provided at least 28 days have elapsed since the first dose.
9. **Varicella vaccine.** (Minimum age: 12 months)
   - Administer the second dose routinely at age 4 through 6 years. However, the second dose may be administered before age 4, provided at least 3 months have elapsed since the first dose.
   - For children aged 12 months through 12 years the minimum interval between doses is 3 months. However, if the second dose was administered at least 28 days after the first dose, it can be accepted as valid.
10. **Hepatitis A vaccine (HepA).** (Minimum age: 12 months)
    - Administer to all children aged 1 year (i.e., aged 12 through 23 months). Administer 2 doses at least 6 months apart.
    - Children not fully vaccinated by age 2 years can be vaccinated at subsequent visits
    - HepA also is recommended for older children who live in areas where vaccination programs target older children, who are at increased risk for infection, or for whom immunity against hepatitis A is desired.
11. **Meningococcal vaccine.** (Minimum age: 2 years for meningococcal conjugate vaccine [MCV4] and for meningococcal polysaccharide vaccine [MPSV4])
    - Administer MCV4 to children aged 2 through 10 years with persistent complement component deficiency, anatomic or functional asplenia, and certain other conditions placing tham at high risk.
    - Administer MCV4 to children previously vaccinated with MCV4 or MPSV4 after 3 years if first dose administered at age 2 through 6 years. See *MMWR* 2009;58:1042–3.

The Recommended Immunization Schedules for Persons Aged 0 through 18 Years are approved by the Advisory Committee on Immunization Practices (**http://www.cdc.gov/vaccines/recs/acip**), the American Academy of Pediatrics (**http://www.aap.org**), and the American Academy of Family Physicians (**http://www.aafp.org**).

Department of Health and Human Services • Centers for Disease Control and Prevention

FIGURE 51–1   Recommended Immunization Schedule for Persons Aged 0 Through 6 Years—United States, 2010.

The table below provides catch-up schedules and minimum intervals between doses for children whose vaccinations have been delayed. A vaccine series does not need to be restarted, regardless of the time that has elapsed between doses. Use the section appropriate for the child's age.

Vaccine	Minimum Age for Dose 1	Minimum Interval Between Doses			
PERSONS AGED 4 MONTHS THROUGH 6 YEARS		Dose 1 to Dose 2	Dose 2 to Dose 3	Dose 3 to Dose 4	Dose 4 to Dose 5
Hepatitis B[1]	Birth	4 weeks	8 weeks (and at least 16 weeks after first dose)		
Rotavirus[2]	6 wks	4 weeks	4 weeks[2]		
Diphtheria, Tetanus, Pertussis[3]	6 wks	4 weeks	4 weeks	6 months	6 months[3]
Haemophilus influenzae type b[4]	6 wks	4 weeks if first dose administered at younger than age 12 months / 8 weeks (as final dose) if first dose administered at age 12–14 months / No further doses needed if first dose administered at age 15 months or older	4 weeks[4] if current age is younger than 12 months / 8 weeks (as final dose)[4] if current age is 12 months or older and first dose administered at younger than age 12 months and second dose administered at younger than 15 months / No further doses needed if previous dose administered at age 15 months or older	8 weeks (as final dose) This dose only necessary for children aged 12 months through 59 months who received 3 doses before age 12 months	
Pneumococcal[5]	6 wks	4 weeks if first dose administered at younger than age 12 months / 8 weeks (as final dose for healthy children) if first dose administered at age 12 months or older or current age 24 through 59 months / No further doses needed for healthy children if first dose administered at age 24 months or older	4 weeks if current age is younger than 12 months / 8 weeks (as final dose for healthy children) if current age is 12 months or older / No further doses needed for healthy children if previous dose administered at age 24 months or older	8 weeks (as final dose) This dose only necessary for children aged 12 months through 59 months who received 3 doses before age 12 months or for high-risk children who received 3 doses at any age	
Inactivated Poliovirus[6]	6 wks	4 weeks	4 weeks	6 months	
Measles, Mumps, Rubella[7]	12 mos	4 weeks			
Varicella[8]	12 mos	3 months			
Hepatitis A[9]	12 mos	6 months			
PERSONS AGED 7 THROUGH 18 YEARS					
Tetanus, Diphtheria / Tetanus, Diphtheria, Pertussis[10]	7 yrs[10]	4 weeks	4 weeks if first dose administered at younger than age 12 months / 6 months if first dose administered at 12 months or older	6 months if first dose administered at younger than age 12 months	
Human Papillomavirus[11]	9 yrs	Routine dosing intervals are recommended[11]			
Hepatitis A[9]	12 mos	6 months			
Hepatitis B[1]	Birth	4 weeks	8 weeks (and at least 16 weeks after first dose)		
Inactivated Poliovirus[6]	6 wks	4 weeks	4 weeks	6 months	
Measles, Mumps, Rubella[7]	12 mos	4 weeks			
Varicella[8]	12 mos	3 months if person is younger than age 13 years / 4 weeks if person is aged 13 years or older			

1. **Hepatitis B vaccine (HepB).**
   - Administer the 3-dose series to those not previously vaccinated.
   - A 2-dose series (separated by at least 4 months) of adult formulation Recombivax HB is licensed for children aged 11 through 15 years.
2. **Rotavirus vaccine (RV).**
   - The maximum age for the first dose is 14 weeks 6 days. Vaccination should not be initiated for infants aged 15 weeks 0 days or older.
   - The maximum age for the final dose in the series is 8 months 0 days.
   - If Rotarix was administered for the first and second doses, a third dose is not indicated.
3. **Diphtheria and tetanus toxoids and acellular pertussis vaccine (DTaP).**
   - The fifth dose is not necessary if the fourth dose was administered at age 4 years or older.
4. **Haemophilus influenzae type b conjugate vaccine (Hib).**
   - Hib vaccine is not generally recommended for persons aged 5 years or older. No efficacy data are available on which to base a recommendation concerning use of Hib vaccine for older children and adults. However, studies suggest good immunogenicity in persons who have sickle cell disease, leukemia, or HIV infection, or who have had a splenectomy; administering 1 dose of Hib vaccine to these persons who have not previously received Hib vaccine is not contraindicated.
   - If the first 2 doses were PRP-OMP (PedvaxHIB or Comvax), and administered at age 11 months or younger, the third (and final) dose should be administered at age 12 through 15 months and at least 8 weeks after the second dose.
   - If the first dose was administered at age 7 through 11 months, administer the second dose at least 4 weeks later and a final dose at age 12 through 15 months.
5. **Pneumococcal vaccine.**
   - Administer 1 dose of pneumococcal conjugate vaccine (PCV) to all healthy children aged 24 through 59 months who have not received at least 1 dose of PCV on or after age 12 months.
   - For children aged 24 through 59 months with underlying medical conditions, administer 1 dose of PCV if 3 doses were received previously or administer 2 doses of PCV at least 8 weeks apart if fewer than 3 doses were received previously.
   - Administer pneumococcal polysaccharide vaccine (PPSV) to children aged 2 years or older with certain underlying medical conditions, including a cochlear implant, at least 8 weeks after the last dose of PCV. See *MMWR* 1997;46(No. RR-8).
6. **Inactivated poliovirus vaccine (IPV).**
   - The final dose in the series should be administered on or after the fourth birthday and at least 6 months following the previous dose.

   - A fourth dose is not necessary if the third dose was administered at age 4 years or older and at least 6 months following the previous dose.
   - In the first 6 months of life, minimum age and minimum intervals are only recommended if the person is at risk for imminent exposure to circulating poliovirus (i.e., travel to a polio-endemic region or during an outbreak).
7. **Measles, mumps, and rubella vaccine (MMR).**
   - Administer the second dose routinely at age 4 through 6 years. However, the second dose may be administered before age 4, provided at least 28 days have elapsed since the first dose.
   - If not previously vaccinated, administer 2 doses with at least 28 days between doses.
8. **Varicella vaccine.**
   - Administer the second dose routinely at age 4 through 6 years. However, the second dose may be administered before age 4, provided at least 3 months have elapsed since the first dose.
   - For persons aged 12 months through 12 years, the minimum interval between doses is 3 months. However, if the second dose was administered at least 28 days after the first dose, it can be accepted as valid.
   - For persons aged 13 years and older, the minimum interval between doses is 28 days.
9. **Hepatitis A vaccine (HepA).**
   - HepA is recommended for children aged older than 23 months who live in areas where vaccination programs target older children, who are at increased risk for infection, or for whom immunity against hepatitis A is desired.
10. **Tetanus and diphtheria toxoids vaccine (Td) and tetanus and diphtheria toxoids and acellular pertussis vaccine (Tdap).**
    - Doses of DTaP are counted as part of the Td/Tdap series
    - Tdap should be substituted for a single dose of Td in the catch-up series or as a booster for children aged 10 through 18 years; use Td for other doses.
11. **Human papillomavirus vaccine (HPV).**
    - Administer the series to females at age 13 through 18 years if not previously vaccinated.
    - Use recommended routine dosing intervals for series catch-up (i.e., the second and third doses should be administered at 1 to 2 and 6 months after the first dose). The minimum interval between the first and second doses is 4 weeks. The minimum interval between the second and third doses is 12 weeks, and the third dose should be administered at least 24 weeks after the first dose.

Department of Health and Human Services • Centers for Disease Control and Prevention

FIGURE 51–2 Catch-up Immunization Schedule for Persons Aged 4 Months Through 18 Years Who Start Late or Who Are More Than 1 Month Behind—United States, 2010.

Preterm Infants

Preterm infants born to mothers who are negative for the hepatitis B surface antigen (HBsAg) should have hepatitis B immunization delayed until they weigh at least 2 kg or they are about to be discharged from the hospital. At the chronologic age of 2 months (including those infants still hospitalized), the infant should be given the immunizations routinely scheduled for that age.

Preterm infants who are born to mothers who test positive for HBsAg should receive hepatitis B immune globulin within 12 hours of birth and concurrent hepatitis B vaccine (in the appropriate dose per package insert) at a different site. If the maternal HBsAg status is unknown, the vaccine should be given in accordance with the protocol for a mother who tests positive for HBsAg (Pickering, et al., 2009). In addition, preterm infants who have chronic respiratory disease should receive the influenza vaccine annually in the fall beginning at age 6 months.

Immunosuppressed Children

Children who are immunosuppressed or immunodeficient are at risk for actually contracting the disease or experiencing serious adverse effects from live-bacteria or live-virus vaccines. Live vaccines are therefore contraindicated. In general, experience with vaccine administration to an immunosuppressed or immunodeficient child is limited. Efficacy is suboptimal because their ability to develop immunogenicity to a specific agent is altered owing to a depressed immune system. Theoretical considerations are the only guide because experiential data are lacking or adverse consequences have not been reported.

Children with a deficiency in antibody-synthesizing capacity cannot respond to vaccines. These children should receive regular doses of immune globulin, usually intravenous immune globulin, that provide passive protection against many infectious diseases. Specific immune globulins (e.g., varicella-zoster immune globulin) are available for postexposure prophylaxis for some infections. An exception appears to be the judicious use of live-virus varicella vaccine in children with acute lymphocytic leukemia in remission in whom the risk of natural varicella outweighs the risk from the attenuated vaccine virus. This vaccine may be obtained from the manufacturer on a compassionate use protocol for patients ages 12 months to 17 years who have acute lymphocytic leukemia in remission for at least 1 year.

Children with Transplants

Transplant recipients (e.g., bone marrow transplant recipients) should also be viewed in a special light. Some experts elect to reimmunize all children without serologic evaluation, and others, because of the limited amount of data, recommend that immunization protocols be developed for these children in conjunction with experts in the fields of infectious disease and immunology. Information about the use of live-virus vaccines in organ transplant recipients is also limited. Only inactivated poliovirus vaccine should be given to transplant recipients and their household contacts.

Children Taking Corticosteroids

Children receiving corticosteroids also need careful consideration and thorough review of their medical history, including a review of the underlying disease, the specific dose and schedule of corticosteroids prescribed, and current immunization status, which includes an evaluation of risk factors relative to infectious disease. In general, children who have a disease (which suppresses the immune response) and who are receiving either systemic or locally administered corticosteroids (which also suppress the immune response) should not be given live-virus vaccines except in special circumstances. The guidelines for administering a live-virus vaccine to patients receiving corticosteroid therapy are based on the dosage in relation to the child's weight in kilograms and the duration of corticosteroid therapy. The following treatments do not contraindicate administration:

1. Topical therapy or local injections of corticosteroids
2. Physiologic maintenance doses of corticosteroids
3. Low or moderate dosage of systemic corticosteroids (<2 mg/kg/d of prednisone [Deltasone] or its equivalent or <20 mg/d or on alternate days if the child weighs >10 kg)

Special consideration should be given if high-dose corticosteroids are prescribed. Administration of high-dose corticosteroids (≥2 mg/kg/day of prednisone or its equivalent or ≥20 mg/d if the child weighs >10 kg) given daily or on alternate days for 14 days or less preempts administration of live-virus vaccines until the treatment is discontinued. Some experts recommend delaying immunization until 2 weeks after discontinuation of therapy.

Patients who receive high doses of systemic corticosteroids—daily or on alternate days for 14 days or more—should not receive live-virus vaccines until steroid therapy has been discontinued for at least 1 month. In addition, if clinical or laboratory evidence of systemic immunosuppression results from prolonged application, live-virus vaccines should not be administered until corticosteroid therapy has been discontinued for at least 1 month.

Children with Seizures

Infants and children with a personal or family history of seizures are at increased risk for having a convulsion after receiving either pertussis (as DTaP) or measles (as MMR) vaccine. Seizures are usually brief, self-limited, and generalized and occur in conjunction with fever (Pickering, et al., 2009). However, in the case of DTaP vaccine administered during infancy, administration may coincide with or hasten the inevitable recognition of a seizure-related disorder, such as infantile spasms or epilepsy. This causes confusion about the role of the pertussis vaccine, and in this instance, pertussis immunization should be deferred until a progressive neurologic disorder is excluded or the cause of the seizure diagnosed.

Measles immunization, however, is usually given at an age when the cause and nature of the seizure activity have been established. Therefore, measles immunization should not be deferred in children with a history of one or more seizures.

Adolescents

Adolescents continue to be adversely affected by vaccine-preventable disease, including varicella, hepatitis B, measles, HPV, and rubella. In November 1996, the CDC issued recommendations for immunizing adolescents. Recommendations for adolescents at ages 11 and 12 aim to improve the vaccine coverage and to establish routine visits to health care providers. These strategies reflect the recommendations of the ACIP, AAP, American Academy of Family Physicians, and American Medical Association. In addition to providing an opportunity for administering needed vaccines, such as hepatitis B, varicella, second dose of MMR, tetanus and diphtheria booster, and HPV, this visit provides an opportunity to render other recommended preventive services, including health behavior guidance; screening for biomedical, behavioral, and emotional conditions; and delivery of other health services. For more information, see **Figure 51.3**.

IMMUNIZATION RECOMMENDATIONS FOR ADULTS

Immunization prophylaxis is as important for adults as it is for children. However, the practice of routinely reviewing and updating the vaccination status of adults remains an issue. Obstacles that affect vaccination rates include the following:

1. The practitioner's limited knowledge of specific recommendations
2. The patient's reluctance or refusal to be vaccinated
3. Liability and reimbursement issues

As a result, many adults continue to be affected adversely by vaccine-preventable diseases such as varicella, hepatitis B, measles, and rubella. The ACIP and the CDC recommend that an overall review of vaccine status should be completed on all adults at age 50. **Figure 51.4** summarizes risk factors and recommendations for adult immunizations.

DISEASE-SPECIFIC VACCINE RECOMMENDATIONS

Pneumococcal Vaccine 23-Valent

Pneumococcal infection causes an estimated 5,000 deaths annually in the United States, accounting for more deaths than any other vaccine-preventable bacterial disease. *Streptococcus pneumoniae* colonizes the upper respiratory tract and can cause disseminated invasive infections, including bacteremia and meningitis, pneumonia and other lower respiratory tract infections, and upper respiratory tract infections, including otitis media and sinusitis. The pneumococcal vaccine protects against invasive bacteremic disease, although existing data suggest that it is less effective in protecting against other types of pneumococcal infections.

In April 1997, the ACIP recommended that pneumococcal vaccine be used more extensively, particularly for identified high-risk populations (**Box 51.2**). Two available vaccines include 23 purified capsular polysaccharide antigens of *S. pneumoniae*. These replaced the earlier 14-valent vaccines in 1983. If an elderly patient's vaccination status is unknown, he or she should receive one dose of the vaccine. There are no data to support revaccination beyond two doses.

Response to Vaccine

Antibodies develop within 2 to 3 weeks in healthy young adults; immune responses are not consistent among all 23 serotypes in the vaccine. Antibody concentrations and responses to individual antigens tend to be lower in the following populations:

- The elderly
- People with alcoholic cirrhosis, chronic obstructive pulmonary disease, type 1 diabetes mellitus, Hodgkin's disease, or asthma
- People who smoke
- People with chronic renal failure requiring dialysis, renal transplantation, or nephrotic syndrome
- People with acquired immunodeficiency syndrome or HIV infection

Special Circumstances

Antibody response is diminished or absent in people who are immunocompromised or who have leukemia, lymphoma, or multiple myeloma. The antibody levels to most pneumococcal vaccine antigens remain elevated for at least 5 years in healthy adults.

A more rapid decline (within 3–5 years) occurs in certain children who have undergone splenectomy after trauma and in those who have sickle cell disease. Antibody concentrations also decline after 5 to 10 years in elderly people, those who have undergone splenectomy, patients with renal disease requiring dialysis, and people who have received transplants. A lower antibody response or rapid decline in antibody levels is also noted in patients with Hodgkin's disease and multiple myeloma. At least 2 weeks should elapse between immunization and the initiation of chemotherapy or immunosuppressive therapy.

Revaccination is recommended once for patients who are age 2 or older, who are at highest risk for serious pneumococcal infection, and who are likely to have a rapid decline in antibody levels provided that 5 years have elapsed since receiving the first dose of vaccine.

Pneumococcal Conjugate Vaccine

In June 2000, the U.S. Food and Drug Administration licensed a heptavalent pneumococcal conjugate vaccine, PCV7 (Prevnar). This vaccine is recommended for universal use in children age 23 months and younger. The number of doses for the primary series varies with the age of the child at the first dose.

Children ages 24 to 59 months who are at high risk for invasive pneumococcal infection and who have not been previously immunized should also receive 23-valent vaccine to

Recommended Immunization Schedule for Persons Aged 7 Through 18 Years—United States • 2010
For those who fall behind or start late, see the schedule below and the catch-up schedule

Vaccine ▼ Age ►	7–10 years	11–12 years	13–18 years	
Tetanus, Diphtheria, Pertussis[1]		Tdap	Tdap	Range of recommended ages for all children except certain high-risk groups
Human Papillomavirus[2]	see footnote 2	HPV (3 doses)	HPV series	
Meningococcal[3]	MCV	MCV	MCV	
Influenza[4]	Influenza (Yearly)			
Pneumococcal[5]	PPSV			Range of recommended ages for catch-up immunization
Hepatitis A[6]	HepA Series			
Hepatitis B[7]	Hep B Series			
Inactivated Poliovirus[8]	IPV Series			Range of recommended ages for certain high-risk groups
Measles, Mumps, Rubella[9]	MMR Series			
Varicella[10]	Varicella Series			

This schedule includes recommendations in effect as of December 15, 2009. Any dose not administered at the recommended age should be administered at a subsequent visit, when indicated and feasible. The use of a combination vaccine generally is preferred over separate injections of its equivalent component vaccines. Considerations should include provider assessment, patient preference, and the potential for adverse events. Providers should consult the relevant Advisory Committee on Immunization Practices statement for detailed recommendations: http://www.cdc.gov/vaccines/pubs/acip-list.htm. Clinically significant adverse events that follow immunization should be reported to the Vaccine Adverse Event Reporting System (VAERS) at http://www.vaers.hhs.gov or by telephone, **800-822-7967.**

1. **Tetanus and diphtheria toxoids and acellular pertussis vaccine (Tdap).** (Minimum age: 10 years for Boostrix and 11 years for Adacel)
   - Administer at age 11 or 12 years for those who have completed the recommended childhood DTP/DTaP vaccination series and have not received a tetanus and diphtheria toxoid (Td) booster dose.
   - Persons aged 13 through 18 years who have not received Tdap should receive a dose.
   - A 5-year interval from the last Td dose is encouraged when Tdap is used as a booster dose; however, a shorter interval may be used if pertussis immunity is needed.
2. **Human papillomavirus vaccine (HPV).** (Minimum age: 9 years)
   - Two HPV vaccines are licensed: a quadrivalent vaccine (HPV4) for the prevention of cervical, vaginal and vulvar cancers (in females) and genital warts (in females and males), and a bivalent vaccine (HPV2) for the prevention of cervical cancers in females.
   - HPV vaccines are most effective for both males and females when given before exposure to HPV through sexual contact.
   - HPV4 or HPV2 is recommended for the prevention of cervical precancers and cancers in females.
   - HPV4 is recommended for the prevention of cervical, vaginal and vulvar precancers and cancers and genital warts in females.
   - Administer the first dose to females at age 11 or 12 years.
   - Administer the second dose 1 to 2 months after the first dose and the third dose 6 months after the first dose (at least 24 weeks after the first dose).
   - Administer the series to females at age 13 through 18 years if not previously vaccinated.
   - HPV4 may be administered in a 3-dose series to males aged 9 through 18 years to reduce their likelihood of acquiring genital warts.
3. **Meningococcal conjugate vaccine, quadrivalent (MCV4).** (Minimum age: 2 years)
   - Administer MCV4 at age 11 through 12 years with a booster dose at age 16 Years.
   - Administer 1 dose at age 13 through 18 years if not previously vaccinated.
   - Persons who received their first dose at age 13 through 15 years should receive a booster dose at age 16 through 18 years.
   - Administer 1 dose to previously unvaccinated college freshmen living in a dormitory.
   - Administer 2 doses at least 8 weeks apart to children aged 2 through 10 years with persistent complement component deficiency and anatomic or functional asplenia, and 1 dose every 5 years thereafter.
   - Persons with HIV infection who are vaccinated with MCV4 should receive 2 doses at least 8 weeks apart.
   - Administer 1 dose of MCV4 to children aged 2 through 10 years who travel to countries with highly endemic or epidemic disease and during outbreaks caused by a vaccine serogroup.
   - Administer MCV4 to children at continued risk for meningococcal disease who were previously vaccinated with MCV4 or meningococcal polysaccharide vaccine after 3 years (if first dose administered at age 2 through 6 years) or after 5 years (if first dose administered at age 7 years or older).

4. **Influenza vaccine (seasonal).**
   - Administer annually to children aged 6 months through 18 years.
   - For healthy nonpregnant persons aged 7 through 18 years (i.e., those who do not have underlying medical conditions that predispose them to influenza complications), either LAIV or TIV may be used.
   - Administer 2 doses (separated by at least 4 weeks) to children aged younger than 9 years who are receiving influenza vaccine for the first time or who were vaccinated for the first time during the previous influenza season but only received 1 dose.
   - For recommendations for use of influenza A (H1N1) 2009 monovalent vaccine. See MMWR 2009;58(No. RR-10).
5. **Pneumococcal vaccines.**
   - A single dose of 13-valent pneumococcal conjugate vaccine (PCV13) may be administered to children aged 6 through 18 years who have functional or anatomic asplenia, HIV infection or other immunocompromising condition, cochlear implant or CSF leak. See MMWR 2010;59(No. RR-11).
   - The dose of PCV13 should be administered at least 8 weeks after the previous dose of PCV7.
   - Administer pneumococcal polysaccharide vaccine at least 8 weeks after the last dose of PCV to children aged 2 years or older with certain underlying medical conditions, including a cochlear implant. A single revaccination should be administered after 5 years to children with functional or anatomic asplenia or an immunocompromising condition
6. **Hepatitis A vaccine (HepA).**
   - Administer 2 doses at least 6 months apart.
   - HepA is recommended for children aged older than 23 months who live in areas where vaccination programs target older children, who are at increased risk for infection, or for whom immunity against hepatitis A is desired.
7. **Hepatitis B vaccine (HepB).**
   - Administer the 3-dose series to those not previously vaccinated.
   - A 2-dose series (separated by at least 4 months) of adult formulation Recombivax HB is licensed for children aged 11 through 15 years.
8. **Inactivated poliovirus vaccine (IPV).**
   - The final dose in the series should be administered on or after the fourth birthday and at least 6 months following the previous dose.
   - If both OPV and IPV were administered as part of a series, a total of 4 doses should be administered, regardless of the child's current age.
9. **Measles, mumps, and rubella vaccine (MMR).**
   - If not previously vaccinated, administer 2 doses or the second dose for those who have received only 1 dose, with at least 28 days between doses.
10. **Varicella vaccine.**
   - For persons aged 7 through 18 years without evidence of immunity (see MMWR 2007;56[No. RR-4]), administer 2 doses if not previously vaccinated or the second dose if only 1 dose has been administered.
   - For persons aged 7 through 12 years, the minimum interval between doses is 3 months. However, if the second dose was administered at least 28 days after the first dose, it can be accepted as valid.
   - For persons aged 13 years and older, the minimum interval between doses is 28 days.

The Recommended Immunization Schedules for Persons Aged 0 through 18 Years are approved by the Advisory Committee on Immunization Practices (http://www.cdc.gov/vaccines/recs/acip), the American Academy of Pediatrics (http://www.aap.org), and the American Academy of Family Physicians (http://www.aafp.org). http://www.pediatrics.org/cgi/content/full/127/2/387 accessed

Department of Health and Human Services • Centers for Disease Control and Prevention

FIGURE 51-3   Recommended Immunization Schedule for Persons Aged 7 Through 18 Years—United States, 2010.

Recommended Adult Immunization Schedule
UNITED STATES · 2010
Note: These recommendations *must* be read with the footnotes that follow
containing number of doses, intervals between doses, and other important information.

Figure 1. Recommended adult immunization schedule, by vaccine and age group

VACCINE ▼ AGE GROUP ►	19–26 years	27–49 years	50–59 years	60–64 years	≥65 years
Tetanus, diphtheria, pertussis (Td/Tdap)[1,*]	Substitute 1-time dose of Tdap for Td booster; then boost with Td every 10 yrs				Td booster every 10 yrs
Human papillomavirus (HPV)[2,*]	3 doses (females)				
Varicella[3,*]	2 doses				
Zoster[4]				1 dose	
Measles, mumps, rubella (MMR)[5,*]	1 or 2 doses		1 dose		
Influenza[6,*]	1 dose annually				
Pneumococcal (polysaccharide)[7,8]	1 or 2 doses				1 dose
Hepatitis A[9,*]	2 doses				
Hepatitis B[10,*]	3 doses				
Meningococcal[11,*]	1 or more doses				

*Covered by the Vaccine Injury Compensation Program.

For all persons in this category who meet the age requirements and who lack evidence of immunity (e.g., lack documentation of vaccination or have no evidence of prior infection)	Recommended if some other risk factor is present (e.g., on the basis of medical, occupational, lifestyle, or other indications)	No recommendation

Report all clinically significant postvaccination reactions to the Vaccine Adverse Event Reporting System (VAERS). Reporting forms and instructions on filing a VAERS report are available at www.vaers.hhs.gov or by telephone, 800-822-7967.

Information on how to file a Vaccine Injury Compensation Program claim is available at www.hrsa.gov/vaccinecompensation or by telephone, 800-338-2382. To file a claim for vaccine injury, contact the U.S. Court of Federal Claims, 717 Madison Place, N.W., Washington, D.C. 20005; telephone, 202-357-6400.

Additional information about the vaccines in this schedule, extent of available data, and contraindications for vaccination is also available at www.cdc.gov/vaccines or from the CDC-INFO Contact Center at 800-CDC-INFO (800-232-4636) in English and Spanish, 24 hours a day, 7 days a week.

Use of trade names and commercial sources is for identification only and does not imply endorsement by the U.S. Department of Health and Human Services.

Figure 2. Vaccines that might be indicated for adults based on medical and other indications

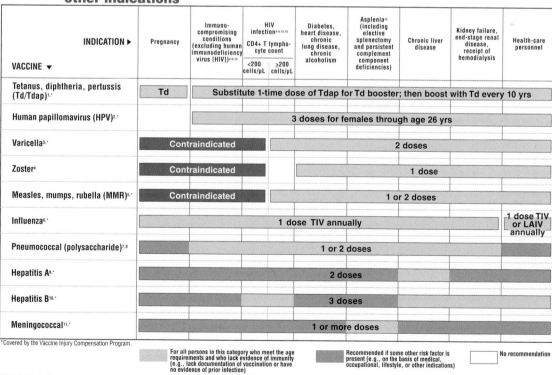

INDICATION ► VACCINE ▼	Pregnancy	Immuno-compromising conditions (excluding human immunodeficiency virus [HIV])[3–5,13]	HIV infection[3–5,12,13] CD4+ T lymphocyte count <200 cells/µL	HIV infection[3–5,12,13] CD4+ T lymphocyte count ≥200 cells/µL	Diabetes, heart disease, chronic lung disease, chronic alcoholism	Asplenia[12] (including elective splenectomy and persistent complement component deficiencies)	Chronic liver disease	Kidney failure, end-stage renal disease, receipt of hemodialysis	Health-care personnel
Tetanus, diphtheria, pertussis (Td/Tdap)[1,*]	Td	Substitute 1-time dose of Tdap for Td booster; then boost with Td every 10 yrs							
Human papillomavirus (HPV)[2,*]		3 doses for females through age 26 yrs							
Varicella[3,*]	Contraindicated			2 doses					
Zoster[4]	Contraindicated			1 dose					
Measles, mumps, rubella (MMR)[5,*]	Contraindicated			1 or 2 doses					
Influenza[6,*]	1 dose TIV annually								1 dose TIV or LAIV annually
Pneumococcal (polysaccharide)[7,8]	1 or 2 doses								
Hepatitis A[9,*]	2 doses								
Hepatitis B[10,*]	3 doses								
Meningococcal[11,*]	1 or more doses								

*Covered by the Vaccine Injury Compensation Program.

For all persons in this category who meet the age requirements and who lack evidence of immunity (e.g., lack documentation of vaccination or have no evidence of prior infection)	Recommended if some other risk factor is present (e.g., on the basis of medical, occupational, lifestyle, or other indications)	No recommendation

These schedules indicate the recommended age groups and medical indications for which administration of currently licensed vaccines is commonly indicated for adults ages 19 years and older, as of January 1, 2010. Licensed combination vaccines may be used whenever any components of the combination are indicated and when the vaccine's other components are not contraindicated. For detailed recommendations on all vaccines, including those used primarily for travelers or that are issued during the year, consult the manufacturers' package inserts and the complete statements from the Advisory Committee on Immunization Practices (www.cdc.gov/vaccines/pubs/acip-list.htm).

The recommendations in this schedule were approved by the Centers for Disease Control and Prevention's (CDC) Advisory Committee on Immunization Practices (ACIP), the American Academy of Family Physicians (AAFP), the American College of Obstetricians and Gynecologists (ACOG), and the American College of Physicians (ACP).

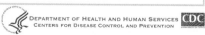

DEPARTMENT OF HEALTH AND HUMAN SERVICES
CENTERS FOR DISEASE CONTROL AND PREVENTION

(continued)

Footnotes

Recommended Adult Immunization Schedule—UNITED STATES · 2010

For complete statements by the Advisory Committee on Immunization Practices (ACIP), visit www.cdc.gov/vaccines/pubs/ACIP-list.htm.

1. Tetanus, diphtheria, and acellular pertussis (Td/Tdap) vaccination

Tdap should replace a single dose of Td for adults aged 19 through 64 years who have not received a dose of Tdap previously.

Adults with uncertain or incomplete history of primary vaccination series with tetanus and diphtheria toxoid-containing vaccines should begin or complete a primary vaccination series. A primary series for adults is 3 doses of tetanus and diphtheria toxoid-containing vaccines; administer the first 2 doses at least 4 weeks apart and the third dose 6–12 months after the second; Tdap can substitute for any one of the doses of Td in the 3-dose primary series. The booster dose of tetanus and diphtheria toxoid-containing vaccine should be administered to adults who have completed a primary series and if the last vaccination was received ≥10 years previously. Tdap or Td vaccine may be used, as indicated.

If a woman is pregnant and received the last Td vaccination ≥10 years previously, administer Td during the second or third trimester. If the woman received the last Td vaccination <10 years previously, administer Tdap during the immediate postpartum period. A dose of Tdap is recommended for postpartum women, close contacts of infants aged <12 months, and all health-care personnel with direct patient contact if they have not previously received Tdap. An interval as short as 2 years from the last Td is suggested; shorter intervals can be used. Td may be deferred during pregnancy and Tdap substituted in the immediate postpartum period, or Tdap can be administered instead of Td to a pregnant woman.

Consult the ACIP statement for recommendations for giving Td as prophylaxis in wound management.

2. Human papillomavirus (HPV) vaccination

HPV vaccination is recommended at age 11 or 12 years with catch-up vaccination at ages 13 through 26 years.

Ideally, vaccine should be administered before potential exposure to HPV through sexual activity; however, females who are sexually active should still be vaccinated consistent with age-based recommendations. Sexually active females who have not been infected with any of the four HPV vaccine types (types 6, 11, 16, 18 all of which HPV4 prevents) or any of the two HPV vaccine types (types 16 and 18 both of which HPV2 prevents) receive the full benefit of the vaccination. Vaccination is less beneficial for females who have already been infected with one or more of the HPV vaccine types. HPV4 or HPV2 can be administered to persons with a history of genital warts, abnormal Papanicolaou test, or positive HPV DNA test, because these conditions are not evidence of prior infection with all vaccine HPV types.

HPV4 may be administered to males aged 9 through 26 years to reduce their likelihood of acquiring genital warts. HPV4 would be most effective when administered before exposure to HPV through sexual contact.

A complete series for either HPV4 or HPV2 consists of 3 doses. The second dose should be administered 1–2 months after the first dose; the third dose should be administered 6 months after the first dose.

Although HPV vaccination is not specifically recommended for persons with the medical indications described in Figure 2, "Vaccines that might be indicated for adults based on medical and other indications," it may be administered to these persons because the HPV vaccine is not a live-virus vaccine. However, the immune response and vaccine efficacy might be less for persons with the medical indications described in Figure 2 than in persons who do not have the medical indications described or who are immunocompetent. Health-care personnel are not at increased risk because of occupational exposure, and should be vaccinated consistent with age-based recommendations.

3. Varicella vaccination

All adults without evidence of immunity to varicella should receive 2 doses of single-antigen varicella vaccine if not previously vaccinated or the second dose if they have received only 1 dose, unless they have a medical contraindication. Special consideration should be given to those who 1) have close contact with persons at high risk for severe disease (e.g., health-care personnel and family contacts of persons with immunocompromising conditions) or 2) are at high risk for exposure or transmission (e.g., teachers; child-care employees; residents and staff members of institutional settings, including correctional institutions; college students; military personnel; adolescents and adults living in households with children; nonpregnant women of childbearing age; and international travelers).

Evidence of immunity to varicella in adults includes any of the following: 1) documentation of 2 doses of varicella vaccine at least 4 weeks apart; 2) U.S.-born before 1980 (although for health-care personnel and pregnant women, birth before 1980 should not be considered evidence of immunity); 3) history of varicella based on diagnosis or verification of varicella by a health-care provider (for a patient reporting a history of or presenting with an atypical case, a mild case, or both, health-care providers should seek either an epidemiologic link with a typical varicella case or to a laboratory-confirmed case or evidence of laboratory confirmation, if it was performed at the time of acute disease); 4) history of herpes zoster based on diagnosis or verification of herpes zoster by a health-care provider; or 5) laboratory evidence of immunity or laboratory confirmation of disease.

Pregnant women should be assessed for evidence of varicella immunity. Women who do not have evidence of immunity should receive the first dose of varicella vaccine upon completion or termination of pregnancy and before discharge from the health-care facility. The second dose should be administered 4–8 weeks after the first dose.

4. Herpes zoster vaccination

A single dose of zoster vaccine is recommended for adults aged ≥60 years regardless of whether they report a prior episode of herpes zoster. Persons with chronic medical conditions may be vaccinated unless their condition constitutes a contraindication.

5. Measles, mumps, rubella (MMR) vaccination

Adults born before 1957 generally are considered immune to measles and mumps.

Measles component: Adults born during or after 1957 should receive 1 or more doses of MMR vaccine unless they have 1) a medical contraindication; 2) documentation of vaccination with 1 or more doses of MMR vaccine; 3) laboratory evidence of immunity; or 4) documentation of physician-diagnosed measles.

A second dose of MMR vaccine, administered 4 weeks after the first dose, is recommended for adults who 1) have been recently exposed to measles or are in an outbreak setting; 2) have been vaccinated previously with killed measles vaccine; 3) have been vaccinated with an unknown type of measles vaccine during 1963–1967; 4) are students in postsecondary educational institutions; 5) work in a health-care facility; or 6) plan to travel internationally.

Mumps component: Adults born during or after 1957 should receive 1 dose of MMR vaccine unless they have 1) a medical contraindication; 2) documentation of vaccination with 1 or more doses of MMR vaccine; 3) laboratory evidence of immunity; or 4) documentation of physician-diagnosed mumps.

A second dose of MMR vaccine, administered 4 weeks after the first dose, is recommended for adults who 1) live in a community experiencing a mumps outbreak and are in an affected age group; 2) are students in postsecondary educational institutions; 3) work in a health-care facility; or 4) plan to travel internationally.

Rubella component: 1 dose of MMR vaccine is recommended for women who do not have documentation of rubella vaccination, or who lack laboratory evidence of immunity. For women of childbearing age, regardless of birth year, rubella immunity should be determined and women should be counseled regarding congenital rubella syndrome. Women who do not have evidence of immunity should receive MMR vaccine upon completion or termination of pregnancy and before discharge from the health-care facility.

Health-care personnel born before 1957: For unvaccinated health-care personnel born before 1957 who lack laboratory evidence of measles, mumps, and/or rubella immunity or laboratory confirmation of disease, health-care facilities should consider vaccinating personnel with 2 doses of MMR vaccine at the appropriate interval (for measles and mumps) and 1 dose of MMR vaccine (for rubella), respectively.

During outbreaks, health-care facilities should recommend that unvaccinated health-care personnel born before 1957, who lack laboratory evidence of measles, mumps, and/or rubella immunity or laboratory confirmation of disease, receive 2 doses of MMR vaccine during an outbreak of measles or mumps, and 1 dose during an outbreak of rubella.

Complete information about evidence of immunity is available at www.cdc.gov/vaccines/recs/provisional/default.htm.

6. Seasonal Influenza vaccination

Vaccinate all persons aged ≥50 years and any younger persons who would like to decrease their risk of getting influenza. Vaccinate persons aged 19 through 49 years with any of the following indications.

Medical: Chronic disorders of the cardiovascular or pulmonary systems, including asthma; chronic metabolic diseases, including diabetes mellitus; renal or hepatic dysfunction, hemoglobinopathies, or immunocompromising conditions (including immunocompromising conditions caused by medications or HIV); cognitive, neurologic or neuromuscular disorders; and pregnancy during the influenza season. No data exist on the risk for severe or complicated influenza disease among persons with asplenia; however, influenza is a risk factor for secondary bacterial infections that can cause severe disease among persons with asplenia.

Occupational: All health-care personnel, including those employed by long-term care and assisted-living facilities, and caregivers of children aged <5 years.

Other: Residents of nursing homes and other long-term care and assisted-living facilities; persons likely to transmit influenza to persons at high risk (e.g., in-home household contacts and caregivers of children aged <5 years, persons aged ≥50 years, and persons of all ages with high-risk conditions).

Healthy, nonpregnant adults aged <50 years without high-risk medical conditions who are not contacts of severely immunocompromised persons in special-care units may receive either intranasally administered live, attenuated influenza vaccine (FluMist) or inactivated vaccine. Other persons should receive the inactivated vaccine.

7. Pneumococcal polysaccharide (PPSV) vaccination

Vaccinate all persons with the following indications.

Medical: Chronic lung disease (including asthma); chronic cardiovascular diseases; diabetes mellitus; chronic liver diseases, cirrhosis; chronic alcoholism; functional or anatomic asplenia (e.g., sickle cell disease or splenectomy [if elective splenectomy is planned, vaccinate at least 2 weeks before surgery]); immunocompromising conditions including chronic renal failure or nephrotic syndrome; and cochlear implants and cerebrospinal fluid leaks. Vaccinate as close to HIV diagnosis as possible.

Other: Residents of nursing homes or long-term care facilities and persons who smoke cigarettes. Routine use of PPSV is not recommended for American Indians/Alaska Natives or persons aged <65 years unless they have underlying medical conditions that are PPSV indications. However, public health authorities may consider recommending PPSV for American Indians/Alaska Natives and persons aged 50 through 64 years who are living in areas where the risk for invasive pneumococcal disease is increased.

8. Revaccination with PPSV

One-time revaccination after 5 years is recommended for persons with chronic renal failure or nephrotic syndrome; functional or anatomic asplenia (e.g., sickle cell disease or splenectomy); and for persons with immunocompromising conditions. For persons aged ≥65 years, one-time revaccination is recommended if they were vaccinated ≥5 years previously and were younger than aged <65 years at the time of primary vaccination.

9. Hepatitis A vaccination

Vaccinate persons with any of the following indications and any person seeking protection from hepatitis A virus (HAV) infection.

Behavioral: Men who have sex with men and persons who use injection drugs.

Occupational: Persons working with HAV–infected primates or with HAV in a research laboratory setting.

Medical: Persons with chronic liver disease and persons who receive clotting factor concentrates.

Other: Persons traveling to or working in countries that have high or intermediate endemicity of hepatitis A (a list of countries is available at wwwn.cdc.gov/travel/contentdiseases.aspx).

Unvaccinated persons who anticipate close personal contact (e.g., household contact or regular babysitting) with an international adoptee from a country of high or intermediate endemicity during the first 60 days after arrival of the adoptee in the United States should consider vaccination. The first dose of the 2-dose hepatitis A vaccine series should be administered as soon as adoption is planned, ideally ≥2 weeks before the arrival of the adoptee.

Single-antigen vaccine formulations should be administered in a 2-dose schedule at either 0 and 6–12 months (Havrix), or 0 and 6–18 months (Vaqta). If the combined hepatitis A and hepatitis B vaccine (Twinrix) is used, administer 3 doses at 0, 1, and 6 months; alternatively, a 4-dose schedule, administered on days 0, 7, and 21–30 followed by a booster dose at month 12 may be used.

10. Hepatitis B vaccination

Vaccinate persons with any of the following indications and any person seeking protection from hepatitis B virus (HBV) infection.

Behavioral: Sexually active persons who are not in a long-term, mutually monogamous relationship (e.g., persons with more than one sex partner during the previous 6 months); persons seeking evaluation or treatment for a sexually transmitted disease (STD); current or recent injection-drug users; and men who have sex with men.

Occupational: Health-care personnel and public-safety workers who are exposed to blood or other potentially infectious body fluids.

Medical: Persons with end-stage renal disease, including patients receiving hemodialysis; persons with HIV infection; and persons with chronic liver disease.

Other: Household contacts and sex partners of persons with chronic HBV infection; clients and staff members of institutions for persons with developmental disabilities; and international travelers to countries with high or intermediate prevalence of chronic HBV infection (a list of countries is available at wwwn.cdc.gov/travel/contentdiseases.aspx).

Hepatitis B vaccination is recommended for all adults in the following settings: STD treatment facilities; HIV testing and treatment facilities; facilities providing drug-abuse treatment and prevention services; health-care settings targeting services to injection-drug users or men who have sex with men; correctional facilities; end-stage renal disease programs and facilities for chronic hemodialysis patients; and institutions and nonresidential daycare facilities for persons with developmental disabilities.

Administer or complete a 3-dose series of HepB to those persons not previously vaccinated. The second dose should be administered 1 month after the first dose; the third dose should be administered at least 2 months after the second dose (and at least 4 months after the first dose). If the combined hepatitis A and hepatitis B vaccine (Twinrix) is used, administer 3 doses at 0, 1, and 6 months; alternatively, a 4-dose schedule, administered on days 0, 7, and 21–30 followed by a booster dose at month 12 may be used.

Adult patients receiving hemodialysis or with other immunocompromising conditions should receive 1 dose of 40 μg/mL (Recombivax HB) administered on a 3-dose schedule or 2 doses of 20 μg/mL (Engerix-B) administered simultaneously on a 4-dose schedule at 0, 1, 2 and 6 months.

(continued)

11. Meningococcal vaccination

Meningococcal vaccine should be administered to persons with the following indications.

Medical: Adults with anatomic or functional asplenia, or persistent complement component deficiencies.

Other: First-year college students living in dormitories; microbiologists routinely exposed to isolates of *Neisseria meningitidis*; military recruits; and persons who travel to or live in countries in which meningococcal disease is hyperendemic or epidemic (e.g., the "meningitis belt" of sub-Saharan Africa during the dry season [December through June]), particularly if their contact with local populations will be prolonged. Vaccination is required by the government of Saudi Arabia for all travelers to Mecca during the annual Hajj.

Meningococcal conjugate vaccine (MCV4) is preferred for adults with any of the preceding indications who are aged ≤55 years; meningococcal polysaccharide vaccine (MPSV4) is preferred for adults aged ≥56 years. Revaccination with MCV4 after 5 years is recommended for adults previously vaccinated with MCV4 or MPSV4 who remain at increased risk for infection (e.g., adults with anatomic or functional asplenia). Persons whose only risk factor is living in on-campus housing are not recommended to receive an additional dose.

12. Selected conditions for which *Haemophilus influenzae* type b (Hib) vaccine may be used

Hib vaccine generally is not recommended for persons aged ≥5 years. No efficacy data are available on which to base a recommendation concerning use of Hib vaccine for older children and adults. However, studies suggest good immunogenicity in patients who have sickle cell disease, leukemia, or HIV infection or who have had a splenectomy. Administering 1 dose of Hib vaccine to these high-risk persons who have not previously received Hib vaccine is not contraindicated.

13. Immunocompromising conditions

Inactivated vaccines generally are acceptable (e.g., pneumococcal, meningococcal, influenza [inactivated influenza vaccine]) and live vaccines generally are avoided in persons with immune deficiencies or immunocompromising conditions. Information on specific conditions is available at www.cdc.gov/vaccines/pubs/acip-list.htm.

FIGURE 51–4   Recommended Adult Immunization Schedule—United States, 2010.

expand the serotype coverage. Indications for children age 24 months and older who are considered to be at moderate or low risk remain under investigation because current data are insufficient to recommend routine administration.

Influenza Vaccine

Influenza and pneumonia are the sixth leading cause of death in the United States and fifth in older adults. Fatalities from influenza begin to rise in midlife and are highest in persons with chronic disease. Measures available to reduce the incidence of influenza include immunoprophylaxis with inactivated (killed virus) vaccine and chemoprophylaxis. Before the influenza season gets under way, vaccination of people at risk and those likely to transmit influenza to at-risk populations is the most effective measure. The vaccine is associated with a decrease in influenza-related respiratory illness in all age groups, decreased hospitalization and death in people at high risk, decreased incidence of otitis media in children, and decreased work and school absenteeism. Influenza vaccine is recommended in anyone age 6 months and older.

Two types of influenza vaccine are available—inactivated virus and live attenuated vaccine (in the form of nasal spray). The live virus is recommended for those ages 5 to 49 and is contraindicated in patients who are immunocompromised and require a protected environment, health care workers, and household members who are in close contact with the immunocompromised individual. If a live virus is given, the patient should not have contact with those who are immunocompromised for 7 days.

Groups at Risk

People at increased risk for influenza-related complications include:

1. Those age 50 and older
2. Children ages 6 to 23 months
3. Adults and children with pulmonary disease, including asthma
4. Adults and children who have required regular medical follow-up or hospitalization during the preceding year because of chronic metabolic diseases (including diabetes mellitus), renal dysfunction, hemoglobinopathies, or immunosuppression (including immunosuppression caused by medications or HIV infection)
5. Children and teenagers on long-term aspirin therapy who might be at risk for development of Reye syndrome after influenza
6. Women in the second or third trimester of pregnancy during the influenza season
7. Persons who live with or care for persons at high risk, including health care workers and household contacts (including children from birth to age 23 months)

Transmission of Influenza

Just as immunizing people in groups at high risk for flu and its complications is important, so too is immunizing those who are most likely to transmit the disease. Groups that can transmit influenza to people at high risk include health care workers (in hospital and outpatient settings and in emergency response service),

---

BOX 51.2

Recommendations for the Use of Pneumococcal Vaccine

Groups for Which Vaccination Is Recommended

People age 65 y and older

People ages 2–64 y with chronic cardiovascular disease, chronic pulmonary disease, asthma, or diabetes mellitus and people who smoke

People ages 2–64 y with alcoholism, chronic liver disease, or cerebrospinal fluid leaks

People ages 2–64 y with functional or anatomic asplenia

People ages 2–64 y living in special environments or social settings

Immunocompromised People

Immunocompromised people age 2 y and older, including those with HIV infection, leukemia, lymphoma, Hodgkin's disease, multiple myeloma, generalized malignancy, chronic renal failure, or nephrotic syndrome; those receiving immunosuppressive chemotherapy (including corticosteroids); and those who have received an organ or bone marrow transplant employees of nursing homes and chronic care facilities who have contact with patients or residents, employees of assisted living and other residences for people in high-risk groups, providers of home care to people at high risk (e.g., visiting nurses, volunteers), household contacts of high-risk individuals, and providers of essential community services. Additional populations for consideration include people with HIV infection, breast-feeding mothers, people traveling to foreign countries, students or other people in institutional settings, and the general populace who want to reduce the likelihood of contracting influenza.

The current 2- to 3-month time frame over which patients are traditionally immunized is too short to fully implement immunization recommendations and inconsistent with the duration of influenza activity. Health care providers and patients should reevaluate their approach to influenza vaccination and recognize the need to extend the immunization time period into January and beyond. To increase influenza immunization rates, the CDC and other professional societies recommend an expanded immunization season, with vaccination offered at every opportunity between October and May.

Antibody development after vaccination can take as long as 2 weeks in healthy adults and as long as 6 weeks in children—or 2 weeks after the second dose. Most persons recommended for influenza vaccination should receive a single dose each year. The exception is children ages 6 months to 9 years who are receiving an influenza vaccine for the first time. They should receive 2 doses administered at least 1 month apart. No influenza vaccine is currently approved for children age 6 months and younger; these vulnerable infants should be protected indirectly through the vaccination of close contacts.

Chemoprophylaxis with antiviral agents, amantadine (Symmetrel), rimantadine (Flumadine), zanamivir (Relenza), and oseltamivir (Tamiflu) can also be helpful. When administered within 48 hours of the onset of illness, they can reduce the severity and shorten the duration of illness in otherwise healthy people. Tamiflu can be used in the prevention of influenza in adults and children age 13 and older. For more information, see **Table 51.1**.

Meningococcal Vaccine

Approximately 3,000 cases of meningococcal diseases occur in the United States each year, with a fatality rate of 10% despite antibiotic therapy early in the illness. During 1991 to 1998, the highest rate occurred among infants younger than age 12 months. Meningococcal vaccine is recommended for everyone age 4 and older.

Human Papillomavirus Vaccine

Quadrivalent HPV vaccine provides protection against the four types of HPV most commonly associated with clinical diseases, including types 6 and 11, which account for over 95% of genital warts, and types 16 and 18, believed to be responsible for approximately 70% of cases of cervical cancer. The vaccine is recommended for females ages 9 to 26. It can be given to immunocompromised women, but the immune response may be reduced. Pregnant women should not receive the HPV vaccine, even if the series has been started before pregnancy. It can be administered to lactating women.

Ideally, the vaccine should be administered before potential exposure to HPV through sexual contact. The vaccine is a series of three doses. The second dose is administered 1 to 2 months after the first dose, and the third dose is administered 6 months after the first dose.

Rotavirus Vaccine

Rotavirus is the most common cause of severe gastroenteritis in children younger than age 5.

Before rotavirus vaccines were available in the United States, more than 200,000 children younger than age 5 received care in hospital emergency departments for rotavirus disease each year, and 55,000 to 70,000 young children were hospitalized.

TABLE 51.1	Recommended Daily Dose for Anti-Influenza Treatment and Prophylaxis				
		Age Group (y)			
Antiviral Agent	**1–9**	**10–13**	**14–64**	**≥65**	
amantadine (Symmetrel)					
Treatment	5 mg/kg/d up to 150 mg in 2 divided doses	100 mg bid	100 mg bid	≤100 mg/d	
Prophylaxis	5 mg/kg/d up to 150 mg in 2 divided doses	100 mg bid	100 mg bid	≤100 mg/d	
rimantadine (Flumadine)					
Treatment	NA	NA	100 mg bid	100 or 200 mg/d	
Prophylaxis	5 mg/kg/d up to 150 mg in 2 divided doses	100 mg bid	100 mg bid	100 or 200 mg/d	
zanamivir (Relenza)					
Treatment	NA	10 mg bid	10 mg bid	10 mg bid	
Prophylaxis	NA	NA	NA	NA	
oseltamivir (Tamiflu)					
Treatment	NA	NA	75 mg bid	75 mg bid	
Prophylaxis	NA	NA	NA	NA	

NA, not applicable.

From Centers for Disease Control and Prevention. (2010e). Prevention and control of influenza: Recommendations of Advisory Committee on Immunization Practices (ACIP). *Morbidity and Mortality Weekly Report, 59* (RR-08), 1–62.

Rotavirus is very contagious. People who get a rotavirus infection shed large amounts of the virus in their feces. The disease spreads when infants or young children get rotavirus in their mouth. This happens through contact with the hands of other people or objects (such as toys) that have been contaminated with small amounts of rotavirus.

The first dose of the rotavirus vaccine can be given as early as age 6 weeks and needs to be given before an infant is age 15 weeks. Children should receive all doses of rotavirus vaccine before they are age 8 months.

ADVERSE EVENTS ASSOCIATED WITH VACCINES

Risks of vaccination vary from inconvenient to severe and life-threatening. Common vaccine side effects (e.g., fever and local irritation to DTaP vaccine) are usually mild to moderate in severity and without permanent consequences. However, serious side effects and adverse reactions are possible, although the occurrence of an adverse event does not prove causation by the vaccine (i.e., the adverse event may be caused by factors other than the vaccine).

Reporting of adverse events is important because it may provide clues to unanticipated adverse reactions. It is important to interview the patient or guardian regarding any side effects after past immunizations. Any unexpected, reported, and observed event that required medical attention soon after the administration should be described in detail in the patient's medical record and reported using the Vaccine Adverse Events Reporting System (VAERS).

The VAERS is a result of the National Childhood Injury Act of 1986, which made provisions for health care providers to report occurrences of certain adverse events and to maintain permanent immunization records. Pertinent information to be reported includes a detailed description of the event (signs and symptoms reported and observed) and the time from administration of vaccine to presentation of signs and symptoms.

Pertinent patient history information should be noted regarding any existing physician-diagnosed allergies, medical conditions, and birth defects as well as any illness at the time of vaccine administration. In addition, information about the vaccine must be included. Documentation should identify the type of vaccine, the manufacturer, lot number, site and route of administration, and any previous doses received.

Staff members from the VAERS contact the provider (reporter) to follow up about the patient's condition at 60 days and at 1 year after the initial reporting of adverse events. **Box 51.3** contains the VAERS form.

CONTRAINDICATIONS TO VACCINATIONS

The primary contraindications to vaccine administration are acute febrile illness, allergy to a vaccine component, or history of hypersensitivity/anaphylactic reaction to vaccine constituents. **Figure 51.5** includes a detailed listing of contraindications by vaccine. The four main types of hypersensitivity reactions include:

1. Allergic reactions to egg-related antigens (e.g., MMR, yellow fever)
2. Mercury sensitivity in some recipients of vaccines or immune globulin
3. Antibiotic-induced allergic reactions (e.g., inactivated or oral poliovirus vaccine—trace streptomycin, neomycin, and polymyxin B; MMR, including single or combined with varicella—trace neomycin)
4. Hypersensitivity to other vaccine components, including the infectious agent

Acute febrile illness suggesting a moderate to severe illness is sufficient reason to defer vaccination until the person recovers. Guidelines in this instance are based on the provider's assessment of the illness and the vaccines scheduled for administration.

The rationale for withholding vaccination in moderate to severe illness, with or without fever, is that evolving signs and symptoms associated with the illness may be difficult to distinguish from the reaction to the vaccine. Minor illness (minor respiratory, gastrointestinal, or other illness) and low-grade fevers are not contraindications to immunization. The benefit of the immunization at the recommended age, regardless of the presence of mild illness, outweighs the risk of vaccine failure (Pickering, et al., 2009).

Pregnancy is an additional contraindication to the administration of live-virus vaccines. In some cases, immunization of immunodeficient and immunosuppressed children is contraindicated. (See the preceding discussions on immunocompromised children.)

PATIENT AND PROVIDER EDUCATION AND ISSUES

Patient and health care provider/practitioner education, updates on immunization protocols, and established office systems with designated areas of responsibility are significant factors in improving immunization rates. Office routines and systems should incorporate pediatric immunization standards (**Box 51.4**) and facilitate use of all possible opportunities to review and update the immunization status of each patient. Tickler systems, chart reminders, and flow sheets that identify needed immunizations clearly and visibly are useful adjuncts to patient care.

A team approach to staff involvement also helps to enhance vaccination rates. Support staff should be aware of immunization needs when scheduling return or preventive visits as well as visits for illness or minor health problems. Visual reminders on the patient's chart or visit-encounter form can be used to alert the practitioner to review specific vaccine needs or requests. **Box 51.5** presents recommendations related to the immunization schedule, and **Box 51.6** offers answers to frequently asked questions about immunization.

BOX 51.3

Vaccine Adverse Event Reporting System Form

VAERS

VACCINE ADVERSE EVENT REPORTING SYSTEM
24 Hour Toll-Free Information 1-800-822-7967
P.O. Box 1100, Rockville, MD 20849-1100
PATIENT IDENTITY KEPT CONFIDENTIAL

For CDC/FDA Use Only

VAERS Number _____

Date Received _____

Patient Name:	Vaccine administered by (Name):	Form completed by (Name):
Last First M.I.	Responsible Physician _____	Relation ☐ Vaccine Provider ☐ Patient/Parent
Address	Facility Name/Address	to Patient ☐ Manufacturer ☐ Other
_____	_____	Address (if different from patient or provider)
_____	_____	_____
_____	_____	_____
City State Zip	City State Zip	City State Zip
Telephone no. (___)_____	Telephone no. (___)_____	Telephone no. (___)_____

1. State	2. County where administered	3. Date of birth __/__/__ mm dd yy	4. Patient age	5. Sex ☐ M ☐ F	6. Date form completed __/__/__ mm dd yy

7. Describe adverse events(s) (symptoms, signs, time course) and treatment, if any

8. Check all appropriate:
☐ Patient died   (date __/__/__ mm dd yy)
☐ Life threatening illness
☐ Required emergency room/doctor visit
☐ Required hospitalization (_____ days)
☐ Resulted in prolongation of hospitalization
☐ Resulted in permanent disability
☐ None of the above

9. Patient recovered ☐ YES ☐ NO ☐ UNKNOWN

10. Date of vaccination __/__/__ mm dd yy   Time_____ AM/PM

11. Adverse event onset __/__/__ mm dd yy   Time_____ AM/PM

12. Relevant diagnostic tests / laboratory data

13. Enter all vaccines given on date listed in no. 10

	Vaccine (type)	Manufacturer	Lot number	Route/Site	No. Previous Doses
a.	_____	_____	_____	_____	_____
b.	_____	_____	_____	_____	_____
c.	_____	_____	_____	_____	_____
d.	_____	_____	_____	_____	_____

14. Any other vaccinations within 4 weeks prior to the date listed in no. 10

	Vaccine (type)	Manufacturer	Lot number	Route/Site	No. Previous doses	Date given
a.	_____	_____	_____	_____	_____	_____
b.	_____	_____	_____	_____	_____	_____

15. Vaccinated at:	16. Vaccine purchased with:	17. Other medications
☐ Private doctor's office/hospital ☐ Military clinic/hospital	☐ Private funds ☐ Military funds	
☐ Public health clinic/hospital ☐ Other/unknown	☐ Public funds ☐ Other/unknown	

18. Illness at time of vaccination (specify)	19. Pre-existing physician-diagnosed allergies, birth defects, medical conditions (specify)

20. Have you reported this adverse event previously?	☐ NO ☐ To health department ☐ To doctor ☐ To manufacturer	Only for children 5 and under

22. Birth weight _____ lb. _____ oz.	23. No. of brothers and sisters

21. Adverse event following prior vaccination (check all applicable, specify)

	Adverse Event	Onset Age	Type Vaccine	Dose no. in series
☐ In patient	_____	_____	_____	_____
☐ In brother or sister	_____	_____	_____	_____

Only for reports submitted by manufacturer/immunization project

24. Mfr./ imm. proj. report no.	25. Date received by Mfr./imm. proj.
26. 15 day report? ☐ Yes ☐ No	27. Report type ☐ Initial ☐ Follow-Up

Health care providers and manufacturers are required by law (42 USC 300ss-25) to report reactions to vaccines listed in the Table of Reportable Events Following Immunization. Reports for reactions to other vaccines are voluntary except when required as a condition of immunization grant awards.

Form VAERS-1(poa)

Guide to Contraindications and Precautions to Commonly Used Vaccines* (Page 1 of 2)

Vaccine	Contraindications	Precautions[1]
Hepatitis B (HepB)	• Severe allergic reaction (e.g., anaphylaxis) after a previous vaccine dose or to a vaccine component	• Moderate or severe acute illness with or without fever • Infant weighing less than 2000 grams (4 lbs, 6.4 oz)[2]
Rotavirus (RV5 [RotaTeq], RV1 [Rotarix])	• Severe allergic reaction (e.g., anaphylaxis) after a previous vaccine dose or to a vaccine component	• Moderate or severe acute illness with or without fever • Immunosuppression • Pre-existing chronic gastrointestinal disease • Previous history of intussusception
Diphtheria, tetanus, pertussis (DTaP) **Tetanus, diphtheria, pertussis (Tdap)**	• Severe allergic reaction (e.g., anaphylaxis) after a previous vaccine dose or to a vaccine component • Encephalopathy (e.g., coma, decreased level of consciousness, prolonged seizures) not attributable to another identifiable cause within 7 days of administration of previous dose of DTP or DTaP	• Moderate or severe acute illness with or without fever • Guillain-Barré syndrome (GBS) within 6 weeks after a previous dose of tetanus toxoid-containing vaccine • History of Arthus-type hypersensitivity reaction following a previous dose of tetanus and/or diphtheria toxoid-containing vaccine: defer vaccination until at least 10 years have elapsed since the previous dose • Progressive or unstable neurologic disorder, uncontrolled seizures or progressive encephalopathy: defer vaccination with DTaP or Tdap until a treatment regimen has been established and the condition has stabilized For DTaP only: • Temperature of 105° F or higher (40.5° C or higher) within 48 hours after vaccination with a previous dose of DTP/DTaP • Collapse or shock-like state (i.e., hypotonic hyporesponsive episode) within 48 hours after receiving a previous dose of DTP/DTaP • Seizure or convulsion within 3 days after receiving a previous dose of DTP/DTaP • Persistent, inconsolable crying lasting 3 or more hours within 48 hours after receiving a previous dose of DTP/DTaP
Tetanus, diphtheria (DT, Td)	• Severe allergic reaction (e.g., anaphylaxis) after a previous vaccine dose or to a vaccine component	• Moderate or severe acute illness with or without fever • GBS within 6 weeks after a previous dose of tetanus toxoid-containing vaccine • History of Arthus-type hypersensitivity reactions following a previous dose of tetanus and/or diphtheria toxoid-containing vaccine: defer vaccination until at least 10 years have elapsed since the previous dose For Td only: In adults, unstable neurologic condition; in teens, progressive neurologic disorder
***Haemophilus influenzae* type b (Hib)**	• Severe allergic reaction (e.g., anaphylaxis) after a previous vaccine dose or to a vaccine component • Age younger than 6 weeks	• Moderate or severe acute illness with or without fever
Inactivated poliovirus vaccine (IPV)	• Severe allergic reaction (e.g., anaphylaxis) after a previous vaccine dose or to a vaccine component	• Moderate or severe acute illness with or without fever • Pregnancy
Pneumococcal (PCV or PPSV)	• Severe allergic reaction (e.g., anaphylaxis) after a previous vaccine dose or to a vaccine component	• Moderate or severe acute illness with or without fever
Hepatitis A (HepA)	• Severe allergic reaction (e.g., anaphylaxis) after a previous vaccine dose or to a vaccine component	• Moderate or severe acute illness with or without fever • Pregnancy
Measles, mumps, rubella (MMR)[3]	• Severe allergic reaction (e.g., anaphylaxis) after a previous vaccine dose or to a vaccine component • Pregnancy • Known severe immunodeficiency (e.g., hematologic and solid tumors; receiving chemotherapy; congenital immunodeficiency; long-term immunosuppressive therapy[4]; or patients with HIV infection who are severely immunocompromised)	• Moderate or severe acute illness with or without fever • Recent (within 11 months) receipt of antibody-containing blood product (specific interval depends on product)[5] • History of thrombocytopenia or thrombocytopenic purpura

Technical content reviewed by the Centers for Disease Control and Prevention, February 2010.   www.immunize.org/catg.d/p3072a.pdf • Item #P3072a (2/10)

Immunization Action Coalition • 1573 Selby Ave. • St. Paul, MN 55104 • (651) 647-9009 • www.immunize.org • www.vaccineinformation.org

(continued)

833

Vaccine	Contraindications	Precautions[1]
Varicella (Var)[3]	• Severe allergic reaction (e.g., anaphylaxis) after a previous vaccine dose or to a vaccine component • Substantial suppression of cellular immunity[5] • Pregnancy	• Moderate or severe acute illness with or without fever • Recent (within 11 months) receipt of antibody-containing blood product (specific interval depends on product)[5] • Receipt of specific antivirals (i.e., acyclovir, famciclovir, or valacyclovir) 24 hours before vaccination, if possible; delay resumption of these antiviral drugs for 14 days after vaccination.
Influenza, injectable trivalent (TIV)	• Severe allergic reaction (e.g., anaphylaxis) after a previous vaccine dose or to a vaccine component, including egg protein	• Moderate or severe acute illness with or without fever • History of GBS within 6 weeks of previous influenza vaccine
Influenza, live attenuated (LAIV)[3]	• Severe allergic reaction (e.g., anaphylaxis) after a previous vaccine dose or to a vaccine component, including egg protein • Possible reactive airways disease in a child age 2 through 4 years (e.g., history of recurrent wheezing or a recent wheezing episode) • Pregnancy • Known severe immunodeficiency (e.g., hematologic and solid tumors; receiving chemotherapy; congenital immunodeficiency; long-term immunosuppressive therapy[4]; or patients with HIV infection who are severely immunocompromised) • Certain chronic medical conditions[6]	• Moderate or severe acute illness with or without fever • History of GBS within 6 weeks of previous influenza vaccine • Receipt of specific antivirals (i.e., amantadine, rimantadine, zanamivir, or oseltamivir) 48 hours before vaccination. Avoid use of these antiviral drugs for 14 days after vaccination. • Close contact with an immunosuppressed person when the person requires protective isolation
Human papilloma-virus (HPV)	• Severe allergic reaction (e.g., anaphylaxis) after a previous vaccine dose or to a vaccine component	• Moderate or severe acute illness with or without fever • Pregnancy
Meningococcal, conjugate (MCV4) **Meningococcal, poly-saccharide (MPSV4)**	• Severe allergic reaction (e.g., anaphylaxis) after a previous vaccine dose or to a vaccine component	• Moderate or severe acute illness with or without fever For MCV4 only: • History of GBS (if not at extremely high risk for meningococcal disease)
Zoster (Zos)	• Severe allergic reaction (e.g., anaphylaxis) after a previous vaccine dose or to a vaccine component • Substantial suppression of cellular immunity[5] • Pregnancy	• Moderate or severe acute illness with or without fever • Receipt of specific antivirals (i.e., acyclovir, famciclovir, or valacyclovir) 24 hours before vaccination, if possible; delay resumption of these antiviral drugs for 14 days after vaccination.

Footnotes

1. Events or conditions listed as precautions should be reviewed carefully. Benefits of and risks for administering a specific vaccine to a person under these circumstances should be considered. If the risk from the vaccine is believed to outweigh the benefit, the vaccine should not be administered. If the benefit of vaccination is believed to outweigh the risk, the vaccine should be administered. Whether and when to administer DTaP to children with proven or suspected underlying neurologic disorders should be decided on a case-by-case basis.

2. Hepatitis B vaccination should be deferred for preterm infants and infants weighing less than 2000 g if the mother is documented to be hepatitis B surface antigen (HBsAg)-negative at the time of the infant's birth. Vaccination can commence at chronological age 1 month. For infants born to women who are HBsAg-positive, hepatitis B immunoglobulin and hepatitis B vaccine should be administered at or soon after birth, regardless of weight.

3. LAIV, MMR, and varicella vaccines can be administered on the same day. If not administered on the same day, these vaccines should be separated by at least 28 days.

4. Substantially immunosuppressive steroid dose is considered to be 2 weeks or more of daily receipt of 20 mg or more (or 2 mg/kg body weight or more) of prednisone or equivalent.

5. For details, see CDC. "General Recommendations on Immunization: Recommendations of the Advisory Committee on Immunization Practices (ACIP)" at www.cdc.gov/vaccines/pubs/acip-list.htm.

6. For details, see CDC. "Prevention and Control of Influenza: Recommendations of the Advisory Committee on Immunization Practices (ACIP)" at www.cdc.gov/vaccines/pubs/acip-list.htm.

*Adapted from "Table 5. Contraindications and Precautions to Commonly Used Vaccines" found in: CDC. "General Recommendations on Immunization: Recommendations of the Advisory Committee on Immunization Practices (ACIP)." *MMWR* 2006; 55(No. RR-15), p. 10–14.

FIGURE 51–5   Guide to Contraindications and Precautions to Commonly Used Vaccines.

Standards for Pediatric Immunization Practices

Standard 1. Immunization services are readily available.

Standard 2. No barriers or unnecessary prerequisites to the receipt of vaccines exist.

Standard 3. Immunization services are available free or for a minimal fee.

Standard 4. Providers use all clinical encounters to screen and, when indicated, immunize children.

Standard 5. Providers educate parents and guardians about immunization in general terms.

Standard 6. Providers question parents or guardians about contraindications and, before immunizing a child, inform them in specific terms about the risks and benefits of the immunizations their child is to receive.

Standard 7. Providers follow only true contraindications.

Standard 8. Providers administer simultaneously all vaccine doses for which a child is eligible at the time of each visit.

Standard 9. Providers use accurate and complete recording procedures.

Standard 10. Providers co-schedule immunization appointments in conjunction with appointments for other child health services.

Standard 11. Providers report adverse events after immunization promptly, accurately, and completely.

Standard 12. Providers operate a tracking system.

Standard 13. Providers adhere to appropriate procedures for vaccine management.

Standard 14. Providers conduct semiannual audits to assess immunization coverage levels and to review immunization records in the patient populations they serve.

Standard 15. Providers maintain up-to-date, easily retrievable medical protocols at all locations where vaccines are administered.

Standard 16. Providers operate with patient-oriented and community-based approaches.

Standard 17. Vaccines are administered by properly trained individuals.

Standard 18. Providers receive ongoing education and training on current immunization recommendations.

From Centers for Disease Control and Prevention. (1993). Standard for pediatric immunization practices: Recommended by National Vaccine Advisory Committee (ACIP). *Morbidity and Mortality Weekly Report, 42* (RR-5), 1–13.

Immunization Schedule Tips

Restarting Vaccine Series

With the exception of oral typhoid vaccine, it never is necessary to restart a vaccine series because the interval has been prolonged—although every effort should be made to adhere to the recommended schedule.

Vaccines Given Too Soon

These will not be accepted at school entry and revaccination will be recommended.

Lack of Written Vaccination Record

An attempt should be made to verify vaccination status. If no record can be verified, the child should be considered unimmunized and should be revaccinated as appropriate for age.

Hepatitis B

In the case of an *interrupted* or *incomplete* series, resume the series; do not repeat or restart. Dose should be appropriate in accord with the manufacturer's instructions. The *third dose* should be given at least 2 mo after the second dose and at least 4 mo after the first dose, but not before 6 mo of age.

PPD/MMR

PPD can be done before or at the same time as the measles vaccine is administered. Give PPD 4 to 6 wk after measles vaccine, if measles is given first, because measles can reduce the reactivity of PPD. This reduction in reactivity is due to mild suppression of cell-mediated immunity, which can lead to false-negative test results.

DtaP

The fourth dose can be given if a child is ≥12 mo of age and 6 mo have elapsed since DTaP dose 3 (especially if the child is unlikely to return at 15 to 18 mo of age). The fifth dose should be given at 4 to 6 y. Children should not receive more than six doses of diphtheria or tetanus-containing toxoid before their seventh birthday. No pertussis-containing vaccines are licensed for use in people ≥7 y of age.

HIB

No HIB vaccine should be given to infants younger than 6 wk of age and is not recommended after age 5 y. Minimum age for last HIB is 12 mo, if at least 2 mo have passed since the previous dose. DTaP/HIB combination products should not be used for primary series (2, 4, 6 mo of age).

Varicella

Dosage for people 12 mo and older: Single 0.5-mL dose subcutaneously suffices for protection 12 mo to 12 y. People 13 y of age and older should receive two 0.5-mL doses at least 4 wk apart.

BOX **51.6**

Questions and Answers About Immunization

Q. How long should the vaccination needle be?

A. Subcutaneous injections for children and adults: ⅝ to ¾ in., 23- to 25-gauge needle.

Intramuscular injections for infants and children: minimum needle length of ⅞ in. for anterolateral thigh and minimum of ⅝ in. for deltoid injection; for adults: 1 to 1½ in. needle (Humiston & Atkinson, 1998).

Q. What are the immunization recommendations for children of parents or household residents who were never vaccinated for polio?

A. If the unvaccinated or inadequately vaccinated person resides in the household, an all-IVP schedule is recommended for the child. Parents and household contacts may receive IVP too.

Q. Which HIB vaccines are the best?

A. Different manufacturers' products are considered interchangeable for the primary series and the booster. However, no HIB vaccine is recommended for infants younger than 6 wk of age. If it is given, it may make the child incapable of responding to subsequent doses.

Q. Are there special recommendations if someone in the family or household has an immune system problem?

A. Yes. The person receiving a polio vaccine should receive only IPV (not OPV because the virus is shed in the stool for up to 6 wk). Other live vaccines and all inactivated vaccines may be given as usual.

Q. What are some special concerns related to pregnancy?

A. There are no contraindications to immunization of a household member if another household member is pregnant. However, if a woman in the household wants to become pregnant and also wants to be vaccinated, she should wait to become pregnant at least 1 mo after receiving mumps, measles, varicella and 3 mo after receiving rubella.

Q. What happens if someone has an extra vaccination?

A. Extra doses of live vaccine do not appear to have adverse consequences and they may boost immunity. Extra doses of inactivated vaccines can induce very high antibody titers. If these people are revaccinated, large local inflammatory reactions may ensue.

Q. Is it harmful to receive vaccines simultaneously?

A. No evidence exists that simultaneous administration of vaccines reduces vaccine effectiveness or increases adverse events.

Q. What are the implications of an error, such as previous administration of a vaccine at the wrong site, in a wrong dose, by a wrong route?

A. Unfortunately, they do not count. Only full doses in acceptable sites should be counted. Revaccinate according to age. The exception to the rule is live vaccines (MMR, varicella), which are recommended to be administered subcutaneously—intramuscular administration of these vaccines is not likely to decrease immunogenicity. *Note:* Reducing or dividing doses of any vaccine including those to preterm or low-birth-weight infants is not indicated.

Q. What is the recommended way to administer multiple injections to infants?

A. The recommended approach is to place the vaccine most likely to cause a local adverse reaction (e.g., DTaP) in one leg and the two less reactive in different sites in the other leg.

Q. How effective is the varicella vaccine?

A. Effectiveness is 70% to 90% protection against infection with 95% protection against severe disease. Protection persists at least 7 to 10 y. The risk of transmission appears low but somewhat higher if the vaccinee develops a varicella-like rash after vaccination. Recommend that vaccinees avoid contact with immunocompromised people when the rash is present.

Q. Why is the MMR vaccine given twice?

A. The second dose is given because 2% to 5% of people do not develop immunity after the first dose, and 95% of the people who did not respond to the first dose respond to the second.

Note: Birth before 1957 is generally considered evidence of rubella immunity; laboratory evidence of immunity is recommended. Combined MMR vaccine is the drug of choice if vaccination is needed.

Q. What is the standard dosing schedule for hepatitis B vaccine?

A. There is no standard dose. That is why it is so important to read the package insert for hepatitis B vaccine carefully. The formulations vary and the appropriate microgram dose must be selected.

Q. What should be done if the patient spits out the dose of OPV?

A. There is no definite rule regarding how much can be spit out before repeating the dose. If in the judgment of the person administering the vaccine a substantial amount was spit out, regurgitated, or vomited, another dose can be administered within 5 to 10 min at the same visit. If the repeated dose is not retained, neither dose should be counted. OPV should be readministered at the next visit (Humiston & Atkinson, 1998).

Vaccines should be stored in the office in sufficient amounts to meet the needs of the patients. Staff should have specific assignments to monitor stock levels, lot numbers, and expiration dates. Vaccines should be stored according to the manufacturer's recommendations with a back-up system to identify times when power outages may have affected vaccines, particularly during nonbusiness hours. Methods can range from plugging in a digital clock in the same outlet to use of alarm systems on the freezer or refrigerator. An inexpensive method of detecting a power outage uses a cup of ice with a penny or other coin placed on top of the ice. The length of a power outage may be judged by how far the coin sinks in the previously completely frozen ice. If power outages occur, the pharmaceutical manufacturer should be contacted for information about vaccine use, revised expiration dates, or unusable vaccine. Staff members should not automatically assume that vaccine should be discarded.

A central log book, maintained by date and time and including lot numbers and expiration dates of the vaccines, is recommended. Used with patient schedule information and chart documentation, the log book helps identify patients should a pharmaceutical company notify the office of a vaccine recall or a need to reimmunize patients receiving a specific lot of vaccine.

In addition, practice decisions need to be made regarding immunization screening processes to be used for all populations. A focus on adolescent and adult populations as well as infants and children is critical. Current recommendations include routine screening at ages 11, 12, and 50. An interim process for high-risk people in combination with aforementioned recommended screenings provides the best mechanism for implementing a comprehensive immunization program.

Several Web sites provide vaccine information: www.aap.org, www.cdc.gov/nip, www.cdc.gov/nvpo, www.immunizationinfo.org.

Case Study 1

J. V. is a 45-year-old woman, married with no children. She presents on October 10 for a follow-up visit for type 2 diabetes mellitus diagnosed 2 months ago. Her history is significant for the following:

- Type 2 diabetes mellitus controlled with diet and exercise
- Recent graduation from a physical therapy program and working in a pediatric hospital
- Immunization status: routine childhood immunizations received with the exception of varicella and hepatitis B. She does not recall having chickenpox. Her last tetanus shot was 11 years ago.

1. In assessing and treating J. V., what is your plan to update her immunizations?
2. What factors would you consider most important and why?
3. Which vaccines would be a priority and why?

Case Study 2

L. L. is a 10-month-old Hispanic boy who presents in November for the first time. He has not had any contact with the health care system since he was 2 months old. He lives in a house with seven people and poor sanitation. The only immunizations that he has had are hepatitis B (two shots), one HIB, one DTaP, one IPV, and one Prevnar.

1. What immunizations would you administer at this visit?
2. When would you schedule his next visit and what immunizations would you give at that visit?

BIBLIOGRAPHY

*Starred references are cited in the text.

American Academy of Pediatrics, Committee on Infectious Diseases. (1999). Poliomyelitis prevention: Revised recommendations for use of inactivated and live oral poliovirus vaccines. *Pediatrics, 103,* 171–172.

Centers for Disease Control and Prevention. (2009). National, state and local area vaccination coverage among adolescents aged 13-17 years—United States, 2009. *Morbidity and Mortality Weekly Report, 59*(32), 1018–1023.

*Centers for Disease Control and Prevention. (2010a). http://www.cdc.gov/vaccines/recs/schedule/child-schedule.htm, accessed September 17, 2010.

*Centers for Disease Control and Prevention. (2010b). http://www.cdc.gov/vaccines/recs/schedule/adult-schedule.htm, accessed September 17, 2010.

*Centers for Disease Control and Prevention. (2010c). http://cdc.gov/vaccines/recs/vac-admin/contraindications-vacc.htm, accessed September 17, 2010.

Centers for Disease Control and Prevention. (2010d). FDA licensure of bivalent human papillomavirus vaccine (HPV2, Cervarix) for use in females and updated HPV vaccination recommendations from the Advisory Committee on Immunization Practices (ACIP). *Morbidity and Mortality Weekly Report, 59*(20), 626–629.

Centers for Disease Control and Prevention. (2010e). Prevention and control of influenza with vaccines: Recommendations of the Advisory Committee on Immunization Practices (ACIP). *Morbidity and Mortality Weekly Report, 59*(RR-08), 1–62.

Centers for Disease Control and Prevention. (2010f). Updated recommendations for prevention of invasive pneumoccal disease among adults using the 23-valent pneumococcal polysaccharide vaccine. *Morbidity and Mortality Weekly Report, 59*(34), 1102–1106.

Cox, T., Mahoney, M., Saslow, D., & Mosicki, A. (2008). ACS releases guidelines for the HPV vaccine. *American Family Physician, 77*(6), 852–863.

Dempsey, A. & Freed, G. (2008). Human papilloma virus vaccine: Expected impacts and unresolved issues. *Journal of Pediatrics, 152*(3), 305–309.

Haber, G., Malow, R., & Zemet, G. (2007). The HPV vaccine mandate controversy. *Journal of Pediatric and Adolescent Gynecology, 20*(6), 325–331. http://www.pediatrics.org/cgi/content/full/127/2/387, accessed October 4, 2011.

Humiston, S., Atkinson, W. (1998). 1998 immunization schedule changes and clarifications. *Pediatric Annals, 27*(6), 338–348.

*Pickering, L., Baker, C., Kimberlin, D., & Long, S. (Eds.). (2009). *The 2009 red book: Report of the Committee on Infectious Diseases* (26th ed.). Elk Grove Village, IL: American Academy of Pediatrics.

Poland, G., & Johnson, D. (2008). Increasing influenza vaccination rates: The need to vaccinate throughout the entire influenza season. *American Journal of Medicine, 121*(7, Suppl. 2), S3–S10.

Trimble, C., & Frazer, I. (2009). Development of therapeutic HPV vaccines. *The Lancet Oncology, 10*(10), 975–980.

Smoking Cessation

Cigarette smoking is a chronic condition. Like sufferers of other chronic conditions, many cigarette smokers cycle through periods of remission (i.e., periods of abstinence from cigarette use) and relapse (i.e., periods of active cigarette use). Similar to other chronic conditions, cigarette smoking contributes to morbidity and mortality, and it is the leading cause of preventable morbidity and mortality in the United States (Centers for Disease Control and Prevention [CDC], 2008c).

The CDC estimates that in the United States, cigarette smoking and second-hand exposure to cigarette smoke results in at least 443,000 premature deaths annually: approximately 269,000 among American men and 174,000 among American women. Lung cancer, ischemic heart disease, and chronic obstructive pulmonary disease (COPD) are the three leading causes of smoking-related deaths (CDC, 2008c).

Smoking accounts for at least 30% of all cancer deaths and nearly 90% of all lung cancer deaths. Smoking also increases the risk of cancer of the nasopharyngeal tract, esophagus, stomach, pancreas, bladder, and cervix and acute myeloid leukemia (American Cancer Society, 2010).

In addition to the variety of cancers, smoking is a major risk factor for cardiovascular diseases, such as ischemic heart disease and aortic aneurysm, cerebrovascular disease, and peripheral arterial disease. It is estimated that each year as many as 30% of all deaths related to ischemic heart disease in the United States may be attributable to cigarette smoking and that smoking doubles the risk of ischemic stroke (Ockene & Houston, 1997). Furthermore, smoking increases the risk of acute respiratory infections. It is also a major risk factor for the development of COPD and is estimated to account for at least 75% of COPD-related deaths (CDC, 2008b).

In the United States, the total economic burden of smoking is estimated to be $193 billion annually, with costs for medical expenditures for care of smoking-related illnesses of approximately $96 billion and costs related to lost earnings and loss of productivity of approximately $97 billion (CDC, 2008c).

An estimated 43.4 million adults in the United States smoke cigarettes (CDC, 2008a). According to the CDC (2008c), more men than women in the United States smoke (22.3% of adult males compared to 17.5% of adult females). Among racial and ethnic populations in the United States, Asians have the lowest rates of cigarette use (9.6%), while American Indians/Alaska natives had the highest rates (36.4%) (CDC, 2008a). Smoking rates vary by age group as well, with the lowest rates among those older than age 65 (8.3%) and higher rates among those younger than age 65 (21% to 23%) (CDC, 2008a). Current smoking among U.S. high school students is estimated to be 19.5% in 2009, down from as high as 36.4% in 1997 (CDC, 2010). It has been estimated that every day, approximately 4,000 children and adolescents smoke their first cigarette, and every day 1,200 children and adolescents become daily smokers (Fiore, et al., 2008). Although 70% of smokers report that they would like to quit, only 47% are likely to be successful; however, many who attempt to quit smoking do not use recommended cessation methods and most relapse within the first week of quitting (CDC, 2008c; Fiore, et al., 2008). The U.S. Department of Health and Human Services/Public Health Service guidelines (DHHS/PHS) recommend that all health care professionals, including physicians, pharmacists, nurses, and others, ask about and document their patients' smoking status (Fiore, et al., 2008). The 2008 DHHS/PHS guidelines urge clinicians to treat tobacco use disorder as a chronic disease similar in many respects to other diseases such as hypertension, diabetes mellitus, and hyperlipidemia and to provide patients with appropriate advice and pharmacotherapy (Fiore, et al., 2008).

PATHOPHYSIOLOGY

Nicotine is the addictive substance in cigarette smoke. It is absorbed and distributed to most tissues of the body, where it binds with nicotinic receptors and produces its physiologic effects on the heart, brain, and other organ systems. Nicotine is a ganglionic cholinergic receptor agonist whose pharmacologic effects are highly dose dependent. These effects include central and peripheral nervous system stimulation and depression, respiratory stimulation, skeletal muscle relaxation, epinephrine release by the adrenal medulla, peripheral vasoconstriction, and increased blood pressure, heart rate, carbon monoxide, and oxygen consumption (Doering, et al., 2007). In addition, nicotine increases dopamine levels in the central nervous system, thus stimulating the rewards system and reinforcement of its use (O'Brien, 2006). Activation of nicotine receptors in the brain produces relaxation, decreases stress and anxiety, and improves concentration and reaction times (Benowitz, 2010). Cessation of smoking leads to depressed mood, irritability, difficulty concentrating, and anxiety. Smokers use nicotine to experience the rewarding effects and to avoid the unpleasant effects of nicotine withdrawal.

A common endocrine and metabolic effect of nicotine is weight loss. Smokers tend to weigh 2.4 to 4.5 kg less than non-smokers (Molarius, et al., 1997). Additional endocrine effects include increased risk of osteoporosis and earlier menopause (Benowitz, 2008). Finally, smoking alters the liver's metabolic effects by inducing hepatic (cytochrome P450) enzymes. These effects on hepatic enzymes result in the increased metabolism of certain medications, such as theophylline and acetaminophen, and substances such as caffeine.

DIAGNOSTIC CRITERIA

Chronic nicotine ingestion may lead to physical and physiologic dependence and tolerance to some of its pharmacologic effects. Nicotine dependence disorder has been defined as a form of substance abuse that can lead to clinically important impairment of distress (American Psychiatric Association [APA], 2000). The key features required for the diagnosis of nicotine dependence are continued use despite wanting to quit, prior attempts at quitting, persistent use in the face of physical illness, tolerance, and presence of withdrawal symptoms (APA, 2000). **Box 52.1** highlights the APA criteria for nicotine dependence (and withdrawal). Another clinical assessment tool for nicotine dependence is the Fagerstrom Test for Nicotine Dependence, which assesses a patient's level of nicotine dependence in part by determining the time to first cigarette of the day (Heatherton, et al., 1991). Nicotine has a relatively short half-life, and nicotine-dependent smokers may experience significant discomfort on waking unless they quickly have their first cigarette (Mallin, 2002). The number of cigarettes smoked per day and the time to first cigarette both have been shown to correlate with the degree of nicotine dependence. Therefore, the use of the Fagerstrom test is recommended (**Box 52.2**), in addition to the APA criteria for diagnosis of nicotine dependence among smokers.

BOX **52.1**

APA Criteria for Dependence and Withdrawal

Dependence

Nicotine dependence is a maladaptive pattern of substance use, leading to clinically important impairment or distress, as manifested by three or more of the following at any time in a 12-month period:

1. Tolerance occurs, as defined by either of the following: a need for markedly increased amounts of the substance to achieve intoxication or the desired effect, or a markedly diminished effect with continued use of the same amount of the substance.
2. Withdrawal occurs, as manifested by either of the following: the characteristic withdrawal syndrome for the substance, or the taking of the same (or a closely related) substance to relieve or avoid withdrawal symptoms.
3. The substance is often taken in larger amounts or for a longer period than was intended.
4. There is a persistent desire or unsuccessful efforts to cut down or control substance abuse.
5. A great deal of time is spent in activities necessary to obtain the substance (e.g., visiting multiple doctors or driving long distances), use the substance (e.g., chain smoking), or recover from its effects.
6. Important social, occupational, or recreational activities are given up or reduced because of substance abuse.
7. The substance use is continued despite the knowledge that there is a persistent or recurrent physical or psychological problem likely to have been caused or exacerbated by the substance (e.g., current cocaine use despite the recognition of cocaine-induced depression, or continued drinking despite the recognition that an ulcer was made worse by alcohol consumption).

Withdrawal

Withdrawal symptoms may be initiated and characterized by the following:

1. Daily use of nicotine for at least several weeks.
2. Abrupt cessation of nicotine use, or reduction in the amount of nicotine used, followed within 24 h by four or more of the following:
   a. Dysphoric or depressed mood
   b. Insomnia
   c. Irritability, frustration, or anger
   d. Anxiety
   e. Difficulty concentrating
   f. Restlessness
   g. Decreased heart rate
   h. Increased appetite or weight gain
3. The symptoms cause clinically significant distress or impairment in social, occupational, or other important areas of functioning.
4. The symptoms are not due to a general medical condition and are not better accounted for by another mental disorder.

Reprinted with permission from the *Diagnostic and Statistical Manual of Mental Disorders,* Fourth Edition, Text Revision (Copyright 2000, American Psychiatric Association).

BOX 52.2

Fagerstrom Tolerance Test for Nicotine Dependence

Write the number of the answer that is most applicable on the line to the left of the question.

_____ 1. How soon after you awake do you smoke your first cigarette?
   0. After 30 min
   1. Within 30 min

_____ 2. Do you find it difficult to refrain from smoking in places where it is forbidden such as the library, theater, or doctor's office?
   0. No
   1. Yes

_____ 3. Which of all the cigarettes you smoke in a day is the most satisfying?
   0. Any other than the first one in the morning
   1. The first one in the morning

_____ 4. How many cigarettes a day do you smoke?
   0. 1–15
   1. 16–25
   2. >26

_____ 5. Do you smoke more during the morning than during the rest of the day?
   0. No
   1. Yes

_____ 6. Do you smoke when you are so ill that you are in bed most of the day?
   0. No
   1. Yes

_____ 7. Does the brand you smoke have low, medium, or high nicotine content?
   0. Low
   1. Medium
   2. High

_____ 8. How often do you inhale the smoke from your cigarette?
   0. Never
   1. Sometimes
   2. Always

Scoring Instructions: Add up your responses to all the items. Total scores should range from 0 to 11, where 7 or greater suggests physical dependence to nicotine.
TOTAL SCORE: _____

Reprinted with permission from Heatherton, T. F., Kozlowski, L. T., Frecker, R. C., et al. (1991). The Fagerstrom Test for Nicotine Dependence: A revision of the Fagerstrom Tolerance Questionnaire. _British Journal of Addictions, 86_(9), 1119–1127.

Patients who are addicted to nicotine may experience withdrawal symptoms. Onset of these symptoms usually occurs within 24 hours and may last for days or weeks or longer (Henningfield, et al., 2009). Nicotine withdrawal is associated with a well-described syndrome characterized by irritability, awakening from sleep, anxiety, impaired concentration, impaired reaction time, restlessness, drowsiness, confusion, increased appetite, and weight gain (Shiffman, et al., 2004; Henningfield, et al., 2009). Tobacco status should be asked about and documented for all patients at every visit. The DHHS/PHS expert panel recommends that tobacco use status be adopted as a new vital sign to be assessed along with blood pressure, temperature, pulse, and respiration rates (Fiore, et al., 2008).

INITIATING DRUG THERAPY

The DHHS/PHS guidelines recommend that all clinicians aggressively motivate and assist their smoking patients to quit (Fiore, et al., 2008). The expert panel's analysis of various studies and trials have found that a wide variety of clinicians can effectively implement these strategies and such interventions as brief as 3 minutes can increase the cessation rate significantly (Fiore, et al., 2008). Such interventions should be made by clinicians in patients unwilling to attempt to quit at the time of inquiry because such interventions increase motivation and the likelihood of future attempts (Fiore, et al., 2008). The panel reminds clinicians that effective treatment of tobacco dependence now exists and that every patient should receive at least minimal treatment every time he or she visits a clinician. The first step in this process, identification and assessment of tobacco use status, separates patients into three treatment categories:

1. Patients who use tobacco and are willing to quit should be treated using the 5 As: Ask, Advise, Assess, Assist, and Arrange (**Box 52.3**).
2. Patients who use tobacco but are unwilling to quit at the time of inquiry should be treated with the 5 Rs of motivational interventions: Relevance, Risks, Rewards, Roadblocks, and Repetition (**Box 52.4**).
3. Patients who have quit using tobacco recently should be provided relapse-prevention treatment. Clinicians should reinforce the patient's decision to quit, review the benefits of quitting, and assist the patient in resolving any residual problems arising from quitting (Fiore, et al., 2008).

Once the diagnosis of nicotine dependence is made, the next step is to assess the patient's readiness to change (Mallin, 2002). The five-step transtheoretical stages of change (SOC) model is useful for assessing the patient's readiness to quit. The SOC model identifies smoking behavior change as a process involving movement through a series of five motivational stages (Mallin, 2002):

- Stage 1—Precontemplation: the patient has no intention to quit.
- Stage 2—Contemplation: a smoker is interested in quitting but has no definite plans.

BOX **52.3**

The "5 As" Model for Treating Tobacco Use and Dependence

Ask every patient about tobacco use and record information in patient's medical record at every visit.

↓

Strongly ***advise*** every tobacco user to quit, using a personalized approach.

↓

Assess the patient's willingness to make an attempt to quit.

↓

Assist the patient who is willing to make an attempt to quit by offering medication and providing or referring for smoking cessation counseling.

↓

Arrange for follow-up contact within the first week after the quit date. For patients unwilling to make a quit attempt, address willingness to quit at next visit.

U.S. Department of Health and Human Services, Public Health Service, Agency for Health Care Policy and Research. (2008). *Treating tobacco use and dependence: 2008 update.* Rockville, MD: Author.

- Stage 3—Preparation: the smoker in this stage is planning to quit within the next month and has made a failed attempt to quit during the previous year.
- Stage 4—Action: the smoker makes a serious effort to quit by modifying his or her behavior and environment. During this stage, the patient has abstained anywhere from 1 day to 6 months. After 6 months of abstinence, the patient enters the final stage.
- Stage 5—Maintenance.

The first step in any cessation program should be to target a quit date with the patient. This date should be identified; otherwise the patient may never actually make the attempt to stop smoking. In addition, picking a definite date provides the patient with an obtainable goal and avoids overwhelming the patient with the thought of having to change an entire lifestyle.

Nonpharmacologic approaches to smoking cessation consist of various individual and group behavioral interventions, including self-management, group counseling and support, nicotine fading, and aversion techniques (APA, 1996). Behavioral therapy is based on the theory that learning processes operate in the development, maintenance, and cessation of smoking (APA, 1996). The core feature of behavioral therapies is to educate the patient about the benefits of smoking cessation. When used alone, these interventions have low success rates because

they do not satiate cravings or prevent withdrawal symptoms. However, patients who are highly motivated or who smoke only a few cigarettes a day may benefit the most from these approaches. The APA recommends using multicomponent behavioral therapy as first-line treatment (APA, 1996).

Self-Management

Self-management techniques are commonly used to make patients more aware of their smoking habits and cues. By becoming more familiar with the environment and events that precede smoking a cigarette, patients may be able to interrupt these patterns by avoiding certain situations. If a relapse occurs, the patient should determine what may have triggered the failed attempt and eliminate those factors. Some nondrug methods to enhance smoking cessation and prevent relapse include getting rid of ashtrays, drinking lots of water and breathing deeply between sips, avoiding places with smoke-filled air, making a dental appointment to get teeth cleaned, exercising, calling on friends or family for support and encouragement, eating a balanced diet, chewing gum or a toothpick, and avoiding the routine that causes craving a cigarette, such as drinking coffee every morning with a cigarette (Mallin, 2002). An analysis of self-help programs showed these programs to be relatively ineffective compared to individual, group, or proactive telephone counseling.

Individual and Group Counseling and Support

The DHHS/PHS expert panel emphasized that there is a strong dose-response relationship between the intensity of tobacco dependence counseling and its effectiveness, meaning that the more intensive interventions are, the more effective they are. Person-to-person contact (via individual, group, or proactive telephone counseling) delivered across four or more sessions seems especially effective in increasing abstinence rates. Two types of counseling and behavioral therapies are recommended by the expert panel to be included in smoking cessation interventions:

1. Provision of practical counseling (problem-solving/skills training)
2. Provision of social support as part of treatment (intra-treatment social support)

Group counseling programs help to educate the patient on the risks and benefits of smoking cessation. In addition, the patient is presented with strategies to cope with and avoid situations that may lead to relapse. These programs are intended to keep the patient motivated to quit smoking.

Nicotine Fading

Nicotine fading consists of a slow decrease in the intake of nicotine. This can be accomplished by decreasing the number of puffs taken or the number of cigarettes smoked per day or by switching to a brand of cigarettes that contains less nicotine. However, the success rate of this technique is limited because

---

BOX 52.4

Tobacco Users Unwilling to Quit: The "5 Rs"

Relevance

Encourage patient to discuss why quitting is personally relevant to him or her. Motivational information has the highest impact when it is relevant to a patient's disease status or risk, family or social situation (e.g., having children in the home), health concerns, and other patient factors (e.g., prior quitting experience, personal barriers to cessation).

Risks

The clinician should ask the patient to identify potential negative consequences of tobacco use. The clinician may suggest and highlight the negative consequence that seems most relevant to the patient. The clinician also should emphasize that smoking low-tar/low-nicotine cigarettes or use of other forms of tobacco (e.g., smokeless tobacco, cigars, and pipes) will not eliminate these risks.

Rewards

The clinician should ask the patient to identify potential benefits of stopping tobacco use. The clinicians may suggest and highlight the benefits that seem most relevant to the patient. Examples of rewards include improved health; greater ability to taste food; improved sense of smell; saving money; less smoke-related odors in home, car, clothing; and feeling better physically and improved appearance (less wrinkling/aging of skin and whiter teeth).

Roadblocks

The clinician should ask the patient to identify barriers or impediments to quitting and provide treatment (e.g., problem-solving counseling, medication) that could address barriers. Typical barriers may include: withdrawal symptoms, fear of weight gain, lack of support, depression and being around other tobacco users.

Repetition

The motivational intervention should be repeated every time an unmotivated patient is encountered in a clinical setting. Tobacco users who have failed previous quit attempts should be encouraged by telling them that most people make repeated quit attempts before they are successful.

U.S. Department of Health and Human Services, Public Health Service, Agency for Health Care Policy and Research. (2008). *Treating tobacco use and dependence: 2008 update.* Rockville, MD: Author.

---

the patient can compensate by inhaling more deeply or for longer periods.

Aversion Therapy

Finally, aversion techniques have been used to make smoking less desirable to the patient. The first method, satiation, requires the patient to smoke double or triple the usual amount in a short time. In the second method, rapid smoking, the patient must inhale rapidly every 6 to 8 seconds until the cigarette is finished or the patient is nauseated. The use of these methods is limited because of possible health problems and compliance issues. Aversive smoking procedures (e.g., rapid smoking, puffing) have been shown to be more effective than providing no counseling, but this method is not recommended by the DHHS/PHS expert panel.

Other Emerging Approaches to Counseling

Recently, individually tailored materials have been researched. Tailored materials are designed to address variables specific to the smoker, such as letters mailed to patients, or web-based materials such as interactive Web sites. Some components of tailored therapy have been shown to be effective. Computerized

interventions via the use of E-health and Internet interventions have the potential to reach a larger portion of the smoking population and are inexpensive to deliver. These computer programs collect information from the smoker and use this information to provide tailored feedback and/or recommendations. However, the most effective features of computerized interventions have yet to be identified, and some Web sites may be confusing and may not tailor information to an individual patient's needs. Stepped-care interventions employ the use of low-intensity intervention with progression to more intensive interventions in treatment failures. While each of these interventions is promising, none has been adequately studied to be recommended as standard interventions at this time (Fiore, et al., 2008).

A health care professional who merely advises his or her patient to quit smoking is providing at least minimal assistance in the efforts.

Goals of Drug Therapy

All patients attempting to quit should be encouraged to use effective pharmacotherapies for smoking cessation. Long-term smoking cessation pharmacotherapy should be considered as a strategy to reduce the likelihood of relapse (Doering, et al., 2007). As with other chronic diseases, smoking cessation requires repeated intervention and multiple quit attempts (Fiore, et al., 2008). The most effective treatment of tobacco dependence requires the use of multiple modalities (Fiore, et al., 2008). According to the DHHS/PHS guidelines, clinicians should encourage all patients initiating a quit attempt to use one or a combination of efficacious pharmacotherapies, although pharmacotherapy use requires special consideration in some patient groups (i.e., those with medical contraindications, those who use smokeless tobacco products, pregnant/ breastfeeding women, and adolescent smokers; Fiore, et al., 2008). Long-term abstinence is the ultimate goal of treatment of nicotine dependence. Initial goals include moving smokers from precontemplating to contemplating quitting or taking action to quit and actually attempting to quit.

Drug therapy known as *nicotine replacement therapy* (NRT), the most commonly used pharmacotherapy for smoking cessation, aims to control nicotine levels in the bloodstream so that withdrawal does not occur while the patient is adjusting to life without cigarette smoking. The goal of therapy is to maintain the cessation of smoking for a period that allows the patient to develop preventive strategies to avoid relapse.

The primary mechanism of action by which NRT enhances smoking cessation is to obtain plasma levels of nicotine that can relieve or prevent withdrawal symptoms (Benowitz, 2008). The pharmacokinetic effects underlie the concept of nicotine replacement as an aid to smoking cessation, providing that steady-state levels of nicotine can prevent a smoker from experiencing intense withdrawal while not providing the reinforcing peaks achieved from smoking (Le Houezec, 2003). **Figure 52-1** shows the pharmacokinetic profiles of currently available NRT products. Smokers can, therefore, achieve abstinence by dealing with the various behavioral aspects of smoking. Once abstinence is achieved, the smoker can taper off the nicotine by gradual reduction (Le Houezec, 2003).

One benefit of NRT includes not exposing the smoker to the carcinogens and other toxins in cigarette smoke. NRT is approved by the U.S. Food and Drug Administration (FDA) as an aid to smoking cessation for the relief of nicotine withdrawal symptoms when used as part of a comprehensive behavioral program. The guideline panel identifies seven first-line medications (bupropion SR, nicotine gum, nicotine inhaler, nicotine nasal spray, nicotine patch, nicotine lozenge, and varenicline) (**Table 52.1**). Two second-line medications (clonidine and nortriptyline) are also identified for smoking cessation but are not approved by the FDA. The DHHS/PHS expert panel found in research studies that the abstinence rate with NRT was 1.5 to 2.3 times that of a placebo at 6 months after therapy. It is important that the patient stops smoking completely before initiating treatment, regardless of which formulation is used, as this may increase the patient's risk of nicotine toxicity and relapse. The DHHS/PHS expert panel does not endorse the use of any one NRT over another because of similar effectiveness demonstrated with all products. Patient preference will help guide the clinician's treatment decisions.

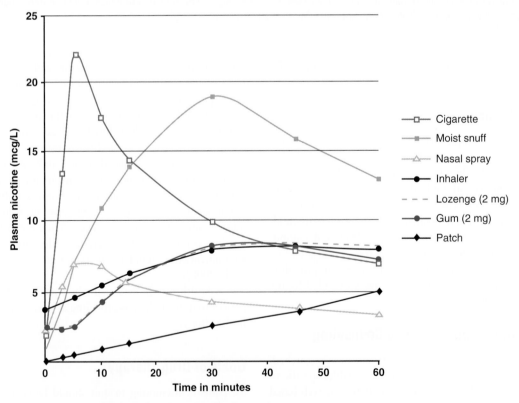

FIGURE 52–1 Pharmacokinetic profiles of nicotine replacement products.

TABLE 52.1   Overview of Selected Agents Used in Smoking Cessation

Generic (Trade) Name and Dosage	Selected Adverse Events	Contraindications	Special Considerations
Nicotine Products			
nicotine patch (various products) ≥10 cigarettes/d: 21 mg for 4 wks, then 14 mg for 2 wks, then 7 mg for 2 wks <10 cigarettes/d: 14 mg for 6 wks, then 7 mg for 2 wks	Cutaneous irritation, GI disturbances, dizziness, headaches	None noted	Patch worn for 16–24 h/d
nicotine patch (Nicoderm CQ) ≥10 cigarettes/d: 21 mg for 6 wks, then 14 mg for 2 wks, then 7 mg for 2 wks <10 cigarettes/d: 14 mg for 6 wks, then 7 mg for 2 wks	Same as above	Same as above	Same as above
nicotine polacrilex gum (Nicorette) Start: 2 mg q1–2h for 6 wks 2 mg q2–4h for 2 wks 2 mg q4–8h for 2 wks Range: 1–24 pieces/d	Sore throat, hiccups, undesirable taste,	Dentures, temporo-mandibular joint disease, dizziness	Gum should be chewed until patient feels a tingling sensation, then "parked" between cheek and gum. Repeat chewing every 15–30 min. When given as monotherapy, patient should chew at least nine pieces each day during first 6 weeks.
nicotine nasal spray (Nicotrol NS) Start: 1–2 sprays in each nasal hourly (one spray = 0.5 mg) Range: 1–40 sprays/day	Nasal irritation, sore throat, dizziness, headache	Hypersensitivity to preservatives Rhinitis, sinusitis	No more than five sprays per hour When given as monotherapy, patient should use at least eight doses each day.
nicotine inhaler (Nicotrol inhaler) Start: six cartridges per day; self-titrated to avoid withdrawal Range: 6–16 cartridges/day	Throat irritation, dizziness, headache, cough	Hypersensitivity to menthol	A minimum of six cartridges must be used for 3–6 wk. Do not use for >6 mo.
nicotine lozenge (Commit) First cigarette within 30 min of waking: 4 mg First cigarette >30 min after waking: 2 mg One lozenge every 1–2 h for first 6 wks, then one every 2–4 h for 2 wks, and one lozenge every 4–8 h for 2 wks.	Hiccups, dyspepsia, dry mouth, and irritation/soreness of the mouth	Those who continue to smoke, chew tobacco, or use other nicotine products	Lozenge should be placed in mouth and allowed to dissolve for about 20–30 min. Do not swallow or chew the lozenge. Occasionally move the lozenge from one side of the mouth to other until completely dissolved.
Non-Nicotine Products			
bupropion (Zyban) Start: 150 mg PO once daily for 3 d, then increase to 150 mg PO bid for 7–12 wk Range: 150–300 mg/d	Headache, dry mouth, insomnia	History of seizures, eating disorders	Patient must set a target quit date the second week of therapy. May be a good agent for initial therapy in smokers with concomitant depression.
varenicline (Chantix) Start: 0.5 mg PO once daily for 3 d, then increase to 0.5 mg PO bid for 4 d, then increase to 1 mg PO bid for 12–24 wks	Neuropsychiatric disturbances such as mood changes, anxiety, suicidal ideation	History of anaphylaxis or skin reactions	Do not start in patients with preexisting psychiatric illness. Patient should set quit date for eighth day of therapy.

Transdermal Patches

Currently, there are two NRT patches on the market, and both products are available without a prescription (**Table 52.1**): Nicoderm CQ and the generic nicotine transdermal patch (formerly Habitrol). Both patches vary slightly in their weaning regimen.

The recommended dosing regimen for Nicoderm CQ patches for patients who smoke more than 10 cigarettes daily is 21 mg for 6 weeks, 14 mg for 2 weeks, and 7 mg for 2 weeks. The recommended dosing regimen for the generic patch (formerly Habitrol) for patients who smoke more than 10 cigarettes daily slightly differs: 21 mg for 4 weeks, 14 mg for 2 weeks, and 7 mg for 2 weeks. For both products, it is recommended that patients who smoke 10 cigarettes or less per day start at a 14-mg patch for 6 weeks and then decrease to a 7-mg patch for 2 weeks. The Nicotrol patch is currently unavailable in the United States but was available by prescription. It is a single-dose, 15-mg patch and is intended for daytime use only as a 16-hour patch.

Both available patches may be worn for 16 to 24 hours and should be applied at the same time each day. The manufacturer for the generic patch (formerly Habitrol) recommends patients wear the patch for 16 hours; only patients who awaken with cigarette cravings are advised to wear the patch for 24 hours. The manufacturer for Nicoderm CQ recommends patients wear the patch for 24 hours and should decrease to 16 hours only if they experience nightmares or other sleep disturbances when wearing the patch for 24 hours. A new patch should then be applied on waking. Only one patch should be applied at a time.

The most common side effects of the transdermal patches include a mild skin reaction with pruritus, burning, and erythema. The skin reactions are usually mild and self-limiting, resolving within 24 hours of removing the patch. Rotating application sites, changing brands, and applying steroid cream may reduce the incidence and severity of these events. While less common, sleep disturbances have been reported with 24-hour patches. When this occurs, it is difficult to distinguish if it is a result of the patch or nicotine withdrawal. If sleep disturbances occur, the patient should be counseled to remove the patch at bedtime and apply a new patch upon waking. Transdermal patches should not be used on patients with systemic eczema, atopic dermatitis, or psoriasis because these patients are more likely to develop skin reactions. Also, the nicotine patch should be avoided in patients with unstable angina or who are immediately post-myocardial infarction or pregnant.

The initial patch should be applied immediately on awakening on the patient's targeted quit date. The application site should be clean and dry before applying the patch. The patient should press the patch onto a hairless portion of the upper outer arms or upper chest and hold it for approximately 10 seconds. To decrease irritation that may occur with the patches, the patient should rotate application sites with each new patch. It is common to experience mild tingling, itching, or burning sensations for the first minute after application. If these symptoms persist for more than 4 days, however, the prescriber should be notified and an alternative method should be used.

If the patch gets wet or if it falls off, a new patch should be applied to a different site, and then removed at the original time the first patch would have been removed. Proper disposal of the patch is important. After the patch is removed, it should be placed in the wrapper from the newly applied patch and discarded responsibly—out of the reach of children and pets.

It is important to advise patients not to use the patch if they use other nicotine-containing products or continue to smoke or chew tobacco unless informed by their physician. Instruct patients not to smoke even if they are not wearing the patch because the nicotine in the skin will be entering the bloodstream for several hours after the patch is removed.

Nicotine Gum

Nicotine polacrilex gum (Nicorette) was the first NRT to be approved and is available without a prescription. The patient should chew the gum slowly until he or she senses a peppery taste or tingling. Then the gum should be "parked" between the cheek and the gingiva to increase absorption. This cycle should be repeated with the same piece of gum approximately every minute for 15 to 30 minutes. The gum is more effective if used on a fixed schedule as opposed to an "as-needed" basis (APA, 1996). This may be explained in part by the fact that one piece of gum stays in the bloodstream for 2 to 3 hours. Therefore, a patient should be advised to chew one pice of gum every 1 to 2 hours, as a fixed schedule will help to ensure consistent nicotine levels in the blood (Hukkanen, et al., 2005). Chewing at least nine pieces a day during the first 6 weeks of attempting to quit has been shown to increase the patient's chance of success. Most patients should use a 2-mg dose, but a 4-mg dose is also available and may be used as the initial dose in the following:

- Patients with a history of severe withdrawal symptoms
- Patients who smoke 25 or more cigarettes per day
- Patients for whom the 2-mg gum failed
- Patients who request it

The initial duration of therapy is 6 weeks regardless of what strength is used. After the first 6 weeks the patient should be slowly weaned off the gum to avoid withdrawal symptoms. The manufacturer of Nicorette gum recommends that the patient chew a piece of gum every 1 to 2 hours during the first 6 weeks of therapy, then decrease to 1 piece of gum every 2 to 4 hours during weeks 7 and 8, and then 1 piece of gum every 4 to 8 hours during weeks 8 to 12. The maximum dose is 24 pieces per day. (See **Table 52.1**.)

The patient should be advised not to smoke while using the gum. In addition, food and fluid should not be taken for at least 15 minutes before and after chewing the gum because certain foods (e.g., coffee, tea, carbonated beverages) cause the saliva to become more acidic and therefore decrease the absorption of the gum. Patients should dispose of the gum and wrapper properly to avoid ingestion by small children and pets.

Common adverse effects of nicotine gum use include jaw muscle aches and fatigue, oral sores, hiccups, belching, throat irritation, and nausea. Some of these events (i.e., hiccups, throat irritation, nausea) result from rapid chewing, leading to excessive nicotine release and absorption. Patient education on the proper use of the gum decreases the incidence of these events.

Nicotine Nasal Spray

The nicotine nasal spray is a prescription product and is marketed under the brand name Nicotrol NS. Compared to other NRT products, nicotine nasal spray has the fastest rate of absorption and thus is the most similar to the onset of the effect that occurs with cigarette smoking (Hukkanen, et al., 2005). This formulation may have a role for patients who fail to quit smoking by using the gum or patch or who are highly dependent smokers who require nicotine replacement at a quicker rate than the gum and patch can provide.

The recommended initial dosage of the nasal spray is one or two 0.5-mg doses in each nostril per hour (1 spray = 0.5 mg nicotine). The dosage may be increased as needed to prevent withdrawal symptoms. The maximum dose is 5 sprays per hour or 40 sprays per day. A minimum of eight doses should be used each day to increase the chance of success. After the initial 6 to 8 weeks of treatment, the dosage should be slowly tapered over the next 4 to 6 weeks. Using the nasal spray for longer than 6 months is not recommended because there is no greater efficacy and it increases the risk of dependence.

Before administering the first dose, the patient must prime the pump. This is accomplished by pumping the medication into a tissue six to eight times until a fine spray appears. If the spray is not used for 24 hours or more, the pump must be primed again. Once the pump is ready for use, the patient must follow the manufacturer's directions. For a summary, see **Box 52.5**. The difference between the nicotine nasal spray and other nasal sprays is that the patient must remember not to sniff or inhale while administering Nicotrol NS. If the spray comes in contact with the mouth, eyes, or skin, the patient should rinse the area immediately with cold water to prevent toxicity. The patient must be aware that it takes approximately 1 week to adjust to the side effects.

Common side effects of the nicotine nasal spray include nose and throat irritation, rhinitis, sneezing, coughing, and watery eyes. These events can occur in more than 75% of patients. The nicotine inhaler is associated with dyspepsia, throat or mouth irritation, oral burning, rhinitis, and cough after inhalation.

Nicotine Inhaler

In 1998, the nicotine inhaler became available as a prescription drug for smoking cessation. The inhaler is thought to improve smoking cessation through two mechanisms. When it is used, it mimics the hand-to-mouth ritual that occurs when smoking a cigarette and it produces a sensation of inhaled smoke on the back of the throat.

The inhaler consists of a mouthpiece and a cartridge. These two separate pieces are pressed together to break the seal on the cartridge. Once the seal is broken, the nicotine-filled air is inhaled into the mouth as a cigarette would be inhaled. The best results have been found when the patient takes shallow, frequent puffs over 20 minutes.

The recommended dose is 6 to 16 cartridges per day. A minimum of six cartridges must be used during the first 3 to 6 weeks of therapy, and therapy should be continued for at least 3 months. After 3 months, the dose should be tapered over the next 6 to 12 weeks. Use of the Nicotrol inhaler should not exceed 6 months. Like the nasal spray, the inhaler must be used regularly for 1 week before the patient adjusts to the side effects. Finally, because the cartridges contain high concentrations of nicotine, they should be stored and disposed of in a place that cannot be accessed by children and pets.

Nicotine Lozenge

The newest formulation of NRT is the nicotine lozenge (formerly Commit, now Nicorette), which was approved by the FDA in October 2002 and is available without a prescription. The nicotine lozenge is available in 2-mg and 4-mg strengths. One study found that treatment with the nicotine lozenge results in significantly greater 28-day abstinence at 6 weeks for the 2-mg (46.0% vs. 29.7%; $p<0.001$) and the 4-mg lozenges compared with a placebo (48.7% versus 20.8%; $p<0.001$; Shiffman, et al., 2002). Similar treatments were maintained for a full year. Use of more lozenges also resulted in reducing cravings and withdrawal (Shiffman, et al., 2002).

The nicotine lozenge helps control cravings by delivering craving-fighting medicine quickly. The lozenge uses a unique method for smokers to determine their degree of physical dependence on nicotine. This indicator is called time to first cigarette (TTFC). With TTFC, those who smoke their first cigarette within 30 minutes of waking are directed to use the

---

BOX 52.5

How to Use a Nicotrol Inhaler

STEP 1: Blow your nose to make sure it is clear.

STEP 2: Tilt your head back slightly and insert bottle tip into nostril as far as it is comfortable.

STEP 3: Breathe in through your mouth and hold your breath.

STEP 4: Press on the bottom of the bottle with your thumb to release one spray. Breathe out through your mouth. Do not sniff or inhale through your nose and do not swallow while spraying. If your nose runs after releasing the spray, gently sniff to keep the spray in your nose. Wait 2–3 min before blowing your nose.

STEP 5: If you are to use one spray in each nostril, repeat steps 2–4 for the other nostril.

STEP 6: Wipe bottle tip and replace the cap.

4-mg strength, whereas those who smoke their first cigarette after 30 minutes of waking are directed to use the 2-mg strength (Shiffman, et al., 2002). It is hypothesized that the TTFC is a better method than number of cigarettes smoked per day as a way of identifying patients who are highly nicotine dependent. This is because some patients may not smoke often each day but are physiologically dependent on nicotine since they develop withdrawal symptoms during prolonged periods without smoking (i.e., upon awakening after no cigarette use while sleeping; Shiffman, et al., 2002). Utilizing TTFC may allow clinicians to identify more patients with physiologic nicotine dependence and recommend higher, more effective doses of NRT. It is recommended that during the first 6 weeks, an individual should take one lozenge every 1 to 2 hours, for at least nine a day. This dosage is then reduced to one lozenge every 2 to 4 hours in weeks 7 to 9, and every 4 to 8 hours in weeks 10 to 12. The recommended length of treatment of therapy for the nicotine lozenge is 12 weeks. Because it delivers 25% more nicotine per dose, the lozenge may be an alternative for patients who report the presence of withdrawal symptoms with the gum (Shiffman, et al., 2002).

The patient should be advised not to eat or drink for 15 minutes before using the nicotine lozenge. The lozenge should be placed in the mouth and sucked on for 20 to 30 minutes to allow the lozenge to slowly dissolve. The lozenge should not be swallowed or chewed. The patient will feel a warm or tingly sensation. Occasionally, the lozenge should be moved from one side of the mouth to the other until it is completely dissolved. Only one lozenge should be used at a time and patients should not use more than five lozenges in 6 hours or more than 20 per day.

The most common side effects of the nicotine lozenge are hiccups, dyspepsia, dry mouth, nausea, and irritation/soreness in the mouth and throat (Shiffman, et al., 2002). These effects mainly occurred in patients who chewed or swallowed the lozenge. Patient education on how to properly administer the lozenge can help decrease these incidences. Finally, because the lozenge looks similar to hard candy, it should be stored and disposed properly to avoid access by children.

Non-Nicotine Therapies

Bupropion

Bupropion is the first non-nicotine product approved for smoking cessation. The drug has been commonly used as an antidepressant under the brand name Wellbutrin SR. It is available by prescription as an aid to smoking cessation under the brand name Zyban SR. The exact mechanism of action is unknown; however, it is believed to be related to dopaminergic or noradrenergic properties. In a randomized double-blind, placebo-controlled trial (Dale, et al., 2001), 27% of patients who received the active drug were abstinent at 6 months compared with 16% of patients taking a placebo ($p<0.001$).

The initial dose of Zyban SR is 150 mg/day for 3 days to decrease the incidence of insomnia. After 3 days, the dose can be increased to 150 mg twice a day for 7 to 12 weeks. Dosages higher than 300 mg/day are not recommended because of the increased risk of seizures. Unlike NRT, Zyban SR therapy should be initiated while the patient is still smoking because the drug takes approximately 1 week to reach steady-state plasma concentrations. The patient should set a target quit date during week 2 of therapy. If the patient has not made significant improvements by week 7 of treatment, the attempt is unlikely to be successful and the medication should be discontinued. Additionally, a patient who successfully quits after 7 to 12 weeks of treatment should be considered for continuation of Zyban SR therapy. Tapering the dose is not required when stopping the medication.

The most common side effects of Zyban SR are dry mouth and insomnia. Insomnia may be reduced by avoiding bedtime administration, but the patient should be counseled to allow 8 hours between the two daily doses. Other adverse events that can occur include nervousness or difficulty concentrating, rash, and constipation. Seizures have also occurred but are very rare (Dale, et al., 2001).

It is important that patients taking Zyban SR participate in behavioral therapy programs that include counseling both during and after therapy. Patients need to be informed not to use Wellbutrin or Wellbutrin SR while taking Zyban SR because these medications all contain bupropion. In addition, monoamine oxidase inhibitors should not be used during or within 14 days of Zyban SR treatment. The interaction between these agents increases bupropion toxicity (i.e., seizures, psychotic changes). Zyban SR should not be chewed or crushed because it will damage the sustained-release formulation, which may increase the risk of overdose and adverse events.

Varenicline

Varenicline is the newest approved agent on the market to aid in smoking cessation. It is available in the United States with a prescription under the brand name Chantix. It aids in smoking cessation by binding to a subunit of the nicotinic acetylcholine receptor. When attached to this subunit, varenicline blocks nicotine's binding to the same subunit and blocks nicotine's effects in the brain (i.e., reward, stimulant, depressant affects). Varenicline is also a partial agonist of the nicotine acetylcholine receptor, so it alleviates withdrawal symptoms produced with smoking cessation. In short, varenicline provides patients attempting to quit some of the rewarding effects felt with smoking while blocking the reinforcement effects of continued nicotine use. In one randomized controlled trial, varenicline given for 12 weeks improved successful quit rates during weeks 9 to 12 when compared to a placebo (43.9% vs. 17.6%, $p<0.001$) and when compared to bupropion (43.9% vs. 29.8%; $p<0.001$; Jorenby, et al., 2006). However, as is the case with many smoking cessation interventions, quit rates during weeks 9 to 52 were lower in all treatment groups but still highest in the varenicline treatment group: 23% varenicline vs. 10.3% placebo ($p<0.001$) and 23% varenicline vs. 14.6% bupropion ($p<0.004$).

To reduce the risk of nausea, varenicline should be titrated over a 1-week period to its effective dose of 1 mg twice daily. The starting dose is 0.5 mg once daily for days 1 to 3, which is then increased to 0.5 mg twice daily for days 4 to 7, and finally increased to the target dose of 1 mg twice daily on day 8. Patients who develop intolerable nausea when taking 1 mg twice daily may have the dose reduced to 1 mg once daily, but a dose titration to 1 mg twice daily should be attempted at a later time. For people with severe renal impairment (creatinine clearance <30 ml/minute), the starting dose is 0.5 mg once daily, which may be titrated to a target dose of 0.5 mg twice daily. Varenicline should be started 1 week before the patient's set quit date. As with other smoking cessation treatments, varenicline should be given along with behavioral counseling.

The most commonly reported adverse events are nausea, constipation, and abnormal dreams. Other side effects are headaches, difficulty concentrating, somnolence, and visual disturbances. There have been several reports of accidents and near-miss accidents while driving or operating heavy machinery in people taking varenicline, which may have been a result of somnolence and visual disturbances. Patients should be counseled not to drive or operate heavy machinery until they know how varenicline will affect them.

Varenicline use has been reported to cause neuropsychiatric symptoms (e.g., mood changes, psychosis, hallucinations, suicidal ideation, suicide attempts, completed suicides). Because of this effect, varenicline should not be prescribed to patients with preexisting psychiatric conditions, and patients who experience any changes in mood or behavior or develop suicidal ideation should stop varenicline and contact their health care provider immediately.

Second-Line Agents: Clonidine and Nortriptyline

Two second-line nonnicotine products are also available to aid in smoking cessation but are not approved by the FDA for smoking cessation. These two products are clonidine and nortriptyline, which are both available only with a prescription. Clonidine therapy has been examined for use in treatment of nicotine addiction because of its availability to reduce withdrawal symptoms in people addicted to narcotics or alcohol (Jones, et al., 2000). Clonidine treatment increased the chance of a successful quit attempt when compared to a placebo (odds ratio 2.1, CI 1.2–3.7; Fiore, et al., 2008). Clonidine therapy is usually started 3 to 7 days before the quit date. Oral clonidine can be given 0.10 mg orally twice daily initially, and the dosage can then be adjusted as tolerated to 0.75 mg/day administered in divided doses (Fiore, et al., 2008). Alternatively, the clonidine transdermal patch can be used at a dosage of 0.1 to 0.2 mg/day. Duration of therapy is for 3 to 10 weeks, during the time acute nicotine withdrawal symptoms would be present. The dose should be tapered over several days in all patients to reduce withdrawal effects from clonidine, but tapering is especially important in patients with hypertension to avoid rebound hypertension and patients with diabetes who may experience relative hypoglycemia (Gourlay, et al., 2008). Those with rebound hypertension should not use clonidine. Common side effects include dry mouth, drowsiness, dizziness, and sedation.

Nortriptyline is another second-line non-nicotine agent that has been effective and well tolerated for the treatment of

addiction to smoking (Da Costa, et al., 2002). Nortriptyline dosage may be started at 25 mg/day and titrated to a target dose range of 75 to 100 mg/day and duration for 12 to 24 weeks (Fiore, et al., 2008). It may double chances of smoking cessation compared to a placebo (odds ratio 1.8, CI 1.2–1.7; Fiore, et al., 2008). Nortriptyline is contraindicated in those with risk of arrhythmias. Common side effects include sedation and dry mouth (Da Costa, et al., 2002).

The DHHS/PHS guidelines recommend the use of these two products as second-line therapy because they are not FDA approved for the treatment of nicotine dependence and withdrawal and because of concerns with the side effect profiles of these agents.

Combination Drug Therapy

Although most of the drugs discussed above have only been approved as single pharmacologic agents, combined treatment may be appropriate for smokers who are unable to quit with monotherapy. Three combinations of nicotine replacement have shown to be safe and effective in smoking cessation and are recommended by the DHHS/PHS expert panel: long-term (>14 weeks) nicotine patch + other NRT (gum or spray); nicotine patch + nicotine inhaler; or nicotine patch + bupropion SR (Fiore, et al., 2008).

An analysis of three studies showed that compared to treatment with nicotine patch monotherapy, combination therapy with long-term nicotine patch and nicotine gum or nicotine spray doubled smoking cessation rates at 6 months (odds ratio 1.9, CI 1.3–2.7; Fiore, et al., 2008). Kornitzer and colleagues studied smoking cessation rates in people given nicotine patch + nicotine gum vs. nicotine patch + a placebo (Kornitzer, et al., 1995). The group receiving the patch + gum was more likely to have continuously abstained from smoking at 3 and 6 months compared to the group receiving the patch alone (34.2% vs. 22.7% at 3 months, $p = 0.027$; 27.5% vs. 15.3% at 6 months, $p = 0.010$). Incidence of side effects was similar in combination and monotherapy groups. A review of four studies found that combination therapy with nicotine patch and nicotine gum reduced withdrawal symptoms in heavy smokers (Okuyemi, et al., 2000). Blondal and colleagues' study results showed the combination of nicotine patch + nicotine spray increased continued smoking cessation at 3 and 6 months when compared to the nicotine patch alone (37% vs. 25%, $p = 0.045$ at 3 months; 31% vs. 16% at 6 months, $p = 0.005$; Blondal, et al., 1999).

An analysis of two studies showed that compared to a placebo, combination therapy with nicotine patch and nicotine inhaler doubled the chances for smoking cessation at 6 months (odds ratios 2.2, CI 1.3–3.6; cessation rate 25.8%; Fiore, et al., 2008). However, this combination may not provide additional benefits over nicotine patch monotherapy. Tonnesen and Mikkelsen found continued abstinence rates were actually lower at 3 and 6 months in the nicotine patch + nicotine inhaler group compared to nicotine patch alone (14.8% vs. 19.2% at 3 months, 8.7% vs. 14.4% at 6 months; Tonnesen & Mikkelsen, 2000). However, interpretation of these results is limited because a direct comparison of cessation rates between the two treatment arms was not performed, and the number of participants in each of the two treatment arms was small (n=104, nicotine patch; n=115, nicotine patch + nicotine inhaler). Adverse events were similar in combination and monotherapy treatment arms. Combination of NRT treatments should be considered for smokers with significant cravings or withdrawal symptoms despite adequate doses of single agents and should be continued for 3 to 6 months (Okuyemi, et al., 2000).

Unlike the other combinations previously described, use of combination therapy with the nicotine patch and bupropion is FDA approved. An analysis of three studies showed that compared to nicotine patch alone, the combination therapy with nicotine patch and bupropion increased the chances for continued smoking cessation at 6 months by 30% (odds ratio 1.3, CI 1.0–2.8; Fiore, et al., 2008). Jorenby and colleagues found that abstinence rates at 6 and 12 months were higher in the bupropion + nicotine patch group compared to patch monotherapy (38.8% vs. 21.3%, $p<0.001$ at 6 months; 35.5% vs. 16.4%, $p<0.001$ at 12 months; Jorenby, et al., 1999). Abstinence rates in the combination group were higher compared to bupropion monotherapy, but these differences were not statistically significant. If this combination is initiated, patients should be started on bupropion 150 mg/day for 3 days, then 150 mg twice daily for 1 to 2 weeks prior to quit date. Transdermal nicotine patch therapy should be added starting on the quit date and treatment continued for 3 to 6 months (Okuyemi, et al., 2000).

Selecting the Most Appropriate Agent

Which therapeutic agent is most effective depends on the patient and the patient's smoking history, among other factors. For a review of the recommended order of treatment and the clinical guidelines for prescribing pharmacotherapy according to the DHHS/PHS guidelines for smoking cessation, see **Tables 52.2** and **52.3** and **Figure 52-2**.

Special Population Considerations

Female patients should be monitored for pregnancy because NRT can harm the fetus. The nicotine gum and lozenge are classified as pregnancy category C (risk cannot be excluded: animal studies have shown an adverse effect on the fetus, but there are no adequate, well-controlled studies in pregnant women), and the patches, nasal spray, and inhaler are classified as category D (positive evidence of risk: studies in humans or post-marketing have demonstrated a risk to the fetus). Zyban SR and varenicline also are classified as category C. These medications should be reserved for patients in whom non-pharmacologic therapy has not worked or those experiencing severe withdrawal symptoms. In pregnant patients, the benefits of using smoking cessation medications should outweigh the risks of smoking.

Nicotine replacement therapy should be used with caution in those patients with cardiovascular disease because it can cause tachyarrhythmia and worsen angina. However, the risks are small compared with the cardiovascular effects of smoking. Nicotine concentrations are higher and delivered more rapidly from cigarettes compared with NRT products.

MONITORING PATIENT RESPONSE

Smoking status must be monitored in all patients. As mentioned, patients starting NRT must stop smoking completely before initiating treatment to avoid nicotine toxicity. Common signs of nicotine toxicity include nausea, vomiting, diarrhea, hypersalivation, abdominal pain, perspiration, dizziness, headache, hearing and visual disturbances, confusion, and weakness. On the other hand, patients beginning treatment with Zyban SR or varenicline must set a quit date after the medication has been taken for at least 1 week (1 week for varenicline and 1 to 2 weeks for Zyban SR).

TABLE 52.2	Recommended Order of Treatment for Smoking Cessation	
Order	**Agents**	**Comments**
First line	All nicotine replacement therapies, bupropion, varenicline	There is evidence showing all of these therapies increase abstinence when compared to a placebo. The patch leads to fewer compliance problems, less patient education time, and greater ease of use. Also, the patch provides continuous nicotine replacement without multiple daily dosing, unlike other forms of nicotine replacement (i.e., gum, lozenge, inhaler, nasal spray). It is recommended that the patch be used routinely in clinical practice unless contraindicated or if the patient has failed the patch.
Second line	Combination therapy	Combination therapy using the patch plus the gum or the patch plus the nasal spray should be considered if patients fail or suffer withdrawal symptoms with the use of the patch alone. In this case, the patch provides continuous nicotine replacement and the gum or spray provides relief of "breakthrough" withdrawal symptoms. The patch plus bupropion may also be considered when a single nicotine replacement agent fails. However, data are limited with regards to the efficacy of adding nicotine replacement therapy to bupropion after the patient has failed bupropion monotherapy.
Third line	Clonidine, nortriptyline	Because of the side effect profile of these agents, they should be reserved for patients who fail first- and second-line therapies.

TABLE 52.3   Clinical Guidelines for Prescribing Pharmacotherapy for Smoking Cessation

Who should receive pharmacotherapy for smoking cessation?	All smokers trying to quit, except in the presence of special circumstances. Special consideration should be given before using pharmacotherapy with selected populations: those with medical contraindications, those smoking fewer than 10 cigarettes/day, pregnant/breast-feeding women, those who use smokeless tobacco, and adolescent smokers.
What first-line pharmacotherapies are recommended?	All seven of the FDA-approved pharmacotherapies for smoking cessation are recommended, including bupropion SR, nicotine gum, nicotine inhaler, nicotine lozenge, nicotine nasal spray, nicotine patch, and varenicline. The clinician should consider the first-line medication regimens that have been shown to be more effective than the nicotine patch alone—varenicline 2 mg/day or the combination of nicotine patch and as-needed use of nicotine gum or nicotine nasal spray.
What factors should a clinician consider when choosing among the seven first-line pharmacotherapies?	Because of the lack of sufficient data to rank-order these seven medications, choice of a specific first-line pharmacotherapy must be guided by factors such as clinician familiarity with the medications, contraindications for selected patients, patient preference, previous patient experience with a specific pharmacotherapy (positive or negative), and patient characteristics (e.g., history of depression, concerns about weight gain).
Are pharmacotherapeutic treatments appropriate for lighter smokers (e.g., 10–15 cigarettes/day)?	If pharmacotherapy is used with lighter smokers, clinicians should consider reducing the dose of first-line NRT pharmacotherapies. No adjustments are necessary when using bupropion SR.
What second-line pharmacotherapies are recommended?	Clonidine and nortriptyline.
When should second-line agents be used for treating tobacco dependence?	Consider prescribing second-line agents for patients unable to use first-line medications because of contraindications or for patients for whom first-line medications are not helpful. Monitor patients for the known side effects of second-line agents.
Which pharmacotherapies should be considered with patients particularly concerned about weight gain?	Bupropion SR and nicotine replacement therapies, in particular nicotine gum and nicotine lozenge, have been shown to delay, but not prevent, weight gain.
Are there pharmacotherapies that should be especially considered in patients with a history of depression?	Bupropion SR and nortriptyline appear to be effective with this population. NRT also provides some help, but varenicline should be used with caution in this population.
Should nicotine replacement therapies be avoided in patients with a history of cardiovascular disease?	No. The nicotine patch in particular is safe and has been shown not to cause adverse cardiovascular effects.
May tobacco dependence pharmacotherapies be used long-term (e.g., 6 months or more)?	Yes. This approach may be helpful with smokers who report persistent withdrawal symptoms during the course of pharmacotherapy, who have relapsed in the past after stopping therapy, or who desire long-term therapy. A minority of individuals who successfully quit smoking use NRT (gum, nasal spray, inhaler) long term. The use of these medications long term does not present a known health risk. Additionally, the FDA has approved the use of bupropion SR, varenicline, and some NRTs for 6-month use.
May pharmacotherapies ever be combined?	Yes. There is evidence that combining the nicotine patch with either nicotine gum or nicotine nasal spray, nicotine patch with nicotine inhaler, and nicotine patch with bupropion increases long-term abstinence rates over a placebo. The use of nicotine patch with either nicotine gum or nicotine nasal spray increases long-term abstinence over the use of a single nicotine replacement product.

U.S. Department of Health and Human Services, Public Health Service, Agency for Health Care Policy and Research. (2008). *Treating tobacco use and dependence: 2008 update*. Rockville, MD: Author.

A follow-up telephone call from the practitioner should occur within 1 week after the patient's scheduled quit date. If the patient is aware of the future call, compliance may be improved. In addition, the follow-up call may help detect ineffective use or adverse events early in the course of treatment. Additional follow-up contacts should occur as needed. If the patient has been successful at the time of the call, the clinician should offer congratulations and additional support.

However, if the patient has relapsed, it is important to reassure the patient that it is not indicative of ultimate failure. Many smokers attempt to quit several times before achieving their goal. The reasons for failure should be identified and eliminated for the next attempt and the patient should be encouraged to try again. Intensification of behavioral counseling may also be warranted. Drug therapy may be prolonged beyond 3 months if the patient develops cravings or feels he or she may relapse

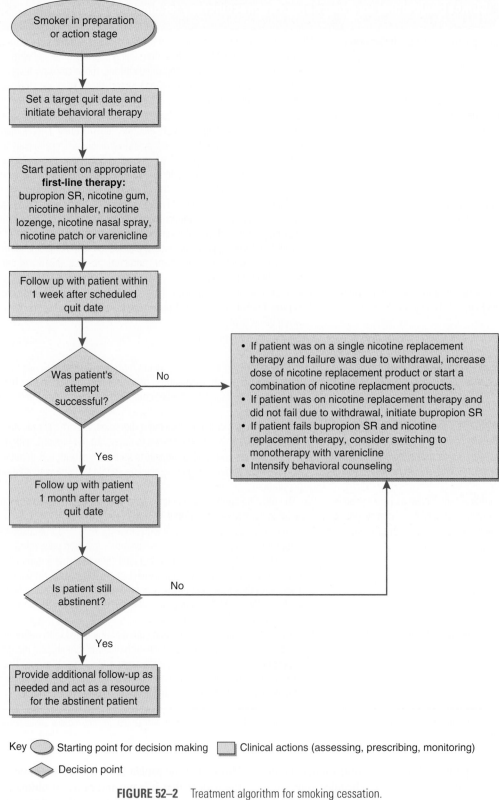

FIGURE 52–2 Treatment algorithm for smoking cessation.

upon discontinuation of therapy. At least one study found that duration of therapy for 6 months or longer was associated with higher quit rates (Steinberg, et al., 2006).

Duration of therapy must be monitored to evaluate if tolerance or physical dependence occurs to NRT. Dependence is most common with the nicotine nasal spray because of its rapid delivery of nicotine. Proper dosage titration and a weaning schedule should be monitored as well to prevent withdrawal symptoms from occurring.

PATIENT EDUCATION

The occurrence of adverse events with any medication has a definite correlation with patient compliance. Therefore, it is important that both the practitioner and patient be aware of the common side effects that may occur when using smoking cessation products. In addition, the patient needs to be informed that tolerance to the adverse effects associated with NRT usually occurs.

Weight gain is a common outcome of smoking cessation and many patients are hesitant to quit for this reason. Many former smokers gain 4 to 5 kg, but as many as 13% gain 11 kg or more (Pisinger & Jorgensen, 2007). The mechanism for this is thought to be a slowing of metabolism. As mentioned earlier, the average smoker weighs 2.4 to 3.0 kg less than the average nonsmoker (Molarius, et al., 1997). Therefore, with the cessation of smoking, the average former smoker should weigh approximately the same as the average nonsmoker. Patients must be informed that weight gain is possible but not significant. In addition, the health risk of increased weight is small compared with continued smoking. The increase in weight can be addressed after the patient has achieved complete abstinence. If weight gain is a major deterrent to treatment, nicotine replacement therapies, particularly nicotine gum and nicotine lozenge, and bupropion may be used since these agents may delay the weight gain.

Furthermore, patient counseling on the proper use of nicotine products including dose and administration can improve efficacy and safety of the medications. Although the important role of pharmacotherapy is addressed, it should be recognized that a sustained reduction in smoking prevalence will require social desirability of limiting access to cigarettes and increasing availability and use of effective cessation interventions. Finally, as the effort to promote smoking cessation interventions is sustained, an increase in quit rates will be expected as well as an ultimate decrease in smoking-related morbidity and mortality among both children and adults.

Case Study

A.P., a 46-year-old white man, has been smoking 1.5 packs of cigarettes per day for the last 28 years. He has a very stressful job as executive of a large marketing company. A.P. and his coworkers frequently go to "happy hour" at the local bar after a long day at work. When he is at home, A.P. has a sedentary lifestyle that consists of lounging by the pool or watching television. He tried to quit smoking "cold turkey" 2 years ago and remained abstinent for approximately 1 year, but has never tried any pharmacologic smoking cessation aids. During his previous attempt to quit, he became very anxious, irritable, and depressed and had trouble sleeping and concentrating at work. He has a medical history of hypertension for the last 10 years and he has not adhered to the therapeutic regimen. His family has been encouraging him to stop smoking for years. He is currently at the doctor's office for his blood pressure checkup and inquires about smoking cessation options.

1. What symptoms experienced by this patient during his previous attempt to quit smoking are consistent with physical dependence to nicotine?
2. What motivational level (stage of change) is this patient in?
3. When A.P. reaches the action stage, what pharmacologic options are available for him?
4. Which smoking cessation aid would you recommend starting in this patient? Why?
5. What adverse events could you see with the product that you chose in the previous question?
6. What are some nondrug methods that may enhance smoking cessation in this patient?

BIBLIOGRAPHY

Starred references are cited in the text.

*American Cancer Society. (2010). *Cancer facts and figures*. Atlanta, GA: Author.

*American Psychiatric Association. (1996). Practice guideline for the treatment of patients with nicotine dependence. *American Journal of Psychiatry, 153*(Suppl. 10), 1–31.

American Psychiatric Association. (2000). *Diagnostic and statistical manual of mental disorders* (4th ed., text revision). Washington, DC: Author.

*Benowitz, N. L. (2008). Tobacco. In L. Goldman (Ed.). *Cecil textbook of medicine* (23rd ed.). Philadelphia: Elsevier.

*Benowitz, N. L. (2010). Nicotine addiction. *New England Journal of Medicine, 362*(24), 2295–2303.

*Blondal, T., Gudmundsson, L. J., Olafsdottir, I., et al. (1999). Nicotine nasal spray with nicotine patch for smoking cessation: Randomized trial with six year follow up. *British Medical Journal, 318*, 285–289.

*Centers for Disease Control and Prevention. (2008a). Cigarette smoking among adults—United States, 2007. *Morbidity and Mortality Weekly Report, 57*(45), 1221–1226.

*Centers for Disease Control and Prevention. (2008b). Deaths from chronic obstructive pulmonary disease—United States, 2000-2005. *Morbidity and Mortality Weekly Report, 57*(45), 1229–1232.

*Centers for Disease Control and Prevention. (2008c). Smoking-attributable mortality, years of potential life lost, and productivity losses — United States, 2000–2004. *Morbidity and Mortality Weekly Report, 57*(45), 1226–1228.

*Centers for Disease Control and Prevention. (2010). Tobacco use among middle and high school students—United States, 2000-2009. *Morbidity and Mortality Weekly Report, 59*(33), 1063–1068.

*Da Costa, C. L., Younes, R. N., & Lourenco, M. T. (2002). Stopping smoking: A prospective, randomized, double-blind study comparing nortriptyline to placebo. *Chest, 122,* 403–408.

*Dale, L. C., Glover, E. D., Sachs, D. P., et al. (2001). Buproprion for smoking cessation. *Chest, 119,* 1357–1364.

*Doering, P. L., Kennedy, W. L., & Boothby L. A. (2007). Substance-related disorders: Alcohol, nicotine, and caffeine. In J. T. Dipiro (Ed.), *Pharmacotherapy: A pathophysiologic approach* (7th ed.). New York: McGraw-Hill.

*Fiore, M. C., Jaen, C. R., Baker T. B., et al. (2008). *Treating tobacco use and dependence: 2008 update.* Clinical Practice Guideline. Rockville, MD: U.S. Department of Health and Human Services, Public Health Service.

Glover, E. D., Glover, P. N., Franzon, M., et al. (2002). A comparison of a nicotine sublingual tablet and placebo for smoking cessation. *Nicotine Tobacco Research, 4,* 441–450.

Gold, P. B., Rubey, R. N., & Harvey, R. T. (2002). Naturalistic, self-assignment comparative trial of bupropion SR, a nicotine patch, or both for smoking cessation treatment in primary care. *American Journal of Addictions, 11*(4), 315–331.

Gourlay, S. G., Stead L. F., & Benowitz, N. (2008). Clonidine for smoking cessation (review). *Cochrane Database of Systematic Reviews, 4,* 1–15.

*Heatherton, T. F., Kozlowski, L. T., Frecker, R. C., et al. (1991). The Fagerstrom Test for Nicotine Dependence: A revision of the Fagerstrom Tolerance Questionnaire. *British Journal of Addictions, 86*(9), 1119–1127.

*Henningfield, J. E., Shiffman, S., Ferguson, S. G., et al. (2009). Tobacco dependence and withdrawal: Science base, challenges and opportunities for pharmacotherapy. *Pharmacology and Therapeutics, 123*(1), 1–16.

*Hukkanen, J., Jacob III, P., & Benowitz, N. L. (2005). Metabolism and disposition kinetics of nicotine. *Pharmacologic Reviews, 57,* 79–115.

Hurt, R. D., Sachs, D. P. L., Glover, E. D., et al. (1997). A comparison of sustained-release bupropion and placebo for smoking cessation. *New England Journal of Medicine, 337,* 1195–1202.

Jones, J. M., Lewis, M. L., & Stembridge, N. Y. (2000). Counseling against cigarette smoking. *US Pharmacist, 23*(2).

*Jorenby, D. E., Hays, J. T., Rigotti, N. A., et al. (2006). Efficacy of varenicline, an α4β2 nicotinic acetylcholine receptor partial agonist, VS. placebo or sustained-release bupropion for smoking cessation. *Journal of the American Medical Association, 296*(1), 56–63.

*Jorenby, D. E., Leischow, S. J., Nides, M. A., et al. (1999). A controlled trial of sustained release buprorion, a nicotine patch, or both for smoking cessation. *New England Journal of Medicine, 340,* 685–691.

*Kornitzer, M., Boutsen, M., Thijs J., et al. (1995). Combined use of nicotine patch and gum in smoking cessation: A placebo-controlled clinical. *Preventive Medicine, 24,* 41–47.

*Le Houezec, J. (2003). Nicotine pharmacokinetics in nicotine addiction and nicotine replacement: A review. *International Journal of Tuberculosis and Lung Disease, 7*(9), 809–810.

*Mallin, R. (2002). Smoking cessation integration of behavioral and drug therapies. *American Family Physician, 65*(16), 1107–1114.

McRobbie, H., & Hayek, P. (2001). Nicotine replacement therapy in patients with cardiovascular disease: Guidelines for health professionals. *Addiction, 96,* 1547–1551.

*Molarius, A., Seidell, J. C., Kuulasmaa, K., et al. (1997). Smoking and relative body weight: An international perspective from the WHO MONICA project. *Journal of Epidemiology and Community Health, 51,* 252–260.

*O'Brien, C. P. (2006). Drug addiction and abuse. In J. L. Burton (Ed.), *Goodman & Gilman's The pharmacological basis of therapeutics* (11th ed.). New York: McGraw-Hill.

*Ockene, I. S., & Houston, N. (1997). Cigarette smoking, cardiovascular disease, and stroke: A statement for healthcare professionals from the American Heart Association. *Circulation, 96,* 3243–3247.

*Okuyemi, K. S., Ahluwalia, J. S., & Harris, K. J. (2000). Pharmacotherapy of smoking cessation. *Archives of Family Medicine, 9,* 270–281.

Patterson, F., Jepson, C., Kaufmann V., et al. (2003). Predictors of attendance in a randomized clinical trial of nicotine replacement therapy with behavioral counseling. *Drug and Alcohol Dependence, 72,* 123–131.

*Pisinger, C., & Jorgensen, T. (2007). Weight concerns and smoking in a general population: The Inter99 study. *Preventive Medicine, 44,* 283–289.

*Shiffman, S., Dresler, C. M., Hajek, P., et al. (2002). Efficacy of a nicotine lozenge for smoking cessation. *Archives of Internal Medicine, 162*(22), 2632–2633.

*Shiffman, S., Dresler, C. M., Rohay, J. M., et al. (2004). Successful treatment with a nicotine lozenge of smokers with prior failure in pharmacological therapy. *Addiction, 99*(1), 83–92.

Shiffman, S., West, R. J., & Gilbert, D. G. (2004). Recommendation for the assessment of tobacco craving and withdrawal in smoking cessation trials. *Nicotine & Tobacco Research, 6*(4), 599–614.

*Steinberg, M. B., Foulds, J., Richardson, D. L., et al. (2006). Pharmacotherapy and smoking cessation at a tobacco dependence clinic. *Preventive Medicine, 42,* 114–119.

*Tonnesen, P., & Mikkelsen, K. L. (2000). Smoking cessation with four nicotine replacement regimes in a lung clinic. *European Respiratory Journal, 16,* 717–722.

Andrew M. Peterson
Henry M. Schwartz

CHAPTER 53

Travel Medicine

In today's world, national and international travel is becoming commonplace, and the need to provide travelers with sufficient information on how to manage their health while in another region is growing as well. Travel medicine is an interdisciplinary specialty area typically focused on the prevention of infections and on patient safety while traveling internationally (Hill, et al., 2006). Within this context, most travel medicine should be performed by a specialist with specific training regarding the infectious and safety risks a patient may be facing while traveling abroad. However, primary care providers (PCPs) will encounter patients traveling domestically as well as internationally, and each will have questions regarding managing their medications during the trip. In this vein, the PCP can supply the traveler with preventive and treatment measures and can ensure that vaccinations, such as hepatitis A, hepatitis B, and other age- and health-status-appropriate vaccinations, are up-to-date. (See Chapter 51 on immunizations.) The PCP can also provide information on safe food and water guidelines, skin and wound care, and precautions against blood-borne disease. Another key element to the discussion could include the potential for contracting exotic infectious diseases such as malaria and dengue fever. While these are typically outside the nonspecialist's scope, discussion by a PCP can help the patient identify the need for a travel medicine specialist.

The PCP should also provide access to additional medications as needed, such as extra prescriptions, particularly when patients travel abroad for extended periods. Further, the PCP should counsel patients on how to manage taking complex drug regimens, particularly when traversing multiple time zones.

The purpose, and thus the organization, of this chapter is to help the PCP deal with routine travel questions posited by patients traveling within the United States, Canada, and Western Europe. As noted earlier, travel to more exotic regions requires the consultation of a travel medicine specialist. **Box 53.1** lists some websites that can help practitioners and patients prepare for travel. For specialists in international travel medicine, go to International Society of Travel Medicine (www.istm.org) and The American Society of Tropical Medicine and Hygiene (www.astmh.org).

GENERAL SAFETY ISSUES IN TRAVEL

One of the key pieces to the effective management of travel-related conditions is being prepared. Pre-travel preparation can include medical evaluations, vaccinations, and the provision of medications and information regarding locations of medical support at the destination. If the travel is short and in country, the risks to the patient are lower than if the travel is extended over a long period (e.g., weeks or months) or if the patient is traveling outside of the native country. Long airplane flights can be problematic, both within and outside the country, due to the potential for developing deep vein thrombosis (DVT) and/or jet lag. There are several steps patients can take before traveling that will help them understand the risks and precautions necessary to minimize the risk. For example, all travelers should ambulate every 2 to 3 hours whether traveling by car, ship, or plane to prevent blood clots from developing. For more recommendations, the Centers for Disease Control and Prevention (CDC) has an extensive website dedicated to travel safety (www.cdc.gov/travel).

Medical Kit

Domestic and international travelers should prepare a medical kit that includes general first-aid materials as well as traveler-specific medications. Prescription medications should be kept in their original labeled containers, kept on the traveler at all times, and not placed in checked luggage. Common over-the-counter medications should remain with the patient as well. These could include analgesics, antidiarrheal agents, antihistamines, and, depending on the destination, sunscreen or insect repellant. See **Box 53.2** for information on sunscreens. The kit should also contain specialized items unique to the planned destination such as chemoprophylaxis for traveler's diarrhea or malaria. See **Box 53.3** for a more comprehensive list.

Medical Care

It is recommended that the traveler purchase travel insurance that will cover medical expenses. These insurance providers also assist in locating medical care at the destination. There exist services for international travel, such as The International

BOX 53.1

Patient and Provider Information Sites Related to Travel Medicine

Centers for Disease Control and Prevention (CDC),
www.cdc.gov/travel
CDC Health Information for International Travel 2012,
www.cdc.gov/travel/page/yellowbook-2012-home.htm
International Association for Medical Assistance to
Travelers,
www.iamat.org
International Society of Travel Medicine,
www.istm.org
Smart Traveler Enrollment Program,
https://travelregistration.state.gov
Transportation Security Administration (TSA),
www.tsa.gov
Travelers with Disabilities and Medical Conditions,
http://www.tsa.gov/travelers/airtravel/
specialneeds/editorial_1374.shtm#3

Association for Medical Assistance to Travelers (www.iamat.org), who can also assist with these services. Travelers should check with their health insurance provider concerning coverage for medical emergencies. Hotels provide assistance in locating medical services for their guests.

International travelers should identify the location of the U.S. embassy at their destination and carry with them the embassy's contact information. Locations of U.S. embas-

sies or consulates can be found on the Bureau and Consular website (http://travel.state.gov). Copies of passports should be maintained in a separate location in case of loss while abroad. The U.S. State Department has a Smart Traveler Enrollment Program that can locate travelers in case of travel emergencies (https://travelregistration.state.gov).

It is important to check travel notices found on the CDC website (http://wwwnc.cdc.gov/travel/) before and during travel. The Transportation Security Administration (TSA) website (www.tsa.gov) assists the traveler with handling items such as medications, continuous positive airway pressure machines, wheelchairs, ostomy supplies, and even service animals.

Vaccinations

One of the primary functions of the PCP is to ensure that the patient is current with his or her vaccinations. This includes age-appropriate vaccinations (Chapter 51) as well as hepatitis A and B vaccinations and other destination-specific immunizations. Region-specific vaccinations vary, and an international travel medicine specialist should be consulted to ensure that required vaccinations are administered. Required vaccinations change, and the up-to-date recommendations are found on the CDC website. Any traveler should consult that website for recommendations for the destination in a timely fashion before departure to ensure safe travel (http://wwwnc.cdc.gov/travel/).

Safe Travel

There are routine procedures that should be followed for safe travel, whether domestic or international. It is important to educate the traveler about these concepts to ensure an event-free trip. All travelers should take a list of medical conditions and current medications in case of an emergency. This should

BOX 53.2

New Labeling Rules for Sunscreens

The U.S. Food and Drug Administration (FDA) states that exposure to the sun can increase the risk of skin cancer and premature skin aging. Primary care practitioners can help educate their patients on proper protection against the harmful effects of the sun's rays.

As background information, there are two types of solar rays: ultraviolet A (UVA) and ultraviolet B (UVB). Both types cause skin cancer, but UVA rays—the most common solar rays reaching the earth—are associated with wrinkling, and UVB rays are associated with sunburn. The sunburn protection factor (SPF) is a scale designed to indicate to the consumer the level of protection against UVB rays, not UVA rays. The new FDA labeling rules will not only include an SPF number, but will require manufacturers to indicate if the product protects against both

UVA and UVB rays (called *broad-spectrum coverage*). Under these new rules, only products labeled as broad spectrum with an SPF of 15 or higher can claim protection against skin cancer and premature aging. The FDA also proposes that sunscreens with an SPF of greater than 50 be labeled as "SPF 50+" because there is no data to show that an SPF higher than 50 produces better results.

In addition to using a broad-spectrum sunscreen with an SPF of 15 or higher, patients should be instructed to:

- limit time in the sun, especially between the hours of 10 AM and 2 PM
- wear clothing to cover exposed skin
- reapply sunscreen at least every 2 hours and more often if swimming or sweating.

Analgesics (acetaminophen or ibuprofen)
Antibacterial ointment
Antidiarrheal medication
Antihistamines
Antiseptic wipes
Bandages
Decongestant
Duplicate prescriptions (in original containers)
Hydrocortisone
Insect repellant (DEET [30% to 35%] and permethrin)
Motion sickness medication
Sleep medication (for jet lag)
Sunscreen (SPF ≥15)
Thermometer

be carried with other identification because this is the first place a health-care agency will look for information if the traveler cannot provide the information.

If special equipment is required, arrangements must be made before travel. Airlines are especially receptive to persons with special needs. Arrangements can be made for wheelchair transport, special meals, and special seating if notified before the flight.

The Traveler with Diabetes

Providers should evaluate possible disruption to a patient's normal routine (such as airport delays, traveling between time zones), availability of medical care, and obtaining medical supplies. Supplies and medication should always be accessible and not placed in checked luggage or in the trunk of a car. Snacks should be packed with the patient's supplies and medications.

Patients should obtain written documentation from their PCP indicating that they have diabetes and then should prepare a list of medications and supplies needed. A medical identification bracelet/necklace should be worn. The information on the bracelet/necklace should state that the patient has diabetes, needs medications, and should contain an emergency contact number. International travelers on insulin should be instructed on possible insulin differences (U-100 vs. U-40 vs. U-80). Patients taking insulin to control their diabetes face a unique situation with respect to timing their doses when they are traveling across time zones. When they arrive at a destination that spans more than three or four time zones, they may be "out of sync" with the local meal times. Traveling east creates a shortened day and may require a reduction in insulin because doses would be administered closer than normal and traveling west creates a longer day, and so insulin doses may need to be increased. However, this seemingly simple and workable rule of "westward = more insulin; eastward = less insulin" may not always hold true. See **Box 53.4** for a sample travel schedule.

The current TSA guidelines allow patients to carry on syringes/needles, lancets, insulin, glucose meters, and insulin pumps (TSA, 2011). Patients should inform the TSA agent that they have diabetes and are carrying diabetes supplies.

Assume that a male patient takes 10 units of long-acting insulin and 10 units of regular in the morning and 8 units of long-acting insulin and 10 units of regular in the evening. The patient is flying round trip from Philadelphia to London with the following basic itinerary:

Monday – 7:55 PM departure and 6:50 AM arrival
Saturday – 11:20 AM departure and 3:20 PM arrival

Monday—Depart from New York at 7:55 PM. The traveler takes the normal evening dose before dinner. The patient arrives Tuesday morning at 6:50 AM, London time. The total travel time has been 6 hours and 55 minutes. Since only 6 hours have elapsed, yet the patient is adjusting to London time, he should take ½ of his morning long-acting dose PLUS the full regular dose with breakfast, and then in the evening, take half of the long-acting dose PLUS the full regular dose with dinner. On Wednesday, the patient

should resume his regular pre-travel schedule. If the travel includes layovers or if there are snacks and small meals, additional insulin may be required.

Saturday—Depart from London at 11:20 AM. On the return flight the following Saturday, the traveler takes his usual morning dose with breakfast and gets on the 11:20 AM flight. The travel time is 8 hours, and the patient arrives at 3:20 PM. If there is a small meal or snack offered during the flight, additional regular insulin should be taken. The patient can resume his regular schedule at dinner that evening. If this travel involves a layover or if the patient will be eating a full meal, then he should take ½ of the long-acting dose PLUS the full regular dose with that meal. When the patient eats dinner later that evening, he should take half of the long-acting dose PLUS the full regular dose with dinner. The patient can resume his normal insulin schedule Sunday morning.

Information on what can be carried on board an airplane can be found on the following website: http://www.tsa.gov/travelers/airtravel/specialneeds/editorial1374.shtm#3.

The Traveler with a Pulmonary or Cardiovascular Condition

The traveler with a chronic disease should see his or her PCP to ensure that travel is possible. The PCP should provide the patient with documentation stating the medical condition, medication prescribed, and any required supplies for treatment (e.g., portable oxygen or nebulizers). As with the other conditions noted, the patient should be instructed to wear a medical identification bracelet/necklace with the condition, medications, and an emergency contact number.

The traveler with a cardiovascular condition should consider where to obtain supplemental oxygen, have a self-management plan for adjusting medications, obtain an electrocardiogram, and know current DVT precautions before traveling. For patients with pacemakers, defibrillators, and other implanted medical devices, it is recommended to carry a medical device identification card. It is important for the traveler who requires oxygen to be sure that the portable tank provides enough oxygen for the trip, taking into consideration layovers, flight delays, and the trip to and from the airport. The capacity of portable tanks prevents many oxygen-dependent persons from traveling long distances. Oxygen also must be available when the traveler arrives at the destination. Many other countries have little regulation about smoking. The person with oxygen must be cognizant of anyone smoking around them because of the hazards involved.

The traveler with a pulmonary condition planning to travel by airplane should check with the TSA for requirements related to transporting oxygen or nebulizers and traveling with implanted medical devices (www.tsa.gov/travelers/). The U.S. Food and Drug Administration requires any person traveling with oxygen to submit a letter from the provider stating the need for its use. Further, the patient should also consider where to obtain supplemental oxygen, develop a self-management plan in case of an exacerbation (asthma, chronic obstructive pulmonary disease), and identify appropriate DVT precautions before traveling.

The Pregnant Traveler

Pregnant travelers should be given consent to travel by their obstetrician. Review of the patient's itinerary is important to evaluate pre-travel needs, such as vaccines, health insurance, and available medical care at the travel destination. Travel for the patient can include travel by car, plane, train, or ship.

Pregnant travelers should try to limit travel by car to no more than 6 hours per day. One of the greatest risks for travelers is motor vehicle accidents. Patients should be instructed to wear seat belts at all times and make frequent stops to get out and walk and move to prevent DVT. Air travel is usually safe up to 32 to 36 weeks' gestation, but travelers need to check with individual airlines for specific restrictions on travel. Patients should be instructed to get up and stretch during long flights.

When sitting, seat belts should be worn at all times. Patients who experience motion sickness can be prescribed an antiemetic if appropriate. Refer to Chapter 5 for more information on medication use during pregnancy. The provider should also recommend that the patient remain hydrated and wear comfortable clothing and footwear.

Pregnant travelers should strictly adhere to food and water precautions in developing countries. Patients should be advised not to travel to malaria-endemic areas. Self-treatment with medications should be individually evaluated by the patient's obstetrician before travel. Bacille Calmette-Guerin, measles-mumps-rubella, human papillomavirus, and varicella vaccines; bismuth subsalicylate compounds; doxycycline; and primaquine are contraindicated during pregnancy.

SPECIFIC CONCERNS FOR THE GENERAL TRAVELER

Altitude Sickness

Altitude sickness is a common condition for individuals traveling to altitudes of 2,500 to 3,500 m (8,200 to 11,500 ft). However, for some individuals, altitude sickness can occur at lower altitudes, such as those commonly encountered in the Western U.S. (e.g., Denver, Colorado). The lower level of oxygen at higher altitudes causes headache, fatigue, sleep disturbances, and dyspnea. Chronic exposure to higher altitudes can lead to polycythemia due to the overstimulation of erythropoiesis and the resultant increase in red blood cells. Patients should be instructed to avoid respiratory depressants. To prevent acute altitude sickness, the patient can use a staged ascent over time or take a medication such as acetazolamide for prevention. Acetazolamide is a carbonic anhydrase inhibitor diuretic that decreases the reabsorption of bicarbonates in the proximal tubule of the kidney. The result is metabolic acidosis that stimulates ventilation and improves cerebral blood flow.

Bedbugs

Bedbugs, or Cimicidae, are parasitic insects that typically feed off the blood of warm-blooded animals. The most common type, Cimex lectularius, prefers to feed on human blood. Bedbugs are becoming an increasing problem in the United States, even though they were effectively eradicated after World War II with the use of DDT.

Adult bedbugs are rusty red or mahogany in color, with a flat, oval-shaped body about 1/5-inch long. Bedbugs are nocturnal, feeding at night while a person is asleep. They feed by piercing the skin with their elongated mouthparts, and since the person is asleep, the pinprick-like feeling is typically not noticed. The bedbug injects saliva under the skin, which may lead to large swellings that itch and may become irritated and infected when scratched. Swelling may not develop until a day or more after feeding, and some people do not show symptoms.

Travelers should check for signs of bedbugs in their hotel or dwelling by checking under the sheets and around mattress seams for the bugs or looking for dark spots indicative of dried bug excrement.

Bedbug bites typically do not require treatment unless pruritus is severe or a secondary infection develops. Then, treatment with a topical antibiotic ointment and/or a corticosteroid cream is appropriate. Bedbugs currently are not considered to be disease carriers.

Jet Lag

Jet lag is a physiological condition secondary to an alteration in a patient's circadian rhythm. It results from long-distance travel across multiple time zones, whereby the patient's internal clock is not in sync with the destination time zone. Crossing 1 to 2 time zones typically does not result in jet lag, but crossing 3 or more time zones generally affects individuals. The degree of jet lag is influenced by the direction of travel—traveling east is generally worse than traveling west—as well as the level of hydration and prior travel rest. The symptoms of jet lag include headache, fatigue, irregular sleep pattern, and gastrointestinal changes.

Before traveling across multiple time zones, the patient should get plenty of rest and eat healthy. Adjusting to the future time zone by 1 to 2 hours each 1 to 2 days before travel can also help minimize the severity of jet lag. During travel, particularly air travel, avoiding alcohol and caffeinated beverages and drinking plenty of water helps prevent dehydration, which could worsen the severity of jet lag.

Traveler's Diarrhea

Diarrhea is the most common illness among travelers with upwards of 50% of international travelers contracting the disease (CDC, 2006b). Patients who are immunocompromised (e.g., patients with human immunodeficiency virus, cancer chemotherapy patients) are more susceptible. Further, patients on acid-lowering medications such as omeprazole or ranitidine may also be at risk for traveler's diarrhea (TD) due to the decrease in acid that normally destroys some intestinal flora. Educate all patients in detail on food and water precautions, including avoiding ice cubes.

Bacterial pathogens, such as enterotoxigenic *Escherichia coli*, cause about 80% of TD cases, but there are other bacteria as well as viruses or parasites associated with TD. Most TD cases occur within the first week of travel and the onset is usually quick. It manifests as an increase in stool frequency and a change to a watery consistency. The resolution is usually quick—1 to 2 days—and is rarely life threatening. Other symptoms include nausea, vomiting, and abdominal cramping.

Key to the successful management of TD is educating the traveler on appropriate precautions regarding food and drink intake. Travelers should be advised to avoid eating foods or drinks from street vendors, avoid raw vegetables, and eat only fruit that has a peel (e.g., bananas, oranges). They should also be advised to drink bottled water and maintain hydration at all times. Antimicrobial prophylaxis is not recommended by the CDC (2006b), but the traveler could use bismuth subsalicylate (two tablets four times daily) for up to 3 weeks to help prevent

the illness. See Chapter 30 for further discussion on the prevention and treatment of TD.

INTERNATIONAL TRAVEL CONCERNS

Although the focus of this chapter is on the patient traveling to common destinations, some PCPs will encounter patients with basic questions about some commonly encountered infectious diseases, such as malaria, yellow fever, and dengue fever. The following section will outline some basic information.

Malaria

Malaria causes the most morbidity and mortality of all the parasitic diseases. It is estimated that 350 to 500 million people worldwide are affected by malaria and that 1 million people die from it every year. In the United States, malaria is confined to people who have visited endemic areas, such as Africa, Asia, and Latin America.

Malaria is caused by protozoan parasites of the genus *Plasmodium*. There are four species of plasmodia that produce disease in humans: *P. falciparum, P. vivax, P. ovale,* and *P. malaria. P. falciparum* is the most widespread and dangerous of the four. All species are transmitted by the bite of an infected female Anopheles mosquito.

Appropriate pharmacotherapy begins with the prescription of suppressive drugs before the patient travels to an area where malaria is a health hazard. Suppressive therapy cannot prevent primary infection of the liver because drug therapy does not affect sporozoites. Suppressive therapy does prevent the erythrocytic infection, which causes the symptoms of malaria. However, once the liver has a primary infection, the patient can have an acute attack when he or she is no longer taking suppressive drugs.

Selection of suppressive drug therapy depends on which region the patient intends to visit. In chloroquine-sensitive areas, chloroquine (Aralen) is the drug of choice for suppressive therapy. In chloroquine-resistant areas, mefloquine (Lariam) is the preferred suppressive agent.

Malaria prevention consists of a combination of mosquito-avoidance measures and chemoprophylaxis. Patients traveling to an endemic area should be referred to their PCP or a physician specializing in international health.

Yellow Fever

Yellow fever virus is a single-stranded RNA virus that belongs to the genus *Flavivirus* that causes an acute viral hemorrhagic disease. According to the World Health Organization (WHO), there are an estimated 200,000 cases of yellow fever, causing 30,000 deaths, worldwide each year.

Yellow fever is endemic in tropical areas of Central America, South America, and Africa. Transmission of the virus is by the bite of an infected *Aedes* or *Haemagogus* mosquito. Blood-borne transmission can also occur via transfusion, needle stick, and intravenous drug use.

Preventive measures include administering the yellow fever vaccine and mosquito avoidance measures. Patients traveling to an endemic area should be referred to a physician specializing in international health. Treatment for yellow fever is symptomatic and includes rest, fluids, and use of analgesics for pain and fever. Aspirin and nonsteroidal anti-inflammatory medications should be avoided because of the risk of bleeding.

Dengue Fever

Dengue fever is now endemic in more than 100 countries and widespread in most tropical countries of the South Pacific, Asia, Africa, Caribbean, Latin America, and South America. According to the WHO, more than two fifths of the world's population is now at risk. It is estimated that there may be 50 million cases each year.

Dengue fever is caused by four immunologically related viruses known as *dengue viruses* (DENV-1, DENV-2, DENV-3, and DENV-4). Infection from each dengue virus will produce lifelong immunity for that dengue virus only. Patients may be infected up to four times during their lifetime. Transmission of the viruses is from the bite of an infected *Aedes aegypti* mosquito.

There is no vaccine or drugs that prevent dengue fever. The only prevention is mosquito-avoidance measures. Patients with symptoms of dengue fever should be referred to a physician specializing in international health. There are no specific therapeutic agents for dengue fever. Treatment consists of bed rest and fluids to prevent dehydration. Fever and pain can be controlled by acetaminophen. Severe pain may require opioid analgesics. Aspirin and nonsteroidal anti-inflammatory medications should be avoided due to their anticoagulant properties.

CONCLUSION

After the patient returns from travel, issues may still arise. Rashes that were experienced during travel may have abated, but if they persist after returning (and treatment), the practitioner needs to consider causes other than dermatitis (e.g., worms). Also, TD may continue or even emerge post-travel, and causes should be explored. (See Chapter 30.)

A commonly reported and problematic post-travel issue is fever, with nearly 28% of patients returning from travel seeking out medical care due to fever (CDC, 2011). With a fever, the possibility of malaria must be evaluated urgently and the patient referred to a specialist qualified in treating this disease. It is a rule of thumb that if a fever is present in a patient returning from a malarious area, it should be treated as such until ruled out through appropriate testing.

Preparing and treating patients for the myriad illnesses that can occur during national and international travel is a specialty in itself. However, the PCP must be knowledgeable about and conversant in the language of travel medicine. From managing basic TD to understanding the complexities of preventing and treating malaria, the PCP plays a pivotal role in helping patients cope with today's global society.

BIBLIOGRAPHY

Starred references are cited in the text.

Carroll, D., & Williams, D. C. (2008). Pre-travel vaccination and medical prophylaxis in the pregnant traveler. *Travel Medicine and Infectious Disease, 6*, 259–275.

*Centers for Disease Control and Prevention. (2006a). http://wwwnc.cdc.gov/travel/. Accessed May 28, 2011.

*Centers for Disease Control and Prevention. (2006b). Traveler's Diarrhea. http://www.cdc.gov/ncidod/dbmd/diseaseinfo/travelersdiarrhea_g.htm. Accessed February 18, 2011.

Centers for Disease Control and Prevention. (2010a). *CDC Health Information for International Travel.* Atlanta, GA: Author. http://wwwnc.cdc.gov/travel/yellowbook/2010/chapter-2/malaria.htm. Accessed May 28, 2011.

Centers for Disease Control and Prevention. (2010b). *CDC Health Information for International Travel.* Atlanta, GA: Author. http://wwwnc.cdc.gov/travel/yellowbook/2010/chapter-2/yellow-fever.htm. Accessed May 28, 2011.

Centers for Disease Control and Prevention. (2010c). *CDC Health Information for International Travel.* Atlanta, GA: Author. http://wwwnc.cdc.gov/travel/yellowbook/2010/chapter-2/sunburn.htm. Accessed June 9, 2011.

Centers for Disease Control and Prevention. (2010d). *CDC Health Information for International Travel.* Atlanta, GA: Author. http://wwwnc.cdc.gov/travel/yellowbook/2010/chapter-5/dengue-fever-dengue-hemorrhagic-fever.htm. Accessed May 28, 2011.

*Centers for Disease Control and Prevention. (2011). The post-travel consultation. http://wwwnc.cdc.gov/travel/yellowbook/2010/chapter-4/general-approach-to-the-returned-traveler.aspx. Accessed March 18, 2011.

Chandra, M., & Edelman, S. V. (2003). Have insulin, will fly: Diabetes management during air travel and time zone adjustment strategies. *Clinical Diabetes, 21*, 82–85.

Cooper, M. C. (2006). The elderly travelers. *Travel Medicine and Infectious Disease, 4*, 218–222.

*Hill, D. R., Ericsson, C. D., Pearson, R. D., et al. (2006). The practice of travel medicine: Guidelines by the Infectious Disease Society of America. *Clinical Infectious Diseases, 43*, 1499–1539.

International Association for Medical Assistance to Travelers (www.iamat.org). Accessed August 15, 2011.

International Society of Travel Medicine (www.istm.org). Accessed August 15, 2011.

Neumann, K. (2006). Family travel: An overview. *Travel Medicine and Infectious Disease, 4*, 202–217.

Sack, R. L. (2009). The pathophysiology of jet lag. *Travel Medicine and Infectious Disease, 7*, 102–110.

Schuwerk, M. A., Richens, J., & Zuckerman, J. N. (2006). HIV and travel. *Travel Medicine and Infectious Disease, 4*, 174–183.

*Transportation Security Administration. (2011). Hidden disabilities: Travelers with disabilities and medical conditions. http://www.tsa.gov/travelers/airtravel/specialneeds/editorial_1374.shtm#3. Accessed March 18, 2011.

U.S. Food and Drug Administration. (2011). FDA announces changes to better inform consumers about sunscreen. http://www.fda.gov/NewsEvents/Newsroom/PressAnnouncements/ucm258940.htm. Accessed June 26, 2011.

Weight Loss

Obesity has reached epidemic proportions, affecting more than 400 million adults worldwide (World Health Organization [WHO], 2005). Obesity is a major cause of death in the United States with 112,000 excess due to cardiovascular disease, 15,000 excess due to cancer, and over 35,000 excess due to noncardiovascular, noncancer disease each year compared to healthy weight persons. (National Institutes of Health [NIH], 2010). According to the most recent survey from the National Health and Nutrition Examination Survey (NHANES) for 2007 to 2008, 68% of U.S. adults are overweight (body mass index [BMI] exceeds 25 kg/m^2) and 33.8% are obese, with a BMI exceeding 30 kg/m^2 (Flegal, et al., 2010).

Since 1980, people's weight in the United States has been increasing at an alarming rate. From 1980 to 2008, the frequency of obesity in adults has more than doubled (15% to 34%) and has more than tripled in children and adolescents (5% to 17%). Looking more closely at the youth, 17.4% of U.S. children and adolescents ages 12 to 19, 18.8% ages 6 to 11, and 13.9% ages 2 to 5 are overweight, according to NHANES 2003–2004 (Ogden, et al., 2006). This is compared with 15.5%, 15.3%, and 10%, respectively, in 1999–2000 (Ogden, et al., 2002). Women and minorities have a higher proportion of obesity among the general population.

CAUSES

Researchers attribute the rise in obesity to caloric imbalances. During the 1980s, the effects of modernization combined with an unprecedented abundance of cheap, energy-dense food produced a population that ate more while becoming increasingly sedentary (Taubes, 1998). Xavier Pi-Sunyer, a Columbia University obesity researcher and NIH Obesity Task Force chairperson, stated, "Food is probably cheaper and more available than it ever has been in history." Coupled with the increased food supply is the transformation of our society from a primarily labor-intensive work force during the agricultural age to a more sedate work force during the industrial and information ages. In other words, researchers theorize that Americans have been getting fatter in the last decades of the 20th century because of too much food and too little activity.

Researchers link obesity to the development of chronic debilitating disease states such as heart disease, type 2 diabetes mellitus, and cancer. Because of these links, the WHO and health officials, such as former U.S. Surgeon General C. Everett Coop, have declared obesity a global epidemic (James, et al., 2001; Wickelgren, 1998). These leading health officials claim that obesity is not only hurting the individuals involved but draining the economy as well. In the United States, the NIH claims that overweight/obese people are costing citizens more than $50 billion annually in direct health care costs with an additional $30 billion spent on weight loss products and services (NIH, 1998). Therefore, obesity accounts for over 5% of annual health care costs in the United States.

Genetic Factors

Obesity tends to run in families, suggesting that it may have a genetic cause. However, family members share not only the genes but the diet and lifestyle habits that may contribute to obesity. Separating these lifestyle factors from genetic factors is difficult. Still, growing evidence points to heredity as a strong determinant of obesity.

Environmental Factors

Although genetics may play a role in the development of obesity, the WHO Consultation on Obesity concluded that behavioral and environmental factors are primarily responsible for the dramatic increase in obesity during the past two decades (Racette, et al., 2003). Environment includes lifestyle behaviors, such as what a person eats and how active he or she is. Americans tend toward high-fat diets, often putting taste and convenience ahead of nutritional content when choosing meals. Most Americans also do not get enough exercise.

Psychological Factors

Psychological factors may also influence eating habits. Many people eat in response to negative emotions such as boredom, sadness, anger, and anxiety. Studies in the 1970s found that overeaters may be treating themselves for depression. The key is the chemical serotonin, which is produced by ingestion of starch and which regulates mood. Overeaters may be scrambling to boost their serotonin levels and also their moods.

Other Causes

Some illnesses can cause obesity. These include hypothyroidism, Cushing syndrome, depression, and some neurologic problems. Certain drugs, such as steroids and some antidepressants, may cause excessive weight gain.

PATHOPHYSIOLOGY

Obesity is not a disorder of body weight regulation. Obese people can regulate their weight appropriately, but that regulation is centered at an elevated homeostatic set point. After adolescence, body weight is usually highly stable, increasing slowly by approximately half a pound yearly over the course of a lifetime. Research studies performed on twins and adopted siblings show that genetic factors strongly influence the homeostatic set point of individuals.

Weigle (1990) suggests that body weight is set at the point of balance between various feedback loops regulating adipose mass. The genetic influence could be mediated by circulating factors or factors that regulate satiety. People with a high set point have lower amounts of these factors and thus have to gain relatively more adipose tissue before appetite and energy expenditure balance. The theory is that it is an extraordinarily difficult feat to cure obesity by dietary energy restriction. Most patients who lose weight through dieting regain that weight, indicating that the weight-regulating system is very strong. "Only persons with incredibly strong will power or the ability to tolerate physical discomfort are likely to be successful in this attempt to defeat a homeostatic mechanism" (Weigle, 1990).

When calorie intake exceeds energy expenditure over the long term, the excess energy is stored as fat. Everyone needs a certain amount of stored body fat for energy, heat insulation, shock absorption, and other functions. As a rule, women have more fat than men. Problems arise when men have more than 25% body fat and women more than 30%.

Body fat distribution is an important health consideration that has been widely overlooked by health care practitioners in terms of risk factors for obesity. Many recent research data suggest that it is not only how much fat a person has but also its distribution in the body that affects the risk for disease associated with that fat.

Women typically collect fat in the lower part of the trunk (hips and buttocks), giving their body a pear shape. Men usually build up fat in the upper trunk and intra-abdominal regions, giving them more of an apple shape. Excess body fat, particularly when distributed in the intra-abdominal region, increases the risk of hypertension, coronary artery disease, type 2 diabetes, gallbladder disease, sleep apnea, gout, and certain types of cancer (National Institute of Diabetes and Digestive and Kidney Diseases [NIDDK], 2000).

Diagnostic Criteria

The standard for body fat measurement is densitometry, which determines the density of a body submersed in water. However, the cost and technical requirements limit its usefulness in the clinical setting. The following paragraphs describe measurements more commonly used in clinical practice.

Weight-for-Height Tables

Weight-for-height tables usually have a range of acceptable weights for a person of a given height. A problem with using weight-for-height tables is that clinicians disagree about which is the best table to use. Many versions are available, and all cite different weight ranges. Some tables take a person's frame size, age, and sex into account; others do not. A limitation of all weight-for-height tables is that they do not distinguish excess fat from muscle (**Figure 54-1**).

Body Mass Index

The BMI is the measurement of choice for clinicians and researchers studying obesity. Besides its simplicity, which eases use in clinical practice, associations have been demonstrated between BMI and adiposity, disease risk, and mortality (NIDDK, 2000; Racette, et al., 2003). In general, when BMI exceeds 25 kg/m², morbidity and mortality rise proportionally (Sheperd, 2003).

The BMI takes into account both a person's height and weight (BMI = kg/m²). In **Table 54.1**, the mathematics and metric conversions have already been done. To use the table, find the appropriate height in the left-hand column and then move across the row to the given weight. The number at the top of the column is the BMI for that height and weight. **Table 54.2** gives the current guidelines for classification of obesity based on BMI. Similar to the weight-for-height tables, a limitation of BMI is that it does not distinguish excess fat from muscle. Therefore, some muscular people may be mistakenly classified as obese using BMI alone. In addition, it

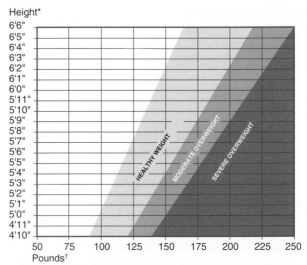

* Without shoes.

† Without clothes. The higher weights apply to people with more muscle and bone, such as many men.

FIGURE 54–1 Height and weight table. (*Source*: Report of the Dietary Guidelines Advisory Committee on the Dietary Guidelines for Americans, 1995, pages 23–24. From *Understanding adult obesity*. National Institute of Diabetes and Digestive and Kidney Diseases online publication.)

TABLE 54.1   Body Mass Index Conversion Chart*

Body Mass Index (kg/m²)

	19	20	21	22	23	24	25	26	27	28	29	30	35	40
Height (inches)	**Body Weight (lbs)**													
58	91	96	100	105	110	115	119	124	129	134	138	143	167	191
59	94	99	104	109	114	119	124	128	133	138	143	148	173	198
60	97	102	107	112	118	123	128	133	138	143	148	153	179	204
61	100	106	111	116	122	127	132	137	143	148	153	158	185	211
62	104	109	115	120	126	131	136	142	147	153	158	164	191	218
63	107	113	118	124	130	135	141	146	152	158	163	169	197	225
64	110	116	122	128	134	140	145	151	157	163	169	174	204	232
65	114	120	126	132	138	144	150	156	162	168	174	180	210	240
66	118	124	130	136	142	148	155	161	167	173	179	186	216	247
67	121	127	134	140	146	153	159	166	172	178	185	191	223	255
68	125	131	138	144	151	158	164	171	177	184	190	197	230	262
69	128	135	142	149	155	162	169	176	182	189	196	203	236	270
70	132	137	146	153	160	167	174	181	188	195	202	207	243	278
71	136	143	150	157	165	172	179	186	193	200	208	215	250	286
72	140	147	154	162	169	177	184	191	199	206	213	221	258	294
73	144	151	159	166	174	182	189	197	204	212	219	227	265	302
74	148	155	163	171	179	186	194	202	210	218	225	233	272	311
75	152	160	168	176	184	192	200	208	216	224	232	240	279	319
76	156	164	172	180	189	197	205	213	221	230	238	246	287	328

*Each entry gives the body weight in pounds for a person of a given height and body mass index. Pounds have been rounded off. To use the table, find the appropriate height in the left-hand column. Move across the row to a given weight. The number at the top of the column is the body mass index for the height and weight. From *Understanding adult obesity*. National Institute of Diabetes and Digestive and Kidney Diseases, U.S. Department of Health and Human Services, http://win.niddk.nih.gov/publications/understanding.htm.

does not take body fat distribution into account, which is an independent predictor of health risk (NIH, 1998).

Waist Circumference

Clinicians are concerned over where fat is located in the body. People whose fat is concentrated mostly in the abdomen are more likely to have many of the health problems associated with obesity. Waist circumference is a marker of abdominal fat and a good predictor of disease risk. Waist circumference is found by measuring the circumference around the waist at the level of the iliac crest (just above the hip bone). A waist

TABLE 54.2   Classification of Obesity by Body Mass Index (BMI)

	BMI (kg/m²)
Underweight	<18.5
Normal	18.5–24.9
Overweight	25.0–29.9
Obesity, class	
I	30.0–34.9
II	35.0–39.9
III (extreme)	≥40

circumference exceeding 40 inches (102 cm) in men and 35 inches (88 cm) in women signifies increased health risk in those who have a BMI of 25 to 34.9 kg/m².

Waist-to-Hip Ratio

Because upper body obesity carries greater risks, patients with central obesity, particularly younger patients, should be targeted for weight reduction. Similar to waist circumference, waist-to-hip ratio is a good indicator of who is at risk based on body fat distribution. However, recent guidelines state that the measurement of waist-to-hip ratio provides no advantage over waist circumference alone (NIH, 2000).

To find someone's waist-to-hip ratio, measure the waist at its narrowest point, and then measure the hips at the widest point. Divide the waist measurement by the hip measurement. Women with waist-to-hip ratio exceeding 0.85 or men with waist-to-hip ratios over 1.0 are at the greatest risk for disease associated with obesity.

INITIATING DRUG THERAPY

Experts generally agree that people who are 20% or more overweight, especially the extremely obese (BMI ≥ 40 kg/m²), can gain significant health benefits from weight loss. Many obesity experts believe that people who are less than 20% above their healthy weight should try to lose weight if they have any of the following risk factors:

- Family history of certain chronic diseases
- Preexisting medical conditions
- High waist-to-hip ratio

People with close relatives who have had heart disease or diabetes are more likely to have these problems if they are obese. High blood pressure, high cholesterol levels, or elevated glucose levels are all warning signs of some obesity-associated diseases. Finally, people whose weight is concentrated around their abdomen may be at greater risk for heart disease, diabetes, or cancer than people of the same weight whose fat is concentrated in the thighs and buttocks.

There are no "magic cures" for obesity. The most successful strategies include calorie reduction, increased physical activity, and behavior therapy designed to improve eating and physical activity habits (Nonas, 1998). Many guidelines advise physicians to have their patients try lifestyle therapy for at least 6 months before embarking on physician-prescribed drug therapy. Weight-loss drugs approved by the U.S. Food and Drug Administration (FDA) for long-term use may be tried as part of a comprehensive weight-loss program that includes dietary therapy and physical activity in carefully selected patients (BMI 30 kg/m^2 without additional risk factors, BMI 27 kg/m^2 if the patient has other risk factors including type 2 diabetes, high blood pressure, dyslipidemia, coronary artery disease, or sleep apnea) who had been unable to lose weight or maintain weight loss with nondrug therapies (**Table 54.3**).

Goals of Drug Therapy

Goals of therapy are to reduce body weight and maintain a lower body weight for the long term (NIH, 2000). A modest weight loss of 5% to 10% can lead to beneficial effects on cardiovascular risk factors associated with obesity including improvements in glycemia, blood pressure, and plasma lipid profiles. Recent studies have also shown that modest weight loss may help prevent or delay the appearance of type 2 diabetes and hypertension (Vidal, 2002). Data also suggest that voluntary modest weight loss is associated with a 25% reduction in total mortality in patients with type 2 diabetes (Williamson, et al., 2000). Proper food choices and regular aerobic exercise are preferable ways of attaining this weight

TABLE 54.3	Overview of Agents Prescribed for Weight Loss		
Generic (Trade) Name and Dosage	Selected Adverse Events	Contraindications	Special Considerations
Amphetamines			
dextroamphetamine (Dexedrine, Dextrostat) Start: 5–10 mg 30–60 min before meals Range: 5–30 mg	Palpitations, tachycardia, CNS stimulation, dry mouth	MAO inhibitors, hyperthyroidism, glaucoma, symptomatic cardiovascular disease or moderate–severe hypertension Same as above, but safety in people <12 y not established	Schedule II drug Do not crush or chew sustained-release dosage form.
methamphetamine (Desoxyn) Start: 5 mg 30–60 min before meals Range: 20–25 mg/d	Same as above	Same as above	Same as above
Appetite Suppressants			
diethylpropion (Tenuate, Tenuate Dospan) Start: 25 mg ac or 75 mg daily (long acting)	Palpitations, tachycardia, CNS stimulation, dry mouth	MAO inhibitors, hyperthyroidism, glaucoma, symptomatic cardiovascular disease or moderate–severe hypertension Same as above, but safety in people <12 y not established	Schedule IV drug
phendimetrazine (Bontril) Start: 17.5–35 mg 2 or 3 times daily, 1 h before meals Range: 35–105 mg daily Long acting: 105 mg every morning before breakfast	Same as above	Same as above	Schedule III drug
phentermine (Adipex-P) 18.75–37.5 mg daily	Headache, insomnia, nervousness, CNS stimulation	Same as above	Schedule IV drug
Lipase Inhibitor			
orlistat (Xenical, Alli) Rx: 120 mg tid with meals OTC: 60 mg tid with meals	Oily spotting, flatus with discharge, fecal urgency, fatty/oily stool	Chronic malabsorption syndrome or cholestasis Safety in people <12 y not established	May decrease absorption of fat-soluble vitamins (A, D, E, K)

loss as opposed to calorie restriction. When body weight drops below the set point by exercise, energy expenditure appears to adapt to the new weight, unlike weight loss by calorie restriction, which elicits strong counter-regulatory mechanisms (Weigle, 1990).

The 2000 guidelines published by the NIH (NIH, 2000) suggest that an initial weight loss goal of 10% over 6 months is reasonable. This should be accomplished through a reduction of caloric intake by 500 to 1,000 kcal/d, resulting in a rate of loss of 1 to 2 lb (0.45–0.9 kg) per week.

Eating behavior, like mood and personality, is thought to be the result of a mixture of neurotransmitters in the brain. Pharmacological approaches to weight loss may be more effective than attempts at behavioral therapy, just as antidepressants have been found in general to be more effective for treating clinical depression than psychotherapy. Amphetamines were once a popular prescription drug for weight control; however, one of the many complaints associated with their use was that all the weight that had been lost during drug therapy was regained after the drug was discontinued. Americans spent at least $467 million on prescription drugs in 1996 and another $32 million on over-the-counter (OTC) diet aids such as pills and herbal therapies (Wickelgren, 1998; **Box 54.1**).

Obesity must be treated as a chronic medical condition in the same way that hypertension is a chronic medical condition (**Figure 54-2**). Seen in this light, weight gain after drug discontinuation is no different from rising blood pressure after the discontinuation of antihypertensive medication. The pharmaceutical industry is very much aware of the marketing potential of a pill that would help combat the lifelong challenge of obesity. Much research time and money have been put into the development of such a pill during the 1990s. Lifelong drug therapy for obesity and the drug risk factors involved are factors that have yet to be addressed by researchers, whose studies have been over the short term (24 months being the longest). At present, drug therapy is used during the weight-loss phase of treatment, with drug safety beyond 2 years of total treatment not yet established. Therefore, it is critical not only to lose weight, but also to maintain the weight loss through changes in lifestyle and dietary habits.

Amphetamines

These agents are not widely used in the treatment of obesity primarily because of their high risk of abuse and high risk of cardiovascular side effects. As Schedule II (C-II) agents, there are often restrictions on the amount and duration of therapy, and some states even prohibit these drugs from being prescribed for weight loss. Nonetheless, they have been and may continue to be used for weight-loss purposes, although they remain a last line of therapy for the obese patient.

The two forms of amphetamines are dextroamphetamine (Dexedrine, Dextrostat) and methamphetamine (Desoxyn). Although each agent exerts similar effects, their potency varies, and therefore the dosing for each varies.

BOX 54.1

Alternative Weight-Loss Therapies

Stimulant Herbs: Coffee (200 mg tid)

Coffee contains the stimulant caffeine, which increases the basal metabolic rate. It also seems to depress appetite and has mild antidepressant and diuretic effects. Despite the availability over the counter, caffeine is not very popular for diet therapy because large doses must be taken, often with unpleasant side effects: insomnia, irritability, jitters, and elevated blood pressure.

Diuretic Herbs

Herbs with diuretic properties—buchu, celery seed, dandelion, juniper, parsley, and uva ursi—are used as a short-term strategy. In this way, diuretics can help people lose several pounds of "water weight." But the body senses the increased water loss diuretics cause and reacts with increased thirst to replace lost fluids. If diuretics continue to be ingested, the body eventually adjusts and retains water despite them. Herbal diuretics do not play a major role in permanent weight control.

Psyllium

Psyllium is the seed of the plantain plant. It is rich in a spongy fiber called *mucilage*. When psyllium comes in contact with water, its mucilage absorbs the fluid and expands substantially. In the stomach, psyllium expansion can produce feelings of fullness. Psyllium seed is sold in bulk in health food stores and herb shops. It is also available in a familiar product, the bulk-forming laxative Metamucil.

Hot, Spicy Herbs

Red pepper and mustard (1 teaspoon with each meal) are two herbs that give hot foods their heat and that increase the basal metabolic rate. As the basal metabolic rate increases, calories burn faster and weight decreases more rapidly. Another weight-loss benefit of hot spices is associated with thirst. Hot herbs stimulate thirst, so the person drinks more liquids, filling up on water instead of food, which also contributes to weight loss.

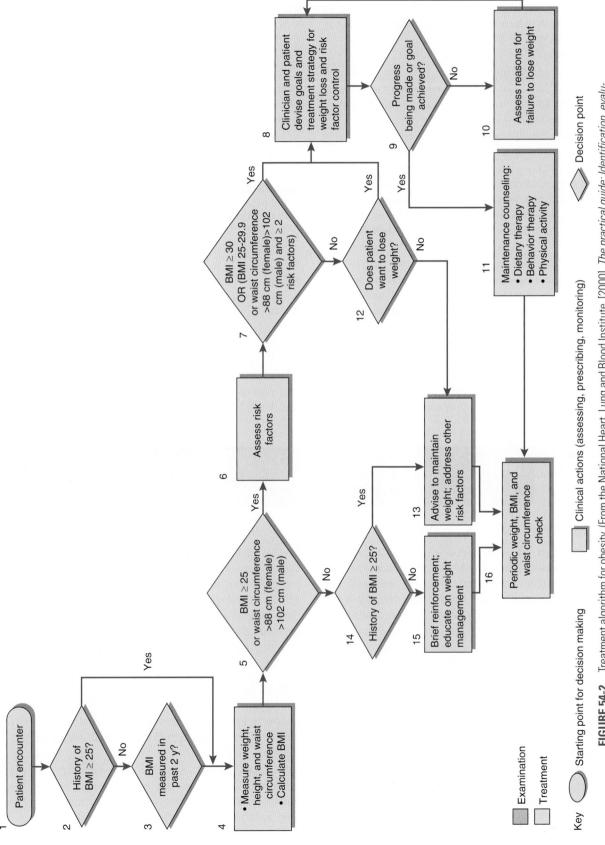

FIGURE 54-2 Treatment algorithm for obesity. (From the National Heart, Lung and Blood Institute. [2000]. *The practical guide: Identification, evaluation and treatment of overweight and obesity in adults* [publication No. 00—4084] Washington, DC: National Institutes of Health.)

Mechanism of Action

The amphetamines cause an increase in the release of norepinephrine from central noradrenergic neurons and possibly a release of dopamine from the mesolimbic system at higher doses. The mechanism of action for weight loss appears to be exerted at the hypothalamic feeding center.

These agents are completely absorbed when administered orally and are widely distributed throughout the body. The plasma half-life varies from approximately 7 hours to more than 30 hours, depending on urinary alkalinization. At an acidic pH, the half-life is short because these agents are protonated in the acidic urine and are not reabsorbed. For every 1-unit increase in pH, the half-life increases by approximately 7 hours (McEvoy, 1999) because of an increase in urinary reabsorption.

Dosage

As a result of the short half-life of these agents, several long-acting dosage forms are available. The dosing of these agents is 5 to 10 mg 30 minutes to 1 hour before meals, and the last dose should be administered more than 6 hours before bedtime to minimize the side effect of insomnia. Because amphetamines display tachyphylaxis, tolerance may occur early on in therapy.

When they are used to treat obesity, these agents should be used at the lowest effective dose with intermittent courses of therapy. The dosage should not exceed 30 mg for dextroamphetamine or 25 mg for methamphetamine. A 3- to 6-week course of therapy followed by an "off" period of half the treatment time (e.g., 4 weeks of drug therapy followed by 2 weeks off, then 4 weeks on) is recommended.

Appetite Suppressants

The nonamphetamine derivatives are considered appetite suppressants. Other terms for these nonamphetamine agents include *anorectics* or *anorexigenics*. These agents (see **Table 54.3**) include diethylpropion (Tenuate), phendimetrazine (Bontril), and phentermine (Adipex-P). They are considered adjuncts to dietary restriction and an exercise program for weight loss. The effects of these agents are often short lived because tolerance may develop to the anorexigenic effect after a few weeks.

In 1992, an article on the long-term effects of a combination of anorexiants and amphetamine-like drugs on weight loss was published (Weintraub, et al., 1992). This article started the "fen-phen" craze of the 1990s. Citing 121 patients losing some 30 pounds each, the study touted the benefits of the combination of products. Each component, fenfluramine and phentermine (hence "fen-phen"), was an FDA-approved drug for treating obesity. However, because of reports of valvular heart disease (Connolly, et al., 1997) and primary pulmonary hypertension (Dillon, et al., 1997), fenfluramine and its dextrorotary congener, dexfenfluramine (Redux), have been voluntarily withdrawn from the market.

Mechanism of Action

The mechanism of action of appetite suppressants works to decrease appetite by stimulating the hypothalamus to release catecholamines, specifically norepinephrine and dopamine. The absorption of these drugs is not affected by food, and the primary route of elimination is renal. The drugs are considered short-acting agents, with half-lives ranging from 1.9 to 9.8 hours. For this reason, these agents are often dosed three times daily, but are also formulated in extended-release products for once-daily dosing. The dosing varies by individual response, but it is recommended to start at the lowest dose and increase based on weight loss and tolerance of adverse events.

Contraindications

All of these agents have a potential for abuse, and as such are classified as Schedule III (C-III) drugs. Caution should be used when prescribing these agents in patients with a history of substance abuse.

Because they lead to increased levels of norepinephrine and dopamine, these agents are contraindicated in patients taking monoamine oxidase (MAO) inhibitors. The combination may cause an increased pressor effect, resulting in hypertensive crisis.

Adverse Events

Adverse events include central nervous system (CNS) stimulation such as insomnia, tremor, and headache. Overstimulation may result in an impairment of ability to perform activities requiring mental alertness (e.g., driving or operating heavy machinery). Occasionally, urinary frequency, blurred vision, and changes in libido may occur.

Other adverse effects include dry mouth and nausea as well as cardiovascular effects such as increases in blood pressure and tachycardia. For this reason, blood pressure and heart rate should be monitored on a biweekly or monthly basis, and even more frequently in patients with preexisting hypertension. Caution should also be used when these agents are prescribed for patients with diabetes. The decrease in caloric intake may decrease a patient's blood glucose level, requiring adjustment of insulin or oral hypoglycemic agents.

Lipase Inhibitor: Orlistat

Orlistat (Xenical) differs from previously available weight-loss medications in that it works nonsystemically, acting locally in the gastrointestinal (GI) tract. Orlistat is a GI lipase inhibitor that facilitates weight loss by lowering the absorption of dietary fat, on average by 30%. In research, orlistat users saw small but significant drops in their total cholesterol, LDL, blood pressure, and blood sugar and insulin levels. Absorption of vitamins A, D, and E and β-carotene also was impaired.

The same meta-analysis that looked at the long-term efficacy of sibutramine for weight loss and improving health status also looked at orlistat. The analysis evaluated 16 double-blind, placebo-controlled trials with orlistat that were at least 1 year in duration. Patients taking orlistat lost 2.9% more weight than those taking a placebo. However, in the four studies that looked at a second year of weight maintenance, there was similar weight regain in both the orlistat and placebo groups, although the weight differential between the two treatment groups was maintained (Padwal, et al., 2003; Rucker, et al., 2007). However, it was noted that the orlistat group did decrease blood pressure, fasting glucose, and hemoglobin A1c levels in patients with diabetes or higher levels of total cholesterol, and LDL. In addition, one 4-year study demonstrated that the incidence of diabetes decreased by 37% in patients with impaired fasting glucose (Rucker, et al., 2007).

Dosage

Orlistat is available as a prescription or OTC medication. Prescription orlistat (Xenical) should be administered at a dose of 120 mg three times a day while OTC orlistat (Alli) should be administered at a dose of 60 mg three times a day. The doses should be taken during or up to 1 hour after a meal containing fat. The meal should contain less than 30% fat, and orlistat should not be taken with a meal containing no fat. The maximum daily dose is 360 mg/day. A primary concern with the use of orlistat is the potential for decreased absorption of the fat-soluble vitamins A, D, E, and K. Multivitamins should be taken by all patients taking orlistat, and these should be separated from the orlistat by 2 or more hours to ensure vitamin absorption.

Contraindications/Precautions

Orlistat is contraindicated in patients with chronic malabsorption syndrome or cholestasis. In addition, orlistat is not indicated in patients younger than age 12.

Adverse Events

Because orlistat is not absorbed, the primary side effects of orlistat include diarrhea, fatty stools, and flatulence. Patients should be advised of this because the fatty stools may appear as an oily leakage, particularly after flatus, and may cause embarrassment. Nausea and abdominal pain may also occur. GI effects associated with orlistat worsen with the more fat the dieter eats. However, data suggest that concomitant administration of natural fiber (psyllium mucilloid) may significantly reduce the self-reported frequency and severity of GI side effects associated with orlistat (Cavaliere, et al., 2001). Caution should be used in patients taking oral warfarin (Coumadin) because orlistat may inhibit the absorption of vitamin K, resulting in an increased international normalized ratio.

Rarely, orlistat can result in hepatotoxicity. Patients should be advised to stop using orlistat and contact their health care provider if they experience any signs or symptoms of liver injury, such as fatigue, fever, jaundice, brown urine, nausea, vomiting, and abdominal pain.

Other Medications

Some antidepressant, antiseizure, and diabetes medications have been studied for use in weight loss. The use of these medications for weight loss is considered an "off-label" use.

Antidepressants Many antidepressant medications have the unexpected side effect of weight loss. It is not clear how it aids in weight loss; it may limit appetite, or it may increase the basal metabolic rate. Because some people overeat when depressed, it may reduce food consumption secondary to depression. Studies of the antidepressants usually have found that patients lost moderate amounts of weight for up to 6 months. However, most studies indicate patients who lost weight while taking antidepressants tended to regain weight while they were still on drug therapy. The exception to this is bupropion (Wellbutrin), in which one study demonstrated weight loss maintenance for up to 1 year.

Antiseizure medications Two antiseizure medications have demonstrated weight loss: topiramate (Topamax) and zonisamide (Zonegran). These are currently being studied to better evaluate their potential use in the treatment of obesity.

Diabetes medications Metformin (Glucophage) has demonstrated the ability to help people with type 2 diabetes and obesity lose weight. It is uncertain how it works to promote weight loss, but it appears to decrease appetite.

The choice of one agent over another has not been well studied in controlled trials. The choice can be influenced by the formulary of the patient's health maintenance organization or the cost to the patient. Each agent may help curb a patient's appetite, but, as noted earlier, these agents are used only as adjuncts to therapy.

Selecting the Most Appropriate Agent

The selection of the most appropriate agent for treating an obese patient depends on a number of factors. Previous use of anorexiants or other weight-loss agents is essential to determine which agent the patient considers to be effective. In addition, the clinician must assess the abuse or dependency potential of the patient because of the controlled nature of the approved prescription agents. The side effect profile must be considered, particularly in patients with hypertension, arrhythmia, or stroke.

All pharmacotherapeutic treatment should be anchored with appropriate dietary restrictions and counseling as well as physical activity. The decreases in caloric intake and the increases in caloric expenditure associated with these behaviors are essential to the effective weight reduction associated with medications. It is important to keep in mind that the amount of weight loss obtained will vary with each individual, but it appears to be no more than 10% of initial weight no matter which agent is selected (Weigle, 2003).

First-Line Therapy

Orlistat has FDA approval for long-term maintenance of weight loss and should be considered for first-line therapy.

Second-Line Therapy

Appetite suppressants may be considered for second-line therapy, but caution regarding addiction and adverse effects must be taken into consideration.

Third-Line Therapy

No single agent is considered a third-line therapy, but surgery is often considered in patients with a BMI of 40 kg/m^2 or higher in whom dietary, physical, and pharmaceutical therapies have failed or in those with a BMI of 35 kg/m^2 or higher with obesity-related comorbidities.

Special Population Considerations

Smokers

Smoking in itself is a risk factor for cardiovascular disease. The additional burden of obesity places the obese smoker in a much higher risk category for long-term cardiovascular effects. Coupled with this is the increase in metabolism induced by smoking. The obese patient, who then quits smoking, runs the risk of gaining weight or thwarting efforts at weight loss. Special attention should be paid to this category of patient. A much greater level of attention should be paid to the lifestyle changes these patients need to make, and a continued reinforcement of the need for abstinence from smoking versus weight loss should be emphasized.

Ethnicity

There appears to be no specific relationship between ethnicity and response to drug therapy for weight loss. However, dietary changes and lifestyle changes, when offered, must be offered within the patient's cultural context.

Socioeconomic Status

Although obesity is a chronic disease with many adverse health consequences, it is a physical disability that is intensely stigmatized in our society. Many people, including some health care professionals, do not view obesity as a condition that deserves medical intervention or sympathy. Studies have shown a striking inverse relationship between obesity and socioeconomic status in the developed world, particularly among women (Gortmaker, et al., 1993). A research study performed by Gortmaker and colleagues found that being overweight during adolescence has a particularly detrimental effect on socioeconomic achievement. They studied the relationship between being overweight and education attainment, marital status, household income, and self-esteem in 10,039 randomly selected people ages 16 to 24 in 1981.

To assess the social consequences of obesity, the investigators compared disability from obesity with that associated with other forms of chronic illness. Seven years later, the overweight women were less educated, less likely to have been married, and had lower household incomes and 10% higher rates of household poverty than women who had not been overweight, independent of baseline socioeconomic status and aptitude test scores (Gortmaker, et al., 1993). Similar trends were also found among men, but the relationship was weaker. It has been said that obesity is due to low socioeconomic status, yet the results of this study indicate that the inverse is also true: low socioeconomic status is influenced by obesity (Gortmaker, et al., 1993).

MONITORING PATIENT RESPONSE

One of the most painful aspects of obesity may be the emotional suffering it causes. American society places great emphasis on physical appearance, often equating attractiveness with slimness, especially in women. The messages, intended or not, make overweight people feel unattractive. Therefore, obese individuals may suffer from social stigmatization, discrimination, and low self-esteem, which may also lead to depression. The social stigma of being obese has created a $40-billion-a-year weight-loss industry that preys on Americans' desire to be thin with weight-loss treatments, such as diets and dietary foods that are clearly ineffective, counterproductive, and associated with adverse effects.

Certain drugs that are used to treat conditions such as psychosis, depression, epilepsy, and diabetes can cause marked weight gain (Weigle, 2003). This may lead to decreased patient compliance with therapy or increased risk of adverse health outcomes. Newer drugs that treat these conditions are available, which cause less weight gain or even weight loss. Therefore, the patient's medication history should be monitored and adjusted as needed.

The patient should be monitored for weight loss, decreases in BMI, and changes in waist-to-hip ratios. In addition, patients taking appetite suppressants, serotonin and norepinephrine reuptake inhibitors, or amphetamines should have their blood pressure monitored at least monthly, if not biweekly. Weight loss should not be faster than 1 to 2 lb/wk over a sustained period, usually 6 or more months. During this period, empiric evidence (NIH, 1998) suggests that frequent visits to a health care practitioner, with reinforcement of dietary and lifestyle changes, improve weight loss and maintenance of weight loss.

PATIENT EDUCATION

Patients should be educated that obesity is more than just a cosmetic problem. It is a health hazard. Someone who is 40% overweight is twice as likely to die prematurely as an average-weight person. This effect is seen after 10 to 30 years of being obese. Research evidence indicates that a sedentary lifestyle confers an even greater risk than being overweight (Wickelgren, 1998).

Dieting as a way of weight loss is not only ineffective but risky. Severely energy-restricted or unbalanced diets are linked to deficiency syndromes, gallstones, arrhythmias, and sudden cardiac death. Even balanced diets lead to chronic fatigue, impaired concentration, cold intolerance, mood changes, and malaise as weight drops below the set point. Cycles of dietary deprivation followed by refeeding ("yo-yo" dieting) may contribute to hypertension, congestive heart failure, and peripheral edema. Yo-yo dieting may enhance metabolic efficiency, thus promoting weight gain. It may also lead to low self-esteem as the dieter fails either to lose weight or maintain weight loss (Weigle, 1990).

Patients should be educated on the fact that obesity has been linked to several serious medical conditions, such as diabetes, heart disease, high blood pressure, and stroke. It is also associated with higher rates of certain types of cancer. Obese men are more likely than nonobese men to die from cancer of the colon, rectum, and prostate. Obese women are more likely than nonobese women to die from cancer of the gallbladder, breast, uterus, cervix, and ovaries.

For more information regarding obesity, practitioners and patients should contact the following organizations or visit their Web sites. The Web site addresses listed below will direct people to the obesity section of the organization's Web site:

The Obesity Society
8630 Fenton Street
Suite 814
Silver Spring, MD 20910
301-563-6526
www.obesity.org

Centers for Disease Control and Prevention
1600 Clifton Road
Atlanta, GA 30333
800-232-4636
www.cdc.gov/obesity/

National Institutes of Health
9000 Rockville Pike
Bethesda, MD 20892
301-496-4000
http://health.nih.gov/topic/obesity

WHO Regional Office for the Americas
525 23rd Street, NW
Washington, DC 20037
202-974-3000
www.who.int/health_topics/obesity/en/

The Surgeon General
Office of the Surgeon General
5600 Fishers Lane
Room 18-66
Rockville, MD 20857
301-443-4000
www.surgeongeneral.gov/topics/obesity/

Case Study

A. P. is a 34-year-old woman who comes into your clinic looking for a medication to help her lose weight. She states that she has tried several times to lose weight but seems to gain it back within months after stopping her dieting. She tried fen-phen a few years ago with some success, but stopped the drug therapy when she heard about the heart problems. She informs you that she has had a follow-up test and that there were no problems found with her heart.

Your workup reveals a normal, young, well-developed woman in no acute distress. She is 66 inches tall and weighs 179 lb. She has no abnormal laboratory values, including a cholesterol level of 187 mg/dL. Her blood pressure is somewhat elevated at 138/87. She has no other pertinent medical history, no allergies to medications, and she takes only birth control pills. She does not smoke or drink alcohol. She works as a secretary in an office. She has a BMI of 29 kg/m².

DIAGNOSIS: OBESITY

1. What would be a good weight goal for A. P.? What BMI?
2. What dietary and lifestyle changes should be recommended to A. P.?
3. What drug therapy would you prescribe? Why?
4. What would you monitor for and how often would you monitor these parameters?
5. Describe one or two drug–drug or drug–food interactions for the selected agent.
6. What patient education would you provide based on the prescribed therapy?
7. Describe one or two adverse reactions for the selected agent that would cause you to change therapy.
8. If one of these occurred, what would be the choice for the second-line therapy?
9. What OTC or alternative medications would be appropriate for this patient?

BIBLIOGRAPHY

*Starred references are cited in the text.

Campfield, L. A., Smith, F. J., & Burn, P. (1998). Strategies and potential molecular targets for obesity treatment. *Science, 280,* 1383–1387.

Camuzzie, A. C., & Allison, D. B. (1998). The search for human obesity genes. *Science, 280,* 1374–1377.

Carek, P. J., et al. (1997). Management of obesity: Medical treatment options. *American Family Physician, 55*(2), 551–558, 561–562.

*Cavaliere, H., Floriano, I., & Medeiros-Neto, G. (2001). Gastrointestinal side effects of orlistat may be prevented by concomitant prescription of natural fibers (psyllium mucilloid). *International Journal of Obesity Related Metabolic Disorders, 25,* 1095–1099.

*Connolly, H. M., Crary, J. L., McGoon, M. D., et al. (1997). Valvular heart disease associated with fenfluramine-phentermine (Fen-phen). *New England Journal of Medicine, 337,* 581–588.

*Dillon, K. A., Putnam, K. G., & Avorn, J. L. (1997). Death from irreversible pulmonary hypertension associated with short-term use of fenfluramine and phentermine (Letter). *Journal of the American Medical Association, 278,* 132.

Duke, J. (1997). *The green pharmacy.* Emmaus, PA: Rodale Press.

Expert Panel on the Identification, Evaluation, and Treatment of Overweight and Obesity in Adults. (1998). Executive summary of the clinical guidelines on the identification, evaluation and treatment of overweight and obesity in adults. *Archives of Internal Medicine, 158,* 1855–1867.

*Flegal, K. M., Carroll, M. D., Ogden, C. L., et al. (2010). Prevalence and trends in obesity among U.S. adults 1999–2008. *Journal of the American Medical Association, 303,* 235–241.

*Gortmaker, S. L., et al. (1993). Social and economic consequences of overweight in adolescence and young adulthood. *New England Journal of Medicine, 329,* 1008–1012.

Hebel, S. K. (Ed.). (1999). Anorexiants. *Drug facts and comparisons.* St. Louis: Facts and Comparisons.

Hill, J. O. (1998). Environmental contributions to the obesity epidemic. *Science, 280,* 1371–1373.

Hollander, P. (2003). Orlistat in the treatment of obesity. *Primary Care in Clinical and Office Practice, 30,* 427–440.

*James, P. T., Leach, R., Kalamara, E., et al. (2001). The worldwide obesity epidemic. *Obesity Research, 9*(Suppl. 5), S228–S233.

Kiberstis, P. A., & Marx, J. (1998). Regulation of body weight. *Science, 280,* 1363.

Lexi-Comp Online™, Lexi-Drugs Online™, Hudson, Ohio: Lexi-Comp, Inc.; 2010; August 11, 2010.

*McEvoy, G. K. (Ed.). (1999). *AHFS drug information 99.* Bethesda, MD: American Society of Health-System Pharmacists.

Micromedex® Healthcare Series [intranet database]. Version 2.0. Greenwood Village, CO: Thomson Healthcare.

*National Institute of Diabetes and Digestive and Kidney Diseases. (2000). Overweight, obesity, and health risk. *Archives of Internal Medicine, 160,* 898–904.

*National Institutes of Health. (1998). *Clinical guidelines on the identification, evaluation, and treatment of overweight and obesity in adults.* (NIH Publication No. 98-4083). Bethesda, MD: Author. Available at http://www.nhlbi.nih.gov/guidelines/obesity/ob_gdlns.pdf. Accessed August 4, 2010.

*National Institutes of Health. (2000). *The practical guide: Identification, evaluation and treatment of overweight and obesity in adults.* (NIH Publication No. 00-4084). Bethesda, MD: Author. Available at http://www.nhlbi.nih.gov/guidelines/obesity/prctgd_c.pdf. Accessed August 4, 2010.

National Institutes of Health. (2007a). *Do you know the health risks of being overweight?* (NIH Publication No. 03-4098). Bethesda, MD: Author.

Available at http://www.niddk.nih.gov/health/nutrit/pubs/health.htm. Accessed August 4, 2010.

National Institutes of Health. (2007b). *Prescription medications for the treatment of obesity* (NIH Publication No. 97-4191). Bethesda, MD: Author. Available at http://www.niddk.nih.gov/health/nutrit/pubs/presmeds.htm. Accessed August 4, 2010.

National Institutes of Health. (2008). *Understanding adult obesity* (NIH Publication No. 01-3680). Bethesda, MD: Author. Available at http://www.niddk.nih.gov/health/nutrit/pubs/unders.htm #tables. Accessed August 4, 2010.

*National Institutes of Health. (2010). *Overweight and obesity statistics.* (NIH Publication No. 04-4158). Bethesda, MD: Author. Available at http://www.nhlbi.nih.gov/guidelines/obesity/ob_home.htm. Accessed August 11, 2010.

*Nonas, C. A. (1998). A model for chronic care of obesity through dietary treatment. *Journal of the American Dietetic Association, 98*(Suppl. 2), S16–S22.

*Ogden, C.L., Carroll, M.D., Curtin L.R., et al. (2006). Prevalence of overweight and obesity in the United States, 1999–2004. *Journal of the American Medical Association, 295,* 1549–1555.

*Ogden, C. L., Flegal, K. M., Carroll, M. D., et al. (2002). Prevalence and trends in overweight among U.S. children and adolescents 1999–2000. *Journal of the American Medical Association, 288,* 1728–1732.

*Padwal R., Li, S. K., & Lau, D. C. (2003). Long-term pharmacotherapy for obesity and overweight. *Cochrane Database of Systematic Reviews,* CD004094.

*Racette, S. B., Deusinger, S. S., & Deusinger, R. H. (2003). Obesity: Overweight prevalence, etiology, and treatment. *Physical Therapy, 83,* 276–288.

*Rucker, D., Padwal, R., Li, S. K., et al. (2007). Long term pharmacotherapy for obesity and overweight: Updated meta-analysis. *British Medical Journal, 335,* 1194–1199.

*Sheperd, T. M. (2003). Effective management of obesity. *Journal of Family Practice, 52,* 34–42.

*Taubes, G. (1998). As obesity rates rise, experts struggle to explain why. *Science, 280,* 1367–1368.

*U.S. Department of Health and Human Services. (2001). *The Surgeon General's call to action to prevent and decrease overweight and obesity.* Rockville, MD. Available at http://www.surgeongeneral.gov/topics/obesity/calltoaction/factsheet03.pdf. Accessed August 11, 2010.

U.S. Department of Health and Human Services. (2010). *The Surgeon General's vision for a healthy and fit nation fact sheet.* Rockville, MD. Available at http://www.surgeongeneral.gov/library/obesityvision/obesityvision_factsheet.html. Accessed August 10, 2010.

*Vidal, J. (2002). Updated review on the benefits of weight loss. *International Journal of Obesity, 26*(Suppl. 4), S25–S28.

*Weigle, D. S. (1990). Human obesity: Exploding the myths. *Western Journal of Medicine, 153,* 421–428.

*Weigle, D. S. (2003). Pharmacological therapy of obesity: Past, present, and future. *Journal of Clinical Endocrinology and Metabolism, 88,* 2462–2469.

*Weintraub, M., et al. (1992). Long-term weight control: National Heart, Lung, and Blood Institute–funded multi-modal intervention study—Conclusions. *Clinical Pharmacology and Therapeutics, 51,* 642–646.

*Wickelgren, I. (1998). Obesity: How big a problem? *Science, 280,* 1364–1367.

*Williamson, D. F., Thompson, T. J., Thun, M., et al. (2000). Intentional weight loss and mortality among overweight individuals with diabetes. *Diabetes Care, 23,* 1499–1504.

*World Health Organization. (2005). *Obesity and overweight: Fact sheet.* Available at: http://www.who.int/mediacentre/factsheets/fs311/en/print.html. Accessed August 4, 2010.

Yaes, R. J. (1993). Futility and avoidance: Medical professionals in the treatment of obesity. *Journal of the American Medical Association, 270,* 1423.

Women's Health

Contraception

Contraception is the inhibition of pregnancy by a process, device, or method. The U.S. Food and Drug Administration (FDA) first approved oral contraception (OC), the use of hormones to prevent pregnancy, in the 1960s, and the last law prohibiting its use in the United States was overturned in 1973 (Speroff & Darney, 2000). Regardless of the type used, one of contraception's major benefits is its potential impact on the rate of unplanned pregnancies. Current estimates are that approximately half of all pregnancies in the United States are unintended. Of these, about 42% are aborted (Espey, et al., 2008). Unintended pregnancies that continue, including both unwanted and mistimed pregnancies, are positively associated with late-entry prenatal care, low birth weight, child abuse or neglect, and behavioral problems in children. One way a decrease in unintended pregnancies may be achieved is through the increased awareness of contraception and the various available options.

The widespread use of contraception in health care in the United States has expanded opportunities for women. Its use has allowed women to take on roles beyond (or in addition to) motherhood. Contraception has increased women's ability to decide when pregnancy and subsequent child-rearing will occur.

Data from 1995 illustrated that 93% of women in the United States between ages 15 and 44 years used some form of contraception. Studies have shown that age and desire for future pregnancy greatly influence a woman's method of choice. Reversible forms of contraception are the regimens of choice among most women planning future pregnancies. Oral, transdermal, and vaginal hormonal contraception are a first choice because return of fertility after discontinuing use is expected. At 48 months after discontinuing this regimen, 82% of patients ages 30 to 34 have given birth. Among women ages 25 to 29, the pregnancy rate is 92% at the same time after discontinuation (Speroff & Darney, 2000).

PHYSIOLOGY

A woman's ability to reproduce begins after she has completed the developmental stage of puberty. The average age of the onset of puberty is 11.2 years, whereas the length of time for the completion of this process is 4 years. Menarche, the last

step in the pubertal process, is when menses commences. The average age for menarche is 12.7 years.

The cause or trigger for the onset of puberty is not completely understood. It is thought that a decreased sensitivity of the hypothalamus and pituitary glands to already circulating sex hormones results in an increased production of luteinizing hormone (LH) and follicle-stimulating hormone (FSH). Increased LH and FSH further stimulate the gonadal response of increased secretion of estrogen, progesterone, and testosterone. LH subsequently surges, inciting the release of ova. In the absence of fertilization, menses ensues.

A woman's menstrual cycle can be described in terms of either the follicular or luteal phase. In addition, in each of these phases, endometrial, ovarian, and pituitary hormone-secreting changes occur. These two major phases and the physiologic changes occurring in each are illustrated in **Figure 55-1**.

The endometrial changes can be subdivided. Menstruation, occurring on days 1 to 4 of the menstrual cycle, is the shedding of the endometrial lining. The next three phases are the proliferative phase (day 4 or 5 through ovulation), the secretory phase (immediately after ovulation), and the implantation phase (approximately days 21 to 27). During these phases, the endometrial lining is prepared for implantation of a fertilized ovum. In the event that an ovum does not implant, the next phase, endometrial breakdown, begins once again.

Relative to the ovarian changes that occur during the menstrual cycle, three major subdivisions can be identified: the follicular, ovulatory, and luteal phases. During the follicular phase, a dominant follicle is produced that will be released and await possible fertilization. The regulatory hormone largely responsible for this portion of the ovarian phase of the menstrual cycle is FSH. FSH stimulates the conversion of androgens to estrogen in the granulosa cells of the ovaries. Stimulation by FSH contributes to the development of a dominant follicle that produces further estrogen. The overall increase in estrogen production stimulates development of the glandular epithelium of the uterine lining, increases cervical mucus production and reduces the viscosity of this mucus, and increases vaginal pH.

Opposing the normal negative feedback mode of the menstrual cycle, in which high concentrations of estrogen inhibit the release of FSH and LH, the eventual peak in estrogen in this late follicular phase stimulates a surge in LH. The

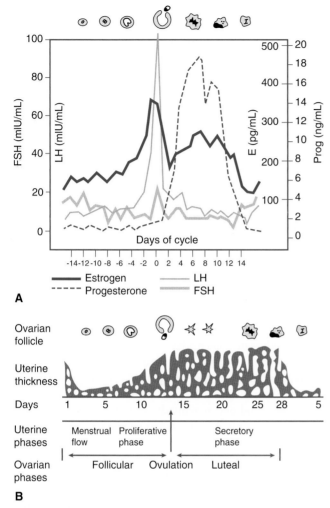

FIGURE 55–1 Comparison of the phases of the reproductive cycle. **A.** Plasma hormone concentrations in the normal female reproductive cycle. **B.** Ovarian events and uterine changes during the menstrual cycle. (From Bullock, B. A., & Henze, R. L. [2000]. *Focus on pathophysiology.* Philadelphia: Lippincott Williams & Wilkins, p. 1100.)

LH surge is subsequently responsible for the final maturation, release, and rupture of the dominant follicle. Follicular rupture and ovulation occur approximately 24 to 36 hours after the beginning of the LH surge and encompass the ovulatory phase of the menstrual cycle.

After the ovulatory phase, the luteal phase of the menstrual cycle enables the implantation of a fertilized ovum and maintenance of the uterine lining. The corpus luteum that remains after the follicle ruptures, releasing the ovum, secretes progesterone and 17-β-estradiol. The secretion of these hormones increases the secretory activity of the endometrial glands. Cervical mucus also increases in viscosity. In the event that pregnancy occurs, the life of the corpus luteum is extended to continue production of these hormones. In the absence of pregnancy, the corpus luteum dies, estrogen and progesterone levels decline, and menstruation occurs.

INITIATING DRUG THERAPY

Given the normal menstrual cycle, pregnancy can be inhibited by preventing fertilization, manipulating hormones of the menstrual cycle such that ovulation never occurs, or interfering with implantation. Contraceptive options may be nonpharmacologic or pharmacologic. **Table 55.1** identifies these options and the failure rates of each.

Nonpharmacologic options include periodic abstinence, barrier devices, and intrauterine devices (IUDs) and systems. Periodic abstinence, which means avoiding sexual intercourse during the period of maximum fertility, includes several assumptions. First, the viability of sperm in the female reproductive tract is 2 to 7 days. Second, the life span of the ovum is 1 to 3 days. It is assumed, therefore, that the period of maximum fertility occurs in the 5 days before ovulation and ends on the day of ovulation. Prediction of ovulation is important in recognizing the dates to avoid sexual intercourse. Several methods may be incorporated into the periodic abstinence method to identify better the time of ovulation. Examples include the use of ovulation predictor kits, monitoring of basal body temperature, and testing of cervical mucus. The increase in progesterone concentration just before the LH surge is accompanied by a 0.4°F to 0.8°F increase in basal body temperature. The woman measures her body temperature orally with a basal thermometer just before arising from bed daily. She also may observe cervical mucus as a guide to predicting ovulation. Midcycle cervical mucus, just before ovulation, is clear, thin, and stringy. Peak mucus production occurs on the day of ovulation. After this, the mucus becomes sticky and wet. Intercourse, with a low presumed risk of pregnancy, is permitted beginning on the fourth day of this sticky, wet mucus.

Other nonpharmacologic options for the prevention of pregnancy include the use of barrier devices such as condoms, diaphragms, and cervical caps. These options vary not only

TABLE 55.1	Contraceptive Options and Rates of Failure
Contraceptive Method	**Failure Rates**[*]
Cervical cap	9%–32%
Combination oral contraceptive pills	0.3%–8%
Condom and spermicides	2%–21%
Depot medroxyprogesterone acetate	0.3%–3%
Diaphragm and spermicides	6%–18%
Intrauterine device	0.6%–2%
Mirena	0.5%–3%
Ortho-evac patch	0.3%
Periodic abstinence	1%–25%
Progesterone mini pills	0.5%–3%
Sterilization	0.1%–0.4%

*Ranges may vary depending on typical or perfect use.

in their efficacy rates but in their abilities to prevent sexually transmitted infections (STIs). The male latex condom helps to prevent the spread of human papillomavirus and many other STIs. It is the only contraceptive option clinically proven to prevent the spread of the human immunodeficiency virus (HIV). The female condom has been shown to act as a barrier to most STIs. However, limitations include its cost, decrease in spontaneity, and improper placement.

The diaphragm and cervical cap are both devices that require fitting by a health care provider. The woman can insert a diaphragm up to 6 hours before intercourse and must leave it in place for at least 6 hours (but no more than 24 hours) after intercourse. The diaphragm has been shown to reduce the risk of cervical gonorrhea, pelvic inflammatory disease (PID), and tubal infertility secondary to STIs. It is not, however, effective against HIV infection, and urinary tract infections are twice as common in diaphragm users compared with nonusers. Comparably, the cervical cap may be left in place for a total of 48 hours. It must remain in place, however, for at least 8 hours after sexual intercourse. Like the diaphragm, it has not been shown to afford any protection against HIV infection.

The third major type of nonpharmacologic contraception is the IUD. Although its mechanism of action is not clearly understood, it is thought to prevent pregnancy through production of a "spermicidal intrauterine environment." The intrauterine environment is rendered unreceptive to sperm or the implantation of a fertilized ovum should fertilization occur. Progesterone-implanted intrauterine systems have also begun to be used. In addition to the proposed mechanism of the IUD, the continued release of progesterone contributes to the contraceptive action of this device through production of viscous cervical mucus, which further impedes the sperm's ability to reach the ovum.

Goals of Drug Therapy

In addition to, or in place of, the nonpharmacologic contraceptive options available, pharmacologic options do exist. The primary mechanism by which these agents prevent pregnancy is through manipulation of the normal menstrual cycle, effects on cervical mucus, or both. Estrogen plus progesterone or progesterone alone is used to interfere with the process of ovulation, conception, or both. Optimal contraception features, as defined by the World Health Organization include:

- safety
- effectiveness
- convenience
- regular bleeding episodes
- rapid reversibility.

Combined (Estrogen and Progestin) Oral, Transdermal, and Vaginal Contraceptives

These prescription methods use a "combination" of two hormones—estrogen and progesterone. All combination methods work primarily by preventing ovulation. They are highly effective when taken every day, with perfect use failure rates of less than 1%. However, the typical failure rate of combination birth control pills is 3% to 8% and much higher in some populations. They also have several noncontraceptive benefits, including reducing the risk of endometriosis, ovulatory pain, ovarian cysts, benign breast disease, premenstrual syndrome, premenstrual dysphoric disorder, and ovarian and endometrial cancer. They also might improve acne, hirsutism, and other manifestations of polycystic ovary syndrome. The improvement occurs secondary to an increase in the level of sex-hormone-binding globulin, which reduces circulating free testosterone and ameliorates many androgenic effects.

The combination contraceptive agents contain estrogen, usually in the form of ethinyl estradiol. Doses of estrogen range from 20 to 35 mg; 98% of all prescribed OCs contain less than 35 mg of estrogen, and even OCs with as little as 20 mg of estrogen are considered effective. Pills with low estrogen content are considered safer than higher-dose OCs for certain patients, including perimenopausal women, those with a family history of heart disease, and smokers younger than age 35 (although women who take OCs and smoke remain at an increased risk of myocardial infarction [MI] and stroke due to OC-associated changes in coagulation factors). Progesterone is in the form of desogestrel, ethynodiol diacetate, levonorgestrel, norethindrone, norethindrone acetate, norgestimate, or norgestrel. A synthetic progesterone (drospirenone [DRSP]) is also available. It has antiandrogenic and antimineralocorticoid properties. It is associated with less water retention than other progesterones, less negative emotional affect, and less appetite increase after 6 months of use.

The mechanism of action of combination contraceptive agents is the suppression of the pituitary gonadotropins FSH and LH by the continued high concentrations of circulating estrogen and progesterone. The suppression of LH, primarily by the progesterone component, inhibits the LH surge responsible for ovulation. Progesterone also exerts its influence through its effects on increasing cervical mucus viscosity, thus impairing sperm transport. FSH suppression, largely through estrogen's influence, prevents the selection and emergence of a dominant follicle. Therefore, the combination of estrogen and progesterone inhibits selection of a dominant follicle and ovulation.

In addition to their influence on the reproductive cycle, the hormones used in OC pills (OCPs) exert other actions. All forms of progesterone exhibit some estrogenic, androgenic, or anabolic activity. For example, highly androgenic forms of progesterone affect lipid and carbohydrate metabolism and promote the appearance of acne, weight gain, and hirsutism. As such, practitioners should consider the various progesterone formulations relative to their androgenic effects when choosing an OCP regimen. The least androgenic forms include the newer, third-generation progesterones desogestrel and norgestimate. In addition to their relative lack of androgenic side effects, they are also more potent than the other progesterones norethindrone, norethindrone acetate, ethynodiol diacetate, and norgestrel.

Knowledge of the differences in the progesterone formulations becomes important when managing (or prospectively avoiding) certain side effects of OCPs.

A common myth is that OCPs reduce the effectiveness of antibiotics or vice versa. In fact, the only antibiotic that may reduce pill effectiveness is rifampin, an antibiotic reserved for specific circumstances and not commonly used. Similarly, many believe that anticonvulsants reduce the efficacy of OCs, an unlikely association. Although anticonvulsants may reduce the level of serum hormones, they have not been observed to be associated with increased incidence of ovulation or accidental pregnancy.

Many options exist when choosing an OC regimen for a patient. In general, combination OCPs are divided into monophasic, biphasic, and triphasic combinations. **Tables 55.2** and **55.3** list the available formulations. Monophasic combinations provide a set amount of estrogen and progesterone daily for 21 days. Placebo or nothing is given on days 22 to 28, the days during which a woman menstruates. The monophasic combinations may be useful in managing adverse effects such as breakthrough vaginal bleeding. Also, women who are sensitive to fluctuations in hormone levels that occur with the biphasic and triphasic OCPs may respond more positively to the monophasic formulations. Side effects, including breast tenderness, nausea, headaches, and bloating, are usually limited to the first 1 to 2 months of use, but may discourage continuation. A backup method of birth control, such as condoms, should be used for the first week after pills are started. Few clinical differences have been noted among the myriad different pill formulations (monophasic, biphasic, triphasic, different generation progestins, and other formulations), so it is reasonable to prescribe a generic monophasic pill containing 30 to 35 mcg of estrogen for most patients.

A variation to the traditional monophasic OCP has been introduced. This formulation provides a constant amount of estrogen and progesterone daily on days 1 to 21. The woman takes placebo tablets on days 22 to 23. On days 24 to 28, a lower dose of estrogen alone is given. The rationale for providing estrogen on days 24 to 28 is to help manage problems in women who may have exhibited symptoms of estrogen deficiency during the traditional week-long placebo period. This includes, for example, women who experience rebound headaches in the absence of estrogen during days 22 to 28.

The biphasic and triphasic OCP combinations were developed to mimic more closely the normal fluctuations in hormones experienced during the menstrual cycle. Changes in the estrogen or progesterone components occur every 7 to 10 days in these products. The phasic OCPs have not been shown to have any proven advantages in efficacy over the monophasic products. The major difference between the biphasic and triphasic regimens and the monophasic regimens is the net amount of progesterone delivered per cycle. The biphasic and triphasic regimens contain, in general, less progesterone. (See **Tables 55.2** and **55.3**.) Therefore, for women experiencing progesterone-related side effects, changing to a regimen containing lower doses of a product with less androgenic effects may be most beneficial.

Extended-cycle OCPs are now available. During the standard 7-day hormone-free interval that occurs with the use of low-dose estrogen formulations, the function of the hypothalamic-pituitary-ovarian axis recovers rapidly, and this increases the risk of ovarian follicle development, ovulation with unintended pregnancy, and increased spotting due to endogenous estradiol production. Fluctuating hormone levels allow endometrial buildup and can exacerbate premenstrual symptoms and menstrual headaches by creating hormone excess and withdrawal states. Extended-cycle OCPs with a shorter or eliminated hormone-free interval reduce the risk of these unwanted effects by preventing endogenous estradiol production while still providing highly effective and safe contraception.

When initiating therapy for patients, a contraceptive regimen is started relative to the woman's menstrual cycle. One can either initiate a day 1 start or a Sunday start regimen. Women who follow a day 1 start regimen begin the contraceptive agent on the first day of their period, regardless of the day of the week. Likewise, women who follow Sunday start regimens

TABLE 55.2	Monophasic Contraception
Brand Name	**Hormonal Components**
Alesse, Aviane, Lessina	20 μg EE, 0.1 mg levonorgestrel
Brevicon	35 μg EE, 0.5 mg norethindrone
Apri, Desogen, Ortho-cept	30 μg EE, 0.15 mg desogestrel
Kelnor 1/35	35 μg EE, 1 mg ethynodiol diacetate
Levlen, Nordette, Portia	30 μg EE, 0.15 mg levonorgestrel
Loestrin 1/20	20 μg EE, 1.0 mg norethindrone acetate
Loestrin 1.5/30	30 μg EE, 1.5 mg norethindrone acetate
Lo-Ovral, Crysette	30 μg EE, 0.3 mg norgestrel
Norethin 1/35E	35 μg EE, 1 mg norethindrone
Norinyl 1 + 35	35 μg EE, 1 mg norethindrone
Notrel 0.5/35	35 μg EE, 0.5 mg norethindrone
Ocella, Yasmin	30 μg EE, 3 mg drospirenone
Ortho-Cyclen	35 μg EE, 0.25 mg norgestimate
Ortho-Novum 1/35, Notrel	35 μg EE, 1 mg norethindrone
Ortho-Novum 1/50, Norinyl 1+50	50 μg EE, 1 mg norethindrone
Ovcon 35	35 μg EE, 0.4 mg norethindrone
Ovcon 50	50 μg EE, 1 mg norethindrone
Ovral	50 μg EE, 0.5 mg norgestrel
Seasonale	30 μg EE, 0.15 mg levonorgestrel
Yaz	20 μg EE, 3 mg drospirenone
Extended Cycle	
Jolessa, Seasonale	30 μg EE, 0.15 mg levonorgestrel
Lybrel	20 μg EE, 0.09 mg levonorgestrel

EE, ethinyl estradiol.

TABLE 55.3	Biphasic and Triphasic Oral Contraceptive Pills
Brand Name	**Hormonal Components**
Biphasic Oral Contraceptive Pills	
Kariva, Mircette	20/10 µg EE, 15 mg desogestrel
Ortho-Novum 10/11	35/35 µg EE, 0.5/1 mg norethindrone
Triphasic Oral Contraceptive Pills	
Cyclessa, Velivet	25/25/25 30 µg EE, 0.1/0.125/0.15 mg desogestrel
Estrostep	20/30/35 µg EE, 1 mg norethindrone acetate
Ortho-Novum 7/7/7, Nortrel 7/7/7	35/35/35 µg EE, 0.5/0.75/1 mg norethindrone
Ortho Tri-Cyclen, Tri-Previfem, Tri-Sprintec	35/35/35 µg EE, 0.18/0.215/0.25 mg norgestimate
Tri-Levlen, Triphasil, Enpresse	30/40/30 µg EE, 0.05/0.075/0.125 mg levonorgestrel
Tri-Norinyl, Aranelle	35/35/35 µg EE, 0.5/1/0.5 mg norethindrone
Triphasil	30/40/30 µg EE, 0.05/0.075/0.125 mg levonorgestrel
Extended Cycle	
Seasonique	30/10/30 µg EE, 0.15 mg levonorgestrel

EE, ethinyl estradiol.

begin the OCP pack on the Sunday directly after the onset of menses. This means that the woman will not menstruate on a weekend, which is desirable to many patients. OCP packs are produced with the Sunday start regimen in mind. In the event that a patient is a day 1 start, the pharmacist places a special label on the pack noting the beginning day of the pack and the end. The situation in which the day 1 versus Sunday start becomes an issue is relative to missed doses, which is discussed later in the chapter.

Another form of contraception is the transdermal patch containing 75 mcg of ethinyl estradiol and 6 mg of norelgestromin. The hormones are absorbed through the skin. The patch can be applied to the abdomen, buttocks, upper outer arm, or upper torso on clean, dry, healthy skin free of lotions. The patient can bathe, shower, or swim while wearing the patch. A new patch is applied each week, worn for 7 days, and removed and replaced with a new patch. During the fourth week, no patch is worn. The first patch should be applied on the first day of menses and a new one on the same day the next week. Detachment has been shown in only 5% of cases, but if it becomes loose or falls off, it must be replaced with a new patch. If the patch is off for more than 24 hours, a new cycle is started and backup methods of birth control used for the next 7 days.

The most frequent complaint from users of the patch is reactions at the application site. Women who weigh more than 198 lb may experience a higher failure rate and should use a different form of contraception.

Combination contraceptive vaginal rings are also available. The NuvaRing is a flexible transparent device inserted into the vagina by the patient. It releases 15 mcg of ethinyl estradiol and 120 mcg of etonogestrel daily. It is removed after 3 weeks for 1 week and a new ring is inserted. Lower hormonal doses are required with the vaginal ring because

there is no hepatic or gastrointestinal (GI) interference. It can remain in place during bathing, swimming, and intercourse.

It has been shown that there is a mean of 5.88 cycles for conception following discontinuation of combined OC (Stenchever, et al., 2001).

Progestin-Only Hormonal Contraceptives

Progesterone alone to prevent pregnancy may be used in the dosage formulations of oral tablets, intramuscular injections, or subdermal implants. Regardless of the formulation, they are the hormonal contraceptive options of choice in women who cannot take or cannot tolerate estrogen-containing formulations. They are a better choice for women with problems, such as high blood pressure or smoking over age 35, which may be negatively impacted by estrogen-containing pills. The progestin-only pill is often recommended for breast-feeding women. In ease of administration, compliance, and efficacy, however, the formulations vary greatly.

The progesterone-only contraceptive pill, commonly referred to as the *mini-pill*, contains a very low dose of progesterone. **Table 55.4** lists the available formulations and active components of each. The mini-pills do not consistently sup-

TABLE 55.4	Progesterone-Only Oral Contraceptive Pills
Brand Name	**Hormonal Component**
Micronor, Camila, Errin, Nor-QD	0.35 mg norethindrone
Ovrette	0.075 mg norgestrel

press the pituitary gonadotropins LH and FSH. Their primary effect is exerted through changing the endometrial and cervical mucus environments. The time from dosing to changes in the cervical mucus is 2 to 4 hours. The impermeability of the mucus declines 22 hours after the dose. Therefore, to help ensure maximum efficacy, it is imperative that the woman take the pill at exactly the same time daily. Recommendations are that if the dose is more than 3 hours late, the woman should use a backup form of contraception. When beginning the mini-pill, the woman should start on the first day of menses and use backup contraception for the first 7 days. The woman takes the mini-pill daily without a placebo week, as is exercised with the combination OCPs.

The FDA approved the use of intramuscularly injected medroxyprogesterone acetate (depo MPA) in 1992. The dose of depo MPA used suppresses ovulation in addition to affecting cervical mucus. Depo MPA is dosed every 13 weeks and is a good choice for women for whom daily compliance with a combination or progesterone-only OCP is an issue. When beginning depo MPA, recommendations are that it be given within the first 5 days of the onset of menses. It can be given to women postpartum and to those who are breast-feeding. Subsequent doses must be given no later than 13 weeks from the prior dose to ensure efficacy. If a woman presents later than 13 weeks for her next injection, the provider needs to determine that the patient is not pregnant before administering the drug.

Depo-Provera is safe for women with a history of cardiovascular disease, stroke, thromboembolism, or peripheral vascular disease. It is ideal for women with hemoglobinopathies, such as sickle cell disease, because these women will likely notice a decrease in painful hemolytic crises.

In addition to the positive compliance effects of this dosage formulation, women wishing future pregnancy also frequently prefer depo MPA. On discontinuation of depo MPA, 70% of women conceive within the first year and 90% within 24 months. Limitations to the use of depo MPA include the occurrence of menstrual changes in most women and episodes of unpredictable bleeding lasting more than 7 days. The latter problem occurs more commonly in the first few months of therapy. Depo-Provera reduces serum estradiol levels, and this can adversely affect bone health. Bone loss was reversible with discontinuation of Depo-Provera. The practitioner should recommend that Depo-Provera users exercise regularly and increase their intake of calcium and vitamin D.

The Intrauterine System

Another form of contraception is intrauterine systems (IUSs). One is Mirena, which is inserted by the clinician into the patient's uterine cavity to prevent pregnancy. It contains levonorgestrel, which is released at 20 mg/day into the uterine lining; it thickens the cervical mucus, suppresses ovarian function, and inhibits sperm movement. It also thins the uterine lining, making it an unfavorable environment

for implantation. The IUS is approved for as long as 5 years of continuous use. Because the IUS contains no estrogen component, it is appropriate for women in whom estrogen is contraindicated. The IUS may also be an effective treatment for women with dysmenorrhea, menorrhagia, and anemia and may serve as an effective transition from contraception to hormone replacement therapy. Little maintenance is required. The patient must check the string after each menstrual period to ensure that it is still in place. For women who choose to become pregnant, the device can be removed by the clinician at any time; no waiting period is required before conception, and IUS use is not associated with a decline in fertility. This system has been shown to lessen dysmenorrhea and bleeding.

Also available is the standard copper-containing IUD, but greater dysmenorrhea and bleeding are associated with this system.

Implanon

Implanon is a contraceptive device that is implanted subdermally in the upper arm and remains active for 3 years. It consists of a single rod that contains etonogestrel, which is the same progestin used in the NuvaRing. Implanon has been available for more than 10 years but has been widely marketed in the United States only since 2007.

Like other progestin-only contraceptives, Implanon works by blocking the LH surge, thereby preventing ovulation. It also thickens the cervical mucus and thins the endometrial lining. Unlike other progestin-only methods, Implanon causes estradiol to gradually increase to normal endogenous levels after an initial decrease. Implanon is extremely effective in preventing pregnancy and has an efficacy rate similar to that associated with sterilization or use of an IUD. Women experience a quick return to normal cycles after implant removal, and there have been no reports of infertility after removal. Implantation and removal of Implanon require training, but they can be performed as simple office procedures.

Implanon may cause irregular bleeding. It is contraindicated in women being treated with CYP3A-inducing or CYP3A-inhibiting medications. Inducers of CYP3A might decrease the efficacy of Implanon and lead to unintended pregnancy, and inhibitors of CYP3A might increase serum etonogestrel levels and cause toxicity. It is also contraindicated in women with active liver disease or active venous thromboembolism. Progestin-only methods of contraception have long been considered safe to use in women with an increased risk of venous thromboembolism (e.g., women who smoke or have hypertension, diabetes mellitus, migraine headaches, or a history of venous thromboembolism).

Emergency Contraception

Two forms of emergency contraception (or "morning-after contraception") are available. There is only one dedicated product available in the United States, a high-dose progestin that may be used to prevent pregnancy for up to 5 days after an act of unprotected intercourse. This high-dose progestin is most effective the earlier it is used and may prevent 87% of pregnancies. It is packaged as two pills—the first taken as soon after unprotected intercourse as possible, the second taken 12 hours later. There is evidence that both tablets of this high-dose progestin may be administered as one dose with no decrease in efficacy. Nausea and vomiting is unusual with progestin-only methods. This form of emergency contraception is thought to work primarily by preventing ovulation and will not disrupt an established pregnancy. It is available over the counter for women over age 17 and requires a prescription for women age 17 and younger.

In addition to the traditional prospective form of preventive contraception, the use of combination OCPs also has been studied in preventing pregnancy after coitus has occurred. The FDA has approved the Yuzpe regimen, 100 mg of ethinyl estradiol plus 1 mg of norgestrel or 0.5 mg of levonorgestrel within 72 hours of unprotected intercourse, to be repeated in 12 hours, as emergency contraception. This is not widely used now that there are specific formulations available. Providers must be aware of the formulation prescribed, such that the dosage strength equals that which has been approved. Monophasic regimens are recommended. If a biphasic or triphasic regimen is chosen, however, the patient must be aware of which tablets and how many she needs to take. Also, practitioners must stress the importance of not using the placebo tablets.

Although the exact mechanism of action of emergency contraception is not clear, several mechanisms have been proposed. These include inhibition or delay of ovulation, alteration of the endometrium, interference with implantation of the fertilized egg, and interference with tubal transport of sperm or egg.

Common side effects include nausea and vomiting. Recommendations are that if the patient vomits within 4 hours of the dose, she should repeat the dose.

Another regimen studied as emergency contraception is the progestin-only regimen. This regimen uses 0.75 mg of levonorgestrel within 72 hours of unprotected intercourse, followed by the same dose 12 hours later. In a clinical trial comparing its use with the Yuzpe regimen, the progestin-only group exhibited a pregnancy rate of 1.1% compared with 3.2% in the Yuzpe group. In addition, the levonorgestrel-only regimen resulted in significantly lower rates of nausea, vomiting, dizziness, and fatigue.

Regardless of the regimen chosen, a woman should menstruate within 21 days. If she does not, the clinician should instruct her to follow up with her provider to determine whether pregnancy has occurred. In addition, the practitioner should take this opportunity to discuss other forms of contraception so that emergency contraception does not become the woman's routine method of pregnancy prevention.

Nausea and vomiting are the most common adverse effects after treatment with the Yuzpe regimen. Other common adverse effects include fatigue, breast tenderness, headache, abdominal pain, and dizziness. Levonorgestrel alone is better tolerated than the Yuzpe regimen. According to the American College of Obstetricians and Gynecologists and the World Health Organization, there are no absolute medical contraindications to the use of emergency contraception with the exception of pregnancy. The daily dose of steroidal hormones provided in these products is high; however, they are taken for only a short time, and thus, the contraindications cited for cyclical combination OCPs are not thought to apply. There is no evidence of increased risk or confirmed safety in women who have contraindications to daily use of OCs.

Drug Interactions

Any agent that increases GI motility or causes diarrhea may reduce the plasma concentration of ethinyl estradiol by decreasing its absorption. Agents, such as ascorbic acid, that inhibit sulfation of ethinyl estradiol in the GI tract may increase the bioavailability of ethinyl estradiol and lead to an increase in estrogenic adverse effects.

Ethinyl estradiol is metabolized by the cytochrome P450 (CYP) 3A4 enzyme pathway. Drugs known to induce CYP3A4 (phenytoin, primidone, barbiturates, carbamazepine, ethosuximide, topiramate, methsuximide, rifampin, and griseofulvin) can lead to decreased plasma ethinyl estradiol levels and may cause failure of emergency contraception. Reports suggest that the enterohepatic circulation of ethinyl estradiol is decreased in women taking antibiotics, which may lead to a decrease in systemic concentrations of ethinyl estradiol. Ethinyl estradiol may interfere with the metabolism of other compounds. It can inhibit microsomal enzymes, which may slow the metabolism of other drugs (i.e., analgesic anti-inflammatory drugs such as antipyrine, antidepressant agents, theophylline, and ethanol), increasing their plasma and tissue concentrations and increasing the risk of adverse effects. There is a potential interaction between warfarin and levonorgestrel given as an emergency contraceptive. The proposed mechanism is the displacement of warfarin by levonorgestrel from the FIS binding site of human alpha$_1$-acid glycoprotein, the main transport protein for drugs in the plasma. This potential interaction should be considered so that the patient's international normalized ratio levels can be monitored because the Yuzpe regimen for emergency contraception generally would not be recommended in women with a history of deep vein thrombosis who are receiving anticoagulant therapy.

Selecting the Most Appropriate Agent

With the wide variety of forms of hormonal contraception, many questions exist about which agent should be used first and for whom. **Table 55.5** addresses some of these issues and is provided as a guide to the prescription of hormonal contraception.

TABLE 55.5	Treatment Order for Available Hormonal Contraceptive Agents

Clinical Scenario	Therapeutic Options
Women wish to use hormonal contraception—adolescents; perimenopausal women; postpartum, nonlactating women with no other medical risks	Any OCP less than 50 mcg EE either continuous or cyclic
History of: • smoking and over age 35 • uncontrolled hypertension • undiagnosed abnormal vaginal bleeding • diabetes with vascular complications or more than 20 years' duration • deep vein thrombosis or pulmonary embolism or history of ischemic heart disease • Headaches with focal neurological symptoms • History of breast cancer • Active viral hepatitis or cirrhosis	Consider progestin-only OCPs, Depo-Provera, Implanon, or IUD.
History of cholestasis with OCP use or pregnancy	
Endometriosis	Monophasic continuous therapy
Postpartum, lactating	Progesterone-only mini-pill
Noncompliance	Depot medroxyprogesterone acetate *or* levonorgestrel subdermal implants
Breakthrough bleeding—first half of cycle	Change to combination pill with higher estrogen content in first half of cycle.
Breakthrough bleeding—second half of cycle	Change to combination pill with higher progestin content in second half of cycle.

Data from Zieman, M., Hatcher, R., Cwiak, C., et al. (2010). *A pocket guide to managing contraception.* Tiger, GA: Bridging the Gap Foundation.

MONITORING PATIENT RESPONSE

Therapeutic drug monitoring of hormonal contraception includes, primarily, monitoring for adverse effects and preventing complications from their use. Before using any of the hormonal regimens, all sexually active patients should receive a gynecologic examination with Papanicolaou smear to observe cervical cytology. They also should have a thorough physical examination before beginning use, including information such as blood pressure and weight. A lipid panel, including baseline total cholesterol, high-density lipoprotein cholesterol, and triglyceride levels may be especially important in women with other risk factors for heart disease. Identification of blood glucose control before and after initiating hormonal contraception is important in women with diabetes mellitus.

In addition to the initial workup and physical examination, it is also important to maintain a high index of suspicion for adverse effects associated with the use of either the estrogen or progesterone components, or both, in women receiving hormonal contraception. It is estimated that 25% to 50% of women discontinue hormonal contraception within the first 12 months of use because of physical side effects. Therefore, it is important to look for these side effects and know how to manage them. **Box 55.1** identifies side effects related to excess estrogen and progesterone.

Side effects due to insufficient estrogen and progesterone, such as breakthrough bleeding, also may occur. In the first half of the menstrual cycle, breakthrough bleeding is likely due to

insufficient estrogen; in the second half of the cycle, it is likely due to insufficient progesterone. Therefore, practitioners can simplify management by adding supplemental estrogen or progesterone when appropriate or changing to a new regimen with higher estrogen or progesterone as necessary.

PATIENT EDUCATION

Poor outcomes secondary to the use of hormonal contraception may include treatment failures, potentially life-threatening side effects, or side effects beyond those commonly expected. Treatment failures frequently are related to compliance with the regimen. In the case of combination OCs, guidelines exist that explain what to do in the event of a missed pill (or pills) to help ensure continued contraceptive efficacy. **Table 55.6** illustrates these guidelines. Another cause of treatment failure includes drug interactions that may affect the efficacy of the hormonal contraceptive. Agents proven to reduce circulating estrogen concentrations, therefore affecting efficacy, include rifampin (Rifadin), phenytoin (Dilantin), and carbamazepine (Tegretol). Recommendations to reduce the risk of treatment failure relative to these agents include the use of higher daily doses of estrogen (50 mg ethinyl estradiol) or use of progesterone-only options.

Patients can best avoid life-threatening side effects of the hormonal contraceptives, especially combination OCs, if they follow the contraindications to their use. **Box 55.2** identifies

Causes of Side Effects of Hormone Contraception

Too Much Estrogen

Heavy bleeding
Cystic breasts
Breast enlargement
Breast tenderness
Dysmenorrhea
Bloating
Premenstrual edema
Gastrointestinal symptoms
Premenstrual headache
Premenstrual irritability
Cervical exstrophy

Too Little Estrogen

Bleeding (spotting) early
  in cycle
Too-light bleeding
Bleeding throughout the
  cycle
Amenorrhea

Too Much Progestin

Increased appetite
Candidiasis
Depression
Fatigue
Cervicitis

Too Little Progestin

Bleeding fewer days
Bleeding (spotting) late
  in cycle
Heavy bleeding
Delayed-withdrawal
  bleeding
Bloating
Dysmenorrhea
Premenstrual edema
Gastrointestinal
  symptoms
Premenstrual headache
Premenstrual irritability

TABLE 55.6 **Guidelines for Missed Pills**

Number of Missed Pills	Recommended Action
One pill	Take missed pill as soon as possible and resume schedule; back-up method of contraception is not necessary.
Two 30–35 μg pills	Take missed pill as soon as possible and resume schedule; back-up method of contraception is not necessary.
Two 20 μg pills More than two pills	Follow directions for more than two pills. Take pill and continue taking a pill daily. Use condom or abstinence for 7 days. If missed in week 3, finish active pills in current pack and start a new pack the next day (skip current inactive pills). If missed pills in first week and had sex, use emergency contraception (EC), then resume taking pills the next day after EC.

to their use (Schesselman, 1995). Clinicians should consider these increased risks when deciding on an initial contraceptive regimen for a patient.

Many women are unaware of the health risks and side effects of the various forms of hormonal contraception. Likewise, 25% of women are unaware that the use of combination contraceptive agents imparts benefits in addition to the prevention of pregnancy. Some of these benefits include a 50% to 60% reduction in ovarian cancer risk with 5 years of use. This benefit persists for up to 10 or more years after discontinuation. In addition, 50% to 60% reductions in PID risk

absolute contraindications to the use of combination OCs. In addition, the acronym *ACHES* is useful in teaching patients about the potential severe side effects that may occur with the use of OCPs. Clinicians should instruct patients to call their primary care provider if any of the following occur:

- Severe **A**bdominal pain (indicative of gallbladder disease)
- **C**hest pain (potentially related to pulmonary embolism or MI)
- **H**eadache (relative to stroke, hypertension, or migraine)
- **E**ye problems (relative to stroke or hypertension)
- **S**evere leg pain (indicative of deep vein thrombosis)

It is crucial to relay this information to the patient. Early recognition and treatment of these adverse events saves lives.

The increased risk of certain types of cancer has been linked to the use of hormonal contraception, especially combination OCPs. Data from 1995 illustrate that, per 100,000 users of combination OCPs, 151 cases of breast cancer, 125 cases of cervical cancer, and 41 cases of liver cancer could be attributed

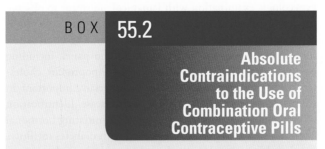

Absolute Contraindications to the Use of Combination Oral Contraceptive Pills

- Thrombophlebitis, thromboembolic disorders, cerebral vascular disease, coronary occlusion*
- Markedly impaired liver function
- Breast cancer (known or suspected)
- Abnormal vaginal bleeding in the absence of a diagnosed cause
- Pregnancy
- Smokers older than age 35

---

*Includes a past history or other situations that may put the patient at risk for developing these conditions.

BOX **55.3**

Noncontraceptive Benefits of Combined Oral Contraceptives

- Decreased iron deficiency anemia
- Decreased dysmenorrhea
- Decreased dysfunctional uterine bleeding
- Decreased incidence of ovarian cysts
- Improvement in acne
- Decreased incidence of pelvic inflammatory disease
- Decreased risk of osteoporosis
- Decreased incidence of endometrial cancer
- Decreased risk of benign breast disease

and 30% to 50% reductions in the occurrence of menstrual disorders have been observed with combination agents.

Another benefit of OCPs is their use in other indications. For example, 60% to 94% of women with endometriosis who are treated with daily monophasic contraceptive agents for 6 to 9 months experience symptomatic improvement. After treatment, a 5% to 10% annual recurrence rate of the disease is noted. Benefits of contraceptive agents are listed in **Box 55.3**.

Several Web sites contain patient information on contraception: www.contraception.net, http://www.nlm.nih.gov/medlineplus/birthcontrol.html, and www.plannedparenthood.org.

Case Study

J .L., a 27-year-old account executive, presents to the Family Medicine office for her annual checkup with her primary care provider. She has no significant past medical history. Her medications include calcium carbonate 500 mg orally twice a day and a multivitamin daily. She exercises regularly. Her family history is significant for cardiovascular disease (her father had an MI at age 54 and died of a further MI at age 63). She notes that she has been dating her current partner for approximately 5 months. She is interested in a reliable form of contraception. After discussing the various contraceptive options, she decides that an OC would best fit her needs.

1. Before prescribing an OCP regimen, what tests or examinations would you like to perform?
2. Identify three different OCP regimens that could be chosen for J.L. Note their differences and why you chose them.
3. Identify the potential side effects that need to be relayed to J.L. Note especially those effects for which J.L. should seek immediate medical care.

BIBLIOGRAPHY

*Starred references are cited in the text.

Ahern, R., Frattarelli, L., Delto, J., & Kaneshire, B. (2010). Knowledge and awareness of emergency contraception in adolescents. *Journal of Pediatric and Adolescent Gynecology, 23*(5), 273–278.

Bonnema, R., Mcnamara, M., & Spencer, A. (2010). Contraceptive choices in women with underlying medical conditions. *American Family Physician, 82*(6), 621–628.

Espey, E., Ogburn, T., & Fotieo, D. (2008). Contraception: What every internist should know. *Medical Clinics of North America, 92*(5), 1037–1058.

Lara-Torre, E. (2009). Update in adolescent contraception. *Obstetrics and Gynecology Clinics, 36*(1), 119–128.

Plastino, K., & Sulak, P. (2008). New forms of contraception. *Obstetrics and Gynecology Clinics, 35*(2), 185–197.

Prine, L. (2007). Emergency contraception, myths and facts. *Obstetrics and Gynecology Clinics, 35*(2), 127–136.

*Schesselman, J. J. (1995). Net effects of oral contraceptive use on the risk of cancer in women in the United States. *Obstetrics and Gynecology 85,* 793–801.

Spencer, A., Bonnema, R., & McNamara, M. (2009). Helping women choose appropriate hormonal contraception: Update on risks, benefits and indications. *American Journal of Medicine, 122*(6), 497–506.

*Speroff, L., & Darney, P. (2000). *A clinical guide for contraception* (3rd ed.). Philadelphia: Lippincott Williams & Wilkins.

Steinauer, J., & Autry, A. (2007). Extended cycle combined hormonal contraception. *Obstetrics and Gynecology Clinics, 34*(1), 43–55.

*Stenchever, M. A., Droegemuller, W., Herbst, A. L., et al. (2001). *Comprehensive Gynecology* (4th ed.). St. Louis: Mosby.

U.S. Department of Health and Human Services. (2001). *Healthy people 2010.* McLean, VA: International Medical Publishing.

Yen, S., Saah, T., & Adams Hillard, P. (2010). Intrauterine devices and adolescents: An underutilized opportunity for pregnancy prevention. *Journal of Pediatric and Adolescent Gynecology, 23*(3), 123–128.

*Zieman, M., Hatcher, R., Cwiak, C., et al. (2010). *A pocket guide to managing contraception.* Tiger, GA: Bridging the Gap Foundation.

Menopause and Menopausal Hormone Therapy

Menopause is the permanent cessation of menstruation resulting from loss of ovarian function. It is an endocrinopathy resulting from failure of the ovary to produce estrogen. Menopause is not an acute condition but rather a gradual transition from perimenopause to menopause and finally postmenopause. The perimenopause, that period from the first changes in ovarian function (which can be identified only in the laboratory) to final menstruation, can range from 2 to 8 years.

Healthy women typically spend one third of their lives in a menopausal state. The postwar baby boom of the 1940s and 1950s has led to an absolute increase in the over-50 population. Every day, over 5,000 women enter menopause. American women today can expect to live beyond age 80. The median age of menopause in the United States is between ages 49 and 51, with a range of ages 41 to 59, so the average life expectancy of a woman reaching menopause is approximately 30 more years. Factors that contribute to menopause at an earlier than average age include a history of irregular menses before the perimenopause, African American heritage, cigarette smoking, and weight reduction diets. Approximately 4% of women undergo a nonsurgical menopause before age 40.

The increased incidence of chronic disease in postmenopausal women appears to be influenced by decreased levels of estrogen or progesterone. The probability of developing coronary heart disease is 46%; stroke, 20%; hip fracture, 15%; breast cancer, 10%; colorectal cancer, 6%; and endometrial cancer, 2.6%. Postmenopausal women have a 1.4- to 3-fold increased risk of Alzheimer's disease over men.

PHYSIOLOGY

Menopause involves an age-related loss of ovarian function and a resulting decrease in estrogen secretion by the ovarian follicular unit. The ovary produces 17-β-estradiol, the major circulating estrogen. At birth, approximately 1 to 2 million ovarian follicles are present. By age 45, the number drops to approximately 10,000.

At middle perimenopause, the woman herself notices changes in her menstrual pattern. The menstrual pattern can change in one or all of three different ways as a result of unstable maturation of ovarian follicles. The time span from the first day of one menstrual period to the first day of the next may increase, the amount of blood lost and the number of days of bleeding may increase or decrease, or menstrual cycles may become anovulatory.

Amenorrhea in menopause results from the remaining follicles becoming resistant to the effect of follicle-stimulating hormone (FSH). The ovaries begin with a large number of follicles that atrophy during the reproductive years at a steady rate until there are too few to produce significant amounts of estradiol. During the perimenopause, estradiol and progesterone production declines. The reduction in hormone levels reduces the negative-feedback loop of the hypothalamic-pituitary system, which leads to a rise in FSH levels.

Estrogen has an impact on many body tissues and systems: bone, teeth, brain, eyes, vasomotor, heart, colon, and urogenital. Ovarian failure causes changes in many organ systems, but the changes are subtle and usually not distressing to women. The most noticeable change is amenorrhea. This is the change in reproductive function that all women experience. After 1 year of amenorrhea, women are considered postmenopausal.

Morbidity in the older woman seems to result from decreased hormone production. There is an unfavorable alteration in lipid profile and in the endothelium and vasoreactivity, predisposing postmenopausal women to cardiovascular disease, which increases in incidence after menopause because of increasing serum lipid levels. Coronary heart disease develops in approximately half of postmenopausal women; 30% die as a result and 20% have a stroke.

Most women seek treatment for menopausal symptoms such as vasomotor symptoms, insomnia, and mood changes. Approximately 85% of women experience vasomotor responses in the form of hot flashes or flushes, which are transient sensations ranging from warmth to intense heat that can last from 30 seconds to several minutes. Hot flashes are not linked to decreasing estrogen levels; rather, they are thought to be caused by gonadotropin-releasing factors that affect the autonomic nervous system, which leads to vasomotor instability. They are the most annoying consequences of menopause for many women. They can disrupt sleep. In addition, women experience vaginal atrophy and vaginal dryness, which can be very bothersome for sexually active women.

There is atrophy of the genitourinary system as a result of menopause. The vagina, vulva, urethra, and bladder have a large number of estrogen receptors. As estrogen levels decrease, there is the potential for urinary and sexual dysfunction. The vulva loses collagen, adipose tissue, and the ability to retain water. There is a shortening and narrowing of the vagina; the walls become thin and pale and elasticity decreases. Vaginal secretions decrease, thereby decreasing vaginal lubrication. The urethra may become irritated as well.

Osteoporosis, a progressive decrease in bone mass leading to potential fractures, is common. Approximately 1.3 million osteoporosis-related fractures are estimated to occur yearly in postmenopausal women.

INITIATING DRUG THERAPY

The treatment of menopause has a long and interesting history; bloodletting, purgatives, and powdered ass penis have all been tried to relieve the symptoms of menopause (Utian, 1997). Today, an increasing number of women are using behavioral changes and herbs to manage menopausal symptoms. Women who reduce intake of refined carbohydrates, caffeine, and alcohol report a reduction in hot flashes. Wearing only cotton clothing and maintaining low environmental temperatures make many women more comfortable during hot flashes.

The phytoestrogens, those estrogens obtained from food, are being marketed in oral form under the trade name of Promensil. Phytoestrogens are also found in a number of common foods (**Box 56.1**). Phytoestrogens appear to block estrogen stimulation of the breast and uterus, but they must be used for 4 to 6 weeks, before improvement is noticed.

Hormone therapy should be used to treat symptoms associated with menopause and not to prevent other diseases. The decision making on the use of menopausal hormone therapy (MHT) rests with the individual patient and provider. Women who choose MHT should have a thorough personal and family medical history to delineate health risk factors that may be affected by hormones. They should have a clear rationale for treatment, usually alleviation of menopausal symptoms such as hot flashes, and should take the lowest dose that provides control of symptoms. The decision to continue MHT should be revisited yearly, and therapy should be discontinued when symptoms resolve—usually in 1 to 3 years after menopause (Lund, 2008).

Women are also turning to other herbs for managing menopause (**Table 56.1**) such as soy or black cohosh.

Estrogen decreases the frequency of night sweats and periods of wakefulness during the night, reduces sleep latency (time between going to bed and falling asleep), and improves sleep in postmenopausal women with sleeping difficulty. Estrogen regimens reduce frequency and intensity of hot flashes by 70% and 90%, respectively, with 3 months of therapy.

About 1 year after menopause, a woman often experiences vulvovaginal symptoms, including vaginal dryness, itching, and burning. These symptoms increase in intensity the further a woman is from menopause. There is a loss of collagen and adipose tissue in the vulva, loss of the protective covering of the clitoral glans, and thinning and loss of elasticity of the vaginal surface. In the Women's Health Initiative (WHI) HOPE (Health, Osteoporosis, Progestin, Estrogen) study, women taking conjugated equine estrogen (CEE) or CEE with medroxyprogesterone acetate (MPA) at all doses had a significant increase in vaginal cells (Utian et al., 2001).

Women with low levels of estrogen are more likely to report sexual problems from vaginal dryness, pain, and burning during intercourse. Hormone therapy can reverse these symptoms. It is recommended that a topical therapy be used if these are the presenting symptoms.

An increase in irregularity of periods and symptoms of hypoestrogenism signal perimenopause. Treatment of perimenopause reflects a consideration of waning but still present fertility, and contraception must be considered. A combination hormone contraceptive has the dual advantage of alleviating hypoestrogenic symptoms and providing contraception.

Studies of Hormone Replacement

The WHI was a large, 8- to 10-year study of healthy, postmenopausal women with an observational component of 93,700 women and a randomized controlled component of 68,000 women. The randomized part had three arms—hormone therapy (estrogen alone, estrogen plus progestin, and placebo), a low-fat diet, and calcium plus vitamin D. The estrogen used was continuous-combined CEE 0.625 mg daily and 2.5 mg MPA daily. The estrogen plus progestin arm was stopped early (after about 5.2 years). This group also had increased risk of coronary events, stroke, pulmonary embolism, and invasive breast cancer. The thought is that because there was an increased incidence of invasive breast cancer, MHT promotes the growth of existing breast cancer rather than causing cancer. There was a reduced risk of colorectal cancer and hip fractures. Many of the risks appeared in year 1 (coronary and venous thromboembolic events) and year 2 (stroke). It was determined based on the data that the risk–benefit profile of estrogen plus progestin was such that its use for primary prevention of chronic conditions was not validated and it should not be prescribed to prevent chronic conditions. The study was stopped in 2002.

BOX 56.1

Food Sources of Phytoestrogens

Soybeans and soy products
Cashews
Peanuts
Oats
Corn
Wheat
Apples
Almonds

TABLE 56.1	Herbal Treatment of Menopausal Symptoms		
Menopausal Symptom	Herbal Treatment	Usual Dose	Adverse Events and Contraindications
Hot flashes	Black cohosh (*Cimicifuga*)	40–200 mg/d; not to be taken for >6 mo	Not to be used during pregnancy Potential side effects: GI disturbances, hypotension
	Isoflavins (soy) Rose tea	20–40 mg/d	Flatulence
Mood swings	St. John's wort (*Hypericum*)	300 mg tid	Do not take with any antidepressant. May cause sun sensitivity

Based on the best available evidence, hormones are used as therapy to treat menopausal symptoms or as a means of helping to avoid or minimize the risk of certain diseases. MHT effectively relieves the most common menopausal symptoms, and the absolute risk of cardiovascular disease and cancer is low when these drugs are used for short periods. In addition, MHT may be appropriate in the prevention or management of osteoporosis, the most common metabolic disease in the United States, and one that is linked directly to declining serum estrogen levels. The results of the WHI study cannot be generalized to a population of women in early menopause because the WHI was designed to evaluate MHT in an older population of aging postmenopausal women. Patients in the WHI were much older, with an average age at randomization of 63 (range, ages 50 to 79), were excluded if they suffered severe menopausal symptoms, and were required to be off MHT before beginning the study. Critics argue that the study of patients in this age group is not clinically useful because most patients who initiate MHT do so during the early menopausal transition when symptoms are greatest. Many subanalyses focusing on the younger cohort of the WHI have failed to find adverse cardiac outcomes among this subset. In fact, women in their 50s who took estrogen appear to have less coronary artery calcification than controls.

Quality of life (QOL) data have been reported for the estrogen plus progestin arm of the WHI. Approximately 16,600 women completed surveys at baseline and year 1. About 1,500 women completed surveys at year 3. At year 1 there was statistically significant improvement in sleep disturbance, physical functioning, and bodily pain as compared with the placebo group. However, the differences were so small that there is a question about clinical significance. There was no significant difference at year 3. In women reporting moderate to severe vasomotor symptoms, those taking estrogen plus progestin had significant improvement in the severity of hot flashes and night sweats.

In the HOPE study, healthy postmenopausal women ages 40 to 65 were randomly assigned to treatment with CEE alone (0.625, 0.45, or 0.3 mg daily), CEE plus MPA (0.625/2.5, 0.45/2.5, 0.45/1.5, or 0.3/1.5 mg daily), or a placebo. Over 13 cycles, women in all active treatment groups had a significant reduction in vasomotor symptoms. In women taking CEE alone, benefit increased with increased dosage. In women taking CEE plus MPA, the benefit was comparable with all doses.

The Heart and Estrogen/Progestin Replacement Study trials (HERS) were conducted to determine if estrogen and progestin therapy alters the risk of coronary heart disease events in postmenopausal women. The drugs were CEE and MPA and placebo. There were more coronary heart disease events in the first year but fewer in years 4 and 5. In HERS, there was an increase in deep vein thromboembolism and pulmonary embolism and biliary tract surgery. There was no cardiac protection in women with previously diagnosed coronary heart disease.

The Postmenopausal Estrogen/Progestin Interventions (PEPI) trial studied healthy women ages 45 to 64. They were randomly assigned to treatment with different hormone regimens (CEE, cyclic CEE plus MPA, continuous CEE plus MPA, or cyclic CEE plus micronized progesterone). The women in the placebo group lost bone mineral density (BMD) at the spine and hip. Women who took hormone therapy gained BMD in the spine and hip.

The benefit of hormone therapy is dose related, and U.S. Food and Drug Administration (FDA) guidance should be followed in using MHT at the lowest dose and for the shortest duration possible, although evidence from randomized, controlled trials supporting this guideline is unavailable. Several estrogen and progestin formulations are available, and there is no strong evidence that one formulation is superior to another. Hormones delivered via a transdermal patch are associated with a lower risk of venous thromboembolism compared to oral formulations. A reasonable starting dose of estrogen for women who are having hot flashes is 0.025 mg of transdermal estradiol, 0.5 mg of oral estradiol, or 0.3 mg of CEE. Although it is reasonable to believe that the transdermal route of administration of estrogen avoids first-pass hepatic metabolism and therefore may reduce thromboembolic risk, no randomized controlled trials to support this concept have been published.

If these products are prescribed solely for vaginal symptoms, health care providers are advised to consider the use of topical vaginal products (gel or cream applied locally).

Studies of Nonhormonal Therapy for Hot Flashes

There has been an evaluation of nonhormonal therapy for hot flashes because of the controversy about MHT. Anecdotal improvement was seen in hot flashes in women using agents that inhibit neuronal uptake of serotonin. Relief was found with fluoxetine (Prozac, Sarafem), venlafaxine (Effexor), and paroxetine (Paxil) (Loprinzi, et al., 1998). Based on these observations, clinical trials were conducted with venlafaxine and paroxetine. In the venlafaxine pilot, 12.5 mg twice a day was used. There was an approximately 50% decrease in hot flashes. A pilot study using paroxetine 20 mg showed a reduction in hot flashes of about 65% (Stearns, et al., 2000).

Further study was done with venlafaxine (extended release) at doses of 37.5 mg, 75 mg, and 150 mg. This was a 4-arm double-blind, placebo-controlled study. There was a 37% reduction in hot flashes with 37.5 mg compared to a 61% reduction with 75 and 150 mg. There was improvement in libido and QOL scores in the venlafaxine groups (Loprinzi, et al., 2000).

Recommendations on Use of HRT

The U.S. Preventive Services Task Force (2002) recommends against the routine use of estrogen and progestin for prevention of chronic conditions in postmenopausal women. MHT has benefits and harms. The benefits are the increase in BMD, decrease in the risk of fracture, and decrease in the incidence of colorectal cancer. The harms are increased risks for breast cancer, venous thromboembolism, coronary heart disease, stroke, and cholecystitis.

The Endocrine Society issued conclusions on the use of MHT with level of evidence A (Santen, 2010):

- "Standard-dose" estrogen used with or without a progestogen is associated with marked reduction in frequency and severity of hot flashes. For many women, lower doses of estrogen are also effective.
- For symptoms of vaginal atrophy, very low doses of vaginal estradiol are effective.
- Symptoms of overactive bladder may be reduced by estrogen given vaginally or systemically.
- Vaginal estrogen is associated with lower rates of recurrent urinary tract infections.
- For women in late postmenopause, estrogen given with or without a progestogen is as effective as bisphosphonate therapy for preventing early postmenopausal bone loss and increasing bone mass.
- Use of estrogen alone and estrogen plus a progestogen is associated with a lower incidence of hip and vertebral fractures.
- For osteoporotic women older than age 60, tibolone is associated with significantly lower rates of vertebral and nonvertebral fractures.
- Treatment with the selective estrogen receptor modulator raloxifene is associated with increased BMD and lower rates of vertebral, but not hip, fractures.
- Use of MHT containing estrogen plus a progestogen is linked to a lower risk of colon cancer.
- Raloxifene is associated with a lower risk of breast cancer.
- Mammographic density is increased in women taking estrogen alone or with a progestogen.
- Sexual function is improved by physiologic amounts of transdermal testosterone, but not by dehydroepiandrosterone.
- Risk for venothrombotic episodes is approximately doubled in women using MHT, and this risk is multiplicative with baseline risk factors such as age, increased body mass index, thrombophilias, surgery, and immobilization.
- Use of raloxifene is associated with an increased incidence of venothrombotic episodes.
- Raloxifene is not associated with any increase in stroke risk.
- In older women with preexisting vascular disease, hormone use does not reduce stroke incidence.
- Although continuous estrogen plus a progestogen does not cause endometrial cancer, estrogen alone without a progestogen is associated with an increased incidence of endometrial cancer.
- The risk of gallbladder disease is increased in women using estrogen alone or with a progestogen.

MHT started after age 60 does not improve memory (Santen, 2010). Women ages 50 to 59 who start MHT a short time after onset of menopause appear to benefit versus women who begin MHT after age 60. Women in the short-time group using MHT for 5 years have a 90% decrease in menopausal symptoms, including hot flashes and overactive bladder (Santen, 2010).

The decision to prescribe MHT should be a joint one between the provider and the patient. When discussing MHT, the women must be informed of the risks. Many women choose pharmacotherapy to relieve the symptoms of menopause. MHT should be prescribed at the lowest possible dose to prevent vasomotor symptoms.

In prescribing MHT, a complete and thoughtful history and physical examination are conducted. The standard family and personal history should be augmented with questions about the woman's gynecologic history, menopausal symptoms, and attitudes toward menopause and her goals in using MHT.

The routine physical examination should also include the patient's measured height, a gynecologic examination, and clinical breast examination. Investigative studies should include a pregnancy test, mammogram, and Papanicolaou (Pap) smear. Conditions that predispose women to increased risk of endometrial cancer include a lifelong history of irregular menses, polycystic ovary disease, or a recent history of irregular menses occurring closer than 21 days apart or menses lasting longer than 10 days. These women should have an endometrial biopsy before beginning MHT.

Low-dose oral contraceptives can be used to prevent and control symptoms until the patient reaches menopause and to ensure prevention of conception because these women are still fertile. To check if the patient taking oral contraceptives is menopausal, FSH levels can be determined on the last hormone-free day. Oral contraceptives are contraindicated in smokers older than 35 years of age. Oral contraceptives are discussed in Chapter 55.

If the choice is to use MHT, it should be individualized. Individual needs should be assessed and menopausal symptoms evaluated.

All continuous MHT regimens can cause breakthrough bleeding. About 30% of all women who are recently menopausal have some breakthrough bleeding; this decreases with women who are more than 3 years postmenopausal. Amenorrhea usually occurs within 1 year of initiating therapy.

Data from the WHI show that short-term use of combined estrogen and progestin increases the incidence of breast cancer and abnormal mammograms. Those women in the study taking MHT were diagnosed at a more advanced stage of breast cancer. The risk is increased less than 1 per 100 women over baseline.

Goals of Drug Therapy

The goal of hormone therapy is treatment of menopausal symptoms. It is no longer to prevent long-term chronic conditions, especially heart disease. MHT generally refers to treatment with estrogen and progestin used in women with an intact uterus and MHT refers to treatment with estrogen alone, used in women who have no uterus.

Estrogen

In the postmenopausal woman, short-term estrogen therapy at the lowest possible dose is the choice for treating symptoms such as hot flashes, vaginal dryness, and sleep disturbances. It is not to be used for prevention of coronary heart disease. Therapy for 1 to 4 years seems to outweigh the risks, but therapy for longer than 4 years is questionable. If these products are prescribed solely for vaginal symptoms, health care providers are advised to consider the use of topical vaginal products (gel or cream applied locally).

No other method provides such consistent and complete relief of menopausal symptoms as MHT. Use the lowest possible dose. Doses as low as 0.3 mg have been shown to provide effective relief from hot flashes and vaginal discomfort. Transdermal doses of estradiol as low as 12.5 μg have been effective.

MHT comes in nonoral forms. These forms seem to better mimic the release of hormones as the ovaries would produce if they were still functional. There are transdermal options with steady-state pharmacokinetics and less hepatic metabolism. There is not an increase in C-reactive protein seen with these as with oral therapy. Vaginal rings containing estrogen are another option.

Dosage

For the management of moderate to severe vasomotor symptoms, the dose for CEE, esterified estrogen, and estropipate is 0.3 to 0.625 mg/d, with 0.3 the recommended dose. The 17-β-estradiol oral dose is recommended at 0.25 to 0.5 mg and the 17-β-estradiol patch 0.025 mg/d. Estrogen can be taken continuously or on a cyclic schedule with 1 week off per month. The lowest dose that controls symptoms is recommended. It does takes longer to achieve maximal benefit with a low dose.

Local products for vaginal symptoms include vaginal estradiol ring (Estring 0.0075 mg/d) and estradiol acetate (Femring 0.05 and 0.10 mg/d). The rings are inserted every 3 months. Additionally there are vaginal topical preparations and 17-β-estradiol suppositories (Vagifem 0.025) and cream (Estrace vaginal cream, 2 to 4 gm/d for 1 to 2 weeks, then 1 to 2 g/d for 1 to 2 weeks, then 1 g one to three times weekly), and CEE (Premarin vaginal cream 0.5 to 2 g daily for 3 weeks on and 1 week off). Dienestrol (Ortho Dinestrol Vaginal Cream 1 to 2 applicatorful/day for 1 to 2 weeks, then half the dose for 1 to 2 weeks, then 1 applicatorful one to three times weekly) is another vaginal cream available. Local products have the lowest systemic absorption.

Adverse Events

To avoid serious adverse events, the practitioner does not prescribe MHT if it is absolutely contraindicated. (**Box 56.2** lists the absolute and relative contraindications.)

Adverse events include intolerance to contact lenses from steepening of corneal curvature, headache, depression, gallbladder disease, nausea, vomiting, abdominal cramps, increased blood pressure, thromboembolic disease, breakthrough bleeding, edema, breast cancer, and breast tenderness.

The results of the WHI showed that for every 10,000 women taking MHT for 1 year, there was an increase of

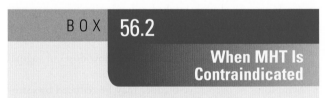

BOX 56.2

When MHT Is Contraindicated

ABSOLUTE CONTRAINDICATIONS

- Known or suspected breast cancer
- Known or suspected endometrial cancer
- Undiagnosed genital bleeding
- Acute liver disease
- Active thromboembolic disease or history of thromboembolic disease
- Known or suspected pregnancy

RELATIVE CONTRAINDICATIONS

- Chronic liver dysfunction
- Uncontrolled or poorly controlled hypertension
- Acute intermittent porphyria

eight strokes, seven cases of coronary heart disease, eight more invasive breast cancers, and eight additional pulmonary embolisms. There was a decreased incidence of six colorectal cancers and five fewer hip fractures.

Interactions

Drug interactions with CEE include increased effects of corticosteroids and decreased levels of estrogen with barbiturates, phenytoin (Dilantin), and rifampin (Rifadin). Patients taking phenytoin excrete estrogen more quickly. There can be increases in thyroxine and serum triglyceride levels. An increased dose is needed in smokers because only half the serum level achieved in nonsmokers is reached. Alcohol increases the circulating levels of estrogen.

Progestin

Progesterone is secreted by the corpus luteum. It acts on the endometrium to change proliferative endometrial tissue to secretory tissue. Progesterone is given as a part of MHT to women with an intact uterus. It decreases the risk of estrogen-induced irregular bleeding, endometrial hyperplasia, and carcinoma. It is not needed in women without a uterus.

Progestins may increase the risk of breast cancer above that with estrogen alone. However, women who have a uterus must take progestogens to protect against endometrial cancer and hyperplasia. The progestogens tend to attenuate the positive cardiovascular effects of estrogen. This shows a need to use the lowest possible dose of progestin other than MPA. Some are more metabolically inert (micronized progesterone, trimegestone, drospirenone).

The PEPI trial showed that CEE with cyclic micronized progesterone had the best lipid profile of any of the combined regimens. Micronized progesterone and norethindrone acetate (NETA) have better side effect profiles than MPA.

The progesterone studied in the WHI study was medroxyprogesterone. Micronized progesterone showed the best lipid profile in the PEPI trial, so it may be the best preparation to use. Another option is NETA.

Dosage

The recommended daily dose is 0.5 to 5 mg for a woman with an intact uterus. The lowest dose is recommended. One study showed that NETA doses as low as 0.1 mg were effective in providing endometrial protection when combined with oral 17-β-estradiol 1.0 mg. The standard dose of NETA is 0.5 mg (Kurman, et al., 2002).

Contraindications

Thrombophlebitis, hepatic disease, breast cancer, undiagnosed vaginal bleeding, pregnancy, and lactation contraindicate progesterone use. Cautious use is recommended with epilepsy, migraine, asthma, and cardiac or renal dysfunction.

Adverse Events

Adverse events include bloating, abdominal cramping, edema, irritability, weight gain, headache, breakthrough bleeding, breast tenderness, and acne.

Combination Products

Products that combine estrogen and progestin provide ease of administration and include CEE/MPA, estradiol/norgestimate, and ethinyl estradiol/NETA.

Testosterone

The slight decrease in testosterone production that accompanies menopause can cause a significant decrease or complete loss of libido in some women. For these women, testosterone can be added to MHT in doses of 1.25 to 2.5 mg methyltestosterone. The adverse events of testosterone in these doses are hirsutism, voice change, and a decrease in the high-density lipoprotein cholesterol level. Long-term use is associated with the risk of hepatocellular neoplasm, increased edema, and possible elevation of cholesterol level. The only indication for treatment is severe vasomotor disturbances and decreased libido.

The most frequent treatment choice is either Estratest, which is 1.25 mg esterified estrogen and 2.5 mg methyltestosterone, or Estratest H.S., which is 0.625 mg esterified estrogen and 1.25 mg methyltestosterone. Estratest H.S. may be used safely as long as lipid levels are normal. Estratest, with its 1.25 mg esterified estrogen, is a high dose of estrogen and should be used only for short periods. Topical testosterone, which has recently received a great deal of attention in the lay press, is not commercially available in the United States.

Nonhormonal Therapy

The most effective alternatives to MHT for the relief of vasomotor symptoms are the selective serotonin reuptake inhibitors (SSRIs) venlafaxine (Effexor) and paroxetine (Paxil). They have been shown to significantly reduce hot flashes in randomized trials, with venlafaxine 75 mg and paroxetine 20 mg or paroxetine CR 12.5 mg and 25 mg having the greatest effect.

Venlafaxine (Effexor), extended release, is the best studied nonhormonal therapy for hot flashes. It is recommended that therapy start at 37.5 mg/d for 1 week. If hot flashes are controlled at that dose, then it is maintained. If they are not controlled, the dose should be increased to a maximum of 150 mg daily. Also recommended is paroxetine (Paxil) 10 to 20 mg daily. Results are usually seen in 1 to 2 weeks.

Sertraline has been shown to decrease vasomotor symptoms at 50 mg/d.

It has been shown that gabapentin (Neurontin) in doses of 900 to 2,400 mg divided into three doses a day can alleviate hot flashes. Clonidine 0.1 mg also can reduce vasomotor symptoms.

TABLE 56.2 **Overview of Selected Agents Used to Treat Menopausal Symptoms**

Generic (Trade) Name and Dosage	Side Effects	Contraindications	Special Considerations
Oral menopause hormone therapy			
conjugated equine estrogen (CEE) (Premarin) Usual daily dose 0.3–0.65 mg Doses available: 0.3, 0.45 and 0.625 mg	Nausea, vomiting, break- through bleeding, edema, weight changes, swollen/ tender breasts, hypertension, depression, hair loss, changes in libido	Estrogen-dependent neoplasia Thrombophlebitis or thromboembolic disorder Pregnancy Undiagnosed vaginal bleeding	May cause GI upset, so take with food
estradiol (Estrace) 1 mg/d	Same as above	Same as above	Same as above
Combination products			
CEE and MPA (Prempro) Doses 0.5/1.5, 0.4/1.5, 0.625/2.5, 0.625/5 mg	Same as above	Same as above	Same as above
ethinyl estradiol & norethindrone acetate (NETA)			
Femhrt 1/5 5 mcg/1 ng	Same as above	Same as above	Same as above
estradiol (NETA) 1 mg/0.5 ng	Same as above	Same as above	Same as above
(Estratest) esterified estrogen 1.25 mg and methyltestosterone 2.5 mg (Estratest H.S.) esterified estrogen 0.625 mg and methyltestosterone 1.25 mg Taken daily for 3 wk then 1 wk off	Liver function changes, nausea, breakthrough bleeding, edema, weight gain, hypertension, depression, intolerance to contact lenses, changes in libido, viriliza- tion, jaundice, gallbladder disease	Breast or endometrial cancer, undiagnosed genital bleed- ing, thromboembolic dis- ease, pregnancy, lactation	Report any adverse events immediately. May take at bedtime to prevent nausea
Progestins			
medroxyprogesterone (Amen, Curretab, Cycrin, Provera) 2.5–10 mg either daily or cyclic	Vision changes, migraine, porphyria, depression, insomnia, jaundice, nausea, thrombophlebitis, pulmo- nary embolism, increased blood pressure, breakthrough bleeding, breast tenderness, rash, hirsutism, increased weight, decreased glu- cose tolerance	Thrombophlebitis, hepatic dis- ease, breast cancer, undi- agnosed vaginal bleeding, pregnancy, lactation Caution in epilepsy, migraine, asthma, cardiac dysfunction	Report any adverse events immediately. May take at bedtime to prevent nausea
norethindrone acetate (NETA) Aygestin dose 2.5–10 mg/d	Same as above	Same as above	Same as above
Transdermal Menopause Hormone Therapy			
estradiol (Alora, Estraderm, Vivelle) Change transdermal patch twice a wk Alora—0.05, 0.075, 0.1 mg/d Vivelle—0.0375, 0.05, 0.075, 0.1 mg/d	Irritation at application site, head- ache, breakthrough bleeding, nausea, abdominal cramps	Undiagnosed abnormal vaginal bleeding, thromboembolic disorder, pregnancy, breast or estrogen-dependent tumor	Apply to clean, dry area on lower abdomen, hips, or buttocks (not breast or waist- line). Rotate application sites. Use 3 wk on and 1 wk off in patient with intact uterus; continuous in patient without uterus.
estradiol (Climara)—0.025, 0.0375, 0.05, 0.075, 0.1 mg Change transdermal patch once a week 0.05, 0.075, 0.1 mg/d	Same as above	Same as above	Same as above
estradiol and NETA (CombiPatch)	Same as above	Same as above	Apply to clean, dry area on lower abdomen, hips, or buttocks (not breast or waistline).

TABLE 56.2	Overview of Selected Agents Used to Treat Menopausal Symptoms (*Continued*)		
Generic (Trade) Name and Dosage	**Side Effects**	**Contraindications**	**Special Considerations**
Change transdermal patch twice a wk (0.05 mg estradiol and 0.14 mg norethindrone, 0.05 mg estradiol and 0.25 mg norethindrone)			Combination therapy
Vaginal Hormones			
estradiol 0.01% (Estrace Vaginal Cream) Initially 2–4 g/d for 1–2 wk, then 1–2 g/d for 1–2 wk; maintenance dose: 1 g, 1–3 times/wk (3 wk on and 1 wk off)	Uterine bleeding, vaginal candidiasis	Breast or estrogen-dependent cancer, thrombophlebitis, undiagnosed genital bleeding, pregnancy, lactation, impaired liver function	Need to take progestin if uterus present
Estring (vaginal ring) 0.0015/d ring into vagina; replaced every 90 d	Headache, leukorrhea, back pain, urinary tract infection, vaginitis, vaginal pain, abdominal pain, bacterial growth	Same as above	Remove while treating vaginitis. Reevaluate every 3–6 mo.
Femring 0.05, 0.1/d			
Premarin vaginal cream 0.625 mg/g 0.5–2 g/d	Nausea, vomiting, breakthrough bleeding, edema, weight changes, swollen/tender breasts, hypertension, depression, hair loss, changes in libido	Same as above	Therapeutic regimen consists of 3 wk on therapy and 1 wk off.

Selecting the Most Appropriate Agent

For women who have had a hysterectomy, the only component needed for MHT is estrogen. The patient needs to decide which estrogen delivery method—transdermal, vaginal, or oral—is desirable for her. Transdermal estrogen is easy to use, which increases compliance. Some women, however, find the concept of a transdermal patch aesthetically unpleasing and they may select an oral estrogen. Both dosage forms have the same effect of reducing hot flashes and preventing osteoporosis. Oral agents have a greater impact on lipid levels. The oral and transdermal products are discussed in **Table 56.2.**

Estrogen must be combined with progestin to prevent endometrial hyperplasia and the possibility of endometrial carcinoma in a woman with an intact uterus. Currently, the only progestin approved by the FDA for oral MHT is MPA.

The woman who has not had a hysterectomy must also select a delivery method for MHT—oral, transdermal, or vaginal—and must also decide if she wants to use cyclic, continuous, or continuous combined MHT.

Progestin exposure should be minimized. Women using MHT who receive MPA 5 or 10 mg every 3 months have only slightly higher rates of hyperplasia (1.5%) (Doren, 2000). In one study, women on lower-dose estrogen, CEE 0.3 mg daily plus MPA 10 mg daily for 14 days every 6 months, the rate of endometrial hyperplasia was only 1.6% (Ettinger, et al., 2001), suggesting that quarterly or biyearly progestin schedules are almost as effective as monthly or continuous regimens at preventing endometrial hyperplasia, although more study needs to be done.

Short-term use is recommended. Risk of breast cancer does not substantially increase until after 5 years and most women's menopausal symptoms abate within 5 years after onset of menopause.

For women with vasomotor symptoms with contraindications to MHT, or who choose not to use MHT, venlafaxine or paroxetine are recommended alternatives.

Administration Options

Oral therapy is the most popular, but therapy is available in transdermal and vaginal preparations as well. Transdermal estrogen is recommended if it is desirable to avoid the first-pass phenomenon in women who have liver disease or who are prone to gallbladder disease. Vaginal preparations are used to relieve genitourinary symptoms associated with menopause.

First-Line Therapy

For a woman with an intact uterus, the most popular regimen is continuous combined oral therapy. Continuous use of estrogen and progestin prevents withdrawal bleeding.

Second-Line Therapy

If the woman cannot tolerate oral estrogen because of intolerance to pills or gastrointestinal upset, or compliance issues, transdermal or vaginal preparations are recommended. The transdermal and vaginal routes, which bypass the liver, are also preferred for women who smoke or who have a history of gallbladder disease, fibrocystic breast disease, thrombophlebitis, elevated triglyceride levels, migraines, or hypertension. Additionally, nonhormonal therapy, such as SSRIs, can be used.

Third-Line Therapy

If vasomotor symptoms are intolerable, estrogen doses can be increased to the next higher dose. If the woman experiences decreased libido, methyltestosterone can be added at a dose of 1.2 to 2.5 mg/d. If this therapy is used, the practitioner must monitor liver function and electrolyte levels every 3 to 6 months. See **Table 56.3** and **Figure 56-1** to review the order of therapy.

MONITORING PATIENT RESPONSE

The patient should be seen 2 months after starting therapy and then in 6 months to check response to therapy, blood pressure, and side effects. After that, annual visits are required.

The health status of a woman on MHT must be evaluated annually. The woman should have an annual clinical breast examination and mammogram if she is older than age 40. Annually, the patient's medical history should be reviewed for the past year, including questions about vaginal bleeding. Any woman on continuous combined MHT who has vaginal bleeding beyond the first year of treatment should be evaluated with an endometrial biopsy. The physical examination should include:

- height measurement to screen for osteoporosis
- weight measurement to screen for obesity
- blood pressure evaluation to screen for cardiovascular disease
- clinical breast examination and review of procedures for breast self-examination
- full pelvic examination, including a Pap smear.

Prescriptions for MHT should not be renewed without a full annual history and physical. Encouraging new MHT users to call the practitioner at the end of 3 months of therapy helps the patient to discuss any concerns or problems with MHT.

At each visit, the risks and benefits of MHT must be discussed and documented. At that time it should be a mutual decision whether to continue or stop the therapy.

Discontinuing MHT should be done gradually. It may be done in several ways. The patient may begin to skip more days between doses or the dose may be decreased at 4- to 6-week intervals.

More than 75% of women discontinue MHT in less than 1 year because of undesirable side effects. Another influence is that the woman may not feel any different when taking the medication. Education is an important aspect of prescribing MHT.

PATIENT EDUCATION

Drug Information

Several options are available for the postmenopausal woman with vasomotor symptoms. If she decides to begin MHT, the decision must be an informed decision. To make an informed decision, the patient must be provided with detailed information on the risks and benefits of therapy and other options available. It is also important to understand the side effects and that there may be monthly bleeding. Key teaching points include:

- The patient must be aware that it may be 4 weeks or more before symptoms disappear.
- MHT can be taken with food or at bedtime to prevent nausea.
- The patient should be taught how to perform a monthly breast self-examination.
- The patient should be familiar with danger signs of adverse events—abnormal vaginal bleeding, pain in the calf or chest, shortness of breath, coughing blood, severe headache, jaundice, breast lump, and vision changes. These should be reported immediately to the health care provider.

Assess the presence and severity of menopausal symptoms and how they impair the patient's QOL. Discuss all reasonable treatment options and prescribe MHT at the lowest dose for the shortest period.

When using hormonal products for the treatment of symptoms of vulvar and vaginal atrophy, use topical preparations.

TABLE 56.3	Recommended Order of Therapy	
Order	**Agents**	**Comments**
First line	MHT short-term for treatment of menopausal symptoms at the lowest therapeutic dose for the shortest period. Therapy can be oral, transdermal, or vaginal. Combination therapy must be used for a woman with an intact uterus.	At each visit the risk/benefits must be discussed and a mutual decision made whether to continue therapy.
Second line	If vasomotor symptoms are not controlled, higher estrogen doses can be used for a short period.	
Third line	If there is contraindication to MHT or if the decision is made not to use this therapy, consider SSRIs for treatment relief or alternative therapies. If the women experience decreased libido, testosterone can be added at a dose of 1.2–2.5 mg of methyltestosterone.	If testosterone is used, liver function and electrolytes must be monitored every 3–6 mo.

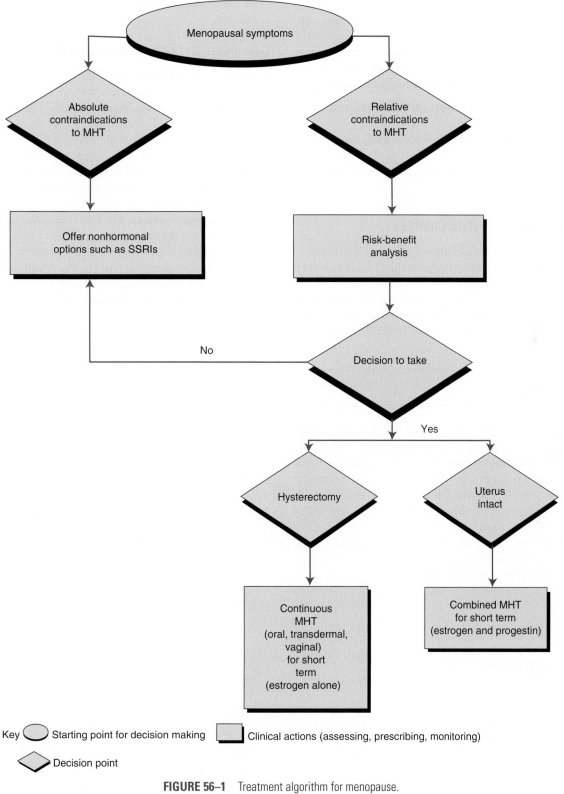

FIGURE 56–1 Treatment algorithm for menopause.

Perform an annual risk–benefit assessment.

If discontinuing MHT, taper it. Reduce the estrogen component and maintain the progestin component. Taper MHT for at least 4 weeks. If the patient develops vasomotor symptoms, return to the previous dose and continue therapy.

Patient information sources for menopause include:

- Harvard Women's Health Watch: www.health.harvard.edu/newsletters
- The National Council for Reliable Health Information: www.ncrhi.org/main.htm
- The North American Menopause Society: www.menopause.org.

Nutritional and Lifestyle Changes

The woman in menopause who is symptomatic needs to be instructed to wear loose, cotton clothing. Environmental adjustments may be helpful, such as keeping the temperature lower. A reduction in the intake of caffeine, simple carbohydrates, and alcohol also helps. She should go to bed just to sleep and have sex. If she is unable to sleep, she should leave the bed and read or do some other activity that is relaxing.

Complementary and Alternative Medicine

A randomized trial of vitamin E showed that the treatment group had one less daily hot flash (Barton, et al., 1998). Some clinical trials have shown improvement of hot flashes with soy and black cohosh and some have shown no improvement (Faure, et al., 2002; Quella, et al., 2000).

Soy, chickpeas, and other legumes contain isoflavins, which exhibit estrogenic properties. They can provide some symptom relief, although their effectiveness in menopause is still being investigated.

Black cohosh is also used to treat menopause. It purportedly induces vaginal maturation and improves hot flashes. However, no long-term scientific data are available currently.

Rose tea has shown to reduce the symptoms of dysmenorrhea and menopause. It is made from the buds or the leaves of *Rosa gallica*. The calyx of the rose contains vitamins A, B, C, E, K, and P, with C having the highest concentration.

Case Study

E.P., a 51-year-old Asian woman who is 68 inches tall and weighs 130 pounds, presents complaining of amenorrhea for the past 8 months. She wakes up at least 5 times a night with hot flashes and experiences them at least 10 times a day. She is very uncomfortable and sleep deprived. At the visit a Pap smear is done and a mammogram is negative. Her FSH level is 32 international units/mL. She has no family history of breast cancer, but her mother has osteoporosis.

1. List specific goals for treatment of E.P.
2. What drug therapy would you prescribe? Why? For how long?
3. What are the parameters for monitoring success of the therapy?
4. Discuss patient education and counseling necessary in this situation.
5. List two adverse reactions of the prescribed therapy.
6. What would be the choice for second-line therapy if E.P. could not tolerate the treatment of choice and symptoms were still present?
7. What alternative therapy may be suggested?
8. What dietary and lifestyle modifications should be made?
9. Describe contraindications to MHT.

BIBLIOGRAPHY

Starred references are cited in the text.

*Barton, D., Loprinzi, C., Quela, S., et al. (1998). Prospective evaluation of vitamin E for hot flashes in breast cancer survivors. *Journal of Clinical Oncology, 16,* 495–500.

*Doren, M. (2000). Hormonal replacement regimens and bleeding. *Maturitas, 34,* S17–S23.

*Ettinger, B., Pressmen, A., & VanGessel, A. (2001). Low-dosage esterified estrogens opposed by progestin at 6 month intervals. *Obstetrics and Gynecology, 98,* 205–211.

*Faure, E., Chantre, P., & Mares, P. (2002). Effects of a standardized soy extract on hot flushes: A multicenter, double-blind randomized, placebo-controlled study. *Menopause, 9,* 329–334.

Gold, E. B., Sternfield, B., Kelsey, J. L., et al. (2000). Relationship of demographic and lifestyle factors to symptoms in a multi-racial/ethnic population of women 40 to 55 years of age. *American Journal of Epidemiology, 152,* 463–473.

Grady, D. (2003). Postmenopausal hormones—Therapy for symptoms only. *New England Journal of Medicine, 348,* 1835–1837.

Grady, D., Yaffe, K., Kristof, M., et al. (2002). Effects of postmenopausal function on cognitive function: The Heart and Estrogen/progestin Replacement Study. *American Journal of Medicine, 113,* 543–548.

Guttosa, T. J. (2000). Gabapentin's effect on hot flashes and hypothermia. *Neurology, 54,* 2161–2163.

Hackley, B., & Rousseau, M. E. (2004). Managing menopausal symptoms after the Women's Health Initiative. *Journal of Midwifery Women's Health, 49*(2), 87–95.

*Kurman, R. J., Felix, J. C., Archer, D. F., et al. (2002). Norethindrone acetate and estradiol-induced endometrial hyperplasia. *Obstetrics and Gynecology, 96,* 373–379.

LeBlanc, E. S., Janowsky, J., Chan, B. K., et al. (2001). Hormone replacement therapy and cognition: Systematic review and meta-analysis. *Journal of the American Medical Association, 285,* 1489–1499.

*Loprinzi, C. L., Kugler, J. W., Sloan, J. A., et al. (2000). Venlafaxine in management of hot flashes in survivors of breast cancer: A randomized controlled trial. *Lancet, 356,* 2059–2063.

*Loprinzi, C. L., Pisansky, T. M., Fonseca, R., et al. (1998). Pilot evaluation of venlafaxine hydrochloride in the therapy of hot flashes in cancer survivors. *Journal of Clinical Oncology, 16,* 2377–2381.

Loprinzi, C. L., Sloan, J. A., Perez, E. A., et al. (2002). Phase III evaluation of fluoxetine for treatment of hot flashes. *Journal of Clinical Oncology, 20,* 1578–1583.

*Lund, K. (2008). Menopause and the menopausal transition. *Medical Clinics of North America, 92*(5), 1253–1271.

Mattox, J., & Shulman, L. (2001). Combined oral hormone replacement therapy formulations. *American Journal of Obstetrics and Gynecology, 185,* S38–S46.

Mulnard, R. A., Cotman, C. W., Kawas, C., et al. (2000). Estrogen replacement therapy for treatment of mild to moderate Alzheimer's disease: A randomized controlled trial: Alzheimer's Disease Cooperative Study. *Journal of the American Medical Association, 283,* 1007–1015.

*Quella, S. K., Loprinzi, C. L., Barton, D. L., et al. (2000). Evaluation of soy phytoestrogens for the treatment of hot flashes in breast cancer survivors. A North Central Cancer Treatment Group Trial. *Journal of Clinical Oncology, 18,* 1068–1074.

Rao, S., Singh, S., Parker, M., & Sugumaran, R. (2008). Health maintenance for postmenopausal women. *American Family Physician, 78*(5), 583–591.

Rapp, S. R., Espeland, M. A., Shumaker, S. A., et al. (2003). Effect of estrogen plus progestin on global cognitive function in postmenopausal women. The Women's Health Initiative Memory Study: A randomized controlled trial. *Journal of the American Medical Association, 289,* 2663–2672.

Reed, S., Newton, K., LaCroix, A., et al. (2007). Night sweats, sleep disturbances and depression associated with diminished libido in late menopausal transition and early postmenopause: Baseline data from the Herbal Alternatives for Menopause Trail (HALT). *American Journal of Obstetrics and Gynecology, 196*(6), 1–7.

*Santen, R. J. (2010). Postmenopausal hormone therapy: An Endocrine Society scientific statement. *Journal of Clinical Endocrinology and Metabolism, 7*(Suppl. 1), S1–S66.

Shifren, J. L., Braunstein, G. D., Simon, J. A., et al. (2000). Transdermal testosterone treatment in women with impaired sexual function after oophorectomy. *New England Journal of Medicine, 343,* 682–688.

*Stearns, V., Isaacs, C., Rowland, J., et al. (2000). A pilot trial assessing the efficacy of paroxetine hydrochloride (Paxil) in controlling hot flashes in breast cancer survivors. *Annals of Oncology, 11,* 17–22.

*U.S. Preventive Services Task Force. (2002). Postmenopausal hormone replacement therapy for primary prevention of chronic conditions: Recommendations and rationale. *Annals of Internal Medicine, 137*(10), 834–839.

*Utian, W. H. (1997). Menopause: A modern perspective from a controversial history. *Maturitas, 26*(2), 73–82.

*Utian, W. H., Shoupe, D., Bochman, G., et al. (2001). Relief of vasomotor symptoms and vaginal atrophy with lower doses of conjugated equine estrogen and medroxyprogesterone acetate. *Fertility Sterility, 75,* 1065–1079.

Weismiller, D. (2009). Menopause. *Primary Care: Clinics in Office Practice, 36*(1), 199–226.

Writing Group for the PEPI Trial. (1995). Effects of estrogen or estrogen/progestin on heart disease risk factors in post menopausal women. *Journal of the American Medical Association, 273,* 199–208.

Writing Group for the Women's Health Initiative. (2002). Risks and benefits of estrogen plus progestin in healthy postmenopausal women. *Journal of the American Medical Association, 288,* 321–333.

Zoorob, R., Sidani, M., Williams, J., & Grief, S. (2010). Women's health: Selected topics. *Primary Care, 37*(2), 369–387.

Osteoporosis

Osteoporosis is a progressive systemic disease characterized by a decrease in bone mass and microarchitectural deterioration of bone tissue, resulting in bone fragility and increased susceptibility to fractures. Osteoporosis, or low bone mass (osteopenia), is estimated to occur in approximately 44 million Americans, 80% of whom are women. Direct medical costs for the treatment of osteoporotic fractures are at least $15 billion annually (in 2002 dollars). Fracture risk in men is substantial, with one in three osteoporotic fractures occurring in men after age 50. In the United States, the direct costs of osteoporotic fractures are estimated at around $18 billion annually (Burge, 2007).

Bone fracture is the major cause of mortality and morbidity in patients with osteoporosis. The most common fractures are vertebral compression fractures and fractures of the distal radius and proximal femur. One in two women and one in eight men older than age 50 will have an osteoporosis-related fracture in their lifetimes.

CAUSES

The three types of osteoporosis are postmenopausal, senile, and secondary (**Box 57.1**). Many risk factors are associated with osteoporosis (**Box 57.2**).

Skeletal growth and the majority of bone mass are achieved during the first two decades of life, with bone density peaking around age 30. Between age 30 and menopause, bone mass remains relatively stable. At menopause, women have a period of 5 or more years during which there is an accelerated rate of bone loss. Some women lose up to 5% of their bone mass per year during this time.

PATHOPHYSIOLOGY

Two types of bone are discerned at the macroscopic level: cortical bone and trabecular bone. Cortical bone has a dense structure, whereas trabecular bone has a spongy appearance. Long bones have a thick outer layer of cortical bone and a thin inner layer of trabecular bone, whereas short bones consist of mostly trabecular bone with a thin layer of cortical bone.

Bone is in a constant state of remodeling (re-forming). Osteoblasts are responsible for bone formation, osteoclasts

for bone resorption. A balance is normally achieved between osteoblast and osteoclast activity. When bone resorption occurs at a faster rate than bone remodeling, osteoporosis is the result because the bones then become brittle and prone to fracture. Bone loss is greater in trabecular bone than in cortical bone.

Maximal mineral content of cortical bone occurs between the second and fourth decades of life, followed by a slow decline. In general, women have less bone mass than men, so even a small loss is more significant in women. Cortical bone loss in women is approximately 3% per decade until menopause, when the rate of bone loss accelerates to 9% per decade. Women lose approximately 15% of trabecular bone during the first 5 to 7 years after menopause. The rate returns to normal approximately 20 years after menopause. Generalized bone loss in men occurs at a rate of approximately 4% per decade throughout life.

Diagnostic Criteria

Medical history and a drug history are essential in the diagnosis. Bone mineral density (BMD) is related to bone mass at maturity and subsequent bone loss. Dual-energy x-ray absorptiometry (DEXA) scan measures BMD and is used to diagnose osteoporosis. A BMD of −1 to −2.5 standard deviations (SD) signifies osteopenia. A BMD of −2.5 SD, or lower than the mean for a normal 30- to 35-year-old woman, is diagnostic of osteoporosis. Screening is recommended for:

- all women older than age 65
- younger perimenopausal or postmenopausal women and men who have any medical condition or are taking medication associated with bone loss
- any adult older than age 50 with a fracture
- anyone being treated for osteoporosis
- men age 50 and older.

For every 1 SD decrease in bone mass, the relative risk of fracture increases by 1.5 to 3 SD.

The guidelines use fracture-risk calculations derived from a new computerized model developed by the World Health Organization (WHO). FRAX®, or "WHO Fracture Risk Assessment Tool," is a free online tool. It assesses the likelihood a patient will experience an osteoporotic fracture within 10 years. FRAX considers 10 risk factors in addition to the BMD T score so it will aid in the decision-making process of

BOX 57.1
Types of Osteoporosis

TYPE I: POSTMENOPAUSAL OSTEOPOROSIS

Occurs in postmenopausal women between ages 51 and 75

Decreased estrogen causes an accelerated rate of bone loss, especially trabecular bone loss.

The most common fractures are of the vertebrae and distal femur. There is also tooth loss.

TYPE II: SENILE OSTEOPOROSIS

Occurs in men and women older than age 70

There is a proportional loss of cortical and trabecular bone.

The most common fractures are hip, pelvic, and vertebral.

TYPE III: SECONDARY OSTEOPOROSIS

Occurs in men and women at any age

Secondary to other conditions such as drug therapy and other diseases

BOX 57.2
Risk Factors for Osteoporosis

Female sex
Older age
Asian or white race
Family history
Petite stature
Low body weight
Amenorrhea
Menopause (either natural or surgical) without hormone replacement
Sedentary lifestyle
Low calcium intake
Excess alcohol intake
Smoking
Excess caffeine intake
Low testosterone level in men
Drugs
    Thyroid replacement drugs
    Lithium
    Glucocorticoids
    Anticonvulsants
    Chemotherapy
    Heparin
    Cyclosporin
    Depot medroxyprogesterone (Depo-Provera)
    Tamoxifen, before menopause
    Pioglitazone (Actos) and rosiglitazone (Avandia)
Disease states
    Anorexia/bulimia
    Cushing's syndrome
    Thyrotoxicosis
    Rheumatoid arthritis
    Type 1 diabetes mellitus
    Thalassemia

who to treat. The risk factors are age, gender, fracture history, parental hip fracture history, oral steroid therapy, low body mass index, femoral neck BMD, secondary osteoporosis, current smoking, and alcohol intake. FRAX is available for download at http://www.shef.ac.uk/FRAX/.

INITIATING DRUG THERAPY

Prevention of osteoporosis should begin early in life with adequate intake of calcium and vitamin D. Children ages 9 to 18 should consume 1,300 mg of calcium daily. Adults ages 19 to 50 need 1,000 mg of calcium per day, and those age 51 and older require 1,200 mg each day. Because it is difficult to ingest that amount, supplements are usually needed. Weight-bearing exercise enhances bone mass and thereby helps prevent osteoporosis. Alcohol intake should be minimal, and those who smoke should stop.

Drugs used for the prevention and treatment of osteoporosis decrease bone resorption. They are called resorption-inhibiting drugs and include estrogens, bisphosphonates, calcitonin, and selective estrogen receptor modulators (SERMs). When these drugs are given, the rate of bone resorption decreases within weeks and the rate of bone formation increases within months. Remodeling spaces fill in, and an increase of BMD of 5% to 10% occurs with treatment. This process takes 2 to 3 years.

The National Osteoporosis Foundation (NOF) recommends that healthcare providers should consider U.S. Food and Drug Administration (FDA)-approved medical therapies in patients with:

1. Low bone mass (T score from −1.0 to −2.5 at the femoral neck, total hip, or spine) and 10-year probability of hip fracture of 3% or more or a 10-year probability of any major osteoporosis-related fracture of 20% or more.
2. T score of 2.5 or less at the femoral neck, total hip, or spine after appropriate evaluation to exclude secondary causes.
3. Low bone mass (T-score from −1.0 to −2.5 at the femoral neck, total hip, or spine) and secondary causes associated with high fracture risk (such as glucocorticoid use or immobilization).
4. A hip or vertebral (clinical or morphometric) fracture.
5. Other prior fractures and low bone mass (BMD T score from −1.0 to −2.5 at the femoral neck, total hip, or spine).

Goals of Drug Therapy

The goals of drug therapy are minimizing bone loss, delaying the progression of osteoporosis, and preventing fractures and fracture-related morbidity and mortality. Once osteoporosis is diagnosed and drug therapy is started, it is continued for life. **Table 57.1** provides an overview of the drugs used in treatment.

Calcium Supplements

Sufficient calcium is necessary for the prevention of osteoporosis. Postmenopausal women should take 1,200 to 1,500 mg of calcium a day. Calcium is absorbed most effectively when taken in small amounts throughout the day. Patients should not take calcium with meals that are high in fiber or with bulk-forming laxatives because such materials decrease absorption.

The over-the-counter (OTC) antacid Tums is an excellent and inexpensive source of calcium.

Most brand-name calcium products are absorbed easily in the body. If the product information does not state that it is absorbable, how well a tablet dissolves can be determined by placing it in a small amount of warm water for 30 minutes, stirring occasionally. If it hasn't dissolved within this time, it probably will not dissolve in the stomach. Chewable and liquid calcium supplements dissolve well because they are broken down before they enter the stomach. Calcium carbonate is absorbed best when taken with food. Calcium citrate can be taken any time. Calcium, whether from the diet or supplements, is absorbed best by the body when it is taken several times a day in amounts of 500 mg or less, but taking it all at once is better than not taking it at all.

TABLE 57.1	Overview of Selected Agents Used to Prevent or Treat Osteoporosis		
Generic (Trade) Name and Dosage	**Selected Adverse Events**	**Contraindications**	**Special Considerations**
Bisphosphonates			
alendronate (Fosamax) Prevention: 5 mg/d or 35 mg once a wk Treatment: 10 mg/d or 70 mg once a wk	GI upset, abdominal pain, gastroesophageal reflux disease, esophagitis, headache	Esophageal abnormalities, inability to be upright for 30 min, hypocalcemia, creatinine clearance <30	Swallow whole. Take with 8 oz of water 30 min before eating or drinking. Sit or stand for 30 min after taking (do not lie down until after eating). Calcium supplements and aluminum- or magnesium-containing antacids may interfere with absorption, so should be given at a different time.
risedronate (Actonel) 5 mg/d or 35 mg once a wk	Arthralgia, GI disturbances, headache, abdominal pain, rash, edema, chest pain, bone pain, dizziness, leg cramps, infection	Same as above	Same as above This drug is more tolerable for patients with GI problems than alendronate.
ibandronate (Boniva) 2.5 mg PO daily or 150 mg PO once a mo or 3 mg/3 mL IV every 3 mo	Same as above	Same as above	If taken monthly, take the same day each mo. IV medication is given in a bolus over 15–30 sec.
zoledronic acid (Reclast) 5 mg/100 mL once a y	Same as above	Same as above	Infusion must be given over at least 15 min.
Selective Estrogen Receptor Modulators			
raloxifene (Evista) 60 mg qd	Hot flashes, leg cramps	Pregnancy, history of thromboembolic events	Medication is to be stopped 72 h before surgery or prolonged immobilization.
Other			
calcitonin (Miacalcin) 200 U (1 spray) daily 100 U IM or SC daily	Rhinitis, GI upset, back pain, facial flushing (with injection)	Allergy to salmon or fish products, lactation Caution in renal deficiencies	Perform periodic nasal examinations to check for ulceration. Stop if nasal ulceration results. Switch nostrils each day. Injection recommended at bedtime because of possible facial flushing and nausea
Hormone Modifiers			
teriparatide (Forteo) 20 mcg daily SC	Hypercalcemia, dizziness, hyperuricemia, leg cramps, nausea, arthralgia	Paget's disease, previous bone radiation, skeletal malignancy, hypercalcemia, hyperparathyroidism; caution with kidney stones	Used in women with a high risk of fracture or who have failed other therapies

While calcium supplements are a satisfactory option for many people, certain preparations may cause side effects, such as gas or constipation, in some individuals. If simple measures such as increased fluids and fiber intake do not solve the problem, another form of calcium should be tried. Also, it is important to increase supplement intake gradually; take 500 mg/d for a week, then add more calcium slowly.

Vitamin D is responsible for the maintenance of an adequate concentration of calcium and phosphorus in the extracellular fluid. It also works with parathyroid hormone to regulate calcium movement across the gastrointestinal (GI) tract. The recommendation is 800 to 1,000 international units of vitamin D_3.

Menopausal Hormone Therapy

The Women's Health Initiative confirmed that estrogen, with or without progesterone, slightly reduced the risk of hip and vertebral fractures but found that this benefit did not outweigh the increased risk of stroke, venous thromboembolism, coronary heart disease, and breast cancer, even for women at high risk for fractures. Lower doses of conjugated equine estrogen and estradiol have been shown to improve BMD, but the reduced risk of fracture has not been demonstrated and the safety is unknown. The FDA recommends hormone therapy for osteoporosis only in women with moderate or severe vasomotor symptoms, using the lowest effective dose for the shortest time. (See Chapter 56 for a discussion of menopausal hormone therapy.)

Mechanism of Action

Estrogen prevents menopausal osteoporosis. Estrogen receptors are found on osteoclasts. When estrogen binds to these receptors, chemical mediators are secreted that decrease the activity of osteoclasts, causing decreased bone resorption. Estrogen slows bone loss significantly for at least as long as treatment continues. Practitioners should consider estrogen therapy for all estrogen-deficient women without contraindications. Hormone replacement therapy in women who have had a hysterectomy is estrogen alone, but in women with an intact uterus, practitioners must add progestin to prevent endometrial cancer. When treatment stops, bone mass decreases at a rate similar to that in postmenopausal women who are not taking menopausal hormone therapy.

Transdermal hormone therapy is not effective for treating osteoporosis because it takes at least 12 months to be effective. Practitioners can, however, prescribe it for prevention.

Contraindications

Contraindications to estrogen include pregnancy, active or past history of thrombophlebitis or thrombolytic disorders, estrogen-dependent neoplasia, and undiagnosed genital bleeding.

Bisphosphonates

Alendronate (Fosamax), risedronate (Actonel), ibandronate (Boniva), and zoledronic acid (Reclast) are bisphosphonates used for preventing and treating osteoporosis.

Mechanism of Action

These drugs inhibit bone resorption and increase bone density. They are deposited in the bone at sites of mineralization and in resorption lacunae. The bone resorption and fracture rate declines, whereas bone density increases. In studies of alendronate, an increase in bone mass was shown in the spine and hip, with a 48% decrease in the rate of vertebral compression fractures. Bone turnover increases to previous levels after 6 to 9 months when the patient takes alendronate for 6 months and then stops. If the patient takes alendronate for 6 years, no decrease in bone mass is noted for 2 years after therapy stops. These drugs have been used successfully for prevention and treatment of decreased bone mass as a result of long-term use of glucocorticoids.

In large, randomized, controlled trials, alendronate showed consistent increases in BMD irrespective of the severity of the underlying bone density levels, and it reduced the incidence of both vertebral and nonvertebral fractures (Cummings, et al., 1998; Liberman, et al., 1995). Among women with osteoporosis, the incidence of symptomatic vertebral fractures was decreased by 44% over 4 years and clinical fractures were reduced by 36% (Cummings, et al., 1998). Risedronate similarly reduced the incidence of vertebral fractures by 41% over 3 years (Harris, et al., 1999) and reduced hip fractures by 40% in elderly women who had low BMD but not in women who had risk factors alone (McClung, et al., 2001).

Dosage

The dosage for alendronate is 5 mg/d for prevention and 10 mg/d for treatment. It has also been approved for use once a week at 35 mg for prevention and 70 mg for treatment. Intestinal absorption of the drug is poor, so patients should take it on awakening with 8 ounces of water and 30 minutes before consuming any food or other drink. The dosage for risedronate is 5 mg/d or 35 mg once a week for prevention and treatment. The dosage for ibandronate is 2.5 mg daily or 150 mg once a month. There is also a 3 mg/3 mL solution for intravenous (IV) use every 3 months. Zoledronic acid is an IV medication given once a year. The dose is 5 mg/100 mL.

Contraindications

Bisphosphonates are not prescribed to patients with a history of esophageal problems, gastritis, or peptic ulcer disease. Adverse events include GI disturbance, esophagitis, diarrhea, and abdominal pain. Absorption increases with intravenous administration of ranitidine. Bisphosphonates should be prescribed with caution when the patient also is using nonsteroidal anti-inflammatory drugs. Absorption decreases when these drugs are taken with food, calcium, or iron, so patients should take the medication at different times from these substances (i.e., at least 30 minutes before or after taking food or liquid nourishment).

Adverse Events

Alendronate can cause esophagitis, usually within the first month of therapy. Ways to diminish esophagitis as well as to increase drug absorption include taking alendronate and rise-dronate with 8 ounces of water and remaining upright for 30 minutes after administration. Risedronate has fewer harsh effects on the GI system.

Calcitonin

Salmon calcitonin (Miacalcin) is another drug used in treating osteoporosis.

Mechanism of Action

Calcitonin works by inhibiting the action of osteoclasts. It is available in injectable form and as a nasal spray. It is not effective in preventing bone loss early in the postmenopausal period, but studies have shown that it increases bone mass in the spine and decreases the risk of vertebral compression fractures. Calcitonin also has an analgesic effect on pain associated with vertebral compression fractures.

In one study of postmenopausal women who used cal-citonin daily, new vertebral fractures were decreased by 33% compared with placebo, though only a small increase was noted in BMD (Chesnut, et al., 2000).

Dosage

The intranasal dosage of calcitonin is 200 U/d. The patient should alternate nostrils each day. The injectable dosage is 100 U subcutaneously or intramuscularly each day.

Adverse Events

An adverse event with the use of nasal calcitonin is rhinitis. The nasal mucosa should be inspected every 6 months for ulceration. Injection can cause local irritation. With both inhalation and injection, GI upset, flushing, rash, and back pain may occur. Recommendations are for patients to perform injections at bedtime because facial flushing and nausea may occur.

Selective Estrogen Receptor Modulators

SERMs are indicated for treating and preventing osteoporosis. They reduce the risk of vertebral fractures but do not appear to have an effect on hip fractures.

Mechanism of Action

SERMs mimic the effects of estrogen on bones without rep-licating the stimulating effects of estrogen on the breasts and uterus. They decrease bone resorption and bone turnover. These agents also decrease total cholesterol and low-density lipoprotein cholesterol levels.

Dosage

Raloxifene (Evista) is the only available SERM. The dose is 60 mg/day. Supplemental calcium and vitamin D are recommended.

Contraindications

Raloxifene is contraindicated in women who are lactating or who may become pregnant. It is also contraindicated in women who have a history of thromboembolic events. The patient must discontinue the drug 72 hours before prolonged immobilization, such as surgery requiring bed rest.

Adverse Events

Adverse events include hot flashes, GI distress, flu-like symp-toms, leg cramps, deep vein thrombosis, and arthralgias. When taken with cholestyramine, absorption is disrupted.

Hormone Modifiers

Hormone modifiers contain recombinant human parathyroid hormone (PTH). Teriparatide (Forteo) is the only PTH recom-binant currently available.

Mechanism of Action

PTH is the primary regulator of calcium and phosphate metabolism and regulates bone metabolism, renal tubular reabsorption of calcium and phosphates, and intestinal cal-cium absorption. It stimulates new bone formation in trabe-cular and cortical bone surface by preferential stimulation of osteoblastic activity over osteoclastic activity. This causes an increase in skeletal mass and an increase in markers of bone formation and resorption and bone strength.

A study showed women using teriparatide had an increased density of the spine of 10% to 14% and of the hip of 5%. In 18 months, vertebral fractures were reduced 60% to 70% and nonvertebral fractures 55% (Dempster, et al., 2001). It has been shown that teriparatide can prevent back pain in women with osteoporosis for up to 18 months beyond the end of treatment.

Dosage

Teriparatide is the only agent in this class currently. It is admin-istered subcutaneously at a dosage of 20 mcg daily. This is used in women at high risk for fracture or those who have failed to respond to or who are intolerant of other therapies.

Contraindications

Teriparatide is contraindicated in the following circumstances: Paget's disease, children, previous bone radiation therapy, his-tory of skeletal malignancy, metabolic bone disease, hypercal-cemia (which is usually transient), and hyperparathyroidism. It should be used cautiously in patients with a history of kidney stones.

Adverse Events

Teriparatide may increase calcium levels and increase the risk of digoxin toxicity if used together. Common adverse events include dizziness, nausea, leg cramps, arthralgia, and hyperuricemia.

Selecting the Most Appropriate Agent

The patient needs to take calcium and vitamin D in addition to any other drug selected. Results of the DEXA scan guide the provider's decision in selecting therapy for osteoporosis. If the T score is less than –1 SD from the norm, the patient is said to have no osteoporosis or osteopenia, but calcium intake and weight-bearing exercise are encouraged. A T score below –1 SD or less than –2.5 SD from the mean indicates osteopenia, and treatment with calcium and vitamin D should begin. Also, the practitioner should consider preventive resorption-inhibiting therapy. The risk of fracture almost doubles for each BMD decrease of 1 SD. The DEXA scan should be repeated in 2 years or sooner

if the patient experiences menopause. The NOF recommends pharmacologic treatment if the T score is below –2 SD from the mean, if the T score is –1.5 with other risk factors for osteoporosis or fracture, and if the woman is older than age 70 with multiple risk factors, especially previous fractures (**Figure 57-1**).

First-Line Therapy

Raloxifene or bisphosphonate therapy is used for prevention; bisphosphonates are used for treatment (**Table 57.2**). Patients should also take calcium and vitamin D supplementation. Treatment decisions are based on patient history. For instance, if the patient has a history of esophagitis, alendronate is not

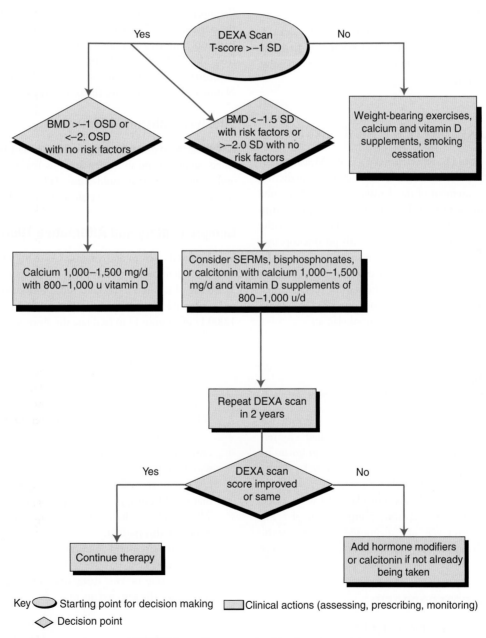

FIGURE 57–1 Treatment algorithm for osteoporosis.

TABLE 57.2	Recommended Order of Prevention and Treatment for Osteoporosis	
Order	**Agents**	**Comments**
First line	Prevention: raloxifene, alendronate, ibandronate, zoledronic acid, or risedronate plus calcium and vitamin D Treatment: raloxifene, alendronate, risedronate, ibandronate, zoledronic acid, or calcitonin	Treatment may be lifelong.
Second line	Addition of hormone modifiers or calcitonin if not being taken	

the best choice; if the patient has a history of thromboembolic disease, raloxifene is not the appropriate therapy.

Second-Line Therapy

Calcitonin or a hormone modifier is recommended for second-line therapy in women who have failed to respond to first-line therapy or who cannot tolerate hormone replacement therapy, bisphosphonates, or SERMs.

MONITORING PATIENT RESPONSE

The DEXA scan should be repeated every 2 years. Measurement of the density of the proximal femur is most helpful in predicting fractures, and measurement of the density of the lumbar spine is most effective in measuring the response to therapy. Within 2 years, resorption-inhibiting drugs increase the BMD of the lumbar spine by 5% to 10% in women with postmenopausal osteoporosis, causing the incidence of fractures to decrease by 50% (Cummings, et al., 1993; Melton, et al., 1993). Follow-up is recommended 1 to 2 months after the start of therapy, then every 3 to 6 months if the patient has osteoporosis. Follow-up is necessary every year if the therapy is prophylactic.

PATIENT EDUCATION

Drug Information

Bisphosphonates should be taken with 8 ounces of water, and the patient should remain upright for 30 minutes after administration. Information about osteoporosis can be obtained from the NOF website (http://www.nof.org) or the National Institutes of Health Osteoporosis and Related Bone Disease National Resource Center (http://www.osteo.org).

Lifestyle/Nutritional Changes

A well-balanced diet is important, as are weight-bearing exercises. Safety strategies are necessary, such as removing unstable rugs and keeping items that could cause a fall out of the way. Smoking cessation is essential. Excessive alcohol intake should be avoided.

Complementary and Alternative Therapy

Supplemental calcium and vitamin D are important adjuncts to therapy. Patients without osteopenia or osteoporosis should ingest 1,200 mg of calcium a day, and those with osteopenia or osteoporosis should ingest more—1,500 mg calcium daily and 800 to 1,000 U of vitamin D to facilitate the absorption of calcium.

Case Study

J.S., a 72-year-old woman of Asian descent, has just transferred to your practice. She had a hysterectomy 8 years ago and has not been on hormone replacement therapy. She is 5 ft, 2 inches and weighs 102 lb. She has had a sedentary lifestyle (she was a secretary and retired 2 years ago). She drinks four glasses of wine a day. Her mother died at age 62 from complications of a hip fracture. J.S.'s sister was just diagnosed with metastatic breast cancer. You prescribe a DEXA scan, and the T score is –2.6 SD.

DIAGNOSIS: OSTEOPOROSIS

1. List specific goals of therapy for J.S.
2. What drug therapy would you prescribe? Why?
3. What are the parameters for monitoring the success of the therapy?
4. Discuss specific patient education based on the prescribed therapy.
5. List one or two adverse reactions for the selected agent that would cause you to change therapy.
6. What OTC or alternative medicines might be appropriate for this patient?
7. What dietary and lifestyle changes might you recommend?
8. Describe one or two drug–drug or drug–food interactions for the selected agent.

BIBLIOGRAPHY

Starred references are cited in the text.

*Burge, R. (2007). Incidence and economic burden of osteoporosis. *Journal of Bone Mineral Research, 22*(3), 465–475.

*Chesnut, C. H. III, Silverman, S., Andriano, K., et al. (2000). A randomized trial of nasal spray salmon calcitonin in postmenopausal women with established osteoporosis: The Prevent Recurrence of Osteoporotic Fractures Study. PROOF Study Group. *American Journal of Medicine, 109,* 267–276.

Compston, J. (2010). Osteoporosis: Social and economic impact. *Radiologic Clinics of North America, 48*(3), 477–482.

*Cummings, S. R., Black, D. M., Thompson, D. E., et al. (1998). Effect of alendronate on risk of fracture in women with low bone density but without vertebral fractures: Results from the Fracture Intervention Trial. *JAMA, 280,* 2077–2082.

*Dempster, D. W., Cosman, F., & Kurland, E. S. (2001). Effects of daily treatment with parathyroid hormone on bone microarchitecture and turnover in patients with osteoporosis: A paired biopsy study. *Journal of Bone Mineral Research, 16,* 1846–1853.

*Harris, S. T., Watts, N. B., Genant, H. K., et al. (1999). Effects of risedronate treatment on vertebral and nonvertebral fractures in women with postmenopausal osteoporosis: A randomized controlled trial. Vertebral Efficacy with Risedronate Therapy (VERT) Study Group. *JAMA, 282,* 1344–1352.

Kaufman, J., & Goemaere, S. (2008). Osteoporosis in men. *Best Practice and Research in Clinical Endocrinology and Metabolism, 22*(5), 787–812.

Lash, R., Nicholson, J., Velez, L., et al. (2009). Diagnosis and management of osteoporosis. *Primary Care: Clinics in Office Practice, 36*(1), 181–198.

Lewiecki, E. M. (2008). Prevention and treatment of osteoporosis. *Obstetrics and Gynecology Clinics, 35*(2), 301–315.

*Liberman, U. A., Weiss, S. R., Broll, J., et al. (1995). Effect of oral alendronate on bone mineral density and the incidence of fractures in postmenopausal osteoporosis. The Alendronate Phase III Osteoporosis Treatment Study Group. *New England Journal of Medicine, 333,* 1437–1443.

*McClung, M. R., Geusens, P., Miller, P. D., et al. (2001). Effect of risedronate on the risk of hip fracture in elderly women. *New England Journal of Medicine, 344,* 333–340.

*Melton, L. J., Atkinson, E. J., O'Fallon, W. M., et al. (1993). Long-term fracture prediction by bone mineral assesses at different skeletal sites. *Journal of Bone Mineral Research, 8,* 1227–1233.

Simon, L. (2007). Osteoporosis. *Rheumatic Disease Clinics of North America, 33*(1), 149–176.

Sweet, M., Sweet, J., Jeremiah, M., & Galazka, S. (2009). Diagnosis and treatment of osteoporosis. *American Family Physician, 79*(3), 193–200.

Vaginitis

Vaginitis is one of the most common gynecologic complaints. The most common causes of vaginitis are vulvovaginal candidiasis, bacterial vaginosis, and *Trichomonas vaginalis*. The presentation is often vaginal or perineal itching, burning, vulvar or vaginal irritation, and abnormal vaginal discharge. Many women may be asymptomatic. Other causes of vaginal irritation or inflammation include allergic reactions and atrophic changes in the vaginal mucosa.

CAUSES

Candidiasis

Most vaginal yeast infections are caused by *Candida albicans*, although other organisms, such as *Candida tropicalis* and *Candida glabrata*, are seen, especially in recurrent candidiasis. Colonization of Candida at other sites, such as the oral mucosa and the gastrointestinal (GI) tract, may be associated with recurrent vaginitis. Candidal vaginitis is often accompanied by vulvitis, so the term *vulvovaginal candidiasis* (VVC) may better describe this disorder.

Behavioral factors may cause VVC. Sexual factors, in particular orogenital sex, may contribute to the introduction of microorganisms or cause microtrauma to the vulva and vestibule. Contraceptive practices may contribute to VVC; oral contraceptives, use of a diaphragm and spermicide, and the use of an intrauterine device are associated with an increased risk of infection.

Bacterial Vaginosis

Bacterial vaginosis (BV) is a polymicrobial vaginal infection that occurs when the hydrogen peroxide–producing lactobacillus normally present in the vagina diminish, allowing other bacteria to proliferate. Bacteria, such as *Gardnerella vaginalis*, *Prevotella* species, *Mobiluncus* species, and *Mycoplasma hominis*, are responsible for BV. Although the cause of BV is not well understood, some studies suggest that causes may include complications of pregnancy and infections associated with gynecologic procedures, pelvic inflammatory disease, and cervical intraepithelial neoplasia. It is unclear whether BV is only sexually transmitted.

Although BV in the past frequently has been ignored, it is considered the most common form of vaginitis and affects approximately 30% of women. The prevalence of BV among U.S. women ages 14 to 49 is about 29% (Koumans, et al., 2007).

Because most women who have BV exhibit no or minor symptoms, there is a tendency to overlook this condition. Sociodemographic factors associated with BV include younger age, being non-Hispanic black or Mexican American, having less than a high school education, living at or near the federal poverty level, and douching. Sexual risk factors, such as being sexually active, age of first sexual intercourse, and having multiple male lifetime sexual partners, particularly over the past year, all are risk factors for BV. In lesbian women, female partners of women who have BV have a higher incidence of BV. Despite the sexual risk factors associated with BV, however, BV is considered sexually associated but not sexually transmitted. While infection is rare in women who have never been sexually active, treatment of male sex partners has not proven to be beneficial in preventing recurrence.

Trichomoniasis

T. vaginalis, an anaerobic protozoan, is one of the most commonly sexually transmitted organisms. Practitioners have long recognized that some asymptomatic women may harbor the organism. The organism, which can apparently survive in the environment for several hours, may be transmitted by contact, particularly with moist objects (e.g., underclothing and towels). Increased numbers of sexual partners, a recent new sexual partner, or early initiation of sexual activity (younger than age 16) is associated with an increased prevalence. Up to 86% of trichomoniasis infections may be asymptomatic. Trichomonads can live for a limited length of time on moist surfaces and may be transmitted by fomites, such as towels or sexual toys.

Allergies and Irritants

Conditions or products that irritate the vulva or the vaginal epithelium or local allergic reactions may produce symptoms similar to those of infectious vaginitis. Examples of irritants include vaginal lubricants, condoms, spermicides, and feminine hygiene products. Women who have other atopic skin conditions may experience vaginal and vulvar manifestations as well.

Atrophy

Low levels of estrogen in a postmenopausal woman may lead to atrophy of the vaginal epithelium and subsequent irritation and inflammation, which also may predispose the woman to vaginitis.

PATHOPHYSIOLOGY

A review of the normal physiology of the vaginal environment forms the basis for understanding the possible causes and pathophysiology of vaginitis. In postpubertal women, both anaerobic and aerobic bacteria make up the normal vaginal flora. These include potential pathogens, such as *Staphylococcus*, *Streptococcus*, and *Bacteroides* species, and nonpathogens, such as lactobacilli and diphtheroids. *C. albicans* is a saprophytic fungus that is a normal vaginal inhabitant in 15% to 25% of women.

One of the most important factors in the defense against infection is an acidic vaginal pH, which may be influenced by the acidic by-products produced by the normal vaginal flora. Hydrogen peroxide–producing strains of lactobacilli in vaginal secretions have been associated with protection against some vaginal infections as well. Therefore, variables that alter the vaginal pH or destroy lactobacilli may predispose a woman to vaginal infection. Among these variables are pregnancy, diabetes, sexual activity, hormonal changes, antibiotic therapy, and the use of feminine hygiene products. The thickness of the vaginal epithelium may also influence antimicrobial defenses.

DIAGNOSTIC CRITERIA

Candidiasis (VVC)

Symptoms of VVC include intense pruritus and erythema, dysuria, and a thick, white, curdlike vaginal discharge that tends to adhere to the vaginal walls. Diagnosis is made on the basis of presenting complaints, physical findings, and observation of pseudohyphae on potassium hydroxide (KOH) wet mount slide. Gram's stain and culture of the vaginal discharge are other methods that may be employed in the diagnosis of VVC. Vaginal cultures can confirm the diagnosis and identify the species of *Candida* causing infection. Since 10% to 20% of women harbor *Candida* in the vagina, it is not recommended that asymptomatic women be treated. If the vaginal pH is tested, the value in candidiasis is usually less than 4.5. *Candida* may also be identified on Papanicolaou (Pap) smears of symptomatic or asymptomatic women. VVC may be classified as complicated or uncomplicated (**Box 58.1**).

Bacterial Vaginosis

Routine cultures are not helpful in diagnosing BV because up to 50% of women who harbor *G. vaginalis* vaginally are asymptomatic. When symptomatic, a woman may complain of a fishy odor, yellow or grayish discharge, and vaginal irritation. A yellow discharge increases the likelihood of BV fourfold, but also can indicate a trichomonas infection. A white discharge makes BV less likely. A clinical diagnosis of BV requires three out of four Amsel

---

BOX 58.1

CDC Classification of Vulvovaginal Candidiasis (VVC)

Uncomplicated VVC

Sporadic or infrequent vulvovaginal candidiasis

or

Mild to moderate vulvovaginal candidiasis

or

Likely to be *C. albicans*

or

Non-immunocompromised women

Complicated VVC

Recurrent vulvovaginal candidiasis

or

Severe vulvovaginal candidiasis

or

Non-*albicans* candidiasis

or

Women with uncontrolled diabetes, debilitation, or immunosuppression, or those who are pregnant

---

criteria, which are 92% sensitive but only 77% specific. Amsel criteria are abnormal grayish homogenous discharge, vaginal pH greater than 4.5, positive amine or "whiff test" ("fishy" odor with KOH applied to discharge), and more than 20% positive clue cells (epithelial cells surrounded by adherent coccobacilli) on microscopy (**Box 58.2**). Treatment reduces symptoms, yet recurrences are common, with 23% at one month and 58% at 12 months.

Trichomoniasis

Patients with vaginitis caused by *Trichomonas* organisms report a profuse, frothy, yellowish vaginal discharge, vaginal and vulvar irritation, dysuria, and dyspareunia. Microscopic identification of the motile organism on a wet-mount slide usually confirms the diagnosis. *Trichomonas* organisms may also be

---

BOX 58.2

Diagnostic Tests for Bacterial Vaginosis

Affirm VPIII (Becton-Dickinson, Sparks, Maryland)
FemExam test card (Cooper Surgical, Shelton, Connecticut)
Pip Activity TestCard (Litmus Concepts, Inc., Santa Clara, California)

CDC, 2002.

identified on a Pap smear. Because the organism may be recovered from male partners of infected women, this form of vaginitis is considered to be sexually transmitted.

Occasionally, asymptomatic women are diagnosed with trichomoniasis by routine Pap smear, which is reported to be 57% sensitive and 97% specific. If symptomatic, trichomoniasis presents as vaginal itching, burning, vaginal discharge (frequently profuse, yellowish-green, and malodorous), or postcoital bleeding. Trichomonads often appear in motion on a vaginal secretion saline wet mount, "swimming" with the flagella in a jerking or tumbling action. The sensitivity of detecting trichomonads on saline wet mount is estimated at 62% with a specificity of 97% and a positive predictive value of 75%. Culture is very sensitive (95%) and specific (greater than 95%), but delays diagnosis and is not routinely performed.

Allergic Vaginitis

Vaginitis resulting from allergy or irritants may be characterized by pruritus, discharge, and dyspareunia. The diagnosis often relies on exclusion. Although vaginal discharge may be increased, the secretions, when examined microscopically, do not harbor candidal organisms, trichomonads, or clue cells.

Atrophic Vaginitis

Vaginitis associated with atrophy of the vaginal walls produces pruritus, discharge, dryness, and dyspareunia. Physical examination reveals thinning of the vaginal walls with a characteristic shiny-smooth appearance. Introduction of the speculum into the vaginal introitus may cause bleeding. Microscopic examination reveals no candidal organisms, trichomonads, or clue cells.

INITIATING DRUG THERAPY

When considering pharmacotherapy for vaginitis, the practitioner explores lifestyle choices that may predispose the patient to infection or inflammation. Questions to ask regard the use of douches or other feminine hygiene products, sexual practices and partners, the possible relationship between sexual activity and appearance of symptoms, and recent antibiotic or oral contraceptive use. The practitioner should perform a thorough assessment to identify other possible irritants or complaints.

Before choosing a plan of therapy, the practitioner and patient also need to consider the issue of recurrent infection. In the case of recurrent VVC (four or more symptomatic episodes annually), the practitioner should be alert to the possibility of diabetes, and the need for screening should be discussed. In the case of recurrent trichomonal infection, sex partners should be examined and treated if they are found to be transmitting the organisms. It also is not uncommon for BV to recur.

Goals of Therapy

The primary goal of therapy in treating infectious vaginitis is eradication of the offending organism. The primary goals of therapy for allergic vaginitis include reducing inflammation and avoiding irritants. Addressing the hypoestrogenic state of postmenopausal women with hormone replacement therapy alleviates the symptoms of atrophic vaginitis. (Refer to Chapter 56 for a discussion of these treatment options.)

Another important goal of therapy is relief of symptoms. Vaginitis can cause considerable discomfort, both physically and emotionally. Women with vaginitis often experience embarrassment and even fear, particularly of the implications of a sexually transmitted disease. The frustration associated with recurrent infection may lead women to repeated attempts to self-treat, which delays proper evaluation by their primary care provider. For more information on self-treatment, see **Box 58.3**.

In the treatment of BV, additional goals of therapy include reduction of the risk of complications following gynecological procedures (e.g., abortion and hysterectomy) and reduction in the risk of acquiring other sexually transmitted infections. Adverse pregnancy outcomes have been associated with BV and trichomoniasis. The treatment of asymptomatic women with BV is not recommended, but some specialists recommend that women at high risk for preterm delivery be screened and treated for BV during the first prenatal visit.

Topical Azole Antifungals

Topical vaginal preparations for treating VVC include the following azoles: clotrimazole, butoconazole, tioconazole, miconazole,

---

BOX | **58.3**

Self-Diagnosis and Self-Treatment of Vaginitis

Studies assessing the accuracy of self-diagnosis of vaginal symptoms found the incidence of misdiagnosis to be high (Ferris, Dekle, & Litaker, 1996; Njirjesy, Weitz, Grody, & Lorber, 1997). In both studies, women were self-treating symptoms that they attributed to vulvovaginal candidiasis with OTC antifungals (Ferris, et al., 1996; Njirjesy, et al., 1997) and other OTC alternative medicines (Njirjesy, et al., 1997).

Although misuse of these pharmaceuticals rarely causes adverse reactions, a delay in diagnosis of infections such as pelvic inflammatory disease, bacterial vaginosis, or urinary tract infections could have significant consequences. Furthermore, repeated use of these medications unsuccessfully by women before their visit to the provider can make accurate assessment of the symptoms and physical findings difficult.

and terconazole. Treatment duration with these agents varies from 1 to 3 to 7 days. Response to treatment varies according to the duration of therapy. Types of topical preparations include creams, ointments, tablets, and suppositories. Oral fluconazole is also available for treatment in a one-time dose.

Time Frame for Response

The cure rates for topically applied azoles have long been established at between 80% and 90%. It can take up to 3 days to see the effect of the medications. These preparations are considered to be more effective than the antifungal nystatin (Mycostatin). **Table 58.1** lists the azole drugs currently available by prescription or without a prescription. In the case of VVC, only women who were previously diagnosed with this form of vaginitis should choose to self-treat with an over-the-counter (OTC) medication. Practitioners should advise women whose symptoms persist or recur within 2 months of self-treatment to seek medical care. In general, the only contraindication to

the topical antifungals is hypersensitivity to the azole or components of the cream or gel.

Adverse Events

Topical azoles seldom cause systemic adverse events, although they may cause local irritation. Unfortunately, these effects may be difficult to distinguish from the conditions for which they are being used. Less common events may include penile irritation of the sex partner, abdominal cramps, or headache.

Interactions

Since these preparations are oil-based, they may weaken latex condoms and diaphragms.

Oral Azole Antifungal Agents

Fluconazole, the only oral azole to be recommended by the Centers for Disease Control and Prevention (CDC) for treating

TABLE 58.1 Overview of Antifungal Agents

Generic (Trade) Name and Dosage	Selected Adverse Events	Contraindications	Special Considerations
OTC Preparations			
butoconazole 2% cream (Femstat) 1 applicatorful intravag. qhs for 3 d	Vaginal irritation, skin rash, hives	Allergy	Oil-based; might weaken latex condoms and diaphragms
butoconazole 2% cream (sustained-release) 1 applicatorful hs × 3 d			Refer to product labeling for more information.
clotrimazole 1% cream (Gyne-Lotrimin, Mycelex-G) 1 applicatorful intravag. qhs for 7–14 d	Same as above	Same as above	Same as above
clotrimazole 100-mg vaginal tablets (Gyne-Lotrimin, Mycelex-G) 1 tab intravag. qhs for 7 d or 2 tabs intravag. qhs for 3 d	Same as above	Same as above	Same as above
miconazole 2% cream (Monistat 7) 1 applicatorful intravag. qhs for 7 d	Same as above	Same as above	Same as above
miconazole 200-mg suppository (Monistat 3) 1 suppository intravag. qhs for 3 d	Same as above	Same as above	Same as above
miconazole 100-mg suppository (Monistat 7) 1 suppository intravag. qhs for 7 d	Same as above	Same as above	Same as above
tioconazole 6.5% ointment (Vagistat) 1 applicatorful intravag. qhs, single dose	Same as above	Same as above	Same as above
Prescription Preparations			
terconazole 0.4% cream (Terazol 7) 1 applicatorful intravag. qhs for 7 d	Same as above	Same as above	Same as above
terconazole 0.8% cream (Terazol 3) 1 applicatorful intravag. qhs for 3 d	Same as above	Same as above	Same as above
terconazole 80 mg suppositories (Terazol 3) 1 suppository intravag. qhs for 3 d	Same as above	Same as above	Same as above
fluconazole 150-mg tablet (Diflucan) 1 tablet orally, single dose	Headache, abdominal pain, nausea Rare: hepatic injury	Same as above	May interact with oral hypoglycemics, anticoagulants, cyclosporine, rifampin, theophylline, calcium channel antagonists, cisapride, astemizole, phenytoin, protease inhibitors, tacrolimus, terfenadine, trimetrexate

CDC recommendations, 2006.

uncomplicated VVC, is available by prescription in a single 150-mg dose. It is as effective as topical azoles. The findings of a study evaluating the acceptance of single-dose oral fluconazole by patients and physicians showed that most participants believed the drug to be effective in relieving or alleviating the symptoms of VVC. Oral fluconazole maintenance therapy for recurrent VVC should be extended for 6 months, but caution should be used with long-term ketoconazole therapy since hepatotoxicity may occur.

Contraindications

Contraindications to oral azole antifungals include known hypersensitivity to these azoles and the concomitant use of drugs with which they interact.

Time Frame for Response

Because patients treated with oral antifungals may not obtain relief of symptoms for 2 or 3 days, they may need to use an OTC antifungal cream for a few days. Failure to respond necessitates reevaluation.

Adverse Events

The most commonly reported adverse events noted in patients treated with oral fluconazole are headache, nausea, and abdominal pain. Ketoconazole and itraconazole can cause GI disorders, headache, and pruritus. Hepatotoxicity may also occur, especially with ketoconazole. Liver enzyme levels may need to be monitored, especially with long-term use. Adverse effects tend to be dose-related. Interactions may occur because oral azoles are cytochrome P450 inhibitors.

Antibacterials/Antibiotics

Metronidazole (Flagyl) may be used orally or intravaginally for treating BV. Oral metronidazole 500 mg twice daily for 7 days is the standard treatment for BV, and only the oral form is effective in treating trichomonal infection. Tinidazole 2 g in a single dose is also used. (See **Table 58.2** for specific dosages.) Topical clindamycin cream 2% (Cleocin) should be used in patients who are allergic to metronidazole. Clindamycin 300 mg twice daily may also be used orally for a 7-day course. It is contraindicated in patients with hypersensitivity to it or to other preparations containing lincomycin. Cleocin Ovules intravaginally are also effective if inserted at bedtime for 3 nights.

Contraindications

Metronidazole is no longer thought to be teratogenic, and therefore it is not contraindicated in the first trimester of pregnancy. It is contraindicated, however, in patients with a known hypersensitivity to it or other nitroimidazoles.

Adverse Events

Metallic taste, headache, and GI distress are common side effects of metronidazole. To avoid the disulfiram-like effect of nausea and vomiting, patients must not consume alcohol during treatment and for 24 hours after treatment stops.

TABLE 58.2	CDC* Recommendations for Treating Bacterial Vaginosis		
Generic (Trade) Name and Dosage	**Selected Adverse Events**	**Contraindications**	**Special Considerations**
Recommended Regimens			
metronidazole 500 mg tablets (Flagyl) 1 tab PO bid for 7 d	Metallic taste, headache, GI distress	Allergy (No longer contraindicated in pregnancy)	Avoid alcohol during therapy and for 24 h after stopping (will cause nausea and vomiting). May potentiate the anticoagulant effects of warfarin and other anticoagulants
clindamycin 2% cream (Cleocin) 1 applicatorful intravag. qhs for 7 d Clindamycin ovules 100 g intravaginally once hs for 3 d	Vaginal irritation, skin rash, hives	Allergy	Oil-based; may weaken latex condoms and diaphragms Refer to product labeling for more information.
metronidazole gel 0.75%. (MetroGel) 1 applicatorful intravag. bid for 5 d	Vaginal irritation, skin rash, metallic taste, GI distress	Same as above	Although blood levels are lower than with the use of oral metronidazole, alcohol still should be avoided.
clindamycin 300-mg tablets (Cleocin) 1 tablet orally bid for 7 d	GI distress	Same as above	None

*CDC recommendations as of 2006.

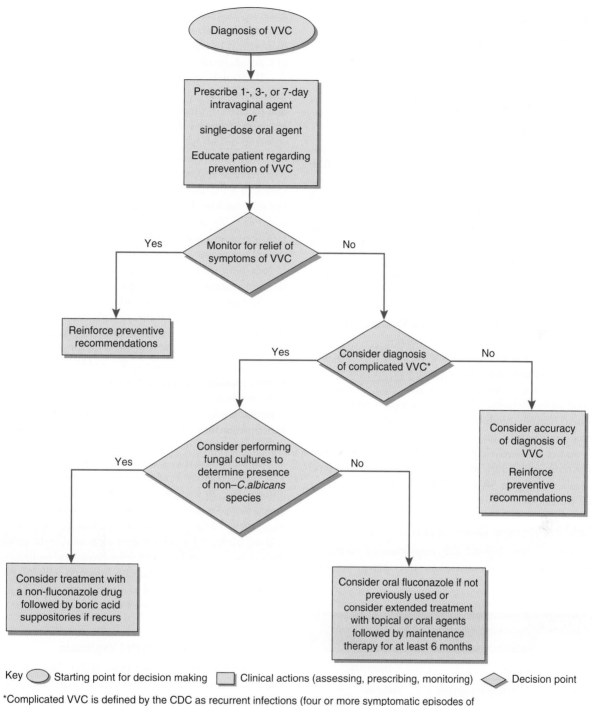

FIGURE 58–1 Treatment algorithm for vaginitis known as vulvovaginal candidiasis (VVC).

*Complicated VVC is defined by the CDC as recurrent infections (four or more symptomatic episodes of VVC per year), immunocompromised patient, severe infection, non–*C.albicans* species.

Interactions

Metronidazole may potentiate the anticoagulant effect of warfarin (Coumadin) and other oral anticoagulants. Although some animal studies have linked metronidazole to cancer, no current evidence indicates that the drug has a similar effect on humans.

Estrogens

Treatment of atrophic vaginitis consists of systemic estrogen replacement or topical estrogen creams administered externally or intravaginally. Refer to Chapter 56 for a complete discussion of these therapies.

Anti-Inflammatories

Mild topical steroid preparations can be used on a short-term or episodic basis. Careful monitoring of the patient's response is advised.

Selecting the Most Appropriate Agent

First-Line Therapy: Candidiasis

In an attempt to guide therapeutic options, the CDC classifies VVC as either uncomplicated or complicated. (See **Box 58.2**.)

OTC topical antifungals are typical first-line therapy of uncomplicated VVC and can be used before the patient seeks professional treatment. Women experiencing typical symptoms such as pruritus and vaginal discharge can obtain relief of symptoms promptly without the expense of a visit to the practitioner. Appropriate therapy consists of 1 to 7 days of treatment with the topical antifungals. It is recommended that self-treatment with OTC antifungals be reserved for women who have been previously diagnosed with VVC and who have not experienced a recurrence within 2 months.

Single-dose oral antifungals are an alternative first-line therapy in uncomplicated VVC, especially because the ease of administration may ensure therapeutic adherence. Fluconazole is the oral azole of choice. The patient's sex partners need not be treated because candidiasis is not sexually transmitted. However, consideration may be given to treating male sex partners of women with recurrent infection. Male sex partners who have symptoms of balanitis may benefit from the use of topical antifungals. See **Figure 58-1** and **Table 58.3** for an overview of VVC treatment.

Second-Line Therapy: Candidiasis

If symptoms persist beyond the recommended course of therapy with first-line agents, second-line therapy involves assessing for possible recurrent VVC or infection with non–*albicans Candida*, such as *C. glabrata*. Vaginal cultures should be obtained to confirm the diagnosis and identify the species of Candida involved.

If an oral antifungal was not the first-line therapy, the practitioner may opt to treat with oral fluconazole as second-line therapy or extend the course of topical or oral therapy. It has been suggested that 7- to 14-day treatment with topical agents or a 150-mg dose of oral fluconazole repeated 3 days later may achieve remission in patients with recurrent VVC. Maintenance regimens are recommended for patients with recurrent VVC and include clotrimazole (500-mg suppositories once weekly), ketoconazole (100-mg dose once daily), fluconazole (100- to 150-mg dose once weekly), or itraconazole (100-mg dose once monthly). These maintenance therapies should be continued for 6 months. Hepatotoxicity may occur in long-term treatment with ketoconazole, and these patients should be monitored accordingly.

Second-line therapy for patients with non-*albicans* VVC consists of 7- to 14-day treatment with a non-fluconazole azole drug followed by boric acid suppositories (600 mg in a gelatin capsule intravaginally once daily for 14 days), if the infection recurs. Topical flucytosine 4% and nystatin 100,000-unit vaginal suppositories are additional options in the treatment of non-*albicans* VVC. However, consultation with a specialist is recommended. Women who are immunocompromised also benefit from the prolonged therapy (7 to 14 days) with either topical or oral agents.

In complicated cases, a second dose of oral fluconazole 150 mg given at day 3 yields an 80% cure rate versus 67% with a single dose. In women who have more than four infections a year, a 7- to 14-day course of oral fluconazole may be needed to suppress the *Candida*. Suppression therapy with fluconazole 150 mg weekly for 6 months controls symptomatic episodes in 90% of women, and one half have prolonged symptom relief. A treatment failure may indicate infection with *C. glabrata*, which does not respond well to azoles. Boric acid 600-mg capsules given intravaginally for 14 days may be effective.

First-Line Therapy: Bacterial Vaginosis

Oral metronidazole (500 mg twice daily) 7-day therapy has long been considered standard first-line treatment for BV. However, the CDC (2006) also recommends topical clindamycin cream 2% (intravaginally for 7 days) or metronidazole gel 0.75% (intravaginally for 5 days) as acceptable first-line therapy. Alternative regimens for first-line therapy include clindamycin 300 mg twice daily orally for a 7-day course or clindamycin ovules 100 g intravaginally at bedtime for 3 days. Once-daily dosing with metronidazole 750-mg extended-release tablets has been approved by the U.S. Food and Drug Administration for the treatment of BV, but data are not available regarding the efficacy of this regimen (CDC, 2006). Treatment of sex partners is not recommended because clinical trials have not shown a relationship between treatment of partners and recurrence of BV. See **Figure 58-2** and **Table 58.4** for an overview of treatment.

TABLE 58.3	Recommended Order of Treatment for Vulvovaginal Candidiasis	
Order	**Agents**	**Comments**
First line	OTC topical antifungals *or* Single-dose oral antifungal	Patients may self-treat before visit with practitioner.
Second line	Single-dose oral antifungal *or* Extend course of therapy of topical or oral antifungal *or* Maintenance therapy with an oral or topical antifungal *or* Boric acid suppositories	If not used as first line. Vaginal cultures to determine presence of non-*albicans* candidiasis

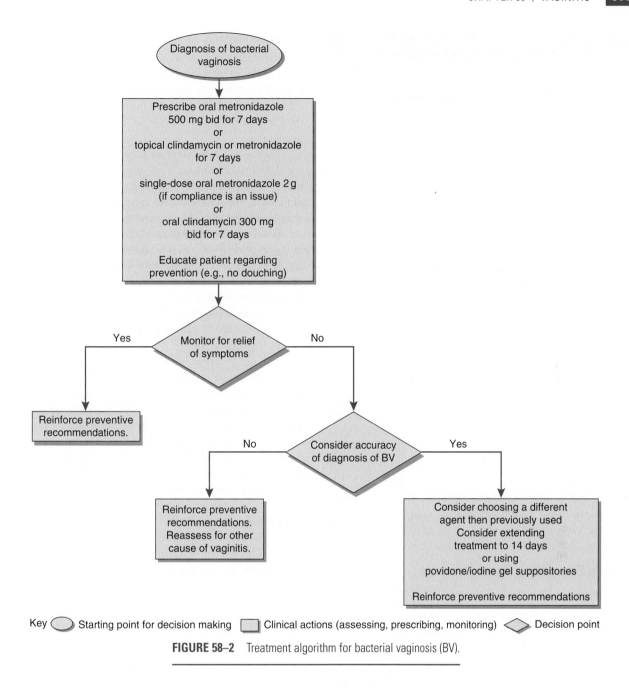

FIGURE 58–2 Treatment algorithm for bacterial vaginosis (BV).

Second-Line Therapy: Bacterial Vaginosis

Treatment reduces symptoms, yet recurrences are common, with 23% at 1 month and 58% at 12 months. Recurrent BV should be treated. One randomized trial for persistent BV indicated that metronidazole gel 0.75% twice per week for 6 months after completion of a recommended regimen was effective in maintaining a clinical cure for 6 months (Sobel, et al., 2006). Clinical trials indicate that a woman's response to therapy and the likelihood of relapse or recurrence are not affected by treatment of her sex partner(s). Therefore, routine treatment of sex partners is not recommended.

First-Line Therapy: Trichomoniasis

Only one treatment regimen is considered to be clinically efficacious for trichomoniasis: metronidazole or tinidazole given as a single 2-g dose. An alternative regimen is metronidazole 500 mg twice daily for 7 days. Treatment of male sex partners (who are usually asymptomatic) is recommended, and patients and their partners should avoid intercourse until they have completed therapy and are symptom-free. Patients should be cautioned to avoid alcohol, as previously described. See **Figure 58-3** and **Table 58.5** for an overview of treatment.

TABLE 58.4	Recommended Order of Treatment for Bacterial Vaginosis	
Order	**Agents**	**Comments**
First line	Oral metronidazole *or* clindamycin cream 2% *or* metronidazole gel 0.75% *or* clindamycin orally *or* clindamycin ovules	Traditionally used as first line
Second line	Extend duration of above agents *or* povidone–iodine gel suppositories *or* choose different agent	*May* be effective

Second-Line Therapy: Trichomoniasis

Some strains of *T. vaginalis* can have diminished susceptibility to metronidazole but respond to tinidazole or higher doses of metronidazole. Tinidazole has a longer serum half-life and reaches higher levels in genitourinary tissues than metronidazole. If treatment fails and reinfection is excluded, the patient can be treated with metronidazole 500 mg orally twice daily for 7 days or tinidazole 2 g in a single dose. For patients failing either of these regimens, clinicians should consider treatment with tinidazole or metronidazole at 2 g orally for 5 days.

Special Population Considerations

Pediatric

Before menarche, when estrogen levels are low, the vaginal epithelium is thin and the vaginal pH tends to be between 6.0 and 7.0. These conditions create a vaginal environment that is more susceptible to invading anaerobic bacteria if the child is exposed. Infections may be sexually transmitted or caused by contamination with fecal flora, and the possibility of sexual abuse must be considered. Poor hygiene and the use of vaginal irritants such as bubble baths and other products may also contribute to infections in the prepubertal child. Because of the high vaginal pH of the prepubertal child, candidiasis usually does not occur.

Postmenopausal Women

The decline in estrogen levels that occurs in the postmenopausal woman produces conditions similar to those in prepubertal children, and these conditions predispose the woman to infection and atrophy. As noted previously, the practitioner needs to be aware that atrophic vaginitis is a common cause of vaginal symptoms, and accurate diagnosis is essential.

Pregnant Women

Because vaginitis may occur during pregnancy, therapeutic goals include relieving symptoms and avoiding complications. Depending on the cause of vaginitis, therapy aims to achieve one or both of these goals. Refer to **Box 58.4** for the CDC recommendations for the treatment of vaginitis in pregnancy.

Physiologic conditions of pregnancy increase the risk of VVC. For treatment of VVC during pregnancy, the CDC recommends that only topical azoles be used for a 7-day course of therapy. The most effective agents are butoconazole, clotrimazole, miconazole, and terconazole.

Because adverse pregnancy outcomes have been reported in patients with BV, it is recommended that women who are at high risk (i.e., those who have previously delivered a premature infant) and who are asymptomatic should be treated. Symptomatic BV in women at low risk (no history of premature delivery) should be treated to relieve symptoms. Oral metronidazole and clindamycin may be used in both groups. (See **Table 58.3**.)

The use of topical agents is not recommended because of reports of adverse events, such as premature birth. Although the use of oral metronidazole in pregnancy had long been controversial, multiple studies have found no relationship between birth defects and the use of metronidazole during pregnancy. Follow-up of high-risk pregnant women who have been treated for BV is recommended 1 month after completion of treatment to ensure a successful response.

Trichomonas infections have been associated with preterm delivery. Symptomatic infections during pregnancy can be treated with metronidazole. Asymptomatic pregnant women who have incidentally noted trichomonads should not be treated. The severity of a woman's symptoms needs to be balanced against the risk that metronidazole therapy may increase preterm delivery.

MONITORING PATIENT RESPONSE

Diagnosis and management of vaginitis can be frustrating for both the patient and the practitioner, especially in patients with chronic symptoms and recurrent infections. Symptoms may recur or persist despite adherence to prescribed therapy. The practitioner should consult an expert if the patient fails to respond to current treatment recommendations.

The use of fungal cultures to assess response to therapy and to identify the offending candidal species is beneficial in assessing and treating patients with recurrent VVC. Fungal cultures play a role in detecting non-*albicans* candidal infections that may require second-line therapy.

Practitioners need to individualize the plan of care with each patient. They also need to maintain current knowledge of research regarding alternative therapies and to inform patients of findings. In many situations, yogurt and similar products may cause no harm and may provide patients with a perception of control over a frustrating condition.

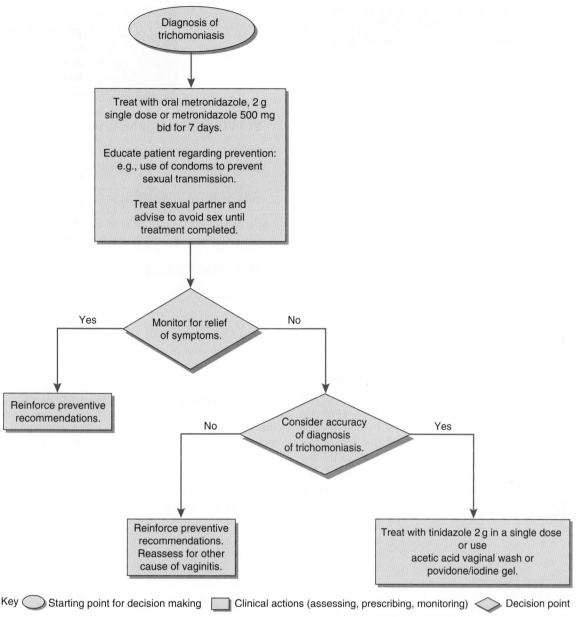

FIGURE 58–3 Treatment algorithm for vaginitis resulting from *Trichomonas* organisms.

Because of the increased risk of postoperative infectious complications associated with BV, some specialists suggest that before performing surgical abortion or hysterectomy, providers should screen for and treat women with BV in addition to providing routine prophylaxis. However, more information is needed before recommending treatment of asymptomatic BV before other invasive procedures. Routine treatment of sex partners is not recommended because studies have shown that treatment of partners does not reduce the incidence of recurrence or relapse.

PATIENT EDUCATION

Drug Information

Metronidazole and tinidazole can cause nausea and vomiting if alcohol is ingested during therapy and up to 24 to 72 hours after therapy stops. Patients should be instructed to adhere to the directions included with the product. In patients taking oral azole and oral antibiotic medications, the practitioner should reinforce the importance of following directions

TABLE 58.5	Recommended Order of Treatment for Trichomonal Infection	
Order	Agents	Comments
First line	Metronidazole Single dose of 2 g	
Second line	Extend the course of metronidazole *or* Acetic acid vaginal wash or povidone–iodine solutions	*May* be effective

BOX 58.4

CDC Recommendations for Treatment of Vaginitis in Pregnancy

VULVOVAGINAL CANDIDIASIS

Topical azole therapies, *only*, for 7 days (most effective: butoconazole, clotrimazole, miconazole, terconazole)

BACTERIAL VAGINOSIS

Recommended: metronidazole 250 mg PO tid for 7 days *or* clindamycin 300 mg PO bid for 7 days

TRICHOMONIASIS

Metronidazole 2 g orally single dose

Data are current for 2006.

carefully and completing the full course of antibiotic therapy even if symptoms subside earlier.

Lifestyle Changes

The patient should avoid tight-fitting clothing, should wear undergarments that allow adequate vaginal ventilation, and should avoid douches and other feminine hygiene products that may alter the normal vaginal pH. The possibility that sexual activity may be associated with the onset of symptoms should be discussed, and the patient should be instructed to monitor these patterns. The patient should use condoms to protect against sexually transmitted disease. Because the use of antibiotics and oral contraceptives may be factors that predispose patients to vaginitis, other treatment options should be explored.

Complementary and Alternative Medicine

Ingesting yogurt (or other commercially available products containing *Lactobacillus acidophilus*) to promote vaginal recolonization may be effective in preventing VVC. The true benefit of colonization with lactobacilli as protection against VVC or BV, however, has not been established. The treatment of BV with nonvaginal lactobacilli or douching has not been shown to be effective.

Case Study

R.S. is a 32-year-old woman who seeks treatment for a vaginal discharge that she has had for the past month. She is sexually active and has had the same partner for the past 6 months. She reports noticing an odor, especially after sexual intercourse. Her history reveals that she has been using a commercial douche on a biweekly basis during the past year for hygienic purposes in an attempt to prevent vaginal infections. She denies any other associated symptoms. The physical examination reveals a white vaginal discharge. Microscopic examination of the vaginal discharge shows clue cells, and the pH is 5.5.

DIAGNOSIS: BACTERIAL VAGINOSIS

1. List specific goals of treatment for this patient.
2. What drug therapy would you prescribe? Why?

3. What are the parameters for monitoring the success of the therapy?
4. Discuss specific patient education based on the prescribed therapy.
5. List one or two adverse reactions for the selected agent that would cause you to change therapy.
6. What would be the choice for second-line therapy?
7. What OTC or alternative medications would be appropriate for this patient?
8. What dietary or lifestyle changes should be recommended?
9. Describe one or two drug–drug or drug–food interaction for the selected agent.

BIBLIOGRAPHY

Starred references are cited in the text.

Allsworth, J., & Peipent, J. (2008). Prevalence of bacterial vaginosis: 2001–2004: National Health and Nutritional Survey data. *Obstetrics and Gynecology, 109*(1), 114–120.

Biggs, W., & Williams, R. (2009). Common gynecological infections. *Primary Care: Clinics in Office Practice, 36*(1), 33–51.

*Centers for Disease Control and Prevention. (2006). Sexually transmitted treatment guidelines, 2006. *Morbidity and Mortality Weekly Reports, 55*(RR-11), 1–93.

Ferris, D. G., Dekle, C., & Litaker, M. (1996). Women's use of over the counter antifungal medications for gynecological symptoms. *Journal of Family Practice, 42,* 595–600.

*Koumans, E., Steinberg, M., Bruce, C., et al. (2007). Prevention of bacterial vaginosis in the United States 2001–2004 associated with symptoms, sexual behavior and reproductive health. *Sexually Transmitted Diseases, 34*(1), 844–869.

Njirjesy, P., Weitz, M. V., Grody, M. H. T., & Lorber, B. (1997). Over the counter and alternative medicines in the treatment of chronic vaginal symptoms. *Obstetrics and Gynecology, 90,* 50–53.

Nyirjesy, P. (2008). Vaginovulvar candidiasis and bacterial vaginosis. *Infectious Disease Clinics of North America, 22*(9), 637–652.

Risser, J., Risser, W., & Risser, A. (2008). Epidemiology of infections in women. *Infectious Disease Clinics of North America, 22*(4), 581–599.

*Sobel, J. D., Ferris, D., Schwebke, J., et al. (2006). Suppressive antibacterial therapy with 0.75% metronidazole vaginal gel to prevent recurrent bacterial vaginosis. *American Journal of Obstetrics and Gynecology, 194,* 1283–1289.

Workowski, K. A., & Berman, S. M. (2006). Sexually transmitted diseases treatment guidelines. *MMWR Recommendations and Report, 55*(RR-11), 1–94.

Integrative Approach to Patient Care

CHAPTER 59

Samir K. Mistry
Joshua J. Spooner

The Economics of Pharmacotherapeutics

As little as 100 years ago, health insurance in the United States was scarce. Although President George Washington signed a law establishing prepaid health care in 1798, health insurance plans were slow to develop. Traditionally, patients paid health care providers and hospitals directly for their services on a fee-for-service basis. This system worked well for patients in times of good health; however, a serious injury or illness could leave the patient facing financial ruin.

The goal of this chapter is to provide a brief review of pharmacoeconomics, educate the reader about the methods used by managed care organizations (MCOs) to manage health care expenditures, explain how these methods are developed and implemented, and review how MCOs evaluate the practices of contracted providers. Understanding the rationales, benefits, and limitations associated with MCOs can be a factor in helping practitioners select appropriate drug therapy for their patients.

ORIGINS OF MANAGED CARE

Modern health insurance's origins can be traced to 1929, when the Baylor University Hospital in Dallas began to offer 1,500 school teachers up to 21 days of hospital care a year for $6 per person (Starr, 1982). Other groups also entered into agreement to prepay for Baylor's services. Shortly thereafter, several other Dallas-area hospitals followed suit and offered similar plans. Other early health insurance plans included the Kaiser Health Plans (early to mid-1930s) and the Group Health Association in Washington, DC (1937). As the country slid into the Depression and hospital revenues plummeted by 75% per patient, hospitals began to rely on insurance payments for a greater proportion of their operating budget (Starr, 1982).

Most health plans offered indemnity insurance (also known as *fee-for-service insurance*), in which patients paid for health care expenses out of their own pockets and then requested reimbursement from the insurer (often 80%). Unfortunately, indemnity insurance did little to control health care expenditures because physicians and hospitals received payments proportional to the volume of services they provided. Concerned with the rising cost of providing health care, insurance providers sought a way to slow the increases in expenditures. After extensive lobbying and negotiations in Congress, President Richard Nixon signed the federal Health Maintenance Organization (HMO) Act into law on December 29, 1973. This act encouraged the growth of managed care by providing grants and loans to develop HMOs, overturned restrictive state laws regulating health providers, defined a basic package of services that HMOs were required to offer, and established procedures by which HMOs could become federally qualified. The act also provided other support for the expansion of HMOs.

Because HMOs could be cost effective without reducing the quality of care, they were an attractive health insurance alternative for employers. The rate of enrollment in HMOs grew rapidly during the 1980s and 1990s and rivaled preferred provider organizations as the leading source of health insurance in the United States in the late 1990s before undergoing a decline in enrollment in the next decade (Kaiser Family Foundation, 2010b). The federal government encouraged Medicare recipients to enroll in HMOs to manage the health care costs of beneficiaries; HMOs were reimbursed on a prospective basis by the government. The states soon followed suit, offering HMO-based options to Medicaid recipients.

OVERVIEW OF PHARMACOECONOMICS

One of the most important aspects of managed care pharmacy involves the MCOs' emphasis on economics in the decision-making process. *Pharmacoeconomics* is the description and analysis of the costs of drug therapy to health care systems and society (Bootman, et al., 2004). Because they evaluate both cost and human data, studies on pharmacoeconomics are important tools for MCOs in making drug therapy decisions. To provide an overview, some different pharmacoeconomic study designs are described in the following sections.

Cost–Benefit Analysis

A cost–benefit analysis is used to determine the overall cost of a particular intervention or protocol by evaluating all pertinent data and converting the data to a monetary end point (e.g., U.S. dollars or E.U. Euros). Most often, this type of analysis is used to compare two different programs that also have different units for end points because the data can then be converted to one common unit (usually the dollar). The limitation to this analysis involves the evaluation of "intangible" end points or data that cannot be equated to a monetary value.

Cost Minimization Analysis

A cost minimization analysis evaluates the cost of two or more interventions with equivalent components or end points and determines which intervention is least costly. The most appropriate use for such analyses involves situations in which every aspect of compared interventions is identical except the cost of the intervention. Because efficacy and safety are identical, the cost of each intervention becomes the differential outcome. The outcomes of these analyses are also expressed in a monetary end point.

Cost-Effectiveness Analysis

A cost-effectiveness analysis may help determine the best program or intervention, where the desired outcome is a combination of both a monetary end point and a nonmonetary end point relative to an improvement in health (e.g., life expectancy, blood glucose measurements). An example of this would be dollars per life-year saved.

Cost–Utility Analysis

A cost–utility analysis, which is closely related to a cost-effectiveness analysis, measures data in terms of quality of life. Quality of life is an assessment of a patient's well-being and social functioning, which can assist practitioners in determining a patient's response to drug therapy (Bootman, et al., 2004). Along with traditional clinical results (e.g., laboratory values, blood pressure, serum glucose level), a cost–utility analysis provides a more complete evaluation of a patient's progress and compares the cost of an intervention or program in terms of more intangible end points, rather than dollars. These analyses predominantly use quality-adjusted life-years (QALYs) gained as a major outcome. The QALY is symbolic of healthy years of life and is the unit of measurement that encompasses outcomes (e.g., morbidity and mortality) in preferential sequence. This method has been very successful in evaluating various procedures compared with drug therapy in which a patient's quality of life is the chosen outcome (Bootman, et al., 2004).

Pharmacoeconomic research compares cost and consequence with respect to pharmaceutical products and their impact on individuals, the health care system, and society. Such parameters are seldom analyzed in most studies.

FORMULARIES AND PHARMACY AND THERAPEUTICS COMMITTEES

An evaluation of American health expenditures identified $2.3 trillion in total health care spending in 2008, three times the $714 billion spent in 1990 (Centers for Medicare and Medicaid Services, 2010). Of this $2.3 trillion in health expenditures, 10% was spent on prescription drugs. Although this represents a small portion of overall health care expenditures, it has been identified by many MCOs as a target for intervention due to large annual increases in prescription drug spending. Prescription drug spending increased 5.1% in 2009 (IMS Health, 2010), an increase from the 3% growth observed in 2008 (Hartman, 2010).

Formularies

One of the most effective methods by which an MCO can improve the quality of care provided to patients and mitigate the increasing costs of providing a prescription benefit is by implementing a formulary. Also known as a *preferred drug list*, a medication formulary is simply a list of preferred medications approved for use within an HMO, third-party payer, or pharmacy benefit manager (Navarro, et al., 2008). Formularies are usually organized by therapeutic area and medication class, with the formulary status and reimbursement category listed for each medication.

Formularies encourage the use of medications considered to be safer, more clinically effective, or more cost-effective than other medications within the same therapeutic category. When an MCO wants to limit the use of a drug for a specific reason (safety, efficacy or cost), the formulary allows the flexibility to implement restrictions or limitations. Examples of such restrictions include prior authorizations, step therapies, quantity limitations, and tiered copayments.

Evolution of Formularies

The use of formularies can be traced back to 1925, when the physicians and pharmacists of Syracuse University Hospital collaborated to establish a formulary system to monitor drug use and reduce therapeutic duplication (the unnecessary use of two or more medications to treat the same condition) in its drug therapy program (Sonnedecker, 1976). By the 1960s, formularies were being implemented in hospitals throughout the country with the guidance of the *American Hospital Formulary Service*, a prominent set of formulary development materials published by the American Society of Hospital Pharmacists. Following the HMO Act of 1973, many HMOs adopted the hospital formulary to monitor medication use. Formularies were initially used by managed care as an inventory control mechanism for staff-model HMOs (Navarro, et al., 2008), but they have evolved into effective tools for monitoring and regulating medication utilization for all types of MCOs.

Structure of Formularies

Although formats may differ among plans, a formulary usually contains the same fundamental information. Formularies usually begin with a basic plan summary and detail key points of reference, then proceed to the list of drugs. The drugs are most often categorized within their respective therapeutic classes with the therapeutic classes listed in alphabetic order. The order of the drugs within each therapeutic class can vary but are often listed alphabetically, either in complete alphabetical order (generic and brand drugs intermixed) or generic drugs listed before brand-name drugs. Additional information usually detailed for each drug includes the brand/generic status; the drug's relative cost, which is most often symbolized by relative $ signs; co-pay tier; and any potential utilization management programs. An example of a formulary is shown in **Table 59.1**. A "formulary medication" is a drug that is covered (reimbursed) by the health plan; formulary medications can be subdivided into different groups such as preferred and nonpreferred agents. "Preferred" agents are drugs that the health plan would prefer the practitioner to prescribe, due to safety, efficacy, and/or relative cost. "Nonpreferred" drugs are not the preferred drugs of the health plan, but will nonetheless be covered by the plan at a higher out-of-pocket cost. Most formularies have different tiered co-pays for preferred and nonpreferred drugs, in which preferred drugs have a lower cost tiered co-pay than the nonpreferred drugs. "Nonformulary medications" are drugs that are not covered in or are excluded from the formulary; health plans generally do not publish nonformulary medications on their formularies. Prescribers must usually provide exception justification for a patient to receive reimbursement for nonformulary medications.

Formularies can be grouped into three different categories: closed, open, and tiered formularies. Closed formularies limit clinicians to prescribing from a limited list of preferred agents (Troy, 1999). Open formularies usually do not involve a preferred group of agents; instead, they allow the prescriber to select any covered medication. Tiered formularies are essentially the compromise between closed and open formularies. Tiered formularies are open formularies that set different co-pay tiers for generic, preferred, and nonpreferred medications (Navarro, et al., 2008).

Impact of Formularies on Patients

The price that consumers pay for prescription medications varies from plan to plan. Patients are commonly required to pay a portion of the cost of the prescription, also known as the *co-payment*, or *co-pay*. Co-pay amounts can differ from plan to plan and by geographic region. Closed and open formularies usually only have two co-pays: one for generic drugs and brand drugs, respectively. Tiered formularies have more than two co-pays, and each tier is related to a co-pay amount. Tiered formularies usually have three tiers: generic drugs, preferred brand drugs, and nonpreferred brand drugs.

Most co-pays are set to cover up to a 1-month supply of medication (28 to 34 days of therapy, depending on the health plan). Thus, a patient who received a prescription for a 7-day course of therapy of prednisone for an acute allergic reaction would likely have the same co-payment as a patient who received a prescription for a 30-day course of therapy of prednisone for chronic use.

Some plans may allow patients to get more than a 1-month supply of medication at a time for a maintenance medication (medications used for chronic conditions). For maintenance medications, most health plans allow patients to receive a 90-day supply of medication. Health plans usually charge patients three co-pays for a 90-day supply (three 1-month supply co-pays). For example, if a patient paid a $10 co-pay for a 1-month supply, then the 90-day supply would cost $30. Health plans often offer reduced co-payments as an enticement for patients to order their maintenance medications from a mail-order pharmacy service; a 90-day supply of medication might only cost the patient one or two co-payments instead of three.

In the rigid formulary systems in the 1990s, a two-tiered prescription co-payment system was used by most health plans and pharmacy benefits manager (PBM); the lower co-payment tier was used for generic medications, whereas the higher co-payment tier was used for formulary brand-name medications. Nonformulary medications were rarely covered by health plans or PBMs without prior approval; if granted, the prescription would fall into the higher co-payment tier. Nonformulary medications that were not approved by the health plan were not covered; either the patient paid the full retail price for the prescription, or the prescription was switched to a formulary agent by the prescribing physician.

Fueled by increasing prescription costs and charges of restrictions of care (Flanagan, 2002; Horn, et al., 1998; Talley, 1997), health plans and PBMs abandoned the two-tiered formulary

TABLE 59.1	Example of a Formulary				
Drug Name	**Brand/Generic**	**Relative Cost**	**Tier**	**Edits**	
Drug A	Generic	$	Tier 1		
Drug B	Generic	$	Tier 1	QL	
Drug C	Brand	$$	Tier 2	QL, ST	
Drug D	Brand	$$	Tier 2		
Drug E	Brand	$$$	Tier 3	ST	
Drug F	Brand	$$$$	Tier 3	PA	
Drug G (Specialty Injectable)	Brand	$$$$$$	Tier 4	QL, ST	

Key: PA = Prior Authorization   Tier 1 = Generic
     QL = Quantity Limits   Tier 2 = Preferred Brand Drug
     ST = Step Therapy   Tier 3 = Nonpreferred Brand Drug
                Tier 4 = Specialty Injectable

system in favor of three- and four-tiered systems (PBM News, 2001). Within these formulary systems, the first two tiers are set up the same as the previous two-tiered system, with the first (lowest) tier co-payment reserved for generic products and the second tier co-payment reserved for preferred brand-name products. Agents in the third tier are the nonpreferred brand-name products; the co-payment is substantially higher than the second tier co-payment. Some plans include a fourth tier to their formulary for lifestyle drugs (impotence medications, wrinkle creams, hair restoration medications, etc.) with the highest prescription co-payments. Three- and four-tiered formularies have introduced value considerations to patients: Do they value a specific third-tier product enough to pay the higher co-payment or will a second-tier product (with a lower co-payment) be suitable for their needs? The multiple-tiered co-payment has been proven to successfully move patients to products in the first and second tiers of the formulary without restricting access to prescription products (Fairman, et al., 2003).

Functions of Formularies

Formularies have been used to promote the safe, efficacious, and cost-effective use of medications. Formularies' main functions are to promote the use of generic medications, incentivize the use of preferred brand drugs over nonpreferred brand drugs, or completely prevent the prescribing of nonformulary drugs. MCOs also implement policies or programs with their formularies to promote appropriate drug utilization and the use of generic drugs and preferred brand drugs prior to nonpreferred and nonformulary drugs. Examples of such policies or programs include generic substitution, therapeutic interchange, dispensing limitations around quantity, duration of therapy, age and gender, prior authorization, step therapy, and medical necessity.

Generic Substitution

A highly effective method of reducing the cost of the pharmacy benefit is generic substitution. Generic substitution is the process of dispensing an appropriate generic equivalent of a prescribed brand-name drug. Prescribing generic products can reduce the cost of providing prescription medications for patients by 10% to 25% without reducing the quality of care (Navarro, et al., 2008). Generic substitution has been supported by cost minimization analyses; as the brand and generic agents are considered identical in composition and activity, cost becomes the contributing factor for an agent's selection.

As noted in Chapter 1, a generic drug is considered equal, or bioequivalent, to a brand-name drug and must undergo stringent testing and comply with specific criteria established by the U.S. Food and Drug Administration (FDA). The FDA has set certain therapeutic equivalence evaluation codes to show the relative bioequivalence of generic agents to the brand-name drugs (FDA, 2010). There are two basic rating codes: A and B. The "A" rating indicates that the drug is considered therapeutically equivalent to other pharmaceutically equivalent products.

The "B" rating indicates that the agent is not therapeutically equivalent to other pharmaceutically equivalent agents. Both A- and B-rated drugs are further differentiated based on dosage form. An "AB" rating states that the product's bioequivalence problems have been resolved, and evidence exists supporting the bioequivalence to pharmaceutically equivalent agents.

An example of generic substitution is dispensing the diuretic furosemide when the prescriber writes the prescription for Lasix, and the prescriber has not indicated that the brand-name product is medically necessary. In such a situation, the pharmacist is filling the prescription with an FDA-approved, bioequivalent form of the brand-name drug. Some insurance plans may allow the patient or physician to request the brand-name agent, but this often results in a higher co-payment for the patient (Navarro, et al., 2008). The increase in co-payment may be as large as the difference in cost to the health plan between the brand and generic agents.

To maximize generic substitution, plans may use restrictive strategies such as "dispense as written" (DAW) blocks. A DAW code describes the rationale for the drug's selection and is entered into the prescription claim by the pharmacist before it is transmitted to the health plan for adjudication. There are DAW codes for "substitution permissible" (DAW 0), "dispense as written" (DAW 1), "patient requests brand" (DAW 2), as well as other choices to provide a rationale for the chosen agent. A health plan can require that the patient receive an acceptable generic substitution for a brand-name product unless a suitable DAW code has been entered. A DAW code of 7 is used for products with a narrow therapeutic index. Due to the risk of disrupting the level of drug in the patient's blood, drugs with a narrow therapeutic index may not have to be automatically substituted for an equivalent generic agent. A DAW of 7 informs the health plan that either the physician, pharmacist, or patient has elected to continue use of the brand-name product. Drugs in this category include warfarin (Coumadin) and digoxin (Lanoxin).

Therapeutic Interchange

Therapeutic interchange is defined as the procedure of dispensing prescribed medications that are chemically different but deemed therapeutically similar to the medication prescribed (American Society of Consultant Pharmacists, 2010). In general, therapeutic interchange involves the substitution of drugs that are different chemical compounds but are considered to exert the same therapeutic effect and have similar toxicity and side effect profiles (e.g., angiotensin receptor blockers [ARBs]: substitution of generic losartan [Cozaar] for Benicar). The use of therapeutic interchange has increased significantly because of a large influx of new medications that do not offer any therapeutic advantages over existing therapies but are priced much higher than the established products. These medications are commonly known as *me too drugs*. Some popular examples of therapeutic categories that contain me too drugs include proton pump inhibitors (PPIs), HMG CoA reductase inhibitors (statins), ARBs, and bisphosphonates.

Pharmaceutical manufacturers offer rebates to health plans to compete for preferred status on formularies, which lowers the prescription benefit cost. Controversies tend to arise when discounts are used to exchange one drug over another when the drugs are in different classes. If a therapeutic interchange involves two drugs of the same therapeutic class, it can be considered an example of therapeutic minimization because the only difference between the two agents is cost (assuming that the relative safety/efficacy data for the two agents are similar).

Therapeutic interchange is used for reasons other than controlling costs, including promoting the use of agents associated with fewer drug–drug interactions (e.g., substitution of fluconazole [Diflucan] for ketoconazole [Nizoral]), or of agents with a more convenient dosing schedule (e.g., once-daily enalapril [Vasotec] instead of two- to three-times daily captopril [Capoten]). These interventions may prevent unnecessary drug–drug interactions or enhance medication compliance, which could, in turn, improve care and decrease overall health care costs.

In the retail pharmacy setting, therapeutic interchange must be verified and accepted by the prescribing practitioner. In the institutional setting, therapeutic interchange does not necessarily require a prescriber's approval if the institution's pharmacy and therapeutics (P&T) committee approves the specific interchange protocol (Chase, et al., 1998). The American Medical Association (AMA) endorses the practice of therapeutic interchange in settings that have an organized medical staff and a functioning P&T committee (AMA, 1994).

Drug Dispensing Limitations

Limitations about dispensing drugs are developed and implemented to promote appropriate prescribing of medications and are often structured around FDA-approved labeling and evidence-based medical data. Examples of drug limitations include drug quantity limits, duration of therapy limits, age limits, and gender limits. Drug quantity limitations are used to promote the appropriate quantity of medication that should be prescribed. There are two main types of quantity limits: quantity per filled prescription and quantity per days. Quantity per filled prescription limits are implemented for drugs that are prescribed for short-term use, such as analgesics and antibiotics. An example of such a quantity limit would be limiting the prescribing of ondansetron (used for the short-term prevention of nausea and vomiting) to four tablets per prescription. Quantity per days limits are utilized for chronically used (maintenance) medications. An example of this type of quantity limit would be limiting the prescribing of simvastatin to one tablet per day. Duration of therapy limits are implemented to manage how long a drug should be used, especially for medications that are not considered maintenance medications. An example of a duration of therapy limit would include a 3-month duration of therapy limit for the prescribing of onychomycosis antifungal agents. Age limitations prevent the use of medications either above or below what is recommended by the FDA. An example of an age limit would be to prevent the use of oseltamivir for members younger than age 1. Gender limits prevent the use of medications for a gender when prescribing would not be safe and/or appropriate, an example of which would prevent prescriptions of oral contraceptives for males.

Prior Authorization and Step Therapy Programs

Prior authorization refers to the approval process that health plans may require for certain medications before they will be covered. The primary purpose of a prior authorization process is to control the use of and prevent the overuse of nonformulary, hazardous, or inappropriately prescribed medications. Prior to the recent move by health plans toward increasingly open formularies with three and four tiers of co-payments, health plans would require prior authorizations for most nonformulary drugs, expensive drugs, newly approved drugs, and drugs with less expensive alternatives (Navarro, et al., 2008). Over 75% of commercial health plans used prior authorization programs in 2010 (Takeda Pharmaceuticals, 2010), and prior authorizations are used by a majority of the states in their Medicaid programs (National Conference of State Legislatures, 2010).

The criteria for approval of each drug undergoing the prior approval process will depend on the drug, the patient, the disease state involved, and the prescribing practitioner. Some prior authorizations may require a diagnosis along with pertinent laboratory values, whereas others may require a patient to fail therapy with certain drugs that are indicated to treat the same disease as the restricted agent. Other criteria may include patient demographics, such as age or gender limits, or prescriber limits, where only specific specialty types are allowed to prescribe for certain medications (e.g., only allowing dermatologists to prescribe isotretinoin).

The usual chain of events involving prior authorization starts with a patient presenting a pharmacist with a prescription for a newly prescribed medication. The pharmacist, after submitting a claim and having it rejected, learns that the medication requires prior authorization (often from a message sent with the rejected claim). The pharmacist or patient then contacts the prescriber, tells the prescriber that the medication prescribed requires prior authorization, and requests that the prescriber contact the MCO to explain why the patient requires that medication. Prescribers can decide to either contact the MCO and pursue prior authorization, or they may choose not to pursue prior authorization and select an alternative agent. MCOs often accept prior authorization requests from practitioners by mail, fax, telephone, or internet. Completing the prior authorization process may result in the drug's approval for use in that patient, or the MCO may again reject the claim and offer a list of alternative medications that are covered by the plan.

If the prescriber knows that the drug requires prior authorization, the necessary paperwork can be completed to have the drug approved for the patient before the patient enters the pharmacy. Problems arise when the patient and prescriber are unaware of which agents on the MCO's formulary require prior authorization. This confuses many patients, possibly leading them to think that the prescriber ordered the wrong medication or the pharmacist made an error in filling the prescription (Lisi, 1997).

Step therapy programs are utilization management programs that are a version of prior authorization, in which they promote the use of one drug before another (Navarro, et al., 2008). There are two main types of step therapy programs: those driven by cost-effectiveness and those that promote more clinically effective medications before less effective medications. The cost-effectiveness step therapy programs promote the use of cost-effective generic medication before the use of an expensive branded medication. They can be implemented using drugs within the same therapeutic class or different categories. An example of a step therapy within a therapeutic class would be to require the use of a generic PPI, such as omeprazole, before the approval of a branded PPI like AcipHex. An example of a step therapy using different categories would be to require the use of metformin before the approval of thiazolidinediones like Actos and Avandia. Step therapy programs implemented for the purpose of promoting clinical effectiveness are usually based on practice guidelines or evidence-based medical data. An example of this type of program would be to require the use of nasal corticosteroids or nonsedating antihistamines before the approval of leukotriene inhibitors for the treatment of allergic rhinitis.

MCOs have increased their efforts to prospectively review prescriptions requiring prior authorization during the claim adjudication process. When a pharmacy sends a claim for a prior authorization drug to the PBM for adjudication, the PBM can review the patient's prescription claim history and the claim itself to determine if the prior authorization criteria have been met. This step can decrease the number of rejected prescription claims and minimize the time and efforts of prescribers, pharmacists, and patients in obtaining prior authorizations. When initiated effectively by informing practitioners of the drug's status and the preapproval process, prior authorization can become a very efficient mechanism for controlling costs and drug use.

Medical Necessity

Some MCOs use the term *medical necessity* interchangeably with *prior authorization*. In most settings, a drug considered a medical necessity is a nonformulary drug that is usually extremely expensive and that may have less expensive alternatives or is indicated only for rare disorders (Glassman, et al., 1997; Roy-Byrne, et al., 1998). Some MCOs make medical necessity drugs available only after failure of drug therapy with a drug requiring prior authorization. MCOs carefully evaluate drugs before classifying them as medical necessity drugs, knowing that the drugs will be restricted if they are covered. Like the criteria for medications requiring prior authorization, the criteria for coverage vary from drug to drug.

PHARMACY AND THERAPEUTICS COMMITTEE

Structure and Function

A P&T committee is a group that meets periodically to review and revise the MCO's formulary. The committee is composed primarily of physicians and pharmacists and may also include nurses, nurse practitioners, physicians' assistants, drug information personnel, and members of the administration. The physicians on the committee often comprise a diverse group from various fields of practice, with general practitioners and specialists represented. The committee is a well-balanced mix of practitioners who can view health care policies from different perspectives and provide sound recommendations.

Formulary Management

The main responsibilities of a P&T committee are to revise the formulary, create and implement medication policies, and provide education for practitioners. Formulary reviews include evaluating new medications for formulary consideration, periodic drug class reviews, and utilization analyses. A major goal of the P&T committee is to provide cost-effective, clinically safe, and effective therapy. Frequent formulary revisions are needed for several reasons: the introduction of new products into the marketplace, modifications to a product's labeling to include new treatment indications, emerging research indicating a previously unknown benefit or risk of therapy, changes in consensus disease treatment guidelines, and changes in the brand/generic status of a product or other pricing concerns.

The inclusion and exclusion of agents is a time-intensive process for P&T committees. As such, many P&T committees elect to delay their consideration of a new product until it has a sufficient body of evidence to perform a review. P&T committees may consider a wide variety of information when evaluating a new product, including peer-reviewed clinical trials, adverse event/safety data, patient-oriented health outcomes (e.g., the ability of an antihypertensive to reduce the risk of myocardial infarctions, not merely to lower blood pressure), the FDA-approved product labeling for the new agent, quality of life research, and pharmacoeconomic data (**Box 59.1**). The committee must consider the issue of bias when evaluating results provided by any research sponsored by the pharmaceutical manufacturer. Literature that includes data comparing the new agent with an agent currently used to treat the same disorder is prized by P&T committees for its utility in comparing one drug with another. If the new agent offers a clinical, safety, or economic advantage to existing formulary agents, the P&T committee may place the agent on the formulary, and can do so by adding the new product with or without removing an existing product or products. Further, committees can add the drug to the formulary unconditionally or may recommend implementation of certain restrictions on the coverage

Information Considered by a Pharmacy and Therapeutics Committee When Reviewing a Product for the Formulary

FDA-APPROVED INDICATIONS

1. Pharmacology / mechanism of action
2. Pharmacokinetic / pharmacodynamic data
3. Dosing and administration, including special monitoring or drug administration requirements
4. Adverse effect profile, warnings, precautions, contraindications, and black box warnings
5. Drug interactions (with other drugs, foods, or medical conditions)
6. Clinical evidence: clinical trials, health outcomes research, retrospective database analyses, quality of life research
7. Risks versus benefits regarding clinical efficacy and safety of a particular drug relative to other drugs with the same indication
8. Pharmacoeconomic data and modeling
9. Off-label uses
10. Cost comparisons against other drugs available to treat the same medical condition(s)
11. Source of supply and reliability of manufacturer and distributor

(prior authorization, quantity limitations, step therapy) of the new agent to allow its inclusion in the formulary.

Because of the increase in prescription drug spending by health plans, cost now plays a more significant role in formulary status, although cost should be considered only after safety and efficacy data are evaluated. To promote a drug's addition to a formulary, pharmaceutical manufacturers may offer prescription volume-dependent rebates to MCOs as incentives.

Development of Disease Management Programs or Treatment Protocols

Another responsibility of a P&T committee is to develop or approve disease management programs or treatment protocols for the MCO. These programs and protocols provide useful recommendations for practitioners treating various diseases. They may be based on current consensus practice guidelines, or they may be developed by the P&T committee using current clinical data. A main purpose of guidelines or algorithms is to minimize treatment variations and improve patient outcomes while reducing costs (Navarro, et al., 2008).

ENSURING FORMULARY AND PRACTICE GUIDELINE COMPLIANCE

One of the primary reasons that MCOs develop formularies and practice guidelines is to help lower the cost of the prescription drug benefit. Unfortunately, merely printing and distributing formularies and algorithms often is not enough to alter prescribing practices. Patients and pharmacists may also be wary of the formulary system, failing to understand both its necessity and utility. While educational programs (including seminars, newsletters, provider peer-to-peer communications, and one-on-one meetings) are useful, these tools alone do not ensure improved formulary compliance. MCOs have developed a variety of payment and reimbursement strategies to improve compliance. The following sections describe the ways that MCOs evaluate formulary and treatment guideline compliance and how MCOs use different levels of payments to improve compliance.

Prescriber Incentives for Compliance

MCOs can monitor compliance to the formulary and treatment protocols with a variety of tools. Many MCOs use the level of peer compliance to determine the amount of a prescriber's or practice's year-end incentives. Prescribers can be eligible for financial incentives if their compliance to the formulary or treatment protocols meets the threshold established by the MCO (Navarro, et al., 2008).

Some MCOs may tie a portion of a provider's compensation to the level of compliance. If a practitioner fails to follow treatment protocols closely and inexplicably high prescription costs result, an MCO may withhold a portion of the provider's compensation. In a capitated plan, the provider receives a fixed, predetermined, per-member payment by the MCO to provide services for members, regardless of how much or how frequently a member uses service. Providers can reap financial reward if they can provide services at a cost lower than their level of payment but are responsible for all costs if expenses should rise above their level of payment. While capitation remains a frequently utilized tool by MCOs to manage medical costs (Kaiser Family Foundation, 2010a), few (if any) health plans utilize a capitated pharmacy benefit.

Evaluating Compliance: Percentage Formulary Compliance

The simplest way for an MCO to evaluate formulary compliance is to determine the prescriber's percentage of prescriptions for generic and branded formulary products. Although this method is useful for determining formulary compliance (e.g., the use of generic and branded formulary ARBs compared with nonformulary-branded ARBs), it does not evaluate the quality of prescribing; just because a formulary agent is prescribed does not make the prescription appropriate. It may be more important to determine if the prescriber is following consensus disease treatment guidelines. A prescriber who prescribes a formulary agent but is not following treatment guidelines has the same percentage formulary compliance as a prescriber who uses a different and potentially less expensive or more appropriate formulary medication by following treatment guidelines. Also, prescribers who use medically necessary or appropriate nonformulary drugs are penalized in this system. Many MCOs have initiated programs to evaluate the quality of physician prescribing by implementing physician profiling programs, where clinicians evaluate questionable prescribing with the physicians.

Because of the aforementioned limitations with percentage formulary compliance, MCOs also use another tool to evaluate compliance: per-member–per-month (PMPM) reports.

Health Care Trend Reporting

When analyzing health care trends for an MCO, many variables are reviewed and factored in to evaluate and justify the trends during any particular year. The PMPM reports are a unit of measure related to each enrollee for each month. When used to evaluate prescribing practices, average PMPM prescription costs are determined for each provider. Theoretically, prescribers who adhere to formulary and practice guidelines will achieve lower PMPM prescription costs than their peers who do not. This is not a foolproof method to evaluate compliance because a small number of patients requiring expensive therapy (e.g., chemotherapy, antipsychotics) can substantially increase a prescriber's PMPM amount. More frequently, MCOs use PMPM reports to evaluate prescription costs for a specific disease. An example of a disease-specific PMPM report appears in **Table 59.2**. Although prescriber A is responsible for the highest dollar expenditure on antihyperlipidemics, his PMPM prescription cost is close to the average of the prescriber's peers. On the other hand, despite prescriber C's low overall dollar expenditure on lipid agents, his PMPM prescription cost is the highest.

Another factor that is considered in evaluating health care trends is drug cost. Monitoring the rate of increase in drug cost has become a significant factor in overall health care spending. As the prices of prescription medications increase, MCOs are adjusting their overall plan designs to compensate for that increase. These adjustments may include changes in product status on drug formularies, implementation of prior authorization and step therapy programs for expensive products, increases in member co-payments, or increases in member premiums.

Improving Formulary Compliance

In addition to prescribers, MCOs have an opportunity to improve formulary and practice guideline compliance by providing financial incentives or disincentives to other players: the prescription dispenser (pharmacist) and the prescription recipient (patient). These financial incentives include bonuses, differential reimbursement rates, and different levels of prescription co-payment.

Pharmacist Reimbursement

An MCO can influence pharmacists as a secondary step in limiting the use of nonformulary medications. As a part of the contracting process, MCOs may impose requirements on pharmacies if the pharmacy wishes to serve members of the plan. MCOs can require that pharmacies dispense generic products when available, unless the physician requires the prescription to be DAW or the medication has a narrow therapeutic index (e.g., phenytoin [Dilantin], warfarin). Many states already require automatic generic substitution when applicable. To reduce wasted or unused medication, MCOs often impose a limit on the amount of medication that a community pharmacist can dispense—usually no more than 1 month's worth at a time. Once a patient is stabilized on a maintenance dose for medications used to treat chronic illnesses (e.g., hypertension, hyperlipidemia), MCOs may require that patients receive a 3-month supply of medication from a mail-order pharmacy; this can be done at a lower expense to the MCO.

Pharmacies that are successful in increasing formulary compliance or reducing member pharmacy costs may be eligible for bonuses or they may receive a higher reimbursement rate. Alternatively, pharmacies that fail to meet the requirements of the contract may receive a lower reimbursement rate or have their contract terminated altogether. MCOs frequently audit the claims of pharmacies with a higher-than-average number of DAW orders to ensure that the prescriber does in fact require the brand-name drug be dispensed to the patient.

Patient Prescription Co-Payment

The impact of prescription co-payment on patients was reviewed earlier in this chapter. In summary, as formularies have progressively become more open, health plans have responded by using differential co-payments in an effort to encourage patients to use lower-cost generic or preferred brand products. Patients who are hesitant to pay a high prescription co-payment when lower priced alternatives are available frequently ask their physician to prescribe the product with the lower co-payment; the physician will often comply with the

TABLE 59.2	Per-Member–Per-Month (PMPM) Prescription Costs for Patients Receiving Antihyperlipidemic Therapy		
Prescriber	**Number of Member Months**	**Lipid Prescription Costs ($)**	**PMPM Prescription Costs ($)**
A	561	45,183	80.54
B	240	18,818	78.41
C	285	25,639	89.96
D	496	36,248	73.08
E	357	30,780	86.22
F	489	40,223	82.31

patient's request if they believe the change can be made without adversely affecting the outcome of care.

CURRENT ISSUES IN MANAGED CARE

One cause of discontent among health care purchasers is the cost of insurance premiums, which began to rise at a rate greater than that of inflation starting in the mid-1990s. The average family premium cost nearly $14,000 in 2010, with covered workers paying 30% of the premium (Kaiser Family Foundation, 2010b). Some of this price increase can be attributed to increasing expenditures for medications, which increased 5.1% in 2009 (IMS Health, 2010). The increase in expenditures for prescription drugs is the effect of three factors: rising use, rising prices, and the increased availability of novel medications. The influence of direct-to-consumer advertising, manufacturer pricing policies, and prescription drug coverage through Medicare Part D on the rising cost of health care continues to be debated. This much remains clear: if prescription drug spending continues to increase as projected (Posler, et al., 2007), MCOs will have to modify the extent to which they cover prescription drugs through coverage limits, establishing more rigid formulary systems, and increased cost shifting to consumers.

In March 2010, the U.S. Congress passed the Affordable Care Act, more commonly known as the Healthcare Reform Bill. The premise for the act was to ensure accountability to MCOs, lower health care costs, improve quality of care, and provide improved consumer choice for health care services (U.S. Department of Health and Human Services, 2010). The provisions of the reform act are proposed to be implemented over a 4-year period beginning in 2010, with the majority of regulations implemented in 2014. The act will work toward improving consumers' access to and quality of health care, including improving access to Medicaid coverage, decreasing out-of-pocket costs to Medicare-eligible members, and extending coverage for younger adults under the insurance held by their parents/guardians. Regulations targeted for MCOs, employers, and other payers will be implemented to prevent inappropriate denial of coverage, promote preventive care, and improve the standards of coverage and quality of care provided. Other regulations will also be implemented to lower health costs, prevent waste, and improve overall quality of patient care. As the Act faces challenges in its funding and implementation, the regulations and timelines noted here may be modified or eliminated in the future.

Despite its critics and shortcomings, managed care is likely to remain the leading manner of financing and delivering health care in the United States. Through more effective communication and cooperation, practitioners and MCOs may some day resolve their conflicting issues. It is imperative for practitioners and MCOs to understand each other's role in health care. Although practitioners and MCOs have quite different responsibilities in health care, both groups share a common goal: the delivery of high-quality care to patients.

BIBLIOGRAPHY

Starred references are cited in the text.

Academy of Managed Care Pharmacy. (2009). *A format for the submission of clinical and economic evidence of pharmaceuticals in support of formulary consideration.* Alexandria, VA: Author.

*American Medical Association. (1994). AMA policy on drug formularies and therapeutic interchange in inpatient and ambulatory patient care settings. *American Journal of Hospital Pharmacy, 51,* 1808–1810.

*American Society of Consultant Pharmacists. (2010). Guidelines for implementing therapeutic interchange in long-term care. Public Policy Guidelines: http://www.ascp.com/resources/policy/upload/Gui97-Therapeutic%20Interchange.pdf. Accessed March 24, 2011.

*Bootman, J. L., Townsend, R. J., & McGhan, W. F. (2004). Introduction to pharmacoeconomics. In J. L. Bootman, R. J. Townsend, & W. F. McGhan (Eds.), *Principles of pharmacoeconomics* (3rd ed.). Cincinnati, OH: Harvey Whitney Books.

Campbell, G., & Sprague, K. L. (2001). The state of drug decision-making: Report on a survey of P&T committee structure and practices. *Formulary, 36,* 644–655.

*Centers for Medicare and Medicaid Services. (2010). Office of the Actuary, National Health Statistics Group. National health care expenditures data. Washington, DC: Author.

*Chase, S. L., Peterson, A. M., & Wardell, C. J. (1998). Therapeutic-interchange program for oral histamine H_2-receptor antagonists. *American Journal of Hospital Pharmacy, 55,* 1382–1386.

*Fairman, K. A., Motheral, B. R., & Henderson, R. R. (2003). Retrospective, long-term follow-up study of the effect of a three-tier prescription drug co-payment system on pharmaceutical and other medical utilization and costs. *Clinical Therapeutics, 25,* 3147–3161.

Fins, J. J. (1998). Drug benefits in managed care: Seeking ethical guidance from the formulary? *Journal of the American Geriatrics Society, 46,* 346–350.

*Flanagan, J. (2002). HMO light and tight plan will restrict access to care and provide fewer patient protections. The Foundation for Taxpayer and Consumer Rights. www.consumerwatchdog.org/healthcare/pr/pr002772. php3. Accessed March 4, 2004.

Fullerton D. S., & Atherly D. S. (2004). Formularies, therapeutics, and outcomes: New opportunities. *Medical Care, 42*(4 Suppl.), 39–44.

*Glassman, P., Jacobson, P., & Asch, S. (1997). Medical necessity and defined coverage benefits in the Oregon health plan. *American Journal of Public Health, 87,* 1053–1058.

*Hartman, M. H. (2010). Health spending growth at a historic low in 2008. *Health Affairs. 29,* 147–155.

*Horn, S. D., Sharkey, P. D., & Phillips-Harris, C. (1998). Formulary limitations and the elderly: Results from the Managed Care Outcomes Project. *American Journal of Managed Care, 4,* 1105–1113.

*IMS Health. (2010). Press release: IMS Health reports U.S. prescription sales grew 5.1 percent in 2009, to $300.3 billion. Norwalk, CT: Author.

*Kaiser Family Foundation. (2010a). Medicaid and managed care: Key data, trends, and issues. (Publication No. 8046). Washington, DC: Author.

*Kaiser Family Foundation. (2010b). Employer health benefits 2010 annual survey. (Publication No. 8085). Menlo Park, CA: Author.

Keech, M. (2001). Using health outcomes data to inform decision-making. *Pharmacoeconomics, 19,* 27–31.

*Lisi, D. (1997). Ethical issues for pharmacists in managed care. *American Journal of Health-System Pharmacy, 54,* 1041–1045.

Luce, B. R., Lyles, A. C., & Rentz, A. M. (1996). The view from managed care pharmacy. *Health Affairs, 15,* 168–176.

Lyles, A., & Palumbo, F. B. (1999). The effect of managed care on prescription drug costs and benefits. *Pharmacoeconomics, 15*(2), 129–140.

Monane, M., Nagle, B., & Kelly, M. (1998). Pharmacotherapy: Strategies to control drug costs in managed care. *Geriatrics, 53*(9), 53–63.

*National Conference of State Legislatures. (2010). State Pharmaceutical Assistance Programs 2010. http://www.ncsl.org/default.aspx?tabid=14334. Denver, CO: Author.

Navarro, R. (Ed.). (1998). *Pharmacy benefit report: Trends and forecasts.* East Hanover, NJ: Novartis Pharmaceuticals.

Navarro, R. P., & Cahill, J. A. (1999). The U.S. health care system and the development of managed care. In R. P. Navarro (Ed.). *Managed care pharmacy practice* (pp. 3–28). Gaithersburg, MD: Aspen Publishers.

*Navarro, R. P., Dillon, M. J., & Grzegorczyk, J. E. (2008). Role of drug formularies in managed care organizations. In R.P. Navarro (Ed.). *Managed care pharmacy practice* (2nd ed., pp. 233–252). Sudbury, MA: Jones and Bartlett Publishers.

*PBM News. (2001, Fall). Use of multiple-tier plan designs continue to increase. (On-line). http://www.pbmi.com/pbmnews/V6N4_plandesigns.html. Accessed February 16, 2005.

Penna, P. M. (2002). AMCP format for formulary submissions: Who is using them, who will be evaluating them, and what regulatory concerns do they raise? International Society for Pharmacoeconomics and Outcomes Research Seventh International Meeting, Arlington, VA.

*Posler, J. A., Truffer, C., Smith, S. A., et al. (2007). Health spending projections through 2016: Modest changes obscure Part D's impact. *Health Affairs, 26,* W242–W253.

*Roy-Byrne, P., Russo, J., Rabin, L., et al. (1998). A brief medical necessity scale for mental disorders: Reliability, validity, and clinical utility. *Journal of Behavioral Health Services and Research, 25,* 412–424.

*Sonnedecker, G. (1976). *Kremer's and Urdang's history of pharmacy.* Madison, WI: American Institute of the History of Pharmacy.

*Starr, P. (1982). *The social transformation of American medicine.* New York: Basic Books.

Sweet, B. T., Wilson, M. W., Waugh, W. J., et al. (2002). Building the outcomes-based formulary. *Disease Management and Health Outcomes, 10,* 525–530.

*Takeda Pharmaceuticals. (2010). 2010–2011 prescription drug benefit cost and plan design report (Publication TAK-00299R1). Scottsdale, AZ: Pharmacy Benefit Management Institute.

*Talley, C. R. (1997). Managed care backlash. *American Journal of Health-System Pharmacy, 54,* 1049.

*Troy, T. (1999). Defining your firm's formulary. *Managed Healthcare,* 25–37.

*U.S. Department of Health & Human Services. (2010). Understanding the Affordable Care Act: About the Law. http://www.healthcare.gov/law/about/index.html. Accessed December 2, 2010.

*U.S. Food and Drug Administration. (2010). Orange Book: Approved drug products with therapeutic equivalence evaluations. Rockville, MD: United States Department of Health and Human Services.

Integrative Approaches to Pharmacotherapy—A Look at Complex Cases

The cases presented in each of the chapters on disorders were designed to help the learner think through the process of evaluating the drug therapy needed for a patient. The cases were simple ones, typically involving a single problem related to the disorders discussed in that chapter. This chapter, however, uses cases involving patients with multiple problems, which forces the learner to assess the problems and prioritize them. When faced with multiple problems in a single patient, the practitioner then must decide among a variety of treatment options. This level of complexity is reflective of real-life situations and requires a systematic approach to the patient to manage the complexities.

THE COMPLEXITY OF PATIENTS

The reality of life is that patients are complex individuals with multiple competing issues and priorities. Patients have economic, social, emotional, and cultural issues that affect their medical conditions.

Medications are expensive, with the 2009 average prescription price for a branded medication being $155.45 and generic medication $39.73 (National Association of Chain Drug Stores, 2009). Nearly two thirds of elderly patients use medications on a daily basis with an average of eight prescription medications per person in the elderly (Chrischilles et al., 1992). The monthly cost alone could range from $240 to $640, clearly prohibitive for some patients without a prescription drug coverage plan. The selection, then, of treatment options must consider the cost of the treatment, because if patients cannot afford the treatment they will not follow the plan.

In addition, the social and emotional impact of a diagnosis must be considered. Patients requiring insulin injections to maintain adequate blood sugar levels need assistance in making the lifestyle change necessary to incorporate the injections as well as the monitoring into their daily routine. The emotional reminder of "illness associated with chronic medication-taking behavior" must be addressed at the initial and subsequent visits. Last, culturally accepted treatment options are important considerations; injectable medications containing human blood products (e.g., albumin) may not be acceptable to patients who

are of the Jehovah's Witness faith. In another vein, Asian cultures view illness as an inevitable consequence of life and, as a result, may not seek care or may refuse treatment.

GENERAL OVERVIEW OF METHODS FOR ASSESSING PATIENTS AND DRUG THERAPY

One of the more common methods for organizing medical information is the problem-oriented medical record (POMR). Each of the patient's medical problems is identified and prioritized in order of importance. The order of the problems depends on the acuity and severity of the situation. Typically, the most severe and acute problems are listed first, followed by the chronic conditions, and then problems requiring preventive measures (e.g., smoking cessation).

In addition to the prioritized problem list, the POMR system uses the "SOAP" note technique for organizing information associated with each problem. The acronym *SOAP* stands for (S)ubjective, (O)bjective, (A)ssessment, and (P)lan. The subjective and objective components are the data that support the identification of the prioritized problem. The subjective data refer to information provided by the patient (or other individual) that cannot be independently verified. The objective data often are laboratory data or health assessments (e.g., blood pressures) performed or observed by the practitioner.

The information needed in this part of the SOAP note includes the chief complaint, history of the present illness, past medical history, family and social history, medication history, the results of the review of systems, and physical examination and laboratory results. This data collection is key in the assessment of the patient.

The assessment section of the SOAP note integrates the subjective and objective information and is where the practitioner delineates the potential diagnosis related to the problem. The rationale for the diagnosis should be included as well as an indication of the severity and acuity of the problem. The last portion of the note is the therapeutic plan. In this section, the practitioner may include additional diagnostic tests necessary to confirm or rule out the suspected diagnosis. This diagnostic plan may also include referral to other practitioners as necessary. The other portion of the plan section should include information about changes in therapeutic plans such as adding/deleting drug therapy, identifying desired outcomes, and monitoring parameters.

Anticipating Problems

One of the key elements to a good practitioner is the ability to plan for unintended consequences. A patient may become noncompliant with a medication due to an adverse event and not report the event or the noncompliance to you, before your next scheduled visit. The result is the patient forgoes treatment for an identified problem for an unknown period of time. When confronted, the patient will admit to the noncompliance but indicate that he did not "want to bother you" with the problem. Upfront discussions regarding the potential consequences (adverse reactions, noncompliance) will help reduce the frequency of these types of encounters. As a practitioner, you should always consider what you will do if your patient has a drug reaction, takes an interacting drug, or even stops taking the drug.

Other Information Needed Before Prescribing

When taking a medication history, the practitioner needs to assess specific information related to drug therapy. An inventory of patient-reported allergies is vital to a good medication history. These allergies include an assessment of drug allergies. A patient may report a symptom as an allergy, but the clinician must assess the validity of the report. For example, a patient may report abdominal discomfort as an allergy to erythromycin, but in reality, the reported symptom is an adverse effect of the drug. This type of report is not a true allergy and would not preclude the patient from receiving that drug or a related drug. However, the practitioner must consider the impact the symptom has on the patient's willingness to take a prescribed medication. If the patient was prescribed a medication that would cause distress, the patient is less likely to take it.

Food allergies are also important to assess. Reports of allergies to shellfish or other iodine-containing foods are important to know when prescribing medications such as intravenous contrast dyes.

Further, within this section of the patient history, the practitioner must not only assess prescription medication use, but also obtain a good history of nonprescription and complementary and alternative medication use. In 2007, 38% of adults and 12% of children used natural products as part of their personal treatment plan (National Center for Complementary and Alternative Medicine, 2007). The most commonly used products were echinacea (40.3%), ginseng (24.1%), and gingko biloba (21.1%; Barnes, et al., 2004). The potential for drug–drug and drug–disease interactions with these and other agents exists and must be considered as part of the treatment plan.

Questions

As noted earlier, each disorder chapter had a simple case with a series of questions designed to help you work through the pharmacotherapeutic approach to the patient. These nine questions are indicative of a thought process that should be followed when developing the pharmacotherapeutic aspect of the care plan. The following real-life cases are more complex than those in the disorder chapters and are designed to help the learner integrate the treatment plan for patients with multiple disorders. We use the same nine questions, in varying forms, to exemplify the thought process. The answers provided may not be the only "right" answers. Other choices of drug therapy may clearly be available, or as time progresses, we may learn that there are better choices due to new drug development and new research on existing drugs. We encourage you to use this process to help you think through the problem, not just come up with an answer.

Case 1: Diabetes/Lipids/HTN/CAD with Microalbuminuria

J. S. is a 52-year-old white man who is an accountant who was diagnosed with type 2 diabetes mellitus 5 years ago. He has not been controlled with diet or three different diabetic medications. He also has osteoarthritis of his right knee and a strong family history of coronary artery disease (CAD). He comes to the office complaining of frequent urination, blurry vision, and fatigue. He travels two times a month for business, sometimes internationally. He does not regularly check his blood sugar. J.S. also complains of erectile dysfunction.

Weight: 250 lb
Height: 70 inches
BP: 136/84
Pulse: 72
Current medications:
> Metformin 850 mg BID, glipizide 10 mg daily and
>   repaglinide 1 mg with each meal
> Naproxen 500 mg bid, as needed

Lab values:
Glucose 260 mg/dL
HbA$_{1c}$ 8.9%
Total cholesterol 250 mg/dL
LDL 140 mg/dL
HDL 30 mg/dL
Triglycerides 280 mg/dL
Creatinine 1.0 mg/dL
BUN 14 mg/dL
AST 15
ALT 20
Urine microalbumin +

Issues: J. S. has type 2 diabetes mellitus. In addition, he is obese, has hyperlipidemia, hypertension, and microalbuminuria. All of these factors must be considered in determining which medications are appropriate for J. S. He also has erectile dysfunction. J. S. travels with his job.

List specific goals for treatment for J. S.

One of the primary goals for J. S. is to lower his risk of developing complications associated with metabolic syndrome. These include microvascular complications such as retinopathy, neuropathy, nephropathy, and the macrovascular complications of heart attack, stroke, and death. Preventing these are the long-term goals. The intermediate goals for J. S. are as follows:

Maintaining fasting blood glucose at <120 mg/dL
Maintaining HbA$_{1c}$ at <6.5%
Preventing complications of diabetes mellitus
Prevention of cardiovascular morbidity and mortality by reducing blood pressure to <120/80
Reducing total cholesterol to <200 mg/dL
Reducing low-density lipoprotein (LDL) to <70 mg/dL

What drug therapy would you prescribe? Why?

J. S. has uncontrolled type 2 diabetes while on oral medications. Since he failed a trial of three oral medications, initiation of insulin may be appropriate at this time. Consider discontinuing the repaglinide and starting 10 units daily of a basal insulin, such as Lantus, to begin and then bring the patient back within 2 weeks to recheck the fasting blood glucose and adjust accordingly. Each additional unit of insulin is expected to bring the blood sugar down an additional 30 mg/dL.

Blood pressure control may be an issue with J. S. Because of the presence of albuminuria, it is recommended that J. S. receive an angiotensin-converting enzyme (ACE) inhibitor or angiotensin receptor blocker (ARB) to protect kidney function. The addition of either of these agents is appropriate.

Hyperlipidemia is also a problem with J. S. His total cholesterol should be under 200 mg/dL with his LDL less than 70 mg/dL. His high-density lipoprotein (HDL) level should be more than 40 mg/dL. A statin should be started at the lowest therapeutic dose.

Since he is complaining of erectile dysfunction, a thorough cardiac history must be taken. After the results are determined, consideration may be given to adding a phosphodiesterase type 5 (PDE5) inhibitor such as sildenafil.

What are the parameters for monitoring success of the therapy?

Success of therapy for diabetes mellitus is determined by measurement of HbA$_{1c}$ every 3 months. If the HbA$_{1c}$ level does not show a downward progression, the dosage of the insulin should be increased.

Success of therapy for hypertension is measured by blood pressure readings. Ideally, blood pressure for a diabetic patient should be under 120/80 mm Hg. For the hyperlipidemia, maximal effects are seen by 4 to 6 weeks after starting drug therapy. Therefore, fasting lipid panel results should be reviewed approximately 6 weeks after starting or titrating drug therapy. If no changes are made in therapy, a fasting lipid panel test should be repeated at 3 and 6 months and yearly thereafter if the patient has achieved the LDL cholesterol goal.

Discuss specific patient education based on the prescribed therapy.

Patient education includes teaching the signs and symptoms of hypoglycemia and dietary modifications for lowering blood sugar and cholesterol. Consideration should be given to having J. S. see a dietitian to review specific changes in his diet to meet the therapeutic lifestyle changes needed to maximize drug therapy efficacy.

Additional discussion should focus on the potential side effects of these agents. If J. S. experiences muscle aches and pains, he should seek attention to rule out rhabdomyolysis secondary to the statin. Similarly, ACE-inhibitor cough, while not life-threatening, is a common side effect, and J. S. should monitor for it. The practitioner should discuss how to manage his insulin therapy across time zones. With the frequent travel J. S. engages in, learning how to manage this aspect of his drug regimen is crucial to long-term success. If J. S. is flying east, then he loses time and may decrease food intake, thus decreasing his insulin needs; flying west is the reverse. Also inform J. S. that he should carry his medicine on his person and inform the screener that he is carrying insulin syringes and blood sugar testing materials (e.g., lancets). With respect to the sildenafil, he should be cautioned not to consume high-fat meals and if the erection lasts for 4 hours or more, to seek immediate care.

List one or two adverse reactions for the selected agent that would cause you to change therapy.

If J. S. is taking an ACE inhibitor and developed a cough, it would be appropriate to switch to an ARB.

If myalgias occur, this could be a side effect of the statin. Sometimes lowering the dose or switching to another statin may rectify this. Additionally, creatine kinase (CK) should be measured to see if it increases. Patients may experience myalgias, however, without increased CK. If the symptoms persist on another statin, ezetimibe (Zetia) may be considered.

What would be the choice for second-line therapy?

If J. S.'s blood glucose is not controlled or if his HbA$_{1c}$ is above 6.5%, consider increasing the dose or re-add repaglinide if previously discontinued or add a short-acting insulin at meals.

If his blood pressure is not at an appropriate level, a second antihypertensive agent may be added. A diuretic is often very effective in combination with other drug therapy.

If lipids have not reached therapeutic levels, ezetimibe can be added to the current statin for further reduction.

What over-the-counter or alternative medications would be appropriate for J. S.?

Aspirin 81 mg daily is recommended for prophylaxis of heart attack or stroke. Higher doses than this can slightly increase the risk of a peptic ulcer and offer little additional benefit. Fish oil is recommended for hyperlipidemia. Also, omega-3 fatty acids can be added.

What lifestyle changes would you recommend to J. S.?

J. S. needs to reduce his weight. This can be accomplished by dietary changes and increased exercise. If he has a high sodium intake, reducing this to 2,000 mg or less daily can help to reduce his blood pressure. J. S. is encouraged to follow a low-fat diet to reduce his cholesterol and reduce his risk for a major cardiac event. Fat intake should be restricted to 25% to 35% of total calories.

Describe one or two drug–drug or drug–food interactions for the selected agent.

There may be a decreased antihypertensive effect with non-steroidal anti-inflammatory drugs (NSAIDs) and antihypertensive agents, so blood pressure must be carefully monitored. Some statins have an interaction with grapefruit. Grapefruit can increase the 3-hydroxy-3-methylglutaryl-coenzyme A (HMG CoA) inhibitor levels. Sildenafil interacts with nitrates, so if angina develops, the sildenafil should be discontinued if nitrates are added to the regimen.

Case 2: Elderly/Statin/Warfarin Comes Down With an Infection

M.T. is a 66-year-old woman with a chief complaint of generalized feeling poor and a 24-hour history of dysuria, urinary frequency, and urgency. She has had recent sexual activity. She has a 1-year history of atrial fibrillation. She also has type 2 diabetes and hypercholesterolemia. She had a hysterectomy 3 years ago.

Her medications include simvastatin, 40 mg qd; diltiazem extended release, 180 mg bid; sotalol, 80 mg bid; warfarin, 7.5 mg qd; metformin, 850 mg bid; calcium carbonate, 1,000 mg qd.

Most recent pertinent labs:
INR 2.2   Creatinine 1.3 mg/dL
All others WNL

Physical exam: unremarkable except for urinalysis: WBC 10–15 cells/hpf, RBCs, 1–5 cells/hpf, bacteria 2–5/hpf, nitrite negative
Allergies: NKDA

Diagnosis: Acute uncomplicated urinary tract infection (UTI)

What specific goals do you have for M. T.'s current condition?

The goals of treatment for M.T. include eradication of the urinary bacteria and a return to a normal urinary habit and evaluation of the confusion.

What drug therapy would you prescribe? Why?

A variety of drug choices are available for M.T. Antibiotic therapy is the mainstay of treatment because UTIs are typically bacterial in nature. One of the most common organisms causing an uncomplicated UTI is *Escherichia coli*. The first-line therapy for treating this type of organism in a UTI is typically sulfamethoxazole–trimethoprim (Bactrim). This agent concentrates well in the urine and has good activity against *E. coli*. Often, a single-day or a 3-day treatment regimen of double-strength sulfamethoxazole–trimethoprim is sufficient to eradicate the organism. However, in patients with diabetes, single-dose treatment is not recommended. There are some reports of an increasing resistance to this agent, which may be endemic to a geographical region (Butler, et al., 2004).

In the case of M.T., however, sulfamethoxazole–trimethoprim may not be the best first choice. Due to her atrial fibrillation, she is receiving warfarin as venous thromboembolism (VTE) prophylaxis. The drug–drug interaction between warfarin and sulfamethoxazole–trimethoprim can lead to an increased international normalized ratio (INR). Although her INR is 2.2 (within the desired range of 2 to

3), the protein binding displacement of warfarin caused by the sulfamethoxazole component can lead to unacceptable changes in the coagulation factors. This would place M.T. at risk for a minor or a major bleed, particularly if she were to inadvertently injure herself through a fall. Instead, she would be a candidate for a fluoroquinolone antibiotic such as levofloxacin or ciprofloxacin. Due to her being on a fixed income, ciprofloxacin is a good choice due to its generic availability and lower cost.

Consideration should be given to the appropriate dose of ciprofloxacin. For uncomplicated UTIs, the dose is typically 500 mg BID orally for 7 days. Typically, a fluoroquinolone dose adjustment should be made for patients with renal dysfunction (estimated creatinine clearance [CrCl] <50 mL/minute). However, because the drug concentrates well in the urine and the dose is low to begin with, the adjustment is not necessary for UTIs until the CrCl is 20 mL/minute or less.

What are the parameters for monitoring success of the drug therapy?

The primary parameter would be a resolution of the symptoms. M.T. should return to a normal urinary habit within 48 to 72 hours after initiation of antibiotic treatment. A repeat urinalysis after treatment ends would confirm bacterial eradication, but often is unnecessary if symptoms resolve. If the confusion persists after resolution of the infection, M.T. should be referred for a neurological evaluation.

Discuss specific patient education based on the prescribed therapy.

The patient should be educated on the need for taking ciprofloxacin for the entire 7 days even if the symptoms begin to resolve. Information regarding increasing water/fluid intake should also be part of the patient education process.

Describe one or two drug–drug or drug–food interactions for ciprofloxacin.

The patient should also be advised not to take the ciprofloxacin with chelating agents such as iron supplements, magnesium- or aluminum-containing antacids, or zinc products. If M.T. needs to take one or more of these, then the ciprofloxacin should be taken 2 hours before or after the agent.

Further, quinolones have been reported to enhance the effects of warfarin anticoagulation when administered concomitantly. No specific dosage adjustments are needed with either medication, but the INR should be monitored closely to prevent bleeding complications.

List one or two adverse reactions for the ciprofloxacin that would cause you to change therapy.

Many side effects can be associated with quinolone antibiotics. Common ones include gastrointestinal (GI), neurologic, and cardiac disturbances. The GI effects such as vomiting and diarrhea put her at risk for dehydration, worsening her metabolic state. The neurologic effects such as seizures, delirium, and abnormal coordination put her at risk for falls and the development of a major bleed.

What would be the choice for the second-line therapy?

An alternative agent is sulfamethoxazole–trimethoprim, but due to the warfarin, it may not be the best choice. If unsuccessful, urine cultures would be the best method to help direct appropriate treatment based on microbiological sensitivities.

What over-the-counter or alternative medications would be appropriate for M. T.?

There are no over-the-counter or complementary/alternative medications appropriate to treat M.T.'s infection. The practitioner should discourage the use of these types of medications, particularly those that may interact with her warfarin.

What dietary and lifestyle changes should be recommended for M. T.?

M.T. should be encouraged to drink plenty of water, particularly while taking the antibiotic. The water helps to flush the bacteria out of the system. Also, M.T. should be encouraged to urinate when she has the urge; she should not hold back on urination because this may increase bacterial growth.

Case 3: Postmenopausal/Hypothyroid/Osteoporosis

L.L. is a 56-year-old white woman who has not menstruated for 1 year. She is waking up at night with hot flashes and consequently is tired all of the time. During the day she has 8 to 10 hot flashes and is very uncomfortable. She wants to do something about the hot flashes. Her gynecologic exam and Pap smear are normal, and you order a dual-energy x-ray absorptiometry (DEXA) scan.
PMH: Hypothyroidism
Medications: Vitamin C 1,000 mg daily
Synthroid 112 mcg daily
Ibuprofen as needed for back pain
Multivitamin daily
Weight: 115 lb
Height: 5 ft 6 inches (she was 5 ft 8 inches 2 years ago)
BP: 118/76
DEXA scan: t score of –2.6 left hip and –2.0 lumbar spine
TSH: 7.4
Issues: L.L. is postmenopausal and is symptomatic for hot flashes. She also has osteoporosis. Another area of concern is poor control of hypothyroidism.

List specific goals for treatment for L. L.

For L.L., there are two types of outcomes desired: humanistic and clinical. The humanistic outcomes relate to the quality of life. In the short run, this would mean a reduction in the menopausal symptoms for L.L. and an improvement in the symptoms related to poor thyroid control or depression. In the long run, the clinical goal would be to prevent the development of fractures. L.L.'s DEXA scan results show that she is at risk for fractures, and if she continues on this course, the risk will only increase. Therefore, goals of therapy include:

- reduction of menopausal symptoms
- prevention of fracture
- maintenance of thyroid function at normal levels
- resolution of feelings of depression.

What drug therapy would you prescribe? Why?

L. L. should be prescribed a low-dose combination of hormone therapy including estrogen and progesterone because she has an intact uterus. A dose of 0.3 mg estrogen and 1.5 mg progesterone is acceptable. She should be kept on this therapy for the shortest possible time just for relief of menopausal symptoms.

Alendronate (Fosamax) 70 mg is a suitable choice for osteoporosis. It is given once a week.

L. L.'s Synthroid dose must be increased because she is still hypothyroid. An increase to 100 μg will be made.

What are the parameters for monitoring success of the therapy?

Patient history of menopausal symptom relief is the key to determining if hormone therapy is successful. L. L. should return in 2 months to check response to hormone replacement therapy (HRT) and blood pressure. It is recommended that L. L. stay on HRT for the shortest possible time to prevent cardiac events.

L. L.'s thyroid-stimulating hormone (TSH) level should be rechecked in 6 to 8 weeks. If it is within normal levels, the dose of Synthroid should remain at 100 μg. At this time, the patient should be evaluated for continuing signs of depression. If she still complains of depression, then consideration should be given to counseling and/or drug therapy. TSH levels should be monitored in 6 months and then yearly if it is stable.

A DEXA scan should be repeated every 2 years to ensure effectiveness of therapy. There should be little to no change in the DEXA scan results during therapy with alendronate. Compliance should also be checked.

Discuss specific patient education based on the prescribed therapy.

L. L. must be told that it may take at least 4 weeks of HRT before she notices a significant change in menopausal symptoms. It is important that she be taught the correct method for performing a monthly breast self-exam and to report any palpable masses. Any abnormal vaginal bleeding is to be reported immediately.

Thyroid medications should be taken 1 hour before or 4 hours after any other medications, especially calcium and iron supplements. It needs to be stressed that L. L. will require life-long thyroid replacement.

Alendronate must be taken at least 30 minutes before any other food or liquid (except what is used to take the medicine). L. L. should remain in a sitting or standing position for at least 30 minutes after ingestion to prevent damage to the esophagus.

List one or two adverse reactions for the selected agent that would cause you to change therapy.

Adverse reactions of HRT include GI upset and elevated blood pressure. Adverse reactions of Synthroid include palpitations and nervousness. If this occurs, the TSH level needs to be checked because it indicates too high a dose of Synthroid. An adverse event associated with alendronate is severe GI upset.

What would be the choice for second-line therapy?

Use of a transdermal hormone patch can reduce menopausal symptoms and many side effects. If the patch does not contain progesterone, supplemental progesterone must be given to prevent uterine hyperplasia.

Calcitonin would be a second-line therapy for osteoporosis for L. L. A selective estrogen receptor modulator would not be appropriate with HRT because the combination increases the risk of clots.

What over-the-counter or alternative medications would be appropriate for L. L.?

Black cohosh can be used in place of HRT with some relief of symptoms. Calcium at a dose of 1,500 mg with 800 to 1,000 units of vitamin D is recommended for postmenopausal women in addition to the alendronate, but should be taken at least 2 hours after the alendronate because it can interfere with absorption.

What lifestyle changes would you recommend to L. L.?

L. L. should wear cool clothing to diminish the hot flashes. Weight-bearing exercises are important in the patient with osteoporosis because they build bone mass.

Describe one or two drug–drug or drug–food interactions for the selected agent.

Synthroid absorption is decreased if given with calcium products and should be taken 1 hour before or 4 hours after calcium. Antacids can decrease absorption of alendronate.

Case 4: Asthma/ADHD/Allergies With Exacerbation of Allergy

N.J. is an 11-year-old boy with a 5-year history of attention deficit hyperactivity disorder (ADHD) and a 7-year history of asthma. He also experiences perennial allergic rhinitis. N. J.'s mother is bringing him into your office due to an exacerbation of this allergy. The symptoms he presents with include increased cough and runny nose and sneezing. He has no other medical history. The following is his current list of medications:

Concerta 36 mg every morning
Albuterol inhaler, 2 puffs as needed (uses one to two times a day)
Singulair 5 mg PO daily
Zyrtec 5 mg PO daily

List specific goals of treatment for N.J.

The obvious goal is to decrease the coughing and other allergic symptoms. However, it is not clear if the cough is a secondary manifestation of the uncontrolled asthma or as a result of the rhinorrhea associated with the allergies. Therefore, an additional goal would be to improve the asthma control. Specific goals related to asthma would be a decrease in the frequency of use of the albuterol inhaler.

What drug therapy would be appropriate for N.J.? Why?

The National Asthma Education and Prevention Program update of 2007 recommends that all persons with persistent asthma be prescribed a low-dose inhaled corticosteroid controller balancing the availability on the patient's formulary and the convenience of administration (BID versus QID). He should also remain on the Singulair daily and the albuterol as needed.

What are the parameters for monitoring success of the therapy?

For the allergies, a reduction in the rhinorrhea, and if appropriate, a decrease in the cough would be good clinical markers of success. For the asthma, the primary indicator would be a decreased use of the short-acting β agonist to less than twice weekly as well as improved lung function such as improved peak flow readings or improved exercise tolerance.

Discuss specific patient education based on the prescribed therapy.

An investigation of the potential changes in the household or other environmental changes should be part of the workup. Discussion with the mother and child regarding triggers is a key to preventing these exacerbations.

Finally, the patient needs to be educated about the use of this agent as a long-term controller and not a symptom reliever. The inhaled corticosteroid is not intended to relieve acute symptoms of asthma. The clinician should also observe N.J.'s use of the inhaler to assure proper technique.

List one or two adverse reactions for the selected agent that would cause you to change therapy.

When considering alternative therapy, a thorough review of the use of short-acting β_2 agonists must also be considered because these will also produce palpitations, chest pain, and tachycardia. Further, an increasing need for short-acting β_2 agonists or a perceived lack of benefit of short-acting β_2 agonists may be a sign of seriously worsening asthma, and the patient should notify the clinician immediately.

What would be the choice for the second-line therapy for treating N.J.?

If N.J.'s symptoms are not resolved, a second-line therapy would be to move up to moderate-dose corticosteroid with or without the Singulair. Alternatively, a long-acting beta-agonist such as salmeterol can be added to the regimen.

What over-the-counter or alternative medications would be appropriate for N.J.?

For treating the rhinorrhea, over-the-counter antihistamines may be used additively, but the sedating effects need to be taken into consideration.

What dietary and lifestyle changes should be recommended for N.J.?

Avoidance of allergen triggers should be considered one of the primary lifestyle changes. Removal of carpets from the bedroom, keeping pets out of rooms in which N.J. spends time, and washing sheets/linens in hot water weekly are some of the strategies for reducing environmental allergens. Exposure to second-hand smoke should also be minimized.

Case 5: Depression/GERD

M.M. is a 60-year-old African American man who presents with a 3-month history of lack of sleep because he awakens every 2 hours and cannot get back to sleep. He lacks desire to do anything that he previously enjoyed, has an increased appetite, and does not want to leave his house. It is an effort for him to go to work every morning. Additionally, he says that when he eats anything, he gets burning in his stomach and esophagus and is awakened at night with indigestion.

Social history: Married for 35 years to the same woman. Two grown children. His 15-year-old dog died 3 months ago. He took the dog everywhere with him. He smokes 1/2 pack of cigarettes a day.

BP: 126/80
P: 76
Weight: 204 lb
Height: 67 inches
Rest of physical exam: WNL
Labs:
   TSH 3.4
   PSA 0.6
   Cholesterol 212 mg/dL
   LDL 128 mg/dL
   HDL 40 mg/dL
Issues: M.M. has symptoms of depression. Insomnia is an issue. He also has the symptoms of new-onset gastroesophageal reflux disease (GERD).

List specific goals for treatment for M. M.

The goals of therapy for M. M. relate to quality of life as well as clinical goals. Relieving the depressive symptoms should help M. M. enjoy life and feel better, but the time frame for response is 4 to 6 weeks, provided the initial therapy works. This should be discussed with M. M. as therapy is initiated. A depression scale, such as the Hamilton Depression Scale (HAM-D), might be given to determine a baseline level of depression and as a means of monitoring progress as treatment continues. A specific goal might be a 50% decrease or better from the baseline HAM-D score.

However, relief of indigestion and providing adequate sleep are more immediate goals that should be achievable within the first week of therapy. Progress on these short-term goals is likely to help M. M. continue with the therapy for relieving the long-term problem of depression. Therefore, specific goals are:

- relief of symptoms of depression
- provision of adequate sleep
- relief of reflux symptoms
- smoking cessation.

What drug therapy would you prescribe for M. M.? Why?

Paroxetine is a good choice because it promotes better sleep. It is best to give this agent in the evening due to slight sedative effects. If another agent is on formulary at a substantially lower cost, such as sertraline, it can be prescribed and taken in the morning. Typically, a sleeping aid is prescribed in patients such as M. M., but the sedative effects of paroxetine might be sufficient. If the insomnia persists after 4 to 6 weeks, an additional hypnotic may be considered. A proton pump inhibitor (PPI) would be a reasonable choice for relief of his GERD now, and if it persists after 3 months, endoscopy would be indicated.

What are the parameters for monitoring success of the therapy?

Follow-up history is the best way to monitor therapy for depression. Readministration of a depression scale with an improved score would indicate successful therapy. Also, indication of 8 hours of sleep a night demonstrates successful therapy. Patient-reported frequency and severity of GERD episodes is a good tool to determine success of therapy for GERD.

Discuss specific patient education based on the prescribed therapy.

The overall premise is the promotion of "good sleep habits," which include setting a routine bedtime, instituting regular exercise habits, using the bed for sleeping only, and getting in bed only when ready for sleep. Occasional completion of a sleep log is an important tool for the clinician to evaluate the effectiveness of therapy.

Lifestyle changes are as important as drug therapy in managing GERD. Discussion with the patient and family should cover the following important dietary changes: avoidance of excess alcohol and food intake; decreased amounts of chocolate and spicy, fried, or fatty foods; and avoidance of the recumbent position for at least 3 hours after meals. Because these recommended changes involve many activities or foods that are pleasurable for the patient, they should be eliminated gradually—one at a time. A nutritionist can be consulted to help the patient learn to choose and prepare less problematic foods.

Additional measures include teaching the patient to elevate the head of the bed approximately 4 to 6 inches (using blocks); to avoid tight, restrictive clothing; and to lose weight if necessary.

The patient needs to be counseled on the risks of continued smoking. The patient's readiness for change must be ascertained, and he needs to be educated on the poor health consequences associated with continued smoking.

List an adverse reaction for the selected agents that would cause you to change therapy.

If M. M. complains of decreased libido from the paroxetine, then consideration should be given to lowering the dose or changing to a non–selective serotonin receptor inhibitor. This is particularly important if it becomes upsetting to him because he and his wife have a very satisfying sexual relationship.

What would be the choice for second-line therapy?

Lowering the dose of paroxetine might help with the side effects. However, if this is not possible, bupropion is an appropriate choice for second-line therapy for the depression, particularly as it relates to sexual side effects.

What over-the-counter or alternative medications would be appropriate for M. M.?

Some patients, especially those with delayed sleep phase insomnia, may benefit from the administration of exogenous melatonin; however, further study is necessary.

Aloe vera juice may help in the healing of gastrointestinal tract irritation. Other herbs, such as catnip, fennel, ginger, and marshmallow root, as well as papaya juice, may help stop heartburn. Licorice is used to treat both heartburn and stomach and esophageal ulcers.

What lifestyle changes would you recommend to M. M.?

Lifestyle modifications are essential for the patient with GERD. Although drug therapy will help reduce the level of acid in the stomach and promote healing, lifestyle changes will aid in preventing the symptoms from returning. These lifestyle changes include dietary changes, such as avoiding irritating foods like caffeine, alcohol, and spicy foods. Further, refraining from eating at least 3 hours before bedtime and elevating the head of the bed by at least 6 inches will help reduce nighttime symptoms. Weight loss will also reduce the frequency of GERD symptoms. Lastly, smoking cessation will reduce the frequency of GERD symptoms.

The overall premise is the promotion of "good sleep habits," which include setting a routine bedtime, instituting regular exercise habits, using the bed for sleeping only, and getting in bed only when ready for sleep. Occasional completion of a sleep log is an important tool for the clinician to evaluate the effectiveness of therapy.

Describe one or two drug–drug or drug–food interactions for the selected agents.

Paroxetine is an inhibitor of the cytochrome P450 (CYP) 2D6 system and might increase the serum concentrations of cough suppressants such as dextromethorphan and codeine,

so care must be taken when using these agents during cough/cold season. The PPIs omeprazole, lansoprazole, and pantoprazole are inhibitors of the CYP2C19 system and would increase levels of drugs such as diazepam, phenytoin, or amitriptyline.

Case 6: Acute Care Visit Scheduled for a Cold; Discovered to Have Hypertension

J.F. is a 41-year-old white male who presents with a cold that he has had for about 4 days. He has a runny nose, cough that is annoying, and periodic headache. He has not tried any over-the-counter medicines. He wants an antibiotic for the cold because he is going skiing this weekend.

While in the office he says he needs a note saying he is well enough to use the gym. He has no known health problems but has not seen a health professional in over 4 years. **Social history:** Single. Elementary school teacher. Multiple sexual partners. Strong family history of heart disease. His father and uncle died before age 50 of an acute myocardial infarction. Does not smoke. Drinks socially but may have 10 beers on the weekend.

Physical exam:
BP 150/100
P 70 RRR
Weight 250 lb
Height 70 inches
Nasal mucosa red and swollen
Ears normal
No lymphadenopathy
Lungs clear to auscultation
Issues: J. F. presents with symptoms of a viral upper respiratory infection. He wants antibiotics for a quick fix. He also wants clearance for the gym. Physical exam shows that he is overweight and has hypertension. He also has a strong family history of heart disease at an early age.

List specific goals for treatment for J. F.

The cold appears to be viral in nature. Symptoms of a cold consist primarily of clear nasal discharge, sneezing, nasal congestion, cough, low-grade fever (below 102°F), scratchy or sore throat, mild aches, chills, headache, watery eyes, tenderness around the eyes, full feeling in the ears, and fatigue. Symptoms usually resolve in approximately 1 week, but they may linger for 2 weeks.

Specific goals are:

- relief of symptoms
- reduction of the risk of complications
- prevention of spread to others.

The fact that J. F. has an elevated blood pressure is concerning, especially in light of his family history. At this time, clearance for the gym cannot be given until there is further cardiac testing completed.

There are other issues that need to be addressed, such as his alcohol intake and multiple sexual partners.

What drug therapy would you prescribe for J. F.? Why?

Nonpharmacologic alternatives to treating the common cold are the first line. For example, rest allows the body to gain strength and be more effective in defending itself against the pathogen. The body can then dictate the increase in activities. An alternative to decongestants and expectorants is increasing water or juice intake. This assists in liquefying tenacious secretions, making expectoration easier, soothing scratchy, sore

throats, and relieving dry skin and lips. Saline gargles also are effective for soothing sore throats.

Coughing caused by chest congestion can cause a muscular chest pain. Menthol rubs can soothe this ache and open airways for some congestion relief. Menthol lozenges also have been effective in soothing scratchy throats and clearing nasal passages. Saline nasal flushes are also effective for clearing nasal passages without the rebound side effect. Petrolatum-based ointments for raw and macerated skin around the nose and upper lip ease the drying effects of dehydration and the use of multiple tissues.

Other measures, such as drinking chicken soup, taking a hot shower, or using a room humidifier, may prove helpful. Inhaling warm, moist heat helps raise the temperature of the nasal mucosa to at least 37°C, a temperature at which the virus does not replicate so readily.

Expectorants, including water, increase the output of respiratory tract fluid by decreasing the adhesiveness and surface tension of the respiratory tract and by facilitating removal of viscous mucus. The effect is noted within 1 to 2 hours.

J. F.'s symptoms appear viral in nature so an antibiotic is not indicated at this time. Decongestants are not recommended for J. F. because of his elevated blood pressure.

What are the parameters for monitoring success of the therapy?

Follow up is the best way to monitor therapy. Acute sinusitis often results from progression of the common cold (5% to 10% of cases). J. F. should be seen back in 1 week to evaluate symptoms.

At that time his other issues, such as blood pressure, multiple sexual partners, and alcohol intake, need to be addressed.

If the infection has failed to resolve or improve after 7 to 10 days, he may have sinusitis. Major symptoms include facial pain, pressure, congestion, fullness, obstruction, blockage, or discharge with a temperature greater than 38° C. Purulent drainage in the middle meatus may be a strong indicator of acute sinus disease; however, nasal purulence does not differentiate viral from bacterial infection. Symptoms may include headache, fatigue, dental pain, halitosis, otalgia, or cough. Other symptoms include toothache and a poor response to decongestants. There is usually edema of the mucous membranes upon examination and tenderness over the sinus areas upon percussion.

Characteristic signs are purulent, green or yellow nasal discharge and abnormal sinus illumination. Acute bacterial sinusitis is a consideration in patients who report cold symptoms lasting more than 8 days or with prolonged nasal obstruction or a cold that seems to have gotten better but returns with more severe symptoms.

Discuss specific patient education based on the prescribed therapy.

J.F. needs to be educated not to take decongestants that might increase his blood pressure. He should increase fluids and humidity for symptom relief. If symptoms do not get better within 1 to 2 weeks he needs to follow up. Education should be included as to how to prevent spread of germs.

However, J.F. needs to schedule a visit within 1 to 2 weeks to address his other issues. He needs a cardiac workup and probably an antihypertensive. Since his hypertension is presumed to be stage 1, the recommended antihypertensive is a thiazide diuretic.

List one or two adverse reactions for the selected agent that would cause you to change therapy.

Adverse reactions from expectorants include drowsiness, headache, and GI symptoms. Decongestants are not used because they can increase blood pressure.

What would be the choice for second-line therapy?

An antibiotic would be considered if symptoms do not resolve in 1 to 2 weeks since it has probably become sinusitis.

The recommended length of antibiotic therapy for acute bacterial sinusitis is at least 14 days, or 7 days beyond the resolution of symptoms, whichever is longer. Amoxicillin is appropriate for the initial treatment of acute, uncomplicated, mild sinusitis in patients with no recent antibiotic use. Antimicrobial agents with more broad-spectrum activity may be indicated as initial therapy for patients who have more severe infection, comorbidity, risk factors for bacterial resistance, or who have not responded to amoxicillin therapy. These agents include amoxicillin and clavulanic acid, the newer quinolones (e.g., levofloxacin, gatifloxacin, moxifloxacin), and some second- and third-generation cephalosporins (cefdinir, cefuroxime-axetil, and cefpodoxime proxetil). Patients who are allergic to penicillin may be treated with a macrolide, trimethoprim-sulfamethoxazole, tetracyclines, or clindamycin.

If J.F.'s blood pressure is not controlled on the diuretic, it is recommended to start a second antihypertensive agent in addition to the diuretic.

What over-the-counter or alternative medications would be appropriate?

Increased humidification is recommended. Also, J.F. should increase fluid intake to loosen secretions. A hot shower helps to relieve sinus congestion.

What dietary and lifestyle changes should be recommended?

J.F. needs to decrease sodium intake because of his elevated blood pressure. He needs to lose weight and increase physical activity after a cardiac evaluation.

J.F. needs counseling in safe sexual practices, such as the use of condoms. These issues can be handled at another visit when he follows up.

Case 7: Adolescent with Dysmenorrhea/Acne and Sexually Active

S.S. is a 16-year-old presenting with severe dysmenorrhea. She began menstruating at age 13. Her periods have been irregular. Each month she misses a day of school because of severe cramps and heavy bleeding with her menses. She also has a moderate case of acne, which is very disturbing to her. She has tried topical preparations and antibiotic therapy for the acne without results. She has no history of gallbladder disease, migraine headaches, or chest pain.

Social history: S.S. is a sophomore in high school. She is sexually active but does not use condoms. She has had two sexual partners, although now she is in a monogamous relationship with senior at her high school. She lives with her mother and younger brother. She does not smoke or drink.

Issues: S.S. has dysmenorrhea that affects her quality of life. In addition, she has acne, which is disturbing to her self-image. S.S. is sexually active and does not use condoms. This puts her at risk for pregnancy and sexually transmitted infections.

List specific goals for treatment.

Goals of treatment for S. S. relate to quality of life as well as clinical goals. Relief of dysmenorrhea is paramount. It will decrease absences from school and improve overall well-being. Additionally, treatment of acne is important because that affects her self-image.

Another goal is prevention of pregnancy and sexually transmitted infections (STIs). Therefore, specific goals are:

- relief of dysmenorrhea
- treatment of acne
- prevention of pregnancy
- prevention of STIs.

What drug therapy would you prescribe? Why?

NSAIDS can be used for treatment of dysmenorrhea. However, oral contraceptives (OCs) are the drug of choice for S. S. since she is sexually active and has acne unresponsive to other treatment. OCs prevent pregnancy, reduce the risk of endometriosis, ovulatory pain, dysmenorrhea, ovarian cysts, benign breast disease, premenstrual syndrome, premenstrual dysphoric disorder, and ovarian and endometrial cancer. They also might improve acne. The improvement occurs secondary to an increase in the level of sex-hormone-binding globulin, which reduces circulating free testosterone and ameliorates many androgenic effects. It is reasonable to prescribe a generic monophasic OC pill containing 30 to 35 mcg of estrogen.

In addition, S. S. should receive Quadrivalent human papillomavirus (HPV) vaccine. This provides protection against the four types of HPV most commonly associated with clinical diseases. It is recommended for females ages 13 to 26. It is a series of three doses.

Ideally, vaccine should be administered before potential exposure to HPV through sexual contact. The second dose is administered 1 to 2 months after the first dose, and the third dose is administered 6 months after the first dose.

What are the parameters for monitoring success of therapy?

Follow-up history is the best way to monitor success of the OCs for dysmenorrhea. Resolution of acne can be determined by examination of the skin.

Discuss specific patient education based on the prescribed therapy.

OCs can have either a day 1 start or a Sunday start regimen. Women who follow a day 1 start regimen begin the contraceptive agent on the first day of their period, regardless of the day of the week. Likewise, women who follow Sunday start regimens begin the OC pill pack on the Sunday directly after the onset of menses. This means that the woman will not menstruate on a weekend, which is desirable to many patients. S. S. may experience some breakthrough bleeding for the first 3 months of therapy.

OCs should be taken at the same time every day. It can be recommended to place them with S. S.'s toothbrush so she takes them when she brushes her teeth. If a pill is missed, S. S. should follow this regimen:

One pill	Take missed pill as soon as possible and resume schedule; back-up method of contraception is not necessary.
Two 30–35 mg pills	Take missed pill as soon as possible and resume schedule; back-up method of contraception is not necessary.
Two 20 μmg pills	Follow directions for more than two pills.
More than two pills	Take pill and continue taking a pill daily.
	Use condom or abstinence for 7 days.
	If missed in week 3, finish active pills in current pack and start a new pack the next day (skip current inactive pills).
	If missed pills in first week and had sex, use emergency contraception (EC) then resume taking pills the next day after EC.

It is imperative to discuss the use of condoms to prevent STIs. OCs prevent pregnancy, but not STIs.

List adverse reactions for the selected agent that would cause you to change therapy.

If S. S. had prolonged breakthrough bleeding, a change in hormone content would be considered. In the first half of the menstrual cycle, breakthrough bleeding is likely due to insufficient estrogen; in the second half of the cycle, it is likely due to insufficient progesterone. Therefore, changing to a new regimen with higher estrogen or progesterone is recommended.

CONCLUSION

These are a few examples of the decision-making process in prescribing medications. Most patients do not present with just one diagnosis and are taking several medications, and these factors must be considered in deciding on the best pharmacologic approaches. The intent of these examples is to help the reader understand *possible* solutions to some common problems. Not all the problems are addressed fully, nor would they be in real life. The complexity of patients requires the practitioner to begin to judge which problems should be addressed first and with what therapy. As the relationship between the practitioner and the patient continues, other problems can be addressed.

BIBLIOGRAPHY

Starred references are cited in the text.
*Barnes, P. M., Powell-Griner, E., McFinn, K., et al. (2004). Complementary and alternative medication use among adults; United States, 2002. *Advance Data from Vital and Health Statistics, 343.*

*Butler, K. H., Reed, K. C., & Bosker, G. (2004). New diagnostic modalities, alterations in drug resistance patterns, and current antimicrobial treatment guidelines for the hospital and outpatient setting. Part I: Diagnosis, evaluation, and principles of antibiotic selection. Clinical Consensus Reports. http://www.ahcpub.com/ahc_root_html/ccr/uti_pt1.html. Accessed September 25, 2004.

*Chrischilles, E. A., Foley, D. J., Wallace, R. B., et al. (1992). Use of medications by persons 65 and over: Data from the established populations for epidemiologic studies of the elderly. *Journal of Gerontology, 47,* M137–M144.

*National Association of Chain Drug Stores. (2009). National association of chain drug stores. http://www.nacds.org/wmspage.cfm?parm1=6536#pharmpricing. Accessed January 21, 2011.

*National Asthma Education and Prevention Program, National Heart, Lung and Blood Institute, National Institutes of Health (2007). *Expert Panel Report III: Guidelines for the diagnosis and management of asthma. Update on selected topics.* Bethesda, MD: U.S. Department of Health and Human Services.

*National Center for Complementary and Alternative Medicine (2007). http://nccam.nih.gov/news/camstats/2007/camsurvey_fs1.htm. Accessed January 19, 2011.

Note: Page numbers followed by "f" denote figures; those followed by "t" denote tables; and those followed by "b" denote boxes.